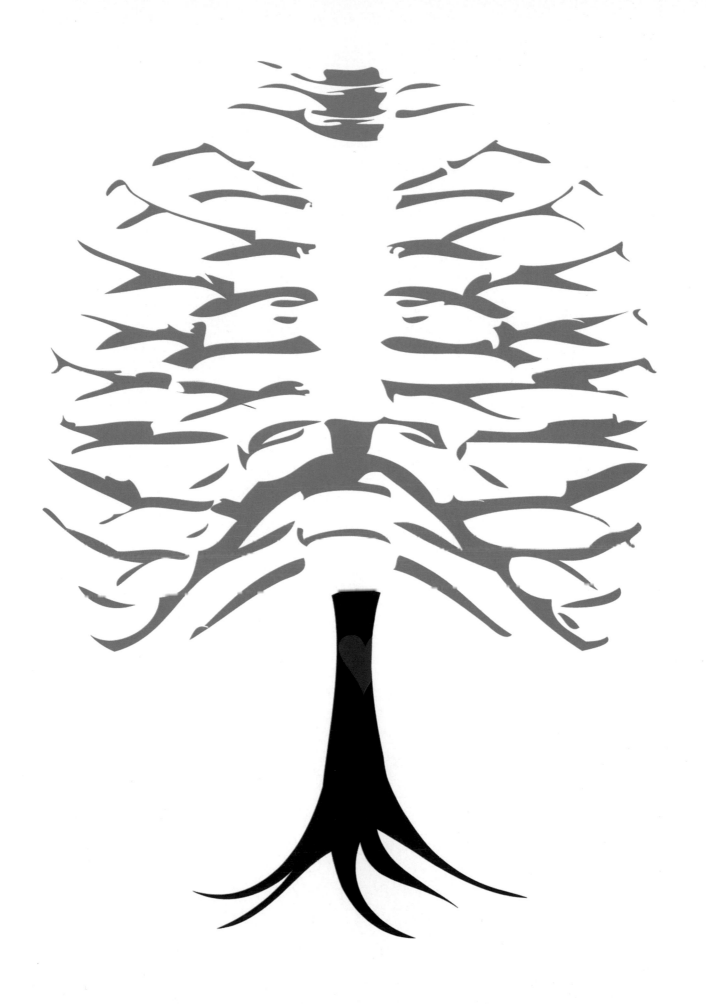

Cardiothoracic Surgery in the Elderly

Mark R. Katlic

Editor

Cardiothoracic Surgery in the Elderly

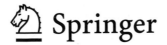 Springer

Editor
Mark R. Katlic, MD
Department of Thoracic Surgery
Geisinger Wyoming Valley Medical Center
1000 East Mountain Drive
Wilkes-Barre, PA 18711
USA
mrkatlic@geisinger.edu

ISBN 978-1-4419-0891-9   e-ISBN 978-1-4419-0892-6
DOI 10.1007/978-1-4419-0892-6
Springer New York Dordrecht Heidelberg London

Library of Congress Control Number: 2011925567

To Dee, forever young

Foreword

This important and timely book reflects the thoughtful work of pioneers in geriatric surgery. It encompasses their knowledge of the science related to geriatric surgery, and their reflections and guidance on the rapidly accumulating knowledge related to improving the health and surgical care of seniors.

Two background points serve as a basis for this foreword.

First: Moving into the category of older person or "senior" is highly variable. Most persons slip into this category subtly, although all too often there is a precipitous decline in one's physical status as might occur, for example, following an acute illness or surgery. Certainly the threshold to be an older person is not 65 on average but more typically about 75–80 years.

Second and key to the importance of this book: Why are seniors different from the surgeon's point of view? Seniors as a group are among the most vulnerable surgical patients and not simply "wizened versions of your standard 30 year old" as a nationally renowned general surgeon, the late Dr. James Thompson, wrote [1]. The vulnerability of this group is not unlike that of the very young, the recognition of which gave rise to the development of experts in pediatric surgery beginning 7 or 8 decades ago. The senior patient, however, is at increased risk from the perturbation of a surgical operation for different reasons than the very young. In the very old patient, the surgeon must consider three major factors: variable age-related decline in physiological reserve, the high likelihood of the presence of multiple chronic diseases, and heterogeneity.

Physiological losses begin at around the age of thirty and progress imperceptibly – except in high performance athletes and a few others requiring maximum physiological functions – and on average become an important clinical factor at around age 80. These changes affect every body system and if these charges are not appreciated by the surgeon they can impact adversely procedural outcomes. Anesthetic or drug toxicity, volume depletion, functional losses, and other postoperative complications easily result.

Multiple chronic diseases are nearly always present. Chronic diseases in the same individual add complexity to any surgical intervention. Associated with the presence of multiple diseases is the use typically of multiple medications with the increased potential for side effects and drug–drug interactions. There simply is no room for imprecise treatment that may initiate a major drug reaction or an exacerbation of an existing illness. Such outcomes can precipitate clinical deterioration, poor surgical outcomes, and even death.

Heterogeneity is a hallmark among older persons. The variability of physiological losses within an individual and the variable pattern of chronic disease and disease severities create universal heterogeneity among elderly surgical patients. Indeed, one 85-year old patient undergoing a thoracic operation is unlike any other patient. This heterogeneity requires that the surgical team have enormous insight, judgment, and individualization of preoperative, operative, and postoperative management.

Increasingly surgeons are operating on the very old, even those who are age 90 years and above. Age is never, in and of itself, a contraindication for surgery. As our editor, Dr. Mark Katlic, has written, "the senior patient can tolerate operations but not complications [2]."

Indeed, once a complication develops it often leads to a spiral of deterioration with one problem developing after another resulting in death or a major loss of function and permanent dependency (a clinical sequence colloquially referred to as the "slippery slope"). Anticipation of this complex situation mandates that the surgeon and his or her team provide individualized precise pre-, intra- and postoperative management to achieve an acceptable outcome. Helping the surgeon and the surgical team achieve such goals is the purpose of this book, achieved with significant, pertinent pointers.

Already seniors dominate the American healthcare system with only about 13 % of the population accounting for nearly half of heathcare expenditures. In the 2006 National Hospital Discharge Survey, nearly 40 % of hospital admissions were for individuals age 65 and older [3]. In data derived from this national survey, seven of the most common cardiac or thoracic surgical procedures were disproportionally done in seniors: 55% and 23% of these seven common procedures were performed in patients older than 65 and 75 years of age, respectively. In 2000, according to the U.S. Census (www.uscensus.gov) there were 16.5 million Americans 75 years or older. To further emphasize the need for geriatrics in surgical care, the US Census Population Projections predict that those individuals age 85 years and older in the United States will increase in size more rapidly than any other age cohort of our society: In 2030 and 2050, 8.7 and 19 million individuals, respectively, are estimated to be in this age group. This cohort of seniors aged 85 and older are certainly the most vulnerable group for surgical procedures. A continuing increase in the age of patients undergoing surgery portends higher rates of complications, longer lengths of stay, and increasing costs. The so-called "demographic imperative" means that all surgeons will have considerable experience in caring for patients who are in their 80s and 90s. Unfortunately, most practicing surgeons have had no formal training in the geriatric aspects of their discipline. Many currently active surgeons, however, have learned by experience and hunting through the literature for practical clinical knowledge regarding the cardinal principles and pitfalls in performing surgery and caring postoperatively for the old/old.

This comprehensive book will help those cardiovascular thoracic surgeons in training and those already in practice obtain this needed current knowledge. Indeed, this book provides a scholarly review of the constantly expanding knowledge base about cardiovascular and thoracic surgery in seniors. The book follows a logical sequence covering general aspects of care, cardiac surgery, and thoracic surgery. Chapters are focused on common, devastating and often missed complications of surgical care in the seniors. These include delirium, depression, pressure sores, functional losses, incontinence, volume depletion, and asymptomatic or atypical complications – myocardial infarction, postoperative diarrhea, urinary track infections and pneumonia. Each is expertly reviewed. Strategies to help the surgeon and the surgical team anticipate, recognize, and effectively prevent or manage such problems are discussed and the evidence basis for such strategies is provided.

This book is particularly timely and the first to review the substantial body of knowledge that has been developed in recent years related to geriatric cardiothoracic surgical problems. It builds on the many peer reviewed scientific articles concerning the care of the elderly patient. Indeed, such geriatric-specific papers have increased dramatically in recent years. This documentation of the growth in the peer reviewed literature concerning geriatric aspects of care is a reflection of a national effort by many pioneers. The annual growth from 44 articles focused on care of the seniors in 1960 to over 43,000 in 2007 is impressive [4] and suggests that in the coming years such articles will accumulate logarithmically.

A portion of the scholarship on which this book is based flows from research done under the auspices of the Geriatrics for Specialists Initiative (GSI) of the American Geriatrics Society (AGS), an initiative that reflects and in some ways initiated a national effort to improve the surgical care of seniors [5]. The GSI began in 1994 as a national effort to encourage and help specialty leaders to begin responding to the need for more geriatrics knowledge in their fields. Visionary academic geriatrician leaders led initially by the late Dennis W. Jahnigen, then by David H. Solomon, spirited the program with the continuing help of surgical specialty leaders, leaders from the AGS and foundation sponsors: The John A. Hartford Foundation and the

Atlantic Philanthropies. Over the years the program has evolved into a highly functional and collaborative multispecialty organization of leaders representing the specialties of Emergency Medicine, Anesthesiology, General Surgery, Thoracic Surgery, Ear, Nose and Head and Neck Surgery, Urology, Gynecology, Ophthalmology, Orthopedic Surgery, and Physical Medicine and Rehabilitation. Two overarching organizations, the American College of Surgeons and the American Medical Association, are also its members. The ten specialty organizations represent the care of the surgical patient throughout a hospital stay: emergency department to anesthesiology to surgery to rehabilitation. Those who joined this cause were those larger specialties that potentially might provide a broader impact in medical education. The GSI now has a well-organized structure with a governing council of leaders representing each participating organization, a robust scientific meeting held annually with the national meeting of the AGS, informational and an educational web-site, www.americangeriatrics.org/specialists/, where details about its accomplishments and other resource information is readily available.

Since the beginning of the specialty of geriatric medicine many years ago and its substantive establishment as a formal academic discipline in the 1980s, many thought that there would be ample geriatricians to assist and work with surgeons in the care of the very old. While this is happening in a very few locations, nationally, the number of geriatricians are actually now decreasing dramatically. This phenomena of inadequate numbers of geriatricians has been documented by surveys of the Association of Directors of Academic Geriatrics Programs (ADGAP), www.ags/adgap and in the Institute of Medicine report of April 2008 [6], available online at www.iom.workforce. The bottom line is this: all surgeons must become fully competent in the special needs of their very old patients as geriatrician colleagues are few and far between.

This valuable textbook arrives when most needed. It catalogs well the expanding knowledge basis for achieving successful surgical outcomes in the very old and it provides for cardiovascular/thoracic surgeons a most useful resource.

John R. Burton, MD

References

1. Thompson JC. Introduction (Symposium on Surgery in the Elderly). *J Am Coll Surg.* 199: 760–1; 2004.
2. Katlic MR. *Principles and Practice of Geriatric Surgery.* In: Rosenthal RA, Zenilman ME, Katlic MR, eds. Principles and Practice of Geriatric Surgery. New York: Springer; 2001, pp. 92–104.
3. DeFrances CJ, Lucas CA, Buie VC, Golosinsky A. 2006 National Hospital Discharge Survey. National Health Statistics Reports: No. 5. Hyattsville, MD: National Center for Health Statistics, 2008.
4. Rich MW, Hustey F, Sun B, Carpenter C. Geriatric Literature Review: Revisited. *J Am Geriatr Soc* 57: 585–7; 2009.
5. Solomon DH, Burton JR, Lundebjerg NE, Eisner J. The new frontier: Increasing geriatrics expertise in surgical and medical specialties. *J Amer Geriat Soc.* 2000; 48:702–4.
6. Institute of Medicine. *Retooling for an aging America: Building the health care workforce.* National Academies. Washington: The National Academies Press; 2008.

Preface

The aging of the population will be the greatest force affecting health care – affecting society as a whole – in our lifetime. Already the elder group is experiencing near-exponential growth, with the most explosive growth in the over 85 years subset. In addition, the conditions that require cardiothoracic surgery (atherosclerosis, lung and esophageal cancer, degenerative valve disease, dysrhythmia) increase in incidence with increasing age. Cardiothoracic surgeons *are* geriatric surgeons.

My own interest in geriatric surgery is over 30-years old. As a surgical resident at the Massachusetts General Hospital I cared for several hundred-year-old patients and retrospectively reviewed the records of several others. All survived operation and lived one or two years, one even taking an around the world cruise. I published these results in 1985 and went on to edit books on geriatric surgery. This is the first devoted to cardiothoracic surgery.

Our chapter authors were encouraged to keep their focus on the elderly and not to simply reproduce a general chapter on cardiac or thoracic surgery. To that end, for example, Cleveland's chapter on Preoperative Evaluation discusses nutrition, delirium, disability, and advanced directives as opposed to cardiopulmonary fitness. Weigel and her coauthors have added elements of Comprehensive Geriatric Assessment to their presurgery routine. Every reader will benefit from chapters on Nursing/Models of Care, Delirium, Ethics, Wound Healing, Neurologic and Cognitive Changes, Medication Usage, Palliative Care, and many others. Despite my study in the field for decades I have learned from each chapter in our book.

Ageism exists in Society, in Medicine, and in Surgery, but not in these pages. Our authors' unflinching reviews of the results of cardiothoracic surgery in the elderly are based on data and not prejudice. No cohorts' physiologic reserve and list of comorbidities varies as much, for a given chronologic age, as our subjects'. In some cases, older patients do experience greater mortality or stay longer in the hospital or cost more than younger counterparts but this is far from universal: many groups have shown that excellent results are attainable with compulsive attention to detail.

A brief note about our logo: the oak tree, like the model from my own yard (Fig. 1a) represents strength and elegance and endurance throughout long life. I asked my neighbor, designer Tracey Selingo, to incorporate a stylized thorax in its branches. The colorful and whimsical heart carved into the trunk was her idea (Fig. 1b). And to my editors at Springer, Executive Editor Paula Callaghan and Developmental Editor Portia Bridges: what a delight it has been to work together, now on two books. Portia, especially, has been the backbone of this project; she is one of the best.

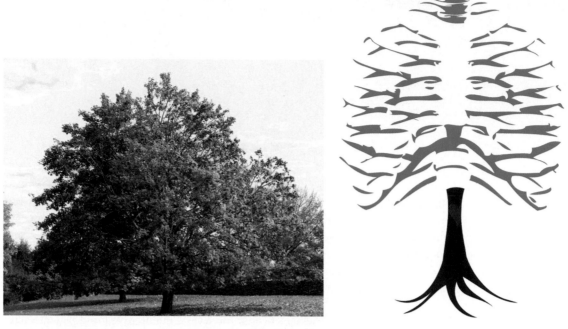

Fig. 1 (**a**) Katlic oak tree, model for logo; (**b**) cardiothoracic surgery in the elderly logo

What could be more difficult – and thereby more rewarding – than successfully performing medicine's most complex procedures on our highest risk patients? A man or a woman who is a consistently good geriatric surgeon is likely to be a consistently good surgeon. So, let us all become good geriatric surgeons.

Wilkes-Barre, PA   Mark R. Katlic

Contents

Contributors

James H. Abernathy, III, MD, MPH, FASE
Department of Anesthesia and Perioperative Medicine,
Division of Cardiothoracic Anesthesiology, Medical University of South Carolina,
25 Courtenay Dr., Suite 4200, MSC 240, Charleston, SC 29425, USA
abernatj@musc.edu

Naveed Z. Alam, MD, FRCSC
Department of Surgery, St. Vincent's Hospital, Melbourne, Victoria 3065, Australia

Luciana Armaganijan, MD
Department of Medicine, McMaster University, 237 Barton Street East,
Hamilton, ON L8L2X2, Canada
luciana_va@hotmail.com

Wilbert S. Aronow, MD
New York College of Medicine, Macy Pavillion, Valhalla, NY 10595, USA
wsaronow@aol.com

Tawfik Ayoub, MD
Department of Anesthesiology, Keck School of Medicine,
University of Southern California, Los Angeles, CA 90275, USA

Christopher J. Barreiro, MD
Division of Cardiac Surgery, The Johns Hopkins Hospital, 600 N. Wolfe Street,
Blalock 618, Baltimore, MD 21287, USA
cbarrei1@jhmi.edu

William A. Baumgartner, MD
Department of Surgery, Division of Cardiac Surgery, The Johns Hopkins Hospital,
Baltimore, MD 21205, USA
wbaumgar@jhmi.edu

Jack M. Berger, MS, MD, PhD
University of Southern California, Keck School of Medicine,
1500 San Pablo Street, Los Angeles, CA 90033, USA
jmberger@usc.edu

Sarah E.Billmeier, MD
Department of Surgery, Brigham and Women's Hospital, 75 Francis Street,
Boston, MA 02115, USA
sbillmeier@partners.org

F. Charles Brunicardi, MD
Michael E. DeBakey Department of Surgery, Baylor College of Medicine,
Houston, TX 77030, USA

Marie Boltz, PhD
Hartford Institute for Geriatric Nursing, New York University College of Nursing,
New York, NY 10003, USA

Margarita T. Camacho, MD
Department of Cardiothoracic Surgery, Newark Beth Israel Medical Center,
201 Lyons Avenue, Suite G-5, Newark, NJ 07112, USA
mcamacho@sbhcs.com

Elizabeth A. Capezuti, PhD
Hartford Institute for Geriatric Nursing, New York University College of Nursing,
726 Broadway, 10th Floor, New York, NY 10003, USA
ec65@nyu.edu

Stephen D. Cassivi, MD, MSc, FRCSC
William J. von Liebig Transplant Center, Mayo Clinic, Rochester, MA, USA

Chiara Cattabiani, MD
Department of Internal Medicine and Biomedical Sciences Section of Geriatrics,
University of Parma, Parma 43100, Italy

Gian Paulo Ceda, MD
Department of Internal Medicine and Biomedical Sciences Section of Geriatrics,
University of Parma, Parma 43110, Italy

Su Min Chang, MD, FACC
Department of Cardiology, Methodist DeBakey Heart and Vascular Center,
Weill Medical College of Cornell University, Houston, TX 77030, USA

Joseph C. Cleveland, Jr., MD
Department of Surgery, University of Colorado Health Sciences Center,
12631 East 17th Avenue, Aurora, CO 80045, USA
joseph.cleveland@ucdenver.edu

Alberto de Hoyos, MD
Department of Cardiothoracic Surgery, Northwestern Memorial Hospital,
Chicago, IL 60611, USA

Geoffrey P. Dunn, MD, FACS
Department of Surgery and Palliative Care, Hamot Medical Center,
2050 South Shore Dr., Erie, PA 16505, USA
gpdunn1@earthlink.net

Maqsood M. Elahi, MD, FACS
Wessex Cardiovascular Center, Division of Developmental Origins of Health & Disease,
Institute of Developmental Sciences, School of Medicine, University of Southampton,
MP-887, General Hospital, Tremona Road, Southampton, SO16 6YD,
United Kingdom
manzoor_elahi8@yahoo.com

M. Kate Elfrey, DO
Department of Internal Medicine, Johns Hopkins Bayview Hospital,
Baltimore, MD 21224, USA

Christopher G. Engeland, PhD
University of Illinois at Chicago, College of Dentistry,
Chicago, IL 60612, USA
engeland@uic.edu

David A. Etzioni, MD, MSHS
Departments of Colorectal Surgery and Preventive Medicine,
Keck School of Medicine, University of Southern California, 1411 Eastlake Avenue,
Suite 7418, Los Angeles, CA 90033, USA
etzioni.david@gmail.com

Juan J. Fibla, MD
Lung Transplant Program, William J. von Liebig Transplant Center, Mayo Clinic,
200 First Street SW, Rochester, MN 55905, USA
fibla.juan@mayo.edu

Raja M. Flores, MD
Mount Sinai Medical Center, 1275 York Avenue, New York, NY 10021, USA
floresr@mskcc.org

William H. Frishman, MD, MACP
Department of Medicine, Westchester Medical Center,
Rosenthal Professor of Medicine, NY Medical College, Valhalla, NY 10595, USA

Praveen K. Gajendrareddy, BDS, PhD
Department of Periodontics, College of Dentistry, Chicago, IL 60612, USA

Arnar Geirsson, MD
Yale University School of Medicine, 333 Cedar Street,
FMB 121, New Haven, CT 06520, USA
arnar.geirsson@yale.edu

Carl I. Gonzales II, MD
Department of Surgery, Stony Brook University School of Medicine,
Stony Brook, NY 11794, USA
Carl.Gonzalez@stonybrook.edu

Robert A. Guyton, MD
Division of Cardiothoracic Surgery, Emory University Hospital, Atlanta, GA 30308, USA

Rose E. Hardin, MD
Department of Heart, Lung and Esophageal Surgery Institute,
University of Pittsburgh Medical Center,Pittsburgh, PA 15213, USA
hardinre@upmc.edu

Keenan A. Hawkins, MD, FCCP
Division of Pulmonary and Critical Care Medicine, Northwestern University Feinberg
School of Medicine, Chicago, IL 60611, USA
khawkins@nmff.org

Jeff S. Healey, MD, MSc
Department of Medicine, McMaster University, Hamilton, Ontario L8L2X2, Canada

Susan M. Hecker, MD, MPH
Division of Cardiothoracic Surgery, Medical University of South Carolina,
25 Courtenay Drive, Suite 710, Charleston, SC 29425, USA

Brannon R. Hyde, MD
Department of Surgery, University of Kentucky, A301 KY Clinic,
Lexington, KY 40536-0284, USA
brhy222@uky.edu

Michael T. Jaklitsch, MD
Department of Surgery, Brigham and Women's Hospital, Boston, MA 02115, USA

Sean M. Jeffery, PharmD
Pharmacy (119), VA Connecticut Healthcare System, West Haven,
CT, 06516, USA;
Department of General Internal Medicine, Dartmouth Hitchcock Medical center,
Lebanon, NH, 03755, USA

Ravi Kalhan, MD, MS, FCCP
Division of Pulmonary and Critical Care Medicine, Northwestern University Feinberg
School of Medicine, Chicago, IL 60611, USA

Marshall B. Kapp, JD, MPH
Florida State University, FSU Center for Innovative Collaboration in Medicine and Law,
Tallahassee, FL 32306-4300, USA
kapp@siu.edu

Mark R. Katlic, MD
Department of Thoracic Surgery, Geisinger Wyoming Valley Medical Center,
1000 East Mountain Drive, Wilkes-Barre, PA 18711, USA
mrkatlic@geisinger.edu

Lois A. Killewich, MD, PhD
Department of Surgery, University of Texas Medical Branch, Galveston, TX 77555, USA

Hongsoo Kim, PhD, MPH
Graduate School of Public Health, Seoul National University, Seoul, 110-799, South Korea

Joshua Kindelan, MD
Northwestern University, Feinberg School of Medicine,
Chicago, Illinois Fellow, Division of Cardiothoracic Surgery, USA
joshua.kindelan@yahoo.com

Anne C. Kolker, BS, MA, MD
Department of Anesthesia, Memorial Sloan Kettering Cancer Center,
1275 York Avenue, New York, NY 10065, USA
kolkera@mskcc.org

Anai Kothari, BS
Department of Surgery, Division of Cardiothoracic Surgery,
University of Wisconsin School of Medicine and Public Health, Madison, WI 53792, USA

John C. Kucharczuk, MD
Division of Thoracic Surgery, Hospital of the University of Pennsylvania,
Philadelphia, PA 19104, USA

Corey J. Langer, MD
Department of Medicine, Division of Hematology and Oncology,
Hospital of the University of Pennsylvania, Philadelphia, PA 19104, USA

Ticiana Leal, MD
Department of Medicine, University of Wisconsin Hospitals and Clinics,
600 Highland Avenue, Mail Code 5669, Madison, WI 53792-5669, USA
tbleal@medicine.wisc.edu

Stephen H. Little, BSc, MD, FRCPC, FACC, FACE
Department of Cardiology, Methodist DeBakey Heart and Vascular Center,
Weill Medical College of Cornell University, Houston, TX 77030, USA

Joseph LoCicero, III, MD
Department of Surgery, SUNY Downstate, 1158 Church Street,
Mobile, AL 36604, USA
lociceroj@comcast.net

Noelle K. LoConte, MD
Department of Medicine, University of Wisconsin Hospital and Clinics,
Madison, WI 53792, USA

James D. Luketich, MD
Heart, Lung and Esophageal Surgery Institute, University of Pittsburgh Medical Center,
Pittsburgh, PA 15213, USA

Marcello Maggio, MD, PhD
Department of Internal Medicine and Biomedical Sciences, Section of Geriatrics,
University of Parma, Parma 43100, Italy
marcellomaggio2001@yahoo.it

Richard A. Marottoli, MD, MPH
Department of Geriatric Medicine, Yale School of Medicine,
VA Connecticut Healthcare System, 950 Campbell Ave, West Haven, CT 06516, USA
richard.marottoli@ynhh.org

Douglas J. Mathisen, MD
Department of Surgery, Division of Thoracic Surgery, Massachusetts General Hospital,
Blake 1570, 55 Fruit Street, Boston, MA 02114, USA
dmathisen@partners.org

J. Riley McCarten, MD
Department of Neurology, University of Minnesota Medical School, VA Medical Center,
One Veterans Drive, Minneapolis, MN 55417, USA
mccar034@umn.edu

Edwin C. McGee, Jr., MD
Department of Cardiac Surgery, Northwestern Memorial Hospital,
Bluhm Cardiovascular Institue, Chicago, IL 60611, USA
emcgee@nmh.org

Jay Menaker, MD
Department of Surgery, University of Maryland Medical Center, R. Adams Cawley Shock
Trauma Center, Baltimore, MD 21201, USA
jmenaker@umm.edu

Daniel L. Miller, MD
Section of General Thoracic Surgery, Emory University School of Medicine,
1365 Clifton Road, Atlanta, GA 30322, USA
dlmill2@emory.edu

Rita A. Mukhtar, MD
Department of General Surgery, University of California, 513 Parnassus Avenue,
S321, San Francisco, CA 94143, USA
Rita.Mukhtar@ucsfmedctr.org

Ashok Muniappan, MD
Department of Surgery, Division of Thoracic Surgery, Massachusetts General Hospital,
Boston, MA 02114, USA

Carlos G. Musso, MD
Department of Nephrology, Hospital Italiano de Buenos Aires, Gascon 450, C1181
Ciudad de Buenos Aires, Argentina
carlos.musso@hospitalitaliano.org.ar

Faisal Nabi, MD, FACC
Department of Cardiology, Weill Medical College of Cornell University,
Methodist DeBakey Heart and Vascular Center,
Houston, TX 77030, USA
FNabi@tmhs.org

Katie S. Nason, MD, MPH
Department of Heart, Lung and Esophageal Surgery Institute,
University of Pittsburgh Medical Center, Pittsburgh, PA 15232, USA

Eric W. Nelson, DO
Department of Anesthesiology and Perioperative Medicine,
Medical University of South Carolina, Charleston, SC 29425, USA

Dimitrios O. Oreopoulos, MD, PhD, FRCPC, FACP, FRCPS (Glasgow)
Department of Medicine, University of Toronto, Toronto, ON, M5T 2S8, Canada

Jayeshkumar Patel, MD
Department of Anesthesiology, USC University Hospital, Los Angeles, CA 90033, USA

Roshini C. Pinto-Powell, MD
Department of Internal Medicine, Dartmouth Hitchcock Medical Center,
Dartmouth Medical School, Lebanon, NH 03755, USA

John A. Primomo, MD
Michael E. DeBakey Surgery Department, Baylor College of Medicine,
Houston, TX 77030, USA

Philip A. Rascoe, MD
Division of Cardiothoracic Surgery, Texas A&M University Health Science Center
College of Medicine, Scott & White Memorial Hospital and Clinic,
Olin E. Teague Central Texas VA Medical Center,
Temple, TX 76508, USA
rascoe@uphs.upenn.edu

James L. Rudolph, MD, SM
Geriatric Research, Education, and Clinical Center,
Boston, MA 02130, USA
jrudolph@partners.org

Ronnie A. Rosenthal, MD
Department of Surgery, Yale University School of Medicine,
VA Connecticut Healthcare System, West Haven, CT 06516, USA
ronnie.rosenthal@yale.edu

Robert M. Sade, MD
Division of Cardiothoracic Surgery, Medical University of South Carolina,
Charleston, SC 29425, USA
sader@musc.edu

Thomas M. Scalea, MD
R. Adams Cawley Shock Trauma Center, University of Maryland Medical Center,
Baltimore, MD 21201, USA

Vaughn A. Starnes, MD
Department of Surgery, Keck School of Medicine, University of Southern California,
Los Angeles, CA 90033, USA

Dipan J. Shah, MD, FACC
Department of Cardiology, Methodist DeBakey Heart and Vascular Center,
Weill Medical College of Cornell University, Houston, TX 77030, USA

Jo-Anne O. Shepard, MD
Department of Radiology, Division of Thoracic Imaging and Intervention,
Massachusetts General Hospital, 55 Fruit Street, Founders 202, Boston, MA 02114, USA
jshepard@partners.org

Vadim Sherman, MD, FRCSC, FACS
Michael E. DeBakey Surgery Department, Baylor College of Medicine,
Houston, TX 77030, USA
vsherman@bcm.tmc.edu

Kerry J. Stewart, EdD
Department of Medicine/Cardiology, Johns Hopkins Bayview Medical Center,
Baltimore, MD 21224, USA

Pierre R. Theodore, MD
Department of Adult Cardiothoracic Surgery, University of California,
San Francisco, CA 94115, USA

Vinod H. Thourani, MD
Division of Cardiothoracic Surgery, Department of Surgery, Emory University Hospital,
550 Peachtree Street, Emory University Hospital Midtown, 6th Floor Medical Office Tower,
Cardiac Surgery, Atlanta, GA 30308, USA
vthoura@emory.edu

Sandra C. Tomaszek, MD
William J. von Liebig Transplant Center, Mayo Clinic, Rochester, MN 55905, USA

Patricia Ursomanno, PhD
Division of Cardiac Surgery, New York University Langone Medical Center,
New York, NY 10016, USA

Huber R. Warner, PhD
College of Biological Sciences, University of Minnesota, St. Paul, MN 55108, USA
warne033@centurylink.net

Tracey L. Weigel, MD
Department of Surgery, University of Wisconsin Hospitals and Clinics,
Madison, WI 53792, USA

Jared Weiss, MD
Thoracic, Head and Neck Cancer Programs,
Division of Hematology/Oncology, 170 Manning Drive,
Room 3115, Campus Box 7305, Chapel Hill, NC 27599, USA
jared_weiss@med.unc.edu

Ilene C. Weitz, MD
Jane Anne Nohl Division of Hematology and Center for Study of Blood Disorders,
University of Southern California, Keck School of Medicine,
Norris Comprehensive Cancer Center, Los Angeles, CA 90033, USA
warne033@centurylink.net

Glenn Whitman, MD
Department of Surgery, Division of Cardiac Surgery, Johns Hopkins Medical Institutes,
Baltimore, MD 21287, USA

Melissa L. Wong
Department of Cardiothoracic Surgery, Newark Beth Israel Medical Center, New York,
NJ 07112, USA

Cameron D. Wright, MD
Department of Thoracic Surgery, Massachusetts General Hospital,
32 Fruit Street, Blake 1570, Boston, MA 02114-2698, USA
wright.cameron@mgh.harvard.edu

Carol C. Wu, MD
Department of Radiology, Division of Thoracic Imaging and Intervention,
Massachusetts General Hospital, 55 Fruit Street, Founders 202, Boston, MA 02114, USA

Kenton J. Zehr, MD
Professor of Surgery, Texas A & M Health Sciences Center College of Medicine,
Director, Division of Cardiothoracic Surgery & Center for Aortic Disease,
Scott & White Clinic, 2401 S. 31st Street, Temple, TX 76508, USA
KZEHR@swmail.sw.org

Michael E. Zenilman, MD
Department of Surgery, Johns Hopkins Medicine, Bethesda, MD 20814, USA
mzenilm1@jhmi.edu

Susan J. Zieman, MD, PhD
National Institute on Aging, National Institutes of Health,
7201 Wisconsin Ave, Suite 3C307, Bethesda, MD 20892, USA
susan.zieman@nih.gov

Joseph B. Zwischenberger, MD
Department of Surgery, University of Kentucky, Lexington, KY 40536, USA

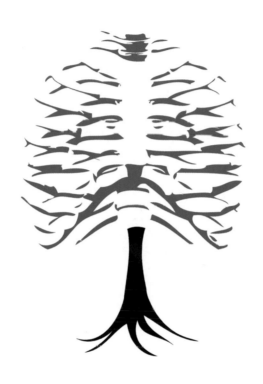

Chapter 1
Invited Commentary

Ronnie A. Rosenthal

Citations regarding the negative impact of old age on clinical outcomes can be found as far back as the beginning of the medical literature itself. The hieroglyphic sentence below from the Papyrus Prisse (1580 B.C.), quoted in the Edwin Smith Papyrus which is thought to be among the oldest surviving documents in the surgical literature, decries the vicissitudes of growing old by stating "To be an old man is evil for people in every respect [1]" (Invited Commentary Fig. 1.1). At the time of that writing, attaining a 25th year of life was an accomplishment achieved by only the heartiest of persons. Over the ensuing 3,500 years, mean life expectancy increased very slowly, on average 0.7 years per century, reaching 47 years in western countries by 1900 A.D. Then, thanks to the advent of public health measures, modern medicine, and lifestyle modification in the following one century alone, life expectancy increased an additional 30 years. "Old" now is very different in many ways from "old" back then. But while the time point at which one becomes "old" has changed, the fact that old age has negative consequences has not. In fact, recent advances have created a population living longer with diseases that would have proven fatal in the past. Over the next several decades, as the baby boom generation reaches "old age," the medical profession will be faced with a huge number of octogenarians and nonagenarians, many with chronic diseases, expecting to not only live longer, but also to do so in an active and productive manner. Many of these older patients will find themselves needing the services of a surgeon; they will require cataract removal, total joint replacement, resection for cancer, and coronary and peripheral revascularization. The need to analyze when, how, by whom, and on whom these procedures should be performed, as well as how to pay for them, has only recently begun to attract the attention of healthcare providers and healthcare policymakers.

In 2007, in response to this tsunami of aging potential patients in the United States, the Institute of Medicine (IOM) convened The Committee on the Future Health Care Workforce for Older Americans, to "probe these challenges and to set out a course of action that will improve our nation's readiness to care for an aging population. The committee conducted a thorough analysis of the forces that shape the health care workforce, including education, training, modes of practice, and the financing of public and private programs [2]." In April 2008, the IOM issued its report entitled "Retooling for an Aging America: Building the Health Care Workforce," in which the following three-pronged approach was recommended:

1. Increase geriatric competence in all providers
2. Increase recruitment and retention of geriatric specialists
3. Redesign models of care

Textbooks such as this one are an essential part of the effort to increase geriatric expertise in those who will care for our older surgical patients.

As a student of "geriatric surgery" since my PGY 4 resident experiences 30 years ago in a small community hospital

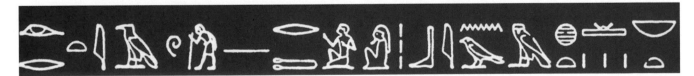

Fig. 1.1 This hieroglyphic sentence, "To be an old man is evil for people in every respect", appears in the Edwin Smith Surgical Papyrus (17th century B.C.) (Reprinted with permission from Gruman [1])

R.A. Rosenthal (✉)
Department of Surgery, Yale University School of Medicine,
VA Connecticut Healthcare System, West Haven, CT 06516, USA
e-mail: ronnie.rosenthal@yale.edu

M.R. Katlic (ed.), *Cardiothoracic Surgery in the Elderly*, DOI 10.1007/978-1-4419-0892-6_1,
© Springer Science+Business Media, LLC 2011

adjacent to a large nursing home facility (where staff surgeons could somehow translate mental status changes into acute cholecystitis with none of the usual signs or symptoms present), I am heartened by the growing national interest in learning more about how to care for older patients in general and older surgical patients in particular. Even my fellow residents, who in 1981 thought that geriatric surgery meant caring for sacral pressure ulcers, now realize that there is a whole additional set of principles and rules of practice that need to be defined and followed when undertaking major surgical intervention for older persons. Prior focus on only the treatment of the surgical disease is now tempered by considerations of maintenance of function, quality of life, and the patient's goal of care. Previous acceptance of "sundowning" as the norm for an old person after surgery is now replaced by a concerted effort to identify, prevent, and treat delirium. Advanced directives and palliative care are no longer viewed as preparations for and admissions of failure, but rather appropriate considerations for persons with life-threatening disease in advanced age.

In few other surgical specialties, the issues of geriatric surgery have become more distinct than in cardiac surgery. Cardiovascular disease is a leading cause of death among the elderly and has been for the last century, even as life expectancy has increased. With the advent of minimally invasive methods to revascualrize the heart, the number of coronary artery bypass procedures (CABGs) done per year has fallen, while the age, comorbidity, and complexity of disease in patients requiring surgery have increased. These changes now leave the highest-risk patients in need of highest risk and most costly interventions. Isn't performing CABG in the elderly then an expensive prescription for failure? No, because cardiovascular surgery is specifically designed to improve function, rather than just treat disease and therefore issues of quality of life, not just prolongation of life, dominate both the risk benefit and cost benefit discussions. In a wonderful study of the cost-effectiveness of coronary artery bypass grafting in octogenarians, Sollano et al. [3] compared outcomes and cost per quality life year saved of CABG versus medical therapy. Three- and 4-year survival for patients treated with surgery was 80 and 69% compared to 64 and 32%, respectively, for those treated medically. Quality of life in five domains, pain, activity, mobility, self-care, and depression/anxiety, was also better in the surgery group. And finally, the cost per quality life year saved was approximately $10,400, less than the cost for many common procedures such as screening mammography.

In the chapters that follow, the authors will define the principles and discuss the issues involved in providing the highest quality care for older patients requiring cardiac and thoracic surgery. While much remains yet to be studied, these chapters provide an excellent foundation upon which to further build our knowledge and skills.

References

1. Gruman GJ, editor. Roots of modern gerontology and geriatrics. New York, NY: Ayers; 1979.
2. Committee on the Future Health Care Workforce for Older Americans, Institute of Medicine. Retooling for an Aging America: Building the Health Care Workforce. Washington, D.C.: The National Academies. 2008. http://www.nap.edu/catalog/12089.html.
3. Sollano JA, Rose EA, Williams DL, et al. Coat-effectiveness of coronary artery bypass surgery in octogenarians. Ann Surg. 1998;228:297–306.

Chapter 2
The Epidemiology and Economics of Cardiothoracic Surgery in the Elderly

David A. Etzioni and Vaughn A. Starnes

Abstract Cardiothoracic surgery is performed primarily in older individuals. Within the United States and globally, the numbers of these older individuals will increase dramatically in the near future, driving enormous changes in the amount, profile, and delivery of health care. In this chapter we analyze recent trends in the patterns of treatment provided by cardiothoracic surgeons. While incidence rates for coronary artery bypass procedures have declined, other procedures have not changed significantly in frequency. With the forecasted increases in the number of older individuals there is good reason to believe that the volumes of cardiothoracic procedures that are performed will rise significantly, even if incidence rates continue to decline. Cardiothoracic surgeons should meet the challenges engendered by these changes through ongoing innovation and a continued focus on quality of care and clinical outcomes.

Keywords Coronary artery bypass • Open heart surgery • Elderly • Health manpower • Appropriateness • Epidemiology • Health care costs • Economics

Introduction

The disease processes which call upon the skill of a cardiothoracic surgeon are predominantly found in older individuals. Atherosclerotic coronary artery disease (CAD), valvular disorders, and neoplastic disorders are all primarily afflictions of the elderly. The primary focus of a cardiothoracic surgeon is to care for these problems in the manner which optimizes patient outcomes, and it is this focus which has earned the field respect and status. In the chapters that follow, the clinical considerations of treating a patient who is older relative to one who is younger are explored. With this chapter, we take a step away from the clinician-patient relationship and explore the epidemiologic, economic, and pragmatic ramifications of cardiothoracic surgery in a population that is increasingly elderly. In the interest of providing insights which have depth and detail, these analyses will focus primarily on the United States (US) population.

Demographics: The Aging Population

"Demography is destiny"

August Comte

Over the next two decades, the US population is poised to undergo an unprecedented change. The "aging" population – often mentioned but rarely explained – is a demographic shift that results from several distinct demographic phenomena. First, we are living longer. Based on data from the US Centers for Disease Control, an individual born in 2004 has a life expectancy of 77.8 years, compared to less than 50 years one century ago [1]. Second, the baby boomers are entering retirement age. Between 1946 and 1964 the US saw a remarkable rise in the number of births relative to the periods before or following. In 2011, the first of the baby boomers enter retirement age, and the proportion of individuals in the US aged 65 years and older will begin to increase rapidly. Another demographic phenomenon is also important to mention: the US population is increasing rapidly. Between 1990 and 2000 the US population increased by 32.6 million (13%), the largest absolute increase of any decade in the country's history.

Taken together, these trends have clear importance for the field of cardiothoracic surgery in determining the base population of potential patients. Between 2010 and 2025, the US population is expected to increase by 40.5 million people (13.1%) (Fig. 2.1a). Increases will be disproportionately higher among older individuals – the numbers of individuals

D.A. Etzioni (✉)
Department of Surgery,
Mayo Clinic Arizona,
5777 E. Mayo Blvd, Phoenix, AZ 85054, USA
e-mail: etzioni.david@mayo.edu

M.R. Katlic (ed.), *Cardiothoracic Surgery in the Elderly*, DOI 10.1007/978-1-4419-0892-6_2,
© Springer Science+Business Media, LLC 2011

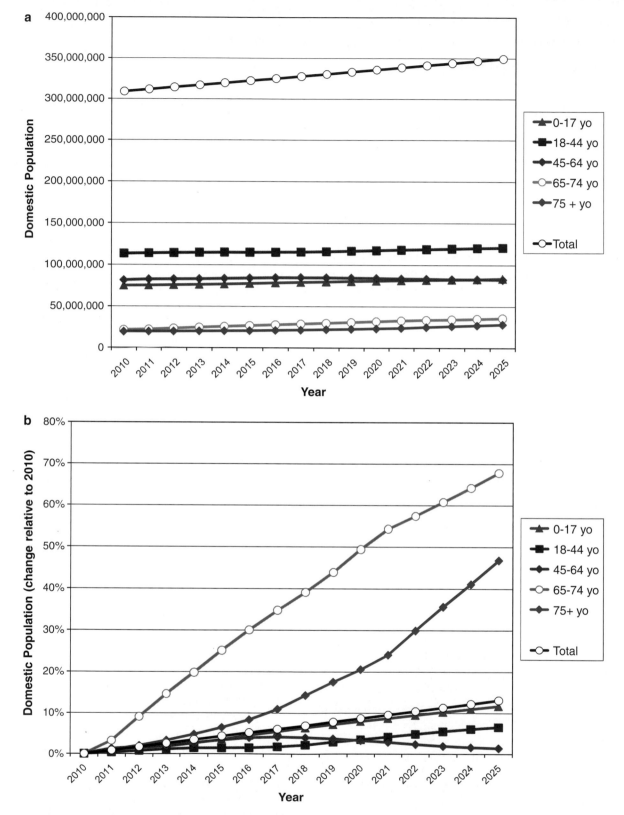

Fig. 2.1 (**a**) US Population, 2010–2025; (**b**) US Population, 2010–2025 (% change relative to 2010)

aged 65–74 will increase by 67.8% and those aged 75+ by 46.7% (Fig. 2.1b).

The US is not alone in experiencing dramatic shifts toward an aging population. Figure 2.2 shows global statis-

tics that illustrate similar emerging trends in the global population. These shifts are predicted to be more dramatic in less developed regions relative to more developed regions.

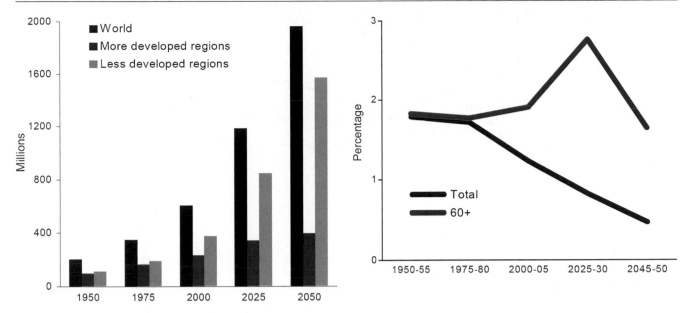

Fig. 2.2 World growth in population aged 60+ years (from the United Nations Department of Economic and Social Affairs Population Division [38])

A Data-Driven Approach

Throughout this chapter, we will use original analyses of existing data in order to provide insight into patterns of cardiothoracic surgical treatment provided within the US. In order to do this, we will rely on two population-based databases of domestic hospital discharges – the National Hospital Discharge Survey (NHDS) and the Nationwide Inpatient Sample (NIS). A brief description of each of these sources of data is therefore important.

The NHDS is managed by the National Center for Health Statistics, and represents an annual sampling of domestic hospital discharges. Each year, 350,000 discharges from approximately 500 hospitals are abstracted based on an approach that is designed to yield information that is representative of all domestic hospitalizations [2]. Within the NHDS, de-identified information about each discharge, including age, sex, race/ethnicity, diagnoses, procedures performed (according to ICD-9 coding scheme), and diagnosis-related grouping (DRG) are reported.

The NIS is published by the Healthcare Cost and Utilization Project through a partnership that is organized by the Agency for Healthcare Research and Quality. Similar to the NHDS, the NIS database contains discharge data including procedure and diagnosis codes (also according to ICD-9 coding scheme). The NIS differs from the NHDS in that it represents much larger sample (approximately eight million records per year), but it does not sample from as broad a range of geographic regions. Also, the regions which contribute discharge data to the NIS have changed significantly over time.

These two datasets are best considered complementary. For analyses of procedures which are performed commonly,

the NHDS data are the most accurate representation of the overall, nationally-representative patterns of treatment. Also, because the NHDS sampling methodology has remained stable over time, it is a better resource for examining temporal trends in procedure rates. The NIS, because of its larger sample size, is a better resource for assessing rates of procedures which occur with lower frequency. We rely on the NIS to yield detailed point estimates for procedural rates which can then be used for the purposes of forecasting, and in situations where a large sample size is required in order to yield more precise estimates. At the time of writing this chapter, the most current data available for each of these datasets was 2006. In Appendix 1 we document the International Classification of Disease, *9th Edition* (ICD-9) procedure codes which we used to ascertain procedures for this analysis.

Historical Rates of Treatment

The number of individuals in the US who undergo cardiothoracic surgical procedures is changing. Within this section we will analyze historical rates of specific types of cardiothoracic surgical procedures – coronary artery bypass grafts (CABGs), valve operations, and pneumonectomies (see Appendix 1 for description of corresponding ICD-9 procedure codes). These three classes of procedures clearly do not represent the breadth of the field; by limiting our analyses to these relatively more common procedures we hope to provide a report that is more detailed while still representative of evolving trends in the entire workload of cardiothoracic surgeons.

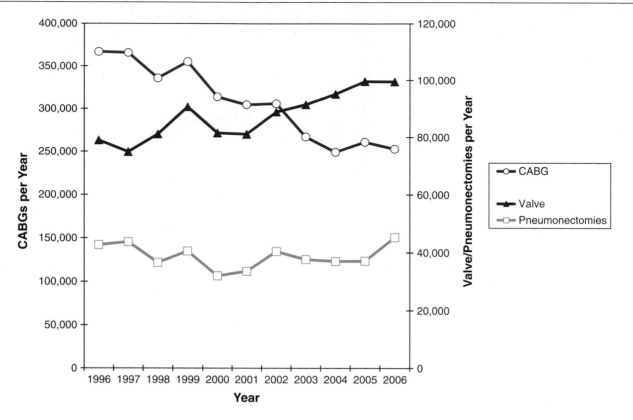

Fig. 2.3 Domestic volume of CABG, cardiac valve replacements, and pneumonectomies; 1996–2006 (from The National Hospital Discharge Survey (NHDS), available at http://www.cdc.gov/nchs/nhds.htm)

Between 1996 and 2006 the numbers of CABG operations performed in the US declined, from 366,000 per year in 1996 to 252,000 in 2006 (31% decrease) (Fig. 2.3). Valve operations and pneumonectomies each increased slightly; valve operations increased from 79,000 per year in 1996 to 99,000 in 2006 (26% increase) and pneumonectomies increased from 66,000 per year 78,000 per year (19% increase). The measurement and tracking of procedural volume is enormously important for policy planning, however, it is important to acknowledge that over the last 10 years, the US population has grown considerably and also aged. To account for these trends, all subsequent figures in this section are "age-adjusted." This method modifies an overall incidence rate to adjust for changes in the demographic makeup (especially age distribution) of a population over time.

The importance of accounting for differences in procedure rates within age groups is best demonstrated in terms of an incidence rate curve for each procedure. Figure 2.4 demonstrates incidence rate curves for several commonly performed cardiothoracic procedures. These incidence rate curves clearly show that it is the elderly population who are the primary patient population for cardiothoracic surgical procedures. Changes in the population of individuals aged less than 40 years old clearly would have little impact on procedure volumes; quite the opposite for the population aged 65 years or older.

It is also useful to analyze how these incidence rates have changed over time (Fig. 2.5a–c). For CABG procedures, the population-based incidence rate has declined from 13.8 procedures per 10,000 population in 1996 to 8.5 in 2006, a 38% reduction (Fig. 2.5a). Decreases were most rapid in the age groups with the highest rates of operation – those aged 60–79 years. Incidence rates were more stable, however, in the oldest age group (80+ years old). By contrast, the incidence rates for valve procedures and pneumonectomies have remained fairly constant (Fig. 2.5b–c).

Forecasting Rates of Treatment

"It's tough to make predictions, especially about the future."

Yogi Berra

What will happen to rates of cardiothoracic surgical procedures in the future? In general, forecasting patterns of treatment is an endeavor which can be labeled better as art than science. The effort needs to be made, however, in order to ensure that the resources available are sufficient to the task at hand. Historically, several methods have been used to project the demand for surgical procedures. While each has

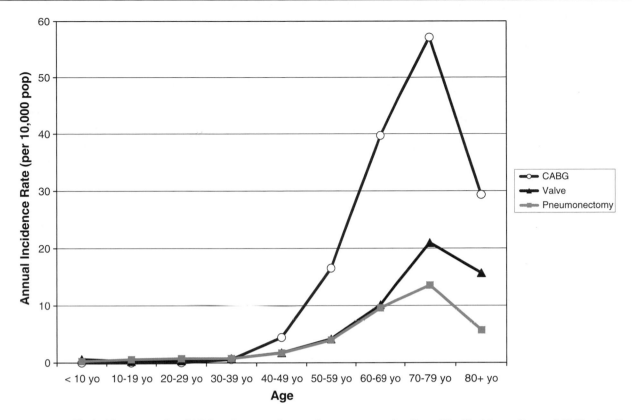

Fig. 2.4 Age-specific incidence rates for CABG, valve operations, and pneumonectomies (from The Healthcare Cost and Utilization Project (HCUP), available at http://www.ahrq.gov/data/hcup/datahcup.htm)

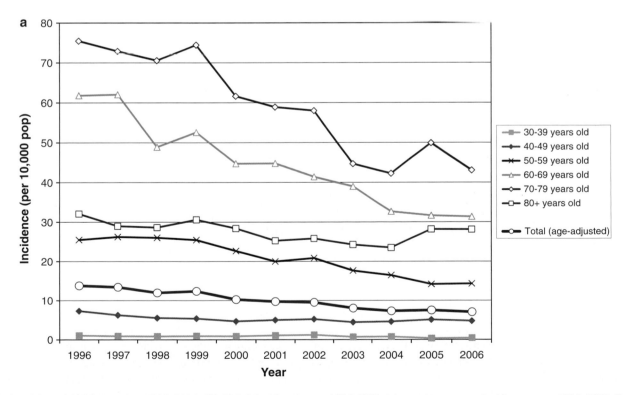

Fig. 2.5 (**a**) CABG incidence rates: 1996–2006; (**b**) CABG incidence rates: 1996–2006; (**c**) pneumonectomy incidence rates: 1996–2006 (from The National Hospital Discharge Survey (NHDS), available at http://www.cdc.gov/nchs/nhds.htm)

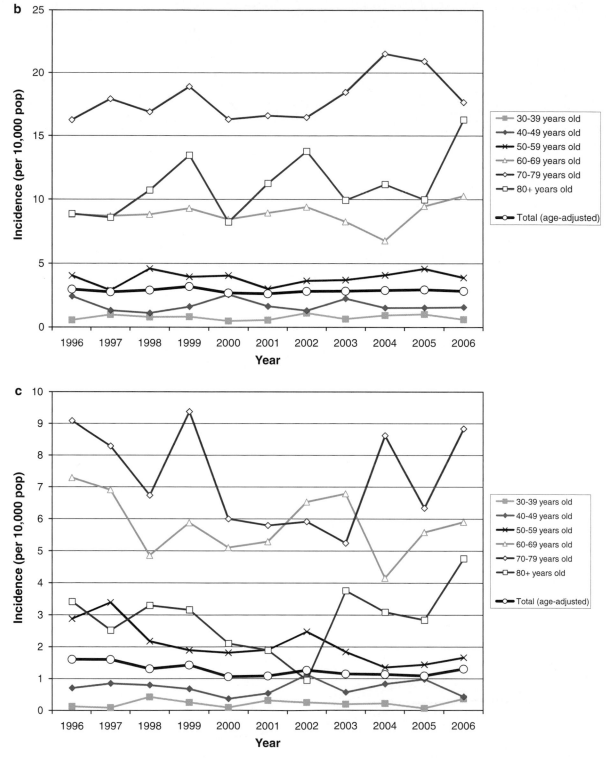

Fig. 2.5 (continued)

its own shortcoming, we will rely on what is best considered a "demands-based model." In this type of model, rates of surgical treatment (numbers of procedure per unit population) are assumed to be constant, and projections are calculated based on changes in demography. It is important to calculate these estimates within specified age groups – as we have shown above, cardiothoracic procedures are predominantly performed in older individuals. For the purposes of calculating projected rates of procedures, we will assume that rates of cardiothoracic procedures will be similar to those in 2006,

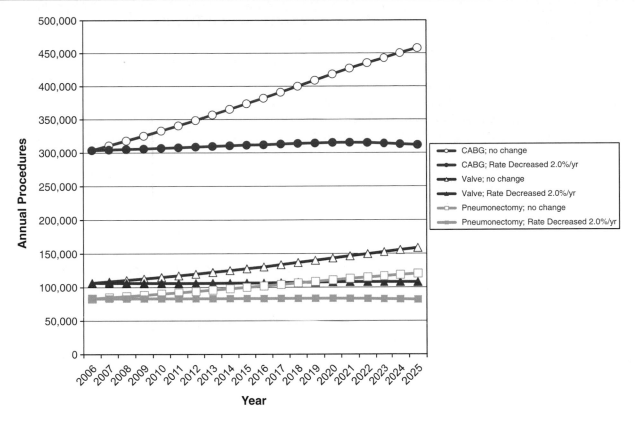

Fig. 2.6 Forecasted volumes of CABGs, valve operations, pneumonectomies; 2006–2025 (from The Healthcare Cost and Utilization Project (HCUP), available at http://www.ahrq.gov/data/hcup/datahcup.htm)

and consider the impact of population growth/aging on rates of treatment.

The results of this basic method are shown below in Fig. 2.6. In addition to calculating estimated procedures with a stable incidence rate, we also computed what would happen if the incidence rate for each procedure decreased by 2.0% per year. With the assumption of stable incidence rate, the number of CABGs is forecasted to increase by over 50% between 2006 and 2025. Similar increases are seen for valve operations and pneumonectomies, with increases of 48 and 44%, respectively. It is also worth noting that even with significant decreases in rates of treatments, the numbers of procedures performed per year is still estimated to increase as a result of population growth and aging.

Determinants of Rates of Treatment

In the preceding discussion, we have focused on the obvious relationship between demographics and the utilization of cardiothoracic surgical procedures. Clearly, however, demography is not the only determinant of the numbers of cardiothoracic procedures performed in any region. This point has

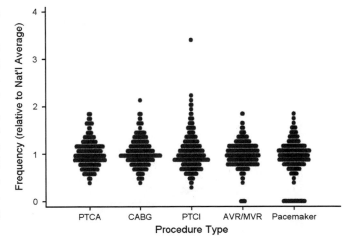

Fig. 2.7 Variation of coronary procedures in hospital referral regions (data from the 2006 Dartmouth health atlas)

been made eloquently and often by health policy researchers from Dartmouth ever since the early 1970s [3]. Their research has demonstrated a significant variation between regions in terms of the rates at which specific procedures are performed. Figure 2.7 shows rates of several types of heart procedures: percutaneous transluminal coronary angiography (PTCA),

CABG, percutaneous transluminal coronary intervention (PTCI), aortic valve replacement/mitral valve replacement (AVR/MVR) within 306 hospital referral regions (HRRs). HRRs are geographic regions which are defined based on patterns of referral for cardiovascular and neurosurgical procedures. Rates of coronary procedures show a significant degree of variation across regions, with many HRRs demonstrating rates that are greater than twice the national average.

What is responsible for these significant variations in rates of procedures? Underlying population-based differences in the prevalence of specific disease processes might explain part of the variation, but this is not believed to be a major explanatory factor. The prevailing explanation is that patterns of treatment and availability of specialists drive the majority of these variations. At some level this is intuitive – an area with few or no cardiologists is likely to have a lower rate of angiography and PTCI. In areas where there is not a shortage of specialists, however, the story becomes much more nuanced and we will devote some time to reviewing current knowledge of the drivers of procedure rates for cardiothoracic surgery. While an exhaustive discussion of these factors is beyond the scope of this chapter, we will focus on several main areas: epidemiologic trends, outcomes in elderly patients, overuse/overuse, payment systems, and the impact of medical technology.

Epidemiologic Trends

In this section we will review recent trends in the epidemiology of atherosclerotic CAD, valvular disease, and lung neoplasms.

Trends in Coronary Artery Disease (CAD)

Patients with atherosclerotic CAD are usually diagnosed on the basis of an acute myocardial infarction (AMI), and we will therefore use data regarding rates of hospitalization for AMI as an estimate of underlying population-based rates of significant CAD. In Fig. 2.8 we show these data. Rates of AMI and CABG are declining at approximately similar rates (AMI decreased by 42.3%, and CABG by 49% between 1996 and 2006). What is driving these significant reductions in rates of hospitalization for AMI? The answer is almost certainly multifactorial, including improved preventive care, early diagnosis of CAD, better cholesterol-lowering medications, and improved medical/surgical interventions.

These successes are reflected in trends regarding the death rate for heart disease in the US. According to data from the American Heart Association, between 1996 and 2006 the

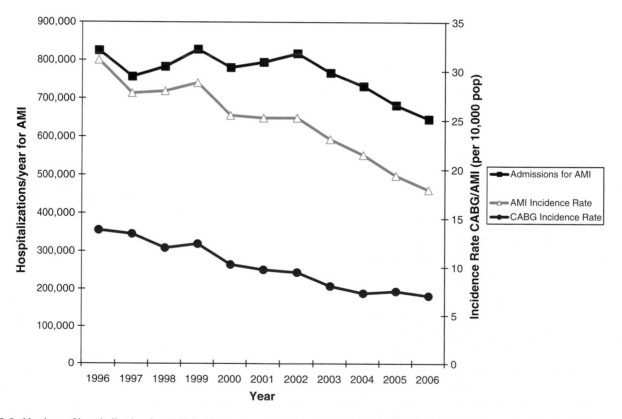

Fig. 2.8 Numbers of hospitalization for AMI; incidence rates of AMI and CABG; 1996–2006 (from The Healthcare Cost and Utilization Project (HCUP), available at http://www.ahrq.gov/data/hcup/datahcup.htm; all incidence rates age-adjusted to 1996 population)

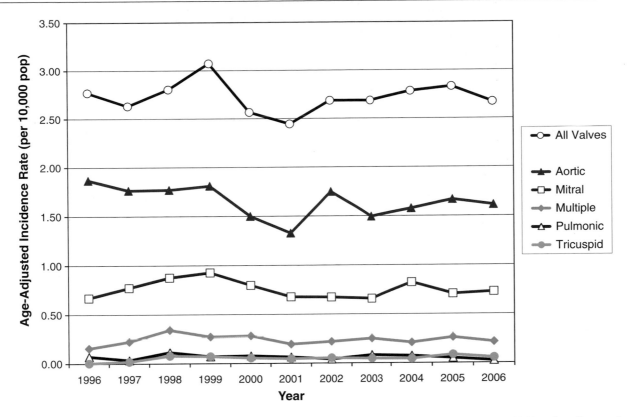

Fig. 2.9 Incidence rates for open heart valve operations (from The National Hospital Discharge Survey (NHDS), available at http://www.cdc.gov/nchs/nhds.htm)

death rate from cardiovascular disease decreased by 29.5% [4]. As a cause of death, heart disease clearly encompasses a broad spectrum of disease processes. These analyses are all important, however, in demonstrating the successes achieved in the US in treating CAD.

Trends in Valvular Heart Disease

As with CAD, it is difficult to estimate an underlying population-based incidence of valvular heart disease. While several studies have attempted to calculate such rates based on claims data [5] or prospective cohort studies [6], differences in the definitions of what constitutes disease make comparison difficult. One study pooled data on 11,911 randomly selected adults and found moderate or severe valvular heart disease in 615 [7]. Extrapolated to the entire US population in the year 2000, this study yielded an estimated 2.5% prevalence.

The etiology of valvular heart disease is evolving rapidly. Rheumatic heart disease is increasingly rare in the US, and rates of surgery for rheumatic valvular disease are declining [8]. Other diseases which reflect the effect of senescence on the aortic and mitral valve systems are becoming more common.

Unfortunately, population-based data sources which accurately capture the underlying cause of valvular disease leading to surgical treatment are not available [9]. In Fig. 2.9 we demonstrate that the overall population-based incidence rates for valve operations requiring open heart surgery (valve replacement or valvuloplasty) are approximately stable over the period from 1996 to 2006.

Trends in Lung Cancer

As a disease process, lung cancer is exquisitely sensitive to a singular risk factor – smoking. Over the last century, the incidence rate of lung cancer among individuals living in the US has peaked and is now falling in males, but has reached a plateau in females (Fig. 2.10). These trends are attributable primarily to underlying changes in rates of smoking. Domestic volumes of pneumonectomies remained fairly constant between 1996 and 2006 (Fig. 2.3).

In Fig. 2.11 we show incidence rates for pneumonectomies according to indication. Rates of resection for lung cancer fell sharply between 1996 and 2000, but have been stable between 2000 and 2006. However, in examining age-specific incidence rates an interesting pattern emerges

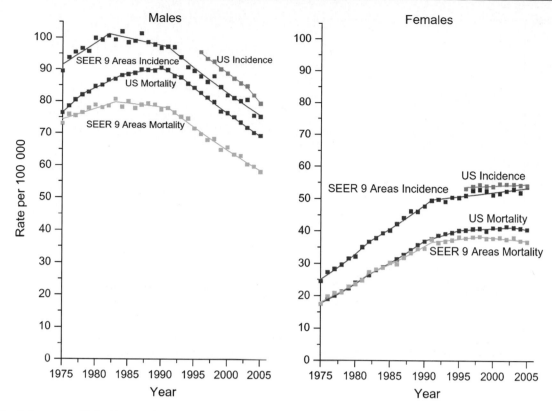

Fig. 2.10 Trends in age-specific incidence and death rates of/from lung cancer by year and gender (from Jemal et al. [39] reprinted with permission)

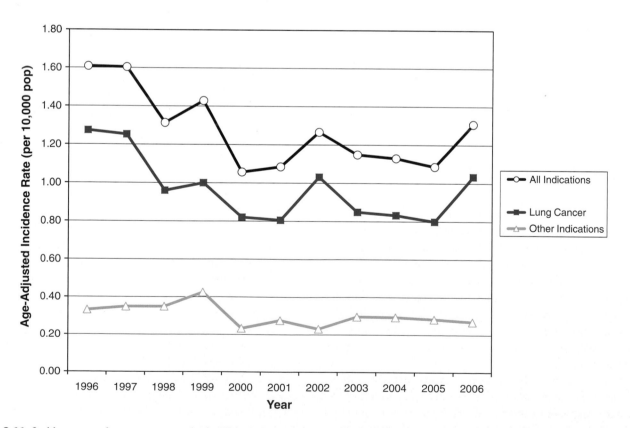

Fig. 2.11 Incidence rates for pneumonectomies in US by indication, 1990–2005 (from The National Hospital Discharge Survey (NHDS), available at http://www.cdc.gov/nchs/nhds.htm)

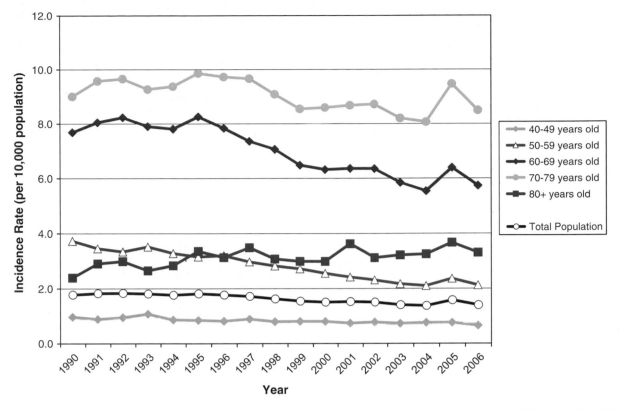

Fig. 2.12 Incidence rates for pneumonectomy for lung cancer in the US, 1990–2005 (from The Healthcare Cost and Utilization Project (HCUP), available at http://www.ahrq.gov/data/hcup/datahcup.htm)

(Fig. 2.12). Incidence rates are declining in younger individuals, but are more constant (if not increasing) in the oldest age groups (70–79 and 80+ years old). These trends are not dramatic, but do raise two related questions which we will explore in the next section. First, what are the outcomes of surgery in very elderly patients? Second – with advances in surgical technique, are these outcomes improving over time?

4.6% for octogenarians and 2.2% for septuagenarians, a rate that was not statistically different from that seen in patients under the age of 70 years (2.4%).

In Fig. 2.13 we analyze trends in hospital mortality for CABG. Overall mortality rates decreased for 4.1% in 1991 to 2.8% in 2006. Improvements were especially dramatic for patients aged 70–79 years, with mortality falling from 5.9 to 3.8%. Unfortunately, this type of analysis is not appropriate for addressing questions regarding which changes in practice are responsible for these improvements.

Outcomes of Cardiothoracic Surgery in Elderly Patients

Overuse and Underuse

The ability of cardiothoracic surgical procedures to render a positive clinical outcome is clearly related to the age of the patient in question. Intuitively, the risks and expense of surgery must be weighed against what is known regarding long-term clinical benefits. The safety of major cardiothoracic surgical procedures in elderly patients is increasingly documented in the surgical literature. In a recent review of 2,985 patients who underwent CABG at the Mount Sinai School of Medicine in New York, 28.6% were 70–79 years of age and 9.4% were 80 years or older [10]. Hospital mortality was

If one assumes that across regions the patterns of treatment provided to patients is *exactly* the same, then inter-region variations in rates of treatment would be attributable entirely to underlying differences in the prevalence of diseases. Few believe this to be the case. In considering how patterns of treatment generate differences in rates of treatment, some nomenclature is useful to organize a review of current knowledge. Toward this goal we will use important terms: underuse and overuse. These terms have been defined elegantly by Chassin et al. and the Institute of Medicine: [11]

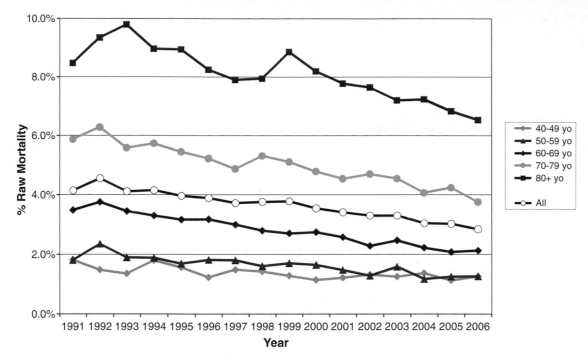

Fig. 2.13 Age-specific and overall hospital mortality rates for CABG; 1991–2006 (from The Healthcare Cost and Utilization Project (HCUP), available at http://www.ahrq.gov/data/hcup/datahcup.htm)

Overuse

Overuse occurs when a health care service is provided under circumstances in which its potential for harm exceeds the possible benefit. Prescribing an antibiotic for a viral infection like a cold, for which antibiotics are ineffective, constitutes overuse.

Underuse

Underuse is the failure to provide a health care service when it would have produced a favorable outcome for a patient. Missing a childhood immunization for measles or polio is an example of underuse.

Few areas of medicine have been as closely scrutinized regarding the presence of overuse and underuse as has the treatment of patients with coronary arterial disease (CAD). Any discussion regarding underuse and overuse necessarily begins with an explicit definition of what constitutes an *appropriate* indication for the procedure. Several groups, most notably the group from RAND/UCLA, have developed a method for synthesizing evidence using expert panelists and an iterative approach to attaining consensus. This method has proven to be highly reproducible and valid, albeit more accurate in assessing underuse than overuse [12, 13]. In Table 2.1 we present a summary of studies performed in the

last 10 years which examine underuse and overuse in the use of coronary angiography and revascularization in the treatment of patients with CAD. This brief review shows a rate of overuse of these procedures that is dramatically less than the rate of underuse.

In order to organize the discussion of overuse and underuse of patients with CAD we turn to a simplistic flow chart (Fig. 2.14). The number of patients who receive surgical treatment is, conceptually, a cross product of steps A, B, and C. Most studies examining the diagnosis and treatment of CAD have ascertained cohorts of symptomatic patients on the basis of presentation with AMI. In the remainder of this section, we will describe evidence that examines underuse and overuse of procedures at each of these steps.

Cardiologic Evaluation

For any one of a number of reasons, the ability of patients to access cardiologic evaluation may be limited. Under-insurance (either no insurance or insured by Medicaid) is an obvious reason. Philbin et al. analyzed a database of New York State hospital discharges where the principal diagnosis was AMI, and found that Medicaid patients were less likely than non-Medicaid patients to undergo coronary angiography, PTCA, and CABG procedures [14]. If under-insurance is a barrier to evaluation, rates of underuse should be lower

Table 2.1 Recent literature examining rates of underuse and overuse of coronary angiography and revascularization

Study	Context	Sample size	Procedure(s) evaluated	Findings
Carlisle et al. [41]	Los Angeles/ multiinstitutional	181 AMI 215 Angiographies	Angiography	22% underuse 3% overuse
Leape et al. [42]	New York/ multiinstitutional	631 Angiographies with CAD	PTCA and CABG after angiography	26% underuse of revascularization
Guadagnoli et al. [16]	HCFA CCP	44,294 AMI	Angiography	39% underuse[a]
Hemingway et al. [20]	London/ multiinstitutional	2,552 Angiographies with CAD	PTCA and CABG after angiography	6% of PTCAs were overuse 2% of CABGs were overuse 34% underuse of PTCA 26% underuse of CABG
Schneider et al. [43]	Medicare	788 PTCAs 709 CABGs	PTCA and CABG after angiography	14% of PTCAs were overuse 10% of CABGs were overuse
Garg et al. [44]	HCFA CCP	9,455 AMI	Angiography	42% underuse
Petersen et al. [15]	VA Medicare	1,665 AMI 19,305 AMI	Angiography Angiography	56% underuse 49% underuse
O'Connor et al. [45]	New England/ multiinstitutional	4,684 CABGS	CABG	1.4% overuse

[a]Figure not published; extracted from figure, therefore represents an approximate value

Fig. 2.14 Treatment of patients with CAD (overuse and underuse)

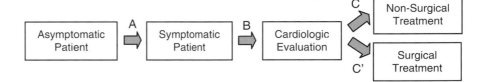

in systems where access to care is more readily available. Petersen et al. examined the treatment provided to patients treated for AMI in the Veterans Health Affairs (VA) and Medicare programs [15]. They found that only 43.9% of VA patients and 51.0% of Medicare patients underwent an angiography that was considered clinically necessary. Even for patients who are insured and/or in integrated health systems there are significant problems with achieving high rates of appropriate evaluation.

The likelihood of coronary angiography is also a function of the degree to which a patient's clinical picture constitutes a mandate for angiography. Guadagnoli et al. analyzed regional variation in rates of angiography using data from the Health Care Financing Administration's Cooperative Cardiovascular Project [16]. They found that regional variations were most affected by differences in the use of angiography for discretionary indications, rather than frank overuse or underuse.

Probably the most important determinant of a patient's likelihood of undergoing coronary angiography during admission for AMI is the availability of the service at the admitting hospital. Theoretically, a patient with a clinical need for angiography would be transferred from a hospital where such services are unavailable to one where the service could be provided. Several investigations have shown,

however, that the hospital capability to perform these procedures has a significant impact on the use of angiography [17]. The timing of arrival at a hospital also appears to have an impact on likelihood of coronary angiography. Kostis et al. examined patients admitted with a first AMI on weekends vs. weekdays and found higher mortality rates and lower use of invasive cardiac procedures for weekend admissions [18].

Surgical vs. Nonsurgical Treatment

The type of treatment (step C, Fig. 2.14) provided to patients after cardiologic evaluation has also been a focus of recent research. Denvir et al. presented standardized patient scenarios to groups of cardiologists and cardiothoracic surgeons in order to better understand their clinical decision-making process [19]. They found that initial agreement between clinicians was quite poor, but improved after open discussion in the context of a multidisciplinary panel. It might be tempting to view these differences in patterns of diagnostic and therapeutic studies as a mere curiosity. The reality is more dramatic, however. Patients who are considered appropriate candidates for CABG have lower rates of mortality when they do undergo CABG compared with patients who do not [20]. Patients who are treated at hospitals where more aggressive coronary angiography is performed have better survival rates [21].

The decision as to which approach is preferred for a specific patient needs to be considered in the context of evidence regarding the relative efficacy of PTCI and CABG. In 2009, Hlatky et al. published a pooled analysis of randomized trials comparing PTCI vs. CABG for multivessel CAD [22]. Their study analyzed 7,812 patients, and found that rates of death or MI after each type of intervention were not significantly different. Specific subgroups of patients did, however, have better results after CABG compared with PTCI — elderly (age ³65 years) and those with diabetes. A similar analysis performed in 2009 by Naik et al. examined outcomes from trials comparing PTCI and CABG for left main CAD [23]. They found no differences in terms of outcomes (mortality, cerebrovascular/cardiovascular events). Both the Naik and the Hlatky studies found higher rates of re-intervention in the PTCI groups. Since Hlatky's analysis, initial (1 year follow-up) results from the Synergy between PCI with Taxus and Cardiac Surgery (SYNTAX) trial have emerged [24]. The finding from this randomized trial of 1,800 patients was that CABG yielded a lower incidence of a composite endpoint including major cardiovascular/cerebrovascular events. Ongoing results from this trial will surely clarify the discussion regarding the indications for CABG vs. PTCI.

Improving the Appropriateness of Care

The interests of public health are well-served by minimizing the rates of underuse and overuse described above. In this section we discuss what is known regarding barriers to improving the appropriateness of treatment for patients with CAD, and possible mechanisms by which to address them.

Perhaps most importantly, a greater degree of professional consensus regarding which types of patients and types of disease are best served by which type(s) of treatment needs to be achieved. The process that arrives at this higher degree of consensus requires significant advances in clinical research, both observational and experimental, in order to provide sufficient evidence. Improving the evidence basis for treatment is only part of the answer, however. Underuse and overuse of cardiologic evaluation and coronary intervention need to be improved through structural mechanisms within the health care delivery system. The most important of these mechanisms is a multidisciplinary panel which involves the input of both cardiologists and cardiothoracic surgeons. Additionally, health care delivery systems should engage in real-time monitoring and reporting of the appropriateness of treatment provided to patients hospitalized with cardiologic conditions. We are not the first to make these recommendations [25–27].

Professional consensus and monitoring mechanisms are only part of the equation; improving access to care is also part of the equation. Patients treated for acute coronary syndrome in hospitals where intervention facilities are not available are less likely to undergo necessary procedures [17]. While this may not be surprising, it is important to envision a system where every patient receives an *appropriate* evaluation and treatment, regardless of initial portal of entry. Such a system may require greater regionalization, expanded capacity, or other more innovative solutions.

Payment Systems

"There are many mechanisms for paying physicians; some are good and some are bad. The three worst are fee-for-service, capitation, and salary."

James C. Robinson, 2001 [28]

Total costs of inpatient hospital care for patients with cardiovascular disease are estimated to be $71.2 billion per year [4]. The average cost for a CABG is over $30,000 [29]. Who pays these considerable costs?

Demonstrated in Fig. 2.15, Medicare is the most important payment source for the majority of open heart procedures

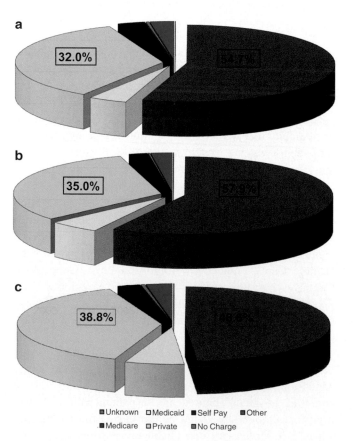

Fig. 2.15 Payment sources for open heart procedures (from The National Institute of Science, available at http://www.nationalinstituteofscience.org/). (**a**) CABG; (**b**) valve; (**c**) pneumonectomy

and almost half of pneumonectomies. Medicare is primarily held by individuals aged 65 years and older, and therefore stands to become an even more important payor as the proportion of patients who undergo these procedures are elderly. How quickly is this proportion going to change? In Fig. 2.16, we estimate the proportion of patients undergoing a CABG procedure who will be in specific age groups, using a methodology similar to that used to generate the forecasts discussed earlier. Based on this approach, patients aged 65 years and older will become a more prominent proportion of patients undergoing CABG. In 2006, those aged 65+ years were 56.7% of the CABG patient population, and by 2025 this proportion is forecasted to increase to 67.3%. Over time, Medicare will become an increasingly important mechanism through which cardiothoracic procedures are reimbursed.

The mechanism by which Medicare reimburses facilities and professionals for surgical procedures is primarily based on a fee-for-service model. Facilities are paid through a prospective payment system (PPS) and professionals based on an estimation of the amount of work required – the relative value unit (RVU). In an era of increased focus on cost containment and clinical effectiveness, payers and providers are seeking other mechanisms that more closely link payment with measurable aspects of quality. We will discuss several of these.

Starting in 2006, Geisinger Health System in central Pennsylvania instituted a PPS within which payments for elective CABG patients encompassed 90 days of follow-up care. This program effectively provided payors with a "guarantee" by covering all expenses resulting from complications incurred during the post-operative period. The effective linkage between efforts to reduce complications and cost savings is intuitive and has the potential to help drive quality improvement. Whether such a system can be expanded to other contexts remains to be seen.

A second, similar system is the Prometheus payment model which works on the payer side of the reimbursement system. Within the Prometheus model, the amount of care required to treat a specific condition is bundled together, along with an estimate of the costs of treating complications – termed "potentially avoidable costs (PACs)." If a health care system can reduce its rate of PACs, then its net reimbursement may be substantially higher. On the other hand, if multiple complications (PACs) occur, an episode of care may engender a lower net income or financial loss.

The same concept is embodied in the "never events" approach taken by the Centers for Medicare and Medicaid

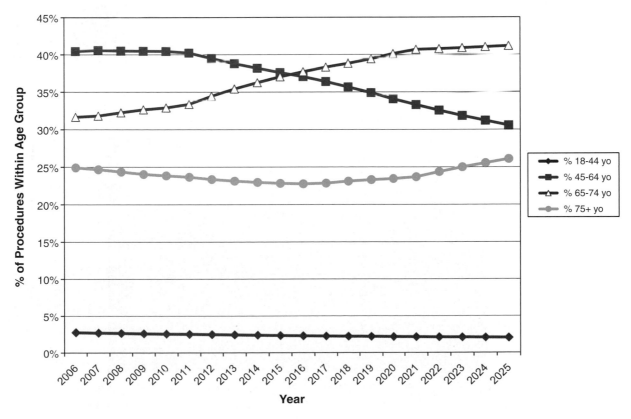

Fig. 2.16 Forecasted changes in payor mix for CABG: 2006–2025 (from The Healthcare Cost and Utilization Project (HCUP), available at http://www.ahrq.gov/data/hcup/datahcup.htm)

Services (CMS). Beginning October 1, 2008, CMS no longer reimburses hospitals for additional costs related to the development of any one of the following 8 PACs:

— Pressure ulcer stages III and IV.
— Falls and trauma.
— Surgical site infection after bariatric surgery for obesity, certain orthopedic procedures, and bypass surgery (mediastinitis).
— Vascular-catheter associated infection.
— Catheter-associated urinary tract infection.
— Administration of incompatible blood.
— Air embolism.
— Foreign object unintentionally retained after surgery.

As these systems evolve, new approaches are sure to emerge. At all levels, major participants in the health care delivery system will be asked to link payment to clinical outcomes [30].

Medical Technology

The impact of evolving medical technology on the epidemiology and economics of cardiothoracic surgical procedures is impossible to predict. It may be useful, however, to draw lessons from other fields which have experienced significant technological shifts.

Laparoscopic techniques have dramatically altered the types and rates of surgical procedures performed by abdominal surgeons. The incidence rate for cholecystectomy increased dramatically as a result of rapid uptake of laparoscopic techniques [31]. This change involved not only an increase in the use of the procedure, but also a change in what was considered an acceptable indication. When the procedure involved a large subcostal incision and a 2–4-day hospital stay, cholecystectomies were primarily performed for acute cholecystitis. With laparoscopic techniques, and lengths of stay often less than 24 h, the procedure is now primarily performed for patients with symptomatic cholelithiasis.

Vascular surgeons have also seen significant changes in the treatment for peripheral arterial disease (PAD). Endovascular procedures are rapidly supplanting open revascularization techniques for the treatment of patients with PAD, in both acute and nonacute contexts [32, 33]. What is most remarkable about this shift, however, is the rapid change in the *types of physicians* who perform endovascular procedures (Fig. 2.17). Vascular surgeons and cardiologists have quickly replaced radiologists as the specialties who are most likely to use endovascular technology for the treatment of PAD.

The lessons for cardiothoracic surgeons are clear. Minimally invasive technologies expand the pool of patients who are appropriate for surgical treatment. With the introduction of techniques for percutaneous valve procedures, there is the potential for a significant increase in the demand for these procedures. Cardiothoracic surgeons should become intimately involved in these technologies, in the same manner that vascular surgeons embraced endovascular approaches.

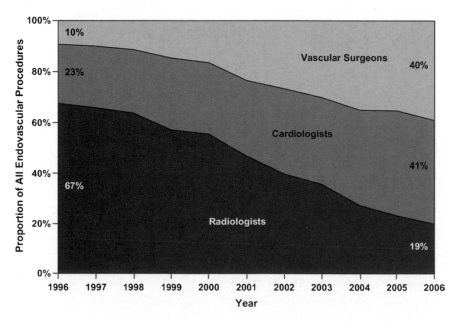

Fig. 2.17 Proportion of endovascular interventions performed by specialty, 1996–2006 (reprinted from Goodney [33] with permission. Copyright 2009, with permission from Elsevier)

Percutaneous valve procedures are only an example – the future will surely present the field of cardiothoracic surgery with many opportunities to be involved in evaluating and applying other new technologies.

The Domestic Supply of Cardiothoracic Surgeons

If the numbers of cardiothoracic procedures performed per year in the US increases, will the workforce be sufficient? In this section, we will consider trends in the numbers of surgeons certified by the American Board of Thoracic Surgeon (ABTS) in order to forecast the numbers of cardiothoracic surgeons in the future. The ABTS was initially formed in 1948, at which time 229 members were certified as founders. In 1949 an additional 15 diplomates were certified, and this number gradually rose, peaking in 1998 with 168 certifications (Fig. 2.18). Since 1998, there has been some decline in the number of certifications per year, with 118 new certifications in 2009.

We estimated the workforce of active ABTS diplomates based on historical data from the ABTS and three basic assumptions: (1) annual certification rate at 2009 levels (118 per year), (2) a 30-year career in practice after certification,

and (3) a 1.0% annual attrition rate. The results of this model are shown in Fig. 2.18. This model shows a decrease from 3,708 to 3,411 surgeons between 2009 and 2025 – a decline of approximately 8%.

The prospect of a workforce of cardiothoracic surgeons which is shrinking and a rising number of procedures raises the possibility of a shortage. If these assumptions hold, how much more work output will be expected per surgeon? We examine the answer to this question in Fig. 2.19. With an assumption of stable incidence rates in the three types of cardiothoracic surgical procedures (CABGs, valve operations, and pneumonectomies), we forecast dramatic increases in the number of procedures per active cardiothoracic surgeon. For CABG, the number would increase 67.5%, and for valve procedures and pneumonectomies, 65.0 and 60.4%, respectively. With an assumption of declining incidence rates, these increases are still significant – 14.1, 12.4, and 9.3% (for CABG, valve procedures, and pneumonectomies). The results we achieve with this simple model parallel those demonstrated by Grover et al who used a methodology similar to ours [34].

Our model's simplicity may underestimate the magnitude of growth in demand relative to supply, especially in its estimation of the effective size of the cardiothoracic surgical workforce. The current workforce of cardiothoracic surgeons

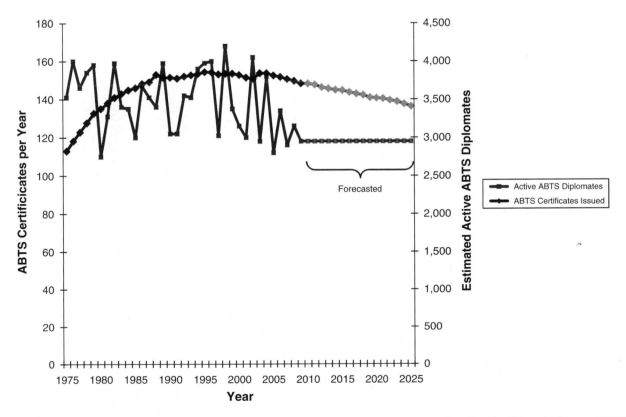

Fig. 2.18 Workforce of ABTS diplomates in the United States with forecast to 2025 (from The American Board of Thoracic Surgery (ABTS))

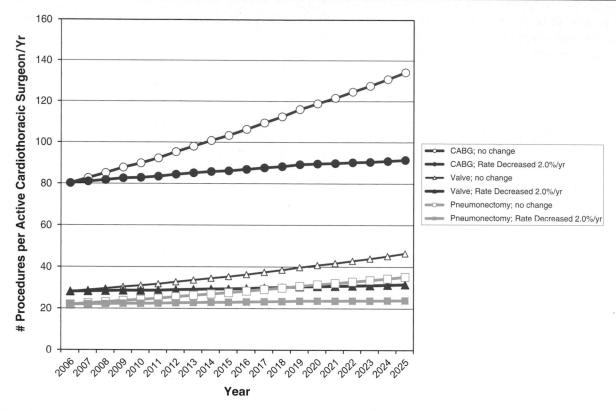

Fig. 2.19 Forecasted changes in numbers of procedures per active cardiothoracic surgeon (from The Healthcare Cost and Utilization Project (HCUP), available at http://www.ahrq.gov/data/hcup/datahcup.htm)

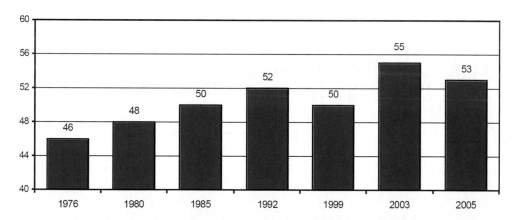

Fig. 2.20 Average age of thoracic surgeons in the US (this graph is reprinted from the 2005 STS/AATS practice survey final results (http: www. sts.org/documents/pdf/2005practsurvFinalResults.pdf) and shows the mean age trend of cardiothoracic surgeons based on longitudinal data from survey respondents. © The Society of Thoracic Surgeons. Used with permission. All rights reserved.) [40]

is increasingly older (Fig. 2.20) may be retiring earlier than in previous generations [35].

Other health policy researchers have forecasted reductions in the amount of work per physician, resulting from an increasing proportion of women in the medical workforce as well as generational changes in work hours [36]. The actual impact of these trends is difficult to estimate.

Conclusion

The field of cardiothoracic surgery is at an inflection point in its trajectory. With the advent of minimally invasive techniques to treat CAD, rates of cardiac procedures have fallen. These changes had an immediate and dramatic impact on the field, demonstrated in the reduced rates of surgical training [37]. Over the next 10–20 years, as a result of profound changes in the US population, the field of cardiothoracic surgery will see a significant increase in its patient base. Even with continued decreases in the population-based incidence rates of heart disease and lung cancer, the numbers of open heart procedures and pneumonectomies that will be performed will increase steadily. Percutaneous techniques for valve repair/replacement also have the potential to significantly expand the demand for heart procedures. Cardiothoracic surgeons need to take a leadership role in developing, testing, and diffusing these technologies. Given the declining numbers of cardiothoracic surgeons trained per year and this new demand, we agree with other health policy researchers in forecasting an increase in the workloads of cardiothoracic surgeons [34].

Demography is not the only driver of destiny, however. The appropriateness and quality of care delivered to patients needs to be examined closely and on an ongoing basis. Many view CABG procedures as discretionary procedures which are over-applied to the population as large, a view which is not grounded in truth. Cardiothoracic surgeons need to be a part of the evolution toward a system which considers the care provided to *all* patients after cardiologic evaluations, not only those deemed appropriate for surgical intervention. The field of cardiothoracic surgery must have a seat at the able where these reforms are generated in order to ensure the best health for the population.

Appendix 1: Cardiothoracic Surgical Procedures

Procedure description	ICD-9 Code(s)
Pneumonectomy	32.xx
Local excision or destruction of lesion or tissue of lung/bronchus	32.0x, 32.2x
Other excision of bronchus	32.1x
Segmental resection of lung	32.3x
Lobectomy of lung	32.4x
Complete pneumonectomy	32.5x
Radical dissection of thoracic structures	32.6x
Other excision of lung	32.9x
Valve repair/replacement	35.xx
Closed heart valvotomy	35.0x
Open heart valvuloplasty without replacement	35.1x
Replacement of heart valve	35.2x
Coronary artery bypass graft	36.xx
Removal of coronary artery obstruction and insertion of stent(s)	36.0x
Bypass anastomosis for heart revascularization; w/wo arterial implant	36.1x, 36.2x
Other heart revascularization	36.3x
Other operations on vessels of heart	36.4x

Italicized procedures considered nonsurgical, excluded from analysis.

References

1. Arias E. United States Life Tables, 2004. National Vital Statistics Reports 2007;56.
2. Dennison C, Pokras R. Design and operation of the National Hospital Discharge Survey: 1988 redesign. Vital Health Stat. 2000;1:1–42.
3. Wennberg J, Gittelsohn A. Small area variations in health care delivery. Science. 1973;182:1102–8.
4. Lloyd-Jones D, Adams RJ, Brown TM, et al. Heart disease and stroke statistics – 2010 update. A report from The American Heart Association. Circulation. 2009;17:17.
5. Bach DS, Radeva JI, Birnbaum HG, Fournier AA, Tuttle EG. Prevalence, referral patterns, testing, and surgery in aortic valve disease: leaving women and elderly patients behind? J Heart Valve Dis. 2007;16:362–9.
6. Singh JP, Evans JC, Levy D, et al. Prevalence and clinical determinants of mitral, tricuspid, and aortic regurgitation (the Framingham Heart Study). Am J Cardiol. 1999;83:897–902.
7. Nkomo VT, Gardin JM, Skelton TN, Gottdiener JS, Scott CG, Enriquez-Sarano M. Burden of valvular heart diseases: a population-based study. Lancet. 2006;368:1005–11.
8. Cosgrove D. View from North America's cardiac surgeons. Eur J Cardiothorac Surg. 2004;26 Suppl 1:S27–30; discussion S-1.
9. Gammie JS, Sheng S, Griffith BP, et al. Trends in mitral valve surgery in the United States: results from the Society of Thoracic Surgeons Adult Cardiac Surgery Database. Ann Thorac Surg. 2009;87:1431–7; discussion 7–9.
10. Filsoufi F, Rahmanian PB, Castillo JG, Chikwe J, Silvay G, Adams DH. Results and predictors of early and late outcomes of coronary artery bypass graft surgery in octogenarians. J Cardiothorac Vasc Anesth. 2007;21:784–92.
11. Chassin MR, Galvin RW. The urgent need to improve health care quality. Institute of Medicine National Roundtable on Health Care Quality. JAMA. 1998;280:1000–5.
12. Shekelle PG, Kahan JP, Bernstein SJ, Leape LL, Kamberg CJ, Park RE. The reproducibility of a method to identify the overuse and underuse of medical procedures. N Engl J Med. 1998;338:1888–95.
13. Shekelle PG, Park RE, Kahan JP, Leape LL, Kamberg CJ, Bernstein SJ. Sensitivity and specificity of the RAND/UCLA Appropriateness Method to identify the overuse and underuse of coronary revascularization and hysterectomy. J Clin Epidemiol. 2001;54:1004–10.
14. Philbin EF, McCullough PA, DiSalvo TG, Dec GW, Jenkins PL, Weaver WD. Underuse of invasive procedures among Medicaid patients with acute myocardial infarction. Am J Public Health. 2001;91:1082–8.
15. Petersen LA, Normand SL, Leape LL, McNeil BJ. Regionalization and the underuse of angiography in the Veterans Affairs Health Care System as compared with a fee-for-service system. N Engl J Med. 2003;348:2209–17.
16. Guadagnoli E, Landrum MB, Normand SL, et al. Impact of underuse, overuse, and discretionary use on geographic variation in the use of coronary angiography after acute myocardial infarction. Med Care. 2001;39:446–58.
17. Ellis C, Devlin G, Matsis P, et al. Acute Coronary Syndrome patients in New Zealand receive less invasive management when admitted to hospitals without invasive facilities. N Z Med J. 2004;117:U954.
18. Kostis WJ, Demissie K, Marcella SW, Shao YH, Wilson AC, Moreyra AE. Weekend versus weekday admission and mortality from myocardial infarction. N Engl J Med. 2007;356:1099–109.
19. Denvir MA, Pell JP, Lee AJ, et al. Variations in clinical decision-making between cardiologists and cardiac surgeons; a case for management by multidisciplinary teams? J Cardiothorac Surg. 2006;1:2.

20. Hemingway H, Crook AM, Feder G, et al. Underuse of coronary revascularization procedures in patients considered appropriate candidates for revascularization. N Engl J Med. 2001;344: 645–54.

21. Selby JV, Fireman BH, Lundstrom RJ, et al. Variation among hospitals in coronary-angiography practices and outcomes after myocardial infarction in a large health maintenance organization. N Engl J Med. 1996;335:1888–96.

22. Hlatky MA, Boothroyd DB, Bravata DM, et al. Coronary artery bypass surgery compared with percutaneous coronary interventions for multivessel disease: a collaborative analysis of individual patient data from ten randomised trials. Lancet. 2009;373: 1190–7.

23. Naik H, White AJ, Chakravarty T, et al. A meta-analysis of 3, 773 patients treated with percutaneous coronary intervention or surgery for unprotected left main coronary artery stenosis. JACC Cardiovasc Interv. 2009;2:739–47.

24. Serruys PW, Morice MC, Kappetein AP, et al. Percutaneous coronary intervention versus coronary-artery bypass grafting for severe coronary artery disease. N Engl J Med. 2009;360:961–72.

25. Pell JP, Denvir MA. Angioplasty, bypass surgery or medical treatment: how should we decide? Heart. 2002;88:451–2.

26. Kravitz RL, Laouri M. Measuring and averting underuse of necessary cardiac procedures: a summary of results and future directions. Jt Comm J Qual Improv. 1997;23:268–76.

27. Taggart DP. PCI or CABG in coronary artery disease? Lancet. 2009;373:1150–2.

28. Robinson JC. Theory and practice in the design of physician payment incentives. Milbank Q. 2001;79:149–77; III.

29. Mark DB, Hlatky MA. Medical economics and the assessment of value in cardiovascular medicine: part II. Circulation. 2002;106: 626–30.

30. Lee PV, Berenson RA, Tooker J. Payment reform – the need to harmonize approaches in Medicare and the private sector. N Engl J Med. 2010;362:3–5.

31. Escarce JJ, Chen W, Schwartz JS. Falling cholecystectomy thresholds since the introduction of laparoscopic cholecystectomy. JAMA. 1995;273:1581–5.

32. Rowe VL, Lee W, Weaver FA, Etzioni D. Patterns of treatment for peripheral arterial disease in the United States: 1996–2005. J Vasc Surg. 2009;49:910–7.

33. Goodney PP, Beck AW, Nagle J, Welch HG, Zwolak RM. National trends in lower extremity bypass surgery, endovascular interventions, and major amputations. J Vasc Surg. 2009;50:54–60.

34. Grover A, Gorman K, Dall TM, et al. Shortage of cardiothoracic surgeons is likely by 2020. Circulation. 2009;120:488–94.

35. Shemin RJ, Dziuban SW, Kaiser LR, et al. Thoracic surgery workforce: snapshot at the end of the twentieth century and implications for the new millennium. Ann Thorac Surg. 2002;73:2014–32.

36. Cooper RA, Getzen TE, McKee HJ, Laud P. Economic and demographic trends signal an impending physician shortage. Health Aff (Millwood). 2002;21:140–54.

37. Salazar JD, Lee R, Wheatley 3rd GH, Doty JR. Are there enough jobs in cardiothoracic surgery? The thoracic surgery residents association job placement survey for finishing residents. Ann Thorac Surg. 2004;78:1523–7.

38. http://www.un.org/esa/population/publications/worldageing19502050/. Accessed 01 Apr 2010.

39. Jemal A, Thun MJ, Ries LA, et al. Annual report to the nation on the status of cancer, 1975–2005, featuring trends in lung cancer, tobacco use, and tobacco control. J Natl Cancer Inst. 2008;100: 1672–94.

40. www.sts.org/documents/pdf/2005practsurvFinalResults.pdf. Accessed 01 June 2010.

41. Carlisle DM, Leape LL, Bickel S, et al. Underuse and overuse of diagnostic testing for coronary artery disease in patients presenting with new-onset chest pain. Am J Med. 1999;106:391–8.

42. Leape LL, Hilborne LH, Bell R, Kamberg C, Brook RH. Underuse of cardiac procedures: do women, ethnic minorities, and the uninsured fail to receive needed revascularization? Ann Intern Med. 1999;130:183–92.

43. Schneider EC, Leape LL, Weissman JS, Piana RN, Gatsonis C, Epstein AM. Racial differences in cardiac revascularization rates: does "overuse" explain higher rates among white patients? Ann Intern Med. 2001;135:328–37.

44. Garg PP, Landrum MB, Normand SL, et al. Understanding individual and small area variation in the underuse of coronary angiography following acute myocardial infarction. Med Care. 2002;40:614–26.

45. O'Connor GT, Olmstead EM, Nugent WC, et al. Appropriateness of coronary artery bypass graft surgery performed in northern New England. J Am Coll Cardiol. 2008;51:2323–8.

Chapter 3
Principles of Geriatric Surgery

Mark R. Katlic

Abstract The world population is aging and the conditions that require cardiothoracic surgery – atherosclerosis, lung and esophageal cancer, degenerative valve disease, dysrhythmia, and others – increase in incidence with increasing age. What do we know about surgery in the elderly that will help us improve our care of these conditions? Six general principles are useful for teaching purposes. These include the fact that the clinical presentation of surgical problems may be subtle or different from that of the general population; the elderly handle stress well but not severe stress due to lack of reserve; preoperative preparation and attention to detail are crucial; when these are lacking, as in emergency surgery, risk dramatically increases; and the results of elective surgery in the elderly are good and do not support prejudice against advanced age. Cardiothoracic surgeons must become students of the physiologic changes that occur with aging and, guided by these few principles, apply this knowledge to daily clinical care. We owe it to our elders to become good geriatric surgeons and in so doing we will become better surgeons to patients of all ages.

Keywords Principles • Reserve • Preoperative • Emergency • Prejudice • Ageism • Complications

With a few obvious exceptions, those of us who are cardiothoracic surgeons must become geriatric surgeons. The population as a whole is aging, with the most explosive growth in the over 85 year group, and the conditions that require cardiac or thoracic surgery (atherosclerosis, lung and esophageal cancer, degenerative valve disease, dysrhythmia, and others) increase in incidence with increasing age. Ferguson and Vigneswaran [1], for example, reported that of all patients requiring major lung resection, the proportion over age 70 rose from 20 to 30% over the last three decades. In Germany, the percentage of similarly aged patients undergoing cardiac

surgery rose from 24.9 to 45.3% in one decade [2]. Over the next 20 years there will be a 67% increase in cancer incidence for older adults, compared with an 11% increase for younger adults [3]. Improving our care of the elderly chest surgical patient – the *raison d'etre* of this book – will become progressively more important to us all.

Admittedly, surgeons have always cared for the elderly, but the definition of "elderly" has changed. A threshold of 50 years was chosen for the 167 patients described in an article in 1907 [4], and 20 years later influential surgeons still wrote that elective herniorrhaphy in this age group was not warranted [5]. Now, though, we are performing complex operations such as esophagectomy and reoperative cardiac surgery in octogenarians, nonagenarians, and occasionally centenarians [6–10]. In addition, the salutary results of such surgery can even influence general sentiment about medical care of the elderly. Linn and Zeppa's study [11] of junior medical students reported that the surgery rotation, in contrast to other clerkships, positively influenced the students' attitudes about aging regardless of the students' career choices, as the elderly surgical patients were admitted and treated successfully.

Surgery therefore has much to offer the geriatric patient, but that patient must be treated with appropriate knowledge and attention to detail. Discussions of physiologic changes in the elderly and results of specific operations comprise the bulk of this book and are not presented here. The author's quarter-century study in this area, in addition to caring for an elderly thoracic oncology population, has led to a distillate of several general principles (Table 3.1) which are relevant to all who care for the aged. These principles are worthwhile chiefly for teaching purposes, as they cannot apply to every patient or every clinical situation. Some principles also apply to surgery in the young patient, but the quantitative differences in the elderly are significant enough to approach qualitative status. Risks of many emergency operations in the young, for example, are indeed greater than the risks of similar elective operations, but the differences are small compared to the threefold increase in the elderly. With respect to these principles the elderly need not be treated as a separate

M.R. Katlic (✉)
Department of Thoracic Surgery, Geisinger Wyoming Valley Medical Center, 1000 East Mountain Drive, Wilkes-Barre, PA 18711, USA
e-mail: mrkatlic@geisinger.edu

M.R. Katlic (ed.), *Cardiothoracic Surgery in the Elderly*, DOI 10.1007/978-1-4419-0892-6_3,
© Springer Science+Business Media, LLC 2011

Table 3.1 Principles of geriatric surgery

I.   The *clinical presentation* of surgical problems in the elderly may be subtle or somewhat different from that in the general population. This may lead to delay in diagnosis

II. The elderly handle stress satisfactorily but handle severe stress poorly because of *lack of organ system reserve*

III. Optimal *preoperative preparation* is essential, because of Principle II. When preparation is suboptimal the perioperative risk increases

IV. The results of elective surgery in the elderly are reproducibly good; the results of emergency surgery are poor though still better than nonoperative treatment for most conditions. The risk of *emergency surgery* may be many times that of similar elective surgery because of Principles II and III

V.   Scrupulous *attention to detail* intraoperatively and perioperatively yields great benefit, as the elderly tolerate complications poorly (because of Principle II)

VI. A patient's age should be treated as a *scientific fact, not with prejudice*. No particular chronologic age, of itself, is a contraindication to operation (because of Principle IV)

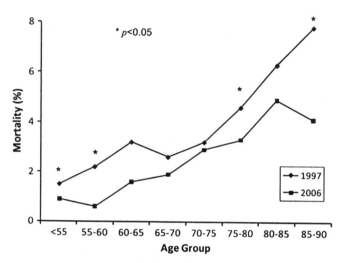

Fig. 3.1 Mortality versus age in aortic valve replacement. Mortality was age dependent in 1997 and 2006. Mortality was less in 2006 than in 1997. *Asterisk* indicates *p* < 0.05 (Reprinted from Brown et al. [13] Copyright 2009, with permission from Elsevier)

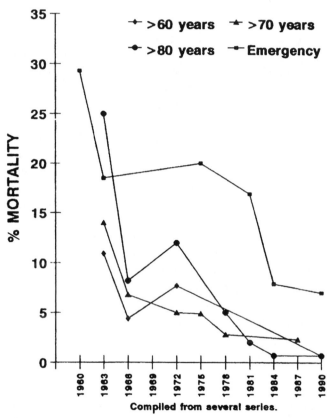

Fig. 3.2 Decline in surgical mortality in elderly over time (emergency always much higher) (Reprinted from Thomas and Ritchie [12] with permission from Wiley-Blackwell)

species but perhaps as a separate genus or order within the same larger group of surgical candidates.

Although our results have generally improved over the years [12, 13], this improvement has not been universal [14, 15] (Fig. 3.1) and emergency surgery is still risky (Fig. 3.2). Understanding these six general principles may help us improve our care of the geriatric patient who requires cardiothoracic surgery.

Principle I: Clinical Presentation

The clinical presentation of surgical problems in the elderly may be subtle or somewhat different from that in the general population. This may lead to delay in diagnosis.

Examples from general surgery illustrate this principle. Classic symptoms of appendicitis are present in a minority of elderly patients, as few as 26% in Horattas' series over 20 years [16] (Table 3.2). Rebound tenderness was present in

fewer than half the patients in another [17] and leukocytosis in only 42.9% in another [18]. Clouding the picture further, objective tests may suggest alternative diagnoses: one in six patients has an elevated bilirubin and one in four has signs of ileus, bowel obstruction, gallstones, or renal calculus on abdominal radiographs [19]. Computed tomograms therefore may alter clinical diagnosis in over 40% of cases of abdominal pain [20, 21]. Even astute diagnosis may not prevent perforation, present in 42–60% of elderly patients despite operation within 24 h of symptom onset [16, 18, 21].

Table 3.2 Classic symptoms of appendicitis are present in a minority of elderly patients, resulting in perforation despite expeditious operation

Twenty-year comparison and compilation

Characteristic	1978–1988 (n=96)	1988–1998 (n=113)	1978–1998 (n=209)
Classic presentation	(19) 20%	(36) 30%	(55) 26%
Delayed presentation (>48 h)	(32) 33%	(36) 30%	(68) 33%
Imaging			
AAS	(81) 84%	(86) 76%	(167) 80%
Sensitivity	(22) 27%	(22) 25%	(44) 26%
CT		(50) 44%	
Sensitivity		(45) 90%	
Correct admitting diagnosis	(49) 51%	(52) 46%	(101) 48%
Surgery within 24 h	(80) 83%	(97) 85%	(177) 85%
Perforation	(60) 72%	(58) 51%	(127) 61%
Complications	(30) 32%	(24) 21%	(54) 26%
Those with perforation	(25) 83%	(15) 72%	(40) 76%
Deaths	(4) 4%	(4) 4%	(8) 4%

Reprinted from Storm-Dickerson [16], Copyright 2003, with permission from Elsevier

Table 3.3 Symptoms of gastroesophageal reflux disease may be different and more subtle in the elderly

	No. (%) of patients		
Symptom	Group A (<65 Years) (n=241)	Group B (≥65 years) (n=63)	p Value
Heartburn	209 (86)	45 (47)	0.001
Dysphagia	92 (38)	28 (35)	0.77
Regurgitation	113 (47)	46 (71)	0.001
Chest Pain	97 (39)	18 (28)	0.13
Cough	89 (37)	42 (67)	0.001
Response to proton pump inhibitors[a]	70	75	0.53

[a]Percentage of patients
Source: Reprinted with permission from Tedesco [33], Copyright © American Medical Association. All rights reserved

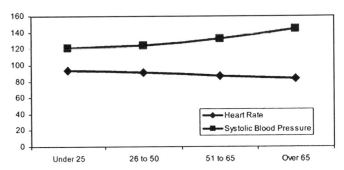

Fig. 3.3 Field heart rate and systolic blood pressure following trauma, by age group, indicating "pseudostability of elderly." (Reprinted from Lehmann et al. [42], Copyright 2009, with permission from Elsevier)

Biliary tract disease is the most common entity requiring abdominal surgery in the elderly, yet the diagnosis is often delayed. More than one-third of patients with acute cholecystitis are afebrile, one-fourth are nontender, and one-third are without leukocytosis [22–24]. Cholangitis may appear only as fever of unknown origin or as confusion [25]. Consequently, the elderly predominate in series of patients with complications of biliary disease (gallbladder perforation, empyema, gangrene, gallstone ileus, and cholangitis) [26], and the complication may result in the first apparent symptom [23, 27]. Saunders et al. [28] reported that abdominal pain was a less prominent symptom and that the bilirubin level was nearly double in elderly patients presenting with bile duct carcinoma, compared to the findings in young patients seen during the same time period.

Peptic ulcer disease may present as confusion, malaise, anemia, or weight loss as opposed to pain [29]; even with perforation pain may be absent or minimal. Rabinovici and Manny [30] found a discrepancy between "severe intraoperative findings" and preoperative objective findings such as heart rate (mean 88/min), temperature (37.2°C), and white blood cell count (10,900/dL). Some have suggested that the elderly and possibly their physicians become tolerant over the years to abdominal pain, loss of energy, and other symptoms, resulting in a delay in diagnosis or an emergency presentation. In Mulcahy et al.'s [31] series of patients with colorectal carcinoma, for example, elderly patients were nearly twice as likely (18%) as younger patients (11%) to present emergently. Elderly patients with perforated diverticulitis are three times more likely to have generalized peritonitis at operation than young patients [32].

Gastroesophageal reflux disease in the elderly is less likely to cause heartburn and more likely to cause regurgitation

or cough (p=001) [33]. In Pilotto et al.'s study of 840 consecutive patients [34], typical heartburn/acid reflux, pain, and indigestion were more likely in the young (p<0.001); older patients more often experienced dysphagia, anorexia, anemia, or vomiting (p<0.001 each) or weight loss (p<0.007) (Table 3.3).

Head and neck disease may also present differently in the elderly. Sinusitis may lead to subtle signs such as delirium or fever of unknown origin [35, 36]; and head and neck cancers are less likely to be associated with smoking (p<0.01) [37] and alcohol use (p<0.001) [37, 38]. Hyperparathyroidism is more likely to cause dementia or skeletal complaints and less likely to cause renal stones [39]. In Thomas and Grigg's series [40] of patients with carotid artery disease, stroke was the most common indication for surgery in octogenarians and was the least common indication in younger patients. Unstable angina is as likely to present with dyspnea, nausea, or diaphoresis as it is with classic chest pain [41].

Lehmann et al. [42] found that "hypotension and tachycardia were unreliable predictors of the need for urgent intervention in the elderly group [of trauma patients]" (Fig. 3.3), and refers to the "pseudostability" of elderly patients with unrecognized shock after traumatic injury.

hemoglobin applies to every patient, but correction of anemia and dehydration do assume greater importance in the elderly because of their general lack of reserve and particularly the physiology of the aged heart and kidney. Among the predictors of an overall good postoperative course in Seymour's series of 288 elderly general surgery patients were a hemoglobin level of more than 11.0 g/dL and absence of volume depletion [73]. Bo et al. [74] found that hemoglobin level was an independent predictor of 1-month mortality as well as length of stay in 294 elderly surgical patients. Contrary to this, Dzankic et al. found that routine blood testing in the elderly surgical patient rarely showed abnormal results and even when abnormal did not correlate with adverse postoperative outcome [75].

Few would argue that pulmonary problems are among the most common perioperative complications in the elderly, in part due to decreased respiratory muscle strength. Nomori et al. [54] showed that following thoracotomy patients older than 70 years experience significant reductions in both maximum inspiratory and expiratory pressures, unlike their younger counterparts; this effect persists for 12 weeks (Fig. 3.8). Although few data exist to support the routine use of preoperative pulmonary conditioning or rehabilitation (Bobbio et al. [76] reported benefit but the number of patients was small), most authors strongly advocate smoking cessation [77] and treatment of bronchitis and reactive airways disease such as asthma [78, 79]. Prophylaxis against deep vein thrombosis (DVT) – clearly a risk in the elderly – [80] and against pulmonary embolism should be routine [81].

The value of preoperative optimization of cardiac function (e.g., via placement of a pulmonary artery catheter) is controversial. Some authors have shown clear benefit [82], whereas others [83, 84], citing methodologic flaws in the former studies, reported no reduction in perioperative morbidity or mortality. These studies do not include exceptionally high risk or very elderly patients, who could well be helped by such treatment. Another unsettled issue concerns the value of aggressive preoperative screening for coronary and carotid artery disease, particularly in patients scheduled for peripheral vascular surgery. Leppo [85] considered age over 70 as one of the several risk factors (the others being a history of angina, congestive heart failure, diabetes mellitus, prior myocardial infarction, and ventricular ectopy), which should trigger further cardiac assessment. Echocardiogram and dobutamine stress testing have been shown to bear incremental value over clinical evaluation [86] (Fig. 3.9).

There is some evidence that performance testing may hold value. Maximal oxygen consumption (VO_2 Max) tests may not be readily available in all hospitals, but reasonable surrogates – stair climbing [87, 88], shuttle walk [89], long distance corridor walk [90], and metabolic equivalent (MET) – have been shown to correlate. Weinstein [91] reported prolonged length of stay following thoracic cancer surgery in those patients with METs ≤4 (equating to calisthenics or walking briskly). The International Society of Geriatric Oncology has studied a standardized preoperative assessment in elderly cancer patient; postoperative complications were associated with poor preoperative performance status and lower score on Instrumental Activities of Daily Livin,g but major complications correlated only with American Society of Anesthesiologists (ASA) Physical Status ≤2 [92] (Table 3.4). However, as Internullo et al. recently concluded, "a practical and reliable individual risk assessment tool is still lacking" [93].

Preoperative antibiotics are not necessary for every type of elective surgery, but researchers agree that advanced age

a

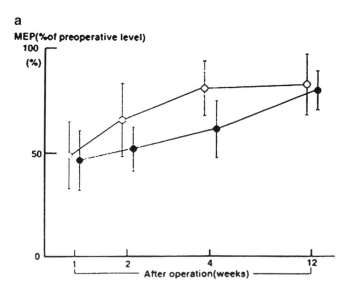

b

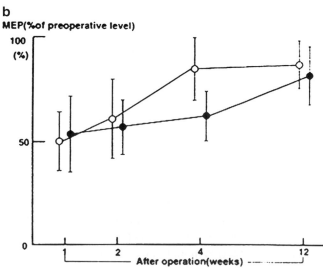

Fig. 3.8 Postoperative changes in mean (**a**) maximum inspiratory pressure (MIP, percent of preoperative level) and (**b**) maximum expiratory pressure (MEP, percent of preoperative level) following pulmonary resection in 36 patients younger than 69 years (*open circles*) and 12 patients older than 70 years (*closed circles*) (Reprinted with permission from Nomori et al. [54], Copyright Elsevier 1996)

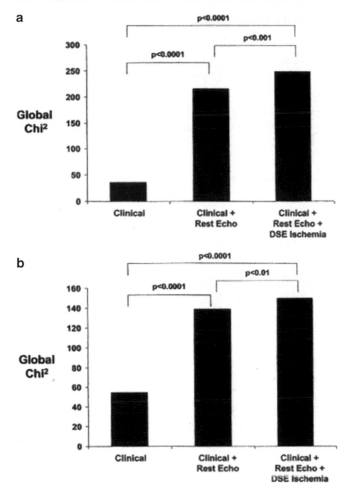

a

b

Fig. 3.9 Incremental value of echocardiogram and dobutamine stress echocardiogram (DSE) over clinical evaluation for prediction of cardiac events (**a**) and all-cause mortality (**b**) in the elderly (Reprinted from Biagini et al. [86] by permission of Oxford University Press)

Table 3.4 Univariate association between components of PACE with 30-day morbidity (any and major complication) adjusted for age sex type and stage of cancer and severity of surgery

Components of PACE	Any complication RR[a]	95% CI	Major complication RR[a]	95% CI
MMS abnormal (<24)	1.23	0.81–1.88	1.08	0.48–2.44
ADL dependent (>0)	1.41	0.95–2.10	1.87	0.95–3.69
IADL dependent (<8)	*1.43*	1.03–1.98	1.65	0.88–3.08
GDS depressed (>4)	1.30	0.93–1.81	1.69	0.93–3.08
BFI mod/severe fatigue (>3)	*1.52*	1.09–2.12	1.24	0.67–2.27
ASA abnormal (≥2)	1.00	0.73–1.38	*1.96*	1.09–3.53
PS abnormal (>1)	*1.64*	1.07–2.52	1.97	0.92–4.23
Satariano's index (1)	1.11	0.78–1.59	1.29	0.68–2.44
Satariano's index (2+)	1.58	0.88–2.85	1.95	0.74–5.18

Components of preoperative assessment of cancer in the elderly (PACE); *MMS* mini mental status; *ADL* activities of daily living; *IADL* instrumental activities of daily living; *GDS* geriatric depression scale; *BFI* brief fatigue inventory; *ASA* American Society of Anesthesiologists Physical Status; *PS* Eastern Cooperative Oncology Group Performance Status *Source*: Reprinted from Audisio et al. [92], Copyright 2008, with permission from Elsevier
[a]Bold italics: significant relationship ($p < 0.05$)

is a risk factor for nosocomial infection. Iwamoto [94] studied 4,380 patients who underwent general anesthesia for thoracic, abdominal, or neurologic surgery and concluded that advanced age is a risk factor for nosocomial pneumonia, especially after thoracic surgery. Age greater than 70 has been shown to be a risk factor for both positive bile cultures ($p < 0.001$) [95] and septic complications of biliary surgery compared to younger patients [96]; antibiotic prophylaxis can reduce these complications [97].

Efforts to improve our elderly patients' preoperative nutritional state would seem desirable – even active, community-dwelling older adults manifest impaired recovery of strength after major surgery [98] – but it is unclear how to do this. Low levels of serum albumin, for example, correlate strikingly with postoperative problems [99] (Fig. 3.10), but cannot be improved to a great degree preoperatively. Souba [100] reviewed the literature on nutritional support and concluded that preoperative support should be reserved for severely malnourished patients scheduled to undergo major elective surgery and then should be provided for no more than 10 days.

In addition to those already cited, a number of surgeons have attributed their improved results in elderly patients to compulsive preoperative preparation. Bittner et al. [101] believed that the significant decrease in mortality after total gastrectomy in septuagenarians (32.0% in 1979 to 4.4% in 1996) was the result of standardized perioperative antibiotics, thromboembolic prophylaxis, "a systemic analysis of risk factors and their thorough preoperative therapy," and

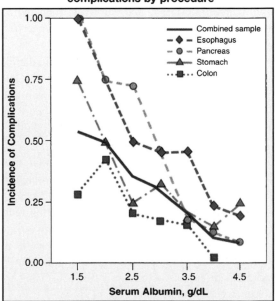

Albumin levels and incidence of surgical complications by procedure

Fig. 3.10 Preoperative albumin level and major postoperative complications (From Kudsk et al. [99] Copyright © 2003. Reprinted by permission of SAGE Publications)

nutritional support for the malnourished. After studying 412 patients who underwent pancreatic resection, Pratt [102] advocates gerontology consultation and intense preoperative preparation in those over age 75, including hyperalimentation and biliary drainage as indicated.

Hypovolemia is tolerated poorly by the elderly patient and it must be corrected. Smoking should stop. Treating other correctable aberrations such as anemia, bronchitis, and hypertension preoperatively increases the elderly patient's chance for a smooth postoperative course.

Principle IV: Emergency Surgery

The results of elective surgery in the elderly are reproducibly good; the results of emergency surgery are poor though still better than nonoperative treatment for most conditions. The risk of emergency surgery may be many times that of similar elective surgery because of Principles II and III.

The results of elective surgery in the elderly are good, frequently indistinguishable from the results in younger counterparts [103–105]. Coyle et al. [106] reported the results of carotid endarterectomy in 79 octogenarians and summarized the results of five other series (634 total patients); mortality and morbidity were similar to those in a younger cohort. Maehara [107] had 0% operative mortality in 77 patients over age 70 who underwent resection of gastric carcinoma, and Jougon et al.'s [108] results for esophagectomy in 89 patients aged 70–84 were identical to those in 451 younger patients. Patients older than 80 years can tolerate profound hypothermic circulatory arrest for ascending and arch aortic surgery [109]. An octogenarian with lung cancer could anticipate mortality and survival after pulmonary lobectomy statistically identical to that of younger patients with similar stage disease [78, 103, 110–112].

Identical operations performed emergently in the elderly, however, carry at least a threefold (and as much as a 10-fold) increased risk [15]. Keller [113], for example, reported 31% morbidity and 20% mortality in 100 patients over age 70 who underwent emergency operations, which is significantly more ($p < 0.0005$) than the 6.8% morbidity and 1.9% mortality following elective operation in 513 similar patients. Elective cholecystectomy can be performed in young and old with the risk of death approaching 0% [27, 114, 115]; the risk of mortality for emergency cholecystectomy increases somewhat in the younger group (1–2%) but increases greatly in the elderly (5–15%) [27]. Surgical priority clearly affects cardiac surgery risk [116, 117]. Elective operative mortality for colorectal surgery is as low as 1.5–3.0%, rising to over 20% for emergency operation [118, 119].

A patient's advanced age therefore weighs in favor of commencing rather than deferring needed elective surgery.

Principle V: Attention to Detail

Scrupulous attention to detail intraoperatively and perioperatively yields great benefit, as the elderly tolerate complications poorly (because of Principle II).

Perioperative blood loss is the *bete noire* of geriatric surgery, as the elderly lack the responsive compensatory mechanisms necessary to restore equilibrium. Fong [64] reported that the only independent predictor of postoperative complications in 138 patients over age 70 who underwent pancreatic resection was intraoperative blood loss exceeding 2 L. This finding has been mirrored in reports from cardiac surgery [120], hepatectomy [121], and neurosurgery. Sisto [122] reported that 6 of 23 octogenarian coronary bypass patients who required reexploration for tamponade died; Logeais [123] found that reoperation for tamponade following aortic valve replacement placed the elderly patient at high risk for mortality ($p < 0.001$). Hemostasis is exceptionally important in the elderly craniotomy patient, possibly because the elderly brain is less likely to expand to obliterate dead space: Maurice-Williams et al. [124] reported that postoperative bleeding following resection of meningioma occurred in 20% of 46 elderly patients and 0% of 38 young patients ($p < 0.05$). In Pratt's series of pancreatic resection patients, intraoperative blood loss was termed the "primary driver of surgical performance; fittingly, it also represents the one factor (physiologic or operative) over which the surgeon has the most control" [102].

Prevention of infection is crucial in the geriatric surgical patient. Kaye [125], in a study of 1,352 elderly patients at Duke University Medical Center, reported nearly four times greater mortality in patients who developed surgical site infection versus those who did not. Older age has been found to be an independent predictor of mortality from *Staphylococcus aureus* bacteremia, with odds of dying doubling for every decade increase in age [126].

Meticulous surgical technique is important in any patient, but it becomes crucial in those of advanced age. Anastomotic leak after esophageal or gastric resection, a dreaded complication in any patient, embodies an exceptional risk of mortality in the elderly [127]; yet this complication can be minimized by careful technique [128, 129]. Only one of Bandoh's [130] elderly patients who underwent gastrectomy for cancer experienced a leak, as did only 2 of 163 patients over age 70 in Bittner's series [101]. Despite having significantly greater preoperative comorbidity, the elderly patients undergoing gastrectomy in Gretschel's series experienced no greater postoperative morbidity [68]. The elderly cardiac surgery patient may benefit from extra care when they have a calcified aorta (e.g., intraoperative ultrasound or modified clamping and cannulation technique) or a fragile sternum (e.g., additional or pericostal wires) [131]. Even endotracheal intubation is riskier in the elderly [132]. Operative speed is less important than technique: in Cohen et al.'s series of 46 nonagenarians undergoing major procedures [10], the duration of operation did not correlate with mortality.

Perioperative monitoring is more important in the elderly, since they may manifest few signs or symptoms of impending problems (see Sect. "Principle I: Clinical Presentation"). Bernstein [133] credits intensive hemodynamic monitoring in his lack of mortality among 78 patients over age 70 who underwent abdominal aortic aneurysmectomy. Such monitoring and intensive care were also emphasized by Alexander et al. [6], who reported excellent results for 59 octogenarians having major upper abdominal cancer operations, and by Lo et al. [134] for 85 elderly patients undergoing adrenal surgery at the Mayo Clinic. As early as 1990 surgeons reported improved outcomes in elderly trauma patients with early invasive monitoring and early intensive management [135, 136]. Giannice [137] credits attention to perioperative care (DVT prophylaxis, antibiotics, monitoring, respiratory care, pain management, and early mobilization) for his group's improved recent results in gynecologic oncology patients.

The elderly patient undergoing lung resection, for example, might have reinforcement of vascular and bronchial closures in addition to compulsive hemostasis and minimization of parenchymal air leaks. He or she would be monitored postoperatively. If she developed an atrial arrhythmia it would be aggressively treated; if he developed tracheobronchial secretions he would promptly undergo therapeutic bronchoscopy.

Zingone et al. found that postoperative complications following cardiac surgery in 355 octogenarians were stronger risk factors for mortality than either preoperative comorbidities or procedural variables. He noted that "the threshold for entering a complicated course may be lower and that for getting out of it higher for the elderly" [138].

We should continue to teach the surgical aphorism, "Elderly patients tolerate operations but not complications" (Table 3.5).

Principle VI: Age Is a Scientific Fact

A patient's age should be treated as a scientific fact, not with prejudice. No particular chronologic age, of itself, is a contraindication to operation (because of Principle IV).

Great biologic variability exists among the elderly, with some octogenarians and nonagenarians proving to be healthier than their sons and daughters. Even an 88-year-old patient has a life expectancy exceeding 4 years [139, 140], so why not offer him resection of his lung cancer? No other treatment is likely to give him those 4 years. Yet even in 2005 this does not always happen: prejudice against the elderly, so-called "ageism" exists.

Despite the fact that elderly patients treated for lung cancer have survival equal to their younger matched counterparts, Nugent et al. [141] found that patients older than 80 years were significantly less likely ($p < 0.05$) to be treated surgically. Kuo et al. [142] similarly reported that octogenarian patients with lung cancer were more likely ($p < 0.01$) to receive only palliative care; when offered chemotherapy they tolerate it [143].

Feasibility of mitral valve repair for degenerative etiology in the elderly is similar (93%) to younger counterparts [144] and, despite a relatively high operative mortality (23%), survivors experience a markedly improved QOL [145] unless burdened by many preoperative conditions [146]. Nevertheless, mitral valve surgery is often denied in these individuals: in the Euro Heart Survey on valve disease the decision to operate was undertaken in 42% of patients aged 70–79 and 15% of patients older than 80 years [147].

Elderly patients with ovarian cancer are less likely to undergo aggressive chemotherapy and surgery [148, 149] despite results equal to the young [150]. Older patients with osteosarcoma are less likely to have limb salvage (56 vs. 90% in younger population) or chemotherapy [151]. Older women with breast cancer are less likely to have had screening mammograms [152, 153], are more likely to present in advanced stages than younger women [153], and are less likely to undergo definitive local therapy [154] and adjuvant therapy; [155] once diagnosed and offered surgery, they tolerate it well [156, 157].

Guadagnoli [158] presented evidence against ageism in the treatment of early breast cancer, but Herbert-Croteau et al. [159] found that only tamoxifen use was similar in women over and under age 70 ($p < 0.41$), while all other

Table 3.5 Importance of postoperative complications in failure of octogenarians to return to normal function following major abdominal surgery

Multivariate analysis of failure to return to premorbid function		
All cases	Odds ratio	95% CI
Emergency operation	2.7	0.99–7.24
ASA III or IV	1.0	0.29–3.56
Comorbidity index >5	1.8	0.48–6.66
Dependence on activities of daily living	1.8	0.42–7.73
Preexisting cardiac disease	1.9	0.69–5.44
Preexisting chronic pulmonary disease	2.0	0.54–7.47
Preexisting cerebrovascular disease	2.0	0.43–9.06
Development of postoperative complications	24.5	3.08–194.88
Elective cases only comorbidity index >5	11.2	1.08–116.26
Development of postoperative complications	10.6	3.08–194.88

Source: Reprinted from Tan et al. [127], with permission from Springer Science+Business Media

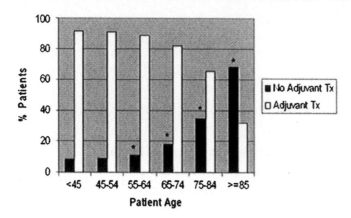

Fig. 3.11 Use of adjuvant therapy by patient age in patients with resected pathologic stage II–III rectal cancer (*Tx* therapy); *asterisk*: compared to patients aged less than 45, *p*<0.001 (Reprinted from Esnaola et al. [167] with permission from Springer Science+Business Media)

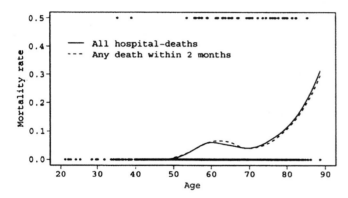

Fig. 3.12 Linear logistic regression analysis of mortality rate by age as a continuous variable for all in-hospital deaths and any death within two months of esophagectomy (Reprinted with permission from Moskovitz et al. [173], Copyright Elsevier 2006)

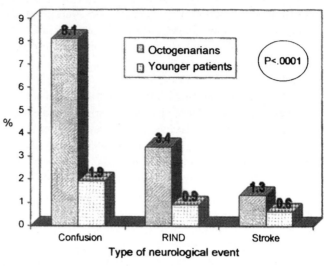

Fig. 3.13 Early postoperative neurologic complications after coronary artery bypass surgery and valve surgery in octogenarians (*RIND* reversible ischemic neurological deficit) (Reprinted from Ngaage [120] Copyright 2008, with permission from Elsevier)

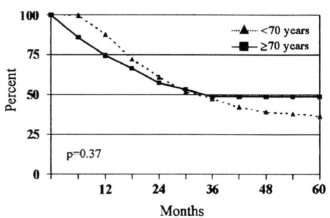

Fig. 3.14 Esophagectomy following neoadjuvant chemoradiation. Kaplan–Meier survival curves (including postoperative deaths) plotted for patients age <70 versus ≥70 years (Reprinted from Ruol et al. [196], with permission from Springer Science+Business Media)

treatments (breast-conserving surgery, radiotherapy, axillary node dissection, and chemotherapy) differed significantly (*p*<0.0001). When elderly patients do receive chemotherapy for breast cancer, they tolerate it [160] and they benefit from it [161, 162]. Even multiagent therapy is feasible in octogenarians with various cancers [163].

In a 2007 editorial, Siu [164] concluded that "ageism is probably the greatest impediment to the enrollment of older patients in trials for cancer therapy."

Elderly patients with colon cancer are less likely to undergo extensive lymph node dissection (*p*<0.0001) [165] and less likely to receive chemotherapy [166, 167] (Fig. 3.11). Few patients with severe osteoarthritis of knee or hip reported that their primary care physician discussed joint replacement [168]. Selection bias in the elderly may also lead to delay in referral for abdominal aortic aneurysm surgery [169] and coronary artery bypass surgery [170].

Even when trauma is recognized and acknowledged by emergency medical services, "providers are consistently less likely to consider transporting elderly patients to a [designated] trauma center" [171].

Some studies do report increased operative mortality [15, 172–174] (Fig. 3.12), increased complications [120, 174, 175] (Fig. 3.13), and increased lengths-of-stay in the elderly [176–180], but overall results do not differ from the young for a wide variety of procedures: neurosurgery [124, 181], head and neck surgery [37, 182–184], carotid endarterectomy [185–188], cardiac surgery [62, 131, 170, 189–193], esophagectomy [93, 108, 128, 194–196] (Fig. 3.14), gastrectomy [6, 107,

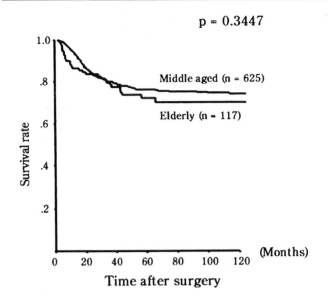

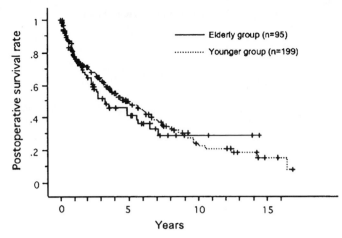

Fig. 3.15 Surgical outcome in elderly (≥75 years) and middle-aged (45–65 years) patients with gastric cancer (Reprinted from Kunisakı et al. [198], Copyright 2006, with permission from Elsevier)

Fig. 3.17 Hepatic resection for hepatocellular carcinoma. Postoperative survival (Kaplan–Meier curves) of elderly and younger patients (Reprinted with permission from Kondo [205])

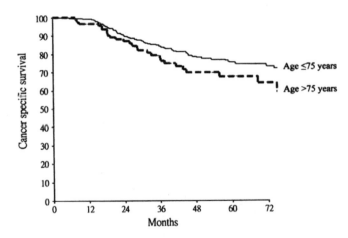

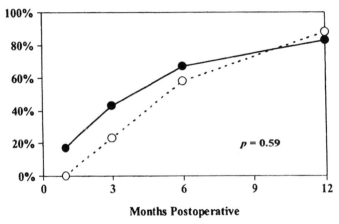

Fig. 3.16 Cancer-specific survival of elderly and younger patients treated for mid to distal colorectal cancer (p = 0.061), n = 612 (Reprinted with permission from Law et al. [201])

Fig. 3.18 Return to normal functional activity after thoracic aneurysm repair depending on age: <70 years (*solid circles*) and ≥70 years (*open circles*); n = 110 (Reprinted with permission from Zierer [221], Copyright Elsevier 2006)

197, 198] (Fig. 3.15), colectomy [199–201] (Fig. 3.16), hepatectomy [64, 121, 202–205] (Fig. 3.17), pancreaticoduodenectomy [64, 206, 207], radical hysterectomy [208], total knee/hip replacement [209–211], microvascular free tissue transfer [212], cardiac transplant [213], lung transplant [214], endovascular surgery [215, 216], gastric bypass [217], laparoscopic colectomy [218], and hernia [219]. Return to preoperative QOL is gratifying after elective surgery for gastric or colorectal disease [220], joint replacement [211], thoracic aneurysm [221] (Fig. 3.18), lung resection [222, 223] (Fig. 3.19), and aortic valve replacement [224, 225] (Fig. 3.20).

For most patients, general medical condition and associated medical problems (Fig. 3.21) are more important than

age. Dunlop et al. [226] studied 8,889 geriatric surgical patients in Canada and concluded that severity of illness on admission was a much better predictor of outcome than was age; Akoh et al. [227] had similar findings in 171 octogenarians undergoing major gastrointestinal surgery. Comorbidities were a greater influence on survival than age in several series of elderly patients with lung cancer [45, 46, 228]. Mehta et al. [229] reported that separation of mitral valve replacement patients into low, medium, and high risk medical groups was more important than stratification by age within these three groups. Within the ASA Physical Status system [230], the ASA status influences results more than age (Fig. 3.22). Bo reported that "the ASA score remains an excellent

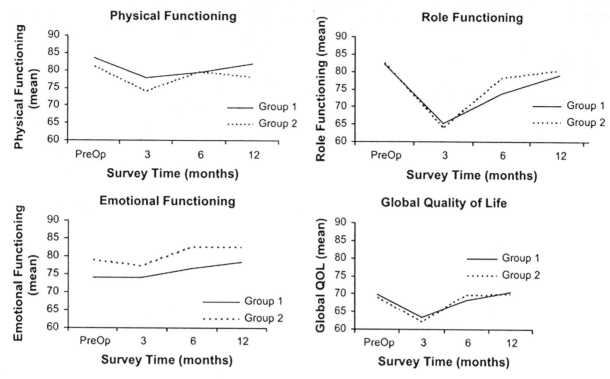

Fig. 3.19 Quality of life (QOL) after pulmonary lobectomy. Mean QOL domain scores plotted as a function of survey time (Reprinted from Burfiend et al. [223], Copyright 2008, with permission from Elsevier)

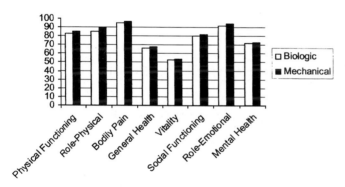

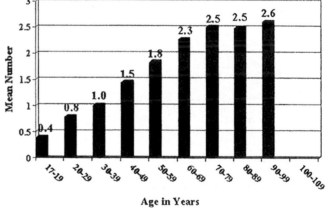

Fig. 3.20 Scores for the domains of the Medical Outcomes Survey Short-Form 36 Health Survey following aortic valve replacement in octogenarians; biologic (*open boxes*) and mechanical (*filled boxes*) valve prostheses; *n*=345 (Reprinted with permission from de Vincentiis et al. [224], Copyright Elsevier 2008)

Fig. 3.21 Mean number of medical risk factors by age in a population (*n*=7,696) of surgical patients (Reprinted with permission from Turrentine et al. [15], Copyright Elsevier 2006)

predictor of mortality in older surgical patients" [74]. For elderly patients undergoing surgery for cancer, the stage of the malignancy also influences outcome more than age [46, 231–234].

Many geriatric surgery patients, including nonagenarians, have survival rates equal to those expected in the general population; even the sobering results of emergency surgery in the elderly are better than the results of nonoperative treatment for the same conditions. A patient's age should therefore be considered but not feared.

Conclusion

Surgical problems abound in the elderly and the numbers of elderly are increasing worldwide. Surgeons must become students of the physiologic changes that occur with aging and, guided by a few general principles, apply this knowledge to daily clinical care. The results of surgery in the elderly do not support prejudice against advanced age.

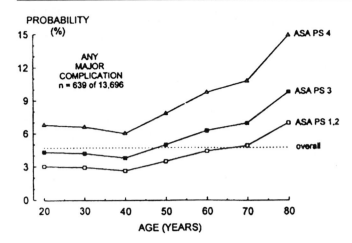

Fig. 3.22 Probability of a major postanesthesia complication based on age and the American Society of Anesthesiologists Physical Status (ASA) system (Reprinted with permission from Muravchick [237])

We owe it to our elders to become good geriatric surgeons and in so doing we will become better surgeons to patients of all ages.

References

1. Ferguson MK, Vigneswaran WT. Changes in patient presentation and outcomes for major lung resection over three decades. Eur J Cardiothorac Surg. 2008;33(3):497–501.
2. Gummert JF, Funkat A, Beckmann A, Hekmat K, Ernst M, Krian A. Cardiac surgery in Germany during 2005: a report on behalf of the German Society for Thoracic and Cardiovascular Surgery. Thorac Cardiovasc Surg. Aug 2006;54(5):362–71.
3. Smith BD, Smith GL, Hurria A, Hortobagyi GN, Buchholz TA. Future of cancer incidence in the United States: burdens upon an aging, changing nation. J Clin Oncol. 2009;27(17):2758–65.
4. Smith OC. Advanced age as a contraindication to operation. Med Rec (NY). 1907;72:642–4.
5. Ochsner A. Is risk of operation too great in the elderly? Geriatrics. 1967;22:121–30.
6. Alexander HR, Turnbull AD, Salamone J, Keefe D, Melendez J. Upper abdominal cancer surgery in the very elderly. J Surg Oncol. 1991;47(2):82–6.
7. Bridges CR, Edwards FH, Peterson ED, Coombs LP, Ferguson TB. Cardiac surgery in nonagenarians and centenarians. J Am Coll Surg. 2003;197(3):347–56; discussion 356–7.
8. Katlic MR. Surgery in centenarians. JAMA. 1985;253(21):3139–41.
9. Ullery BW, Peterson JC, Milla F, et al. Cardiac surgery in select nonagenarians: should we or shouldn't we? Ann Thorac Surg. 2008;85(3):854–60.
10. Cohen JR, Johnson H, Eaton S, Sterman H, Wise L. Surgical procedures in patients during the tenth decade of life. Surgery. 1988;104(4):646–51.
11. Linn BS, Zeppa R. Student attitudes about surgery in older patients before and after the surgical clerkship. Ann Surg. 1987;205(3):324–8.
12. Thomas DR, Ritchie CS. Preoperative assessment of older adults. J Am Geriatr Soc. 1995;43(7):811–21.
13. Brown JM, O'Brien SM, Wu C, Sikora JA, Griffith BP, Gammie JS. Isolated aortic valve replacement in North America comprising 108, 687 patients in 10 years: changes in risks, valve types, and outcomes in the Society of Thoracic Surgeons National Database. J Thorac Cardiovasc Surg. 2009;137(1):82–90.
14. Goodney PP, Siewers AE, Stukel TA, Lucas FL, Wennberg DE, Birkmeyer JD. Is surgery getting safer? National trends in operative mortality. J Am Coll Surg. 2002;195(2):219–27.
15. Turrentine FE, Wang H, Simpson VB, Jones RS. Surgical risk factors, morbidity, and mortality in elderly patients. J Am Coll Surg. Dec 2006;203(6):865–77.
16. Storm-Dickerson TL, Horattas MC. What have we learned over the past 20 years about appendicitis in the elderly? Am J Surg. 2003;185(3):198–201.
17. Elangovan S. Clinical and laboratory findings in acute appendicitis in the elderly. J Am Board Fam Pract. 1996;9(2):75–8.
18. Lau WY, Fan ST, Yiu TF, Chu KW, Lee JM. Acute appendicitis in the elderly. Surg Gynecol Obstet. 1985;161(2):157–60.
19. Horattas MC, Guyton DP, Wu D. A reappraisal of appendicitis in the elderly. Am J Surg. 1990;160(3):291–3.
20. Esses D, Birnbaum A, Bijur P, Shah S, Gleyzer A, Gallagher EJ. Ability of CT to alter decision making in elderly patients with acute abdominal pain. Am J Emerg Med. 2004;22(4):270–2.
21. Sheu BF, Chiu TF, Chen JC, Tung MS, Chang MW, Young YR. Risk factors associated with perforated appendicitis in elderly patients presenting with signs and symptoms of acute appendicitis. ANZ J Surg. 2007;77(8):662–6.
22. Adedeji OA, McAdam WA. Murphy's sign, acute cholecystitis and elderly people. J R Coll Surg Edinb. 1996;41(2):88–9.
23. Hafif A, Gutman M, Kaplan O, Winkler E, Rozin RR, Skornick Y. The management of acute cholecystitis in elderly patients. Am Surg. 1991;57(10):648–52.
24. Parker LJ, Vukov LF, Wollan PC. Emergency department evaluation of geriatric patients with acute cholecystitis. Acad Emerg Med. 1997;4(1):51–5.
25. Chen Y, Zheng M, Hu X, et al. Fever of unknown origin in elderly people: a retrospective study of 87 patients in China. J Am Geriatr Soc. 2008;56(1):182–4.
26. Stewart L, Griffiss JM, Jarvis GA, Way LW. Elderly patients have more severe biliary infections: influence of complement-killing and induction of TNFalpha production. Surgery. 2008;143(1):103–12.
27. Magnuson TH, Ratner LE, Zenilman ME, Bender JS. Laparoscopic cholecystectomy: applicability in the geriatric population. Am Surg. 1997;63(1):91–6.
28. Saunders K, Tompkins R, Longmire W, Jr., Roslyn J. Bile duct carcinoma in the elderly. A rationale for surgical management. Arch Surg. 1991;126(10):1186–90; discussion 1190–1.
29. Hilton D, Iman N, Burke GJ, et al. Absence of abdominal pain in older persons with endoscopic ulcers: a prospective study. Am J Gastroenterol. 2001;96(2):380–4.
30. Rabinovici R, Manny J. Perforated duodenal ulcer in the elderly. Eur J Surg. 1991;157(2):121–5.
31. Mulcahy HE, Patchett SE, Daly L, O'Donoghue DP. Prognosis of elderly patients with large bowel cancer. Br J Surg. 1994;81(5):736–8.
32. Watters JM, Blakslee JM, March RJ, Redmond ML. The influence of age on the severity of peritonitis. Can J Surg. 1996;39(2):142–6.
33. Tedesco P, Lobo E, Fisichella PM, Way LW, Patti MG. Laparoscopic fundoplication in elderly patients with gastroesophageal reflux disease. Arch Surg. 2006;141(3):289–92; discussion 292.
34. Pilotto A, Franceschi M, Leandro G, et al. Clinical features of reflux esophagitis in older people: a study of 840 consecutive patients. J Am Geriatr Soc. 2006;54(10):1537–42.
35. Knutson JW, Slavin RG. Sinusitis in the aged. Optimal management strategies. Drugs Aging. 1995;7(4):310–6.

36. Norman DC, Toledo SD. Infections in elderly persons. An altered clinical presentation. Clin Geriatr Med. 1992;8(4):713–9.

37. Koch WM, Patel H, Brennan J, Boyle JO, Sidransky D. Squamous cell carcinoma of the head and neck in the elderly. Arch Otolaryngol Head Neck Surg. 1995;121(3):262–5.

38. Ehlinger P, Fossion E, Vrielinck L. Carcinoma of the oral cavity in patients over 75 years of age. Int J Oral Maxillofac Surg. 1993;22(4):218–20.

39. Chigot JP, Menegaux F, Achrafi H. Should primary hyperparathyroidism be treated surgically in elderly patients older than 75 years? Surgery. 1995;117(4):397–401.

40. Thomas PC, Grigg M. Carotid artery surgery in the octogenarian. Aust N Z J Surg. 1996;66(4):231–4.

41. Canto JG, Fincher C, Kiefe CI, et al. Atypical presentations among Medicare beneficiaries with unstable angina pectoris. Am J Cardiol. 2002;90(3):248–53.

42. Lehmann R, Beekley A, Casey L, Salim A, Martin M. The impact of advanced age on trauma triage decisions and outcomes: a statewide analysis. Am J Surg. 2009;197(5):571–4; discussion 574–5.

43. Hellmann DB. Eurekapenia: a disease of medical residency training programs? Pharos Alpha Omega Alpha Honor Med Soc. Spring 2003;66(2):24–6.

44. Durso SC. A bipolar disorder: eurekaphoria, then discouragement. Pharos Alpha Omega Alpha Honor Med Soc. Summer 2004; 67(3):49.

45. Birim O, Zuydendorp HM, Maat AP, Kappetein AP, Eijkemans MJ, Bogers AJ. Lung resection for non-small-cell lung cancer in patients older than 70: mortality, morbidity, and late survival compared with the general population. Ann Thorac Surg. 2003;76(6):1796–801.

46. Brock MV, Kim MP, Hooker CM, et al. Pulmonary resection in octogenarians with stage I nonsmall cell lung cancer: a 22-year experience. Ann Thorac Surg. 2004;77(1):271–7.

47. Keagy BA, Pharr WF, Bowes DE, Wilcox BR. A review of morbidity and mortality in elderly patients undergoing pulmonary resection. Am Surg. 1984;50(4):213–6.

48. Au J, el-Oakley R, Cameron EW. Pneumonectomy for bronchogenic carcinoma in the elderly. Eur J Cardiothorac Surg. 1994;8(5):247–50.

49. Miller DL, Deschamps C, Jenkins GD, Bernard A, Allen MS, Pairolero PC. Completion pneumonectomy: factors affecting operative mortality and cardiopulmonary morbidity. Ann Thorac Surg. 2002;74(3):876–83; discussion 883–4.

50. Rostad H, Naalsund A, Strand TE, Jacobsen R, Talleraas O, Norstein J. Results of pulmonary resection for lung cancer in Norway, patients older than 70 years. Eur J Cardiothorac Surg. 2005;27(2): 325–8.

51. Balduyck B, Hendriks J, Lauwers P, Nia PS, Van Schil P. Quality of life evolution after lung cancer surgery in septuagenarians: a prospective study. Eur J Cardiothorac Surg. 2009;35(6):1070–75; discussion 1075.

52. Demmy TL, Plante AJ, Nwogu CE, Takita H, Anderson TM. Discharge independence with minimally invasive lobectomy. Am J Surg. 2004;188(6):698–702.

53. Jaklitsch MT, DeCamp Jr MM. Liptay MJ, et al. Video-assisted thoracic surgery in the elderly. A review of 307 cases. Chest. 1996; 110(3):751–8.

54. Nomori H, Horio H, Fuyuno G, Kobayashi R, Yashima H. Respiratory muscle strength after lung resection with special reference to age and procedures of thoracotomy. Eur J Cardiothorac Surg. 1996;10(5):352–8.

55. Yim AP. Thoracoscopic surgery in the elderly population. Surg Endosc. 1996;10(9):880–2.

56. Cattaneo SM, Park BJ, Wilton AS, et al. Use of video-assisted thoracic surgery for lobectomy in the elderly results in fewer complications. Ann Thorac Surg. 2008;85(1):231–235; discussion 235–6.

57. Patel HJ, Williams DM, Upchurch GR, Jr., et al. A comparison of open and endovascular descending thoracic aortic repair in patients older than 75 years of age. Ann Thorac Surg. 2008;85(5):1597–603; discussion 1603–4.

58. Guller U, Jain N, Peterson ED, Muhlbaier LH, Eubanks S, Pietrobon R. Laparoscopic appendectomy in the elderly. Surgery. 2004;135(5): 479–88.

59. Bergus BO, Feng WC, Bert AA, Singh AK. Aortic valve replacement (AVR): influence of age on operative morbidity and mortality. Eur J Cardiothorac Surg. 1992;6(3):118–21.

60. Salomon NW, Page US, Bigelow JC, Krause AH, Okies JE, Metzdorff MT. Coronary artery bypass grafting in elderly patients. Comparative results in a consecutive series of 469 patients older than 75 years. J Thorac Cardiovasc Surg. 1991;101(2):209–17; discussion 217–8.

61. Lytle BW, Navia JL, Taylor PC, et al. Third coronary artery bypass operations: risks and costs. Ann Thorac Surg. 1997;64(5): 1287–95.

62. Elayda MA, Hall RJ, Reul RM, et al. Aortic valve replacement in patients 80 years and older. Operative risks and long-term results. Circulation. 1993;88(5 Pt 2):II11–16.

63. Fortner JG, Lincer RM. Hepatic resection in the elderly. Ann Surg. 1990;211(2):141–5.

64. Fong Y, Blumgart LH, Fortner JG, Brennan MF. Pancreatic or liver resection for malignancy is safe and effective for the elderly. Ann Surg. 1995;222(4):426–34; discussion 434–7.

65. de Liguori Carino N, van Leeuwen BL, Ghaneh P, Wu A, Audisio RA, Poston GJ. Liver resection for colorectal liver metastases in older patients. Crit Rev Oncol Hematol. 2008;67(3):273–8.

66. Escarce JJ, Shea JA, Chen W, Qian Z, Schwartz JS. Outcomes of open cholecystectomy in the elderly: a longitudinal analysis of 21,000 cases in the prelaparoscopic era. Surgery. 1995;117(2): 156–64.

67. Tsujitani S, Katano K, Oka A, Ikeguchi M, Maeta M, Kaibara N. Limited operation for gastric cancer in the elderly. Br J Surg. 1996;83(6):836–9.

68. Gretschel S, Estevez-Schwarz L, Hunerbein M, Schneider U, Schlag PM. Gastric cancer surgery in elderly patients. World J Surg. 2006;30(8):1468–74.

69. Okada M, Koike T, Higashiyama M, Yamato Y, Kodama K, Tsubota N. Radical sublobar resection for small-sized non-small cell lung cancer: a multicenter study. J Thorac Cardiovasc Surg. 2006;132(4): 769–75.

70. Mery CM, Pappas AN, Bueno R, et al. Similar long-term survival of elderly patients with non-small cell lung cancer treated with lobectomy or wedge resection within the surveillance, epidemiology, and end results database. Chest. 2005;128(1):237–45.

71. Kilic A, Schuchert MJ, Pettiford BL, et al. Anatomic segmentectomy for stage I non-small cell lung cancer in the elderly. Ann Thorac Surg. 2009;87(6):1662–6; discussion 1667–8.

72. Lawrence VA, Hazuda HP, Cornell JE, et al. Functional independence after major abdominal surgery in the elderly. J Am Coll Surg. 2004;199(5):762–72.

73. Seymour DG, Vaz FG. A prospective study of elderly general surgical patients: II. Post-operative complications. Age Ageing. 1989;18(5):316–26.

74. Bo M, Cacello E, Ghiggia F, Corsinovi L, Bosco F. Predictive factors of clinical outcome in older surgical patients. Arch Gerontol Geriatr. 2007;44(3):215–24.

75. Dzankic S, Pastor D, Gonzalez C, Leung JM. The prevalence and predictive value of abnormal preoperative laboratory tests in elderly surgical patients. Anesth Analg. 2001;93(2):301–308, 302nd contents page.

76. Bobbio A, Chetta A, Ampollini L, et al. Preoperative pulmonary rehabilitation in patients undergoing lung resection for non-small cell lung cancer. Eur J Cardiothorac Surg. 2008;33(1):95–8.

77. Vaporciyan AA, Merriman KW, Ece F, et al. Incidence of major pulmonary morbidity after pneumonectomy: association with timing of smoking cessation. Ann Thorac Surg. 2002;73(2):420–5; discussion 425–6.

78. Mizushima Y, Noto H, Sugiyama S, et al. Survival and prognosis after pneumonectomy for lung cancer in the elderly. Ann Thorac Surg. 1997;64(1):193–8.

79. Reilly JJ. Preparing for pulmonary resection: preoperative evaluation of patients. Chest. 1997;112(4 Suppl):206S–8.

80. Goldhaber SZ, Tapson VF. A prospective registry of 5,451 patients with ultrasound-confirmed deep vein thrombosis. Am J Cardiol. 2004;93(2):259–62.

81. Jacobs LG. Prophylactic anticoagulation for venous thromboembolic disease in geriatric patients. J Am Geriatr Soc. 2003;51(10): 1472–8.

82. Berlauk JF, Abrams JH, Gilmour IJ, O'Connor SR, Knighton DR, Cerra FB. Preoperative optimization of cardiovascular hemodynamics improves outcome in peripheral vascular surgery. A prospective, randomized clinical trial. Ann Surg. 1991;214(3):289–97; discussion 298–9.

83. Bender JS, Smith-Meek MA, Jones CE. Routine pulmonary artery catheterization does not reduce morbidity and mortality of elective vascular surgery: results of a prospective, randomized trial. Ann Surg. 1997;226(3):229–36; discussion 236–7.

84. Ziegler DW, Wright JG, Choban PS, Flancbaum L. A prospective randomized trial of preoperative "optimization" of cardiac function in patients undergoing elective peripheral vascular surgery. Surgery. 1997;122(3):584–92.

85. Leppo JA. Preoperative cardiac risk assessment for noncardiac surgery. Am J Cardiol. 1995;75(11):42D–51.

86. Biagini E, Elhendy A, Schinkel AF, et al. Long-term prediction of mortality in elderly persons by dobutamine stress echocardiography. J Gerontol A Biol Sci Med Sci. 2005;60(10):1333–8.

87. Pollock M, Roa J, Benditt J, Celli B. Estimation of ventilatory reserve by stair climbing. A study in patients with chronic airflow obstruction. Chest. 1993;104(5):1378–83.

88. Brunelli A, Refai M, Xiume F, et al. Performance at symptom-limited stair-climbing test is associated with increased cardiopulmonary complications, mortality, and costs after major lung resection. Ann Thorac Surg. 2008;86(1):240–7; discussion 247–8.

89. Win T, Jackson A, Groves AM, Sharples LD, Charman SC, Laroche CM. Comparison of shuttle walk with measured peak oxygen consumption in patients with operable lung cancer. Thorax. 2006;61(1):57–60.

90. Simonsick EM, Fan E, Fleg JL. Estimating cardiorespiratory fitness in well-functioning older adults: treadmill validation of the long distance corridor walk. J Am Geriatr Soc. 2006;54(1):127–32.

91. Weinstein H, Bates AT, Spaltro BE, Thaler HT, Steingart RM. Influence of preoperative exercise capacity on length of stay after thoracic cancer surgery. Ann Thorac Surg. 2007;84(1): 197–202.

92. Audisio RA, Pope D, Ramesh HS, et al. Shall we operate? Preoperative assessment in elderly cancer patients (PACE) can help. A SIOG surgical task force prospective study. Crit Rev Oncol Hematol. 2008;65(2):156–63.

93. Internullo E, Moons J, Nafteux P, et al. Outcome after esophagectomy for cancer of the esophagus and GEJ in patients aged over 75 years. Eur J Cardiothorac Surg. 2008;33(6):1096–104.

94. Iwamoto K, Ichiyama S, Shimokata K, Nakashima N. Postoperative pneumonia in elderly patients: incidence and mortality in comparison with younger patients. Intern Med. 1993;32(4):274–7.

95. Kwon AH, Matsui Y. Laparoscopic cholecystectomy in patients aged 80 years and over. World J Surg. 2006;30(7):1204–10.

96. Landau O, Kott I, Deutsch AA, Stelman E, Reiss R. Multifactorial analysis of septic bile and septic complications in biliary surgery. World J Surg. 1992;16(5):962–4; discussion 964–5.

97. Meijer WS, Schmitz PI, Jeekel J. Meta-analysis of randomized, controlled clinical trials of antibiotic prophylaxis in biliary tract surgery. Br J Surg. 1990;77(3):283–90.

98. Watters JM, Clancey SM, Moulton SB, Briere KM, Zhu JM. Impaired recovery of strength in older patients after major abdominal surgery. Ann Surg. 1993;218(3):380–90; discussion 390–3.

99. Kudsk KA, Tolley EA, DeWitt RC, et al. Preoperative albumin and surgical site identify surgical risk for major postoperative complications. JPEN J Parenter Enteral Nutr. 2003;27(1):1–9.

100. Souba WW. Nutritional support. N Engl J Med. 1997;336(1): 41–8.

101. Bittner R, Butters M, Ulrich M, Uppenbrink S, Beger HG. Total gastrectomy. Updated operative mortality and long-term survival with particular reference to patients older than 70 years of age. Ann Surg. 1996;224(1):37–42.

102. Pratt W, Callery MP, Vollmer Jr CM. Optimal surgical performance attenuates physiologic risk in high-acuity operations. J Am Coll Surg. 2008;207(5):717–30.

103. Myrdal G, Gustafsson G, Lambe M, Horte LG, Stahl E. Outcome after lung cancer surgery. Factors predicting early mortality and major morbidity. Eur J Cardiothorac Surg. 2001;20(4):694–9.

104. Allen MS, Darling GE, Pechet TT, et al. Morbidity and mortality of major pulmonary resections in patients with early-stage lung cancer: initial results of the randomized, prospective ACOSOG Z0030 trial. Ann Thorac Surg. 2006;81(3):1013–19; discussion 1019–20.

105. Cerfolio RJ, Bryant AS. Survival and outcomes of pulmonary resection for non-small cell lung cancer in the elderly: a nested case-control study. Ann Thorac Surg. 2006;82(2):424–9; discussion 429–30.

106. Coyle KA, Smith 3rd RB, Salam AA, Dodson TF, Chaikof EL, Lumsden AB. Carotid endarterectomy in the octogenarian. Ann Vasc Surg. 1994;8(5):417–20.

107. Maehara Y, Oshiro T, Oiwa H, et al. Gastric carcinoma in patients over 70 years of age. Br J Surg. 1995;82(1):102–5.

108. Jougon JB, Ballester M, Duffy J, et al. Esophagectomy for cancer in the patient aged 70 years and older. Ann Thorac Surg. 1997;63(5):1423–7.

109. Shah PJ, Estrera AL, Miller 3rd CC, et al. Analysis of ascending and transverse aortic arch repair in octogenarians. Ann Thorac Surg. 2008;86(3):774–9.

110. de Perrot M, Licker M, Reymond MA, Robert J, Spiliopoulos A. Influence of age on operative mortality and long-term survival after lung resection for bronchogenic carcinoma. Eur Respir J. 1999;14(2):419–22.

111. Okada M, Nishio W, Sakamoto T, Harada H, Uchino K, Tsubota N. Long-term survival and prognostic factors of five-year survivors with complete resection of non-small cell lung carcinoma. J Thorac Cardiovasc Surg. 2003;126(2):558–62.

112. Thomas P, Sielezenff I, Rajni J, Giridicilli R, Fuentes P. Is lung cancer resection justified in patients aged over 70 years? Eur J Cardiothorac Surg. 1993;7:246–51.

113. Keller SM, Markovitz LJ, Wilder JR, Aufses Jr AH. Emergency and elective surgery in patients over age 70. Am Surg. 1987;53(11): 636–40.

114. Bingener J, Richards ML, Schwesinger WH, Strodel WE, Sirinek KR. Laparoscopic cholecystectomy for elderly patients: gold standard for golden years? Arch Surg. 2003;138(5):531–5; discussion 535–6.

115. Tambyraja AL, Kumar S, Nixon SJ. Outcome of laparoscopic cholecystectomy in patients 80 years and older. World J Surg. 2004;28(8):745–8.

116. Tsai TP, Chaux A, Matloff JM, et al. Ten-year experience of cardiac surgery in patients aged 80 years and over. Ann Thorac Surg. 1994;58(2):445–50; discussion 450–1.

117. Tseng EE, Lee CA, Cameron DE, et al. Aortic valve replacement in the elderly. Risk factors and long-term results. Ann Surg. 1997;225(6):793–802; discussion 802–4.

118. Bender JS, Magnuson TH, Zenilman ME, et al. Outcome following colon surgery in the octagenarian. Am Surg. 1996;62(4): 276–9.

119. Spivak H, Maele DV, Friedman I, Nussbaum M. Colorectal surgery in octogenarians. J Am Coll Surg. 1996;183(1):46–50.

120. Ngaage DL, Cowen ME, Griffin S, Guvendik L, Cale AR. Early neurological complications after coronary artery bypass grafting and valve surgery in octogenarians. Eur J Cardiothorac Surg. 2008;33(4):653–9.

121. Menon KV, Al-Mukhtar A, Aldouri A, Prasad RK, Lodge PA, Toogood GJ. Outcomes after major hepatectomy in elderly patients. J Am Coll Surg. 2006;203(5):677–83.

122. Sisto D, Hoffman D, Frater RW. Isolated coronary artery bypass grafting in one hundred octogenarian patients. J Thorac Cardiovasc Surg. 1993;106(5):940–2.

123. Logeais Y, Langanay T, Roussin R, et al. Surgery for aortic stenosis in elderly patients. A study of surgical risk and predictive factors. Circulation. 1994;90(6):2891–8.

124. Maurice-Williams RS, Kitchen ND. Intracranial tumours in the elderly: the effect of age on the outcome of first time surgery for meningiomas. Br J Neurosurg. 1992;6(2):131–7.

125. Kaye KS, Anderson DJ, Sloane R, et al. The effect of surgical site infection on older operative patients. J Am Geriatr Soc. 2009;57(1):46–54.

126. Malani PN, Rana MM, Banerjee M, Bradley SF. Staphylococcus aureus bloodstream infections: the association between age and mortality and functional status. J Am Geriatr Soc. 2008;56(8): 1485–9.

127. Tan KY, Chen CM, Ng C, Tan SM, Tay KH. Which octogenarians do poorly after major open abdominal surgery in our Asian population? World J Surg. 2006;30(4):547–52.

128. Adam DJ, Craig SR, Sang CT, Cameron EW, Walker WS. Esophagectomy for carcinoma in the octogenarian. Ann Thorac Surg. 1996;61(1):190–4.

129. Mathisen DJ, Grillo HC, Wilkins Jr EW, Moncure AC, Hilgenberg AD. Transthoracic esophagectomy: a safe approach to carcinoma of the esophagus. Ann Thorac Surg. 1988;45(2):137–43.

130. Bandoh T, Isoyama T, Toyoshima H. Total gastrectomy for gastric cancer in the elderly. Surgery. 1991;109(2):136–42.

131. Katz NM, Chase GA. Risks of cardiac operations for elderly patients: reduction of the age factor. Ann Thorac Surg. 1997;63(5):1309–14.

132. Minambres E, Buron J, Ballesteros MA, Llorca J, Munoz P, Gonzalez-Castro A. Tracheal rupture after endotracheal intubation: a literature systematic review. Eur J Cardiothorac Surg. 2009;35(6):1056–62.

133. Bernstein EF, Dilley RB, Randolph 3rd HF. The improving long-term outlook for patients over 70 years of age with abdominal aortic aneurysms. Ann Surg. 1988;207(3):318–22.

134. Lo CY, van Heerden JA, Grant CS, Soreide JA, Warner MA, Ilstrup DM. Adrenal surgery in the elderly: too risky? World J Surg. 1996;20(3):368–73; discussion 374.

135. Scalea TM, Simon HM, Duncan AO, et al. Geriatric blunt multiple trauma: improved survival with early invasive monitoring. J Trauma. 1990;30(2):129–34; discussion 134–6.

136. Demetriades D, Karaiskakis M, Velmahos G, et al. Effect on outcome of early intensive management of geriatric trauma patients. Br J Surg. 2002;89(10):1319–22.

137. Giannice R, Foti E, Poerio A, Marana E, Mancuso S, Scambia G. Perioperative morbidity and mortality in elderly gynecological oncological patients (>/= 70 years) by the American Society of Anesthesiologists physical status classes. Ann Surg Oncol. 2004;11(2):219–25.

138. Zingone B, Gatti G, Rauber E, et al. Early and late outcomes of cardiac surgery in octogenarians. Ann Thorac Surg. 2009;87(1): 71–8.

139. http://www.ssa.gov/OACT/STATS/table4c6.html. Period life table, 2000. Actuarial publications, statistical tables. Accessed 8 March 2004.

140. Minino AM, Heron MP, Smith BL. Deaths: preliminary data for 2004. Natl Vital Stat Rep. 2006;54(19):1–49.

141. Nugent WC, Edney MT, Hammerness PG, Dain BJ, Maurer LH, Rigas JR. Non-small cell lung cancer at the extremes of age: impact on diagnosis and treatment. Ann Thorac Surg. 1997;63(1):193–7.

142. Kuo CW, Chen YM, Chao JY, Tsai CM, Perng RP. Non-small cell lung cancer in very young and very old patients. Chest. 2000;117(2):354–7.

143. Fruh M, Rolland E, Pignon JP, et al. Pooled analysis of the effect of age on adjuvant cisplatin-based chemotherapy for completely resected non-small-cell lung cancer. J Clin Oncol. 2008;26(21): 3573–81.

144. Detaint D, Sundt TM, Nkomo VT, et al. Surgical correction of mitral regurgitation in the elderly: outcomes and recent improvements. Circulation. 2006;114(4):265–72.

145. Goldsmith I, Lip GY, Kaukuntla H, Patel RL. Hospital morbidity and mortality and changes in quality of life following mitral valve surgery in the elderly. J Heart Valve Dis. 1999;8(6):702–7.

146. Maisano F, Vigano G, Calabrese C, et al. Quality of life of elderly patients following valve surgery for chronic organic mitral regurgitation. Eur J Cardiothorac Surg. 2009;36(2):261–6; discussion 266.

147. Mirabel M, Iung B, Baron G, et al. What are the characteristics of patients with severe, symptomatic, mitral regurgitation who are denied surgery? Eur Heart J. 2007;28(11):1358–65.

148. Cress RD, O'Malley CD, Leiserowitz GS, Campleman SL. Patterns of chemotherapy use for women with ovarian cancer: a population-based study. J Clin Oncol. 2003;21(8):1530–5.

149. Moore DH. Ovarian cancer in the elderly patient. Oncology (Huntingt). 1994;8(12):21–5; discussion 25, 29–30.

150. Edmonson JH, Su J, Krook JE. Treatment of ovarian cancer in elderly women. Mayo Clinic-North Central Cancer Treatment Group studies. Cancer. 1993;71(2 Suppl):615–7.

151. Longhi A, Errani C, Gonzales-Arabio D, Ferrari C, Mercuri M. Osteosarcoma in patients older than 65 years. J Clin Oncol. 2008;26(33):5368–73.

152. Singletary SE, Shallenberger R, Guinee VF. Breast cancer in the elderly. Ann Surg. 1993;218(5):667–71.

153. Wanebo HJ, Cole B, Chung M, et al. Is surgical management compromised in elderly patients with breast cancer? Ann Surg. 1997;225(5):579–586; discussion 586–9.

154. Freedman RA, He Y, Winer EP, Keating NL. Trends in racial and age disparities in definitive local therapy of early-stage breast cancer. J Clin Oncol. 2009;27(5):713–9.

155. Hurria A, Wong FL, Villaluna D, et al. Role of age and health in treatment recommendations for older adults with breast cancer: the perspective of oncologists and primary care providers. J Clin Oncol. 2008;26(33):5386–92.

156. Swanson RS, Sawicka J, Wood WC. Treatment of carcinoma of the breast in the older geriatric patient. Surg Gynecol Obstet. 1991;173(6):465–9.

157. van Dalsen AD, de Vries JE. Treatment of breast cancer in elderly patients. J Surg Oncol. 1995;60(2):80–2.

158. Guadagnoli E, Shapiro C, Gurwitz JH, et al. Age-related patterns of care: evidence against ageism in the treatment of early-stage breast cancer. J Clin Oncol. 1997;15(6):2338–44.

159. Hebert-Croteau N, Brisson J, Latreille J, Blanchette C, Deschenes L. Compliance with consensus recommendations for the treatment of early stage breast carcinoma in elderly women. Cancer. 1999;85(5):1104–13.

160. Hurria A, Hurria A, Zuckerman E, et al. A prospective, longitudinal study of the functional status and quality of life of older patients with breast cancer receiving adjuvant chemotherapy. J Am Geriatr Soc. 2006; 54(7):1119–24.

161. Silliman RA, Ganz PA. Adjuvant chemotherapy use and outcomes in older women with breast cancer: what have we learned? J Clin Oncol. 2006;24(18):2697–9.

162. Muss HB, Berry DA, Cirrincione CT, et al. Adjuvant chemotherapy in older women with early-stage breast cancer. N Engl J Med. 2009;360(20):2055–65.

163. Choi M, Jiang PQ, Heilbrun LK, Smith DW, Gadgeel SM. Retrospective review of cancer patients > or =80 years old treated with chemotherapy at a comprehensive cancer center. Crit Rev Oncol Hematol. 2008;67(3):268–72.

164. Siu LL. Clinical trials in the elderly – a concept comes of age. N Engl J Med. 2007;356(15):1575–6.

165. Bilimoria KY, Stewart AK, Palis BE, Bentrem DJ, Talamonti MS, Ko CY. Adequacy and importance of lymph node evaluation for colon cancer in the elderly. J Am Coll Surg. 2008;206(2):247–54.

166. Hardiman KM, Cone M, Sheppard BC, Herzig DO. Disparities in the treatment of colon cancer in octogenarians. Am J Surg. 2009;197(5):624–8.

167. Esnaola NF, Stewart AK, Feig BW, Skibber JM, Rodriguez-Bigas MA. Age-, race-, and ethnicity-related differences in the treatment of nonmetastatic rectal cancer: a patterns of care study from the national cancer data base. Ann Surg Oncol. 2008;15(11): 3036–47.

168. Schonberg MA, Marcantonio ER, Hamel MB. Perceptions of physician recommendations for joint replacement surgery in older patients with severe hip or knee osteoarthritis. J Am Geriatr Soc. 2009;57(1):82–8.

169. Chalmers RT, Stonebridge PA, John TG, Murie JA. Abdominal aortic aneurysm in the elderly. Br J Surg. 1993;80(9):1122–3.

170. Blanche C, Matloff JM, Denton TA, et al. Cardiac operations in patients 90 years of age and older. Ann Thorac Surg. 1997;63(6):1685–90.

171. Chang DC, Bass RR, Cornwell EE, Mackenzie EJ. Undertriage of elderly trauma patients to state-designated trauma centers. Arch Surg. 2008;143(8):776–781; discussion 782.

172. Finlayson E, Fan Z, Birkmeyer JD. Outcomes in octogenarians undergoing high-risk cancer operation: a national study. J Am Coll Surg. 2007;205(6):729–34.

173. Moskovitz AH, Rizk NP, Venkatraman E, et al. Mortality increases for octogenarians undergoing esophagogastrectomy for esophageal cancer. Ann Thorac Surg. 2006;82(6):2031–36; discussion 2036.

174. Larusson HJ, Zingg U, Hahnloser D, Delport K, Seifert B, Oertli D. Predictive factors for morbidity and mortality in patients undergoing laparoscopic paraesophageal hernia repair: age, ASA score and operation type influence morbidity. World J Surg. 2009;33(5): 980–5.

175. Leo F, Scanagatta P, Baglio P, et al. The risk of pneumonectomy over the age of 70. A case-control study. Eur J Cardiothorac Surg. 2007;31(5):780–2.

176. Barnett SD, Halpin LS, Speir AM, et al. Postoperative complications among octogenarians after cardiovascular surgery. Ann Thorac Surg. 2003;76(3):726–31.

177. Jarvinen O, Huhtala H, Laurikka J, Tarkka MR. Higher age predicts adverse outcome and readmission after coronary artery bypass grafting. World J Surg. 2003;27(12):1317–22.

178. Lightner AM, Glasgow RE, Jordan TH, et al. Pancreatic resection in the elderly. J Am Coll Surg. 2004;198(5):697–706.

179. Sosa JA, Mehta PJ, Wang TS, Boudourakis L, Roman SA. A population-based study of outcomes from thyroidectomy in aging Americans: at what cost? J Am Coll Surg. 2008;206(3): 1097–105.

180. Mamoun NF, Xu M, Sessler DI, Sabik JF, Bashour CA. Propensity matched comparison of outcomes in older and younger patients after coronary artery bypass graft surgery. Ann Thorac Surg. 2008;85(6):1974–9.

181. Fraioli B, Pastore FS, Signoretti S, De Caro GM, Giuffre R. The surgical treatment of pituitary adenomas in the eighth decade. Surg Neurol. 1999;51(3):261–6; discussion 266–7.

182. Derks W, De Leeuw JR, Hordijk GJ, Winnubst JA. Elderly patients with head and neck cancer: short-term effects of surgical treatment on quality of life. Clin Otolaryngol. 2003;28(5):399–405.

183. Uruno T, Miyauchi A, Shimizu K, et al. Favorable surgical results in 433 elderly patients with papillary thyroid cancer. World J Surg. 2005;29(11):1497–501; discussion 1502–3.

184. Shin SH, Holmes H, Bao R, et al. Outpatient minimally invasive parathyroidectomy is safe for elderly patients. J Am Coll Surg. 2009;208(6):1071–6.

185. Salameh JR, Myers JL, Mukherjee D. Carotid endarterectomy in elderly patients: low complication rate with overnight stay. Arch Surg. 2002;137(11):1284–7; discussion 1288.

186. Durward QJ, Ragnarsson TS, Reeder RF, Case JL, Hughes CA. Carotid endarterectomy in nonagenarians. Arch Surg. 2005;140(7): 625–8; discussion 628.

187. Bremner AK, Katz SG. Are octogenarians at high risk for carotid endarterectomy? J Am Coll Surg. 2008;207(4):549–53.

188. Suliman A, Greenberg J, Chandra A, Barillas S, Iranpour P, Angle N. Carotid endarterectomy as the criterion standard in high-risk elderly patients. Arch Surg. 2008;143(8):736–42; discussion 742.

189. Beauford RB, Goldstein DJ, Sardari FF, et al. Multivessel off-pump revascularization in octogenarians: early and midterm outcomes. Ann Thorac Surg. 2003;76(1):12–7; discussion 17.

190. Chiappini B, Camurri N, Loforte A, Di Marco L, Di Bartolomeo R, Marinelli G. Outcome after aortic valve replacement in octogenarians. Ann Thorac Surg. 2004;78(1):85–9

191. Collart F, Feier H, Kerbaul F, et al. Valvular surgery in octogenarians: operative risks factors, evaluation of Euroscore and long term results. Eur J Cardiothorac Surg. 2005;27(2):276–80.

192. Ferguson TB Jr, Hammill BG, Peterson ED, DeLong ER, Grover FL. A decade of change--risk profiles and outcomes for isolated coronary artery bypass grafting procedures, 1990-1999: a report from the STS National Database Committee and the Duke Clinical Research Institute. Society of Thoracic Surgeons. Ann Thorac Surg. 2002;73(2):480–9; discussion 489–90.

193. Huber CH, Goeber V, Berdat P, Carrel T, Eckstein F. Benefits of cardiac surgery in octogenarians – a postoperative quality of life assessment. Eur J Cardiothorac Surg. 2007;31(6):1099–105.

194. Rice DC, Correa AM, Vaporciyan AA, et al. Preoperative chemoradiotherapy prior to esophagectomy in elderly patients is not associated with increased morbidity. Ann Thorac Surg. 2005;79(2):391–7; discussion 391–7.

195. Ruol A, Portale G, Zaninotto G, et al. Results of esophagectomy for esophageal cancer in elderly patients: age has little influence on outcome and survival. J Thorac Cardiovasc Surg. 2007;133(5): 1186–92.

196. Ruol A, Portale G, Castoro C, et al. Effects of neoadjuvant therapy on perioperative morbidity in elderly patients undergoing esophagectomy for esophageal cancer. Ann Surg Oncol. 2007;14(11):3243–50.

197. Poon RT, Law SY, Chu KM, Branicki FJ, Wong J. Esophagectomy for carcinoma of the esophagus in the elderly: results of current surgical management. Ann Surg. 1998;227(3):357–64.

198. Kunisaki C, Akiyama H, Nomura M, et al. Comparison of surgical outcomes of gastric cancer in elderly and middle-aged patients. Am J Surg. 2006;191(2):216–24.

199. Avital S, Kashtan H, Hadad R, Werbin N. Survival of colorectal carcinoma in the elderly. A prospective study of colorectal

carcinoma and a five-year follow-up. Dis Colon Rectum. 1997;40(5):523–9.

200. Barrier A, Ferro L, Houry S, Lacaine F, Huguier M. Rectal cancer surgery in patients more than 80 years of age. Am J Surg. 2003;185(1):54–7.

201. Law WL, Choi HK, Ho JW, Lee YM, Seto CL. Outcomes of surgery for mid and distal rectal cancer in the elderly. World J Surg. 2006;30(4):598–604.

202. Aldrighetti L, Arru M, Caterini R, et al. Impact of advanced age on the outcome of liver resection. World J Surg. 2003;27(10):1149–54.

203. Cescon M, Grazi GL, Del Gaudio M, et al. Outcome of right hepatectomies in patients older than 70 years. Arch Surg. 2003;138(5): 547–52.

204. Ferrero A, Vigano L, Polastri R, et al. Hepatectomy as treatment of choice for hepatocellular carcinoma in elderly cirrhotic patients. World J Surg. 2005;29(9):1101–5.

205. Kondo K, Chijiiwa K, Funagayama M, Kai M, Otani K, Ohuchida J. Hepatic resection is justified for elderly patients with hepatocellular carcinoma. World J Surg. 2008;32(10):2223–9.

206. Sohn TA, Yeo CJ, Cameron JL, et al. Should pancreaticoduodenectomy be performed in octogenarians? J Gastrointest Surg. 1998;2(3):207–16.

207. Petrowsky H, Clavien PA. Should we deny surgery for malignant hepato-pancreatico-biliary tumors to elderly patients? World J Surg. 2005;29(9):1093–100.

208. Geisler JP, Geisler HE. Radical hysterectomy in patients 65 years of age and older. Gynecol Oncol. 1994;53(2):208–11.

209. Anderson JG, Wixson RL, Tsai D, Stulberg SD, Chang RW. Functional outcome and patient satisfaction in total knee patients over the age of 75. J Arthroplasty. 1996;11(7):831–40.

210. Wurtz LD, Feinberg JR, Capello WN, Meldrum R, Kay PJ. Elective primary total hip arthroplasty in octogenarians. J Gerontol A Biol Sci Med Sci. 2003;58(5):M468–71.

211. Hamel MB, Toth M, Legedza A, Rosen MP. Joint replacement surgery in elderly patients with severe osteoarthritis of the hip or knee: decision making, postoperative recovery, and clinical outcomes. Arch Intern Med. 2008;168(13):1430–40.

212. Malata CM, Cooter RD, Batchelor AG, Simpson KH, Browning FS, Kay SP. Microvascular free-tissue transfers in elderly patients: the leads experience. Plast Reconstr Surg. 1996;98(7): 1234–41.

213. Morgan JA, John R, Weinberg AD, et al. Long-term results of cardiac transplantation in patients 65 years of age and older: a comparative analysis. Ann Thorac Surg. 2003;76(6):1982–7.

214. Mahidhara R, Bastani S, Ross DJ, et al. Lung transplantation in older patients? J Thorac Cardiovasc Surg. 2008;135(2):412–20.

215. Minor ME, Ellozy S, Carroccio A, et al. Endovascular aortic aneurysm repair in the octogenarian: is it worthwhile? Arch Surg. 2004;139(3):308–14.

216. Kpodonu J, Preventza O, Ramaiah VG, et al. Endovascular repair of the thoracic aorta in octogenarians. Eur J Cardiothorac Surg. 2008;34(3):630–4; discussion 634.

217. St. Peter SD, Craft RO, Tiede JL, Swain JM. Impact of advanced age on weight loss and health benefits after laparoscopic gastric bypass. Arch Surg. 2005;140(2):165–8.

218. Chautard J, Alves A, Zalinski S, Bretagnol F, Valleur P, Panis Y. Laparoscopic colorectal surgery in elderly patients: a matched case-control study in 178 patients. J Am Coll Surg. 2008;206(2): 255–60.

219. Gianetta E, de Cian F, Cuneo S, et al. Hernia repair in elderly patients. Br J Surg. 1997;84(7):983–5.

220. Amemiya T, Oda K, Ando M, et al. Activities of daily living and quality of life of elderly patients after elective surgery for gastric and colorectal cancers. Ann Surg. 2007;246(2):222–8.

221. Zierer A, Melby SJ, Lubahn JG, Sicard GA, Damiano Jr RJ, Moon MR. Elective surgery for thoracic aortic aneurysms: late functional status and quality of life. Ann Thorac Surg. 2006;82(2):573–8.

222. Ferguson MK, Parma CM, Celauro AD, Vigneswaran WT. Quality of life and mood in older patients after major lung resection. Ann Thorac Surg. 2009;87(4):1007–12; discussion 1012–3.

223. Burfeind Jr WR, Tong BC, O'Branski E, et al. Quality of life outcomes are equivalent after lobectomy in the elderly. J Thorac Cardiovasc Surg. 2008;136(3):597–604.

224. de Vincentiis C, Kunkl AB, Trimarchi S, et al. Aortic valve replacement in octogenarians: is biologic valve the unique solution? Ann Thorac Surg. Apr 2008;85(4):1296–301.

225. Vicchio M, Della Corte A, De Santo LS, et al. Tissue versus mechanical prostheses: quality of life in octogenarians. Ann Thorac Surg. 2008;85(4):1290–5.

226. Dunlop WE, Rosenblood L, Lawrason L, Birdsall L, Rusnak CH. Effects of age and severity of illness on outcome and length of stay in geriatric surgical patients. Am J Surg. 1993;165(5):577–80.

227. Akoh JA, Mathew AM, Chalmers JW, Finlayson A, Auld GD. Audit of major gastrointestinal surgery in patients aged 80 years or over. J R Coll Surg Edinb. 1994;39(4):208–13.

228. Battafarano RJ, Piccirillo JF, Meyers BF, et al. Impact of comorbidity on survival after surgical resection in patients with stage I non-small cell lung cancer. J Thorac Cardiovasc Surg. 2002;123(2): 280–7.

229. Mehta RH, Eagle KA, Coombs LP, et al. Influence of age on outcomes in patients undergoing mitral valve replacement. Ann Thorac Surg. 2002;74(5):1459–67.

230. Muravchick S. Anesthesia for the elderly. In: Miller RD, editor. Anesthesia. 5th ed. Philadelphia: Churchill Livingston; 2000. p. 2140–56.

231. Barzan L, Veronesi A, Caruso G, et al. Head and neck cancer and ageing: a retrospective study in 438 patients. J Laryngol Otol. 1990;104(8):634–40.

232. Gupta R, Kawashima T, Ryu M, Okada T, Cho A, Takayama W. Role of curative resection in octogenarians with malignancy. Am J Surg. 2004;188(3):282–7.

233. Martin II RC, Jaques DP, Brennan MF, Karpeh M. Extended local resection for advanced gastric cancer: increased survival versus increased morbidity. Ann Surg. 2002;236(2):159–65.

234. Siegelmann-Danieli N, Khandelwal V, Wood GC, et al. Breast cancer in elderly women: outcome as affected by age, tumor features, comorbidities, and treatment approach. Clin Breast Cancer. 2006;7(1):59–66.

235. Muravchick S. Anesthesia for the elderly. In: Miller R, editor. Anesthesia. 5th ed. Philadelphia: Churchill Livingstone; 2000. p. 2140–56.

236. Lakatta EG. Cardiovascular reserve capacity in healthy older humans. Aging (Milano). 1994;6(4):213–23.

237. Muravchick S. Choosing an anesthetic for the elderly patient. Am Rev PAN. 1997;19:117–24.

Chapter 4
Geriatric Models of Care

Elizabeth A. Capezuti, Patricia Ursomanno, Marie Boltz, and Hongsoo Kim

Abstract Although patients aged 65 and over represent about 13% of the US population, they account for 40% of those undergoing surgical procedures in American hospitals. Due to the increased likelihood of comorbidities, older patients also represent a higher rate of postoperative complications that influence morbidity and mortality following major surgery. These problems have led to the development of several geriatric models of care across all health care settings. This chapter provides a brief overview of complications that are more frequently found in older patients, care delivery issues that are addressed by geriatric models of care, and a description of the most commonly employed hospital models.

Keywords Geriatric • Aging • Health services for the aged • Nursing

Introduction

Models of care addressing the unique needs of older hospitalized patients can be traced to the comprehensive geriatric assessment (CGA) programs first developed in the 1970s [1]. CGA programs screen older patients at high risk for geriatric-specific problems, assess for modifiable risk factors, and implement evidence-based strategies consistent with the patient's treatment goals. Over the last 30 years changes in the health care system, coupled with the increasing older adult population, have led to the development of several geriatric models of care across all health care settings. In general, the goals of these geriatric models of care in the hospital focus on [1] the prevention of complications that occur more commonly in older adults and [2] address hospital factors that contribute to complications. This chapter provides a

brief overview of complications that are more frequently found in older patients, care delivery issues that are addressed by geriatric models of care, and a description of the most commonly employed hospital models.

Complications of Older Hospitalized Patients

Although patients aged 65 and over represent about 13% of the US population, they account for 40% of those undergoing surgical procedures in American hospitals [2]. Newer surgical approaches will increase the numbers of older patients receiving cardiac surgery. For example, recent studies have demonstrated that older patients with valvular heart disease can benefit from valve surgery with an improvement in quality of life, and referral should not be delayed until the patient develops heart failure [3, 4]. Based on recent ACC/AHA guidelines [5], the number of elderly patients referred for valve surgery is likely to increase for the symptomatic and asymptomatic patient with left ventricular dysfunction, and many older patients may benefit as much as younger patients from cardiac surgery. These numbers have prompted some to ask if cardiac surgery is now a geriatric specialty [6].

In addition to the high proportion of older patients, the most troublesome finding is that older patients also represent a higher complication rate for certain conditions which subsequently lead to higher health care costs. Age may be viewed as a proxy for multiple chronic diseases. Postoperative complications that are known determinants of short- and long-term survival following major surgery such as myocardial infarction and sepsis are associated with age due to the increased likelihood of comorbidities such as cardiac disease [7].

Older adults are more likely to experience additional types of complications that, in addition to reducing survival, can result in loss of independence and lead to hospital readmission, increased usage of rehabilitation services, and new placement in a nursing home. Physical frailty and cognitive impairment [8, 9] (either chronic dementia and/or delirium)

E.A. Capezuti (✉)
Hartford Institute for Geriatric Nursing, New York University College of Nursing, 726 Broadway, 10th Floor, New York, NY 10003, USA
e-mail: ec65@nyu.edu

M.R. Katlic (ed.), *Cardiothoracic Surgery in the Elderly*, DOI 10.1007/978-1-4419-0892-6_4,
© Springer Science+Business Media, LLC 2011

can further compound an older person's vulnerability to complications during hospitalization [10]. Frailty refers to "decreased reserves in multiple organ systems" [11] that is highly associated (after controlling for age, race, sex, and comorbid illness) with an increased risk for falls, cardiovascular disease, hypertension as well as reduced mobility, decreased functional status, institutionalization, and death [12, 13].

Persons with dementia are more prone to negative outcomes related to disease management and hospitalization. Older patients with dementia hospitalized for exacerbation of a chronic disease have significantly longer lengths of hospital stays (LOS) as compared to older patients without dementia. For example, the LOS of older patient with COPD is 121 days/1,000 persons as compared to older patients with both COPD and dementia, who have a LOS of 361 days/1,000 persons [14]. For those who develop delirium (for both those with and without an underlying chronic dementia) during hospitalization, increased LOS and higher hospital costs are well documented [15]. The complex challenges of those adult patients with cognitive impairment are often not adequately addressed. Table 4.1 provides examples of common behaviors of cognitively impaired persons that can lead to complications.

Although geriatric models of care can improve the overall outcomes and experiences of hospitalization, in general, these programs are designed to target those adverse events that occur more commonly in older patients. Table 4.2

Table 4.1 Behaviors of cognitively impaired patients contributing to high complication rate

Behaviors	Example	Potential complication
Inability to follow directions	Does not use call bell to ask for assistance and gets out of bed without needed assistance	Fall-related injury
Removal of treatments	Pulls out central lines	Hemorrhage
		Infection
		Physical restraints and associated complications
Not able to communicate needs	In pain but not able to verbally communicate this to nurse	Functional decline
Wandering	Leaves unit and exits hospital in gown	Hypothermia
		Other injuries
		Use of physical and chemical restraints that increase likelihood of delirium, falls, fall-related injury, and nutritional problems
Misinterprets visual and auditory cues	Resists staff attempts to assist the patient to get out of bed which is perceived as an assault and then hits staff	Agitation-related injury
		Overuse of psychoactive medication that increase likelihood of delirium, falls, and fall-related injury
Decreases inhibition of inappropriate behaviors	Removes clothing and walk down hallway nude	Agitation-related injury
		Overuse of psychoactive medication that increases likelihood of delirium, falls, and fall-related injury

Source: Data from Silverstein N, Maslow K, editors. Improving hospital care for persons with dementia. New York: Springer; 2006. p. 3–22, cited in Maslow [14]

Table 4.2 Complications in the older surgical patient[a]

Complication	Hospital factors[b]	Clinical outcome	Cost implications
Functional decline	Immobility	Reduced/loss of independence in function (activities of daily living (ADL))	Longer length of stay (LOS)
	Bed rest without medical/surgical indication	Reduced/loss of ambulation	Increased rate of institutional or home-based rehabilitation
	Physical restraint	Pain	Nursing home placement
	Inappropriate medication prescribing	Increased rate of pressure ulcers, falls, fall-related injuries, and development of contractures	
	New psychoactive drug use		
	Obstacles in the hospital physical environment		
Fall-related injury	Immobility	Pain	Medicare will not pay for treatment[c]
	Physical restraint	Fracture requiring surgical intervention	Surgery
	Inappropriate medication prescribing	Reduced/loss of independence in function (ADL)	Longer LOS
	New psychoactive drug use	Reduced/loss of ambulation	Institutional or home-based rehabilitation
	Obstacles in the hospital physical environment		Nursing home placement

(continued)

Table 4.2 (continued)

Complication	Hospital factors[b]	Clinical outcome	Cost implications
Under/ malnutrition	Immobility Inattention to oral care Lack of feeding assistance for those with physical or cognitive impairments	Reduced wound healing Discomfort due nasogastric tube placement Percutaneous enteral access procedures (gastrostomy) Delirium Physical restraint to prevent tube removal Aspiration Functional decline	Longer LOS Surgery Institutional or home-based enteral nutrition therapy
Pressure ulcer	Immobility Physical restraint Under/malnutrition Dehydration	Immobility Sleep deprivation Pain Sepsis Septicemia Surgical debridement Surgical techniques (direct closure, flaps, and skin grafting)	Medicare will not pay for treatment[b] Longer LOS Institutional or home-based skilled nursing treatment
Urinary tract infection (UTI. secondary to catheter use or CAUTI)	Emergency room placement without indication Incontinence treatment No post-surgical monitoring of catheter use	Immobility Pain Delirium Acute pyelonephritis Bacteremia Sepsis Prosthetic joint infection Higher risk for death	Medicare will not pay for treatment[b] Longer LOS Rehospitalization
Delirium	Physical restraint Inappropriate medication prescribing New psychoactive drugs Urinary cathetherization CAUTI Immobility Under/malnutrition Dehydration	Functional decline Persistent cognitive impairment Falls, injuries Undetected infection Sleep deprivation	Longer LOS Rehospitalization Nursing home placement Death

[a]Geriatric syndromes refer to "clinical conditions in older persons that do not fit into discrete disease categories." This may also include other conditions highly associated with aging such as frailty, sleep disorders, self-neglect. For the purpose of this review, these syndromes and potential complications are more narrowly defined

[b]Hospital factors. There is a myriad of patient and hospital factors that contribute to each complication; however, this list provides examples of those specific hospital practices that place the older adults at high risk and which are the focus of geriatric care model interventions

[c]As of October 2008, hospitals do not receive payment for eight hospital-acquired conditions; three of these eight indicated in the table are complications known to occur most frequently in older inpatients and have been found to be reduced when geriatric models of care are employed (fall-related injury, pressure ulcer, and catheter-associated urinary tract infection (CAUTI))

provides a summary of these complications and the clinical and cost outcomes associated with these complications. These complications are often referred to as "geriatric syndromes" which refer to "clinical conditions in older persons that do not fit into discrete disease categories" [16].

A US congressional mandate instituted on August 1, 2007, significantly changed the Inpatient Prospective Payment System that the Centers for Medicare & Medicaid Services (CMS) use to reimburse hospitals [17–19]. As of October 2008, hospitals do not receive payment for eight hospital-acquired conditions; three of these eight are complications that are known to occur most frequently in older inpatients and have been found to be reduced when geriatric models of care are employed [20]. These three complications (fall-related injury, pressure ulcer, and catheter-associated urinary tract infection (CAUTI)) are among the six adverse events or complications specifically associated with hospitalization of older adults. Although there are other geriatric syndromes (e.g., incontinence) and other potential complications associated with older inpatients (e.g., sleep deprivation, inadequate pain management, dehydration, and adverse drug effects), many of these syndromes and complications are either risk factors or outcomes of the following.

Functional Decline

Functional decline refers to the loss of the ability to perform basic activities of daily living (ADL). A systematic review of 30 studies examining correlates of functional decline found that between 15 and 76% of hospitalized elders experience diminished performance in at least one ADL at discharge [21]. Of those with decline at discharge, only half will recover function at 3 months post-discharge, and, for many, this decline will result in permanent loss of independent living [22]. Functional decline is considered a "profound marker of morbidity and mortality" [23] resulting in longer lengths of stay, greater costs, and increased rate of nursing home placement [24].

Although an increasing number of patients over 70 years old are undergoing cardiac surgery with acceptable morbidity and mortality rates, those undergoing traditional cardiac surgery are more likely to experience a prolonged recovery and are unable to return home immediately due to poor functional status outcomes [25, 26]. New technologies in cardiac surgery can reduce the likelihood of functional decline among older cardiac patients. For example, minimally invasive valve surgery (MIVS) has increased in the last decade due to the need to reduce overall surgical trauma, lessen complications, shorten the length of hospital stay, and improve patient recovery. In comparison to traditional sternotomy, studies have demonstrated that MIVS results in comparable morbidity and mortality, similar bypass and cross-clamp times, fewer blood product transfusions, less postoperative pain, and decreased length of hospital stay [27, 28]. The results of a study of 44 heart failure patients 65 years or older undergoing MIVS (both aortic and mitral) at New York University Langone Medical Center indicated fewer postoperative complications, a shortened hospital stay, and a decreased need for inpatient cardiac rehabilitation [29]. More importantly, the older MIVS patients exceeded their preoperative baseline New York Heart Association (NYHA) functional status by the sixth week. The study also utilized the Inventory of Functional Status in the Elderly (IFSITE) [30] measurement to assess specific instrumental ADL (e.g., shopping, laundry) patients were able to perform after undergoing MIVS. All the patients resumed these activities by 6 weeks and most patients demonstrated an improvement of greater than 10% from baseline to 6 weeks. Most notably, the percentage of patients who were able to perform exercise increased from 27.3% at baseline to 93.2% at 6 weeks and meal preparation increased from 59.1% at baseline to 84.1% at 6 weeks. These results are in contrast to studies of traditional sternotomy patients that report that functional status did not return to the preoperative baseline level at 6 weeks and many did not recover functional status even at 6–12 months following cardiac surgery [31].

Fall-Related Injury

Roughly 2–5% of older adults fall during hospitalization [32]. The number of falls per 1,000 patient days is highest in hospital units admitting mostly older adults such as geropsychiatry, rehabilitation, and geriatric medicine. Among hospitalized older adults, falls from bed account for approximately one-third of all falls. Almost one-third of all fall-related injuries occur among persons 85 years of age or older. Approximately 3–10% of falls happening in hospitals result in either serious or minor injuries [33]. Hip fractures, occurring in about 1–4% of hospital falls, are particularly significant because older adults are more likely to suffer from a substantial decline in physical functioning and often require longer periods of active rehabilitation services as compared to younger persons [34].

Under/Malnutrition

Undernutrition and malnutrition are deficiency syndromes caused by inadequate intake or absorption of macronutrients. Malnutrition has long been associated with important adverse outcomes, such as increased morbidity and mortality and decreased quality of life. Weight loss and hypoalbuminemia are both strongly correlated with increased mortality in ill adults [35]. Body weight and body composition have important implications for physical functioning of older persons, and the prevalence of malnutrition in older hospitalized patients has been estimated to be between 40 and 60% [36].

Pressure Ulcers

Pressure ulcers continue to present a major health problem for hospitalized adults with reported nosocomial incidence rates between 0.4 and 38% [37]. Pressure ulcers are highly correlated with age [38]. At least a fifth of pressure ulcers will progress to a more advanced stage of deterioration. Most ulcers develop in the sacrum and coccyx areas with rates higher in patients with mobility impairment. Pressure ulcers remain a major cause of morbidity and are associated with longer LOS. Nosocomial pressure ulcers and their progression in severity during hospitalization have been used as a quality care indicator [39].

Urinary Tract Infection

Approximately 4% of patients with urinary tract infection (UTIs) will develop bacteremia which is known to significantly increase in length of stay and is associated with higher mortality in older patients [40]. The major care-associated practice leading to UTI in older inpatients is the overuse of urinary catheters, defined as catheter use for longer than 2 days [41]. CAUTI is the most common nosocomial infection [42]. A study using a random sample of almost 36,000 Medicare patients undergoing major operations from 2,965 US hospitals reported that 86% had perioperative indwelling urinary catheters and among these 50% had catheters for longer than 2 days postoperatively. These patients' risk of developing a UTI was twice as likely compared to patients with catheterization [43]. Among another sample of approximately 39,000 Medicare patients undergoing major surgery who were discharged to a nursing home found that those patients discharged with catheters were at higher risk for rehospitalization for UTI and death within 30 days than patients who did not have catheters [44]. In addition to infection, catheter use is associated with immobility, delirium, and pain [45].

Delirium

Delirium, a transient state of cognitive impairment, may develop in both cognitively intact and impaired older adults. It is estimated that between 14 and 24% of older persons are admitted to the hospital with delirium, and an additional 6–56% of hospitalized elders will develop delirium during their hospitalization replace especially if they are admitted to an ICU [46]. Postoperative delirium is more likely to occur following hip fracture, cardiac, non-cardiac thoracic, aortic aneurysm, and abdominal surgery. Postoperative delirium is more likely in those deemed vulnerable. Patient vulnerability including presence of previous brain pathology, decreased ability to manage change, impaired sensory function, multiple comorbidities, and changes in pharmacodynamic responses to medications are all suggested possible causes for delirium. In surgical patients, both preoperative (use of narcotic analgesics, history of alcohol abuse, and depression) and perioperative (greater intraoperative blood loss, more postoperative transfusions, postoperative hematocrit less than 30%, and severe postoperative pain) risk factors have been identified for delirium postoperatively [47]. Additionally, hospital practices that lead to iatrogenic events including use of physical restraints, malnutrition, more than three medications, and urinary catheterization are also significantly associated with delirium [48]. There are no significant differences in incidence of postoperative delirium following general versus epidural anesthesia.

Despite high incidence, most delirium goes undetected [49, 50], thus contributing to many negative consequences. Delirium is associated with poor hospital outcomes such as higher mortality rates, increased length of hospital stay, increased intensity of nursing care, greater health care costs as well as increased risk of several adverse outcomes after discharge, including functional decline, persistent cognitive impairment, rehospitalization, and nursing home placement [51].

The occurrence of each of these complications leads to interventions that can often prolong the hospital stay. Following hospital discharge, they frequently contribute to death, institutionalization as well as disproportionately high rehospitalization rates, high emergency department usage, and increased need for rehabilitation therapy services. As illustrated in Table 4.2, the *interrelationships* among these various complications during hospitalization are obvious and also well documented [12]. The data supporting the importance of prevention, early detection, and treatment of these complications in older surgical patients are described in the ACOVE (Assessing Care of Vulnerable Elders) report, Quality Indicators for Hospitalization and Surgery in Vulnerable Elders [52].

Although patient characteristics, especially multiple comorbidities, frailty, and cognitive impairment, may increase vulnerability of older inpatient to negative consequences, the hospital environment plays an independent and significant role in determining staff practice and subsequent patient outcomes such as iatrogenic complications. This has led to the development of geriatric models to address these hospital-based or institutional factors that are likely to contribute to complications among older patients. Effective resolution of these negative consequences is dependent on geriatric models that target both patient and environmental (institutional) risk factors.

Geriatric Care Model Objectives

Although geriatric models of care differ in their approach to prevent complications and address care delivery problems that can contribute to complications, all share a common set of general objectives. Although these objectives could be applied to any patient regardless of age, it is how geriatric care models apply these that are age-specific. Table 4.3 provides examples of processes and interventions to meet these six general objectives.

The six general objectives of geriatric care models are:

Educate health care providers in core geriatric principles. The complications most frequently encountered among older patients are often due to system-level problems. These include inadequate educational preparation of health care providers to recognize age-specific factors that increase risk of complications. All geriatric care models require a coordinator or clinician with advanced geriatric education; however, the

Table 4.3 Geriatric care models: objectives, processes, and interventions

Objective	Examples of processes	Examples of interventions
Educate health care providers in core geriatric principles	Resident training includes required geriatric rotation *or* mandatory geriatric rotation for residents Institutional continuing education includes geriatric-specific training *or* geriatric-specific interdisciplinary continuing education programs Geriatric specialist responsible for geriatric training initiatives	Hospital intranet includes geriatric programming Journal club includes geriatric journals and/or articles focusing on geriatric outcomes Medical, surgical, nursing, and interdisciplinary rounds include geriatric case studies
Target risk factors for complications	Policies, protocols, and documentation system includes assessment tools and practices that identify older adults at risk for complications Assessment tools prompt providers to consult geriatric specialists for evaluation of high risk problems Geriatric specialist provides individual evaluation of risk factors	Electronic medical record (EMR) provides alerts for medications prescribed that are known to increase fall risk EMR prompts providers to document daily cognitive testing results Hospital policy for daily cognitive assessment of at-risk patients Cognitive assessment indicates delirium that leads to geriatric specialist consultation
Incorporate patient (family) choices and treatment goals	Policies and protocols support and documentation system includes forms that elicit patient choices as well as family involvement in care Geriatric nurses are prepared to coordinate an interdisciplinary evaluation and promote development of *informed* patient/family treatment goals and plan of care Palliative care is consulted and provides informed choices to patients/families in situations of life-threatening illness	Admission history includes evaluation of patient's preferences for post-discharge rehabilitation Unlimited visiting hours and bedside recliners encourage family participation in recovery Patient and family preferences for type and degree of family involvement is documented Patient with Alzheimer's disease who is unable to verbally indicate needs is evaluated by palliative care specialist for pain evaluation/treatment
Employ evidence-based interventions	Policies and protocols integrate geriatric-specific implications Education and training for all clinicians include core geriatric content	Hospital protocol for urinary catheter removal within 2 days post-surgery Unit-based mobility program Physical environment reduces injury risk for non-ambulatory patients with dementia such as low-height beds and bedside mats
Promote inter-disciplinary communication	Medical record facilitates patient information across disciplines Processes in place to encourage face-to-face interaction among disciplines Unit-based and hospital wide committee includes geriatric specialist representation	Interdisciplinary team rounds held bi-weekly Programmatic initiatives include all applicable disciplines, e.g., physical and occupational therapy in unit-based mobility program Comanage patients across specialties such as geriatric oncology Collaborate with other programs such as palliative care in providing symptom management
Emphasize discharge planning or transitional care	Documentation system provides comprehensive hospital course information to primary care provider and other post-discharge providers (home care, nursing home, etc.) as well as elicits pertinent information *from* other providers	Patient and caregiver receive comprehensive documentation of hospital treatment, changes in treatment plan, and post-discharge instructions Understanding of instructions is evaluated before discharge Phone follow-up post-discharge to evaluate patient condition and needs

implementation of any model depends on direct care staff with the knowledge and competencies to deliver safe and evidence-based care to older patients. Thus, the coordinator or other geriatric clinician role includes teaching of other staff through rounds, journal clubs, conferences, and other internal institutional educational venues.

Target risk factors for complications. Given the disproportion of certain complications or geriatric syndromes among hospitalized older adults, the clinical focus of all geriatric models is prevention via risk factor reduction and early detection of these problems. Some models may focus on a particular syndrome; however, the interrelationship of these complications and their shared risk factors often result in a reduction of the other geriatric syndromes. Targeting risk factors requires standardized assessment tools known to be valid and reliable for older adults. See the Hartford Institute's Try This and How to Try This series for examples of assessment instruments (http://www.hartfordign.org/trythis). Implementation of geriatric care models often includes institutionalizing these practices such as incorporating these tools in the medical record as well as hospital policies, procedures, and protocols.

Incorporate patient (family) choices and treatment goals. All health care decision should be guided by the patient's choices. Choices range from decisions about activity level and medication use to more complex issues including advance directives. Decisions regarding life-sustaining treatment are often influenced by quality of life considerations balanced by the potential length of life. For family members acting in the best interests of patients who can no longer participate in decision making, this can be a complicated dilemma. Life-sustaining treatments are often employed with very old patients who die in the course of hospitalization although most prefer comfort care. Geriatric models are meant to address this lack of congruence by supporting efforts to provide care that is more consistent with patients' preferences [53]. For this reason, many geriatric models work collaboratively or in conjunction with palliative care programs.

Employ evidence-based interventions. Given that most physicians, nurses, and other health providers have received minimal content in their training regarding geriatrics, it is not surprising that there is a higher complication rate for older hospitalized patients. Advances in geriatric science, similar to other research-based approaches, are not readily employed in hospital care. Problems with polypharmacy, inappropriate medications (e.g., overuse of psychoactive), overuse of restraints, inadequate detection of delirium, depression, and undermanagement of pain are some of the many hospital factors that can contribute to poor outcomes. Thus, geriatric models promote the use of standardized evidence-based protocols.

Promote interdisciplinary communication. Since geriatric syndromes are not just medical problems but represent a complex interaction of medical, functional, psychological, and social issues, other disciplines such as nursing, pharmacy, social work, physical, and occupational therapy are needed. Geriatric care models all include interdisciplinary teams, i.e., an approach that facilitates communication among disciplines.

Emphasize discharge planning (or transitional care). Many older patients will require rehabilitation or skilled nursing services following hospitalization. Almost a quarter of older hospital patients are discharged to another institution such as a rehabilitation hospital or nursing home and more than 10% are discharged with home care [54]. Older adults are more likely to experience problems associated with discharge planning that can lead to delays in discharge and greater use of emergency service use and hospital readmission. Hospital readmission for older patients is most likely associated with medical errors in medication continuity [55, 56], diagnostic

workup, or test follow-up [57]. These poor outcomes are attributed to a lack of coordination among health care providers that can result in unresolved medical issues [58] and deficient preparation of patients and their caregivers to carry out discharge instructions [59]. One study found wide variations among providers in discharge planning effectiveness; the providers cited their lack of knowledge and experience when not making appropriate home care referrals [60]. Thus, geriatric models not only focus on the in-patient experience but also the post-hospital care environment and the care transition following hospital discharge. Two of the six models consider the care transition a primary focus of their programs.

Geriatric Models

There are several types of geriatric models that are currently employed in hospitals throughout the United States. In addition to incorporating the original tenets central to CGA (screen for those at high risk for geriatric-specific problems, assess for modifiable risk factors, and implement strategies consistent with the patient' treatment goals) all also strive to deliver quality care for older adults in a cost-effective manner. CGA assumes that the systematic evaluation of a frail older person by a multidisciplinary health care team will uncover actual or potential health problems. The considerable advances in geriatric health care science over the last 30 years can then be applied to treating or preventing these conditions and thus result in better health outcomes.

Although the specific mode of intervening may differ among the models, they all address both common health problems and care delivery issues. The geriatric model may consider all geriatric syndromes or target specific ones such as delirium or functional decline. Similarly, the geriatric model may be employed as a hospital-wide approach, unit-based intervention, or focus on specific processes of hospitalization such as admission screening or discharge planning. Regardless of the structure of the geriatric model, all facilitate the general objectives listed in Table 4.3. Table 4.4 provides a summary of the clinical foci, unique features, coordination, and interventions for each of the six most commonly employed geriatric models of care.

Geriatric Consultation Service provides a geriatrician, a gero-psychiatrist, a geriatric clinical nurse specialist, or an interdisciplinary team of geriatric health care providers to conduct a CGA or evaluate a specific condition (delirium), symptom (patient dislodges or removes treatment), or situation (adequacy of family support for discharge back to community setting). The consultation may be requested by another primary service for an individual patient or may be

Table 4.4 Core components of six geriatric care models

Model type	Clinical outcome focus[a]	Unique features	Program/team coordination	Interventions[b]
Geriatric Consultation	Primary focus can vary depending on composition of consult team and may be specific to a surgical specialty or procedure	Employed by primary provider request	Individual consultant (geriatrician, geropsychiatrist, or geriatric nurse specialist) *or* Interdisciplinary team that is coordinated by geriatric medicine or psychiatry fellow, geriatric nurse specialist, or an administrative director	Comprehensive geriatric assessment (CGA): medical, psychiatric, functional, and social. Recommends interventions based on consultant discipline (medicine, psychiatry, or team that includes nurses, social workers, and others). Primary provider chooses which recommendation to employ
Acute Care for the Elderly (ACE)	Functional decline	Dedicated unit with explicit admission criteria. Requires interdisciplinary team *and* Redesign of physical environment to accommodate physical and cognitive needs	Unit directed and/or team coordinated by geriatrician, geriatric nurse specialist, administrator, or comanaged by clinician-manager	Physical environment to promote patient mobility, orientation, and staff observation. Interdisciplinary rounds facilitate care coordination and thus: Identify modifiable risk factors for geriatric syndromes and complications. Prevent avoidable discharge delay. Promote timely referrals to disciplines or specialists
Nurses Improving the Care of Health System Elders (NICHE): GRN/ACE	Nursing processes related to all geriatric syndromes and potential complications such as avoiding restraint use, initiating urinary catheter removal	Focus on improving nursing care of all geriatric syndromes. Prepares staff nurses to take active part in geriatric care management including coordinating or facilitating other geriatric models of care	Program implementation by NICHE Coordinator (usually a geriatric nurse specialist). Geriatric Resources Nurses (staff nurses with additional training) implement protocols. Depending on availability, other clinicians (geriatrician, hospitalist, social worker, etc.) work as interdisciplinary team	Nurse-initiated protocols: Restraint and psychoactive drug reduction. Functional mobility. Fall/injury prevention. Pressure ulcer assessment/treatment. Prevention of UTI – early catheter removal. Delirium assessment/treatment. Organizational strategies including measurement schema, performance improvement techniques, and management tools to promote implementation of above protocols
The Hospital Elder Life Program (HELP)	Delirium prevention and early management	Requires use of volunteers	Elder Life Nurse Specialist or Elder Life Specialists coordinates interdisciplinary team (geriatrician, recreation therapy, physical therapy, etc.) and trained volunteers	Delirium risk factor protocols: Mental orientation. Therapeutic activities. Early mobilization. Vision and hearing adaptations. Hydration and feeding assistance. Sleep enhancement
Advanced practice nurse (APN) Transitional Care Model	Reducing complications specific during the transition from hospital to home	Requires APN coordinator to follow patient in hospital and following discharge	APN (nurse practitioner or clinical nurse specialist)	Protocols to assess/intervene with: Medication discrepancies and inappropriate medication usage. Case management and APN surveillance across settings

(continued)

Table 4.4 (continued)

Model type	Clinical outcome focus[a]	Unique features	Program/team coordination	Interventions[b]
The Care Transitions Intervention	Reducing complications specific during the transition from hospital to home, such as prevent post-hospital medication discrepancies, increase likelihood of patient/caregiver detection of worsening condition	Requires nurse transitions coach to follow patient in hospital and following discharge	Transition Coach (nurse or APN) empowers patient and caregiver	Personal Health Record includes data elements essential to promote productive patient-provider encounters across settings Discharge Preparation Checklist to facilitate patient's knowledge of discharge instructions Medication Discrepancy Tool used by transition coach to identify medication issues

[a]All programs are meant to address geriatric syndromes and potential complications. Geriatric syndromes refer to "clinical conditions in older persons that do not fit into discrete disease categories." This may also include other conditions highly associated with aging such as frailty, sleep disorders, and self-neglect. For the purpose of this review, these syndromes and potential complications are more narrowly defined to six of the most common complications

[b]Interventions are guided by the use of standardized assessment tools known to be valid and reliable for older adults. See the Hartford Institute's Try This and How to Try This series for examples of assessment instruments (http://www.hartfordign.org/trythis)

initiated by a hospital policy for all patients who are screened at high risk for geriatric-related complications or are admitted from a home-bound program or a nursing home [61].

Outside of academic medical centers, few hospitals have geriatric departments that can provide geriatricians or a geriatric consultation team. Although geriatric nurse specialists may be more prevalent in hospitals than geriatricians, many function without the benefit of a geriatric team or a geriatrician. Similar to geriatricians, it is difficult to evaluate their effectiveness when their practice is limited to a consultative role in which recommendations may not be followed or institutional resources are not adequately available for staff to implement [62].

Acute Care for the Elderly (ACE) Units are discrete geriatric care-focused units. Originally developed in the 1970s within Veterans Administration Hospitals, Geriatric Evaluation and Management (GEM) Units were meant to provide CGA delivered by a multidisciplinary team with a focus on the rehabilitative needs of older patients. Multidisciplinary team rounds and patient-centered team conferences are considered the hallmarks of care. The core team includes a geriatrician, clinical nurse specialist, social worker as well as specialists from other disciplines providing consultation: occupational and physical therapy, nutrition, pharmacy, audiology, and psychology. GEM units usually have been redesigned to facilitate care of the older patient, which, in contrast to geriatric consultation services, have direct control over the implementation of team recommendations. Research conducted in the 1980s and 1990s have documented significant reductions in functional decline and suboptimal medication use as well as return to home post-discharge and, more recently, decreased rate of nursing home placement [63] among hospitalized veterans on GEMUs compared to general medical units.

Beginning in the 1990s, ACE units have been implemented in non-VA hospitals although they generally focus on more acutely ill patients than GEM units. These units utilize staff with geriatric expertise working collaboratively in an interdisciplinary team (fostered by care processes such as team rounds and family conferences) in a physical environment with adaptations to addresses age-related changes (e.g., flooring to reduce glare and low-height beds to reduce fall-related injury), promote orientation (clocks and calendars), and facilitate staff observation (e.g., alarmed exit doors, windows inserted in walls, and communal space for meals). The interdisciplinary team (led by geriatricians and/or geriatric nurse specialists) aims to facilitate care coordination and thus identify modifiable risk factors for geriatric syndromes and complications, prevent avoidable discharge delay, and promote timely referrals to disciplines/specialist.

Palmer et al. [64] designed the first ACE unit at the University Hospitals of Cleveland. A randomized controlled trial of Acute Care for Elders in an academic medical center reported improved functional status (ADL, instrumental ADLs and ambulation) at discharge of patients hospitalized on the ACE unit compared to those on other units. Fewer patients from the ACE group were discharged to nursing homes. These beneficial effects were achieved without increasing in-hospital or post-discharge costs. There were no significant differences in mortality, length of stay, readmission, or hospital costs between the two groups [65]. In another randomized trial conducted in a community hospital, patients were randomly assigned to either ACE care or a regular care unit. Positive outcomes of the ACE intervention were demonstrated in several processes of care including a reduction in restraint use, days to discharge planning, and use of high-risk medications. They also found benefit in a composite outcome of ADL improvement and nursing home placement, but not in discharge ADL levels alone. There was no significant reduction in length of stay, hospital costs, or mortality in the ACE unit subjects compared to the regular unit subjects [66].

Since one unit cannot provide care for all older patients within a hospital, many hospitals use this unit for patients at highest risk for age-related complications. The unit is an excellent environment for training of all disciplines. ACE staff may also provide consultation throughout the hospital to export ACE principles throughout the health system.

Nurses Improving the Care of Health System Elders (NICHE; http://www.nicheprogram.org) is a national program aimed at system improvement to achieve positive outcomes for hospitalized older adults. NICHE has two main goals: improving the quality of care to patients and improving nurse competence. This is accomplished by "modifying the nurse practice environment with the infusion of geriatric-specific: (a) core values into the mission statement of the institution; (b) special equipment, supplies, and other resources; and (c) protocols and techniques that promote interdisciplinary collaboration" [67]. NICHE includes several approaches, each of which facilitates transfusion of evidence-based geriatric best practices into hospital care. A geriatric nurse specialist as the NICHE Coordinator functions in both a "primary care role (evaluating and managing patients directly) and in a leadership role (teaching and mentoring others and changing systems of care)" [68]. Foundational to NICHE is the Geriatric Resource Nurse Model (GRN) which is an educational intervention model that prepares staff nurses as the clinical resource person on geriatric issues to other nurses on their unit. The GRN model provides staff nurses, via education and modeling by a NICHE coordinator, with specific content for improved knowledge of care management for geriatric syndromes. Clinical protocols and organizational strategies provide necessary tools to apply evidence base practice. For example, in one NICHE orthopedic unit, GRNs received intensive education on the prevention and detection of delirium in a unit where the primary diagnoses were joint replacement and hip fracture repair. Utilizing a combination of standardized assessment of cognition and focused interventions to prevent postop delirium, the unit realized a significant reduction in the incidence of delirium. Other systemic interventions utilized by the GRNs include a revised nursing database and delirium-specific order sets [69].

An evaluation of responses of 9,802 direct care registered nurses from 75 acute care hospitals participating in NICHE found that a positive geriatric nurse practice environment was associated with positive geriatric care delivery. The independent contribution of all three aspects of the geriatric nurse practice environment (resource availability, institutional values, and capacity for collaboration) influences care delivery for hospitalized older adult patients. The study

findings demonstrate that a nurse practice environment that provides adequate geriatric-specific resources (continuing education, education, and specialty services), promotes interdisciplinary collaboration, and fosters patient, family, and nurse involvement in treatment-related decision making is associated with quality geriatric care [64]. In single site studies, NICHE hospitals demonstrate improved clinical outcomes, rate of compliance with geriatric institutional protocols, cost-related outcomes, and nurse knowledge. In a study of eight hospitals nurses reported higher quality of geriatric care following NICHE implementation [70].

NICHE also promotes a unit-based ACE model. The ACE model within NICHE emphasizes: (1) implementation of nurse-driven protocols, (2) geriatric training of all nursing staff, and (3) utilization of geriatric-specific units within a health system's overall geriatric care programming. Similar to other ACE studies, a NICHE-ACE unit in which the majority of the staff nurses were nationally certified in geriatric nursing reported lower fall and pressure ulcer rates, and lower length of stay when compared to overall hospital [71].

Since NICHE is a system-level approach, it provides a structure for nurses to collaborate with other disciplines and to actively participate or coordinate other geriatric care models. For example, in hospitals with a geriatric department or consultation service, GRNs screen for appropriate referrals to these services and can effectively implement geriatric service recommendations with support from the NICHE coordinator. The models enhance NICHE program effectiveness by expanding the scope of geriatric programming within a health system.

The Hospital Elder Life Program (HELP; http://elderlife. med.yale.edu/public/public-main.php) is a program designed to implement protocols that target six delirium risk factors: mental orientation, therapeutic activities, early mobilization, vision and hearing adaptations, hydration and feeding assistance, and sleep enhancement. These protocols were tested in several well-designed clinical trials and demonstrated significant reduction in the incidence of new delirium. Further, among those who did develop delirium, these protocols are associated with a significant reduction of total number of episodes and days with delirium, functional decline, costs of hospital services, and reduction in use of long-term nursing home services [72, 73].

HELP employs geriatric specialists of various disciplines (geriatrician, geriatric nurse specialist, recreation therapy and physical therapy) working together as an interdisciplinary team with trained volunteers. The program is coordinated by Elder Life Specialists, typically an Elder Life Nurse Specialist who has advanced geriatric nursing education and is responsible for implementing nursing-related assessments and tracking of delirium risk factor protocol adherence. The latter depends on the involvement of well-trained and supervised volunteers in patient care interventions [74].

The research-tested protocol was made available to hospitals in 2000. Implementation in many hospitals has been adapted based on hospital resources. This has led to wide variations in adherence to the intervention protocol. Although higher levels of adherence have been associated with lower rates of delirium, these adapted protocols continue to provide positive results [75].

Transitional Care Models

An American Geriatric Society Position Statement defines transitional care as a set of actions designed to ensure the coordination and continuity of health care as patients transfer between different locations or different levels of care within the same location [76]. Older adult patients with complex medical and social needs and their caregivers require assistance to effectively navigate the health care system, including recovery from surgery and return to premorbid health and living arrangements. Two models have emerged that have demonstrated improved outcomes for older adults hospitalized for both medical and surgical interventions.

Advanced practice nurse (APN) transitional care model utilizes APNs whose primary responsibility is to optimize the health of high-risk, cognitively intact older adults with a variety of medical and surgical conditions during hospitalization and for designing and overseeing the plan for follow-up care following discharge [77]. The APN work collaboratively with the older adult, family caregiver, physician, and other health team members and are guided by evidence-based protocols. The same nurse implements this plan after discharge by providing traditional home care services and by phone availability 7 days a week. Three federally funded, randomized, controlled trials consistently demonstrated that this model of care improves older adults' satisfaction, reduces rehospitalizations, and decreases health care costs [78–80].

Care transitions coaching or *Care transitions intervention* (see http://www.caretransitions.org/index.asp) employs a nurse or "transitions coach" to encourage older patients and their family caregivers to assume more active roles during care transitions by facilitating self-management and direct communication between the patient/caregiver and primary care provider. The four content areas or "pillars" of the patient/caregiver intervention are: (1) medication self-management, (2) a patient-centered record, (3) primary care and specialist follow-up, and (4) knowledge of "red flags" warning symptom or sign indicative of a worsening condition [81]. The Personal Health Record includes data elements essential to promote productive patient-provider encounters across settings such as an active health problem list; medications and allergies; a list of warning symptoms or signs that correspond to the patient's chronic illnesses; and a checklist of activities that need to take place before and following discharge This record is maintained by the patient and caregiver with assistance from the transition coach. The 4-week intervention begins in the hospital and continues through home visits and/or phone follow-up after discharge.

Several studies, including a randomized, controlled trial, found that patients who received this intervention had lower all-cause rehospitalization rates 30 and 90 days after discharge compared with control patients. Intervention patients also had lower rehospitalization rates for the same condition that they were admitted for in the index hospitalization at 90 and 180 days than controls. Mean hospital costs were approximately $500 less for patients in the intervention group compared with controls [82].

New Specialty Models

In some hospitals, multiple geriatric models are employed. For example, a hospital may begin with NICHE. The NICHE coordinator, a geriatric nurse specialist, will then become an Elder Life Specialist to implement HELP hospital wide or within a discrete ACE unit. Often the core geriatric interdisciplinary team of any geriatric program screens patients for other related services such as palliative care, rehabilitative services, or pain management programs. Some have developed dual-function units such as merging an ACE unit with a palliative care unit [68].

Others have developed programs that merge geriatrics with other specialties such as hip fracture, trauma, and oncology. These programs incorporate geriatric comanagement of surgical patients with the expectation that involvement of geriatric specialists in care management will avoid iatrogenic problems [83]. These programs have been shown to reduce delirium by over one-third, reduce severe delirium by over one-half, decrease predicted length of stay, readmission rates, complication rates, and mortality [84]. Although we are not aware of any such programs with geriatric comanagement of older cardiac surgery patients, hospitals participating in the NICHE program report that cardiac patients receive geriatric consultation for those demonstrating delirium postoperatively.

Conclusion

Although these models use different strategies, all share common goals of treatment. Each hospital or health system chooses a model based on the unique needs of that hospital's patient population, the resources available (geriatric specialists, bed capacity to support separate unit, volunteers, etc.), and especially senior administrator's commitment to geriatric programming. Since there is no direct reimbursement for many components of these models (interdisciplinary rounds, geriatric nurse specialist, volunteers, etc.), administrators seek external (grants, donor gifts) and internal funding (hospital foundation grants). They are motivated by the model's alignment to the hospitals strategic plan (e.g., excellence in senior care), the institution's mission, patient/family satisfaction, relationship with the community, and costs savings (i.e., reduction of complications). All the models have demonstrated positive outcomes and each have been implemented in at least 50 hospitals; however, this still only represents a small proportion of American hospitals. Each model was originally developed with government and/or foundation support. Future survival of these models may depend on advancing the unique contributions of each within an integrated model that will enhance the hospital experience of the older patient [85, 86].

Another problem influencing geriatric model implementation is availability of geriatric clinicians. Since significant geriatric medicine input is needed for many of these models, they generally are limited to academic medical centers, which only represent a small proportion of US hospitals. All these models require providers with knowledge of core concepts in geriatrics; however, there is a significant shortage of fellowship-trained geriatricians, geriatric psychiatrists, master's prepared geriatric nurse specialists, as well as other disciplines [87]. In addition to efforts to increase the training of geriatric specialists, several initiatives are underway that involve specialty organizations, medical schools, and resident training programs to integrate principles of geriatric care into curriculums and practice [88, 89]. As more geriatrics is being integrated into undergraduate medical training and surgical resident training, knowledge of geriatric care principles and collaboration with geriatric models will enhance outcomes of the older surgical patients. The Council of the Section for Surgical and Related Medical Specialties in the American Geriatrics Society program provides the Geriatrics Syllabus for Specialists, a useful guide (lectures, PowerPoint presentations, etc.) geared toward providing vital information for surgeons caring for older patients as well as faculty leadership training to promote geriatric training and research within their disciplines. The initiative also provides enable surgical professional certifying bodies and societies to build the capacity of their members to provide better care of older adults [90].

Financial and administrative barriers deter the implementation of geriatric models. Medicare payment system focuses on provider-specific reimbursement and thus limits payment for organizational redesign, multidisciplinary teams, or nurse coordinators. The new CMS financial incentives that will not reimburse for nosocomial "never" events such as pressure ulcers, catheter-associated infections, and fall-related injury, may eventually encourage the use of these models [15]. A recent IOM report recommended that "payers should promote and reward the dissemination of those models of care for older adults that have been shown to be effective and efficient" [89]. Incentives suggested included elimination of Medicare's copayment disparity for mental health and enhanced payments for services under these models.

Finally, most of the research documenting complications of the older patient are based on studies combining both medical and surgical patients, thus future research should address the risk factors of these complications specific to surgical patients. Studies are needed that identify complications within specific types of surgical procedures. This may provide important data to tailor models to specific surgical populations. The development of less invasive cardiac procedures such as MIVS will more likely lead to more older adults undergoing surgery, thus geriatric models that can enhance positive outcomes needs to be incorporated in practice.

References

1. Rubenstein LZ. Geriatric assessment programs. In: Capezuti EA, Siegler E, Mezey M, editors. The encyclopedia of elder care. 2nd ed. New York: Springer; 2008. p. 346–9.
2. Older Patients: A Growing Concern for Surgeons and Related Specialists. American Geriatrics Society – Geriatrics For Specialists. http://www.americangeriatrics.org/specialists/involved.shtml. Accessed 2 Nov 2009.
3. Gogbashian A, Sepic J, Soltesz EG, Nascimben L, Cohn LH. Operative and long-term survival of elderly is significantly improved by mitral valve repair. Am Heart J. 2006;151(6):1325–33.
4. Sedrakyan A, Vaccarino V, Paltiel AD, Elefteriades JA, Mattera JA, Roumanis SA, et al. Age does not limit quality of life improvement in cardiac valve surgery. J Am Coll Cardiol. 2003;42(7):1208–14.
5. Bonow RO, Carabello BA, Kanu C, de Leon Jr AC, Faxon DP, Freed MD, et al. ACC/AHA 2006 guidelines for the management of patients with valvular heart disease: a report of the American College of Cardiology/American Heart Association Task Force on Practice Guidelines (writing committee to revise the 1998 Guidelines for the Management of Patients With Valvular Heart Disease): developed in collaboration with the Society of Cardiovascular Anesthesiologists: endorsed by the Society for Cardiovascular Angiography and Interventions and the Society of Thoracic Surgeons. Circulation. 2006;114(5):e84–231.
6. Nashef SAM. Is cardiac surgery now a geriatric specialty? Crit Care Resusc. 2007;9(3):248–50.
7. Khuri SF, Henderson WG, DePalma RG, et al. Determinants of long-term survival after major surgery and the adverse effect of postoperative complications. Ann Surg. 2005;242(3):326–41.
8. Fortinsky RH, Covinsky KE, Palmer RM, Landefeld CS. Effects of functional status changes before and during hospitalization on nursing home admission of older adults. J Gerontol A Biol Sci Med Sci. 1999;54(10):M521–6.
9. Gill TM, Williams CS, Tinetti ME. The combined effects of baseline vulnerability and acute hospital events on the development of functional dependence among community-living older persons. J Gerontol A Biol Sci Med Sci. 1999;54(7):M377–83.

10. Naylor MD, Hirschman KB, Bowles KH, Bixby MB, Konick-McMahan J, Stephens C. Care coordination for cognitively impaired older adults and their caregivers. Home Health Care Serv Q. 2007;26(4):57–78.

11. Ahmed N, Mandel R, Fain MJ. Frailty: an emerging geriatric syndrome. Am J Med. 2007;120(9):748–53.

12. Walston J, Fried LP. Frailty and the older man. Med Clin North Am. 1999;83:1173–94.

13. Fried LP, Tangen CM, Walston J, et al. Frailty in older adults: evidence for a phenotype. J Gerontol. 2001;56A:M146–56.

14. Maslow K. How many people with dementia are hospitalized? In: Silverstein N, Maslow K, editors. Improving hospital care for persons with dementia. New York: Springer; 2006. p. 3–22.

15. Leslie DL, Marcantonio ER, Zhang Y, Leo-Summers L, Inouye SK. One-year health care costs associated with delirium in the elderly population. Arch Intern Med. 2008;168(1):27–32.

16. Inouye SK, Studenski S, Tinetti ME, Kuchel GA. Geriatric syndromes: clinical, research, and policy implications of a core geriatric concept. J Am Geriatr Soc. 2007;55(5):780–91.

17. Centers for Medicare & Medicaid Services. Medicare program: changes to the hospital inpatient prospective payment systems and fiscal year 2008 rates. Fed Regist. 2007;72(162):47129–8175.

18. Pronovost PJ, Goeschel CA, Wachter R. The wisdom and justice of not paying for "preventable complications". JAMA. 2008;299(18): 2197–9.

19. Wald HL, Kramer AM. Nonpayment for harms resulting from medical care: catheter-associated urinary tract infections. JAMA. 2007;298(23):2782–4.

20. Flood KL, Rohlfing A, Le CV, Carr DB, Rich MW. Geriatric syndromes in elderly patients admitted to an inpatient cardiology ward. J Hosp Med. 2007;2(6):394–400.

21. McCusker J, Kakuma R, Abrahamowicz M. Predictors of functional decline in hospitalized elderly patients: a systematic review. J Gerontol A Biol Sci Med Sci. 2002;57(9):M569–771.

22. Covinsky KE, Justice AC, Rosenthal GE, Palmer RM, Landefeld CS. Measuring prognosis and case mix in hospitalized elders. The importance of functional status. J Gen Intern Med. 1997;12:203–8.

23. Thomas DR. Focus on functional decline in hospitalized older adults. J Gerontol A Biol Sci Med Sci. 2002;57(9):M567–8.

24. Inouye SK, Wagner DR, Acampora D, Horwitz RI, Cooney LM, Tinetti ME. A controlled trial of a nursing-centered intervention in hospitalized elderly patients: The Yale Geriatric Care Program. J Am Geriatr Soc. 1993;41:1353–60.

25. Garza JJ, Gantt DS, Van Cleave H, Riggs MW, Dehmer GJ. Hospital disposition and long-term follow-up of patients aged >/=80 years undergoing coronary artery revascularization. Am J Cardiol. 2003;92(5):590–2.

26. Khan JH, McElhinney DB, Hall TS, Merrick SH. Cardiac valve surgery in octogenarians: improving quality of life and functional status. Arch Surg. 1998;133(8):887–93.

27. Sharony R, Grossi EA, Saunders PC, Schwartz CF, Ribakove GH, Culliford AT, et al. Minimally invasive aortic valve surgery in the elderly: a case-control study. Circulation. 2003;108 (Suppl 1): II43–7.

28. Mihaljevic T, Cohn LH, Unic D, Aranki SF, Couper GS, Byrne JG. One thousand minimally invasive valve operations: early and late results. Ann Surg. 2004;240(3):529–34.

29. Ursomanno P. Functional status in the elderly undergoing minimally invasive valve surgery. Unpublished doctoral dissertation, New York University, New York; 2006.

30. DiMattio MJ, Tulman L. A longitudinal study of functional status and correlates following coronary artery bypass graft surgery in women. Nurs Res. 2003;52(2):98–107.

31. King KB, Rowe MA, Kimbel LP, Zerwic JJ. Optimism, coping and long term recovery from coronary artery bypass surgery in women. Res Nurs Health. 1998;21:15–26.

32. Rubenstein LZ. Falls in older people: epidemiology, risk factors and strategies for prevention. Age Ageing. 2006;35 Suppl 2:ii37–41.

33. Rubenstein LZ, Josephson KR. The epidemiology of falls and syncope. Clin Geriatr Med. 2002;18(2):141–58.

34. Magaziner J, Hawkes W, Hebel JR, et al. Recovery from hip fracture in eight areas of function. J Gerontol A Biol Sci Med Sci. 2000;55(9):M498–507.

35. Sullivan DH, Bopp MM, Roberson PK. Protein-energy undernutrition and life-threatening complications among the hospitalized elderly. J Gen Intern Med. 2002;17(12):923–32.

36. Nutrition Screening Initiative. Nutrition State of Principle; 2002. http://www.hospitalmedicine.org/geriresource/toolbox/determine. htm. Accessed 2 Nov 2009.

37. Lyder CH. Pressure ulcer prevention and management. JAMA. 2003;289(2):223–6.

38. Whittington K, Patrick M, Roberts JL. A national study of pressure ulcer prevalence and incidence in acute care hospitals. J Wound Ostomy Continence Nurs. 2000;27(4):209–15.

39. Lyder CH, Preston J, Grady JN, et al. Quality of care for hospitalized medicare patients at risk for pressure ulcers. Arch Intern Med. 2001;161(12):1549–54.

40. Emori TG, Banerjee SN, Culver DH, et al. Nosocomial infections in elderly persons in the United States, 1986–1990· National Nosocomial Infections Surveillance System. Am J Med. 1991; 91(3B):289S–93.

41. Kunin CM. Urinary-catheter-associated infections in the elderly. Int J Antimicrob Agents. 2006;28 Suppl 1:S78–81.

42. Tambyah PA, Maki DG. Catheter-associated urinary tract infection is rarely symptomatic: a prospective study of 1,497 catheterized patients. Arch Intern Med. 2000;160:678–82.

43. Wald HL, Ma A, Bratzler DW, Kramer AM. Indwelling urinary catheter use in the postoperative period: analysis of the national surgical infection prevention project data. Arch Surg. 2008;143(6): 551–7.

44. Wald HL, Epstein AM, Radcliff TA, Kramer AM. Extended use of urinary catheters in older surgical patients: a patient safety problem? Infect Control Hosp Epidemiol. 2008;29(2):116–24.

45. Saint S, Lipsky B, Goold S. Urinary catheters: a one-point restraint? Ann Intern Med. 2002;137(2):125–7.

46. Dubois MJ, Bergeron N, Dumont M, Dial S, Skrobik Y. Delirium in an intensive care unit. A study of risk factors. Intensive Care Med. 2001;27:1297–304.

47. Silverstein JH, Timberger M, Reich DL, Uysal S. Central nervous system dysfunction after noncardiac surgery and anesthesia in the elderly. Anesthesiology. 2007;106(3):622–8.

48. Inouye SK. Prevention of delirium in hospitalized older patients: risk factors and targeted intervention strategies. Ann Med. 2000;32(4):257–63.

49. Inouye SK, Schlesinger MJ, Lydon TJ. Delirium: a symptom of how hospital care is failing older persons and a window to improve quality of hospital care. Am J Med. 1999;106(5):565–73.

50. Inouye SK, Foreman MD, Mion LC, Katz KH, Cooney Jr LM. Nurses' recognition of delirium and its symptoms: comparison of nurse and researcher ratings. Arch Intern Med. 2001;161(20):2467–73.

51. Inouye SK, Rushing JT, Foreman MD, Palmer RM, Pompei P. Does delirium contribute to poor hospital outcomes? A three-site epidemiologic study. J Gen Intern Med. 1998;13(4):234–42.

52. Arora VM, McGory ML, Fung CH. Quality indicators for hospitalization and surgery in vulnerable elders. J Am Geriatr Soc. 2007;55 Suppl 2:S347–58.

53. Somogyi-Zalud E, Zhong Z, Hamel MB, Lynn J. The use of life-sustaining treatments in hospitalized persons aged 80 and older. J Am Geriatr Soc. 2002;50(5):930–4.

54. Coleman EA, Min SJ, Chomiak A, Kramer AM. Posthospital care transitions: patterns, complications, and risk identification. Health Serv Res. 2004;39(5):1449–65.

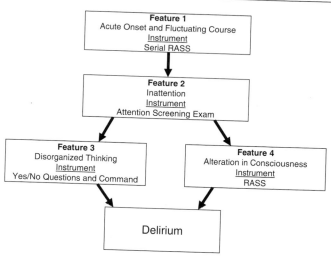

Fig. 5.1 Algorithm of the confusion assessment method. For delirium a patient needs feature 1 (acute onset and fluctuating course), feature 2 (inattention), AND either feature 3 (disorganized thinking) or feature 4 (altered level of consciousness). Below the features are the elements of the CAM-ICU, which can be used to assess the feature (adapted from [1, 9])

Table 5.1 Differentiating delirium and postoperative cognitive dysfunction

Feature	Delirium	POCD
Onset	Acute; early postoperative	Longer-term >3-months
Cognitive domain(s)	Attention	Attention
		Memory
		Executive function
		Visuospatial
Assessment	CAM-ICU; attention screen	Neuropsychological testing
Diagnosis	CAM; DSM-IV	Not defined
Causes	Unknown	Unknown
Morbidity	Decreased functional recovery	Decreased functional recovery
	Nursing home placement	
	Death	

CAM confusion assessment method; *CAM-ICU* confusion assessment method for the intensive care unit; *DSM-IV* diagnostic and statistical manual of mental disorders IV edition; *POCD* postoperative cognitive dysfunction

Because the CAM-ICU has been validated in nonverbal intensive care unit patients, its use in the postoperative cardiac surgery patient would be appropriate [93]. The advantages of the CAM-ICU are that it can be performed and scored in under 90 s by trained nurses or physicians; can be repeated over time to detect fluctuation and changes; and has been associated with ICU outcomes including mortality [10], length of stay [11], and cost [12]. The key elements of the CAM-ICU are the Richmond Agitation and Sedation Scale, a validated measure of consciousness [13], the Attention Screening Exam [14], and five thought questions. This information is used to complete the CAM algorithm for delirium.

Distinction Between Delirium and Postoperative Cognitive Dysfunction

Much work in cardiac surgery has been focused on the assessment of long-term postoperative cognitive dysfunction (POCD). Table 5.1 highlights the distinct features of each of these diagnoses. Delirium is more acute that POCD. First, according to the statement of consensus for neurobehavioral outcomes after cardiac surgery, POCD should be measured at least 3 months postoperatively [15]. Second, delirium is clinical diagnosis, which is to be made at the bedside, while POCD requires sensitive and lengthy neuropsychological tests. Finally, there may be overlap of prolonged delirium and POCD, because attention is required for optimal performance of both [16]. In a study of older, general surgery patients, delirium increased the risk of POCD at 7 days postoperatively, but not at 3 months postoperatively [17]. The causes of delirium have been better elucidated in delirium

[10, 18] than POCD. However, the pathophysiology of both the disorders is poorly understood.

Pathophysiology of Delirium After Cardiac Surgery

There are several potential pathophysiological causes for delirium after cardiac surgery but none has been proven to be causal. The model frequently used to measure and study factors associated with delirium includes a predisposed patient (predisposing factors) being subjected to a series of insults (precipitating factors), which precipitates the delirium [19]. This model is important in the understanding of the etiology of delirium, because baseline vulnerabilities increase the susceptibility to precipitating factors, but are not necessarily pathophysiological for delirium [20]. For example, impaired vision is a risk factor for delirium, but may not be associated with the precipitating factors in cardiac surgery (anesthesia, emboli, hypotension, inflammation, tryptophan release, etc.) [21]. Additionally, one specific insult may not precipitate delirium, but the cumulative effect of several small insults precipitates the delirium. In the older cardiac surgery patient, there can be significant variability in both the predisposing and precipitating factors.

Anticholinergic Burden

Within the CNS, cholinergic receptors play a neuromodulatory role in the processes of attention, reward and reinforcement, and memory [22]. Thus, blockade of the acetylcholine receptor (e.g., anticholinergic activity) can lead to deficits in these cognitive processes. An available assay, anticholinergic activity, measures the blockade of cholinergic receptors [23, 24]. Serum anticholinergic activity has been associated with delirium in the medical, surgical, and nursing home populations [24–26]. This anticholinergic activity is presumed to originate from medications, but some patients carry a high baseline anticholinergic activity level, which may predispose to delirium [21, 24, 27].

Within the operative care of cardiac surgery, many potential medications are delivered, which have anticholinergic activity. Most notably, paralytics used during general anesthesia act on the cholinergic mechanism of the neuromuscular junction resulting in a large anticholinergic load. Meperidine, an opioid analogue, is highly anticholinergic and may predispose to delirium [28]. Medications used for their sedative properties, such as diphenhydramine and amitriptyline, have anticholinergic activity and have been associated with delirium [29, 30]. Many antipsychotics have high anticholinergic activity and may also contribute to delirium [31]. There are several validated ranked summaries of anticholinergic medications for the ambulatory and hospitalized older patient [30–32].

Inflammation

Delirium develops in states of elevated systemic stress such as surgery, infection, trauma, and myocardial infarction. Circulating inflammatory markers are elevated during surgery [33], infection [34], trauma [35], and myocardial infarction [36]. The inflammatory response rises immediately after surgery, but then quickly returns to baseline. IL-6 level, an early pro-inflammatory cytokine, peaks 4–24 h after surgery and is near baseline by 48 h, [37]. IL-10, an anti-inflammatory cytokine, peaks 4–12 h postoperatively and is near baseline by 48 h, [38]. In response to the inflammatory response triggered by early cytokines, such as IL-6 and IL-10, other cytokines peak later in the postoperative course. Tumor necrosis factor-α (TNF-α) will peak 24–36 h postoperatively and return to baseline by about 72 h. C-reactive protein (CRP) is produced in response to IL-6 release, peaks at 24–48 h, will return to near normal levels by postoperative day 7 [37].

Prior work has found that cytokines and chemokines are associated with delirium after cardiac surgery. Several smaller studies have identified increased individual cytokines in patients with delirium, but consistent markers for delirium have not emerged [39, 40]. Additionally, major challenge to the inflammation hypothesis is that peripheral inflammatory cytokines may not represent the central nervous system process. Thus studies that measure brain inflammation via CSF or brain biopsy are needed.

Large Neutral Amino Acids

Serotonin is a key neurotransmitter involved in cognitive processes and serotonin deficiency has been associated with delirium. Tryptophan is a precursor to serotonin production and one of the large neutral amino acids, which all compete for a blood–brain barrier transporter. In catabolic states, the serum ratio of tryptophan to other large neutral amino acids, most notably phenylalanine, is reduced because of the relative frequency in muscle tissue [41]. As a result, less phenylalanine is transported to the central nervous system, and the brain may see a reduced serotonin production [21]. In small cross-sectional studies, the ratio of tryptophan to large neutral amino acids has been associated with delirium [42]. These studies are difficult due to rapidly fluctuating levels of amino acids, which are dependent on catabolism and diet.

Atherosclerosis and Blood–Brain Barrier Compromise

Atherosclerosis in the microvasculature (leukoariosis) of the brain is associated with blood–brain barrier compromise and deficits in attention [43, 44]. Because patients undergoing coronary artery bypass graft surgery have atherosclerosis, these patients are also likely to have increased leukoariosis, and thus, increased blood–brain barrier permeability [45]. This permeability would allow the entry of peripheral inflammatory cytokines, medications, and other circulating molecules into the brain parenchyma and may have impact on the cognitive functioning. Increasing atherosclerosis burden, as measured by aortic arch plaque, carotid stenosis, and the number of vessels bypassed, has been associated with delirium after surgery [46].

Preoperative Assessment for Delirium Risk

Although many preoperative risk factors for delirium have been described in the literature, using a validated delirium prediction rule for delirium after cardiac surgery can help identify those patients most at risk for delirium after cardiac surgery. The validated prediction rule for delirium after cardiac surgery identified four major risk factors: impaired cognitive function, low albumin, preoperative depression, and prior stroke or TIA [47]. Table 5.2 describes the point scoring system for the prediction rule. The incidence of delirium increases with increasing points so that the highest risk group is 4 times more likely to develop delirium than the lowest risk group. To complete the prediction rule, a thorough history and physical combined with cognition and depression screening is required.

Table 5.2 Preoperative prediction rule for delirium after cardiac surgery

Characteristic	Points	Total points	Incidence of postoperative delirium (%)
Cognitive impairment		0	18–19
Severe	2	1	43–47
Mild	1	2	60–63
Depression	1	≥3	86–87
Prior stroke/TIA	1		
Low albumin	1		

Assessment of Preoperative Cognitive Function

Atherosclerosis, a requirement for coronary artery bypass grafting surgery, is not confined to the arteries of the heart and may occur in the extremities, kidneys, neck, and brain. Recent work had found that atherosclerosis in the brain may affect higher order cognitive processes called executive functions [43, 48, 49], which is responsible for attention, insight, abstraction, and planning. Executive function deficit, more so than memory deficit, has been associated with delirium after cardiac surgery [50]. As a result, many patients going to cardiac surgery are cognitively impaired preoperatively [51, 52]. As in most studies of delirium [53], including the prediction rule above, cognitive impairment is the strongest risk factor for delirium. Thus, many have called for preoperative cognitive screening in all cardiac surgery patients, to identify preoperative cognitive deficits [54]. The specific assessment of cognitive function varies widely amongst the studies [55]. Although most studies use the Mini Mental State Examination as a general measure of cognitive function [56], there is a lack of executive function task that may make other assessments more appropriate [57].

Assessment of Depression

In addition to the prediction rule, other studies have identified depression as a risk factor for delirium after cardiac surgery [58]. Although the pathophysiology of this relationship remains to be determined, it is known that depression can interfere in the process of clinical care, because patients are less motivated to complete the needed rehabilitation and may be less likely to resume independent functioning after cardiac surgery. The assessment of depression in older patients is generally performed with the 15 question Geriatric Depression Scale, which assesses depressive symptoms using 15 yes/no questions [59]. The advantage of the GDS is that it can be self-completed by the older patient and scored by the clinician in a short time frame (3 min).

Albumin

Serum albumin is considered as an overall biomarker of function, frailty, and nutrition [60, 61]. In a patient with low albumin, there may be synthesis (liver function), excretion (renal disease), or function (malnutrition, poor social support, poor dietary habits, etc.) deficit. In any of these conditions, the patient undergoing cardiac surgery will require additional thought and planning during the course of the operation and recovery. For example, albumin plays an important role in intravascular volume status and drug binding and thus, intraoperative fluids and medications may need dosage adjustments and monitoring. After the surgery, careful assessment of nutrition intake and education about dietary choices may be needed [62].

Age-Associated Risk Factors Associated with Delirium

Age itself is generally not considered a risk factor for delirium, but many conditions that are associated with age may also be risk factors for delirium. For example, patients with preoperative sensory impairments are more likely to develop delirium [18]. Because older patients are more likely to have decreased hearing abilities (presbycusis), smell (presbyosmia), and vision abilities (presbyopia), they have more difficulty getting sensory inputs into the brain, especially when adaptive aids (glasses, hearing aids, dentures, etc.) are withheld, as is common in the perioperative period. Additionally, age-associated comorbidities may predispose a patient to develop delirium. For example, stroke and transient ischemic attack have increased prevalence with age and was found to be an independent risk factor for delirium [47]. Table 5.3 highlights other predisposing factors, which may be associated with delirium in the cardiac surgery population, but have not been independently validated.

Precipitating Factors for Delirium

Studies of cardiac surgery have inherent variability because of patient factors (age, education, comorbidity), cardiac surgery factors (hypothermia, cardiopulmonary bypass, cross clamp, bleeding), physiologic factors (inflammation, microembolization, blood–brain barrier function), intraoperative factors (anesthesia, cerebral oxygenation, hypotension), perioperative factors (medication, sleep, complications), and postoperative factors (rehabilitation, depression, social supports). Thus, all of the precipitating factors for postoperative delirium have not been fully elucidated. Table 5.3

Table 5.3 Predisposing and precipitating factors associated with delirium after surgery

Predisposing factors	Precipitating factors	
Preoperative	Intraoperative	Postoperative factors
Demographics	*Complexity of operation*	*Early complications of operation*
Increasing age	Operation time	Low hematocrit
Male gender	Cardiopulmonary bypass time	Cardiogenic shock
Comorbidities	Prolonged intubation	Hypoxemia
Impaired cognition	Valve surgery (±CABG)	Prolonged intubation
Dementia	Decreased cardiac output	
Mild cognitive impairment	Shock/hypotension	*Later complications of operation*
Preoperative memory complaint	Unable to wean	Low albumin
Atherosclerosis	*Operative factors*	Abnormal electrolytes
Intracranial stenosis	Low intraoperative temperature	Iatrogenic complications
Carotid stenosis	Benzodiazepine administration	Infection
Peripheral vascular disease	Propofol administration	Liver failure
Prior stroke/TIA	Hemofiltration	Renal failure
Diabetes	Blood transfusion	Sleep-wake disturbance
Hypertension	Microemboli	
Atrial fibrillation		
Psychiatric disease		
Anxiety		
Depression		
Benzodiazepine use		
Function		
Low albumin		
Impaired functional status		
Sensory impairment		
Severe illness		
Preoperative IABP		
Pain		
Electrolyte abnormalities		
Lifestyle factors		
Alcohol		
Sleep deprivation		
Smoking		

highlights preoperative, intraoperative, and postoperative factors, which may be associated with delirium.

Microemboli

Microemboli are felt to be air, organic debris (disrupted atherosclerotic plaque), or thrombus that travels to the brain and cause punctuate ischemia and ultimately cognitive impairment [63]. Although there has been much speculation about "pump-head," an acute change in cognitive function, which is thought to be related to microemboli, a systematic review of microemboli and cognitive function found that most studies did not demonstrate a significant relationship [64]. Additionally, studies of cognitive function with and without cardiopulmonary bypass have not been able to demonstrate a difference in cognitive function, despite several studies demonstrating that cardiopulmonary bypass does generate more microemboli [65, 66]. Logically, efforts

to reduce the number of microemboli should continue, but the assumption of a causative relationship has not been established [67].

Intraoperative Medication

During cardiac surgery, numerous medications with cognitive properties are given to patients. Inhaled anesthetics slow and flatten electrical activity in the brain and have been associated with amyloid deposition and apoptosis [68]. Induction agents, benzodiazepines, and paralytics have significant cognitive properties, which may precipitate delirium [28]. Pain medications may precipitate delirium. Additionally, ionotropic agents such as dopamine and norepinepherine deliver supra-physiologic doses of neurotransmitters, which may travel centrally. Although these are needed for the operation, recognizing the risk and taking preoperative function, albumin, and cognition into account is necessary.

Postoperative Medication

Following cardiac surgery, many patients are given medications, which can impair their cognitive function. For example, in the postoperative intubated patient, sedatives such as benzodiazepines or propofol are given. In these patients, dexmedetomidine used for sedation may cause delirium less frequently [69]. Although pain medication is a requirement following sternotomy, protocols for standing pain medication should be used to treat pain and taper opioid doses. Strong consideration should be given to standing pain medication, especially acetaminophen, which has been shown to lower the opioid load and improve patient reports of pain in a postoperative randomized controlled trial [70]. The advantage of acetaminophen is the limited cognitive properties, compared with opioids. Improved sleep hygiene by nonpharmacological measures such as decreasing environmental noise, creating a relaxing environment, and preserving the circadian rhythm have been shown to improve sleep without medication in older hospitalized patients [71].

Metabolic Abnormalities

The older brain is more susceptible to fluid shifts and electrolyte imbalances compared with the younger brain, and one manifestation of this may be delirium. Because of the intraoperative fluid load, third-spacing, and the associated electrolyte shifts, the brain of older patients may react adversely to these changes. In past work, electrolyte abnormalities (e.g., hyperkalemia, hyponatremia, hypernatremia, hypoglycemia, hyperglycemia) and markers of dehydration (BUN/Cr > 18) were found to be a strong risk factors for delirium after surgery [19, 72, 73]. Additionally, renal function declines 1% per year in older patients, and this effect may be more pronounced in patients with atherosclerosis. Thus, the ability to regulate electrolytes rapidly may be diminished in older patients undergoing cardiac surgery.

Postoperative Environment

After cardiac surgery, patients are transferred to the ICU environment, which is busy, noisy, and light-filled, where patients are approached, assessed, and stimulated constantly. Recent work in the ICU setting found that the environment may contribute to delirium, through sleep deprivation and overstimulation [74]. Although this environment is required in the immediate postoperative period, transfer of medically stable patients to less intense wards should be considered, including those with delirium.

Iatrogenic Events

Complications of hospitalization and surgery can precipitate delirium. For example, a leading identifiable cause of delirium in older inpatients is urinary tract infection associated with catheter use [19]. Preventable medical processes such as deep venous thrombosis, UTI, pressure ulcer, deconditioning, malnutrition, and dehydration should be assessed using a team approach when necessary [62]. Additionally, reduced mobility through formal restraints or informal tethers (i.e., intravenous lines, oxygen tubing, urinary catheters, etc.) can contribute to delirium, loss of function, falls, and increased rehabilitation placement [18].

Prevention of Delirium

Two multi-component studies have demonstrated that delirium can be prevented in operative and medical patients [62, 71]. Both of these studies target moderate and high risk patients, and use modules to improve baseline vulnerabilities. The modules are compared in Table 5.4. Both approaches use, low-tech interventions to prevent delirium. For example, the nonpharmacological sleep protocols involved environmental changes conducive to sleep (i.e., lights off, create a

Table 5.4 Comparison of prevention strategies for delirium

Prevention module	Hip fracture	Medical patients
Cognitive stimulation	Appropriate environmental stimuli protocol	Cognitive stimulation protocol
Improve sensory input	Appropriate environmental stimuli protocol	Vision protocol
		Hearing protocol
Mobilization	Mobilization and rehabilitation protocol	Mobilization protocol
Avoidance of psychoactive medication	Elimination of unnecessary medications protocol	Nonpharmacological sleep protocol
	Pain management protocol	
Fluid and nutrition	Fluid/electrolyte protocol	Rehydration protocol
	Adequate nutrition protocol	
Avoidance of hospital complications	Bowel and bladder protocol	
	Adequate CNS O_2 delivery protocol	
	Postoperative complication monitoring protocol	

relaxing environment, minimizing nighttime interruptions, dedicated time for sleep, etc.), which were successful in reducing psychoactive medication use and, ultimately, delirium. Other key modules include improving sensory input, nutrition, ambulation, and preventing complications.

Haloperidol is a high-potency dopamine antagonist (antipsychotic) medication. In a single site study, prophylactic administration of haloperidol was associated with reduced risk of delirium after hip fracture [75]. A follow-up study comparing high potency antipsychotic, atypical antipsychotic, and placebo in intensive care unit patients found no difference in the rate of delirium. As a result, the practice of prophylaxis with antipsychotics should be avoided at present because of the increased risk of death, delirium, and complications in older patients attributed to antipsychotics [76].

Several recent studies have found that the use of dexmedetomidine for sedation in the ICU setting has a reduced rate of delirium compared with midazolam and lorazepam [77, 78]. Additionally, a randomized trial of intraoperative sedation with dexmedetomidine, propofol, or midazolam found that dexmetometadine was associated with a lower incidence of postoperative delirium [69].

Treatment of Delirium

The treatment of delirium is to identify and treat the underlying causes for delirium. Thus, the clinician is recommended to begin with a broad differential diagnosis and systematically eliminate potential causes. See Table 5.5 for a differential diagnosis of causes of delirium after cardiac surgery. It should be noted that delirium is associated with significant morbidity and mortality, and thus all patients with delirium should be assessed promptly with an interim history, thorough physical exam with a focus on the neurological exam, and necessary laboratory testing.

Cerebral Imaging

Prior work has found that in the absence of focal neurological deficits, a CT has low diagnostic value [79]. MRI scanning in the postcardiac surgery patient is difficulty, because of the acuity of illness, recently implanted hardware (e.g., valves, cardiac stents, grafts, sternal wires, etc.), and the time and cooperation required for scanning. In the patient with delirium, sedation, which can worsen or prolong the delirium, may be needed for imaging [80]. In the patient after cardiac surgery, there will likely be new foci on imaging related to microemboli during the operation [81]. As above the causal link between microemboli and delirium has not been established [64]. Additionally, stroke thrombolysis is

Table 5.5 Differential diagnosis of delirium

Cause	Precipitating factors
Drugs	Anticholinergic
	Antihistamines
	Benzodiazepines
	Centrally acting cardiac medications
	Tricyclic antidepressants
Electrolyte abnormalities	Hypoglycemia
	Hyperglycemia
	Hyponatremia
	Hypernatremia
	Hypocalcemia
Lack of drugs	Pain
	Alcohol withdrawal
	Withdrawal from chronic medications
	Gabapentin
	Antidepressants
	Benzodiazepines
Infection	Urinary tract infection (catheter associated)
	Aspiration pneumonia
	Pressure ulcer
	Line infection
	Wound infection
Reduced sensory input	Restraints
	ICU environment
	Hearing loss
	Vision loss
	Bed rest
Intraoperative	Hypotension
	Embolization
	Delayed effects of anesthesia
	Medications
Urinary retention ± fecal impaction	Medications
	Benign prostatic hypertrophy
Myocardial	Postoperative myocardial infarction
	Pulmonary embolism
	Congestive heart failure
	Graft failure

absolutely contraindicated in the postoperative cardiac surgery patient due to major surgery [82]. Finally, the treatment of infarct in the postoperative patients is identical to the treatment of cardiac disease (e.g., aspirin, statin, blood pressure control, cardiac risk reduction, rehabilitation).

Remove or Minimize Cognitively Active Medications

In the course of perioperative care, many medications with substantial cognitive effects are administered. For example, pain medication or benzodiazepines can precipitate delirium [80, 83]. Paralysis, a component of general anesthesia, is a high anticholinergic load and the inhaled anesthetics precipitate reversible coma or a reduction in brain function. Ionotropic agents infuse supra-physiological doses of neurotransmitters, the cognitive effects of which are not entirely understood. Although all of these treatments are necessary in the context of the operation, they may have variable cognitive properties spanning from delayed recovery to long-term POCD. The important process in the treatment of delirium is to (1) eliminate unnecessary medications, (2) minimize the exposure to that which is necessary for treatment, and (3) to provide supportive care in the postoperative setting for those patients with delirium.

Pain Control

Although opioids may precipitate delirium, uncontrolled pain may also precipitate delirium [84]. As a result, pain should be treated on an individual basis. A previous randomized controlled trial found that standing of acetaminophen reduced opioid load and improved patient reports of pain in operative patients [70]. Preoperative assessment of prior opioid exposure and pain tolerance are important for management of postoperative pain. Patients with opioid tolerance may require additional pain medication postoperatively. Especially in the early postoperative period, the standing treatment of pain is important.

Management of Agitation Associated with Delirium

For patients who develop agitation, a thorough review of the medications and physical exam, including pain assessment is required. If possible to relieve the offending symptom, then this should be attempted (constipation, urinary retention, etc.). If the cause of agitation is not immediately available, nonpharmacologic treatments should be initiated first. For example, elimination of environmental noise, allowing the patient to sleep at night, and reorientation efforts should be attempted. A model of care for the delirious patient found that environmental modifications and staff training could produce reductions in patient agitation, reduction in use of psychoactive medications, with similar length of stay [85]. Another useful resource is the family, which can serve as a reorienting and reassuring stimulus.

Antipsychotics are considered the first line for the management of agitation associated with delirium [30, 76]. Haloperidol at a dosage of 0.5–1.0 mg should be able to achieve effect. If there is no response within 1 h, a repeat dosage may be considered. If there is no effect after 2–3 mg of haloperidol, it is unlikely that the patient is going to respond. Antipsychotics administered in the acute setting have not been demonstrated to have increased mortality, but short term

(6–12 weeks) use of antipsychotics are considered to carry an increased mortality, especially in cognitively impaired patients [86, 87]. Additionally, monitoring electrocardiograms should occur in patients on antipsychotics for more than 1 day due the compromised cardiac condition necessitating surgery and the risk QTc prolongation associated with antipsychotic use age. Finally, early evidence suggests that acute administration of antipsychotics may be associated with oropharyngeal dysphagia, which may further delay the recovery [88].

For patients with contraindications to antipsychotics such as Parkinson's disease, Lewy Body dementia, prior seizures, and prior neuroleptic malignant syndrome, agitation may be better managed with benzodiazepines. In general, benzodiazepines disinhibit patients and patients should be monitored for a paradoxical reaction, where administration of the benzodiazepine results in agitation. Additionally, prior work has shown that benzodiazepines may actually prolong or worsen the course of delirium [80].

References

1. Inouye SK, van Dyck CH, Alessi CA, Balkin S, Siegal AP, Horwitz RI. Clarifying confusion: the confusion assessment method. A new method for detection of delirium. Ann Intern Med. 1990;113(12): 941–8.
2. Wei LA, Fearing MA, Sternberg EJ, Inouye SK. The Confusion Assessment Method: a systematic review of current usage. J Am Geriatr Soc. 2008;56(5):823–30.
3. O'Keeffe ST, Gosney MA. Assessing attentiveness in older hospital patients: global assessment versus tests of attention. J Am Geriatr Soc. 1997;45(4):470–3.
4. Stavros KA, Rudolph JL, Jones RN, Marcantonio ER. Delirium and the clinical assessment of attention in older adults. J Am Geriatr Soc. 2008;56(S1):S199–200.
5. Liptzin B, Levkoff SE. An empirical study of delirium subtypes. Br J Psychiatry. 1992;161:843–5.
6. Inouye SK, Foreman MD, Mion LC, Katz KH, Cooney Jr LM. Nurses' recognition of delirium and its symptoms: comparison of nurse and researcher ratings. Arch Intern Med. 2001;161(20): 2467–73.
7. Levkoff SE, Evans DA, Liptzin B, Cleary PD, Lipsitz LA, Wetle TT, et al. Delirium – the occurrence and persistence of symptoms among elderly hospitalized-patients. Arch Intern Med. 1992;152(2):334–40.
8. Kiely DK, Jones RN, Bergmann MA, Marcantonio ER. Association between psychomotor activity delirium subtypes and mortality among newly admitted post-acute facility patients. J Gerontol A Biol Sci Med Sci. 2007;62(2):174–9.
9. Ely EW, Margolin R, Francis J, May L, Truman B, Dittus R, et al. Evaluation of delirium in critically ill patients: validation of the Confusion Assessment Method for the Intensive Care Unit (CAM-ICU). Crit Care Med. 2001;29(7):1370–9.
10. Pun BT, Ely EW. The importance of diagnosing and managing ICU delirium. Chest. 2007;132(2):624–36.
11. Ely EW, Gautam S, Margolin R, Francis J, May L, Speroff T, et al. The impact of delirium in the intensive care unit on hospital length of stay. Intensive Care Med. 2001;27(12):1892–900.
12. Milbrandt EB, Deppen S, Harrison PL, Shintani AK, Speroff T, Stiles RA, et al. Costs associated with delirium in mechanically ventilated patients. Crit Care Med. 2004;32(4):955–62.

13. Ely EW, Truman B, Shintani A, Thomason JW, Wheeler AP, Gordon S, et al. Monitoring sedation status over time in ICU patients: reliability and validity of the Richmond Agitation-Sedation Scale (RASS). Jama. 2003;289(22):2983–91.

14. Hart RP, Levenson JL, Sessler CN, Best AM, Schwartz SM, Rutherford LE. Validation of a cognitive test for delirium in medical ICU patients. Psychosomatics. 1996;37(6):533–46.

15. Murkin JM, Newman SP, Stump DA, Blumenthal JA. Statement of consensus on assessment of neurobehavioral outcomes after cardiac surgery. Ann Thorac Surg. 1995;59(5):1289–95.

16. Jackson JC, Gordon SM, Hart RP, Hopkins RO, Ely EW. The association between delirium and cognitive decline: a review of the empirical literature. Neuropsychol Rev. 2004;14(2):87–98.

17. Rudolph JL, Marcantonio ER, Culley DJ, Silverstein JH, Rasmussen LS, Crosby GJ, et al. Delirium is associated with early postoperative cognitive dysfunction. Anaesthesia. 2008;63(9):941–7.

18. Inouye SK. Delirium in older persons. N Engl J Med. 2006;354(11): 1157–65.

19. Inouye SK, Charpentier PA. Precipitating factors for delirium in hospitalized elderly persons. Predictive model and interrelationship with baseline vulnerability. JAMA. 1996;275(11):852–7.

20. Inouye SK, Ferrucci L. Elucidating the pathophysiology of delirium and the interrelationship of delirium and dementia. J Gerontol A Biol Sci Med Sci. 2006;61(12):1277–80.

21. Marcantonio ER, Rudolph JL, Culley D, Crosby G, Alsop D, Inouye SK. Serum biomarkers for delirium. J Gerontol A Biol Sci Med Sci. 2006;61(12):1281–6.

22. Hshieh TT, Fong TG, Marcantonio ER, Inouye SK. Cholinergic deficiency hypothesis in delirium: a synthesis of current evidence. J Gerontol A Biol Sci Med Sci. 2008;63(7):764–72.

23. Tune LE, Damlouji NF, Holland A, Gardner TJ, Folstein MF, Coyle JT. Association of postoperative delirium with raised serum levels of anticholinergic drugs. Lancet. 1981;2(8248):651–3.

24. Tune LE. Serum anticholinergic activity levels and delirium in the elderly. Semin Clin Neuropsychiatry. 2000;5(2):149–53.

25. Flacker JM, Cummings V, Mach Jr JR, Bettin K, Kiely DK, Wei J. The association of serum anticholinergic activity with delirium in elderly medical patients. Am J Geriatr Psychiatry. 1998;6(1):31–41.

26. Golinger RC, Peet T, Tune LE. Association of elevated plasma anticholinergic activity with delirium in surgical patients. Am J Psychiatry. 1987;144(9):1218–20.

27. Carnahan RM, Lund BC, Perry PJ, Pollock BG. A critical appraisal of the utility of the serum anticholinergic activity assay in research and clinical practice. Psychopharmacol Bull. 2002;36(2):24–39.

28. Marcantonio ER, Juarez G, Goldman L, Mangione CM, Ludwig LE, Lind L, et al. The relationship of postoperative delirium with psychoactive medications. JAMA. 1994;272(19):1518–22.

29. Agostini JV, Leo-Summers LS, Inouye SK. Cognitive and other adverse effects of diphenhydramine use in hospitalized older patients. Arch Intern Med. 2001;161(17):2091–7.

30. Campbell N, Boustani MA, Ayub A, Fox GC, Munger SL, Ott C, et al. Pharmacological management of delirium in hospitalized adults – a systematic evidence review. J Gen Intern Med. 2009;24(7):848–53.

31. Rudolph JL, Salow MJ, Angelini MC, McGlinchey RE. The anticholinergic risk scale and anticholinergic adverse effects in older persons. Arch Intern Med. 2008;168(5):508–13.

32. Carnahan RM, Lund BC, Perry PJ, Pollock BG, Culp KR. The Anticholinergic Drug Scale as a measure of drug-related anticholinergic burden: associations with serum anticholinergic activity. J Clin Pharmacol. 2006;46(12):1481–6.

33. Holmes JH, Connolly NC, Paull DL, Hill ME, Guyton SW, Ziegler SF, et al. Magnitude of the inflammatory response to cardiopulmonary bypass and its relation to adverse clinical outcomes. Inflamm Res. 2002;51(12):579–86.

34. Slotman GJ. Prospectively validated predictions of shock and organ failure in individual septic surgical patients: the Systemic Mediator Associated Response Test. Crit Care. 2000;4(5):319–26.

35. Perl M, Gebhard F, Knoferl MW, Bachem M, Gross HJ, Kinzl L, et al. The pattern of preformed cytokines in tissues frequently affected by blunt trauma. Shock. 2003;19(4):299–304.

36. Gabriel AS, Martinsson A, Wretlind B, Ahnve S. IL-6 levels in acute and post myocardial infarction: their relation to CRP levels, infarction size, left ventricular systolic function, and heart failure. Eur J Intern Med. 2004;15(8):523–8.

37. Biglioli P, Cannata A, Alamanni F, Naliato M, Porqueddu M, Zanobini M, et al. Biological effects of off-pump vs. on-pump coronary artery surgery: focus on inflammation, hemostasis and oxidative stress. Eur J Cardiothorac Surg. 2003;24(2):260–9.

38. Mahdy AM, Galley HF, Abdel-Wahed MA, el-Korny KF, Sheta SA, Webster NR. Differential modulation of interleukin-6 and interleukin-10 by diclofenac in patients undergoing major surgery. Br J Anaesth. 2002;88(6):797–802.

39. Rudolph JL, Ramlawi B, Kuchel GA, McElhaney JE, Xie D, Sellke FW, et al. Chemokines are associated with delirium after cardiac surgery. J Gerontol A Biol Sci Med Sci. 2008;63(2):184–9.

40. Kudoh A, Takase H, Katagai H, Takazawa T. Postoperative interleukin-6 and cortisol concentrations in elderly patients with postoperative confusion. Neuroimmunomodulation. 2005;12(1):60–6.

41. van der Mast RC, Fekkes D, Moleman P, Pepplinkhuizen L. Is postoperative delirium related to reduced plasma tryptophan? Lancet. 1991;338(8771):851–2.

42. Flacker JM, Lipsitz LA. Large neutral amino acid changes and delirium in febrile elderly medical patients. J Gerontol A Biol Sci Med Sci. 2000;55(5):B249–52; discussion B53–4.

43. O'Sullivan M, Morris RG, Huckstep B, Jones DK, Williams SC, Markus HS. Diffusion tensor MRI correlates with executive dysfunction in patients with ischaemic leukoaraiosis. J Neurol Neurosurg Psychiatry. 2004;75(3):441–7.

44. Hanyu H, Asano T, Tanaka Y, Iwamoto T, Takasaki M, Abe K. Increased blood-brain barrier permeability in white matter lesions of Binswanger's disease evaluated by contrast-enhanced MRI. Dement Geriatr Cogn Disord. 2002;14(1):1–6.

45. Breteler MM, van Swieten JC, Bots ML, Grobbee DE, Claus JJ, van den Hout JH, et al. Cerebral white matter lesions, vascular risk factors, and cognitive function in a population-based study: the Rotterdam Study. Neurology. 1994;44(7):1246–52.

46. Rudolph JL, Babikian VL, Birjiniuk V, Crittenden MD, Treanor PR, Pochay VE, et al. Atherosclerosis is associated with delirium after coronary artery bypass graft surgery. J Am Geriatr Soc. 2005;53(3):462–6.

47. Rudolph JL, Jones RN, Levkoff SE, Rockett C, Inouye SK, Sellke FW, et al. Derivation and validation of a preoperative prediction rule for delirium after cardiac surgery. Circulation. 2009;119(2):229–36.

48. Breteler MM, van Amerongen NM, van Swieten JC, Claus JJ, Grobbee DE, van Gijn J, et al. Cognitive correlates of ventricular enlargement and cerebral white matter lesions on magnetic resonance imaging. The Rotterdam Study. Stroke. 1994;25(6): 1109–15.

49. Tuch DS, Salat DH, Wisco JJ, Zaleta AK, Hevelone ND, Rosas HD. Choice reaction time performance correlates with diffusion anisotropy in white matter pathways supporting visuospatial attention. Proc Natl Acad Sci USA. 2005;102(34):12212–7.

50. Rudolph JL, Jones RN, Grande LJ, Milberg WP, King EG, Lipsitz LA, et al. Impaired executive function is associated with delirium after coronary artery bypass graft surgery. J Am Geriatr Soc. 2006;54(6):937–41.

51. Rankin KP, Kochamba GS, Boone KB, Petitti DB, Buckwalter JG. Presurgical cognitive deficits in patients receiving coronary artery bypass graft surgery. J Int Neuropsychol Soc. 2003;9(6):913–24.

52. Vingerhoets G, Van Nooten G, Jannes C. Neuropsychological impairment in candidates for cardiac surgery. J Int Neuropsychol Soc. 1997;3(5):480–4.

53. Fick DM, Agostini JV, Inouye SK. Delirium superimposed on dementia: a systematic review. J Am Geriatr Soc. 2002;50(10):1723–32.

54. Selnes OA, Zeger SL. Coronary artery bypass grafting baseline cognitive assessment: essential not optional. Ann Thorac Surg. 2007;83(2):374–6.

55. Newman S, Stygall J, Hirani S, Shaefi S, Maze M. Postoperative cognitive dysfunction after noncardiac surgery: a systematic review. Anesthesiology. 2007;106(3):572–90.

56. Folstein MF, Folstein SE, McHugh PR. Mini-mental state. A practical method for grading the cognitive state of patients for the clinician. J Psychiatr Res. 1975;12(3):189–98.

57. Stuss DT, Levine B. Adult clinical neuropsychology: lessons from studies of the frontal lobes. Annu Rev Psychol. 2002;53:401–33.

58. Kazmierski J, Kowman M, Banach M, Pawelczyk T, Okonski P, Iwaszkiewicz A, et al. Preoperative predictors of delirium after cardiac surgery: a preliminary study. Gen Hosp Psychiatry. 2006;28(6):536–8.

59. Yesavage JA, Brink TL, Rose TL, Lum O, Huang V, Adey M, et al. Development and validation of a geriatric depression screening scale: a preliminary report. J Psychiatr Res. 1982;17(1):37–49.

60. Schalk BW, Visser M, Deeg DJ, Bouter LM. Lower levels of serum albumin and total cholesterol and future decline in functional performance in older persons: the Longitudinal Aging Study Amsterdam. Age Ageing. 2004;33(3):266–72.

61. Sullivan DH, Sun S, Walls RC. Protein-energy undernutrition among elderly hospitalized patients: a prospective study. JAMA. 1999;281(21):2013–9.

62. Marcantonio ER, Flacker JM, Wright RJ, Resnick NM. Reducing delirium after hip fracture: a randomized trial. J Am Geriatr Soc. 2001;49(5):516–22.

63. Blauth CI. Macroemboli and microemboli during cardiopulmonary bypass. Ann Thorac Surg. 1995;59(5):1300–3.

64. Martin KK, Wigginton JB, Babikian VL, Pochay VE, Crittenden MD, Rudolph JL. Intraoperative cerebral high-intensity transient signals and postoperative cognitive function: a systematic review. Am J Surg. 2009;197(1):55–63.

65. Motallebzadeh R, Bland JM, Markus HS, Kaski JC, Jahangiri M. Neurocognitive function and cerebral emboli: randomized study of on-pump versus off-pump coronary artery bypass surgery. Ann Thorac Surg. 2007;83(2):475–82.

66. van Dijk D, Jansen EW, Hijman R, Nierich AP, Diephuis JC, Moons KG, et al. Cognitive outcome after off-pump and on-pump coronary artery bypass graft surgery: a randomized trial. JAMA. 2002;287(11):1405–12.

67. Rudolph JL, Martin KK, Pochay VE, Crittenden MD. Exploring variability in the causal link of HITS and cognitive decline. Am J Surg. 2009;198(2):294–5.

68. Xie Z, Dong Y, Maeda U, Moir R, Inouye SK, Culley DJ, et al. Isoflurane-induced apoptosis: a potential pathogenic link between delirium and dementia. J Gerontol A Biol Sci Med Sci. 2006;61(12):1300–6.

69. Maldonado JR, Wysong A, van der Starre PJ, Block T, Miller C, Reitz BA. Dexmedetomidine and the reduction of postoperative delirium after cardiac surgery. Psychosomatics. 2009;50(3):206–17.

70. Schug SA, Sidebotham DA, McGuinnety M, Thomas J, Fox L. Acetaminophen as an adjunct to morphine by patient-controlled analgesia in the management of acute postoperative pain. Anesth Analg. 1998;87(2):368–72.

71. Inouye SK, Bogardus Jr ST, Charpentier PA, Leo-Summers L, Acampora D, Holford TR, et al. A multicomponent intervention to prevent delirium in hospitalized older patients. N Engl J Med. 1999;340(9):669–76.

72. Koster S, Oosterveld FG, Hensens AG, Wijma A, van der Palen J. Delirium after cardiac surgery and predictive validity of a risk checklist. Ann Thorac Surg. 2008;86(6):1883–7.

73. Giltay EJ, Huijskes RV, Kho KH, Blansjaar BA, Rosseel PM. Psychotic symptoms in patients undergoing coronary artery bypass grafting and heart valve operation. Eur J Cardiothorac Surg. 2006;30(1):140–7.

74. Osse RJ, Tulen JH, Bogers AJ, Hengeveld MW. Disturbed circadian motor activity patterns in postcardiotomy delirium. Psychiatry Clin Neurosci. 2009;63(1):56–64.

75. Kalisvaart KJ, de Jonghe JF, Bogaards MJ, Vreeswijk R, Egberts TC, Burger BJ, et al. Haloperidol prophylaxis for elderly hip-surgery patients at risk for delirium: a randomized placebo-controlled study. J Am Geriatr Soc. 2005;53(10):1658–66.

76. Lonergan E, Britton AM, Luxenberg J, Wyller T. Antipsychotics for delirium. Cochrane Database Syst Rev. 2007;(2):CD005594.

77. Pandharipande PP, Pun BT, Herr DL, Maze M, Girard TD, Miller RR, et al. Effect of sedation with dexmedetomidine vs lorazepam on acute brain dysfunction in mechanically ventilated patients: the MENDS randomized controlled trial. JAMA. 2007;298(22):2644–53.

78. Riker RR, Shehabi Y, Bokesch PM, Ceraso D, Wisemandle W, Koura F, et al. Dexmedetomidine vs midazolam for sedation of critically ill patients: a randomized trial. JAMA. 2009;301(5):489–99.

79. Alsop DC, Fearing MA, Johnson K, Sperling R, Fong TG, Inouye SK. The role of neuroimaging in elucidating delirium pathophysiology. J Gerontol A Biol Sci Med Sci. 2006;61(12):1287–93.

80. Breitbart W, Marotta R, Platt MM, Weisman H, Derevenco M, Grau C, et al. A double-blind trial of haloperidol, chlorpromazine, and lorazepam in the treatment of delirium in hospitalized AIDS patients. Am J Psychiatry. 1996;153(2):231–7.

81. Abu-Omar Y, Cader S, Guerrieri Wolf L, Pigott D, Matthews PM, Taggart DP. Short-term changes in cerebral activity in on-pump and off-pump cardiac surgery defined by functional magnetic resonance imaging and their relationship to microembolization. J Thorac Cardiovasc Surg. 2006;132(5):1119–25.

82. Adams Jr HP, Adams RJ, Brott T, del Zoppo GJ, Furlan A, Goldstein LB, et al. Guidelines for the early management of patients with ischemic stroke: a scientific statement from the Stroke Council of the American Stroke Association. Stroke. 2003;34(4):1056–83.

83. Leung JM, Sands LP, Vaurio LE, Wang Y. Nitrous oxide does not change the incidence of postoperative delirium or cognitive decline in elderly surgical patients. Br J Anaesth. 2006;96(6):754–60.

84. Marcantonio ER, Goldman L, Orav EJ, Cook EF, Lee TH. The association of intraoperative factors with the development of postoperative delirium. Am J Med. 1998;105(5):380–4.

85. Flaherty JH, Tariq SH, Raghavan S, Bakshi S, Moinuddin A, Morley JE. A model for managing delirious older inpatients. J Am Geriatr Soc. 2003;51(7):1031–5.

86. Schneider LS, Dagerman KS, Insel P. Risk of death with atypical antipsychotic drug treatment for dementia: meta-analysis of randomized placebo-controlled trials. JAMA. 2005;294(15):1934–43.

87. Wang PS, Schneeweiss S, Avorn J, Fischer MA, Mogun H, Solomon DH, et al. Risk of death in elderly users of conventional vs. atypical antipsychotic medications. N Engl J Med. 2005;353(22):2335–41.

88. Rudolph JL, Gardner KF, Gramigna GD, McGlinchey RE. Antipsychotics and oropharyngeal dysphagia in hospitalized older patients. J Clin Psychopharmacol. 2008;28(5):532–5.

89. The American Psychiatric Association. Diagnostic and statistical manual of mental disorders, fourth edition, text revision. Washington: American Psychiatric Association; 2000.

90. Sockalingam S, Parekh N, Bogoch II, Sun J, Mahtani R, Beach C, et al. Delirium in the postoperative cardiac patient: a review. J Card Surg. 2005;20(6):560–7.

91. Franco K, Litaker D, Locala J, Bronson D. The cost of delirium in the surgical patient. Psychosomatics. 2001;42(1):68–73.

92. Koster S, Hensens AG, van der Palen J. The long-term cognitive and functional outcomes of postoperative delirium after cardiac surgery. Ann Thorac Surg. 2009;87(5):1469–74.

93. Ely EW, Inouye SK, Bernard GR, Gordon S, Francis J, May L, et al. Delirium in mechanically ventilated patients: validity and reliability of the confusion assessment method for the intensive care unit (CAM-ICU). JAMA. 2001;286(21):2703–10.

Chapter 6
Cardiac Rehabilitation in the Elderly

Carl I. Gonzales II and Lois A. Killewich

Abstract Rehabilitation following coronary heart events and procedures results in reduced mortality, improved risk factor profiles, and improved quality of life. The American College of Cardiology and the American Heart Association have published specific guidelines regarding the components of cardiac rehabilitation, which include nutritional counseling, weight management, blood pressure management, lipid management, diabetes management, tobacco cessation, psychosocial management, physical activity counseling, and exercise training. Although the majority of patients undergoing cardiac rehabilitation have been younger than 65 years of age, recent studies demonstrate that cardiac rehabilitation is efficacious for the elderly as well. This chapter includes a complete description of the components of cardiac rehabilitation programs, and provides an overview of the efficacy and benefit of cardiac rehabilitation in the elderly.

Keywords Cardiac rehabilitation • Exercise • Elderly • Risk factor modification • Resistance training • Aerobic exercise • Lipid management • Blood pressure management • Physical activity • Smoking cessation • Diabetes management

In the 1920s, the standard of care for the treatment of patients experiencing myocardial infarction (MI) was 6–8 weeks of bedrest followed by "prolonged" inactive convalescence [1]. This policy continued until the 1940s and 1950s, when a cardiologist named Leonard Goldwater demonstrated that 60–70% of individuals in the Cleveland, Ohio area whom he had followed as cardiac patients returned to work [1]. This led to development of studies in the United States (US) and Great Britain to determine the physical, psychological, and socioeconomic well-being necessary for cardiac patients to return to work, and the methods of achieving this.. By the 1970s, studies had been performed in Sweden [2], and other parts of Europe [1], as well as in the US and Great Britain.

Today, rehabilitation is considered the standard of care for patients after MI, and those undergoing coronary artery bypass grafting (C or percutaneous coronary interventions (PCI), and is supported by the American College of Cardiology (ACC) and the American Heart Association (AHA) [3–5]. In the last decade, the indications for such programs have been expanded to include patients with heart failure (HF) [6, 7], stable angina, peripheral arterial disease, and those undergoing heart valve replacement and heart transplantation [8, 9]. Moreover, rehabilitation no longer consists only of exercise, but includes components of risk factor management, nutritional counseling, and psychosocial assessment. Outcomes are not measured only in physical fitness, but also in improvements in quality of life. Rehabilitation is designed not just to promote recovery from a coronary event or procedure, but also to provide "secondary prevention" for future events [3–5].

Definition of Cardiac Rehabilitation

The US Public Health Service, ACC, AHA, and the American Association of Cardiovascular and Pulmonary Rehabilitation (AACVPR) have jointly defined cardiac rehabilitation as follows:

> Cardiac rehabilitation services are comprehensive, long-term programs involving medical evaluation, prescribed exercise, cardiac risk factor modification, education, and counseling. These programs are designed to limit the physiologic and psychological effects of cardiac illness, reduce the risk of sudden death or re-infarction, control cardiac symptoms, stabilize or reverse the atherosclerotic process, and enhance the psychosocial and vocational status of selected patients. [10]

In general, cardiac rehabilitation (CR) programs are divided into three phases:

Phase I, inpatient CR: "A program that delivers preventive and rehabilitative services to hospitalized patients following an index CVD [cardiovascular disease] event, such as an MI/ acute coronary syndrome."

C.I. Gonzales II (✉)
Department of Surgery, Stony Brook University School of Medicine, Stony Brook, NY 11794, USA
e-mail: Carl.Gonzalez@stonybrook.edu

M.R. Katlic (ed.), *Cardiothoracic Surgery in the Elderly*, DOI 10.1007/978-1-4419-0892-6_6,
© Springer Science+Business Media, LLC 2011

Phase II, early outpatient CR: "A program that delivers preventive and rehabilitative services to patients in the outpatient setting early after a CVD event, generally within the first 3–6 months after the event, but continuing for as much as 1 year after the event."

Phase III, long-term outpatient CR: "A program that provides longer-term delivery of preventive and rehabilitative services for patients in the outpatient setting." [8]

Core Components of CR/Secondary Prevention Programs

The AHA and associates have published what they consider to be the "core components" for CR and secondary prevention programs [5]. These core components include patient assessment, nutritional counseling, weight management, blood pressure management, diabetes management, tobacco cessation, psychosocial management, physical activity counseling, and exercise training. Each component includes a description of evaluation, interventions, and expected outcomes (Tables 6.1 and 6.2) [5].

Patient Assessment

"Patient assessment" includes taking a complete history and performing a physical examination, obtaining a resting 12-lead electrocardiogram, and performing testing as indicated by the other core components (e.g., exercise testing) [5]. The intervention portion includes documentation and development of a treatment plan in conjunction with the patient's primary care provider and possibly, a cardiologist. The patient should be prescribed aspirin, clopidogrel, beta (β)-blockers, lipid-lowering agents, and angiotensin converting enzyme (ACE) inhibitors or angiotensin receptor blockers, as recommended by the ACC/AHA [4]. Recently, the ACC/AHA has also recommended that all coronary patients be considered for an annual influenza vaccination [4]. The primary outcome of this component is a documented treatment plan.

Nutritional Counseling

Eating habits, total daily caloric intake, and dietary content of fat and sodium should be determined. The patient should

Table 6.1 AHA core components of CR/secondary prevention programs

	Evaluation	Interventions	Expected outcomes
Patient assessment	Review history; perform physical examination; assess QoL; obtain resting ECG	Develop plan, communicate it to patient and PCP; ensure patient taking appropriate medications per ACC/AHA guidelines [4]; ensure influenza vaccination	Documented treatment plan, discharge plan, appropriate medications
Nutritional counseling	Assess caloric intake and diet, determine targets	Prescribe new dietary goals, educate patient and family, address compliance and behavioral change	Patient adheres to new diet
Weight management	Measure BMI	If BMI >25, establish weight loss plan (including diet, exercise)	Patient achieves new weight goal
Blood pressure management	Measure BP, determine current treatment and compliance	If SBP 120–139 mmHg or DPB 80–89, provide lifestyle modification. If SBP ≥140 or DBP ≥90, add drug therapy. If CKD, HF, or diabetes, add drug therapy for SBP ≥130 or DBP ≥80	Maintenance of BP at goal
Lipid management	Measure lipid profile, assess treatment and compliance, assess liver function	Provide nutritional counseling, add drug therapy if LDL >100 mg/dL; manage triglycerides to keep non-HDL cholesterol <130 mg/dL	LDL <100 mg/dL, non HDL cholesterol <100 mg/dL
Diabetes management	Identify complications; assess treatment and compliance	Educate patient to management, exercise	FPG 90–130 mg/dL, HbA1c <7%
Tobacco cessation	Determine status, readiness to quit, factors impeding success	Motivate and educate to quit, prevent relapse, use drug therapy if indicated	Patient quits
Psychosocial management	Identify problems, including mental illness, substance abuse	Offer counseling, medical referrals and/or therapy	Emotional/mental well-being
Physical activity counseling	Assess current activity level and motivation	Recommend 30–60 min moderate activity daily	Increased activity, aerobic fitness, body composition, well-being
Exercise training	Perform symptom-limited exercise testing	Develop individualized exercise program (aerobic + resistance)	Increased fitness, body composition, well-being

QoL quality of life; *ECG* electrocardiogram; *PCP* primary care provider; *BMI* body-mass index; *BP* blood pressure; *SBP* systolic blood pressure; *DBP* diastolic blood pressure; *CKD* chronic kidney disease; *HF* heart failure; *LDL* low-density lipoprotein; *non-HDL* non-high-density lipoprotein; *FPG* fasting plasma glucose; *HbA1c* glycosylated hemoglobin
Source: Data from ref [5]

Table 6.2 AHA exercise prescription

	Aerobic	Resistance
Frequency	3–5 days/week	2–3 days/week
Intensity	50–80% exercise capacity	10–15 repetitions per set
Duration	20–60 min	1–3 sets of 8–10 upper and lower body exercises
Modalities	Walking, treadmill, cycling, rowing, stair climbing, arm/leg ergometry	Calisthenics, elastic bands, weights
Other	Warm-up and cool-down	Warm-up and cool-down

Source: Data from ref. [5]

then be prescribed dietary modifications to maintain the fat and cholesterol limits associated with the Therapeutic Lifestyle Change diet [11]. The patient and family should be educated as to the necessary steps to achieve these goals, including compliance strategies and behavioral changes. The expected outcomes are that the patient adheres to the prescribed diet and understands the benefits of doing so.

Weight Management

Body-mass index (BMI) should be determined, and for patients with BMI >25, a plan should be developed to reduce body weight by 5–10%, at a rate of 1–2 pounds per week. The plan should include methods to increase energy expenditure, i.e., exercise. Over time, the patient should reduce weight and be able to maintain his/her weight goal.

Blood Pressure Management

Blood pressure should be measured on two separate occasions in both arms, including orthostatic measurements, and current treatment and compliance should be assessed. The goal is to maintain systolic blood pressure (SBP) ≤120 mmHg and diastolic blood pressure (DBP) ≤80 mmHg. If SBP is 120–139 mmHg and/or DBP is 80–89 mmHg, lifestyle modifications should be recommended. If SBP is ≥140 mmHg and/or DBP is ≥90 mmHg, pharmacologic therapy should be added to lifestyle modifications. If chronic kidney disease (CKD), heart failure (HF), or diabetes mellitus (DM) is present, pharmacologic therapy should be added for SBP ≥130 mmHg and/or DBP ≥80 mmHg.

Lipid management: Fasting measurements of total, high-density lipoprotein (HDL), and low-density lipoprotein (LDL) cholesterol and triglycerides should be obtained. Current treatment and compliance should be assessed. Nutritional counseling consistent with the therapeutic lifestyle change diet [11], and weight management recommendations should be initiated, with the goals of maintaining LDL ≤100 mg/dL and non-HDL ≤130 mg/dL. If lifestyle modifications are not sufficient to achieve these goals, pharmacologic therapy should be initiated. If so, liver function should be measured as recommended by the National Cholesterol Education Program [11]. In patients with DM, it "may be reasonable" to aim for LDL ≤70 mg/dL and non-HDL ≤100 mg/dL.

Management of Diabetes Mellitus (DM)

The presence or absence of DM and its complications, including retinopathy, nephropathy, neuropathy, and atherosclerotic manifestations, should be determined. Fasting plasma glucose (FPG) and glycosylated hemoglobin (HbA1c) should be measured at entry into the program. Interventions should be aimed at maintaining FPG levels of 90–130 mg/dL and HbA1c <7%. Interventions include dietary modifications, drug therapy, and exercise. Specific recommendations are provided for monitoring and treatment of blood glucose during and after exercise.

Tobacco Cessation

Patients' smoking status should be determined, and every effort made to induce patients to quit tobacco use. Psychosocial and medical treatments can be employed. Family support should be encouraged.

Psychosocial Management

Psychosocial issues, including mental illness (depression, anxiety, anger), substance abuse, family/marital discord, and sexual dysfunction, should be determined at entry into the program, and interventions (referral to mental health provider, medical therapy, support groups, self-help strategies) should be implemented to treat these problems. This should involve the primary care provider and family as well as the patient. Patients should learn and take responsibility for behavioral change, relaxation, stress management, and compliance with other therapies.

Physical Activity Counseling

Current levels of daily physical activity should be assessed using both questionnaires and quantitative methods such as pedometers. Patients should be encouraged to perform a minimum of 30–60 min per day of moderate-intensity physical activity most days of the week, through increases in domestic, occupational, and recreational activities.

Exercise Training

Current level of physical fitness and exercise should be assessed, and an individualized program should be developed for each patient to increase physical fitness. Prior to entry into an exercise program, each patient should undergo symptom-limited exercise testing to ensure the patient's safety with regard to cardiac events. Exercise programs should include both aerobic (endurance) and resistance components (Table 6.2) [5].

Performance Measures

In 2007, the ACC and AHA, in conjunction with the American Association of Cardiovascular and Pulmonary Rehabilitation (AACVPR), published "performance measures" addressing the quality of care in CR programs [8]. The purpose of the performance measures is to "provide practitioners with tools for measuring the quality of care and for identifying opportunities to improve." Ultimately, adoption of performance measures should reduce cardiovascular morbidity and mortality, and improve quality of life in patients with CHD. The performance measures are based upon published evidence regarding the methodology and efficacy of CR programs, and are intended to be used for patients who have experienced MI, CABG, PCI, or stable angina within the previous year. Although they do not specifically pertain to patients who have undergone heart valve procedures or transplantation, the writing group felt that they could be applied to these populations as well [8].

Two sets of performance measures were developed. The first pertains to the appropriate referral of patients to a CR program, and the second defines the optimal performance of the program. The measure addressing patient referral was developed because, despite the known benefits and 40 years of use of CR programs, less than 30% of eligible patients are currently referred [12–14]. The second was developed because although the AACVPR provides certification for CR programs, only 37% of programs within the US have sought and attained this certification [15]. The performance measures include those directed toward the structure of a program, and those directed toward processes the program uses.

Performance Measurement Set A address referral, and proposes the following:

1. "All hospitalized patients with a qualifying CVD [cardiovascular disease] event are referred to an early outpatient CR program prior to hospital discharge."
2. "All outpatients with a qualifying diagnosis within the past year who have not already participated in an early outpatient CR program are referred by their healthcare provider." [8]

Performance Measure B addresses the delivery of CR services, and includes both structural and process measures. They are as follows:

Structural measures

1. "A physician medical director is responsible for the program."
2. "An emergency response team with appropriate emergency equipment and trained staff is available during patient care hours."

Process measures

1. "Assessment and documentation of each patient's risk for adverse events during exercise."
2. "A process to assess patients for intercurrent changes in symptoms."
3. "Individualized assessment and evaluation of modifiable CVD risk factors."
4. "Development of individualized risk-reduction interventions for identified conditions, and coordination of care with other healthcare providers."
5. "Evidence of a plan to monitor response and document program effectiveness through ongoing analysis of aggregate data." [8]

All purveyors of CR are encouraged to adopt performance measures to assess their programs' quality and patient care. The AACVPR/ACC/AHA document provides examples of instruments which can be used to implement the performance measures.

Safety of CR

Early in the development of CR, concerns were raised regarding the safety of instituting exercise therapy in patients shortly after a CHD event. Over time, however, multiple studies have demonstrated that exercise performed with appropriate prescription and monitoring is very safe [9, 16, 17]. Protocols recommend that physical rehabilitation be initiated following CHD events after 12–48 h of bed rest [16]. During this phase, activities should be limited to breathing and relaxation exercises, and activities such as sitting, standing, and walking. After 4–6 days, stair climbing can be added. Rehabilitation should be performed using electrocardiographic monitoring, and discontinued if any of the following occur: chest pain, dyspnea, increase in heart rate >20 beats/min, decrease in heart rate >10 beats/min, decrease in blood pressure >10–15 mmHg, increase in SBP >200 mmHg, or increase in DBP >110 mmHg [16].

As patients move to an outpatient setting, it is important to perform a symptom-limited exercise test to determine prognosis and direct further rehabilitation. Symptoms which would warrant discontinuation of the test and set appropriate limits for ongoing rehabilitation include chest pain, increasing dyspnea or cyanosis, decrease in SBP >10 mmHg, increase in SBP >250 mmHg, increase id DBP >115 mmHg, dizziness or near fainting, significant arrhythmia, and ST segment elevation ≥1 mm in leads without pathologic Q waves [16]. The target heart rate (HR) during training can be determined by the following formula:

$$\text{Target HR} = \text{resting HR} + (\text{maximum HR} - \text{resting HR}) \times (40 - 80\%).$$

The presence or absence of symptoms is used to determine where within the 40–80% the target heart rate should fall.

If patients are to undergo outpatient exercise in a home-based environment, they should be trained to monitor their blood pressure and heart rates. Transtelephonic electrocardiographic monitoring can be instituted if available. Appropriate forms of exercise, as described earlier, include treadmill training, bicycle ergometry, and walking [16]. Resistance training can be added progressively; it has been shown to be more beneficial in terms of improving fitness during activities of daily living [18].

Using this type of exercise prescription, CR has been found to be safe. Estimates are that "major" cardiac events such as MI and resuscitated cardiac arrest occur in only 1 of 50,000–100,000 h of supervised exercise. Two fatalities were reported in 1.5 million patient-hours of supervised exercise [3, 19]. A scientific statement published by the AHA in 2007 estimated that the risk of a major cardiac complication such as death, MI, or cardiac arrest was one event in 60,000–80,000 h [20].

Efficacy of CR

Efficacy in Patients with MI, Stable Angina, and After CABG or PCI

Two meta-analyses addressing the efficacy of CR in these patient populations were published in the 1980s [21, 22]. These studies included more than 4,000 patients, and demonstrated that patients randomized to exercise-based CR, experienced statistically significant reductions in both all-cause and cardiac mortality of 20–25% compared to patients treated with "usual care." In 1998, the National Health Service of Great Britain published an analysis of seven systematic reviews in the Health Care Bulletin on Cardiac Rehabilitation [23]. The findings of this analysis were that exercise improved physical aspects of recovery from CHD events and was safe, but as a sole intervention was not sufficient to reduce morbidity and mortality.

Because of the contradictory results, as well as observations that the quality of the studies included in these early reviews and meta-analyses was poor, the Cochrane Collaboration undertook a meta-analysis of additional studies which was published in 2001 [24]. The objective of this analysis was to determine the efficacy of exercise-based CR, compared to usual care in terms of mortality, morbidity, quality of life (QoL), and risk factors in patients with CHD. Thirty-two randomized controlled trials (RCTs) including 8440 patients comprised the meta-analysis. The RCTs included patients who had experienced MI, undergone CABG or PCI, or had angina or CHD defined by angiography. Patients with HF and those who had undergone transplantation or valve procedures were excluded. Studies were grouped according to whether exercise was the only component of the CR program, or whether additional interventions such as dietary and weight management were included with the exercise program ("comprehensive CR").

All-cause mortality was reduced by 27% compared to usual care in the exercise-only CR programs. This reduction was statistically significant (OR 0.74, CI 0.51–0.94). In the comprehensive CR programs, all-cause mortality was reduced to a lesser degree, 13%, and this was not significant (OR 0.87, CI 0.71–1.05). Total cardiac mortality was reduced significantly by both exercise-only and comprehensive CR, by 31 and 26% respectively. However, there were no significant reductions in either sudden cardiac death or recurrent non-fatal MI in either CR program.

There were not enough data to determine if significant reductions occurred in the prevalence of revascularization procedures (CABG and PCI). However, using a combined outcome of mortality, non-fatal MI, and revascularization, both exercise-only and comprehensive CR produced statistically significant 20% reductions in this combined "adverse" outcome.

Comprehensive CR also produced significant improvements in total cholesterol, LDL cholesterol, triglycerides, and blood pressure. No significant improvements in smoking status were identified. Although health-related QoL improved in the comprehensive care programs, patients receiving usual care also showed significant improvements in QoL. The authors of the analysis noted that this finding highlighted the importance of recognizing the "natural course of recovery" after a CHD event.

Two meta-analyses addressing CR programs and their effects on CHD morbidity and mortality were published in the first decade of the twenty-first century [25, 26]. The analysis of Taylor et al. included 48 RCTs and 8,940 patients [25]. These authors found statistically significant reductions in all-cause (OR 0.80, CI 0.68–0.93) and cardiac (OR 0.74, CI 0.61–0.96) mortality with exercise-based CR, and improvements in lipid levels, blood pressure, and smoking cessation. As in the Cochrane analysis [24], there were no reductions in non-fatal MI and revascularization rates. Health-related QoL improved in both the CR and usual groups.

The second analysis included 63 trials and 21,295 patients, covering the period of time from 1966 to 2004 [26]. All-cause mortality was reduced (OR 0.85, CI 0.77–0.94); the effect was significantly greater in studies presenting longer follow-up. In 20 trials reporting 12 month data, the risk ratio was 0.97 (CI 0.82–1.14), while in seven trials reporting 5 year data, the risk ratio was 0.77 (CI 0.63–0.93). The rate of recurrent MI was reduced by 17% at 1 year, and risk factor profiles improved. Significant improvements were also noted in QoL. Benefits were similar in programs that provided exercise only versus those that provided exercise and lifestyle modifications.

The findings of these two more recent meta-analyses highlight two important points with regard to CR programs. First, pharmacologic agents for the treatment of CHD have changed dramatically over the last 10–15 years; in particular with the introduction of antiplatelet agents such as clopidogrel, statins for the treatment of dyslipidemia, angiotensin coverting enzyme (ACE) inhibitors, and angiotensin receptor blockers. It has been speculated that the use of these medications might improve patients' health status to the point that CR would not add benefits above those achieved with medications, and would become unnecessary. However, findings of both recent meta-analyses clearly show that patients in more recent studies (published after 1995), who have received treatment with newer medications, derive the same benefits as those participating in studies prior to the introduction of these agents.

Secondly, it has been suggested that the introduction of PCI for the treatment of CHD might eliminate or reduce the need for CR. To address this, Hambrecht et al. randomized 101 patients with stable angina to 12 months of exercise training or PCI. The exercise training consisted of 20 min per day of bicycle ergometry performed at 70% of maximal heart rate. Both groups received maximal medical therapy.

At the end of the study period, the group randomized to exercise experienced a higher event-free survival than the group randomized to PCI (88 vs. 70% respectively, $P=0.023$). The exercise group also developed a higher exercise capacity and maximal oxygen uptake compared to the PCI group (16% increase, $P<0.001$). Both groups experienced similar improvements in symptom-free exercise tolerance. However, analysis revealed that the cost of PCI ($6956) was almost twice that of the exercise intervention ($3429, $P<0.001$). The authors concluded that exercise training, together with medical management, is an effective alternative approach to interventions in "motivated" patients with stable CHD, and recommended that a large, multi-center trial be undertaken [27].

Although such a trial has not been performed, it seems logical to assume that PCI alone will not provide the comprehensive benefits associated with CR, such as improved lipid and weight management and QoL. Therefore, it is the opinion of these authors that patients should continue to be referred for CR following PCI, rather than considering PCI a replacement for CR.

Efficacy of CR in Heart Failure Patients

The prevalence of HF in the US is increasing steadily, both because of the aging of the population, and the increasing survival rates following MI. The AHA currently estimates that there are 670,000 new cases in the US annually [28]. The prognosis of patients with newly diagnosed HF is poor, with approximately 40% dying in the first year [29]. Hospital admissions and costs are also increasing significantly.

To address these issues, CR has been evaluated for its effectiveness in improving exercise capacity and reducing mortality in heart failure patients. A Cochrane Collaboration review of 29 RCTs published in 2004 showed that CR increased exercise capacity over one year of follow-up [30]. Specific improvements were observed in VO_2max, exercise capacity in watts, exercise duration, and the results of a 6 min walk test. In 2006, van Tol et al. published a study which confirmed the findings of the Cochrane review, and also noted improvements in QoL measured by the Minnesota Living with Heart Failure questionnaire in HF patients who underwent exercise training [31]. An update to the Cochrane review was published in 2010 [6]. The objectives of this update were to determine whether exercise-based interventions for heart failure patients improved mortality, morbidity, hospital admissions, and QoL. Nineteen RCTs including a total of 3,647 patients were reviewed.

Exercise training was not found to confer a significant advantage toward survival in this review, although a nonsignificant trend toward reduced mortality was observed in the trials with longer-term follow-up. There was also a nonsignificant trend towards reduced numbers of patients admitted to hospitals. Admissions related to heart failure specifically were significantly reduced in the exercising patients (RR 0.72, CI 0.52–0.99, $P=0.04$). Health-related QoL was significantly better in patients undergoing exercise compared to controls, and the improvements in QoL noted with exercise were also significant [6].

Efficacy in Patients Undergoing Valve Replacement Procedures

The literature addressing the benefits of CR in patients undergoing procedures for cardiac valves is less extensive. No meta-analyses have been performed, and only a few small trials exist [32–35]. The majority of patients with valvular disorders are significantly deconditioned prior to surgery. Although repair or replacement improves function, most patients are still only able to exercise at approximately 50% of normal controls 6 months postoperatively [36]. Patients undergoing procedures on the aortic valve recover more rapidly and more fully than those undergoing procedures on the mitral valve, particularly if pulmonary hypertension or depressed ventricular function is present prior to surgery [33].

Sire randomized 44 patients undergoing aortic valve replacement to a 1-month postoperative course of exercise therapy or usual care. He observed that physical work capacity was increased significantly in the training group compared to the usual care group at 6 months (38% higher in the training group, $P<0.02$) and 12 months (37% high in the training group, $P<0.025$) [32]. Ueshima et al. randomized 64 patients undergoing valve replacement to exercise or usual care. Both VO_2max and QoL, measured using a questionnaire, were greater in the exercising group than in the controls [35].

Efficacy in Patients Undergoing Cardiac Transplantation

There have also been a few studies addressing the benefits of CR in patients undergoing heart transplantation [37–40]. In general, these studies have involved programs conducted 3–4 times per week for 3–4 months at moderate intensity levels. Overall endurance capacity has been observed to improve in exercising patients by 20–50%. A randomized trial of 27 heart transplant patients was performed by Kobashigawa et al [40]. These investigators found that VO_2max increased significantly in patients randomized to 6 months of aerobic and resistance training (49% increase), compared to control patients randomized to "an unstructured home exercise program" (18% increase, $P=0.01$). A significant increase in workload measured in watts also occurred in the structured exercise group compared to the controls ($P=0.01$).

Summary and Conclusions Regarding Efficacy

The heterogeneity and overall quality of the studies reviewed in meta-analyses of CR to some extent prevent drawing substantial conclusions. However, the preponderance of the data shows that CR reduces all-cause and CHD mortality, improves risk factor profiles, and enhances QoL in patients with MI, stable angina, and those undergoing CABG or PCI. Benefits persist despite the introduction of new therapies with pharmacologic agents and interventions. Comprehensive programs appear more effective overall than exercise alone.

Areas in which additional studies would be beneficial include the use of CR in patients with HF, valve procedures, and transplantation, the benefits of resistance versus aerobic exercise, the benefits in elderly patients (discussed below), women and minorities, and cost.

CR in the Elderly

In the US, patients ≥65 years of age constitute more than half of the population experiencing MI and coronary revascularizations. However, they have generally been underrepresented in CR [10, 41]. In the studies included in the Cochrane review published in 2001, the mean age of participants in the exercise-only arm of rehabilitation was 53.1 years; in those receiving comprehensive rehabilitation it was 56.3 years. Amazingly, many of the studies had an upper limit of participation of 65 years [24].

Elderly patients have lower functional capacity, and higher rates of depression and social isolation compared to younger patients. They are thus at particularly increased risk of disability and loss of independence after CHD events [9, 41]. It has been suggested that their reduced functional status makes them particularly attractive candidates for CR – they have the most to gain [41]. Because of this lack of data, more recent studies have addressed the efficacy of CR in elderly populations [41–55].

Outcomes of CR in the Elderly

Morbidity and Mortality

The relationship between CR and mortality has not been well studied in elderly populations. However, a recent study of 30,161 Medicare beneficiaries (average age = 74 yearsshowed a relationship between numbers of CR sessions attended and risk of death or MI. Patients who attended an average of 36 sessions reduced their risk of death by 47%, and their risk of MI by 31% compared to those who attended only an average of 1 session (Table 6.3) [54]. The findings of a second, much smaller study demonstrated that all-cause mortality was lower (14%) in 37 patients undergoing 6 months of CR compared to

Table 6.3 Risk of death and MI versus number of CR sessions attended

	36 versus 24	36 versus 12	36 versus 1
Death	0.86 (0.77–0.97)	0.78 (0.71–0.87)	0.53 (0.48–0.59)
MI	0.88 (0.83–0.93)	0.77 (0.69–0.87)	0.69 (0.58–0.81)

Source: Data from ref. [54]

Hazards ratio and 95% confidence intervals for patients attending 36 sessions versus lower number of sessions

74 age-matched controls (28%, $P=0.081$) [55]. A single study showed that patients undergoing CR had reduced morbidity, manifested as a lower incidence of rehospitalization at 3 months and 1 year, compared to control subjects (13 vs. 29%, $P<0.04$) [56].

Physical Fitness

Elderly patients undergoing CR were able to increase their physical fitness, measured by VO_2max, estimated exercise capacity, and duration of treadmill walking [41, 43, 47, 53]. Estimated exercise capacity, measured as METS, increased in four studies from a mean of 5.1 METS to 6.6 METS [43, 57–59] following 3 months of CR. In a study performed by Lavie and Milani, the increases experienced by elderly patients (43%) were significantly greater than those experienced by younger patients (32%, $P<0.01$) [58].

Treadmill duration increased significantly in elderly patients treated with 3 months of CR compared to an age-match group that did not exercise (47 vs. 8%, $P<0.001$). In this study, patients who continued to exercise for an additional 9 months maintained the improved fitness at 1 year [60].

In a more recent study, walking distance, measured by a 6-min walk test, increased by approximately 32% in 300 patients undergoing CR with a combined aerobic and resistance training program after cardiac surgery. Walking distances improved in 97% of patients, of whom 26% were >75 years old [61].

For the most part, exercise as part of CR programs has consisted of aerobic training such as bicycle ergometry or treadmill walking. However, in the elderly in particular, resistance training is considered as important as aerobic training because of the presence of sarcopenia, the loss of muscle mass that occurs with aging. By increasing muscle mass and mitigating the effects of sarcopenia, resistance training has been shown to improve walking ability, functional status, and QoL in the elderly [41, 62, 63].

Resistance training was evaluated in a study comparing arm and leg strength in younger and older patients after CHD events. In this study, arm and leg strength improved to similar degrees in the elderly, as compared to the younger patients after 3 months of resistance training [46]. The authors noted that this was particularly significant, given that aerobic activities such as walking are limited by leg strength in the elderly [41].

In a more recent RCT, 42 elderly women with CHD (age >65 years) were randomized to a 6 month program of resistance training or "light yoga and breathing exercises." The primary outcome measurement was performance of 16 activities of daily living compiled in the Continuous Scale Physical Functional Performance test. At the completion of the training program, patients in the training group performed 13 of 16 activities faster or with increased weight carried compared to the controls (all $P<0.05$). Measures of endurance, balance, coordination, and flexibility improved in the training group [64].

Exercise training and physical activity are clearly as important in the elderly population undergoing CR as they are in the younger patients. Resistance training is likely to play a more important role in the elderly, whose overall physical status is much lower at entry.

Risk Factor Therapies

Small improvements have been noted in measures of obesity in patients undergoing CR [43, 52, 58, 59, 65]. In particular, Lavie's group noted 1% decreases in weight and BMI (both $P<0.05$), and a 6% decrease in percentage of body fat ($P<0.001$) in 268 elderly patients with a mean age of 70 ± 4 years [65]. Few studies have been performed to determine the effects of CR, and specifically statin medications, on lipid profiles in the elderly. However, subgroup analyses of larger trials have shown impressive reductions of mortality and non-fatal CHD events [66–68]. For example, the findings of the Scandinavian Simvastatin Survival Study demonstrated that simvastatin decreased CHD mortality by 42% in patients <65 years of age, and by 43% in patients ≥65 years [50, 66]. Furthermore, because the very elderly (≥75 years) are at increased risk for CHD events and death, they experience greater absolute benefits.

Both smoking cessation and hypertension management result in reductions in morbidity in patients >70 years of age undergoing CABG [69, 70]. While smoking cessation reduces mortality, anti-hypertensive treatment in the elderly reduces the risk of stroke, major cardiovascular events, and HF.

Psychosocial Disorders and QoL

Depression is common in the elderly, with a prevalence of 10–15%. Anxiety occurs in up to 20% of older patients [71, 72]. Depression, anxiety, and social isolation have been shown to increase the risk of developing CHD and the risks of morbidity and mortality after a CHD event [73]. In one study, CR resulted in a 50% reduction in the prevalence of depression, as well as a 57% reduction in depression score ($P<0.0001$) [71]. In a second study of the very elderly (age >75 years), CR improved scores of anxiety (−66%), somatization (−42%), depression (−56%), and hostility (−65%) [59].

Quality of life scores also improved in the very elderly (+20%) [59] following CR. Lavie and Milani demonstrated significant improvements in QoL as assessed by the Medical Outcomes Score Short Form-36, including total quality of life (+13%), well-being (+11%), function (+16%), pain (+20%), general health (+8%), energy (+18%), and mental health (+5%) following CR. An RCT demonstrated significant improvements in 7 QoL measures in 50 patients aged 65–84 years randomized to 3 months of exercise+optimal medical therapy, compared to an age-matched group randomized to medical therapy alone [47]. More recently, the ENRICHD trial demonstrated smaller, but still significant, improvements in QoL following a cognitive behavioral intervention alone (without the other components of CR) in elderly CHD patients [74].

Summary and Conclusions

Taken together, published data clearly supports the use of CR in the elderly. In fact, the elderly CHD population appears to gain more from CR than younger participants because of their poorer status prior to entry [41]. CR nterventions should be similar to those used in younger patients, but exercise should include a component of resistance training.

A major barrier to achieving widespread benefits from CR in elderly populations has been the reluctance, or lack of understanding, of physicians to refer elderly patients to CR programs [10, 41]. Future efforts should be directed toward educating these physicians regarding both the safety and efficacy of CR in the elderly.

References

1. Muir JR. The rehabilitation of cardiac patients. Proc Roy Soc Med. 1977;70:655–6.
2. Mulcahy R, Hickey N. The rehabilitation of patients with coronary heart disease. Scand J Rehabil Med. 1970;2:108–12.
3. Leon AS, Franklin BA, Costa F, Balady GJ, Berra KA, Stewart KJ, et al. Cardiac rehabilitation and secondary prevention of coronary heart disease: an American Heart Association scientific statement from the Council on Clinical Cardiology (Subcommittee on Exercise, Cardiac Rehabilitation, and Prevention) and the Council on Nutrition, Physical Activity, and Metabolism (Subcommittee on Physical Activity), in collaboration with the American Association of Cardiovascular and Pulmonary Rehabilitation. Circulation. 2005;111:369–76.
4. Smith SC, Allen J, Blair SN, Bonow RO, Brass LM, Fonarow GC, et al. AHA/ACC guidelines for secondary prevention for patients with coronary and other atherosclerotic vascular disease: 2006 update. Circulation. 2006;113:2363–72.
5. Balady GJ, Williams MA, Ades PA, Bittner V, Comoss P, Foody JM, et al. Core components of cardiac rehabilitation/secondary prevention programs: 2007: a scientific statement from the American Heart Association Exercise, Cardiac Rehabilitation, and Prevention Committee, the Council on Clinical Cardiology; the Councils on Cardiovascular Nursing, Epidemiology and Prevention, and Nutrition, Physical Activity, and Metabolism; and the American Association of Cardiovascular and Pulmonary Rehabilitation. Circulation. 2007; 115:2675–82.
6. Davies EJ, Moxham T, Rees K, Singh S, Coats AJS, Ebrahim S, et al. Exercise based rehabilitation for heart failure. Cochrane Database Syst Rev 2010;(4):CD003331.
7. Hunt SA, Abraham WT, Chin MH, Feldman AM, Francis GS, Ganiats TG, et al. ACC/AHA guideline update for the diagnosis and management of chronic heart failure in the adult: summary article: a report of the American College of Cardiology/American Heart Association Task Force on Practice Guidelines (Writing Committee to Update the 2001 Guidelines for the Evaluation and Management of Heart Failure): developed in collaboration with the American College of Chest Physicians and the International Society for Heart and Lung Transplantation: endorsed by the Heart Rhythm Society. Circulation. 2005;112:1825–52.
8. Thomas RJ, King M, Lui K, Oldridge N, Pina IL, Spertus J, et al. AACVPR/ACC/AHA 2007 performance measures on cardiac rehabilitation for referral to and delivery of cardiac rehabilitation/ secondary prevention services. J Cardiopul Rehabil Prev. 2007;27: 260–90.
9. Wenger NK. Current status of cardiac rehabilitation. J Am Coll Cardiol. 2008;51:1619–31.
10. Wenger NK, Froelicher ES, Smith LK, Ades PA, Berra K, Blumenthal JA, et al. Cardiac rehabilitation: clinical practice guideline. Rockville, MD: US Agency for Healthcare Research and Quality, Department of Health and Human Services. 1995; Clinical Guideline No. 17 (AHCPR 96-0672).
11. National Cholesterol Education Program (NCEP) Expert Panel on Detection, Evaluation, and Treatment of High Blood Cholesterol in Adults (Adult Treatment Panel III). Third report of the National Cholesterol Education Program (NCEP) expert panel on detection, evaluation, and treatment of high blood cholesterol in adults (Adult Treatment Panel III) final report. Circulation. 2002;106:3143–421.
12. Thomas RJ, Miller NH, Lamendola C, Berra K, Hedbäck B, Durstine JL, et al. National survey on gender differences in cardiac rehabilitation programs. Patient characteristics and enrollment patterns. J Cardiopulm Rehabil. 1996;16:402–12.
13. Centers for Disease Control and Prevention (CDC). Receipt of cardiac rehabilitation services among heart attack survivors – 19 states and the District of Columbia, 2001. Morb Mortal Wkly Rep. 2003;52:1072–5.
14. Cortes O, Arthur HM. Determinants of referral to cardiac rehabilitation programs in patients with coronary artery disease: a systematic review. Am Heart J. 2006;151:249–56.
15. Currier DY, Savage PD, Ades PA. Geographic distribution of cardiac rehabilitation programs in the United States. J Cardiopulm Rehabil. 2005;25:80–4.
16. Piotrowicz R, Wolszakiewicz J. Cardiac rehabilitation following myocardial infarction. Cardiol J. 2008;15:481–7.
17. Bethell H, Lewin R, Dalal H. Cardiac rehabilitation in the United Kingdom. Heart. 2009;95:271–5.
18. Fletcher GF, Balady GJ, Amsterdam EA, Chaitman B, Eckel R, Fleg J, et al. Exercise standards for testing and training. A statement for healthcare professionals from the American Heart Association. Circulation. 2001;104:1694–740.
19. Franklin BA, Bonzheim K, Gordon S, Timmis GC. Safety of medically supervised outpatient cardiac rehabilitation exercise therapy: a 16-year follow-up. Chest. 1998;114:902–6.
20. Thompson PD, Franklin BA, Balady GJ, Blair SN, Corrado D, Estes III NA, et al. Exercise and acute cardiovascular events: placing the risks into perspective. A scientific statement from the American Heart Association Council on Nutrition, Physical Activity, and Metabolism and the Council on Clinical Cardiology. Circulation. 2007;115:2358–68.
21. Oldridge NB, Guyatt GH, Fischer ME, Rimm AA. Cardiac rehabilitation after myocardial infarction. Combined experience of randomized clinical trials. JAMA. 1988;260:945–50.
22. O'Connor GT, Buring JE, Yusuf S, Goldhaber SZ, Olmstead EM, Paffenbarger RS, et al. An overview of randomized trials of rehabilitation with exercise after myocardial infarction. Circulation. 1989;80:234–44.

23. NHS Centre for Reviews and Dissemination. Cardiac rehabilitation. Effective health care bulletin. Vol. 4, York: University of York; 1998.

24. Jolliffe J, Rees K, Taylor RRS, Thompson DR, Oldridge N, Ebrahim S. Exercise-based rehabilitation for coronary heart disease. Cochrane Database Syst Rev 2001;(1): CD001800.

25. Taylor RS, Brown A, Ebrahim S, Jolliffe J, Noorani H, Rees K, et al. Exercise-based rehabilitation for patients with coronary heart disease: systematic review and meta-analysis of randomized controlled trials. Am J Med. 2004;116:682–92.

26. Clark AM, Hartling L, Bandermeer B, McAlister FA. Meta-analysis: secondary prevention programs for patients with coronary artery disease. Ann Intern Med. 2005;143:659–72.

27. Hambrecht R, Walther C, Mobius-Winkler S, Gielen S, Linke A, Conradi K, et al. Percutaneous coronary angioplasty compared with exercise training in patients with stable coronary artery disease: a randomized trial. Circulation. 2004;109:1371–8.

28. Lloyd-Jones D, Adams RJ, Brown TM, Carnethon M, Dai S, De Simone G, et al. on behalf of the American Heart Association Statistics Committee and Stroke Statistics Subcommittee. Heart disease and stroke statistics – 2010 update. A report from the American Heart Association. Circulation. 2010;121:e1–170.

29. Cowie MR, Wood DA, Coats AJ, Thompson SG, Suresh V, Poole-Wilson PA, et al. Survival of patients with a new diagnosis of heart failure: a population based study. Heart. 2000;83:505–10.

30. Rees K, Taylor RS, Singh S, Coats AJS, Ebrahim S. Exercise based rehabilitation for heart failure. Cochrane Database Syst Rev 2004;(3):CD003331.

31. van Tol BA, Huijsmans RJ, Kroon DW, Schothorst M, Kwakkel G. Effects of exercise training on cardiac performance, exercise capacity and quality of life in patients with heart failure: a meta-analysis. Eur J Heart Fail. 2006;8:841–50.

32. Sire S. Physical training and occupational rehabilitation after aortic valve replacement. Eur Heart J. 1987;8:1215–20.

33. Gohlke-Barwolf C, Gohlke H, Samek L, Peters K, Betz P, Eschenbruch E, et al. Exercise tolerance and working capacity after valve replacement. J Heart Valve Dis. 1992;1:189–95.

34. Jairath N, Salerno T, Chapman J, Dornan J, Weisel R. The effect of moderate exercise training on oxygen uptake post aortic/mitral valve surgery. J Cardiopulm Rehabil. 1995;15:424–30.

35. Ueshima K, Kamata J, Kobayashi N, Saito M, Sato S, Kawazoe K, et al. Effects of exercise training after open heart surgery on quality of life and exercise tolerance in patients with mitral regurgitation or aortic regurgitation. Jpn Heart J. 2004;45:789–97.

36. Carstens V, Behrenbeck DW, Hilger HH. Exercise capacity before and after cardiac valve surgery. Cardiology. 1983;70:41–9.

37. Niset G, Coustry-Degre C, Degre S. Psychosocial and physical rehabilitation after heart transplantation: 1-year follow-up. Cardiology. 1988;75:311–7.

38. Keteyian S, Shepard R, Ehrman J, Fedel F, Glick C, Rhoads K, et al. Cardiorespiratory responses of heart transplant patients to exercise training. J Appl Physiol. 1991;70:2627–31.

39. Brubaker PH, Brozena SC, Morley DL, Walter JD, Berry MJ. Exercise-induced ventilatory abnormalities in orthotopic heart transplant patients. J Heart Lung Transplant. 1997;16:1011–7.

40. Kobashigawa JA, Leaf DA, Lee N, Gleeson MP, Liu H, Hamilton MA, et al. A controlled trial of exercise rehabilitation after heart transplantation. N Engl J Med. 1999;340:272–7.

41. Pasquali SK, Alexander KP, Peterson ED. Cardiac rehabilitation in the elderly. Am Heart J. 2001;142:748–55.

42. Ades PA, Waldemann ML, McCann WJ, Weaver SO. Predictors of cardiac rehabilitation participation in older coronary patients. Arch Intern Med. 1992;152:1033–5.

43. Lavie CJ, Milani RV, Littman AB. Benefits of cardiac rehabilitation and exercise training in secondary coronary prevention in the elderly. J Am Coll Cardiol. 1993;22:678–83.

44. McConnell TR, Laubach CA. Elderly cardiac rehabilitation patients show greater improvements in ventilation at submaximal levels of exercise. Am J Geriatr Cardiol. 1996;5:15–23.

45. Lavie CJ, Milani RV. Benefits of cardiac rehabilitation and exercise training in elderly women. Am J Cardiol. 1997;79:664–6.

46. Fragnoli-Munn K, Savage PD, Ades PA. Combined resistive-aerobic training in older patients with coronary artery disease early after myocardial infarction. J Cardiopulm Rehabil. 1998;18:416–20.

47. Stahle A, Mattsson E, Ryden L, Unden A-L, Nordlander R. Improved physical fitness and quality of life following training of elderly patients after acute coronary events. Eur Heart J. 1999;20: 1475–84.

48. Lavie CJ, Milani RV. Disparate effects of improving aerobic exercise capacity and quality of life after cardiac rehabilitation in young and elderly coronary patients. J Cardiopulm Rehabil. 2000;20: 235–40.

49. McConnell TR, Laubach CA, Memon M, Gardner JK, Klinger TA, Palm RJ. Age following acute myocardial infarction and bypass revascularization surgery. Am J Geriatr Cardiol. 2000;9:210–8.

50. Williams MA, Fleg JL, Ades PA, Chaitman BR, Miller NH, Mohiuddin SM, et al. Secondary prevention of coronary heart disease in the elderly (with emphasis on patients ≥75 years of age). An American Heart Association scientific statement from the Council on Clinical Cardiology Subcommittee on Exercise, Cardiac Rehabilitation, and Prevention. Circulation. 2002;105: 1735–43.

51. Stewart KJ, Turner KL, Bacher AC, DeRegis JR, Sung J, Tayback M, et al. Are fitness, activity, and fatness associated with health-related quality of life and mood in older persons? J Cardiopulm Rehabil. 2003;23:115–21.

52. Lavie CJ, Milani R. Benefits of cardiac rehabilitation in the elderly. Chest. 2004;126:1010–12.

53. Seki E, Watanabe Y, Shimada K, Sunayama S, Onishi T, Kawakami K, et al. Effects of a phase III cardiac rehabilitation program on physical status and lipid profiles in elderly patients with coronary disease: Juntendo Cardiac Rehabilitation Program (J-CARP). Circ J. 2008;72:1230–4.

54. Hammill BG, Curtis LH, Schulman KA, Whellan DJ. Relationship between cardiac rehabilitation and long-term risks of death and myocardial infarction among elderly Medicare beneficiaries. Circulation. 2010;121:63–70.

55. Onishi T, Shimada K, Sato H, Seki E, Watanabe Y, Sunayama S, et al. Effects of phase III cardiac rehabilitation on mortality and cardiovascular events in elderly patients with stable coronary artery disease. Circ J. 2010;74:709–14.

56. Bondestam E, Breikss A, Hartford M. Effects of early rehabilitation on consumption of medical care during the first year after acute myocardial infarction in patients ≥65 years of age. Am J Cardiol. 1995;75:767–71.

57. Williams MA, Maresh CM, Esterbrooks DJ, Harbrecht JJ, Sketch MH. Early exercise training in patients older than age 65 years compared with that in younger patients after acute myocardial infarction or coronary artery bypass grafting. Am J Cardiol. 1985;55:263–6.

58. Lavie CJ, Milani RV. Effects of cardiac rehabilitation programs on exercise capacity, coronary risk factors, behavioral characteristics, and quality of life in a large elderly cohort. Am J Cardiol. 1995;76:177–9.

59. Lavie CJ, Milani RV. Effects of cardiac rehabilitation and exercise training programs in patients ≥75 years of age. Am J Cardiol. 1996;78:675–7.

60. Ades PA, Waldmann ML, Gillespie C. A controlled trial of exercise training in older coronary patients. J Gerontol. 1995;50:7–11.

61. Macchi C, Fattirolli F, Molino Lova R, Conti AA, Luisi MLE, Intini R, et al. Early and late rehabilitation and physical training in elderly patients after cardiac surgery. Am J Phys Med Rehabil. 2007;86: 826–34.

62. Fiatarone MA, Marks EC, Ryan ND, Meredith CN, Lipsitz LA, Evans WJ. High-intensity strength training in nonagenarians. Effects on skeletal muscle. JAMA. 1990;263:3029–34.

63. Singh MA, Ding W, Manfredi TJ, Solares GS, O'Neill EF, Clements KM, et al. Insulin-like growth factor I in skeletal muscle after weight-lifting exercise in frail elders. Am J Physiol. 1999;277(1 Pt 1): E135–43.

64. Ades PA, Savage PD, Cress ME, Brochu M, Lee NM, Poehlman ET. Resistance training on physical performance in disabled older female cardiac patients. Med Sci Sports Exerc. 2003;35:1265–70.

65. Lavie CJ, Milani RV. Impact of aging on hostility in coronary patients and effects of cardiac rehabilitation and exercise training in elderly persons. Am J Geriatr Cardiol. 2004;13:125–30.

66. Miettinen TA, Pyörälä K, Olsson AG, Musliner TA, Cook TJ, Faergeman O, et al. Cholesterol-lowering therapy in women and elderly patients with myocardial infarction or angina pectoris: findings from the Scandinavian Simvastatin Survival Study. Circulation. 1997;96:4211–8.

67. Lewis SJ, Moye LA, Sacks FM, Johnstone DE, Timmis G, Mitchell J, et al. Effect of pravastatin on cardiovascular events in older patients with myocardial infarction and cholesterol levels in the average range: results of the Cholesterol and Recurrent Events (CARE) Trial. Ann Intern Med. 1998;129:681–9.

68. Sacks FM, Tonkin AM, Shepherd J, Braunwald E, Cobbe S, Hawkins CM, et al. Effect of pravastatin on coronary disease events

in subgroups defined by coronary risk factors: the Prospective Pravastatin Pooling Project. Circulation. 2000;102:1893–900.

69. Hermanson B, Omenn GS, Kronmal RA, Gersh BJ. Beneficial six-year outcome of smoking cessation in older men and women with coronary artery disease: results from the CASS registry. N Engl J Med. 1988;319:1365–9.

70. Gueyffier F, Boutitie F, Boissel JP, Pocock S, Coope J, Cutler J, et al. Effect of antihypertensive drug treatment on cardiovascular outcomes in women and men. A meta-analysis of individual patient data from randomized, controlled trials. The INDANA Investigators. Ann Intern Med. 1997;126:761–7.

71. Milani RV, Lavie CJ. Prevalence and effects of cardiac rehabilitation on depression in the elderly with coronary heart disease. Am J Cardiol. 1998;81:1233–6.

72. Investigators ENRICHD. Enhancing recovery in coronary heart disease patients (ENRICHD): study design and methods. Am Heart J. 2000;139:1–9.

73. Frasure-Smith N, Lesperance F, Talajic M. Depression following myocardial infarction: impact on 6-month survival. JAMA. 1993;270:1819–25.

74. de Leon CF Mendes, Czajkowski SM, Freedland KE, Bang H, Powell LH, Wu C, et al. The effect of a psychosocial intervention and quality of life after acute myocardial infarction: the Enhancing Recovery in Coronary Heart Disease (ENRICHD) clinical trial. J Cardiopulm Rehabil. 2006;26:9–13.

Chapter 7
Legal Aspects of Geriatric Surgery

Marshall B. Kapp

Abstract The provision of cardiothoracic surgery services to older patients takes place within a pervasive legal environment. It is imperative for health care professionals working in this arena to be conversant with the major legal considerations that affect their activities. This chapter surveys two particular relevant areas of legal regulation. First, it discusses medical malpractice litigation, with special concentration on the legal risks confronted in the realm of cardiothoracic surgery for older persons, focusing on the elements of a negligence claim and how the applicable standard of care is established and proven, with notice of the risk management implications. Next, the chapter reviews the elements of the legal doctrine of informed consent. Particular attention is devoted to the question of decisional capacity in older patients and the various potential types of surrogate decision-making that might be employed when an older patient is not able to make autonomous medical choices personally.

Keywords Law • Ethics • Legal • Malpractice • Informed consent • Litigation • Liability • Competency • Regulation • Negligence • Statutes • Attorneys

Introduction

As is true for other medical specialties, cardiothoracic surgery, including surgery performed on older patients, is extensively regulated in the United States in a variety of ways (although this chapter focuses exclusively on medical practice in the United States, many of the legal and ethical considerations discussed later apply to other countries as well) [1]. Under our federal system, governmental regulation of the actual practice (as opposed to the economics) of cardiothoracic surgery occurs for the most part at the state level, mainly through the activities of state medical boards that enforce the licensure and disciplinary provisions of their respective state Medical Practice Acts [2]. The states regulate medical practice under their inherent police power to protect and promote the health, safety, welfare, and morals of the general population and under their *parens patriae* (or parental) authority to protect individuals (including some older people) who are unable to protect themselves from harm. In addition to government regulation, a number of private entities contribute to the oversight of medical practice through their standard-setting and disciplinary activities [3]. These private bodies include hospital medical staffs [4], specialty certification boards [5], and medical specialty societies [6].

A further source of regulation is the American judicial system, under which the courts may be utilized by individual patients who bring private civil malpractice lawsuits to seek financial compensation from particular surgeons and other health care providers for harms that they have wrongfully caused. Particularly egregious behavior (such as patient abuse) may even subject a health care professional to criminal law punishments.

Information about adverse actions taken by any of these regulatory or quasi-regulatory bodies against a physician is collected in the National Practitioner Data Bank (NPDB). The NPDB is maintained by a private contractor for the federal Department of Health and Human Services pursuant to the Health Care Quality Improvement Act of 1986 [7].

This chapter examines two specific areas of legal regulation affecting the practice of cardiothoracic surgery for older patients. These foci are medical malpractice litigation and informed consent requirements (including the problem of older patients with capacity too impaired to make their own health care decisions).

Medical Malpractice

Chest surgeons are at relatively high risk of being named as defendants in medical malpractice actions [8, 9]. Claims brought by (or on behalf of) cardiothoracic surgery patients

M.B. Kapp (✉)
Florida State University, FSU Center for Innovative Collaboration in Medicine and Law, 1115 West Call Street, Tallahassee, FL 32306-4300, USA
e-mail: kapp@siu.edu

M.R. Katlic (ed.), *Cardiothoracic Surgery in the Elderly*, DOI 10.1007/978-1-4419-0892-6_7,
© Springer Science+Business Media, LLC 2011

often involve allegations of delay in surgery, error in surgical technique [10], and health care-acquired infection [11]. Wrong-site surgery also accounts for many legal claims [12], although this should be much less of a problem in the realm of chest surgery than in some other surgery situations. Their legal apprehensions exert a negative toll on many surgeons, for example discouraging a large number of them from admitting their clinical mistakes and apologizing to patients for them [13].

Elements of a Claim

In a typical malpractice lawsuit based on the tort theory of negligence, the plaintiff/patient must prove each of four essential elements in order for the professional liability to be imposed by the court. Failure to establish any one of these elements defeats the plaintiff's entire claim. The four elements of a prima facie negligence claim are as follows: (a) a duty owed; (b) breach or violation of that duty (negligence); (c) damage or injury; and (d) both factual and legal (proximate) causation [14].

Duty/Standard of Care

The surgeon owes a professional duty only to one with whom that surgeon has established a physician/patient relationship. Within that relationship, the legally enforceable duty owed is one of "due care" or "reasonable care under the circumstances." In the medical context, common law (judge-made law) tort doctrine, which is developed incrementally on a case-by-case basis, and applicable state statutes ordinarily require the physician to have and to use the degree of knowledge and skill that is usually possessed and used by competent similar physicians in the same or similar circumstances [15].

The "similar physicians" whose degree of knowledge and skill set the standard of care against which the defendant's conduct will be measured in any particular case are that defendant's peers – that is, practitioners of the same profession and specialty as the person whose actions are being reviewed. Thus, a thoracic surgeon ordinarily is compared with others practicing thoracic surgery. In almost every jurisdiction today, the standard of care drawn from one's professional peers is formulated on a national, rather than just a local, basis.

Fact-finders (ordinarily a jury, otherwise the judge acting in a fact-deciding capacity as well as a decider of legal questions) must determine the applicable standard of care in any particular case. The fact-finders look to a variety of sources for that standard of care. Customary practice prevailing at the time of treatment among a majority or at least a "respectable minority" of the defendant's peers usually carries substantial, but not necessarily conclusive, weight. Relevant statutes and regulations, especially those relating to professional licensure and discipline, are also a part of the equation, as are voluntarily adopted clinical practice guidelines or parameters [16] and professional codes of ethics [17]. "Voluntary" (but nonetheless potentially admissible into evidence at trial) standards of care may be created by professional organizations [18] or by private accrediting or certifying bodies such as the Joint Commission [19] or the Accreditation Association for Ambulatory Healthcare [20]. Additionally, a hospital's internal policies and procedures may be introduced into evidence to help prove the standard of care to which physicians and others practicing within that hospital should be held legally accountable. Medical journal literature, textbooks (learned treatises), and informational materials for medical devices and drugs approved for physician use on patients by the Food and Drug Administration also may be introduced into evidence for the fact-finder's consideration.

As noted earlier, the legal duty owed by health care professionals is reasonable or due care *under the circumstances*. The circumstances influencing the applicable standard of care certainly include the patient's age and related needs and capacities. The surgeon must be thoroughly sensitive to and knowledgeable regarding the patient's particular age-based characteristics that may affect diagnostic or therapeutic decision making and action for an older patient. For example, a patient's age is likely to exert an impact on which drugs are prescribed, the risks they may pose to the patient (especially concerning polypharmacy), and the proper dosages and routes of administration. Further, the ability to factor the patient's age into calculating the risks of mortality and morbidity of proposed surgical interventions is part of the physician's duty of due care in advising the patient.

In a medical malpractice trial, both parties ordinarily attempt to educate the lay (i.e., not medically trained) fact-finder about their respective versions of the applicable standard of care through the testimony of expert witnesses [21]. First, the judge determines as a matter of law whether a particular preferred witness possesses sufficient credentials to be allowed to testify as an expert and present a professional opinion; usually, it means that expert testimony about the standard of care applicable to the performance of a cardiothoracic surgeon may only be provided by another qualified cardiothoracic surgeon. However, there have been a few exceptions, when general surgeons have convinced judges that they have sufficient expertise to qualify as expert witnesses regarding the practice of cardiothoracic surgery. Potential expert witnesses may be drawn by either party from a national pool, since the standard of care is a national rather than a local one. Once a legal decision has been made to allow the jury to hear the expert testimony of a witness on the standard of care to which the defendant should be held accountable, then it is up to the fact-finder to decide how much weight or credibility to attach to the witness' testimony. Lately, the testimony of expert witnesses (mainly those testifying for plaintiffs) in medical malpractice trials has begun to be scrutinized for accuracy by professional organizations and state medical boards [22].

Breach of Duty

The second necessary element the plaintiff must prove in a negligence-based malpractice lawsuit is a breach or violation of the applicable standard of care – the element of negligence. The concept that a defendant may be held legally liable only when shown to be at fault is fundamental to the traditional American tort system. Although there continues to be proposals made to move the handling of medically-caused patient injuries in the direction of some form of no-fault system [23], fundamental alteration of the existing tort system is unlikely in the foreseeable future.

Negligence may occur in any one of three categories. Nonfeasance is fault happening through inaction or omission – failing to do something that should have been done. Misfeasance consists of performing an act that should have been performed, but doing it in a substandard manner. By contrast, malfeasance is the performance of an act that should not have been done in the first place.

In the surgical context, this means that the surgeon is legally obligated to properly assess the patient before surgery, both in terms of the need for surgery in light of viable alternatives and in terms of the likely risks for that patient. Additionally, the surgeon is expected to perform the actual surgery competently. The duty of due care extends to engaging in reasonable preoperative actions to reduce risks, as well as to competent handling of postoperative care involving somatic problems, pain control, and confusion. After hospital discharge, the patient is entitled to adequate follow up care by the surgeon for a reasonable period of time.

Delineating the legally enforceable standard of care becomes a particularly difficult matter in the murky area of surgical innovation. At present, surgical innovation is treated for malpractice litigation purposes as a species either of generally accepted and practiced therapeutic care, on the one hand, or of biomedical research involving human subjects (with its own extensive, distinct web of regulations) [24], on the other hand. Some commentators have suggested that this approach is fair neither to the patients nor to the practitioners, and instead advocate the development of a third, separate legal standard-setting track for innovative activity that is supported by some – but not yet a conclusive – body of evidence [25].

The surgeon may be held personally liable for the consequences of his or her own negligent acts or omissions.

The surgeon also may be held vicariously liable, under the doctrine of *respondeat superior*, for negligent conduct engaged in by an employee of the surgeon (e.g., a nurse employed to assist in caring for patients in the physician's office) while acting within the scope of the staff member's employment. The longstanding "captain of the ship" doctrine in the past was used to hold the surgeon responsible for the negligence of anyone participating in an operation, on the theory that the surgeon as "captain of the ship" ought to be in charge of – and precluded from delegating away responsibility for – everything occurring during the surgery; thus, for example, under this doctrine liability would be imposed on the surgeon for retained instruments, sponges, and needles forgotten in the patient, even though the nurses (not the surgeons) were the ones who personally erred in counting [26]. Although automatic application of the "captain of the ship" doctrine has been widely discredited today as unrealistic in light of the complexity of the modern operating room, courts will look at the surgeon's right of control over staff members and impose vicarious liability when such a right of control (whether or not it actually is exercised) is present.

Thoracic surgery occurs within a hospital or other corporate (either for-profit or not-for-profit) entity such as an ambulatory surgery center. Many patient injuries (including many of those leading to malpractice litigation) are caused by multifaceted health care delivery system failures, rather than by isolated deficiencies in the knowledge, skills, or character of an individual surgeon or other single members of the health care team [27, 28]. The entity within which the surgery takes place may be sued not just derivatively under a vicarious liability rationale for the acts and omissions of its employees, but also directly under a corporate liability theory for systemic negligence that causes patient injury. Health care institutional providers owe independent duties to their patients, including the duty to properly evaluate and supervise the physicians they employ or to whom they grant clinical admitting and treating privileges [29].

Damage or Injury

For the third requisite element of proof in a malpractice action, the plaintiff must produce sufficient evidence that some damage or injury has taken place. In the cardiothoracic surgery context, virtually all filed claims involve an allegation of physical injury, with severity of injury being the most important single factor influencing the decision to sue. Particularly in claims involving older patients, frequently the patient's death is the injury claimed. Often, claims for emotional injuries (suffering) are raised in conjunction with physical injury complaints.

If a meritorious malpractice claim has been established to the jury's satisfaction (i.e., by a preponderance of the evidence), a judgment is entered by the court and the defendant is ordered to pay a specific amount of money damages to the injured plaintiff. Ordinarily, this financial payment is made by the defendant's liability insurance carrier on the defendant's behalf and is reported to the NPDB as an adverse action relating to that physician [30].

The overwhelming percentage of successful malpractice lawsuits involves the awarding of compensatory damages. These dollars are intended to compensate the victim for his or her injuries, to make the victim "whole" again (to the extent that money can accomplish that objective). Pecuniary (also called economic or special) compensatory damages encompass precisely measurable out-of-pocket expenditures or lost opportunity costs, such as extra medical bills, special equipment needs, and forgone wages. By contrast, nonpecuniary (also known as noneconomic or general) damages encompass real – but more subjective and hard to measure – losses, such as pain and suffering.

Punitive or exemplary damages are over and above compensatory amounts. These are rarely awarded in malpractice cases, because these damages are intended to punish defendants for egregious, intentional wrongs (such as patient abuse), and to set an example to deter others from engaging in similar conduct. Negligence is the theoretical basis for most medical practice lawsuits and, by definition, consists of unintentional wrongdoing; therefore, punitive or exemplary damages would not make much sense in the negligence context. However, it is noteworthy that as a strategic maneuver, plaintiffs sometimes include a request for punitive damages in their complaints solely to be able to introduce before the jury what otherwise would be inadmissible evidence concerning the robust financial status of the defendant.

Causation

Frequently, the most difficult element to prove in a malpractice action is that the injury suffered by the patient was caused by the defendant's negligence. This is an especially big hurdle for many older patients to surmount, because often it can be counter argued by the defendant that any adverse results sustained are the product not of physician (or other health care provider) negligence, but rather the natural and probable consequence of the older patient's underlying illness(es).

First, the plaintiff must establish that the physician's negligence was a cause in fact of the injury. Under this requirement, it must be shown either that "but for" (*sine qua non*) the physician's negligence the injury would not have occurred or, alternatively, that the physician's negligence was at least a substantial factor in bringing about the injury.

Moreover, the plaintiff is required to show that the physician's negligence not only was the factual cause of the injury suffered,

but also that it was the most direct or proximate cause of the injury sustained. That is, there can be no intervening, superceding (i.e., unforeseeable) factors that occur to break the causal link between physician negligence and patient injury. Take, for example, the case of a surgeon who performs an operation improperly. As a result of the surgeon's mistake, it is necessary for the patient to undergo additional surgery the next day. On the way from the patient's hospital room to the operating room, the patient falls out of a wheelchair in which he or she was insecurely tied by an orderly, hits the floor, and suffers additional injuries. The surgeon's error the previous day in the operation would be a cause in fact of the new injuries; "but for" the physician's negligence, the patient would not have been in the process of being transported to the operating room and the injuries would not have happened. However, in this scenario, the physician would not be liable for the additional injuries because the orderly's failure to transport the patient properly was an intervening, superceding (i.e., unforeseeable) event that broke the necessary proximate cause link.

Informed Consent

Under the ethical principle of autonomy or self-determination, every adult patient (with no upper age limit) has the right to make personal decisions regarding medical care, including decisions about which diagnostic and treatment interventions to undergo or decline. This ethical principle has been translated into the legal doctrine of informed consent [31]. In their legal formulation, the substantive parts of informed consent doctrine have evolved over time as a product of state common law. Moreover, the majority of states have enacted statutes and promulgated regulations spelling out a jurisdiction's specific details regarding informed consent. It is important to note that, although the patient has the right to decline a particular suggested diagnostic or therapeutic intervention, there exists no correlative right to demand medical tests or treatments that the physician believes to be worthless or even harmful to the patient; indeed, in such circumstances, the physician has an obligation to refuse to accede to the patient's demand [32].

Elements

For a patient's choice about any specific medical intervention to be considered an ethically and legally valid exercise of informed consent, three distinct but interconnected elements must be present. These elements are voluntariness, knowledge or information, and decisional capacity.

Voluntariness

First, the patient's participation in the decisional making process and the ultimate decision must be voluntary. This means it must take place free of force, fraud, duress, intimidation, or any other form of undue constraint or coercion [33].

Information

Second, the patient's medical choice must be adequately knowledgeable or informed. The physician has the responsibility to communicate in understandable nontechnical terms material information about the patient's medical situation (i.e., information that might make a difference to a reasonable patient). According to well-established legal precedent, as well as pertinent state statutes and regulations, specific data items that need to be shared with the patient include the following: the diagnosis, nature, and purpose of the proposed intervention(s); all reasonably foreseeable risks; the likelihood of success; viable alternatives and their reasonably expected benefits and risks; the result expected if the recommended intervention is declined; and the physician's professional recommendation [34].

There are other pieces of information that some commentators and courts have argued should also be included as part of the informed consent litany, namely: complementary and alternative medicine alternatives, which are increasingly popular with older individuals; the cost implications of the proposed intervention for the patient (an item of importance to many older individuals); the particular physician's personal experience in performing, and success rate with, the specific intervention recommended; other provider-specific information (such as a drug or alcohol dependency problem [35] or the physician's age-related deterioration in physical and/or cognitive performance) [36] that might act as enhanced risk factors; the physician's financial incentives arguably impacting the patient's care; the level of uncertainty in the medical community regarding the particular recommended intervention for someone in this specific patient's situation; and the role, if any, that defensive medicine considerations are playing in the health care provider's treatment proposal.

Commenting upon the informed consent process, one set of physician authors has suggested the following:

> Taking the time to discuss the surgery with the older patients and their families promotes a clearer understanding of risk and benefits and will help to reduce the chance of false expectations with surgery. Incorporating the common geriatric care format of patient and family conferences in the surgical environment can be very helpful. In such discussions, it is often apparent that an older patient has a different outlook and acceptance of a specific level of care. Shorter-term goals, such as the quality, not quantity, of life may be most important. Additionally, the tolerance of surgery may be

different than that of a younger person. The understanding that a longer time to recover may be necessary is often best communicated in this forum. It is also important to inform the patient and family that an intermediate-care program may be needed, such as a subacute care center, a rehabilitation unit, or the extended use of home care services [37].

To understate the matter, there is substantial opportunity for improvement in the information communication part of the informed consent process, which ideally should serve as an educational and bonding, as well as a risk management, role [38]. Available evidence indicates that physicians commonly have a poor, if any, understanding of their legal obligations in this arena, and patients often quite inadequately understand the information provided to them [39].

Decisional Capacity

Valid decisions require that there be a capable decision maker. A patient must be cognitively and emotionally able to weight alternatives rationally; autonomous choices cannot be made by a nonautonomous person. The United States legal system begins with a rebuttable presumption that every adult is capable enough to make his or her own medical decisions if provided with sufficient information.

However, for some geriatric patients, this aspect of medical decision making may be problematic. There is a significant and increasing incidence of dementia, depression and other affective disorders, delirium, and other mental health problems such as psychoses among older individuals [40, 41]. Because the severity of mental illness, in terms of cognitive and behavioral impairment and therefore the illness' impact on functional ability, varies for different patients at different times along a continuum [42, 43], there is not an automatic, precise correlation between an older person's clinical diagnosis and a simple, dichotomous determination that the individual definitively does or does not possess sufficient present capacity to personally make important decisions about medical care.

In every case, the attending physician needs to assess, either formally or informally, the particular patient's decisional capacity [44]. Sometimes collaboration or consultation with a psychologist or psychiatrist in this endeavor can be very helpful [45]. A large amount of well-funded psychological and psychiatric research has been undertaken over the past few decades aimed at developing and disseminating new standardized instruments useful for the specific purpose of reliably measuring decision-specific capacity among older individuals [46, 47]. Nonetheless, there exists no single, uniform, scientifically agreed upon standard of legal competence/decisional capacity for making medical decisions. "Although tests can help to measure the patient's ability to make medical decisions, observing the patient's ability to handle the information given is more valuable, and more important, than administering any test" [48].

Questions that should be included in the physician's tacit or explicit inquiry about a patient's decisional capacity are given below:

1. Can the patient make and communicate (in any manner) any choices regarding medical interventions?
2. Can the patient articulate any reasons for the choices made (to indicate that some sort of reasoning process is taking place)?
3. Are the stated or apparent reasons given to explain the patient's choices rational in the sense that the patient starts with a factually accurate understanding of the medical circumstances and can reason logically from those circumstances to a conclusion?
4. Does the patient understand or appreciate the implications, including the foreseeable personal risks and benefits, of the alternatives presented and choices made?

Several considerations should guide the physician's assessment of a patient's decisional capacity. Most importantly, first, capacity is a matter of whether the patient has at least a minimally sufficient (not necessarily a perfect) degree of functional ability, regardless of the clinical diagnosis (which may be central for the purpose of designing the recommended treatment plan) or whether the physician personally agrees or disagrees with the patient's decision. Second, capacity needs to be determined on a decision-specific basis [49]. A patient may be capable of rationally making certain kinds of decisions but not necessarily others. A decision about undergoing cardiothoracic surgery ordinarily involves an array of complex facets concerning significant potential risks, benefits, and alternatives, and thus requires a relatively high level of cognitive/intellectual and emotional capacity on the patient's part.

Decisional capacity is variable, rather than static, over time in many older patients. It may wax and wane in particular cases depending on the environmental factors, such as time of day (for instance, the sundowning phenomenon in the elderly), day of the week, physical setting, presence of acute or transient treatable medical problems, other persons involved in supporting or pressuring the patient's decision, or the patient's reactions to medications. Physicians often can affect their patients' capacity, for better or worse, through the details of their care (e.g., through the choice and timing of medication administration). Physicians should endeavor to communicate with patients and, when possible, time the actual decision-making process around a patient's windows of lucidity.

Additionally, many older persons may be capable of engaging in assisted consent with extra time and effort on the physician's part, especially if a person has supportive family or friends available. For instance, an older patient who cannot process information as swiftly or easily as a younger person still may be able to sufficiently understand the complexities of a proposed treatment if afforded enough emotional support.

Surrogate Decision Making

Even when a patient is determined by the medical team to lack sufficient present capacity to autonomously make specific necessary decisions about recommended interventions, informed consent principles apply nevertheless. What is different is that decisions must be made for that patient by a surrogate or proxy. The modern trend pertaining to all of the various mechanisms of surrogate decision making has been toward the substituted judgment standard. Under this approach, the surrogate is expected to make the same decisions that the patient would make, according to the patient's own priorities and values to the extent they can be ascertained, if the patient were presently able to make and express his or her own authentic decisions. The subjective substituted judgment standard is most consistent with respect for patient autonomy. When it cannot realistically be ascertained what the now-incapacitated patient would have decided if imbued with adequate present capacity, the surrogate is expected to act in a fiduciary or trust agent role and rely on the historic best interests standard. That test mandates that decisions be made in a manner that, in the surrogate's considered judgment, would confer the most benefit and the least burden on the incapacitated individual.

Formal designation of a surrogate with legal authority to act as the patient's surrogate for medical decision-making purposes may be accomplished through several different channels. These mechanisms are outlined later.

Guardianship/Conservatorship

Creation of a guardianship or conservatorship (the precise terminology varies among jurisdictions) is the most legally definitive means of transferring decision-making power to a surrogate without the patient's permission. It entails appointment by a state court of a surrogate (the guardian/conservator) who is empowered to make certain decisions on behalf of an incompetent person (the ward). This legal process happens in response to a petition filed by the family, a health care facility, a financial institution, the local adult protective services (APS) agency, or another "interested" party. The legal proceeding involves review (usually very swift and deferential) by the court of the sworn affidavit or live testimony of a physician who has examined the alleged incompetent person. Most courts strongly prefer to appoint a family member who is willing and able to act as a guardian/conservator; in the absence of a willing and able family members, however, the court may appoint someone else (such as a close friend) or a public (governmental) guardianship program [50] or volunteer guardianship program if those options are locally available.

Creating total, or plenary, guardianship entails an extensive deprivation of an individual's fundamental personal rights. When a deprivation of rights (such as the right to make one's own medical decisions) is involved, there exists a legal and ethical policy that society should intervene only in the least restrictive or least intrusive manner possible consistent with accomplishing the purpose of the intervention. On the basis of this least restrictive alternative doctrine, limited or partial guardianship/conservatorship is preferred whenever feasible over the plenary variety. In every American jurisdiction, courts have been given the statutory authority to limit a surrogate's power in terms of duration and the types of decisions covered.

Durable Power of Attorney

A person may take steps, while still decisionally capable, to anticipate and prepare for his or her eventual incapacity. The individual may do this by voluntarily delegating or directing future medical decision-making power. The Durable Power of Attorney (DPOA) is a legal document, explicitly authorized by state statute, in which a decisionally capable individual (the principal) privately directs, by appointing an agent (the attorney-in-fact, who need not be an attorney at law), the making of medical decisions in the event of future incapacity. The principal may give the agent general or specific instructions to direct future medical decision making, or may make an unrestricted grant of authority.

The DPOA is distinguishable from the regular or ordinary power of attorney. The latter ordinarily is used to delegate power to make arrangements and take actions regarding financial or property affairs, and the agent's authority expires when the principal becomes decisionally incapacitated. In the medical decision-making sphere, therefore, an ordinary power of attorney is pretty much useless.

DPOAs fall into two categories. An immediate DPOA comes into effect immediately on the naming of an agent. In a springing DPOA, by contrast, the legal authority is transferred ("springs") from the patient/principal to the agent only when some specified future event (such as confirmation of the principal's incapacity by an examining physician) has occurred. DPOAs in both of these categories allow for the transfer of decisional authority to an authorized agent, according to the patient's wishes, without any necessity of court approval or oversight.

Family Authority Statutes

In the absence of judicial appointment of a guardian/conservator or the patient's formal designation of an agent, the longstanding medical custom has been for physicians to turn to family members (when available) to function as surrogates for incapacitated patients. This practice has been codified in more than 30 states by legislative enactment of "family consent" statutes that expressly authorize specific relatives, enumerated in a priority order, to make particular kinds of decisions (including medical decisions) for incapacitated persons. This statutory codification of common practice is based on the assumption that family members generally know best the basic values and preferences of their relatives (thus making substituted judgment possible) or, at the least, will act as trustworthy advocates for their relatives' best interests. However, health care professionals must be alert to possible serious conflicts of interest – financial and otherwise – that can render a relative inappropriate to act as a surrogate decision maker for the patient.

Documentation of Patient or Surrogate Consent

Although implied consent (implied by the patient's compliant conduct) is sufficient for medical interventions that are not very intrusive or risky, surgery ought to be done only when the patient (or the patient's authorized surrogate) has indicated consent to the intervention expressly, and specifically in writing. A signed separate consent form does not by itself constitute compliance with legal requirements; the doctrine of informed consent ideally refers to a dynamic shared decision-making process revolving around information provision and interactive communication between the physician and patient (or surrogate) [51]. A signed consent form does not take the place of the requisite process of communication, but it does facilitate proof that the process took place in the event that the sufficiency of informed consent is challenged after the fact. In addition, voluntary accreditation standards with which the physician's affiliated institution complies, such as those of The Joint Commission, may require the use of separate written consent forms for particular categories of medical interventions, certainly including surgery.

Emergency Exception

In the case of life-threatening emergencies, the law excuses noncompliance with the usual informed consent requirements, on the rationale that we generally presume that a patient confronted with such an emergency would consent (if currently able) to medical interventions necessary to preserve that person's life. Reliance on the emergency exception to dispense with obtaining the voluntary, informed, and capable consent of the patient or surrogate prior to initiating an intrusive and risky medical intervention such as cardiothoracic surgery should be strictly limited to situations in which: there is a true life-threatening medical emergency; time is of the essence and delay will greatly diminish the likelihood of success; the patient is unable at the time to make an autonomous decision about medical care; there is not enough time to identify, locate, and consult with a legally authorized surrogate decision maker; there is insufficient time to apply for a court order; and surgery is the least intrusive and risky alternative for accomplishing the goal of prolonging the patient's life.

Institutional Ethics Committees

Standards of the Joint Commission require that hospitals have a mechanism in place for resolving ethical dilemmas about patient care. Ethical dilemmas may arise regarding the propriety of performing cardiothoracic surgery on a particular older patient, especially if the patient is decisionally incapacitated and either there is no one available to act as a surrogate decision maker or the available surrogate demands a course of action that appears to be inconsistent with the patient's substituted judgment and/or best interests.

One mechanism for addressing such disputes is the institutional ethics committee (IEC). The IEC is an internal, interdisciplinary structure set up to help a health care facility or agency and its professional staff deal with difficult treatment decisions in an ethically acceptable way. IECs vary among institutions and agencies in terms of exact size, composition, structure, processes, activities, and place within the organizational bureaucracy. IECs may be involved in such functions as drafting organizational policies, education of staff and the public, and case consultation on a concurrent or retrospective basis.

The involvement of an IEC in any particular case probably has positive legal benefits for the provider organization and its individual health care professionals. Such involvement may reduce unnecessary guardianship petitions, deter possible lawsuits against the organization and its individual health care professionals, and evidence good faith to bolster the providers' defense against any professional malpractice civil action that might be brought in this context.

Conclusion

Cardiothoracic surgeons, other health care professionals, and the institutions and organizations within which older patients are served inevitably and continuously interact with laws and the legal system. These interactions may concern panoply of pertinent topics (e.g., medical records, confidentiality, living wills, Medicare and other financing programs, and so on). This chapter has surveyed a couple of broad arenas within which such interaction is likely to occur and to directly affect every physician who cares for older patients. For personalized attention and advice in particular circumstances, especially pertaining to the detailed law of a specific jurisdiction, specialized legal consultation should be sought from knowledgeable attorneys in private practice, counsel and or risk managers employed or retained by the institutional health provider, the health care professional's liability insurance carrier, and/or an IEC.

References

1. British Medical Association. The ethics of caring for older people. 2nd ed. Oxford: Wiley-Blackwell; 2009.
2. Federation of State Medical Boards. http://www.fsmb.org. Accessed 6 Oct 2009.
3. Jones JW, McCullough LB, Richman BW. Who should protect the public against bad doctors? J Vasc Surg. 2005;41:907–10.
4. Firestone MH. Medical staff peer review in the credentialing and privileging of physicians. In: Sanbar SS, editor. Legal medicine. 7th ed. Philadelphia: Mosby; 2007. p. 17–22.
5. American Board of Thoracic Surgery. http://www.abts.orb/sections/certification/index. html. Accessed 6 Oct 2009.
6. American Association for Thoracic Surgery. http://www.aats.org. Accessed 6 Oct 2009.
7. 42 U.S.C. § 11101.
8. Studdert DM. Management of avoidance of medical malpractice crises? The to choose. Chest. 2008;134:901–2.
9. Luce JM. Medical malpractice and the chest physician. Chest. 2008;134:1044–50.
10. Elefteriades JA, Barrett PW, Kopf GS. Litigation in nontraumatic aortic diseases – A tempest in the malpractice maelstrom. Cardiology. 2008;109:263–72.
11. Guinan JL, McGuckin M, Shubin V, et al. A descriptive review of malpractice claims for health care-acquired infections in Philadelphia. Am J Infect Control. 2005;33:310–2.
12. Kwaan MR, Studdert DM, Zinner MJ, et al. Incidents, pattern, and prevention of wrong-site surgury. Arch Surg. 2006;141:353–8.
13. Hicks TC. The medical malpractice crisis in surgery. Am J Surg. 2008;195:288–91.
14. Harris DM. Contemporary issues in healthcare law and ethics. 3rd ed. Chicago: Health Administration Press; 2008. p. 188–9.
15. Sanbar SS, Warner J. Medical malpractice overview. In: Sanbar SS, editor. Legal medicine. 7th ed. Philadelphia: Mosby; 2007. p. 253–64.
16. Samanta A, Mello MM, Foster C, et al. The role of clinical guidelines in medical negligence litigation: A shift from the Bolam standard? Med L Rev. 2006;14:321–66.
17. American Medical Association, Council on Ethical and Judicial Affairs. Code of Medical Ethics: Current Opinions With Annotations. 2008-2009 ed. Chicago: American Medical Association; 2008.
18. Agency for Healthcare Quality. National Guideline Clearinghouse. http://www.guideline.gov. Accessed 6 Oct 2009.
19. Joint Commission. http://www.jointcommission.org. Accessed 6 Oct 2009.

20. Accreditation Association for Ambulatory Healthcare. http://www.aaahc.org. Accessed 6 Oct 2009.

21. Satiani B. Expert witness testimony: rules of engagement. Vasc Endovasc Surg. 2006;40:223–7.

22. Bal BS. The expert witness in medical malpractice litigation. Clin Orthop Relat Res. 2009;467:383–91.

23. Barringer PJ, Studdert DM, Kachalia AB, et al. Administrative compensation of medical injuries: a hardy parennial blooms again. J Health Polit Policy Law. 2008;33:725–60.

24. 45 C.F.R. part 46.

25. Mastroianni AC. Liability, regulation and policy in surgical innovation: the cutting edge of research and therapy. Health Matrix. 2006;16:351–442.

26. Jackson S, Brady S. Counting difficulties: retained instrument, sponges, and needles. AORN J. 2009;87:315–21.

27. Morris JA, Carrillo Y, Jenkins JM, et al. Surgical adverse events, risk management, and malpractice outcome: Morbidity and mortality review is not enough. Ann Surg. 2003;237:844–52.

28. Mello MM, Studdert DM. Deconstructing negligence: the role of individual and sytem factors in causing medical injuries. Georgetown L J. 2008;96:599–623.

29. Krizek TJ. The impaired surgical resident. Surg Clin North Am. 2004;84:1587–604.

30. Nepps ME. The basics of medical malpractice: a primer on navigating the system. Chest. 2008;134·1051–5.

31. White C, Rosoff AJ, LeBlang TR. Informed consent to medical and surgical treatment. In: Sanbar SS, editor. Legal medicine. 7th ed. Philadelphia: Mosby; 2007. p. 337–43.

32. Hafemeister TL, Gulbrabdsen Jr RM. The fiduciary obligation of physicians to "just say no" if an "informed" patient demands services that are not medically indicated. Seton Hall L Rev. 2009;39:335–86.

33. Garrison M. The empire of illness: competence and coercion in health-care decision making. William Mary Law Rev. 2007;49:781–843.

34. Showalter JS. The law of healthcare administration. 5th ed. Chicago: Health Administration Press; 2008.

35. Park S. A physician's drug use and the duty to disclose provider problems: Why patients should not be treated like houses. J Legal Med. 2009;30:387–407.

36. Blasier RB. The problem of the aging surgeon: when surgeon age becomes a surgical risk factor. Clin Orthop Relat Res. 2009;467:402–11.

37. Malani PN, Vaitkevicius PV, Orringer MB. Perioperative evaluation and management. In: Halter JB, Ouslander JG, Tinetti, et al., editors. Hazzard's geriatric medicine and gerontology. 6th ed. New York: McGraw-Hill; 2009. p. 407–16, 409–10.

38. Brenner LH, Brenner AT, Horowitz D. Beyond informed consent: educating the patient. Clin Orthop Relat Res. 2009;467:348–51.

39. Larobina ME, Merry CJ, Negri JC, et al. Is informed consent in cardiac surgery and percutaneous coronary intervention achievable? ANZ J Surg. 2007;77:530–4.

40. Rosenberg I, Woo D, Roane D. The aging patient with chronic schizophrenia. Ann Longterm Care. 2009;17:20–4.

41. Luijendijk HJ, van den Berg JF, Dekker MJHJ, et al. Incidence and recurrence of late-life depression. Arch Gen Psychiatry. 2008;65:1394–401.

42. Hachinski V. Shifts in thinking about dementia. JAMA. 2008;300:2172–3.

43. Okonkwo O, Griffith HR, Belue K, et al. Medical decision-making capacity in patients with mild cognitive impairment. Neurology. 2007;69:1528–35.

44. Appelbaum PS. Assessment of patients' competence to consent to treatment. N Eng J Med. 2007;357:1834–40.

45. Moye J, Karel MJ, Armesto JC. Evaluating capacity to consent to treatment. In: Goldstein AM, editor. Forensic psychology: emerging topics and expanding roles. Hoboken: Wiley; 2007. p. 260–93.

46. Lai JM, Gill TM, Cooney LM, et al. Everyday decision-making ability in older persons with cognitive impairment. Am J Geriatr Psychiatry. 2008;16:693–6.

47. Chodosh J, Edelen MO, Buchanan JL, et al. Nursing home assessment of cognitive impairment: development and testing of a brief instrument of mental status. J Am Geriatr Soc. 2008;56:2069–75.

48. Drickamer MA, Lai JM. Assessment of decisional capacity and competencies. In: Halter JB, Ouslander JG, Tinetti, et al., editors. Hazzard's geriatric medicine and gerontology. 6th ed. New York: McGraw-Hill; 2009. p. 171–6, 174.

49. Moberg PJ, Rick JH. Decision-making capacity and competency in the elderly: a clinical and neuropsychological perspective. NeuroRehabilitation. 2008;23:403–13.

50. Teaster PB, Wood EF, Lawrence SA, et al. Wards of the state: a national study of public guardianship. Stetson Law Rev. 2007;37:193–240.

51. Karlawish JHT, James BD. Ethical issues. In: Halter JB, Ouslander JG, Tinetti ME, et al., editors. Hazzard's geriatric medicine and gerontology. 6th ed. New York: McGraw-Hill; 2009. p. 399–406.

Chapter 8
Ethical Issues in Cardiothoracic Surgery for the Elderly

Susan M. Hecker and Robert M. Sade

Abstract This is a time of turmoil in the United States health care system. Political discussions center mostly around financial issues, but these issues have serious implications for the elderly population, the fastest growing segment of the general population. What will be done with Medicare is still unknown at this time, but whatever is done will have great impact on health care for the elderly. Information gathered over the last 1–2 decades indicates clearly that cardiothoracic surgery in the elderly is associated with outcomes, including mortality and resource use, that is little different from that of the younger people – higher mortality rates are associated with comorbidities, more frequent in older individuals, not with age. There is a temptation to discount the remaining few years of life of people who have already lived out most of their days, but how is one to determine the value of one life over another?

General ethical problems that affect everyone have particular relevance to the elderly. For example, it is more important for elderly individuals to execute advance directives, as the potential for needing them is closer at hand than it is for younger people. The elderly are more likely to refuse curative care, and when little more can be done for their diseases, they will have need for palliative care. Perioperative management must be much more meticulous in the elderly for both technical and ethical reasons; for example, preoperative planning for changing the goals of treatment if serious complications occur is especially important if we are to avoid marching along the road to futility. The high incidence of dementia in the elderly also raises questions of decision-making capacity when the need for surgery arises, or when they are asked to participate as patient-subjects in clinical investigations. Although there are special ethical concerns for individuals over the age of 70 or 80 years, when they present with a cardiothoracic surgical problem, they become our patients and deserve the best that we can offer them.

R.M. Sade (✉)
Division of Cardiothoracic Surgery, Medical University of South Carolina, 25 Courtenay Drive, Suite 710, Charleston, SC 29425, USA
e-mail: sader@musc.edu

Keywords Ethics • Bioethics • Health care • Philosophy of medicine • Geriatrics • Elderly patients • Cardiothoracic surgery in the elderly • Health care reform • Ancient Greek philosophy • Euthanasia • Physician-assisted suicide • Technological imperative • Health care rationing • Palliative care • Palliative sedation • Medical decision making • Ethics of transplantation • Surrogate decision

> Life is a moderately good play with a badly written third act.
> – Truman Capote.
> In youth we run into difficulties. In old age difficulties run into us.
> – Beverly Sills.

Introduction

Contemporary discourse on the ethics of health care for the elderly has been driven by political partisanship, particularly in the highly publicized attempts by Congress to reform health care. Debate about the rational use of limited health care dollars has degenerated into polemics about greedy insurance and drug companies, negligent physicians, death panels, and socialized medicine, pitting "individual choice" against the "greater good" and feeding fears of lack of access to health care with the uncertainties of growing old and debilitation. As health care sector expenditures move closer to consuming 20% of the US Gross Domestic Product, many seek a framework for understanding how individual needs and wants can be satisfied within the bounds of reasonably available resources. Some see equitable distribution of limited resources as the goal of reform, while others claim that maximizing individual freedom and responsibility is the goal. Arising from those broad goals are myriad disparate strategies. Are health care dollars better spent on prevention to reduce the scourge of disease for the many while reducing or eliminating "big ticket" treatments for the few? Do we pay for all diagnostic tests ordered defensively by litigation-sensitive physicians and by technology-oriented house officers until the well of health care dollars runs dry?

What stage of life should be the focus of health care policy? Perhaps it should be childhood, for our children are the future of our nation and arguably deserve the best of care. For some childhood problems, however, the care can be atrociously expensive and of questionable value, as in the case of the premature neonate with grade IV intracerebral hemorrhage and perforated viscus, who languishes for months in the neonatal intensive care unit, destined for repeated expensive hospitalizations. Alternatively, adult heads of households support families both financially and emotionally–should they be the focal point? The elderly lie at the distant end of the life-stage spectrum. In many ways, they seem to be the least likely candidates for our attention, because they have lived their lives, so perhaps should give way to younger people who have a great deal more living to do.

Consideration of health care for the elderly raises many questions. At what age does one enter elderhood? For that matter, is chronological age a proper factor in medical decision making? In a centrally managed health care system, should policy makers weigh medical needs and associated costs against the elderly's personal resources? In a free-market-based system, individuals decide what services to buy and how much to spend, but should that be allowed in the market for health care? How much should we spend to maintain the quality of life of a septua-, octa-, or nonagenarian? Should any resources at all be expended on the very old for curative care, or should only palliative care be offered after a certain age, as some have proposed? [1]. How do we decide whether to expend X dollars to add an additional 5 years to the end of a long life rather than to spend those X dollars to save, extend, or improve the lives of those in the middle or at the beginning of life? At a more fundamental level, when we ask questions in the first person plural, who is the "we" we are talking about – the vague, shadowy entity we call society, government at the national or some other level, public and private institutions such as hospitals and insurance companies, or we as individuals? [2].

Politicians frame the moral dilemmas facing the health care system in terms of limited financial resources, but the ethical foundations of health care are broader and deeper than suggested by that narrow focus. Financial obligations are largely a contemporary concern and do not define the whole or even a substantial part of health care ethics. The complex reality is this: philosophers have continually refined notions of health, illness, and the obligations of physicians since antiquity. The ancient Greeks emphasized the nature of health and illness, how one should think about them, and what should be the appropriate responses to their various manifestations. Physicians of that time had more theories than prognostic judgment, more prognostic judgment than diagnostic acumen, and more diagnostic acumen than effective treatment. They expended less effort in treating illness

and avoiding death than on prognostication and helping patients to face inevitable mortality. Yet, much in ancient philosophy is relevant today. Perhaps particularly pertinent in considering problems related to the elderly and their situation in life is the philosophy of Stoicism.

Epictetus was a first-century former slave who studied Stoicism and became one of its best-known proponents. For him, death in and of itself is neither good nor bad – it is "an indifferent" [3] (see Fig. 8.1). There is no intrinsic value, positive or negative, in becoming ill or dying. Illness strikes and the patient suffers. Little could be done to arrest this process, so emphasis was on how one should face inevitable disability and death. As a former slave, Epictetus saw clearly that much is outside the control of both the well and the sick. He saw that a key to happiness lay in understanding the difference between those things we can control and those we cannot.

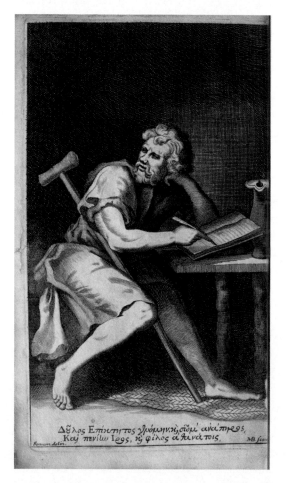

Fig. 8.1 Portrait of Epictetus, from engraved frontispiece of Edward Ivie's Latin translation of Epictetus' Enchiridon, printed in Oxford in 1751. The subscription is an epigram from the Anthologia Palatina (VII 676) and reads: "I was Epictetus the slave, and not sound in all my limbs, and poor as Irus, and beloved by the gods" (Irus is the beggar in the Odyssey) (this image is in the Public Domain; see http://commons. wikimedia.org/wiki/File:Epicteti_Enchiridion_Latinis_versibus_ adumbratum_(Oxford_1715)_frontispiece.jpg)

Focusing on events outside our sphere of influence is exhausting, futile, and leads to unhappiness. We cannot change the inevitability of death; we can only hope to influence how we react when it is imminent. To face the end with courage and forbearance is better than attempting to evade it. Even suicide holds value to the ancient Greeks. Epictetus saw suicide as a window that could be left open, an option to combat the fear or pain of a turbulent end. He cautioned against ending one's life as if one were a capricious child who casts aside a toy when it becomes boring. Life should not be lightly relinquished, but sometimes knowing that the manner or timing of one's end is in one's control can mitigate the unhappiness of illness and the fear of death, a viewpoint held today by those who support assisted suicide [4].

Euthanasia was viewed differently, however. Pythagoras vehemently proscribed the spilling of blood, and Hippocrates famously promoted the concept of avoiding harm when treating patients (see Fig. 8.2). Actively seeking the death of a patient was prohibited, regardless of the worthiness of the underlying intent. To participate in taking another's life would irreparably shatter the foundational trust required by the physician–patient relationship. The potential for abuse of such power would subsequently call into question the character of the physician. Thus, the prescribed behavior of physicians was firmly anchored in treating patients in the best manner possible and avoiding disproportionate harm at all

costs. These views of the ancients capture aspects of human nature and the human condition that have not changed over millennia and continue to guide contemporary physicians in their approaches to illness and death.

The straightforward view of medical ethics by ancient philosophers persists today in the many variations on the themes of the Hippocratic Oath recited by graduating medical students. Over the course of the twentieth century, however, ethics in the health care field has become much more complex. Several subdisciplines of ethics in the health-related professions can be distinguished: bioethics, which broadly addresses relationships among biological sciences, medicine, politics, law, philosophy, and theology; global ethics, which links biology, ecology, medicine, and human values; clinical ethics, which narrowly relates to appropriate care of patients; and medical ethics, which even more narrowly speaks to the professional conduct of physicians.

In the second half of the twentieth century, explosions in scientific discoveries about human physiology and pathological processes and in technologies used to expand our diagnostic and therapeutic capabilities have dramatically changed health-related ethics. Among the most important changes seen in the physician–patient relationship – it is no longer dyadic, as third parties are ubiquitous in health care. Physicians must plan diagnostic strategies, arrange consultations, and implement evidence-based care in the context of multidisciplinary teams, in which responsibilities are frequently diffused.

A convenient way to think about ethics is in terms of principles that can be used to identify and resolve ethical issues; a commonly used set of such principles are the four principles advanced by Beauchamp and Childress, which some have called the Georgetown Mantra: respect for persons, or respect for autonomy, beneficence, nonmaleficence, and justice [5]. These were originally articulated as three rather than four principles (a view we prefer), because beneficence and nonmaleficence were seen as two sides of the beneficence coin in the 1979 Belmont Report, discussed later in this chapter. *Respect for persons* centers around an individual's autonomy, or self-determination, the ability to decide for oneself a course of action. *Beneficence* comprises complementary principles, maximization of benefits, and minimization of harms to the patient. When making decisions for patients, the benefits/harms ratio should always be positive, and the greater the ratio, the better. *Justice* is more difficult to define, because there are many different (and often incompatible) understandings of what justice is. The concept most frequently used in contemporary ethics is distributive justice, or fairness in distributing health care goods and services. This view has been rejected by many – for example, on pragmatic utilitarian grounds [6] and on libertarian grounds [2] – but persists in bioethical and political discussions and debates.

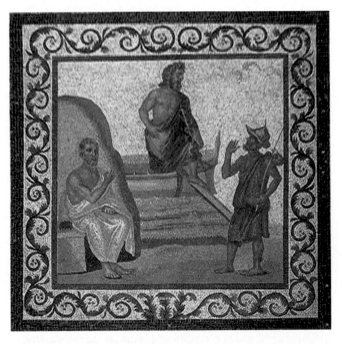

Fig. 8.2 Depiction of Asclepius (*center*) visiting Kos, Hippocrates (*left*), a person from Kos (*right*); floor mosaic, "Kos, Asclepeion" (photo by Dr. Phil. Heinz Schmitz; Creative Commons Attribution ShareAlike 2.5 License; see http://commons.wikimedia.org/wiki/File:HSAsclepiusKos_retouched.jpg)

Further Considerations of Illness and Death in Old Age

Personhood

Who are we during the final stages of our lives, should we be fortunate enough to reach an advanced age? Our notion of self is tied to our achievements and failures, the virtues we have inculcated in ourselves, and the values we have gained and lost. Our selves are determined by the careers from which we have retired or the compilation of jobs that composed our economic lives. We have worked hard, exchanged goods and services with others, and paid taxes. We are members of a family and have loved, married, produced, and reared children from infancy through high school or college education, and have taken pride in being a child, sibling, and parent of loved ones. To a large extent, we have made ourselves into the persons we are, in the context of the social nexus in which we have lived our lives [7].

How we think and act is a product of our choices and experiences and of our conception of ourselves within the world around us [8]. Throughout life, both our world and we ourselves change as we encounter new experiences and adapt to them. As we age, mental acuity declines, yet we can still make choices that correspond with the general character of our prior intact life. Autonomy should be respected, even when decision-making capacity is somewhat diminished. Rarely if ever does dementia stand still, with time, loss of mental acuity progresses most rapidly in those suffering from dementia. Eventually, with increasingly severe loss of mental capacity, the person becomes different from her former self, and begins to make decisions that are incongruous with her life-long character, values, and patterns of decision making. Choices may become random, aimless, and contradictory. At this point, the person has lost the capacity for self-determination that the principle of respect for autonomy is meant to protect. Her ability to achieve her own goals – goals that may no longer exist at all – and participate in life's ordinary activities has been lost. The obligation of others to respect the current choices of the demented person has evaporated – respect for her autonomy must now be expressed through a surrogate.

The Technology Pendulum

As we have noted, Epictetus wrote that the key to happiness is to focus and act upon events that are within our control, and simply accept the events we cannot control. Death can be faced honorably, nobly, and peacefully [3]. For some, death is too great an insult to be easily accepted, whereas for others it comes easily upon the heels of a full life. Western culture has engaged in a struggle against death with an increasingly complex array of treatments and interventions, based upon advancing medical knowledge and technology. The military metaphor of medicine as a war against disease and death has ancient roots, but was reinvigorated in 1971 when President Nixon proclaimed a war on cancer in his State of the Union address, and signed the "National Cancer Act" [9]. Our therapeutic arsenal consisted of aggressive surgical attacks, chemotherapeutic weapons whose toxic side effects had not yet been defeated, and radiation therapies that left patients scarred inside and out (and ironically increased the risk of other malignancies later in life). The later 1970s saw a generalized softening of attitudes and increased interest in such options as alternative medicine and palliative care, redirecting patients' attention from cure to comfort.

The late twentieth and early twenty-first centuries have seen the pendulum swing back toward technologically intense interventions. Several factors have contributed to this effect: therapeutic alternatives have expanded because of new diagnostic modalities, improved chemotherapeutic agents with fewer side effects, advanced surgical techniques, and better postoperative care. In addition, the pharmaceutical industry is at the forefront of medical care; elderly patients are very frequently taking an array of medications to treat their many medical problems.

Rationing Health Care for the Elderly

A particularly controversial view of technological progress has been expressed by Daniel Callahan, an elder statesman of the philosophy of medicine. He argues that we, as a society, have become too captivated by technology and have failed to recognize an important truth: "Aging is a part of life, not just another medical obstacle to overcome" [10]. He has criticized the views that public entitlement programs, specifically, Medicare, should be blind to age and should pay for health care of the elderly by the same standards as everyone else [1]. After achieving certain public policy goals, such as universal health care, curative care should be denied to everyone after a certain age, he says; only palliative care should be offered. He estimated the age at which curative care should no longer be offered to be somewhere in the late 70s or early 80s years of life, based on a "natural life span," which he takes to be an average age at which most people had lived an adequately though not necessarily completely full life.

Callahan's idea of rationing based on age generated a storm of criticism – over 100 critical papers appeared over the next several years – leading to a second edition of the book that added that the subtitle, "With A Response to My Critics" [11]. In this book, he observed that there had been a great deal of success in developing treatments for a variety of illnesses common in the elderly, but the successes were creating the problem of too much technology, so what was needed was "radically slowing up and eventually plateauing the forward march of expensive medical progress." Considering the principles of respect for persons, beneficence, and justice, Callahan's view falls outside of all three: it respects the autonomy of neither patients nor physicians, brings net harms rather than benefits to elderly patients, and treats the elderly unequally.

Palliative Care

Rational goals for optimal medical care are variable and contingent. Whether a patient is deemed to be in the throes of a terminal decline or is merely old, the goals of care may undergo a subtle change. Seeking the next potential cure may become less urgent and its place gradually taken by comfort measures. Instead of the next round of chemotherapy or surgical resection, it is ethically permissible, even laudable, to focus on relieving pain and adequately treating depression. When the patient or family has chosen to redefine the parameters of care, changing from the goal of cure to that of comfort, many options become available. For patients with pain or psychic distress, various kinds and levels of analgesia and sedation can help. Nourishment at the end of live can be provided in a variety of ways. Comprehensive palliative care is multifactorial, whether the need arises from dementia, terminal illness, or simply the gradual decline of old age.

The medical care of patients with dementia is unique, in part because it is a progressive and incurable disease but is not necessarily terminal. The prevalence of dementia is increasing because longevity is increasing. At this time, roughly 1 in 8 persons over 65 years of age suffer from Alzheimer's disease at various stages. The diagnosis is made in a new patient every 70 s. By 2050, new diagnoses will be made every 30 s, because by then over 21% of the population will be older than 65 years of age [12]. The increasing number of the elderly and the reality that dementia inexorably leads both to loss of self-determination and to a requirement for long-term care demonstrate the importance of planning for long-term care, at both the individual and the policy levels.

Planning for decline of decision-making capacity is difficult for individuals because it is difficult to conceive of being incapacitated and thereby to make decisions for an uncertain future. Video depictions of dementia may assist patients in advance care planning by depicting the actual care required, leading to better understanding of the nature of the disease, the care it requires, and less uncertainty about their wishes for future care. In a recent study, after viewing such a video, most individuals opted for comfort care, a small number chose limited care, and no patient chose life-prolonging care when faced with severe dementia [13].

Other Palliative Care Options

When redefining goals as the end of life approaches, other options may allow individuals to deal with pain and anxiety and, in Epictetus' sense, to take control of suffering into their own hands. These options include voluntarily stopping eating and drinking (VSED), palliative sedation, and physician-assisted suicide (PAS) [14]. A mentally competent person who is able physically to take oral nutrition may elect VSED and simply resist eating and drinking. Death comes gradually in 1–3 weeks, by way of dehydration; the more prolonged deaths occur in those who continue to drink fluids. Under those conditions, VSED requires no assistance from caregiver or physician, only the resolve of the patient; under the principle of respect for persons, this is an ethically sound position. Several concerns about VSED remain, however. Hunger or thirst may temporarily increase discomfort, but usually appetites are suppressed in the infirm, and hunger and thirst dissipate. The extended time until death, however, may be unbearable if severe pain, nausea, or anxiety is a prominent feature.

Palliative sedation can be an invaluable tool for end-of-life care when unrelieved distress clouds the patient's last days. There are three levels of sedation [15]. *Ordinary sedation* is used when the patient is normally conscious; sedatives are administered until noxious symptoms abate and the patient is comfortable. The level of adequate sedation is maintained, and if consciousness wanes, doses are reduced or medications changed to preserve awake interaction with reduced anxiety. *Proportionate palliative sedation* for intractable suffering is the next higher level; it is often used to remove the last trace of distress before death. *Palliative sedation to unconsciousness* is the most controversial level of sedation, because the primary goal is unconsciousness, which is an unintended side effect of the other sedation strategies. For severe physical symptoms such as bleeding or an inability to manage oral secretions or "suffering that is predominantly existential or due to the dying patient's need for control," the level of sedation is increased until the patient becomes unresponsive and is kept at that level until death occurs.

VSED and palliative sedation are relatively commonly used for end-of-life care in hospice, but PAS, in which the physician prescribes a lethal dose of a drug, often a barbiturate, is illegal in all states except Oregon and Washington [16]. Although the physician provides the drug, the act of ingesting the lethal dose is completely voluntary. For some, the simple act of having an "outlet" available is enough to regain a modicum of control and comfort. PAS requires that the patient be physically capable of ingesting all of the prescribed pills and absorbing them, because if not, incomplete sedation could occur, and the patient might not die quietly and comfortably as desired, but instead be taken to a hospital for additional unwanted interventions.

PAS generates several ethical dilemmas. Yale Kamisar, a long-time opponent of legalizing PAS on legal grounds, describes three kinds of opposition to PAS [17]. The first posits that PAS is inherently morally wrong. Long-accepted ethical principles state clearly that physicians must not purposely harm patients without compensatory benefits. The second objection is that the relationship between the physician and patient will be fatally compromised if PAS were legalized, because assisting patients in death could foster distrust and misgivings among family members, and physicians could become uncertain of their role as sustainers of life, now become messengers of death. The third camp opposes PAS on grounds of a potential legal slippery slope. Even if an individual case is emotionally compelling, the consequences of legalization are dangerous because a law that begins as a final option for terminally ill patients in uncontrollable pain or suffering may eventually be applied to vulnerable people or those who are not yet truly at life's end. In other words, legalizing PAS opens the door to euthanasia. A fourth position has been offered: PAS is wrong for the first three reasons, but assisted suicide by nonphysicians might not be [18].

Ethical issues posed by the aging process range widely. Contemporary clinical ethics arose from controversies involving human experimentation in the mid-twentieth century, as we will discuss later. Its emphasis on the principles of autonomy, beneficence, and justice requires that patients be given enough information about proposed research or medical interventions to provide informed consent, that the benefits of the research or the medical interventions outweigh the risks, and that the distribution of benefits and burdens is just and equitable. Thus far we have mainly focused upon self-determination and the difficulties inherent in an elderly population, especially given the prevalence of dementia in that group. There are times, however, when the elderly require active care for general medical or surgical problems or cardiothoracic surgical diseases. When the end of life is not imminent, palliation is not an option and decisions must be made about the extent of care to be offered.

Cardiothoracic Surgery in the Elderly

Health care is not intended simply to return the patient to some status quo ante, but to enhance quality of life, understood as including restoration of the vibrancy that was associated with an earlier stage of life [19]. Few medical specialties can enhance quality of life more consistently than cardiothoracic surgery, which often offers the elderly a chance to regain lost vigor. The common thread that emerges from various pathological features of cardiac valve and coronary artery diseases is the patient's inexorable symptomatic decline. Activity levels diminish until quality of life suffers from an inability to participate in the daily activities that make life meaningful. Unlike the degenerative processes of aging, most cardiac diseases are related to a mechanical problem, and once the faulty mechanisms are repaired, bypassed, or replaced, patients fare better. Much encouraging information has become available within the last 20 years on cardiothoracic interventions in the elderly. For octogenarians, the primary goal of cardiac surgery is not longevity; rather, the primary goals are safety, survival, and the "gain of comfort in daily life" [20]. Postoperative quality of life in a study of 136 octogenarians undergoing open heart surgery was generally good: 81% had little to no disability and 93% were symptom-free or nearly so. During a 2½-year average follow-up, 97% of survivors lived either in their own homes or with family. Quality of life in nonagenarians after cardiac surgery is the same as that of an age and disease matched population [21]. The effects of lung surgery on physiological and mental measures of quality of life are not different between elderly and younger patients [22, 23].

Survival after repair of aortic dissections in the elderly in recent reports have been good; operative survival and midterm postoperative survival of patients 70 years of age or older has been comparable with those of patients less than 70 [24] (see Fig. 8.3). In a study that compared operative and nonoperative management of type A dissections in octogenarians surgical repair was associated with lower hospital mortality, but the 5-year survival was the same as those managed medically [25]. This was partly due to decreased physical and mental functioning postoperatively, including intellectual capacity that led postoperatively to an elevated incidence of pneumonia, sepsis, stroke, and complications

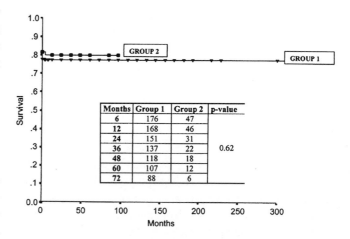

Months	Group 1	Group 2	p-value
6	176	47	
12	168	46	
24	151	31	
36	137	22	0.62
48	118	18	
60	107	12	
72	88	6	

Fig. 8.3 Kaplan-Meier survival curves for patients undergoing repair of aortic dissections, less than 70 years of age (Group 1) and patients 70 or older (Group 2), showing that operative and mid-term postoperative survival was not significantly different between the two groups (reprinted with permission from Chiappini et al. [24], Copyright Elsevier 2004)

from remaining bedridden. Patients survived the surgery, but the relatively poor functional level was not anticipated by patients or their families, who generally believed that benefits of successful surgical management of the dissection paled in comparison to the harms of formerly independent patients sliding into "dementia and diapers" [26].

In general, survival of the very old with life-threatening cardiothoracic disease is better with surgery than without. For example, aortic valve replacement for severe aortic stenosis leads to a much better prognosis than does medical management in patients over 80 years of age: survival with and without valve replacement at 1, 2 and 5 years is 87, 78, and 68% vs. 52, 40, and 22%, respectively [27]. Similar results have been reported by others [28]. Selected nonagenarians who underwent open-heart surgery had a mean survival rate of 5.1 years after surgery and an actuarial survival rate of 67% at 3 years, as good or better than a matched population (see Fig. 8.4).

In elderly patients, early postoperative delirium ranges between 5 and 21%, and after the acute phase, ability to concentrate, memory, and restful sleep suffer [29, 30]. Although cognitive activity often declines after cardiac operations, quality of life is frequently better postoperatively than it was preoperatively [27, 31–33] (see Fig. 8.5). Social support is a positive factor in postoperative recovery. The 6-month mortality rate is lower in elderly patients who have good social or religious attachments than in those who do not have such attachments [34]. Some character traits have a beneficial effect on postoperative quality of life; they include a take-charge

attitude and general optimism. After coronary bypass operations, patients are generally happier, more energetic, more able to perform strenuous activity, and less limited in social interactions than they were preoperatively [33].

The literature on cardiothoracic surgery in the elderly discloses a prevailing theme of greater risk in the elderly than in younger patients. The older the patient, the greater the incidence of comorbidities that increase operative risk; when more risk factors are present, the number of postoperative complications rises, resulting in greater length of stay and total cost of hospitalization [35–37]. Preoperative risk factors for death after valve operations include low ejection fraction, preoperative renal insufficiency, stroke, chronic obstructive pulmonary disease, and renal failure [27, 28, 38, 39], while preoperative predictors of mortality after repair of aortic dissection are new neurologic deficits, cardiac tamponade, shock, and hemodynamic instability at presentation [24, 25, 40] (see Fig. 8.6). Preoperative risk factors for death after coronary artery bypass operations include congestive heart failure on admission, recent myocardial infarction, low ejection fraction, unstable angina, acute renal failure, chronic lung disease, diabetes, and hypertension [41–43]. These risk factors are substantially more prevalent in the elderly population than in younger populations.

A recurring theme in the surgical literature is that older patients are often not offered operations for heart disease until cardiac symptoms have increased, ventricular function has decreased, and the risk of morbidity and mortality has escalated [28, 43, 44]. This fact has led to the conclusion that increased morbidity and mortality rates that have been observed in older age groups in the past are related more closely to comorbidities than to age. In fact, many studies have demonstrated that age alone is not an independent predictor of mortality for several different kinds of cardiothoracic operations [24, 25, 28, 38, 42, 43].

Postoperative complications of cardiothoracic surgery in the elderly are stronger risk factors for hospital death than preoperative comorbidities [45]. Thus, careful preoperative planning, meticulous operative technique, and attentive postoperative care are critically important to optimize survival of the elderly after cardiothoracic surgery. Special steps can be taken to reduce perioperative complications in this age group, taking into account difference in physiology of the elderly compared with younger people and higher rates of comorbidities. In cardiac surgery, epiaortic ultrasound can determine the amount and location of atherosclerotic plaque in the ascending aorta, permitting accurate cannulation to avoid cerebral embolism, and selection of suitable locations for anastomoses [46]. Postoperative strategies for better outcomes in cardiothoracic surgery include maintaining hematocrits higher than 30%, aggressive early extubation, ambulation, and dedicated physical therapy [21].

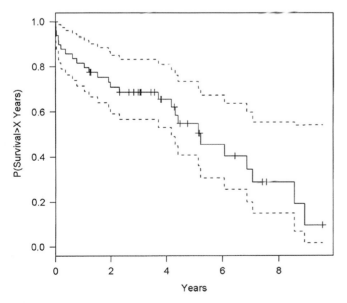

Fig. 8.4 Survival curve (*solid lines, dashed lines* 95% CI) using Kaplan–Meier estimates for 49 nonagenarians who underwent cardiac surgical procedures. Average survival after surgery was 5.1 years (reprinted with permission from Ullery et al. [21], Copyright Elsevier 2008)

Fig. 8.5 Octogenarians in this Swedish study of quality of life after open-heart surgery scored as well or better than the Swedish normal population matched by age and gender. Mean (95% CI) scores for patients who underwent open-heart surgery compared to Swedish normal population matched by age and gender (scores: minimum score = 0; maximum score = 100) (reprinted from Collins et al. [31], Copyright 2002, with permission from Elsevier)

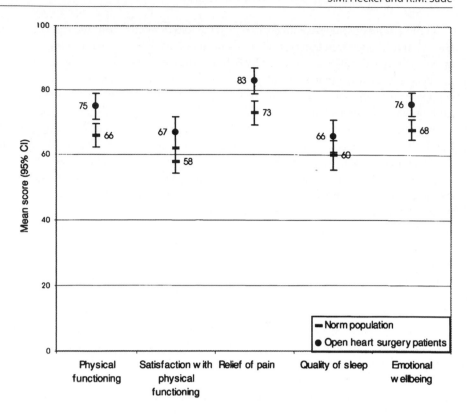

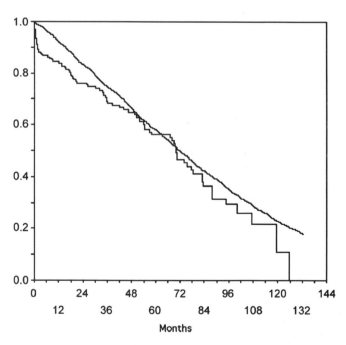

Fig. 8.6 Actuarial survival curve of 215 octogenarians (mean age 83 years) after aortic, mitral, or double valve surgery, compared with same age general population. Mean survival was 84% after 1 year and 56% after 5 years (reprinted from Collart et al. [39], Copyright 2005, with permission from Elsevier)

Preoperative assessment is more important in the elderly than in any other age group, in light of the frequency of comorbid conditions, which often presents atypically so are

less obvious than in younger patients, and compromised capacity for recovery of physiological homeostasis after surgical trauma [47]. Risk assessment prior to heart or lung surgery is also necessary; an instrument is available for assessing cardiac risk [48], and pulmonary risk should be assessed with a series of tests, including spirometry, pulmonary diffusing capacity of the lung for carbon monoxide, room air arterial blood gas, and exercise tolerance tests [47]. Assessment of cognitive function is also of great importance, because elderly patients with dementia, as measured by the mini-mental status examination (MMS), who undergo thoracic surgery, suffer four times the postoperative complication rate of the others [49].

Heart Transplantation in the Elderly

Organ transplantation presents an especially difficult set of ethical problems because organs for transplantation are one of the few truly scarce medical resources. Each year, 6,000–9,000 patients die in the US because of the insufficient number of organs to go around [50]. One of the most difficult and wrenching tasks required of the United Network for Organ Sharing (UNOS) is to develop algorithms for the allocation of organs, knowing that when someone receives an organ, someone else will die because she did not get it.

Three general ethical principles are relevant to organ allocation: autonomy, utility, and justice. Autonomy refers to respect for the decisions individuals make for themselves; utility refers to making choices that provide a net benefit to a community; and justice refers to ensuring that the allocation system is equitable and fair. Unfortunately, when considering various allocation options, these principles often come into conflict, especially utility and justice. The conflict becomes evident when one considers whether a donated heart should be transplanted into a recipient who is 75-years old. A utilitarian will point out that the 75-year old woman has, probably, another 5–10 years to live, while the heart could continue to function for another 20 years, so it would be better to transplant the heart into a younger person who has at least 20 or more years of life expectancy, thus avoiding the waste of 10 years of a functioning heart. The justice-minded will assert that it is not fair to discriminate against a 75-year-old because her life is just as precious as anyone else's, and there is no way of knowing whether she will live for 5 or 25 years, and the same can be said of a younger person who receives the heart – this is clearly unjust discrimination. (Questions of autonomy – the right to refuse an organ, free exchange among competent people, directed donation, and informed decision making – are not at issue here.)

The conflict between utility and justice becomes sharper when it is shown that heart transplantation in carefully selected recipients who are older than 70 years have morbidity and mortality that are similar to younger patients out to 5 years of postoperative follow-up [51] (see Fig. 8.7). As long as these similarities hold true, it is difficult to sustain the argument from utility.

Because of the ethical conflicts inherent in the question of heart transplantation in the elderly, UCLA transplant surgeons have been transplanting donor hearts of such marginal quality that they would not ordinarily be used, into those on an "alternate list," comprising potential recipients who had been excluded from the regular heart transplant list, mostly because they were deemed too old to receive a transplant [52]. Early posttransplant, these patients have done nearly as well as more routine heart recipients, but morbidity and resource use is greater. In one recent study of such an alternate list, median survival was 5 years in patients who were expected to live less than 1 year [53].

This practice raises many questions. Transplant centers are still left with the problem of balancing the death of patients on waiting lists with maximization of posttransplantation survival. If the results of marginal heart transplantation are comparable with those with nonmarginal donor hearts, shouldn't those hearts be used for patients on the regular list who are currently dying without a suitable heart? Robbins has observed that transplant physicians routinely match the risks of donor heart function with parameters of potential recipients [54]. Patients on an alternate list are disadvantaged because they can receive only second-rate hearts, but if the hearts are acceptable, then the potential recipients on the regular list are disadvantaged as they are denied access to acceptable hearts. He goes on to say, "I would continue to advocate responsible stewardship of the limited donor resources and select the best candidates for transplantation *irrespective of patient age* [emphasis ours]." This issue is still unsettled and will remain so until much more information is available about donor heart function and about accurate methods to match donor hearts with the most suitable recipients.

Decision Making for the Elderly with Cardiothoracic Disease

Given these observations about special aspects of risks in cardiothoracic surgery for the elderly, how should a cardiothoracic surgeon choose a particular plan of action when confronted with an elderly patient with cardiothoracic disease that could be amenable to surgery? The Surgical Ethics Program at the University of Chicago's MacLean Center for Clinical Medical Ethics has provided a useful 4-part guide to ethical decision-making in medicine [55]. We have modified the guide to reflect decision making for the elderly in cardiothoracic surgery.

1. *Medical indications*: The Principle of Beneficence
   What critical determinants of postoperative mortality and morbidity are present (e.g., preoperative stroke, renal and respiratory insufficiency, myocardial ischemia, congestive failure, or hemodynamic instability)? *Age alone is NOT a critical determinant of outcome.* What are the goals of treatment? What are the probabilities of success? What are the plans in case of serious complications – has the family discussed and planned for this possibility? (Although as many as 50% of cardiothoracic surgery

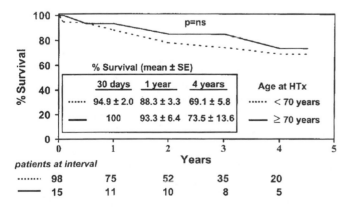

Fig. 8.7 Thirty-day operative survival and actuarial survival up to 4 years for patients <70 years of age (*n*=98) and ≥70 (*n*=15). *ns* not significant; *SE* standard error; *HTX* heart transplantation (reprinted from Blanche et al. [51], Copyright 2001, with permission from Elsevier)

patients prefer to have no information regarding risk of death and 42% want no discussion of risks at all [56], this information is critical for the surgeon to choose appropriate recommendations for the patient and family.)

2. *Patient preferences*: The Principle of Respect for Autonomy
   Is the patient mentally capable of making decisions? If capable, what are the patient's preferences for treatment? Has the patient understood the benefits and risks of alternative treatments, and given consent? If mentally incapacitated, who is the appropriate surrogate/proxy, and is the surrogate using appropriate decision-making standards? Has the patient executed an advance directive, if so, is it currently available? Is the patient unable or unwilling to cooperate with the planned treatment? Does the patient or family prefer to be spared the potentially degrading or disabling effects and side effects of surgical treatment, or do they prefer to minimize regret by "doing everything that can be done," regardless of consequences. (Some families refuse to pay their bills after surgery because of bitter resentment over patients who ended up demented and bedridden, while other families expressed gratitude, even though the patient died during surgery.) [25]

3. *Quality of life*: The Principles of Beneficence and Autonomy
   What was the quality of the patient's life before the current illness, and what is it likely to be during and after treatment? Is she frail and not likely to do well after operation, or is she spry and vigorous with a full, active life, implying that she could survive the surgery and return to her prior state of living? (Several instruments to measure quality of life are available.) [57]. Is there any plan or rationale to avoid surgery? Should plans for palliative care be pursued?

4. *Contextual features*: The Principle of Justice
   Are there other social, economic, or institutional factors at play? Are there family issues that might affect decision making? Are there physician or nursing issues that might affect decision making? Are there economic, religious or cultural issues? Are there problems related to resource allocation? Are there any conflict of interest issues on the part of physicians or the institution? Does the patient have a role as the caregiver of others? Is the family able and willing to provide care for the patient should disabling complications arise?

Advance Directives and Proxy/Surrogate Decision Making

In view of the high incidence of dementia in the elderly, the frequency of incapacity to make medical decisions will be higher in this than in any other age group. If the patient cannot make decisions, the surgeon should be guided by the patient's advance directive, if one exists and is available. The intent of advance directives is to preserve the patient's determination of the medical care they receive – that is, their intent is to respect the patient's autonomy in making medical decisions – if she should become unable to make decisions. Advance directives are of two types: instructional and agent-based. Instructional directives, such as Living Wills, allow the patient to specify her own values, goals, and preferences for end-of-life care. Because Living Wills are executed and signed by the patient, they are "first person" statements, and therefore take precedence over other advance directives. Agent-based directives, such as durable powers of attorney for health care, are much more flexible, allowing the agent to make decisions based on her understanding of the patient's value system or religious preferences.

All 50 states and the District of Columbia have legislation authorizing one or both types of advance directives. When both types are available, it is generally best to execute a durable power of attorney and not execute a Living Will [58]. This is because the Living Will cannot capture all the nuances of future clinical situations and, because it is a first-person statement, its provisions override the agent's judgment, even if the agent is certain that he knows what the patient's decision would have been in these specific circumstances. From the surgeon's viewpoint, it is far better to discuss the clinical situation with someone who knows the patient well rather than for decision making to be inflexibly controlled by a document that might have been completed years earlier [59].

When a patient becomes incapable of making health care decisions, options will be chosen by a proxy or surrogate decision maker. A *proxy* decision maker is a person who was appointed by the patient to act as his agent to make health care decisions in case of incapacitation; this is usually accomplished through a durable power of attorney for health care. In the absence of such an agent, medical decisions are made by a *surrogate* decision maker; the appropriate surrogate is determined by law in nearly all states.

It is important to understand that whether or not an advance directive exists, people should discuss as fully as possible, in advance of any illness, what their end-of-life preferences would be under a variety of clinical circumstances. Such discussions should include the health care agent, if one is appointed, as well as other persons who are likely to be present at a future time of incapacitation.

By both ethical and legal standards, the authority of proxies and surrogates to make decisions is virtually the same as the patient's authority would be if she possessed decision-making capacity. The extent of this authority is stated clearly in the American Medical Association Code of Medical Ethics: "Physicians should recognize the proxy or surrogate as an extension of the patient, entitled to the same respect as the competent patient" [60]. State laws vary as to the extent of authority granted to surrogates/proxies, but virtually all are similar to AMA statement. Thus, if an elderly patient is incapacitated, the surgeon should discuss the details of the patient's illness with the surrogate/proxy decision makers and respect their decisions just as if talking with the patient.

Surrogates/proxies are not free to make any health care decisions they wish. They must use "substituted judgment" in choosing among options; that is, they must make decisions based on their understanding of what the patient would have wanted under the prevailing clinical circumstances. The decision maker may rely on written or oral statements, discussions with the patient when she was competent, or on a general understanding of the patient's value system or religious preferences. If none of these guides to the patient's wishes are available, as in the case of a lifelong mentally disabled patient, proxies/surrogates must use the "best interest" standard in making decisions for the patient; that is, they must make decisions that they believe to be in the patient's best interest [61].

A situation occasionally arises in which the surgeon has reason to believe that the legal decision maker is directing care on the basis of neither substituted judgment nor the patient's best interest, but the proxy/surrogate's interest. For example, if there is a large insurance policy on the patient's life and the proxy/surrogate is a beneficiary, and, further, if an operation is clearly in the patient's best interest but the agent decides that the operation will not be done, the surgeon can challenge the purportedly improper decision and, personally or with the assistance of family members or others, attempt to persuade the questionable decision maker to change the decision. If all attempts at persuasion fail, the final option for the surgeon is to ask the hospital's legal counsel to challenge the proxy/surrogate's competence as

decision maker in a probate court [61]. Fortunately, such a step is rarely necessary.

The Elderly as Research Subjects

As development of new therapeutic agents and technologies accelerated in the second half of the twentieth century, the need grew for subjects, including the elderly, in clinical trials, which were required for studying competing treatments. Until the mid-twentieth century, there were no specific guidelines to aid clinical investigators in designing and implementing clinical trials. Regulation of research came about due in part to two epochal tragedies: the Holocaust of the 1930s and 1940s, which led to the promulgation of the Nuremberg Code and the Declaration of Helsinki, and the Tuskegee Syphilis Trial, which led to the Belmont Report and the Common Rule.

The Nuremberg Code

The atrocities resulting from the Final Plan of the German Third Reich were brought to light soon after the end of World War II, when the Nuremberg Military Tribunals, particularly The Doctors' Trial in 1946–1947, exposed the horrific cruelty and disregard for human suffering of the Holocaust [62] (see Fig. 8.8). The use of prisoners – both German citizens and foreign nationals, who were imprisoned on religious, cultural, and ethnic grounds – as involuntary

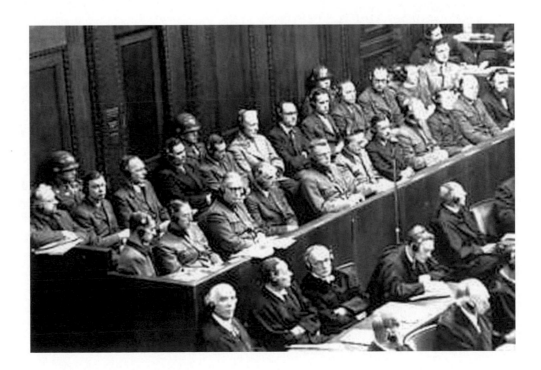

Fig. 8.8 Defendants in *front row* of the dock, defense counsel in *back row*, during the Doctors Trial, which was held in Nuremberg, Germany, from December 9, 1946, to August 20, 1947 (this work is in the public domain in the United States because it is a work of the United States Federal Government under the terms of Title 17, Chapter 1, Section 105 of the US Code, http://www.ushmm.org/research/doctors/charges.htm)

subjects in appalling medical experiments led to the first international code of ethics governing the use of human subjects in medical research: the Nuremburg Code (see Fig. 8.9). Before 1947, no international policy or law existed to govern the conduct of research with respect to ethical treatment of experimental subjects. The facts found by the Tribunals generated international outrage, and the need for protections of experimental subjects was clear. Guidelines were delineated in the Nuremberg Code of 1947, which asserts that medical research can ethically be performed upon human subjects only if subjects participate voluntarily, if they are thoroughly informed and freely consent to well-designed scientific studies in which the risk of harm is low and the benefit is great, and if they can withdraw at any time without penalty [63].

The Declaration of Helsinki

The World Medical Association promulgated the Declaration of Helsinki in 1964 and subsequently amended it eight times, most recently in Seoul, October 2008 [64]. Although the Nuremberg Code responded to a perceived need to condemn

and prohibit war crimes disguised as scientific study, the Declaration of Helsinki took a broader approach, asserting that the "mission of the medical doctor is to safeguard the health of the people," that an obligation of medicine is to ensure progress in medical knowledge, and that some research requires the use of human subjects. Section I of the Declaration overlaps those of the Nuremberg Code, but Parts II and III deal with medical care of patients when they are research subjects. Part II deals with sick people as subjects in studies of their illnesses, while Part III describes the conditions under which nontherapeutic research can be performed with healthy volunteer subjects, by maintaining the basic principles of informed consent, low risk/benefit ratio, and holding welfare of the subject to be of paramount importance.

The Belmont Report

The Tuskegee Syphilis Study began when the few available treatments for syphilis were only marginally effective and not entirely safe [65]. Rural African-American men from Macon, Georgia were recruited and observed for the duration of the study, starting in 1932. Over the next 40 years, the study participants were subjected to painful procedures without treatment even after penicillin became available and was found to offer a reliable cure for syphilis (see Fig. 8.10). A Public Health Service venereal disease investigator queried the Centers for Disease Control in 1966 about the ethical implications of the study, but the study continued unchanged until 1972, when the investigator talked with an Associated Press reporter, who broke the story in the Washington Star.

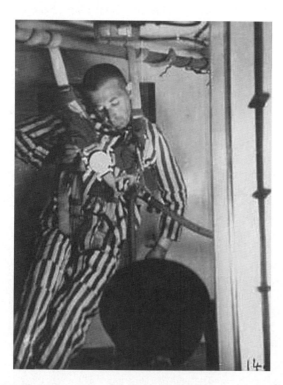

Fig. 8.9 High altitude experiments were carried out in a low-pressure chamber in which atmospheric conditions and pressures prevailing up to 68,000 ft could be duplicated. Here, a prisoner in a compression chamber loses consciousness (and later dies) during an experiment to determine altitudes at which aircraft crews could survive without oxygen. Dachau, Germany, 1942 (this image is in the public domain in the United States because it is a work of the United States Federal Government under the terms of Title 17, Chapter 1, Section 105 of the US Code, http://www.ushmm.org/research/doctors/twoa.htm#A)

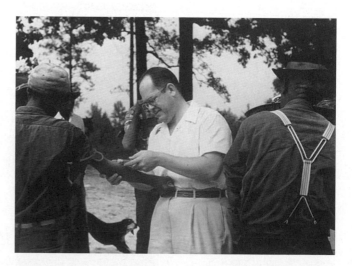

Fig. 8.10 Blood being drawn from subject of Tuskegee study (National Archives and Records Administration, this work is in the public domain in the United States because it is a work of the United States Federal Government under the terms of Title 17, Chapter 1, Section 105 of the US Code, see http://en.wikipedia.org/wiki/Image:Tuskeegee_study.jpg)

The study was terminated the day after the story broke. By that time, however, 128 subjects had died of syphilis or complications, 40 wives were infected, and 19 children were born with congenital syphilis.

Due in part to outcry over this study, the National Commission for the Protection of Human Subjects of Biomedical and Behavioral Research was created; it met at the Belmont Conference Center of the Smithsonian Institution from 1974 to 1978. In 1979, a set of guidelines for clinical investigators was published, "Ethical Principles and Guidelines for the Protection of Human Subjects of Research," generally called the Belmont Report [66]. In 1981, this document served as the basis for federal regulations that prescribed ethical conduct during human subjects research; the regulations were adopted by 16 federal agencies and are therefore referred to as the "Common Rule" [67].

The Elderly as Vulnerable Research Subjects

Protection of vulnerable subjects is a major focus of Belmont, connected particularly to the principle of respect for persons and the principle of justice [68]. Generally, people are in charge of their own lives, making decisions in accordance with their own moral compasses and values. They weigh options, assess risks, and consent or decline to participate as research subjects for their own considered reasons: an altruistic impulse for the betterment of society, their own needs as a patient, or a combination of several motivations. Truly informed consent has always been an elusive target; patients may be compromised by illness, lack of education, fear, inability to understand the English language, belief that they have no option but to comply, or mental disturbances. When enrolling subjects, the researcher must protect vulnerable target populations, such as children, prisoners, and economically disadvantaged persons, who require safeguards beyond those afforded ordinary subjects. Elderly persons are a vulnerable group [69].

In 1974, the National Institute on Aging was established to support studies of the emerging medical and social issues of a population in transition [70]. The complex and heterogeneous geriatric population is the most rapidly expanding segment of society. Among persons older than 70 years of age, 14% have some degree of dementia, and the estimated lifetime risk of developing Alzheimer's dementia is 1 in 5 for women and 1 in 10 for men [12]. Including the elderly in medical research is important because physiologic changes over time mean that conclusions from research on a young, healthy cohort may not apply to the elderly patients [71]. Although it is appropriate for the elderly to participate in clinical research, properly informed consent might be impossible to achieve in the large proportion of those whose mental function has been compromised. Dementia almost always starts insidiously, and the descent into its final stages when autonomous decision making is no longer possible is usually slow. At what point does the investigator decide that truly informed consent is not possible? Is it when the patient-subject cannot find misplaced keys, or only when she cannot recall what keys are used for; when she struggles for a word that is at the tip of her tongue, or only when she cannot remember her own name; when she becomes lost in a familiar office building, or only when she cannot remember where she lives; or when she cannot name the correct date, the sitting US president, or her own children? To place an age-defined limit to research subjects is to risk ageism, because if 10–30% of the elderly population may suffer from various stages of dementia, then the other 70–90% is a heterogeneous mix of robust to weak mental capacity. In research as in clinical medicine, assessment of mental functioning using one of several instruments can help to identify those who no longer have the capacity to consent [49, 57].

A Corollary Principle: Decisional Flexibility

We have shown how ethical principles may be applied to clinical problems in cardiothoracic surgery of the elderly: respect for persons charges surgeons to honor the health care choices made by patients or their surrogates/proxies; beneficence requires surgeons to hold the patient's best interest as the first among many competing interests, seeking to maximize benefit and minimize harm; and justice requires that we treat similarly patients who are similarly situated, regardless of age.

We would add another principle of ethical decision making in cardiothoracic surgery, perhaps best characterized as a corollary of the beneficence principle: decisional flexibility. Once victory in the operating room has been secured, willingness to change direction of care in response to clinical realities is often forgotten, even when the victory turns out to have been Pyrrhic. For example, we are sometimes faced with a patient, frequently elderly, who survived a complex operation but is struggling through a sequence of complications. Hemodynamic instability may lead to renal failure and dialysis, respiratory failure may lead to prolonged ventilation with consequent pneumonia, and cardiogenic shock may lead to multisystem failure. The term "risk of unacceptable badness" has been coined to describe such a course [72].

Hamlet had only two choices – to be or not to be – but now there is a third option, a state of suspension between life and death, in which the patient is severely compromised by a cascade of postoperative complications, reducing life to a state of dependency upon technology, when the original purpose of surgery was to restore independence [73]. The surgeon should look beyond the heroic success in the operating room and see the patient's current situation in the context of clinical circumstances that have evolved since the hopeful preoperative plan was formulated. Even without conscious decision, the target has moved and the surgeon should reevaluate the treatment plan in collaboration with the patient and family, taking into account the new clinical realities. The goal may no longer be saving the patient from a threatening surgical illness, but saving him from the technological imperative – well-meaning but misguided use of technology simply because it is available.

For cardiothoracic surgeons, the idea of backing away from curative efforts is antithetical to training and experience. Our sight is fixed on repairing the problem, and when the cascade of complications is well underway, we treat each new setback with vigor as our elderly patient sinks ever deeper into a quagmire, the probability of meaningful recovery retreats inexorably from possibility, and hubris or gritty determination blinds us to the possibility of unacceptable badness. We must be willing to reevaluate the treatment plans as circumstances evolve, and change course when the possibility of meaningful recovery has disappeared from view.

Older patients may be especially averse to discussion of potential complications of surgery [74], but the need to reevaluate and adjust treatment goals postoperatively should be discussed with the patient and family before the operation during the informational phase of informed consent. As we noted earlier, a positive outlook before an operation is associated with better outcomes, but conversations about the patient's preferences in case of serious complications can facilitate alteration of treatment goals later and do not necessarily preclude positive attitudes. As surgeons, our paramount obligation is to do what is best for our patients, and doing what is best requires modulating plans in accordance with the patient's existing situation, unbound from the constraints of previous decisions. We owe our patients nothing less.

References

1. Callahan D. Setting limits: medical goals in an aging society. New York: Simon and Schuster; 1987.
2. Sade RM. Foundational ethics of the health care system: the moral and practical superiority of free market reforms. J Med Philos. 2008;33(4):461–97.
3. Anagnastopoulos G. Euthanasia and the physician's role: reflections on some views in the ancient Greek tradition. In: Kuczewski MG, Polansky RN, editors. Bioethics – ancient themes in contemporary issues. Cambridge: MIT Press; 2002.
4. Quill T. Death and dignity: making choices and taking charge. New York: Norton; 1993.
5. Beauchamp TL, Childress JF. Principles of biomedical ethics. 5th ed. New York: Oxford University Press; 2001.
6. DeGrazia D. Single payer meets managed competition: the case for public funding and private delivery. Hastings Cent Rep. 2008; 38(1):23–33.
7. Rasmussen DB, Den Uyl DJ. Norms of liberty: a perfectionist basis for non-perfectionist politics. University Park: Pennsylvania State University Press; 2005. p. 268–83.
8. Dworkin R. Life's dominion. New York: Alfred A. Knopf; 1993. p. 218–41.
9. Nixon RM. Statement about the national cancer act of 1971. December 23, 1971. http://www.presidency.ucsb.edu/ws/index.php?pid=3276. Accessed 15 Feb 2010. Accessed 16 Feb 2010.
10. Callahan D. Living and dying with medical technology. Crit Care Med. 2003;31:35.
11. Callahan D. Setting limits: medical goals in an aging society with "a response to my critics. New York: Simon and Schuster; 1995. p. 227.
12. Alzheimer's Association. Alzheimer's disease facts and figures. 2009. http://www.alz.org/national/documents/report_alzfactsfigures2009.pdf. Accessed 16 Feb 2010.
13. Volandes A, Lehman LS, Cook EF, Shaykevich S, et al. Using video images of dementia in advance care planning. Arch Intern Med. 2007;167(8):828–33.
14. Quill T, Lo B, Brock D. Palliative options of last resort: a comparison of voluntarily stopping eating and drinking, terminal sedation, physician-assisted suicide, and voluntary active euthanasia. JAMA. 1997;278(23):2099–104.
15. Quill T, Lo B, Brock D, Meisel A. Last-resort options for palliative sedation. Ann Intern Med. 2009;151:421–4.
16. Jecker NS. Physician-assisted death in the Pacific Northwest. Am J Bioeth. 2009;9(3):1–2.
17. Kamisar Y. Physician-assisted suicide: the problems presented by the compelling, heart wrenching case. J Crim Law Criminol. 1998;88:1121–46.
18. Sade RM, Marshall MF. Legistrothanatry: a new specialty for assisting in death. Perspect Biol Med. 1996;39(3):222–4.
19. Elkinton J. Medicine and quality of life. Ann Intern Med. 1966;64:711–4.
20. Huber C, Goeber V, Berdat P, et al. Benefits of cardiac surgery in octogenarians – a postoperative quality of life assessment. Eur J Cardiothorac Surg. 2007;31:1099–105.
21. Ullery B, Peterson J, Milla F, et al. Cardiac surgery in select nonagenarians: should we or shouldn't we? Ann Thorac Surg. 2008;85:854–61.
22. Brunelli A, Socci L, Refai M, et al. Quality of life before and after major lung resection for lung cancer: a prospective follow-up analysis. Ann Thorac Surg. 2007;84(2):410–6.
23. Salati M, Brunelli A, Xiumè F, et al. Quality of life in the elderly after major lung resection for lung cancer. Interact Cardiovasc Thorac Surg. 2009;8(1):79–83.
24. Chiappini B, Tan ME, Morshuis W, et al. Surgery for acute type a aortic dissection: is advanced age a contraindication? Ann Thorac Surg. 2004;78:585–90.
25. Hata M, Sezai A, Niino T, et al. Should emergency surgical intervention be performed for an octogenarian with type A acute aortic dissection? J Thorac Cardiovasc Surg. 2008;135(5):1042–6.
26. McKneally M. We didn't expect "dementia and diapers". J Thorac Cardiovasc Surg. 2008;135(5):984–5.
27. Varadarajan P, Kapoor N, Bansal R, Pai R. Survival in elderly patients with severe aortic stenosis is dramatically improved by aortic valve replacement: results from a cohort of 277 patients aged >80 years. Eur J Cardiothorac Surg. 2006;30:722–7.
28. Chiappini B, Camurri N, Loforte A, et al. Outcome after aortic valve replacement in octogenarians. Ann Thorac Surg. 2005;78: 85–9.
29. Yildizeli B, Ozyurtkan O, Batirel H, et al. Factors associated with post-operative delirium after thoracic surgery. Ann Thorac Surg. 2005;79:1004–9.
30. Koster S, Hensens A, van der Palen J. The long-term cognitive and functional outcomes of post-operative delirium after cardiac surgery. Ann Thorac Surg. 2009;87:1469–74.

31. Collins SM, Brorsson B, Svenmarker S, et al. Medium-term survival and quality of life of Swedish octogenarians after open-heart surgery. Eur J Cardiothorac Surg. 2002;22:794–801.

32. Bachetta M, Ko W, Girardi L, et al. Outcomes of cardiac surgery in nonagenarians: a 10-year experience. Ann Thorac Surg. 2003;75:1215–20.

33. Duits A, Bocke S, Taams M, et al. Prediction of quality of life after coronary artery bypass graft surgery. Psychosom Med. 1997;59:257–68.

34. Oxman TE, Freeman Jr DH, Manheimer ED. Lack of social participation or religious strength and comfort as risk factors for death after cardiac surgery in the elderly. Psychosom Med. 1995;57(1):5–15.

35. Fernandez J, Chen C, Anolik G, et al. Perioperative risk factors affection hospital stay and hospital costs in open heart surgery for patients >65 years old. Eur J Cardiothorac Surg. 1997;11:1133–40.

36. Kurki T, Hakkinen U, Lauharanta J, et al. Evaluation of the relationship between pre-operative risk scores, post-operative and total length of stay and hospital costs in coronary bypass surgery. Eur J Cardiothorac Surg. 2001;20:1183–7.

37. Barnett S, Halpin L, Speir A, et al. Post-operative complications among octogenarians after cardiovascular surgery. Ann Thorac Surg. 2003;76:726–31.

38. Thourani V, Myung R, Kilgo P, et al. Long-term outcomes after isolated aortic valve replacement in octogenarians; a modern perspective. Ann Thorac Surg. 2008;86:1458–65.

39. Collart F, Feier H, Kerbaul F, et al. Valvular surgery in octogenarians: operative risk factors, evaluation of EuroSCORE and long term results. Eur J Cardiothorac Surg. 2005;27:276–80.

40. Stamou SC, Hagberg RC, Khabbaz KR, et al. Is advanced age a contraindication for emergent repair of acute type A aortic dissection? Interact Cardiovasc Thorac Surg. 2010 [Epub ahead of print]. http://icvts.ctsnetjournals.org/cgi/rapidpdf/icvts.2009.222984v1. Accessed 16 Feb 2010.

41. Acinapura A, Jacobowitz I, Kramer M, et al. Demographic changes in coronary artery bypass surgery and its effect on mortality and morbidity. Eur J Cardiothorac Surg. 1990;4:175–81.

42. Bardakci H, Cheema F, Topkara V, et al. Discharge to home rates are significantly lower for octogenarians undergoing coronary artery bypass graft surgery. Ann Thorac Surg. 2007;83:483–9.

43. Katz N, Chase G. Risks of cardiac operations for elderly patients: reduction of the age factor. Ann Thorac Surg. 1997;63:1309–14.

44. Kirsch M, Guesnier L, LeBesnerais P, et al. Cardiac operations in octogenarians: perioperative risk factors for death and impaired autonomy. Ann Thorac Surg. 1998;66:60–7.

45. Zingone B, Gatti G, Spina A, et al. Early and late outcomes of cardiac surgery in octogenarians. Ann Thorac Surg. 2010;89(2):429–34.

46. Goto T, Baba T, Matsuyama K, et al. Aortic atherosclerosis and post-operative neurological dysfunction in elderly coronary surgical patients. Ann Thorac Surg. 2003;75:1912–8.

47. Jaklitsch M, Billmeier S. Preoperative evaluation and risk assessment for elderly thoracic surgery patients. Thorac Surg Clin. 2009;19(3):301–12.

48. Auerbach A, Goldman L. Assessing and reducing the cardiac risk of noncardiac surgery. Circulation. 2006;113:1361–76.

49. Fukuse T, Satoda N, Hijiya K, Fujinaga T. Importance of a comprehensive geriatric assessment in prediction of complications following thoracic surgery in elderly patients. Chest. 2005;127(3):886–91.

50. Removal reasons by year; Removed from the Waiting List: January, 1995 – March 31, 2009. OPTN: Organ Procurement and Transplantation Network. Available at http://optn.transplant.hrsa.gov/latestData/rptData.asp. Accessed 16 June 2009.

51. Blanche C, Blanche DA, Kearney B, et al. Heart transplantation in patients seventy years of age and older: a comparative analysis of outcome. J Thorac Cardiovasc Surg. 2001;121(3):532–41.

52. Kobashigawa JA, Laks H, Wu G, et al. The University of California at Los Angeles heart transplantation experience. Clin Transpl. 2005:173–85.

53. Russo MJ, Davies RR, Hong KN, et al. Matching high-risk recipients with marginal donor hearts is a clinically effective strategy. Ann Thorac Surg. 2009;87(4):1066–70.

54. Robbins RC. Ethical implications of heart transplantation in elderly patients. J Thorac Cardiovasc Surg. 2001;121(3):434–5.

55. Jonsen AR, Siegler M, Winslade WJ, editors. Clinical ethics, vol. 5. New York: Macmillan; 2002. p. 12.

56. Beresford N, Seymour L, Vincent C, et al. Risks of elective cardiac surgery: what do patients want to know. Heart. 2001;86:626–31.

57. Holmes HM. Quality of life and ethical concerns in the elderly thoracic surgery patient. Thorac Surg Clin. 2009;19(3):401–7.

58. Fagerlin A, Schneider CE. Enough. The failure of the living will. Hastings Cent Rep. 2004;34(2):30–42.

59. Messengers-Rapport BJ, Baum EE, Smith ML. Advance care planning: beyond the living will. Cleve Clin J Med. 2009;76(5):276–85.

60. Council on Ethical and Judicial Affairs. E-8.801 Surrogate decision-making. American Medical Association, Code of medical ethics: current opinions with annotations, 2008–2009. Available at http://www.ama-assn.org/ama/pub/physician-resources/medical-ethics/code-medical-ethics/opinion8081.shtml. Accessed 9 Feb 2010.

61. D'Amico TA, Krasna MJ, Krasna DM, Sade RM. No heroic measures – how soon is too soon to stop? Ann Thorac Surg. 2009;87:11–8.

62. Annas GJ, Grodin MA, editors. The Nazi doctors and the Nuremberg code: human rights in human experimentation. New York: Oxford University Press; 1992. p. 61–144.

63. Annas GJ, Grodin MA, editors. The Nazi doctors and the Nuremberg code: human rights in human experimentation. New York: Oxford University Press; 1992. p. 2.

64. WMA Declaration of Helsinki. Ethical principles for medical research involving human subjects. http://www.wma.net/en/30publications/10policies/b3/index.html. Accessed 14 Feb 2010.

65. Tuskegee Syphilis Experiment. http://en.wikipedia.org/wiki/Tuskegee_syphilis_experiment. Accessed 14 Feb 2010.

66. U.S. National Commission for the Protection of Human Subjects of Biological and Behavioral Research. The Belmont report: ethical principles and guidelines for the protection of human subjects of research. Department of Health, Education, and Welfare (DHEW) Publication No. (OS) 78-0012, Appendix I, DHEW Publication No. (OS) 78-0013, Appendix II, DHEW Publication No. (OS) 78-0014. Washington, DC: U.S. Government Printing Office, 1978. http://ohsr.od.nih.gov/guidelines/belmont.html. Accessed 12 Feb 2010.

67. Protection of Human Subjects, 45 C.F.R.46. 1981, revised 1983, 1991.

68. Levine R. Ethics and regulation of clinical research. 2nd ed. New Haven: Yale University Press; 1988. p. 67–94.

69. Institutional Review Board Guidebook. Chapter VI.). Special classes of subjects. http://www.hhs.gov/ohrp/irb/irb_chapter6ii.htm#g9. Accessed 14 Feb 2010.

70. Levine R. Ethics and regulation of clinical research. 2nd ed. New Haven: Yale University Press; 1988. p. 84.

71. Doerflinger DM. Normal changes of aging and their impact on care of the older surgical patient. Thorac Surg Clin. 2009;19(3):289–99.

72. Cassell J, Buchman TG, Streat S, et al. Surgeons, intensivists, and the covenant of care: administrative models and values affecting care at the end of life. Crit Care Med. 2003;31:1263–70.

73. Gillet G, Hoover D, Crystal S, et al. The RUB. N Z Med J. 2001;114:188–9.

74. Ivarsson B, Larsson S, Luhrs C, Sjoberg T. Extended pre-op information about possible complications at cardiac surgery – do the patients want to know? Eur J Cardiothorac Surg. 2005;28:407–14.

Chapter 9
Acute Pain Control in Geriatric Patients After Cardiac and Thoracic Surgeries

Jack M. Berger, Tawfik Ayoub, and Jayeshkumar Patel

Abstract Inadequately managed pain in elderly patients undergoing thoracic or cardiac surgery can lead to increased morbidity and mortality, increased length of stay in the intensive care unit and the hospital. Even video-assisted procedures or minimally invasive procedures have not eliminated the problem of pain management. Elderly patients are not less sensitive to pain but are more sensitive to the side effects of analgesics and adjuvants, making titration more difficult. Other means of pain control such as the employment of epidural or intrathecal local anesthetics and opioids, paravertebral catheters with the infusion of local anesthetics offer significant benefits in the overall management of these patients. In this chapter, different means of pain control in this population will be reviewed.

Keywords Cardio-thoracic surgery • Acute pain management • Epidural catheters • Paravertebral catheters • Opioid management

In their review article, Brennan, Carr, and Cousins conclude that "because pain management is the subject of many initiatives within the disciplines of medicine, ethics and law, we are at an 'inflection point' in which unreasonable failure to treat pain is viewed worldwide as poor medicine, unethical practice, and an abrogation of a fundamental human right." [1] Attention to the problem of pain control in hospitalized patients was mandated by the Joint Commission for the Accreditation of Healthcare Organizations (JCAHO) in 2000–2002, and the declaration by the US Congress calling 2001–2010 the "*Decade of Pain Control and Research.*" [1] It is clear that this "right" to receive adequate pain management is not more evident than in the postoperative surgical patient (of any age). Yet fear of uncontrolled postsurgical pain continues to be among the primary concerns of many patients about to undergo surgery. [2] Despite increasing research and clinical attention, many adult surgical patients continue to experience moderate to severe pain [3, 4]. However, improvement as a result of the *JAHCO* initiative for better pain management assessment and treatment was reported by Frasco et al., who demonstrated that there has been an increase use of morphine and prophylactic antiemetics in postanesthesia recovery rooms without a concomitant increase in length of stay in the recovery rooms [5].

Cardiothoracic surgery and particularly posterolateral thoracotomy has been described as most debilitating for patients because of pain and consequent respiratory dysfunction [6]. Inadequate control of incisional pain is often complicated by inadequate control of pain from sternal fractures and rib fractures, from sternal retraction leading to costovertebral joint pain, and from chest and mediastinal tube sites. Furthermore, chronic pain develops in 50% of patients who suffer postthoracotomy intercostal nerve injury, of which in 5% the pain is severe and disabling [7–9].

Minimally invasive procedures involving smaller incisions, thought earlier to cause less pain compared with traditional incisions, did not prove to be better [9–11].

The surgical incision lengths are reduced but are relocated to more sensitive regions. Such is the case in minithoracotomy vs. median sternotomy [6].

On the one hand, "Fast track" anesthetic techniques used to permit patients to be extubated in the operating room or the immediate postoperative period require appropriate pain management techniques that will not compromise patient safety or leave patients suffering undue pain. On the other hand, patients who remain intubated and sedated must still be assessed for adequate pain control, admittedly a more difficult task. During emergence from heavy sedation in preparation for extubation, again adequate pain control to permit extubation is of upmost importance.

The ill effects of inadequately treated pain in the acute postoperative period are summarized by Sinatra [12]. Acute pain leads to increased sympathetic activity, which in turn leads to tachycardia and hypertension [12]. The resultant heightened level of sympathetic stimulation increases the level of circulating catecholamines, decreases vagal tone,

J.M. Berger (✉)
University of Southern California, Keck School of Medicine,
1500 San Pablo Street, Los Angeles, CA 90033, USA
e-mail: jmberger@usc.edu

M.R. Katlic (ed.), *Cardiothoracic Surgery in the Elderly*, DOI 10.1007/978-1-4419-0892-6_9,
© Springer Science+Business Media, LLC 2011

and increases oxygen consumption that could result in myocardial ischemia in patients at risk. Inadequate pain control has been shown to result in an increased incidence of atelectasis and significantly lower tissue oxygen levels. Regional blood flow can be impaired, which may increase the risk of postoperative infection [12].

In elderly patients with coronary artery disease, the risk of myocardial infarction is also increased. Furthermore, fear and anxiety resulting from inadequate pain control can impair sleep and rehabilitation. Splinting and shallow breathing can lead to hypoxemia, atelectasis, and pneumonia [12]. Other manifestations include oliguria, ileus, diaphragmatic dysfunction, thromboembolism, and impaired immune response [12–14]. Figure 9.1 shows the relationship of uncontrolled pain and harmful physiologic effects. Less well recognized is the observation that inadequate acute postsurgical pain management can lead to chronic pain syndromes [7, 15, 16].

Without belaboring the point further, it is clear that these pathological effects of acute pain can lead to life threatening consequences and can also lead to chronic "neuropathic pain" states that can affect the quality of the patient's future life through a constellation of maladaptive physical, psychological, family, and social consequences. These chronic neuropathic pain states can be regarded as true disease entities leading to dependence on medication, reduced mobility, loss of strength, disturbances of sleep, and social consequences that can result in dissolution of family relations [17].

These pathological consequences of uncontrolled pain may have even greater consequences in the elderly population [18]. However, there is little merit in separating out the treatment of acute pain in the *elderly population* unless it differs from that provided to younger patients [19]. This begs the questions of whether elderly patients perceive pain

differently from younger patients; and are there changes in nociception that occur with aging? Furthermore, do elderly patients process and respond to nociception differently?

Gagliese and Melzack demonstrated that age did not affect the rating of pain by postsurgical patients [20]. That is to say, tissue injury produces the same intensity of stimulus in an elderly person as in a young person.

However, there are data to suggest that some impairment of Aδ fibers occurs with aging, and therefore impedes the early warning of tissue injury [21]. There are also data that suggest that widespread and substantial changes in structure, neurochemistry, and function occur in the dorsal horn of the spinal cord and central nervous system (CNS) with aging [21]. Multiple studies report reductions in the descending inhibitory modulating systems for nociception in the elderly [21, 22].

Gibson and Ferrell further conclude that the reduced efficacy of endogenous analgesic systems might be expected to result in a more severe pain experience following prolonged noxious stimulation [21]. It is also possible that the documented decline in afferent transmission pathways could be offset by a commensurate reduction in the endogenous inhibitory mechanisms of older persons, with a net result of little or no change in the perceptual pain experience [21].

Figure 9.2 shows the relationship between ascending nociceptive pathways and descending modulating pathways along with the hormonal neurotransmitters involved in descending modulation. This implies that any deficit in endogenous analgesic response (which is stimulus intensity dependant) will become critical, thereby making it more difficult for persons of advanced age to cope with severe or persistent clinical pain conditions [21].

A complete discussion of this issue is beyond the scope of this chapter but suffice to say therefore that *assessment and intervention for pain in the elderly should begin with the assumption that all neurophysiologic processes subserving nociception are intact* [24]. In general, the *pharmacodynamic* actions of drugs (what the drug does to the patient) are unaffected in the normal aging process. The molecular action of morphine is the same in all animals, although dose requirements to produce the same effect may change with age, and the therapeutic window between intended effect and side or adverse effects may be narrowed in the elderly [25, 26]. From a clinical standpoint, it is safer to assume that elderly patients are *not less sensitive* to pain than younger adults, but they are *more susceptible to the side effects of opiate analgesics and therefore require more careful titration of analgesics* [27].

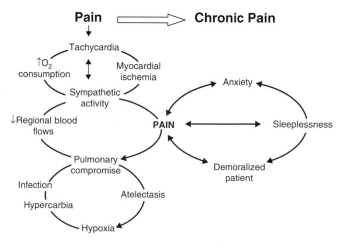

Fig. 9.1 Harmful effects of unrelieved acute pain including postoperative pain. Unrelieved pain can lead to activation of the sympathetic nervous system and cardio-vascular compromise and heightened anxiety. Pulmonary compromise can occur. And it is now clear that chronic pain develops as a consequence of unrelieved pain (modified from Sinatra [12] with permission from Elsevier)

Thoracic Pain Pathways

The chest wall is innervated by the *intercostal nerves*: the ventral branch of each intercostal nerve innervates the anterior chest wall, the posterior branches innervate the posterior

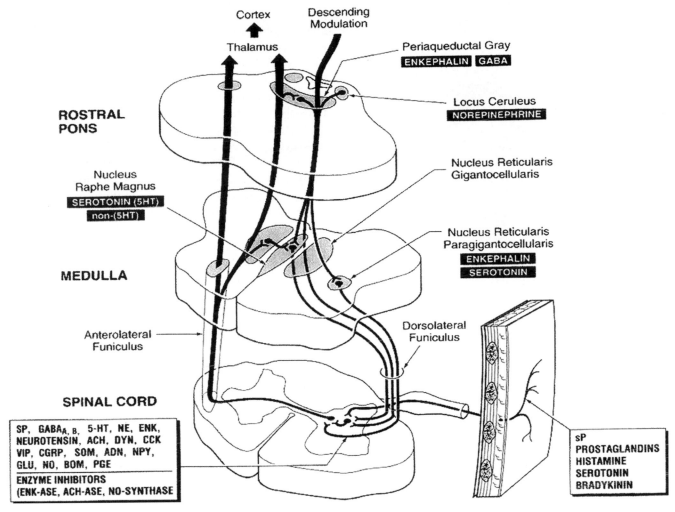

Fig. 9.2 Simplified schema of afferent sensory pathways (*left*) and descending modulatory pathways (*right*). Stimulation of nociceptors in the skin surface leads to impulse generation in the primary afferent. Concomitant with this impulse generation, increased levels of various endogenous algesic agents (substance P, prostaglandins, histamine, serotonin, bradykinin) are detected near the area of stimulation in the periphery. Primary afferent nociceptors relay to projection neurons in the dorsal horn, which ascend in the anterolateral funiculus to terminate in the thalamus. En route, collaterals of the projection neurons activate multiple higher centers, including the nucleus reticularis gigantocellularis (NRG). Neurons from the NRG project to the thalamus and also activate the nucleus raphe magnus (NRM) and periaqueductal gray (PAG) of the midbrain. Descending fibers from the PAG project to the NRM and reticular formation adjacent to the NRM. These neurons activate descending inhibitory neurons, which are located in these regions and travel via the dorsolateral funiculus to terminate in the dorsal horn of the spinal cord. Descending projections also arise from a number of brain stem sites including the locus ceruleus (LC). A number of neurotransmitters are released by afferent fibers, descending terminations, or local interneurons in the dorsal horn and modulate peripheral nociceptive input. These include substance P (SP), gamma aminobutyric acid (GABA), serotonin (5-HT), norepinephrine (NE), enkephalin (ENK), neurotensin, acetylcholine (ACH), dynorphin (DYN), cholecystokinin (CCK), vasoactive intestinal peptide (VIP), calcitonin-gene-related peptide (CGRP), somatostatin (SOM), adenosine (ADN), neuropeptide Y (NPY), glutamate (GLU), nitric oxide (NO), bombesin (BOM) and prostaglandins (PGE). Inhibitors of enzymes such as enkephalinase (ENK-ASE), acetylcholinesterase (ACH-ASE) and nitric oxide synthase (NO-SYNTHASE) may act to modify the action of these neurotransmitter (from Siddall and Cousins [23])

chest wall, and the visceral branches innervate the visceral aspects of the chest. All three branches join together to enter the intervertebral foramina to the spinal canal where they form a dorsal root. Dorsal roots fuse with the spinal cord dorsal horn to enter the CNS [6].

Somatic pain is mediated through partially *myelinated* "Aδ fibers" in the ventral and posterior branches. These fibers are responsible for the early warning system of the body to nociception arising from tissue injury, for example, the surgical incisions and tissue manipulations [6]. Smaller unmyelinated C-fibers are responsible for conducting the postoperative nociceptive signals arising in the "inflammatory soup" of the surgical wound site or sites [28]. Figure 9.3 shows the various viscerotomes and their innervations.

Sympathetic visceral pain is mediated by the *unmyelinated C-fibers* in all three branches; the signal is directed from the intercostal nerve branches through the sympathetic tract, which then pass back to the peripheral nerves to enter the CNS from T-1 to L-2 [6, 28].

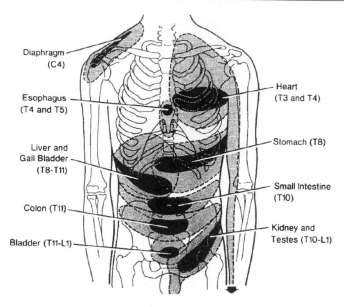

Fig. 9.3 Viscerotomes. Approximate superficial areas to which visceral pain is referred, with related dermatomes in *brackets*. The *dark areas* are those most commonly associated with pain in each viscus. The *gray areas* indicate approximately the larger area that may be associated with pain in the viscus (reprinted with permission from Cousins [29])

Parasympathetic visceral pain is mediated via cranial nerve X: the *vagus nerve*, which enters the CNS through the medulla oblongata, and therefore is not normally affected by the epidural or intrathecal methods of pain control (to be discussed later) [6, 28].

Spinal pain signals cross from the dorsal horn to the contralateral spinal cord structure and then it ascends to the brain via the *Spinothalamic tract*. In the brain, the signal is distributed to numerous structures resulting in cognitive, affective, and autonomic responses to the noxious stimulus. It is well known that the brain does not sense "pain" or nociceptive signals, although it receives and processes these signals from the rest of the body. However, although somatic nociception can be very precisely located by the brain, visceral nociception can be more problematic [28].

And with respect to the heart, the complete absence of "the perception of pain" that can occur in the presence of myocardial ischemia, arteriolar occlusion, myocarditis, early acute endocarditis, valvular ulceration, etc. makes it difficult and yet extremely important to assess for pain in the postcardiac surgery patient [30].

Pain Management Techniques for Thoracic Surgeries

The literature reports indicate that 50% of patients describe pain 1 year after thoracotomy, with many continuing to report pain even years later [31]. Fortunately, the prevalence of

postthoracotomy pain can be reduced, with rates as low as 21% one-year after surgery when perioperative pain is managed aggressively [32]. Surprisingly, video-assisted thoracic surgery (VATS) is associated with a prevalence of chronic pain comparable with that of open procedures [10, 11], with rates of pain ranging from 22 [10] to 63% [11], which is probably due to intercostal nerve and muscle damage resulting from the insertion of the trocars.

Reduction of postoperative complications related to pain is dependent on blocking of nociceptive information from reaching the brain. More importantly, protection of the spinal cord can prevent central sensitization, the process that leads to chronic pain [33]. Noxious input associated with thoracic surgery is conveyed to the CNS along the intercostal, vagus, and phrenic nerves. Irritation of the diaphragm is believed to be the source of the shoulder pain that frequently accompanies thoracic procedures because this pain is ameliorated by blockade of the phrenic nerve [34] but not by blockade of the suprascapular nerve or by thoracic epidural blockade [35].

Intercostal nerve dysfunction resulting from incision, retraction, trocar placement, or sutures is common, and likely plays a significant role in the pain accompanying thoracic surgery [36]. In addition, the necessary action of breathing (incentive spirometry), and the need for enhanced pulmonary toilet (such as coughing), produces an intense and relentless barrage of noxious input to the CNS [37].

For noncardiac thoracic or thoraco-abdominal surgeries, the most effective interventions for pain control are neuraxial and regional analgesic techniques [38]. Furthermore, preventive application of effective analgesic techniques provides protection against the development of chronic pain syndromes [32, 33].

Regional Analgesia

Regional analgesia is the mainstay of pain management for thoracic surgery [39].

Several techniques were adopted each with its' own advantages and disadvantages, but none of them is yet ideal [40].

Epidural Analgesia

Thoracic epidural analgesia is considered the gold standard for postoperative pain relief after thoracotomy and upper abdominal surgeries. It is the most widely used form of regional analgesia for thoracic surgery, but its acceptance for cardiac surgery is not yet established for fear of epidural hematoma formation after heparin administration. Thoracic epidural catheters are usually placed between T-4 and T-10 depending on the incision site and at about 5 cm from the skin to maintain position. Catheters are usually placed with the patient sedated but alert enough to report paresthesias during its placement. A test dose of local anesthetic with epinephrine is usually used to detect intrathecal or intravenous placement. A combination of local anesthetic and opioid is used to activate and maintain analgesia during and after surgery. Activation of the epidural prior to surgical incision provides the benefit of preemptive analgesia. An added intraoperative advantage is the reduction of anesthetic requirement, which promotes faster emergence and reduction of respiratory depression. Administration of an analgesic dose of local anesthetic prior to extubation provides adequate analgesia until the continuous epidural infusion is established either in the postanesthesia recovery area or in the intensive care unit.

In a review article that studied epidural analgesia in management of acute pain, epidural vs. intravenous opioid analgesia were compared: patient satisfaction as determined by visual analog pain score was favorable for epidural analgesia using local anesthetic with or without opioid when compared with parental opioid analgesia. Sedation was less frequent in the epidural group compared with patients receiving patient controlled analgesia (PCA) with morphine [41, 42]. Pruritis was more prevalent for patient receiving epidural analgesia than in patients receiving intravenous PCA. The incidence of nausea and vomiting were equal between both groups. Patients receiving epidural analgesia experienced less pain during coughing when compared with those using PCA analgesia, a property especially important when dealing with postthoracotomy patients [41, 42].

In a large-scale patient survey, the failure rate for epidural analgesia after thoracic epidural catheter placement was 32%. Failure was attributed to dislodgement of the catheters (17%), misplacement of the catheter (11%), and leaks (7%). Unilateral analgesia was reported in 7% of patients [43].

Epidural administration of opioid can be associated with delayed respiratory depression, thus postoperative monitoring of sedation levels and respiratory function must be assured [44]. Most frequently this is done in the setting of an intensive care unit. But healthy volunteer living lung donors, for example, may not require immediate postoperative intensive care, and many thoracic surgery patients can be moved to postoperative surgical wards with their ongoing epidural analgesia after 1 or more days in the intensive care unit. The concurrent use of epidural and intravenous opioid has been blamed for accentuation of respiratory depression, and its use should be done with utmost caution [45].

Certain procedures deserve special considerations, among them "esophagectomy." It is a procedure usually performed in specialized centers. Usually indicated for esophageal tumors, but could have other surgical indications such as esophageal perforation or ruptures. The procedure involves removal of the esophagus through an abdominal and neck incision as in the trans-hiatal approach or a trans-thoracic approach involving an added right lateral thoracotomy. The procedure then involves either a stomach-pull-up or a colon transposition. In both conditions, the stomach or the colon is mobilized into the chest, and the vitality of both organs depends on the limited blood supply through a single artery: the right gastro-epiploic artery in case of the stomach pull-up, and the left colic artery for colon interpositions.

Hypotension arising from the continuous epidural usage could affect the vitality of the stomach or colon in the chest. Furthermore, usage of vasopressors is not advisable, as the vasoconstriction could affect the blood flow through the single arterial supply. It is also important to note that the usage of volume to correct hypotension could be limited by the medical condition of the patient. In such conditions, the surgeon frequently orders the cessation of usage of the epidural and reverts to PCA, which is not ideal to control the pain arising from this type of procedure.

However, epidural analgesia is still used routinely for these procedures and can provide excellent analgesia, permitting early extubation of these patients. Brodner et al. studied the effectiveness of epidural analgesia in 49 patients who underwent thoracoabdominal resection of the esophagus [46]. Epidural catheters were inserted preoperatively at T6–T9, but not utilized intraoperatively, and the patients were managed with general anesthesia. Postoperatively, epidural infusions of 0.125% bupivacaine and 1 µg/ml Sufentanil were infused at 5–10 ml/h with adjustments randomly performed by ICU residents, according to their assessment of the patients' needs.

A second group of 48 patients also had epidural catheters inserted preoperatively at T6–T9 but received an immediate bolus of 10–15 ml of 0.25% bupivacaine and 20–30 µg Sufentanil, with induction of general anesthesia following after a sensory level to T4 was confirmed. During surgery, an infusion was continued with 0.175% bupivacaine and 1 µg/ml Sufentanil at 5 ml/h. Postoperatively, the infusion was continued and adjusted according to the patients' pain levels by members of the acute pain service. The patients also had the opportunity to apply a patient controlled epidural analgesic (PCEA) bolus of 2 ml every 20 min.

Catheters were retained for 5 days in each group. The epidural group subjects were extubated within hours after the conclusion of surgery, while the control group was extubated after 24 h in the ICU. Also, the length of stay in the intensive care unit was decreased by 50% in the epidural group.

Ochroch et al. studied the effect of thoracic epidural analgesia on the recovery of activity and the development of long-term pain after major thoracotomy surgery [32]. One hundred fifty seven patients undergoing thoracotomy were premedicated with midazolam 0–2 mg, and with Fentanyl

0–3 µg/kg for catheter placement. Catheters were placed at T6–T8 and tested with 3 ml 1.5% Lidocaine with 1/200,000 epinephrine. Mispositioned catheters were replaced. Patients were excluded from the study if the catheter could not be placed above T-12. General anesthesia induction included 3 µg/kg Fentanyl.

In Group 1, 6 ml of saline were injected into the epidural catheter followed by an infusion of saline at 8 ml/h starting prior to skin incision. In Group 2, 6 ml of 0.375% bupivacaine with 3 µg/ml Fentanyl were injected as a bolus followed by an infusion of the same mixture at 8 ml/h. If surgery was less or more than the expected surgery, the patients were dropped from the study. At rib approximation, all patients received an epidural bolus of 5 ml of 0.5% bupivacaine with 50 µg fentanyl.

In the postanesthesia care unit (PACU), patients who did not have a band of thoracic anesthesia received 6 ml of 1.5% lidocaine with epinephrine, and those that failed to develop anesthesia were dropped from the study as having an inadequate epidural catheter placement. PCEA was then started with 0.05% bupivacaine and 1 µg/ml Fentanyl at 4 ml/h with 3 ml bolus dose permitted every 10 min. A 30-mg single dose of Ketorolac was administered for chest tube shoulder pain. Catheters were maintained until the chest tube was pulled, and then the patients were converted to oral medications.

The results showed that women tended to have more average, and worst levels of pain than men, but were discharged from the hospital sooner than men. Pain control did not seem to be affected by whether the epidural was activated prior to skin incision or at rib approximation. Long-term pain in both groups was similar at about 21% and correlated with the incidence of preoperative pain. However, this was improved over the 50% level reported in most retrospective studies, indicating that intraoperative activation of epidural analgesia in association with general anesthesia followed by extended *postoperative effective epidural analgesia* does reduce the incidence of chronic pain [32].

If patients do not tolerate epidural local anesthetics, an alternative would be to eliminate the local anesthetic and use a pure hydrophilic opioid epidural analgesic such as hydromorphone, which should not produce hypotension as a secondary effect to analgesia.

More recently, morphine encapsulated within liposomes to provide extended release of the morphine after epidural injection has become available and is commercially known as DepoDur™ (Endo Pharmaceuticals Inc, Chadds Ford, PA). After injection, in physiological conditions, the liposomes degrade to release the morphine slowly [47]. In clinical studies, DepoDur™ was given before surgery as a single epidural injection – without indwelling epidural catheter – and provided pain relief for 48 h, after which time most patients were transitioned to oral analgesics. DepoDur™ has only been approved for lumbar use. Its mechanism of delivery

might promise a longer relief, less break through pain without the cumbersome need for an additional pump, IV pole and extra tubing.

During clinical trials with DepoDur™, the majority of adverse events were typical of opioid medications and consistent with the surgical populations being studied. The use of DepoDur™ for thoracic epidural injection remains to be evaluated for safety and efficacy. Once safety is established, a thoracic single shot epidural with DepoDur™ might be a reasonable analgesic technique for usage during esophagectomy surgery. However, this preparation is designed for use without the simultaneous use of local anesthetics, which can degrade the liposomal structure [48].

Other Regional Anesthetic Techniques

Intercostal Blocks

Multilevel, single shot, intercostal blocks are possible techniques used to block pain from thoracic surgery. These blocks can be placed preemptively or more commonly under direct vision before closure of the surgical site. Local anesthetics are deposited proximally at the inferior border of the corresponding rib. It would offer pain relief until other means could be implemented. In a study comparing continuous epidural analgesia with 0.125% bupivacaine with 2 µg/ml Sufentanil, to multilevel single shot intercostal blocks with 0.5% bupivacaine using visual score analog scales, it could be shown that on the day of surgery, an intercostal block was associated with a lower pain score when compared with epidural anesthesia. However, on the day following surgery, the epidural group had superior pain relief [49].

Extrapleural Analgesia

Prior to closure of the thoracotomy incision, a portion of the parietal pleura is lifted away from the inner chest wall to create an extrapleural pocket. A catheter is introduced percutaneously into this pocket under direct vision. The overlying pleura are sutured closed at the thoracotomy incision site [50]. Percutaneous catheter placement into this space without intraoperative visualization has also been described, albeit with a technical failure rate of 10–30%, and complications in 10% (hypotension, vascular, or pleural puncture) [51, 52]. Many types of catheters can be used [53, 54]. Different types of local anesthetics and concentrations could be used. Most frequently 0.5 or 0.25% bupivacaine, 1% lidocaine, or 0.5% ropivacaine are used. The rate of infusion is generally at 5–7 ml/h for an average adult (0.1 ml/kg/h) [50]. Analgesia to pinprick (~5 dermatomes unilaterally) is similar to a thoracic epidural (bilaterally) [55].

Randomized studies comparing an extrapleural technique with epidural analgesia suggest that outcomes are at least as good, if not better, using an extrapleural approach [56, 57].

Pain relief is somewhat better and narcotic usage somewhat less with an extrapleural catheter, but the differences are not consistent and often not statistically significant. Extrapleural analgesia may preserve forced expiratory volume at 1 s (FEV1) better, but the effect on pulmonary complications is unclear [50].

Randomized studies comparing extrapleural infusions of bupivacaine and lidocaine found no difference in pain relief, need for supplemental opiates, or pulmonary function [58, 59]. More side effects occurred in patients receiving an epidural in studies comparing extrapleural bupivacaine with epidural techniques [57, 60–62].

Extrapleural infusion of bupivacaine has been very well tolerated. Local complications were seen in 0.6% of patients in studies that specifically reported complications (one patient each with transient hypotension and transient Horner's syndrome). Systemic bupivacaine toxicity (confusion) was noted in 0.8% of patients [50]. Average plasma bupivacaine levels during continuous infusion for several days were 3–4 µg/ml (range, 2.1–4.92 µg/ml), which is close to the commonly accepted threshold of 5 µg/ml for CNS toxicity. But these patients did not experience toxicity [54, 55, 61, 63–65]. Maximal levels of 7.48 µg/ml and 10.25 µg/ml have also been reported without toxicity [63, 64].

The explanation may be that the vast majority of plasma bupivacaine during an infusion is bound to serum proteins and is thereby rendered biologically inactive [65]. Attempts to define a toxic plasma level have been unable to do so, and the incidence of toxicity appears to be related to the rapidity of administration [66]. In any case, both epidural and intrapleural techniques are superior to systemic opiates [50].

Interpleural Analgesia

Interpleural administration of local anesthetics is accomplished by introducing a small catheter percutaneously into the pleural space before thoracotomy closure. One or two epidural-type catheters with multiple side holes are generally used, and positioned posteriorly in the paravertebral gutter, spanning several intercostal spaces above and below the incision [50]. Local anesthetics are usually administered in the form of bupivacaine. Intermittent doses are given every 4, 6, or 8 h. Continuous infusion could also be used. The dose of bupivacaine is not consistent, but the most common volume is 20 ml, and the most common concentration is 0.5% [50]. Epinephrine could be added but is not needed. Management of the chest tubes may be important because a large portion (about 30%) of the administered dose drains out the tubes within 15 min.

Randomized studies (mostly double-blind, placebo-controlled) of interpleural local anesthetics after thoracotomy suggest that the benefit of this approach is marginal, at best [50]. No complications owing to interpleural catheter placement have been reported. Systemic bupivacaine toxicity was reported in 5% of patients overall using a constant infusion [62].

Among studies using intermittent dosing, bupivacaine toxicity occurred in 2.1% [66]. Average plasma bupivacaine levels have generally been approximately 1 µg/ml (0.32–2.29 µg/ml) with wide individual variation among patients [66]. The amount of bupivacaine lost in the chest tubes does not seem to correlate with either the plasma levels or the degree of pain relief. The variability in efficacy and toxicity of interpleural analgesia may be related to pleural permeability, inflammation, adhesions, and dilution with blood or effusion [50].

In a study of the use of interpleural catheters for administration of local anesthetics in esophagectomy surgery patients, bupivacaine was found to be effective for the thoracotomy pain but not for the abdominal pain, even with the addition of intravenous PCA morphine [67]. In these types of surgery, epidural analgesia may still be the preferred and the most effective method.

Intravenous Opiates

The use of opioids in pain management has been successfully employed since ancient times. However, physicians still remain reluctant to utilize opioids in elderly patients. Yet in a study conducted by Auburn et al. of 175 elderly patients vs. 875 younger patients who were treated with iv Morphine for postoperative pain in the PACU, there was no increased incidence of adverse side effects noted when a strict titration to pain level protocol was followed. It was not necessary to change the protocol according to age [25].

The most important generalization from physiologic studies of aging is that the basal function of the various organ systems is relatively uncompromised by the aging process per se. However, functional reserve and the ability to compensate for physiologic stress are reduced with aging [68]. With aging there is decreased lean body mass and total body water and an increased proportion of body fat; these alter the volume of distribution and redistribution of drugs and alter their rates of clearance and elimination [68].

There is decreased liver mass and blood flow, which prolongs drug metabolism [69]. There is an age-related decrease in basal metabolic rate of the liver and a decline in albumin production of about 10% [70]. However, overall age-related changes in protein binding do not produce clinical difference in drug transport [71].

Drug biotransformation reactions can either lead to the inactivation of the parent compound, the conversion of an inactive compound to an active one, or result in metabolites that are even more active than the parent active drug. Toxic metabolites are also produced, which depends on rapid excretion to avoid harm to the organism. Drug biotransformation is usually an enzymatic process. Although most tissues have some enzymatic metabolism, most occurs in the liver. Patients with impaired liver function will therefore have altered metabolic capacity for drug elimination [72].

Renal blood flow is also compromised by aging; approximately 10% per decade of life after age 50 with loss of renal parenchyma also [73]. Perioperative metabolic acidosis is relatively common in elderly patients who are less efficient in the renal excretion of acid [68]. Anesthetics, surgical stress, pain, sympathetic stimulation, and renal vasoconstrictive drugs may all compound subclinical renal insufficiency.

The kidney, lungs, GI tract, and skin all have some capacity to metabolize drugs. One of the major enzymatic systems for drug elimination with respect to analgesics and adjuvant analgesics is the cytochrome P450 system of enzymes. Drugs that are administered simultaneously and that are metabolized by the same enzyme system will compete for binding sites and thus can lead to altered blood levels [72].

The elderly have decreased renal function, which increases the risk of nonsteroidal antiinflammatory drug (NSAID) nephrotoxicity and accumulation of metabolites of drugs such as meperidine [73]. There is decreased plasma binding, which increases blood levels of active drugs, opioids, and NSAIDs (even the specific cyclo-oxygenase 2 (COX-2) inhibitors such as Celecoxib (Celebrex®)) [74].

Patient-controlled analgesia (PCA) is a method of pain relief that allows patients to self-administer small doses of opioids on demand, accompanied by the option of a continuous infusion, using a programmable infusion device. Versatile routes (intravenous, subcutaneous, epidural) and pharmacologic agents (morphine, meperidine, hydromorphone, fentanyl) exist for PCA administration [75]. Prior to the advent of PCA, patients primarily received morphine or other opiates either by intramuscular injection or intravenous bolus. However, since the introduction of PCA, many studies have shown its superiority to the older methods.

However, while PCA is now in wide and common use, physicians are still often reluctant to use PCA in older patients. Yet proper pain control is imperative in elderly patients because of higher rates of postoperative confusion, morbidity, and mortality [76]. But PCA was found to be effective in this population with the caveat that the patient is physically or mentally able to operate the machine [76]. It is also advisable to refrain from administering a continuous basal infusion in the elderly population.

Regardless of the method of initial pain control after thoracic or cardiac surgery, there is usually a necessity to convert to oral pain medication for discharge home. Proper and adequate dosing of oral opioids will lead to a more satisfactory transition to home. Below several conversion aides utilized by the authors are presented.

Conversion from Morphine to Transdermal Fentanyl

Remember equi-analgesic principles. A cumulative dose of 60 mg/day of intravenous Morphine or 180 mg/day of oral morphine = 100 µg/h transdermal fentanyl patch, which is changed every 72 h. As with all sustained release opioids, this is for continuous pain that is opiate responsive. You still need to consider breakthrough pain medications, fast onset, short duration, for activity based pain.

Conversion from IV PCA to Control Release Oxycodone in the Postoperative Period

Ginsberg et al. enrolled 189 patients in an open label study, post abdominal, orthopedic, or gynecologic surgeries. Patients with signs of paralytic ileus were excluded. IV Morphine PCA was administered for the first 24 h. Then the patients were converted to controlled release Oxycodone, according to a conversion factor. Most patients were controlled (pain scores ≤4/10 in the first 6 h). Formula: Initial CR Oxycodone mg dose = IV opioid (mg/day) × conversion factor ÷ 2 (for 12 h dosing) [77].

Conversion factors for starting dosing:

Morphine	1.5
Meperidine	0.2
Hydromorphone	10.0

Dosing was adjusted up or down according to available tablet strengths, 10, 20, 40 mg. Immediate release oxycodone was used for breakthrough supplements.

Other conversions
IV Morphine to P.O. Morphine 1:3 ratio (after several days of morphine administration)

24 h IV Morphine × 3 = 24 P.O. Morphine, divided as sustained release morphine in a q8h dosing schedule.
I.V. Morphine to P.O. Methadone

- 24 h I.V. Morphine × 1.2 = 24 h P.O. Methadone after short exposure to Morphine.
- 300 mg/day oral Morphine = 30 mg/day oral Methadone (the higher the morphine dose, the lower the methadone conversion dose due to the presence of acute opioid tolerance).

Other Analgesics

NSAID's, COX-2 inhibitors, and acetaminophen can all be useful adjuvants to pain management in the elderly provided that dosing is carefully monitored since unlike the opiates, these drugs do have organ toxicity.

NSAIDs [78]

The antiprostaglandin effect of NSAIDs can be beneficial during the acute phase of soft tissue injury. This biochemical effect may control an injury's inflammatory response and provide pain relief. The duration of a NSAIDs' analgesic effect may be different than its antiinflammatory effect. Chronic inflammatory disease pain such as arthritis may warrant chronic NSAID therapy.

It is wise to remember that COX-2 specific inhibitors do not affect platelet aggregation and therefore may pose a risk for MI if the patient is taken off aspirin therapy. Since low-dose aspirin is increasingly being used for cardioprotection, it is important to note that coadministration of selective COX-2 inhibitors did not alter this effect [79].

Analgesic Adjuvants

Alpha 2 Agonists

Clonidine and dexmedetomidine are a class of centrally acting α_2-adrenergic agonists. They exhibit an analgesic property through stimulation of the α_2 adrenergic receptor in the substantia gelatinosa of the spinal cord, and sedative properties through agonistic action on the α_2 adrenergic receptors in the locus ceruleus in the brainstem. Activation of the α_2 adrenergic receptors located on sympathetic nerve terminals leads to decrease release of norepinephrine. They potentiate the anesthetic effect of inhalational agents (decrease MAC of inhalational drugs) and potentiate the effect of opioid analgesics. They lack the respiratory depression property of opiates, but may cause hypotension, sedation, and dry mouth.

Preservative-free Clonidine may be used as a component of the epidural infusion or intrathecal injections [80, 81].

Dexmedetomidine is particularly useful during minimally invasive cardiac surgery, where extubation is planned in the operating room. The resultant sedative, analgesic, and hemodynamic effects allow a calm extubation, stable vital signs, and an uneventful transfer to the intensive care unit (Berger, June 2010, unpublished experience).

Cardiac Surgery

Advances in operative therapy and anesthetic techniques have allowed for rapid recovery of patients after cardiac surgery. These advances, along with the increased emphasis on pain control, have highlighted the need for improved strategies of pain management after cardiac surgery [82]. The common cardiac surgeries in the geriatric patient population are CABG, aortic valve replacement, mitral valve repair or replacement, Maze procedure for atrial fibrillation, and repair of thoracic aortic aneurysm/dissection. The surgical incision can be median sternotomy, minimally invasive/mini-thoracotomy or regular thoracotomy (for descending thoracic aortic surgery). Patients experience pain, pressure, or burning sensation in the chest at the incision site and at the chest tube sites, and pain (usually more than chest pain) in the leg or arm at the vein or artery harvest sites.

Early awakening and extubation have brought the problem of postoperative pain management in cardiac surgery into focus [83]. Residual pain 1 year after surgery is reported to be 25% after median sternotomy, emphasizing the role that reduced intercostal nerve disruption and improved stability of the closure may play in reducing chronic pain [84].

The standard practice has been intravenous opiates given as needed followed by conversion to oral pain medications. However, the quest is on to find an ideal postoperative analgesic technique to complement the goal of early extubation and maximize patient satisfaction [83].

Inadequate pain control after coronary artery bypass graft (CABG) surgery and other cardio-thoracic operations can result in both increased morbidity and hospital length of stay [85–88]. Standard management of postoperative pain is with opiate analgesics, such as morphine sulfate. However, opioid effects, such as respiratory depression, nausea, vomiting, decreased gastrointestinal motility, and peripheral vasodilation, can potentially worsen the patient's condition and result in unfavorable outcomes, extended hospital stay, and increased costs [85–89].

As indicated earlier in this chapter, the advantages of intravenous or subcutaneous opiate PCA for cardiac surgery patients include the following: [75]

- Painless routes of administration
- Avoids peaks, valleys, fluctuations, and delays in pain relief
- Provides prompt and lasting comfort
- Flexible, titratable, and individualized therapy
- Potential for fewer opioid-related side effects compared with intermittent bolus administration
- Enhanced sense of control over the pain experience by the patient
- Decreased nursing burden compared with conventional methods

The disadvantages of PCA include the following: [75]

- Requires specialized equipment (the PCA infuser device or "pump")
- Requires patient self-awareness and cognitive understanding of the principles of PCA therapy for safe and effective use
- Potential for operator and/or mechanical errors in programming or delivery

Overall, with good patient selection, PCA can be very effective particularly for sternotomy incision cardiac surgery

Just as with noncardiac thoracic surgeries, studies have advocated the use of epidural or intrathecal anesthetics and/or opioids in cardiac surgery patients [90, 91]. In patients

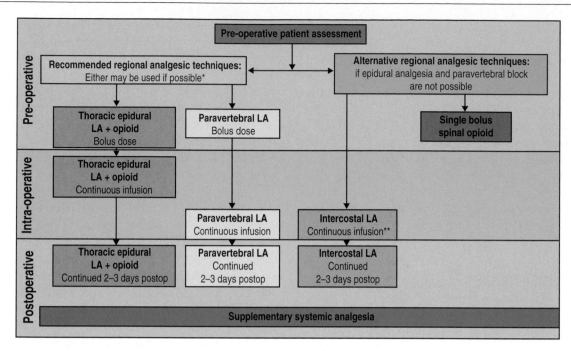

Fig. 9.4 Overall PROSPECT recommendations: regional techniques for post-thoracotomy analgesia. *Asterisk*: either thoracic epidural local anesthetic (LA) opioid or paravertebral block with LA is recommended as the primary analgesic approach; further studies on efficacy and safety are necessary to determine which technique is superior. *Double*

asterisk: if intercostal LA is used, administration by continuous infusion is recommended, despite limited data, because of the requirement for continuous analgesia for the long duration of postthoracotomy pain (reprinted from Joshi [100], with permission from Lippincott Williams & Wilkins)

with severe pain associated with sternal fractures due to the sternal retraction device used during internal mammary artery harvest, epidural analgesia has been shown to be safe and effective; and results in improved postoperative pulmonary function [83]. However, these techniques have not been adopted because of concerns over respiratory depression and epidural hematoma in patients who require full anticoagulation during surgical intervention [82].

Multimodal analgesia, the combination of different modes of delivering analgesia, has been shown to be more effective than single methods of reducing pain. Multiple studies with regional anesthesia strategies in combination with systemic analgesics have demonstrated improved patient outcomes, including decreasing length of hospital stay. [83, 88, 92, 93] Continuous regional infusion of a local anesthetic to the operative site using an elastomeric pump (On Q™ pump) significantly improved postoperative pain control while decreasing the amount of opiate analgesics required in cardiac patients with median sternotomy or thoracotomy incisions [83, 88, 93–96].

These studies also demonstrated that the regional infusion of anesthetic does not increase the incidence of wound complications. Most studies have shown a trend toward a lower infection rate, which has been hypothesized to be due to the antimicrobial action of local anesthetics [97]. Regional anesthetic techniques have been used after minimally invasive cardiac surgery performed through a limited thoracotomy incision [98, 99]. This technique decreased chest wall pain

and had fewer complications compared with those seen in control subjects. These studies demonstrate the safety and efficacy of this technique.

The paravertebral continuous catheter technique for thoracotomy pain is a technique that is gaining popularity because of its effectiveness in controlling unilateral thoracotomy incision pain. The technique is described by Karmakar [100]. Thoracic paravertebral block (TPVB) is the technique of injecting local anesthetic adjacent to the thoracic vertebra close to where the spinal nerves emerge from the intervertebral foramina. This results in ipsilateral somatic and sympathetic nerve blockade in multiple contiguous thoracic dermatomes above and below the site of injection [100]. Catheters can be placed using a similar technique that can then provide a continuous infusion of low concentration local anesthetic. In Fig. 9.4, Joshi and colleagues present a decision tree for the use of various regional anesthetic techniques for management of postthoracotomy pain, which can be useful in the management of these patients [101].

Wound Pump

For median sternotomy incisions, after reapproximation of the sternum with wire sutures, two 20-gauge catheters with multiple side openings are inserted percutaneously and placed

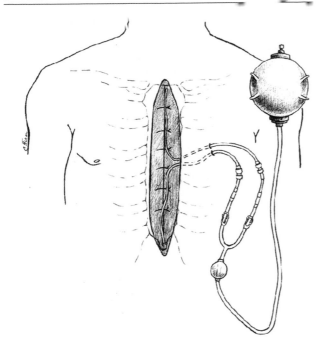

Fig. 9.5 Intraoperative placement of wound catheters and an elastomeric pump (reprinted from Dowling [82] with permission from Elsevier)

directly over the sternum [83]. These catheters can be connected to any type of appropriate pump but are often connected to a pressurized disposable elastomeric pump that contains a flow regulator, which allows for delivery of a local anesthetic (e.g., 0.2% ropivacaine) at predetermined rates (~4 ml/h). These catheters are usually removed after 48 h. This is a straightforward procedure (see Fig. 9.5). After the operation, the elastomeric pump does not require any adjustment or care by physicians or the nursing staff. It can be used for essentially all patients undergoing sternotomy or thoracotomy cardiac surgery, but may not be appropriate for those patients who are anticipated to remain intubated for a prolonged period of time and requiring intravenous sedation [83]. Intercostal nerve blocks are usually performed in combination with this technique for thoracotomy incision. Bilateral intercostal blocks are performed for sternotomy incision. Or as previously mentioned, bilateral paravertebral catheters for continuous local anesthetic infusion can be implemented.

The addition of nonsteroidal antiinflammatory agents (ibuprofen, naproxen sodium) may play an increasing role. However, there are always concerns about bleeding and renal dysfunction with their use, and these drugs often stopped for these reasons [83]. Cox-2 inhibitors (celecoxib) could be useful as described earlier in this chapter for thoracic surgeries. And should a specific Cox-2 inhibitor that is approved for intravenous administration become available, it could be used in the immediate postoperative period with less concerns for bleeding or renal impairment than the currently used Ketorolac.

Intravenous dexmedetomidine infusion has been tried as an adjunct to intravenous opioid with some success. It is an alfa-2 receptor agonist just like clonidine, with a short half-life unlike clonidine. It provides analgesia with side effects of sedation, bradycardia, and hypotension (Berger, June 2010, unpublished experience).

Intravenous ketamine-midazolam infusion has been used to minimize the use of opioids in patients with high tolerance to narcotics (Berger, June 2010, unpublished experience).

On postoperative day two or three, most patients are converted over to oral pain medications, for example, hydrocodone/acetaminophen, acetaminophen/codeine, oxycodone/acetaminophen, etc. Patients at USC University Hospital are given a preoperative cardiac surgery brochure, which describes this process [99].

In addition to the interventions described earlier, there are nonmedication adjuncts to pain relief. When used along with medication, these techniques can dramatically reduce the pain. These are also described for patients in this brochure. Relaxation tapes or Guided Imagery is a proven form of focused relaxation that coaches patients in creating calm, peaceful images in their minds, a "mental escape." Patients can get relaxation tapes from bookstores, hospital gift shops, or can rent them at the library. For best results, patients should practice using the tape or CD before surgery and then use it frequently during recovery while resting.

Surgical Bra and Vest

For women, pain and discomfort may be felt at the incision site due to tension from the weight of the breasts when lying down or standing. Female patients should wear a nonunderwire surgical bra 24 h a day for 1 month after cardiac surgery. Adjustable bras that have velcro closures will support the chest as well as ease pain. Some women may find their own bra more comfortable. Large men may feel more incision support with a surgical vest.

Use of the Pillow

A pillow can splint the incision area and help with pain during coughing and deep breathing exercises. Patients should continue to use the pillow at home to find a more comfortable lying position as well as during coughing and deep breathing exercises to provide support for the chest incision.

Heating Pad

Heating pads can provide significant relief of muscle aches. *They are not to be used on the incision sites.*

Summary

The geriatric patient who presents for thoracic or cardiac surgery must receive careful attention to pain management. But as Cook and Rooke [68] conclude it is clear from a review of the physiologic changes that occur with aging, and that even the fit elderly patient's ability to compensate for perioperative stress is compromised after thoracic or cardiac surgery. The cardiac, pulmonary, neurologic, and neuroendocrine changes that occur with aging make hypotension, low cardiac output, hypoxia, hypercarbia, and disordered *fluid regulation more commonplace in the perioperative period.* Furthermore, because baseline cardiac, pulmonary, renal, and neurologic function is typically adequate in the absence of acute challenges, it can be very difficult to predict the effect of perioperative stress on the older patient [69].

In addition, as Chassery [101] amply reports, postthoracotomy chronic pain occurs frequently and, without prevention, affects more than 50% of patients. He further states and presents data to support the conclusions that this type of chronic pain has significant repercussions on the quality of life for patients and important social costs [101]. Adapting a multimodal perioperative strategy including the use of thoracic epidural catheters and or paravertebral catheters can prevent pain and enhance the effects of other analgesics and adjuvants such as ketamine, gabapentin, and preganbalin [101].

Chassery concludes his report with several "Points To Remember" [101].

• Chronic pain after thoracotomy is defined as a pain persisting for more than 2 months after surgery.
• Chronic pain affects more than 50% of patients after thoracotomy and the neuropathic features of the pain are significant.
• The mechanisms producing acute chronic pain postthoracotomy are associated with intercostal nerve damage and sensitization of the CNS.
• A careful management strategy of anesthesia for patients after thoracotomy should be planned to prevent the development of chronic pain.
• A thoracic epidural associated with a local anesthetic and a lipid-soluble opioid, as well as a paravertebral catheter, remain the chosen techniques for treating acute postthoracotomy pain and preventing pain chronicity.
• VATS allows a reduction in the intensity of acute postoperative pain, but it does not reduce the incidence of chronic pain.

Therefore, failure to appreciate and implement adequate pain control techniques in this patient population will most certainly lead to greater morbidity and mortality after thoracic or cardiac surgery, and represents an abdication of our responsibility as physicians. The availability of techniques to

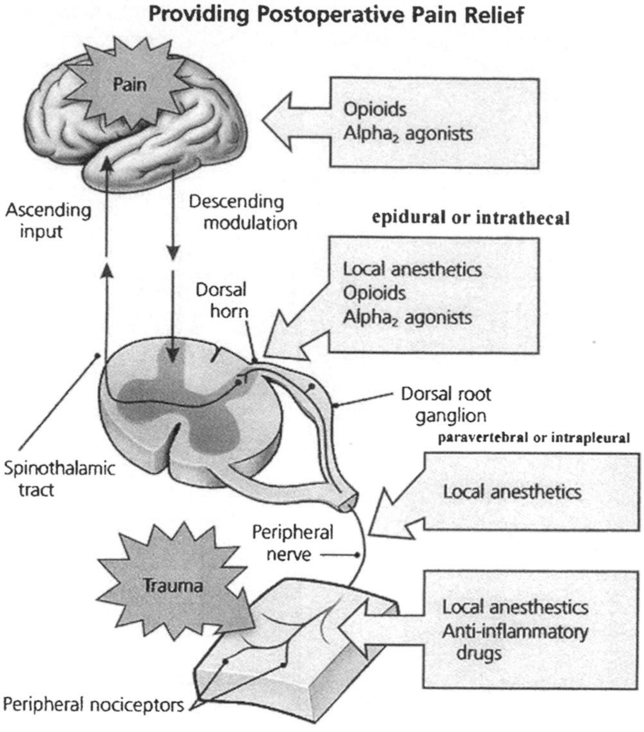

Providing Postoperative Pain Relief

Fig. 9.6 The pain pathway and interventions that can modulate activity at each point (data from Gottschalk [102] and modified with permission from Kehlet [103])

intervene at every level of the nociceptive (*pain*) pathway, as shown in Fig. 9.6, should make uncontrolled pain and chronic pain, conditions of the past.

References

1. Brennan F, Carr D, Cousins M. Pain management: a fundamental human right. Anesth Analg. 2007;105:205–21.
2. Rathmell JP, Wu CL, Sinatra RS, et al. Acute post-surgical pain management: A critical appraisal of current practice. Reg Anesth Pain Med. 2006;31(4 suppl 1):1–42.
3. Gagliese L, Gauthier LR, Macpherson AK, Jovellanos M, Chan YW. Correlates of postoperative pain and intravenous patient-controlled analgesia use in younger and older surgical patients. Pain Med. 2008;3:299–314.
4. Apfelbaum JL, Chen C, Mehta SS, Gan TJ. Postoperative pain experience: Results from a national survey suggest postoperative pain continues to be undermanaged. Anesth Analg. 2003;97(2):534–40.
5. Frasco PE, Sprung J, Trentman TL. The impact of the Joint Commission for Accreditation of Healthcare Organizations pain initiative on perioperative opiate consumption and recovery room length of stay. Anesth Analg. 2005;100:162–8.
6. Stafford-Smith M. McLoughlin T. In: Hensley F, Martin D, Gravlee G, editors. A practical approach to cardiac anesthesia. 4th ed. Philadelphia: Lippincott, Williams & Wilkins; 2008. p. 741–56.
7. Perkins F, Kehlet H. Chronic pain as an outcome of surgery: a review of predictive factors. Anesthesiology. 2000;93:1123–33.

8. Katz J, Jackson M, Kavanagh B, Brian P, Sandler A. Acute pain after thoracic surgery predicts long-term post-thoracotomy pain. Clin J Pain. 1996;12(1):50–5.

9. Macrae WA. Chronic pain after surgery. Br J Anaesth. 2001;87:88–98.

10. Landreneau RJ, Mack MJ, Hazelrigg SR, et al. Prevalence of chronic pain after pulmonary resection by thoracotomy or video-assisted thoracic surgery. J Thorac Cardiovasc Surg. 1994;107:1079–85.

11. Bertrand PC, Regnard JF, Spaggiari L, et al. Immediate and long-term results after surgical treatment of primary spontaneous pneumothorax by VATS. Ann Thorac Surg. 1996;61:1641–5.

12. Sinatra R. Role of COX-2 inhibitors in the evolution of acute pain management. J Pain Symptom Manage. 2002;24(1 suppl):S18–27.

13. Hopf HW, Hunt TK, West JM, et al. Wound tissue oxygen tension predicts the risk of wound infection in surgical patients. Arch Surg. 1997;132(9):997–1004.

14. Page GG, Blakely WP, Ben-Eliyahu S. Evidence that postoperative pain is a mediator of the tumor-promoting effects of surgery in rats. Pain. 2001;90:191–9.

15. Carr D, Goudas L. Acute pain. Lancet. 1999;353:2052–8.

16. Davies HTO, Crombie IK, Macrae WA, Rogers KM. Pain clinic patients in northern Britain. Pain Clin. 1992;5:129–35.

17. Siddall P, Cousins M. Persistent pain as a disease entity: implications for clinical management. Anesth Analg. 2004;99:510–20.

18. Chung F, Mezei G, Tong D. Adverse events in ambulatory surgery: a comparison between elderly and younger patients. Can J Anesth. 1999;46(4):309–21.

19. McCleane G. Pain and the elderly patient, Chapter 1. In: McCleane G, Smith H, editors. Clinical management of the elderly patient in pain. New York: The Haworth Medical Press; 2006.

20. Gagliese L, Melzack R. The assessment of pain in the elderly. In: Lomrang J, Mostofsky D, editors. Handbook of pain and aging. New York: Plenum Press; 1997. p. 69–96.

21. Gibson S, Farrell M. A review of age differences in the neurophysiology of nociception and the perceptual experience of pain. Clin J Pain. 2004;20(4):227–39.

22. Shin S, Eisenach J. Peripheral nerve injury sensitizes the response to visceral distension but not its inhibition by the antidepressant Milnacipran. Anesthesiology. 2004;100(3):671–5.

23. Siddall P, Cousins M. Introduction to pain mechanisms: Implications for neural blockade, chapter 23.1. In: Cousins M, Bridenbaugh P, editors. Clinical anesthesia and management of pain. 3rd ed. Philadelphia: Lippincott-Raven; 1998. p. 687.

24. Berger JM. Acute post-operative pain management in the elderly. In: Rosenthal RA, Zenilman ME, Katlie MR, editors. Principles and practice of geriatric surgery. 2nd ed. New York: Springer; 2010.

25. Auburn F, Monsel S, Langeron O, Coriat P, Riou B. Post operative titration of intravenous morphine in the elderly patient. Anesthesiology. 2002;96:17–23.

26. Daykin A, Bowen D, Daunders D, Norman J. Respiratory depression after morphine in the elderly. Anaesthesia. 1986;41:910–4.

27. Cepeda M, Farrar J, Baumbarten M, Boston R, Carr D, Strom B. Side effects of opioids during short-term administration: effect of age, gender, and race. Clin Pharmacol Ther. 2003;74:102–12.

28. Fine P, Ashburn M. Functional neuroanatomy and nociception, chapter 1. In: Ashburn M, Rice L, editors. The management of pain. New York: Churchill Livingston; 1998. p. 1–16.

29. Cousins MJ. Visceral pain. In: Anderson S, Bond M, Mehta M, Swerdlow M, editors. Chronic non-cancer pain: assessment and practical management. Lancaster: MTP Press; 1987.

30. Malliani A. The conceptualization of cardiac pain as a nonspecific and unreliable alarm system, chapter 4. In: Gebhart G, editor. Visceral pain: progress in pain research and management, vol. 5. Seattle: WA. IASP Press; 1995. p. 63–74.

31. Dajczman E, Gordon A, Kreisman H, Wolkove N. Long-term postthoracotomy pain. Chest. 1991;99:270–4.

32. Ochroch EA, Gottschalk A, Augostides J, et al. Long-term pain and activity during recovery from major thoracotomy using thoracic epidural analgesia. Anesthesiology. 2002;97:1234–44.

33. Latremoliere A, Woolf CJ. Central sensitization: a generator of pain hypersensitivity by central neural plasticity. J Pain. 2009;9:895–926.

34. Scawn ND, Pennefather SH, Soorae A, Wang JY, Russell GN. Ipsilateral shoulder pain after thoracotomy with epidural analgesia: the influence of phrenic nerve infiltration with lidocaine. Anesth Analg. 2001;93:260–4.

35. Tan N, Agnew NM, Scawn ND, et al. Suprascapular nerve block for ipsilateral shoulder pain after thoracotomy with thoracic epidural analgesia: a double-blind comparison of 0.5% bupivacaine and 0.9% saline. Anesth Analg. 2002;94:199–202.

36. Benedetti F, Vighetti S, Ricco C, et al. Neurophysiologic assessment of nerve impairment in posterolateral and muscle-sparing thoracotomy. J Thorac Cardiovasc Surg. 1998;115:841–7.

37. Gottschalk A, Cohen S, Yang S, Ochroch ES. Preventing and treating pain after thoracic surgery. Anesthesiology. 2006;104(3):594–600.

38. Obata H, Saito S, Fujita N, Fuse Y, Ishizaki K, Goto F. Epidural block with mepivacaine before surgery reduces long-term postthoracotomy pain. Can J Anaesth. 1999;46:1127–32.

39. Soto R, Fu ES. Acute pain management for patients undergoing thoracotomy. Ann Thorac Surg. 2003;75:1349–57.

40. Richardson J, Lönnqvist PA. Thoracic paravertebral block. Br J Anaesth. 1998;81:230–8.

41. Mann C, Pouzeratte Y, Bocarra G, et al. Comparison of intravenous or epidural patient-controlled analgesia in the elderly after major abdominal surgery. Anesthesiology. 2000;92(2):433–41.

42. Carli F, Mayo N, Klubien K, Schricker T, Trudel J, Belliveau P. Epidural analgesia enhances functional exercise capacity and health related quality of life after colonic surgery. Results of a randomized trial. Anesthesiology. 2002;97(3):540–9.

43. Viscusi E. Emerging techniques in the management of acute pain: epidural analgesia. Anesth Analg. 2005;101:S23–9.

44. Rawal N, Wattwil M. Respiratory depression after epidural morphine – an experimental and clinical study. Anesth Analg. 1984;63:8–14.

45. Doblar DD, Muldoon SM, Abbrecht PH, Baksoff J, Watson RL. Epidural morphine following epidural local anesthesia: effect on ventilatory and airway occlusion pressure responses to CO_2. Anesthesiology. 1981;55:423–8.

46. Brodner G, Pogatzki E, Van Aken H, et al. A multimodal approach to control postoperative pathophysiology and rehabilitation in patients undergoing abdominothoracic esophagectomy. Anesth Analg. 1998;86:228–34.

47. Howell SB. Clinical applications of a novel sustained-release injectable drug delivery system: DepoFoam™ technology. Cancer J. 2001;7:219–27.

48. DepoDur™(package insert), Bedminster, NJ: EKR Therapeutics Inc; 2007.

49. Wurnig PN, Lackner H, Teiner C, et al. Is intercostal block for pain management in thoracic surgery more successful than epidural anaesthesia? Eur J Cardiothorac Surg. 2002;21:115–9.

50. Detterbeck F. Efficacy of methods of intercostal nerve block for pain relief after thoracotomy. Ann Thorac Surg. 2005;80:1550–9.

51. Conacher ID, Kokri M. Postoperative paravertebral blocks for thoracic surgery. A radiological appraisal. Br J Anaesth. 1987;59:155–61.

52. Lönnqvist PA, MacKenzie J, Soni AK, Conacher ID. Paravertebral blockade. Failure rate and complications. Anaesthesia. 1995;50:813–5.

53. Eng J, Sabanathan S. Site of action of continuous extrapleural intercostal nerve block. Ann Thorac Surg. 1991;51:387–9.

54. Chan VW, Chung F, Cheng DC, Seyone C, Chung A, Kirby TJ. Analgesic and pulmonary effects of continuous intercostal nerve block following thoracotomy. Can J Anaesth. 1991;38:733–9.

55. Perttunen K, Nilsson E, Heinonen J, Hirvisalo EL, Salo JA, Kalso E. Extradural, paravertebral and intercostal nerve blocks for post-thoracotomy pain. Br J Anaesth. 1995;75:541–7.

56. Niamh PC, Andrew DS, Katherine PG. Postthoracotomy paravertebral analgesia: Will it replace epidural analgesia? Anesthesiol Clin. 2008;26(2):369–80.

57. Richardson J, Sabanathan S, Eng J, et al. Continuous intercostal nerve block versus epidural morphine for postthoracotomy analgesia. Ann Thorac Surg. 1993;55:377–80.

58. Barron DJ, Tolan MJ, Lea RE. A randomized controlled trial of continuous extra-pleural analgesia post-thoracotomy: efficacy and choice of local anaesthetic. Eur J Anaes. 1999;16:236–45.

59. Watson DS, Panian S, Kendall V, Maher DP, Peters G. Pain control after thoracotomy: bupivacaine versus lidocaine in continuous extrapleural intercostal nerve blockade. Ann Thorac Surg. 1999;67:825–9.

60. Matthews PJ, Govenden V. Comparison of continuous paravertebral and extradural infusions of bupivacaine for pain relief after thoracotomy. Br J Anaesth. 1989;62:204–5.

61. Bimston DN, McGee JP, Liptay MJ, Fry WA. Continuous paravertebral extrapleural infusion for post-thoracotomy pain management. Surgery. 1999;126:650–7.

62. Richardson J, Sabanathan S, Jones J, Shah RD, Chesma S, Mearns AJ. A prospective, randomized comparison of preoperative and continuous balanced epidural or paravertebral bupivacaine on post-thoracotomy pain, pulmonary function and stress responses. Br J Anaesth. 1999;83:387–92.

63. Kaiser AM, Zollinger A, De Lorenzi D, Largiadèr F, Walter W. Prospective, randomized comparison of extrapleural versus epidural analgesia for postthoracotomy pain. Ann Thorac Surg. 1998;66:367–72.

64. Berrisford RG, Sabanathan S, Mearns AJ, Clarke BJ, Hamdi A. Plasma concentrations of bupivacaine and its enantiomers during continuous extrapleural intercostal nerve block. Br J Anaesth. 1993;70:201–4.

65. Dauphin A, Gupta RN, Young JE, Morton WD. Serum bupivacaine concentrations during continuous extrapleural infusion. Can J Anaesth. 1997;44:367–70.

66. Scott DB. Toxic effects of local anaesthetic agents on the central nervous system. Br J Anaesth. 1986;58:732–5.

67. Francois T, Blanloeil Y, Pillet F, et al. Effect of interpleural administration of bupivacaine or lidocaine on pain and morphine requirement after esophagectomy with thoracotomy: a randomized, double-blind and controlled study. Anesth Analg. 1995;80:718–23.

68. Cook D, Rooke G. Priorities in perioperative geriatrics. Anesth Analg. 2003;96:1823–36.

69. Silverstein J, Bloom H, Cassel C. New challenges in anesthesia: new practice opportunities. Anesthesiol Clin North Am. 1999;17:453–65.

70. Henry C. Mechanisms of changes in basal metabolism during aging. Eur J Clin Nutr. 2000;54:77–91.

71. Grandison M, Boudinot F. Age-related changes in protein binding of drugs: implications for therapy. Clin Pharmacokinet. 2000;38:271–90.

72. Benet L, Kroetz D, Sheiner L. Pharmacokinetics: the dynamics of drug absorption, distribution, and elimination. Chapter 1. In: Hardman J, Limbird L, editors. Goodman & Gilman's the pharmacological basis of therapeutics. 9th ed. New York: McGraw-Hill; 1996. p. 3–28.

73. Epstein M. Aging and the kidney. J Am Soc Nephrol. 1996;7:1106–22.

74. Lewis M. Alterations in metabolic functions and electrolytes, Chapter 7. In: Silverstein J, Rooke GA, Reves J, McLeskey C, editors. Geriatric anesthesiology. 2nd ed. New York: Springer; 2008. p. 97–106.

75. Svarese A. Intravenous and subcutaneous patient-controlled analgesia. In: Wallace M, Staats P, editors. Pain medicine and management: just the facts. New York: McGraw-Hill; 2004.

76. Gagliese L, Jackson M, Ritvo P, Wowk A, Katz J. Age is not an impediment to effective use of patient-controlled analgesia by surgical patients. Anesthesiology. 2000;93(3):601–10.

77. Ginsberg B, Sinatra R, Adler L, Crews J, Hord L, Laurito C, et al. Conversion to oral controlled-release oxycodone from intravenous opioid analgesic in the postoperative setting. Pain Med. 2003;4(1):31–8.

78. Kellet J. Acute soft tissue injuries. A review of the literature. Med Sci Sports Exerc. 1986;18:489–500.

79. Greenberg HE, Gottesdiener K, Huntington M, et al. A new cyclo-oxygenase-2 inhibitor, rofecoxib (VIOXX), did not alter the antiplatelet effects of low-dose aspirin in healthy volunteers. J Clin Pharmacol. 2000;40:1509–15.

80. Mogensen T, Eliasen F, Ejlersen E, Vegger P, Nielsen IK, Kehlet H. Epidural clonidine enhances postoperative analgesia from a combined low-dose epidural bupivacaine and morphine regimen. Anesth Analg. 1992;75:607–10.

81. Lena P, Balarac N, Arnulf JJ, Teboul J, Bonnet F. Intrathecal morphine and clonidine for coronary artery bypass grafting. Br J Anaesth. 2003;90(3):300–3.

82. Dowling R, Thielmeier K, Ghaly A, et al. Improved pain control after cardiac surgery: results of a randomized, double-blind, clinical trial. J Thorac Cardiovasc Surg. 2003;126(5):1271–8.

83. Skubas N, Lichman A, Sharma A, Thomas S. Postoperative pain management, chapter 31. In: Barash PG, Cullen BF, Stoelting RK, editors. Anesthesia for cardiac surgery. 5th ed. Philadelphia: Lippincott Williams & Wilkins; 2006.

84. Kalso E, Mennander S, Tasmuth T, Nilsson E. Chronic post-sternotomy pain. Acta Anaesthesiol Scand. 2001;45:935–9.

85. Scott NB, Turfrey DJ, Ray DA, et al. A prospective randomized study of the potential benefits of thoracic epidural anesthesia and analgesia in patients undergoing coronary artery bypass grafting. Anesth Analg. 2001;93(3):528–35.

86. Gust R, Pecher S, Gust A, Hoffman V, Böhrer H, Martin E. Effect of patient-controlled analgesia on pulmonary complications after coronary artery bypass grafting. Crit Care Med. 1999;27(10):2314–6.

87. Deneuvile M, Bisserier A, Regnard J, Chevalier M, Levasseur P, Herve P. Continuous intercostal analgesia with 0.5% bupivacaine after thoracotomy: a randomized study. Ann Thorac Surg. 1993;55(2):381–5.

88. Roberge CW, McEwen M. The effects of local anesthetics on postoperative pain. AORN J. 1998;68(6):1003–12.

89. Gold BS, Kitz DS, Lecky JH, Neuhaus JM. Unanticipated admission to the hospital following ambulatory surgery. JAMA. 1989;262:3008–10.

90. Mehta Y, Juneja R, Madhok H, Trehan N. Lumbar versus thoracic epidural buprenorphine for postoperative analgesia following coronary artery bypass graft surgery. Acta Anaesthesiol Scand. 1999;43(4):388–93.

91. Chaney M, Furry P, Fluder E, Slogoff S. Intrathecal morphine for coronary artery bypass grafting and early extubation. Anesth Analg. 1997;85(3):706–7.

92. Cheong W, Seow-Choen F, Eu K, Tang O, Heah S. Randomized clinical trial of local bupivacaine perfusion versus parenteral morphine infusion for pain relief after laparotomy. Br J Surg. 2001;80:519–20.

93. Fredman B, Shapiro A, Zohar E, et al. The analgesic efficacy of patient-controlled ropivacaine instillation after cesarean delivery. Anesth Analg. 2000;91(6):1436–40.

94. Klein S, Grant S, Greengrass R, et al. Interscalene brachial plexus block with a continuous catheter insertion system and a disposable infusion pump. Anesth Analg. 2000;91(6):1473–8.

95. Rosenberg H, Renkonen OV. Antimicrobial activity of bupivacaine and morphine. Anesthesiology. 1985;62(2):178–9.

96. Mehta Y, Swaminathan M, Mishra Y, Trehan N. A comparative evaluation of intrapleural and thoracic epidural analgesia for postoperative pain relief after minimally invasive direct coronary artery bypass surgery. J Cardiothorac Vasc Anesth. 1999;13(5):653–5.

97. Dhole S, Mehta Y, Saxena H, et al. Comparison of continuous thoracic epidural and paravertebral blocks for postoperative analgesia after minimally invasive direct coronary artery bypass surgery. J Cardiothorac Vasc Anesth. 2001;15(3):288–92.

98. Cardiothoracic Surgery, University of Southern California, Keck School of Medicine. A patient guide to pain management and medication after heart surgery.

99. Karmakar M. Thoracic paravertebral block: review article. Anesthesiology. 2001;95(3):771–80.

100. Joshi G, Bonnet F, Shah R, et al. A systematic review of randomized trials evaluating regional techniques for postthoracotomy analgesia. Anesth Analg. 2008;107:1026–40.

101. ChasseryC. Thoracic surgery as a model for postoperative acute and chronic pain. Anesthesiology Rounds. 2007;6(1): as presented in the Department of Anesthesiology, Faculty of Medicine , University of Montreal, www.anesthesiologyrounds.ca.

102. Gottschalk A, Smith D. New concepts in acute pain therapy: preemptive analgesia. Am Fam Physician. 2001;63(10):1979–84. (www.aafp.org/afp).

103. Kehlet H, Dahl JB. The value of "multimodal" or "balanced analgesia" in postoperative pain treatment. Anesth Analg. 1993;77:1049.

Chapter 10
Palliative Care in the Elderly

Geoffrey P. Dunn

Abstract During the past two decades, the field of palliative care has matured and organized itself into a recognized specialty of medicine with an increasingly diverse spectrum of settings, including geriatrics and surgery. Palliative care is defined as interdisciplinary care, that aims to relieve suffering, and improve the quality of life for patients and their families with serious or advanced illness. There is no limiting prognostic window for this approach to care, though it is increasingly suitable as the disease progresses. It can be offered as the sole aim of care, or simultaneously with all other appropriate medical treatment. Given its emphasis on symptom control and quality of life, palliative care principles and practice have much to offer elderly patients and their families, anticipating or receiving surgical care for cardiothoracic conditions.

Keywords Surgical palliative care • Palliative care • End-of-life care • Syndrome of imminent demise • Advance directives • Hospice • Communication • Symptom management • Cardiomyopathy • Lung cancer • AICD • Interdisciplinary team

Introduction

During the past two decades, the field of palliative care has matured and organized itself into a recognized specialty of medicine with an increasingly diverse spectrum of settings, including geriatrics and surgery. Although palliative care is rooted in hospice philosophy, it has a much wider scope than terminal illness which is associated with hospice. While hospice care has been limited to patients not planning further disease directed treatment, and who have a life expectancy of less than six months, palliative care is defined as *interdisciplinary care that aims to relieve suffering, and improve the quality of life for patients and their families with serious or advanced illness.* There is no limiting prognostic window for this approach to care, though it is increasingly suitable as disease progresses. It can be offered as the sole aim of care or simultaneously with all other appropriate medical treatment. Given its emphasis on symptom control and quality of life, palliative care principles and practice are especially appropriate for elderly patients and their families anticipating or receiving surgical care for cardiothoracic conditions.

The increasing recognition of the value of the palliative approach to care, reflects a fundamental shift in priorities within the culture of medicine that has been occurring over the past three decades. The dominant imperative of saving or prolonging life has been increasingly tempered by quality of life considerations during this era. This development was presaged by the widespread and growing popularity of home based hospice care in the US, introduced in the mid 1970s. Public awareness of end-of-life issues was further enhanced by judicial decisions ruling on the individual's right to deny medical treatment [1], the debate on physician-assisted suicide, and adverse experiences with end-of-life care [2] that contrasted so sharply with progress in other venues of medical care.

It was not until the mid 1990s that the field of surgery began to direct its attention to quality of life outcomes [3], and only recently have reliable metrics been developed for measuring them. Increasing research, inpalliative care and quality of life related to surgical intervention, has been supported by the American College of Surgeons [4] (Table 10.1), the American Board of Surgery [5], surgical educators [6], and critical care surgeons [7].

Why Palliative Care?

The landmark SUPPORT [2] study of patients with advanced illness, and their families, in acute care hospital settings, demonstrated marked deficiencies in pain management, and communication about patient preferences. Equally sobering

G.P. Dunn (✉)
Department of Surgery and Palliative Care, Hamot Medical Center, 2050 South Shore Dr., Erie, PA 16505, USA
e-mail: gpdunn1@earthlink.net

M.R. Katlic (ed.), *Cardiothoracic Surgery in the Elderly*, DOI 10.1007/978-1-4419-0892-6_10,
© Springer Science+Business Media, LLC 2011

Table 10.1 Statement of principles of palliative care

Respect the dignity and autonomy of patients, patients' surrogates, and
   caregivers

Honor the right of the competent patient or surrogate to choose among
   treatments, including those that may or may not prolong life

Communicate effectively and empathically with patients, their
   families, and caregivers

Identify the primary goals of care from the patient's perspective, and
   address how the surgeon's care can achieve the patient's objectives

Strive to alleviate pain and other burdensome physical and nonphysi-
   cal symptoms

Recognize, assess, discuss, and offer access to services for psychological, social, and spiritual issues

Provide access to therapeutic support, encompassing the spectrum
   from life-prolonging treatments through hospice care, when they
   can realistically be expected to improve the quality of life as
   perceived by the patient

Recognize the physician's responsibility to discourage treatments that
   are unlikely to achieve the patient's goals, and encourage patients
   and families to consider hospice care when the prognosis for
   survival is likely to be less than a half-year

Arrange for continuity of care by the patient's primary and/or
   specialist physician, alleviating the sense of abandonment patients
   may feel when "curative" therapies are no longer useful

Maintain a collegial and supportive attitude toward others entrusted
   with care of the patient

was the recognition that a considerable portion of Medicare expenditure has been for patients during the last 6 months of life, many in a critical care setting with poor quality of life [8]. Moral [9, 10], socioeconomic [11, 12], and clinical outcomes [13, 14] arguments have subsequently been advanced in support of offering palliative care services in the hospital setting, during an era when the demographic pattern is trending towards longer patient survival, including those with multiple, serious, and chronic co-morbidities.

The number of in-hospital palliative care programs has increased linearly from 632 (15% of hospitals) in 2000 to 1,027 (25% of hospitals) in 2003 [15], and has continued to do so since. The critical care setting has proven to be a very successful and rewarding venue for palliative care consultation, because of enhanced communication, more timely clarification of goals, and increased attention to symptom control [16, 17]. In a recent survey of trauma and neurosurgeons at a university-based American College of Surgeons Level 1 trauma center, the respondents believed they were better equipped to manage the consequences of a sudden advanced illness through collaboration with a palliative care service [18].

The Palliative Care Team

An interdisciplinary team is the method of service delivery for all palliative care programs, and has been identified as a core element of palliative care by the National Consensus

Project for Quality Palliative Care [19]. The National Quality Forum [20] subsequently endorsed this. The scope of the team membership is highly variable and flexible, depending on the nature of the facility, the available expertise, and other resources. The core constituents usually include physicians, nurses, social workers, and chaplains, though the contributions of pharmacists, psychologists, physical and occupational therapists, wound care specialists, speech and language pathologists, nutritionists, and volunteers are invaluable. Complementary and alternative therapies are often integrated to the extent they do not conflict or undermine the patient-designated goals of care. Certification in hospice and palliative medicine by respective boards of team members is desirable, though the minimum educational standard for team participation should be a basic understanding of the domains of palliative care (physical, psychological, social, and spiritual), the goals of the Medicare Hospice Benefit (MHB), communication skills, pain and non-pain symptom management, grief, and bereavement.

Indications for Palliative Care Referral

Considerations for referral of elderly cardiovascular surgical patients for palliative care consultation include pre-operative assessment and clarification of goals, assistance with pain and non-pain symptom management, psychosocial family support, assistance in withdrawal of life support, and disposition planning, especially when hospice care is a consideration. When making a referral for palliative care services, it is extremely important to recommend this to the patient and family in a positive, non-defeatist way. Rather than saying, "There is nothing more we can do, so we are just going to make (you/him) comfortable", say, "In order to meet the goals of care we have been discussing [name a few mentioned by patient/family], I would like our palliative care team to visit you" [21]. Emphasis on the team's experience in pain and non-pain symptom management, and its expertise in pinpointing patient-designated goals of care, can follow this introduction. To allay fears of abandonment, reassure the patient/family that palliative care consultation is a supplement to your own on-going involvement.

Clinical Scenarios

The following clinical scenarios have been taken from my consultative practice as a surgeon and a consultant for palliative care during the past 15 years. They represent common themes and problems encountered in clinical palliative care.

Case Scenario 1: Unstable Angina/Cardiomyopathy

Teaching points: communication of bad news, transitioning of goals of care

Mrs. H., an 86-year-old widowed, vivacious white female, living alone in her own home, presented with anginal pain and shortness of breath. Admission chest X-ray showed cephalization of vessels, cardiomegaly, and bilateral pleural effusions consistent with congestive heart failure. Cardiac echo demonstrated global akinesis with an estimated ejection fraction of 15–20%. Serum creatinine was 3.0 mg/dL. A previously performed cardiac catheterization demonstrated coronary disease unfavorable for stenting. Because of this, a cardiothoracic surgeon was consulted for an opinion. A consulting nephrologist expressed concern about the probability of temporary, and possibly permanent hemodialysis following coronary angiography and/or surgery. Following vigorous diuresis, her dyspnea improved, though her serum creatinine increased. Mrs. H's only son who was present during her consultations expressed his strong wish that she undergo any intervention possible to improve her cardiac status, because she was "so 'with it' and otherwise healthy." Sensing Mrs. H's reluctance to undergo catheterization, dialysis, or surgery, her consulting surgeon suggested a meeting with the palliative care team for improving communication about the implications of her condition, and clarification of goals of care.

The surgeon initiated the referral by sitting down next to Mrs. H, and asking her if she would like her son to be present while he made a recommendation. She said she would.

Surgeon: "Because of the complex nature of your condition and the number of individuals involved in your care [gesturing to her son], I recommend you meet with members of our palliative care team because of their ability to communicate with all of us as well as dig deeper about what matters to you and what it will mean for your plan of care. They will also help us control your chest pain and breathlessness as this discussion is taking place."

Shortly after this, a meeting that included Mrs. H, her son, Mrs. H's primary nurse and case manager, and the consulting palliative care physician takes place in a quiet, private setting.

Physician: "Mrs. H, now that you have been here a few days what do you know about your current medical condition"

Mrs. H: "I know I have a bad heart, and that I might need dialysis and surgery."

Physician: "Were you surprised to learn of this?"

Mrs. H: "I wasn't totally surprised. I have had heart trouble before, but this is worse than I thought."

Physician: "What did you learn that meant it was getting worse?"

Mrs. H: "That I might need dialysis and surgery."

Physician: "Are those treatments you would be willing to have?"

Mrs. H: "I don't think so. I have lived a good life and I am ready to see my husband again. We were married 61 years. I just want to be comfortable. Can't you give me something" [laughing].

Son: [Very distraught, looking at his mother] "Mom, do you want to die!"

Mrs. H: "Of course not! I just don't want to be living this way and being a burden to others."

Physician: "If I am correct, Mrs. H, you are saying that wanting to die, and readiness to die have separate meanings?"

Mrs. H: "That is exactly what I am trying to say. I am *ready* to die, but I am in no rush! I just want to be comfortable."

Sensing Mrs. H's son's unresolved tension, the physician asks Mrs. H. if she would mind if he spoke privately with her son to discuss her care further. Both Mrs. H. and her son agree this would be helpful. The physician tells Mrs. H. he will return after the discussion with some recommendations for her care. The discussion continues with the case manger, the son, and the physician:

Physician: "I can see that your mother's decision is upsetting you."

Son: "Well, yes! I don't want to just let her die. She's hardly been sick a day of her life; she was driving just last week, for God's sake, and now you're telling me she's dying!"

Physician: "No one is saying she is dying, but she is more seriously ill than her good spirits let on. Do you want more information about her illness?"

Son: "Mom never complained about anything. I just wished she had done something about this sooner. How sick is she?"

Physician: "Are you the kind of person who likes to know all the facts, or do you want me to focus more on the positive information?"

Son: "I want to know what's going on. The whole truth."

Physician: "I will tell you what we are pretty sure about, as a basis for making our best guess for what is to come. We know she has been increasingly short of breath, and more recently, having chest pain relieved by rest and heart medications. Her physical examination, chest X-ray and echocardiogram findings confirmed our suspicions that her heart is failing, most likely from coronary disease. We also know she previously had moderately severe blockage of her coronary arteries when they were studied several years ago."

Son: "I didn't know about the previous study."

Physician: "As you pointed out, your mother is a private person. She may not have wanted to burden you, just as she has said she doesn't want to in the future."

Son: "How long do you think she has to live?"

Physician: "Before I respond to that we should talk about *how* she prefers to live. She made this part easy for us: She told us she wants to be comfortable. She was very clear earlier about not wanting invasive procedures done, though we can re-confirm that when we speak to her again. Did she ever prepare a document stating her preferences about medical treatments when seriously ill?"

Son: "You mean a 'living will'?"

Physician: "Yes. It's usually made up of two parts: a person designated to make medical decisions on her behalf if she is not capable of doing so herself, and a 'yes' or 'no' check list of medical treatments like attempts at cardiac resuscitation, ventilator support, dialysis, and so on."

Son: "She doesn't have one, but I don't think she wants any of those things."

Physician: "I don't believe most of those things would be consistent with what she has asked for, nor are they likely to improve her quality or even quantity of life. She is not being unreasonable – she is at extremely high risk for a bad outcome with surgery. I wish she were a good candidate."

Son: [fighting tears] "I don't want her to suffer!"

Physician: [placing his hand on the son's shoulder]: "Of course you don't. She is lucky to have you in her corner. I am confident we can keep her comfortable by respecting her wishes and dignity, and using medications to target her bothersome symptoms. To get back to your question, 'How long?' – no one can pinpoint this. Cardiac disease, unlike cancer, is less predictable but it *is* a progressive illness. Patients can plateau for months, or even years, before a new event signals progression. Death can occur suddenly in some patients. Even if her care is focused on comfort rather than increasing survival, we are probably looking at a wide range of time, probably weeks to months, possibly even beyond that.

Son: [clearly saddened, but making good eye contact]: "When can she go home?"

Physician: "I recommend we get back to her to let her know about this discussion, and to make sure we are making her comfortable. With the help of the case manger we can plan her post-hospital care. We wouldn't want her to leave without reassuring her about our commitment to her wishes, and having reliable control of her chest pain and shortness of breath. If she has questions like yours, I will respond to them in the same way I did for you. Are you in agreement with that approach?"

Son: "Yes. And thank you for your honesty."

Physician: "Thank you. We can meet again to discuss other matters, and answer other questions that will come up. Here is my card if you need to leave a message. Let's go see your mother."

The very high rate of Medicare expenditure during the last six months of life of beneficiaries is related to ICU admissions or re-admissions for patients with end-stage disease(s). Even more pressing than the financial burdens imposed on health care systems and families, is the moral imperative of preventing unnecessary suffering related to low-yield highly invasive treatments, frequently in contrast with patients' previous stated preferences. These problems were dramatically brought to light by the landmark SUPPORT [2] study which discovered that up to 85% of patients who had previously expressed their wish to die at home died in hospital. Additionally, half of the patients studied were noted by family members to have uncontrolled, moderate to severe pain in the last days of life. The intervention phase of this study, ongoing nurse clinician notification of the attending physician about enrolled patient's prognosis and preferences, failed to improve the outcomes of pain control and adherence to patient-stated treatment preferences.

Since the time of the study, medical practice has increasingly recognized the role of direct communication between physicians and patients and their families for the achievement of quality of life outcomes. Robert Buckman is widely acknowledged for his pioneering work in elevating the process of clinical communication to the level of skill and recognition it deserves. He introduced a step-wise approach model of communication that can be adapted to both breaking bad news and setting goals of care as in the above vignette [22]. The model requires attention to setting, decorum, appropriate support, clarity of language, and follow-up contingencies. When following this model, the most critical skill in achieving the goal of maintaining the patient/family's trust and hope is the empathic response, which is the ability to identify the emotional response to a statement, i.e., bad news, and then signal to the patient that you have noticed the response and it's connection to it's source as demonstrated in the vignette: "I can see that your mother's decision [to forego life-prolonging treatment] is very upsetting to you."

The safe conduct of an operation is a convenient metaphor for Buckman's stepwise approach to communication (Table 10.2). The giving of unwelcome news is an invasive procedure. The style of communication of adverse news has been shown to have long-term impact on patients and family members. Increased organ donation [23, 24], and post-traumatic stress [25] have been associated with favorable and

Table 10.2 Operation as metaphor for communication

Comparison of Buckman's S-P-I-K-E-S [22] protocol for communication with an operative procedure	
Setting: Where to communicate	Operating room
Perception: What does patient know?	Indications/symptoms
Invitation: What does patient want to know?	Operative permit
Knowledge: Giving the patient the news	Definitive intra-operative intervention (going on bypass, clamping aorta)
Empathic response: Identification of patients' reaction and signaling to him the connection between the reaction and its source.	Assessment of physiologic impact following definitive intervention. (hypotension, hemorrhage)
Summary: Summary of discussion and next steps	Closure of wound, post-operative check

unfavorable assessments of communication, respectively. The American College of Surgeons has recently convened a task force to study patient communication [26].

Case Scenario 2: Post-Operative Multiple System Organ Failure

Teaching points: clarification of goals, withdrawal of life support

Mr. L., an 84-year-old married father of four, underwent an elective aortic valve replacement, that was complicated by a sternal wound infection resulting in SIRS. He subsequently required prolonged ventilator and pressor support, continuous renal replacement therapy, while remaining obtunded except in response to painful stimuli. On the tenth post-operative day the family was asked for permission to perform tracheostomy and percutaneous endoscopic gastrostomy (PEG), because of the anticipated prolonged need for ventilator and nutritional support. Because the family seemed inclined to deny this, despite the surgeon's belief that Mr. L. did not have a terminal illness, but a potential reversible critical illness, a palliative care consultation was arranged to assist with clarification of goals, and possible withdrawal of life support. The patient had no advance directives.

The palliative care consultant reviewed the chart and studies, examined Mr. L, then spoke directly with the surgeon, the intensivist managing the patient's ICU care, and the consulting nephrologist and neurologist. A meeting with the Mr. L's family, his primary ICU nurse, the ICU social worker, and the palliative care physician was then held:

After introductions and explanation of his role in Mr. L.'s care, the physician addresses Mrs. L who has been making medical decisions on her husband's behalf:

Physician: "Mrs. L., can you tell me what you have learned so far about your husband's condition so we are all sure we are making decisions based on the same information?"

Mrs. L.: "Why, certainly. My husband is still on the breathing machine, and now they want to do a tracheostomy and put in a feeding tube. He is on the dialysis machine. They say he is in a coma. Is that what you mean?"

Physician: "Yes. It sounds like you have a pretty good idea about just how sick he is."

Mrs. L.'s son: "Yeah, we know he's really sick, but no one is telling us if he will ever get better."

Mrs. L., doubtful: "Will he get better?"

Mrs. L.'s daughter, angry: "Come on! He never wanted to be like… like this!"

Physician: "I can see how upsetting this is for all of you, to have things not turn out, and to then have to make these types of decisions. I would like to answer the questions each of you has raised [all family members nod affirmatively, daughter crying]. To respond to you, Mrs. L., he could get "better" [gesturing quotation marks], but we have no way of predicting how much. [Looking at the son] What we do know is that getting better will require weeks of critical care at this point, the possibility of permanent dialysis, and even permanent institutionalization if he continues to require ventilator and dialysis support. The chances of survival, not to mention quality of life, are slim based on the number of body systems now in failure. He could survive all of this, but the quality of his life if he does, is much more uncertain. Did he ever leave a record of his preferences in the event of a situation like this one?"

Son: "You mean a living will?"

Physician: "Yes, exactly. 'Advance directives' is another term used to describe this."

Mrs. L.: "No, we were going to do that, but I know he would never want to live this way. [After crying, looks to the physician] What do we do now?"

Physician: "We should talk about how we can make the shift from his current treatment to care that would be in line with his wishes, were he to know what we know about his current condition, and his future prospects for recovery."

Daughter
[others
nodding in
agreement]:   "He would not want it to drag out, but we want him to be comfortable."

Physician: "In responding to this request, we would want to be sure the decision is clear and to the extent possible, one which all of you can support as much as possible. You may need more information or time to discuss what we have already talked about. Some families prefer active participation of their clergy or whomever they trust regarding spiritual matters. By withdrawing life support we mean: the ventilator, dialysis, artificial feeding and hydration, and medications that might prolong his survival but have no immediate impact on his comfort. That usually includes antibiotics, blood thinners, most cardiac drugs, and supplements such as vitamins. Although life support will be withdrawn, care will certainly continue by giving him medication as needed for comfort, and looking after his personal care and dignity."

Son: "How do you stop dialysis and the ventilator and not have him suffer?"

Physician: "We have had much experience with this. Decisions to stop dialysis and ventilator support are quite common in current medical practice, though it's never easy for any of us, even when we strongly agree it is the right decision. Medication is the mainstay we have for assuring ongoing comfort for the patient and his family. In your father's instance, rapid, labored breathing and restlessness are the most likely symptoms to occur that we would want to prevent. We use medicine from the morphine family of medications to prevent rapid and labored breathing. It will also block his feeling of breathlessness even if the underlying cause is not treated. Separate medication is given for restlessness and agitation. Contrary to what you may have heard, stopping dialysis does not cause agony, but a decreasing level of alertness and orientation progressing to a sleep-like state called 'coma' from which he cannot be aroused."

Son: [Nodding his head in acknowledgement but pensive] "Are we 'killing' him if we do this? I don't want him to suffer, and I know he wouldn't want all of this, but I don't want to 'play God'."

Physician: "For most people, this is the most difficult decision they will ever have to make. The courts and the consensus of ethicists, religious and spiritual authorities support an informed and non-coerced individual's right to decline medical treatments even if the treatment could be beneficial. They do not consider this murder or suicide. I should point out that the purpose of medications given for comfort is the relief of burdensome symptoms, not a deliberate attempt to hasten death. If you have someone to whom you turn for religious or spiritual guidance, you may wish to do so to discuss this before making this type of decision."

Mrs. L.:   [Crying, softly] "I think we are 'playing God' by not letting nature take its course. I would like to call our pastor now."

Physician: "I will talk to you again after you have spoken with your pastor before we make any changes in your husband's care. Please take the time you need to contact others whom you would wish to be aware or present."

Decisions to withhold or withdraw life support are common in hospital practice, [27] though infrequent for many primary care, non-hospital based physicians. Prior to discussing a shift in goals from cure and life prolongation to comfort until anticipated death, the prognosis, options of treatment, and goals of care should be discussed with the patient or his surrogate and/or family. The attending physician should lead this discussion or at the very least indicate his involvement and support during this process. The patient's primary nurse, social worker, and chaplain should be invited to participate unless otherwise indicated by the patient. Broaching the subject of withholding or withdrawing medical treatments is less threatening if the goals of care are established first. Once this is done, the *relevance* of treatments is more apparent. Attempts to persuade patients not to pursue an ill-advised intervention on the basis of "futility" arguments are much less helpful and likely to undermine trust in the surgeon. In framing discussions about withholding or withdrawal of life support, the process should never be referred to as "withdrawing care", as this is not only inaccurate, but also heightens the patient's and family's fears of abandonment. In situations when the decision maker seems uncertain about pursuing a treatment course but not ready to change, an agreed upon timed trial of the current course followed by a meeting to jointly assess the impact is helpful.

Ventilator support is the usual primary focus of discussion about withdrawing life support, though the role of other life prolonging treatments (dialysis, artificial hydration and feeding, blood pressure support, blood products, and antibiotics) should be explicitly addressed when considering a shift from life-prolongation to comfort measures until time of death. Automatic implantable cardioverter defibrillators (AICDs) are increasingly present in the list of life prolonging devices to be addressed (see page 22). It is ethical and practical to dispense with all of these interventions once a decision to remove from mechanical ventilator support has been made, instead of the "a la carte" approach of discontinuing interventions in tandem. Interest in or previous decisions about organ donation should be noted though direct discussion with family,and should be referred to the appropriate organ procurement agency.

The RMV discussion should be documented along with the writing of the Do Not Attempt Resuscitation/Do Not Intubate (DNAR/DNI) order. Once a consensus decision has been reached to remove mechanical ventilation (RMV), the goal of care is to establish a peaceful and supportive environment for the patient and family with as much privacy as possible. Small gestures such as inviting the family to bring personal objects from their home (picture, blanket, or pet if permitted) are deeply appreciated, and have been commented upon years later. The family should be advised that prolonged survival can occur following RMV and that future disposition decisions could be required (i.e., nursing home placement, home placement with hospice support). The main anticipated symptoms and their remedies are discussed and while doing so, the family is advised that the purpose of the medications is the relief of burdensome symptoms, not the deliberate hastening of death. A time for RMV is then agreed upon allowing the family to make their social, psychological, and spiritual preparations. Arrangements can be made at this time for the presence of a chaplain at the time of RMV if desired by the family. Family should be welcomed but not expected to be present at the time of extubation and after. The organ procurement agency should be notified of impending RMV at this time when applicable.

At the time of RMV, an experienced physician should be present to manage the occasional patient who has refractory symptoms or unexpected symptoms such as stridor, in addition to his supportive role to staff and family members. The family is informed of the sequence and anticipated symptomatic consequences (if any) of withdrawal. The sequence of clinical maneuvers, medication doses, and other orders are reviewed with the primary nurse, following which a respiratory therapist is called for assistance with RMV. Paralytic agents should be stopped and confirmed reversed following which opioids and anxiolytics are given before extubation until patient appears relaxed, Richmond Agitation Sedation Scale (RASS) Level -3. At the time of extubation, an attempt to "un-medicalize" the venue as much as possible should be made by removing distractions such as the ventilator, serial compression devices, wrist restraints, monitoring leads, etc.) Seating for family attendance should be available.

Following extubation, the family is immediately notified if not at bedside by one of the clinicians in attendance, and privacy for the family and patient is provided to the extent possible. Family should be notified in advance if transfer to a regular nursing floor is anticipated ,and the extubated patient should remain in the critical care setting until consistent symptom relief is assured.

Case Scenario 3: Advanced Carcinoma of the Lung

Teaching points – palliative assessment, disposition planning

Mr. W is a 79-year-old, married, retired engineer referred to the thoracic surgery service for evaluation and management of a recurrent right sided malignant pleural effusion, secondary to a recently diagnosed advanced non-small cell carcinoma of the lung. The patient has declined chemotherapy. His wife has end-stage chronic obstructive pulmonary disease requiring home oxygen therapy. They live in the residence they have owned for 35 years. Both their children live in their community. CT imaging reveals a large right pleural effusion and a right upper lobe mass measuring 6 cm. There is prominent mediastinal adenopathy. After initial introductions, the interview continues:

Surgeon: "Did your oncologist, Dr. Tarceva, explain to you why I would be seeing you?"

W (looking distracted): "Yes. He said you were going to do something about the fluid in my lung."

S : "Yes, he wanted me to see you and give my opinion about what we might be able to do about the fluid around the lung. Before we talk about that specifically, are you having any discomfort now?"

W: "Yes. I have had this pain in my right side [indicating his right lateral chest]."

S : "Can you describe the pain? Is it sharp, is it always there?"

W: "It's sharp. It's always there but there are times it is really bad. When I cough."

S : "Can you rate you pain on a scale of 0–10, 0 being no pain, 10 being the kind of pain you would have if you touched a hot stove?"

W: "I would say about 8."

S : "Has it ever been less than that during the past 24 hours?' W: "Only a little. I would say about 5 or 6."

S : "Would you like some relief before we talk further?"

W (with some relief): "Yes, that would be nice."

The surgeon notes that one 5/325 mg hydrocodone/acetominophen tab has been ordered every 6 h, as needed, for pain. Mr. W last received a dose 2 h previously. No other analgesics are prescribed. His other medications include atenolol 25 mg daily, lovastatin 40 mg daily, enoxaparin 30 mg SQ daily, and a daily vitamin supplement. The surgeon orders oxycodone 10 mg to be given stat and every 4 h. In addition, he orders oxycodone 5 mg by mouth every 2 h, as needed, for breakthrough pain, and a daily stimulant laxative. About an hour and a half after the 10 mg of oxycodone is administered, he returns to Mr. W's room with Mr. W's nurse and finds him much more comfortable, rating his pain at 1 or 2.

Surgeon: "Do you feel better enough to talk a bit about your situation?"

Mr. W.:   "Yes" [pulling himself up in bed and gesturing to a chair]

S :   "Before discussing the specifics about the fluid in your chest, would you tell me what you know about your illness?"

W: *"Well, it isn't good. Dr. Tarceva told me I have two months.* We talked about chemotherapy, but he didn't seem too excited about it and, to tell you the truth, I don't want to go that route. He said I have fluid in my chest, and I should have it taken out. They took some out but it came back."

S :   "Before your diagnosis was made did you notice any changes in how you felt?"

W: "I was feeling fine until about two months ago when I began to have no energy. I then noticed I was losing weight, and had no appetite. I started to feel more and more out of breath even when sitting in the Lazy Boy. This pain I have been having started about a month ago. That's when I began to wonder if something was going on. When I became really short of breath last week, I decided to go to the emergency room. After they ran tests on the fluid from my lung they told me they detected cancer. Everything that had been happening finally made sense but now I am worried about my wife. She has emphysema and has been in the hospital twice during the last year. I have been the one taking care of her."

S :   "I can see why you would worry about her when you are not feeling at all well yourself. How has your mood been?'

W: "OK, all things considered."

S :   "Have you ever had problems with depression or felt depressed?"

W: "Not really – the usual I guess. I have had some down times like everyone else."

S :   "Who helps you out when you need help with your wife or if you were disabled?"

W: "My children. They would do anything to help but I hate to bother them."

S :   "Are your children and your wife aware of your diagnosis?"

W: "Oh, yes. We keep no secrets in our family"

S :   "Is it OK with you if I talk to them about your care in case they call or I run into them?

W: "Definitely. My wife and I have living wills so she needs to know what's going on."

S :   "Tell me more about your living will. Do you have a copy here?"

W: "I don't have it here, but I don't want to live on machines if that's what you mean. If I am terminal what's the use anyway? Does two months sound right to you, too?"

S :   "Would you like to talk more about what's ahead? That way it will be much easier for you to decide about what treatments you would want or don't want. If you would like we could discuss this with others you may want present."

W: "Thanks. I think I would like to talk with you by myself first, and then talk with my family afterwards. You can tell me the truth without sugar-coating."

S :   "I will tell you what we are sure about before venturing any guesses about what we are less sure about. We are sure you have not been feeling well for the past two months. We are sure that you have advanced and incurable lung cancer. We are sure about your treatment preferences so far. [Pauses for a few moments]. We have proven we can make your pain less, and I am pretty sure we can relieve you of your shortness of breath. We are also sure that your main concern is your wife [Pauses for a few moments]. To respond to your earlier question, the usual life expectancy for someone with your diagnosis, if untreated and running its natural course, is in the range of weeks to a couple of months. This is only an educated guess and not a sentence or prophesy. [Mr. W looks down for what seems like an eternity, and then he looks up after a long silence]

The surgeon continues: "I can see this is quite a bit to take in. What helps you through hard times like this?"

W: "My family and my faith in God."

S :   "Can you tell me more about your spiritual beliefs?"

W: "Certainly. I was raised Protestant, but we don't belong to a church. I do believe there is a God and I know things will be alright in the end." [After a long pause, smiling with some puzzlement] Now what do we do?"

S :   "Putting everything I have said together and recognizing your concern for your wife's welfare, I would recommend focusing your medical care on securing your comfort and quality of life to the extent possible, while initiating the planning for your wife's future care. It sounds to me like your children will be important allies in this endeavor and I will be happy to repeat this type of discussion with them with or without you as you prefer [pauses for a few moments]. I would like to get your pain under control using the medications we have just started, I would like to propose a surgical procedure [Video- assisted laparoscopic surgery for pleurodesis] for the drainage of the fluid in your chest which would have very good prospects to prevent it's re-accumulation, and finally, I would like to refer you to a hospice program to assist with your care when you return home. It probably wouldn't be too early to address your wife's future care such as assisted living, or some durable arrangement in which she would have some of the assistance you have provided in the past. Does this plan seem agreeable to you?"

W: "Yes. I would like you to meet my family to discuss everything you have just said."

S [putting his hand on Mr. W's upper arm] "We will be here to help you. I will stop by later to check in."

The palliative assessment, as was performed in this vignette, was not only an interaction that defined goals of care and established a critical baseline for future assessments, but was an important step in establishing trust for this patient, a necessary prerequisite in maintaining hope in the face of life-limiting disease. The palliative assessment could be looked at as a "staging procedure," [28] to determine the degree of distress as well as assets for responding to illness and fostering future hope.

The assessment should touch upon the four basic domains of human experience: physical, psychological, social (and economic), and spiritual. The assessment also allows the surgeon to tackle problems encountered in each domain. The surgeon is not expected to definitively manage any of these problems, but he should at least identify the salient symptoms and issues for future interdisciplinary management. Goal setting is much easier once the problems and aspirations relevant to the patient are identified. This is by no means an exhaustive assessment, though frequently assessment may occur over a series of contacts. The amount of time required to do this is more than offset by the long-term advantages of better symptom control and the engagement of ancillary services.

Before an accurate assessment can be performed, highly distracting symptoms should be acknowledged and treated, as was the case here. The chronic nature of this patient's pain was the reason it was not immediately obvious because the autonomic response to pain with its tell tale signs of sweating, wincing, tachycardia had long been attenuated. This is a common trap leading to the under-recognition of chronic persistent pain ("He doesn't look like he's in pain") may have fooled observers about its severity. The patient was receiving a compound drug containing hydrocodone and acetaminophen which has very limited use for chronic persistent pain because of hydrocodone's analgesic ceiling and the increasing toxicity of acetaminophen when usage exceeds 3,000 mg/24 h. For the degree of patient reported pain, an equianalgesic doubling of his previous pain medication dose was appropriate. In addition, no bowel prophylaxis was

Table 10.3 Medicare Hospice Benefit: eligibility, team, and services [29]

Eligibility for Medicare Hospice Benefit
- Patient is eligible for Medicare Part A
- Two physicians must certify that patient has a condition whose prognosis is associated with a survival of 6 months or less if the illness pursues its natural course. One of the physicians must be the hospice program's medical director
- Patient (surrogate if patient not competent) must sign form electing hospice benefit
- Hospice care must be provided by a Medicare-certified hospice program

Core team members
- Physician
- Registered nurse
- Social worker
- Pastoral (spiritual) or other counselor
- Minimum percentage of non-professional volunteer hours required

Services
- Pain and non-pain symptom management
- Assistance of patient and family with the emotional, social and spiritual aspects of dying
- Provides medications for control of symptoms, medical supplies, and durable medical equipment
- Education of family on care of the patient
- Specialized therapy services (speech, massage, dietary counseling, and physical therapy)
- Home health aide and homemaker services
- Short-term inpatient care (respite care) when pain or symptoms unmanageable at home, or when caregiver needs respite
- Bereavement care for surviving family and friends for 1 year from the date of the death

ordered to prevent opioid-induced constipation. Achieving immediate pain control was a valuable first step in developing trust necessary to prepare the patient for inevitable future challenges.

During this interview, the surgeon responds empathically on several occasions. He also takes the precaution of asking the patient about his preferences in receiving information and assessing his comprehension. When probing the patient's spiritual domain, he avoids the trap of assuming that spiritual needs are met by an individual's profession of a religion or belief (non-belief) system.

He refers the patient appropriately to hospice services, because the patient has identified his preference for comfort-directed care, *and* he is aware of his likely prognosis, which is less than the hospice referral criterion of six months or less of anticipated survival (Table 10.3). It would not have been appropriate to recommend hospice referral without the patient's previous understanding of his likely prognosis and willingness to forego disease-directed treatments.

In the moral tradition of the "post-operative check", the encounter closes as the surgeon reassures the patient of non-abandonment, the cardinal principle of surgical palliative care.

Case Scenario 4: Cardiomyopathy and Delirium

Teaching point – recognition and management of syndrome of imminent demise

Margaret is an 82-year-old woman with advanced cardiomyopathy with an estimated ejection fraction of 10–15%, congestive heart failure, status post implantation of an automatic cardioverter defibrillator, previous cerebrovascular accident, and chronic kidney disease, stage 5 (CKD-5) on chronic hemodialysis. She had been admitted to an acute care facility for confusion and hypotension. Sepsis was subsequently ruled out after an empiric course of antibiotics. A cardiothoracic surgeon has been consulted to replace a non-functioning dialysis catheter. Upon evaluation of the patient in the dialysis unit, the consulting surgeon notes she is lethargic and confused. She denies pain but admits to shortness of breath. Her partner, Bill, is at her bedside and asks if the medicine she been receiving "is making her sleepy". The surgeon verifies that Bill is also Margaret's surrogate for medical decision-making. Bill notes that she has been sleeping much of the time during the past few weeks, and eating or drinking very little. He stated a nurse had told him that the pain medicine she was receiving and her kidney failure could be causing these changes. On physical examination, she is an elderly, chronically ill appearing woman with pallor, blood pressure of 85/50, breathing 30 shallow respirations/min. assisted by a nasal cannula administering 4 L/min oxygen. On chest auscultation she has bilateral basilar rales and an S3 gallop. Mottling is noted in her lower extremities below the knees. The surgeon asks her if she is comfortable to which she responds that she is extremely tired, nods affirmatively to the surgeon's request to speak to her partner to discuss and direct her care, then immediately lapses into sleep.

Bill, sensing the surgeon's
concern : "Is there something going on?"

Surgeon: "Yes, Bill. I would like to talk to you about it."
The surgeon takes Bill to a private room near by and in the presence of Ms. T's nurse, he determines that Bill wants to be given an honest appraisal of what is happening "with no sugar-coating". Bill is well informed about the "end-stage" nature of the Ms. T's medical problems, though he is under the impression she would be going home after a few dialysis treatments.

Surgeon: "Bill, I believe her illness is progressing. It's true, as you mentioned, there are things that can explain why she is so tired and confused that we can reverse, but it is quite likely what you and others have observed are related to her heart condition and can't be reversed."

Bill, after a long pause: "Do you think she is dying?"

Surgeon: "I believe she is."

Surgeon, following a long pause during which Bill becomes tearful while Ms. T's nurse hands him a tissue: "I wish I could blame these changes on her medicine or her kidney failure, but the whole picture looks and feels like something bigger is happening."

Bill, regaining some composure: "How long do you think she has?"

Surgeon: "With the changes I see, I believe it could be as soon as a few hours to several days."

Bill   :   "That soon! She has friends I need to contact."

Bill   :   "Funny. Last night she said she didn't think she was going to get out of the hospital. She has never said anything like that before, even when she had emergency heart surgery. Last week she said she saw her mother. Her mother died 30 years ago. She's been through so much."

Surgeon: "No matter what the time remaining for her is, we will be caring for her. What would she want us to do and not do if she could understand what is happening now? I am not sure how completely she can understand in order to make medical decisions, which is why we need and value your guidance. She has already deferred that to you."

Bill   :   "She doesn't want to be on any machines. I just want her to be comfortable."

S   :   "We will do everything we can to keep her comfortable. I don't believe machines, including further dialysis treatments, would extend her survival at this point, and they are not necessary to keep her comfortable."

Bill   :   "I know she would agree."

Nurse   :   "Should we talk about what we should do about her defibrillator?"

Surgeon: "Thank you for reminding me about that."

Bill
[uneasy]:   "Do you mean turning her heart off?"

Surgeon: "Not at all. Her AICD has two components, one that paces the heart. That part will stay on but won't prolong her dying. There will come a point when the heart will ignore the pacer's reminder to keep beating. The other part, the defibrillator, gives a painful, strong shock when the heart develops certain rhythms that, if unchecked, would lead to immediate death. This part can be programmed off. It doesn't require a procedure. It's done with the same equipment you may have seen when the device was interrogated."

Bill   :   "I certainly don't want her to be getting shocked and neither would she."

Surgeon : "Even more important than what we won't do is what we *will* do for her. I propose we get her back to her room, make sure you and those she wishes have access to her with as much privacy as possible, while we provide her with medicine she will likely require for her comfort. [pause] We will be giving medications similar to morphine when needed, if she says or appears to have pain or breathlessness. You may soon hear a breathing noise that has been described as a "death rattle". It's not drowning. It's actually a small amount of fluid way up here [pointing to his own larynx] around the vocal cords that makes most of the noise. The fluid is normal secretion that accumulates because of her profound weakness. Suctioning does not help this and is extremely uncomfortable. We also will administer a medication to dry the secretions so her breathing won't sound so noisy. This is more for our peace of mind than hers, as the rattle is not distressing her as far as we can tell [long pause]. Does Margaret have any religious or spiritual beliefs we should be mindful and supportive of at this time?"

Bill : "I am going to call her pastor. Thank you for asking."

Nurse : "We support your decisions, Bill. Do you have any other questions?"

Bill : "Not now. I am sure I will have more as soon as soon as you leave."

Surgeon : "Before I write orders that reflect your understanding and agreement, let's go see her to let her know we have talked and see whatever else she may want to know or do."

The biophysical, social, and spiritual implications for management of the syndrome of imminent demise or "active dying" are so significant that all clinicians are advised to include this as a differential consideration in any patient with advanced illness presenting with the following constellation of symptoms: bed bound state, increasing somnolence and/or delirium, diminishing oral intake, dysphagia, and decreasing urine output. In this vignette the reversible causes for the clinical changes were acknowledged, as they should be, in discussions with patients and families. The development of the "death rattle" heralds a more advanced stage of active dying with demise usually occurring within hours to a few days. Coma, signs of brainstem dysfunction (irregular breathing patterns, tachycardia, hypotension, vasomotor changes) are very late signs with death usually ensuing within hours. Fever, when present, is usually due to aspiration pneumonia. This should not be treated with antibiotics in this context. The syndrome can span as little as a few hours up to 2 weeks. The trajectory of the syndrome is more protracted in nutritionally replete and non-septic patients, such as a patient in coma from a stroke for whom the decision has been made to forego artificial nutrition and hydration.

The main symptoms and signs to be anticipated during active dying include labored breathing, oral secretions, pain, and delirium (Table 10.4). It is uncommon for these not to yield to pharmacotherapy, though it is helpful to mention the likelihood of their occurrence and their management in advance. A small percentage of patients will exhibit marked agitated delirium. Intracranial pathology, history of major psychiatric disorder, renal and hepatic failure are risk factors for this highly distressing picture. In extreme cases, permission should be sought for deliberate heavy sedation, but with a clear understanding that the purpose of the sedation is the relief of symptoms and not a deliberate attempt to hasten death.

Common concerns of family include ongoing unrecognized pain for their loved one, what to expect (many believe that gasping for air is common at death, particularly from

Table 10.4 Management of common symptoms and signs during active dying

Symptom/sign	Management
Dyspnea	Morphine 10–15 mg PO/PR or 2–5 mg IV/SC every 5–10 min until relief in the opioid naïve patient. Higher doses necessary for patients on chronic opioid therapy. Hydromorphone is a suitable and alternative opioid
	Anxiolytics (lorazepam) can reduce the anxiety component of dyspnea
	Stop exogenous fluid administration
	Trial of oxygen up to 4–6 L/min via nasal cannula. Masks can worsen agitation. Explain to family that benefits of oxygen almost always limited and patient will need medication for relief
	Fan
Pain	Morphine 10–15 mg PO/PR or 2–5 mg IV/SC every 5–10 min until relief in the opioid naïve patient. Higher doses necessary for patients on chronic opioid therapy
	Explain to family that behavioral cues are used to monitor pain and that pain can occur in an unresponsive patient
Oral secretions	Explanation to family that patient is not "drowning"
	Glycopyrrolate 0.4 mg SQ Q6HR
	Atropine (scopolamine drops or patch) is commonly used in hospice care It can precipitate or worsen delirium
	Stop exogenous fluid administration
	Re-positioning (lateral decubitus)
	Avoid deep suctioning
Delirium	Decrease sensory stimulation (low level light)
	Re-orient patient
	Haloperidol: Start at 0.5–1 mg PO or IV. Titrate up by 2–5 mg per hour per until requirement determined, then give as 2 or 3 divided doses per day
	Anxiolytics (e.g., lorazepam) can worsen agitated delirium in the elderly

pneumonia), should they remain at the bedside, what will occur after death (who will pick up the body, who should be called), and if the dying person can hear. It is unusual when a family cannot be reassured about these concerns by an experienced critical care or hospice nurse. Ideally, the time of active dying should not be a medicalized event, but a time during which medical support allows the full experience and expression of the social, psychological, and spiritual domains of the patient and family during this unique time.

Conclusion

Because of the successful reach of cardiothoracic surgery into the elderly population, a concurrent strategy and set of tactics for the relief of distress and promotion of quality of life are necessary, not only because of the afflictions of illness but also the natural consequences of aging. Cardiothoracic surgeons, with the help of interdisciplinary teams, can assume a leadership role in meeting these growing expectations, while enjoying the profound and privileged sense of personal satisfaction that follows the effective response to their most basic humanitarian impulses.

References

1. *Cruzan v Director, Missouri Department of Health*, 497 DS 261 (1990).
2. The SUPPORT Clinical Investigators. A controlled trial to improve care for seriously ill hospitalized patients. The study to understand prognoses and preferences for outcomes and risks of treatments (SUPPORT). JAMA. 1995;274(20):1591–8.
3. Velanovich V. Quality of life studies in general surgical journals. J Am Coll Surg. 2001;193(3):328–96.
4. American College of Surgeons' Palliative Care Task Force and Committee on Ethics. Statement of principles of palliative care. Bull Am Coll Surg. 2005;90(8):34–5.
5. American Board of Surgery. Surgery, Booklet of Information 2008–2009. Philadelphia: American Board of Surgery. p. 8. www.absurgery.org. Accessed 23 Sept 2009.
6. American College of Surgeons, Division of Education. Surgical Education and Self-Assessment Program (SESAP)13. Chicago: American College of Surgeons; 2007. p. 624–9.
7. Tilden LB, Williams BR, Tucker RO, MacLennan PA, Ritchie CS. Surgeons' attitudes and practices in the utilization of palliative and supportive care services for patients with a sudden advanced illness. J Pall Med. 2009;12(11):1037–42.
8. Hoover DR, Crystal S, Kumar R, Sambamoorthi U, Cantor JC. Medical expenditures during the last year of life: findings from the 1992-1996 Medicare current beneficiary survey. Health Serv Res. 2002;37:1625–42.
9. Singer PA, Martin DK, Kelner M. Quality end-of-life care: patients' perspectives. JAMA. 1999;281(2):163–8.
10. Steinhauser KE, Christakis NA, Clipp EC, McNeilly M, McIntyre L, Tulsky JA. Factors considered important at the end of life by patients, family, physicians, and other care providers. JAMA. 2000;284:2476–82.
11. Smith TJ, Coyne P, Cassel B, Penberthy L, Hopson A, Hager MA. A high volume specialist palliative care unit and team may reduce in-hospital end of life care cost. J Pall Med. 2003;6(5):699–705.
12. White KR, Stover KG, Cassel JB, Smith TJ. Nonclinical outcomes of hospital-based palliative care. J Healthc Manag. 2006;51:260–73.
13. Casarett D, Pickard A, Bailey FA, Ritchie C, Furman C, Rosenfeld K, et al. Do palliative consultations improve patient outcomes? J Am Geriatr Soc. 2008;56:593–9.
14. Gade G, Venohr I, Conner D, McGrady K, Beane J. Richardson RH, Williams MP, Liberson M, Blum M, penna R. Impact of an inpatient palliative care team: a randomized control trial J Palliat Med. 2008;11:180–90.
15. Morrison RS, Maroney-Galin C, Kralovec PD, Meier DE. The growth of palliative care programs in United States hospitals. J Pall Med. 2005;8(6):1127–34.
16. Mosenthal AC, Murphy PA. Trauma care and palliative care: Time to integrate the two. J Am Coll Surg. 2003;197:509–16.
17. Mosenthal AC, Murphy PA. Interdisciplinary model for palliative care in the trauma and surgical intensive care unit: Robert Wood Johnson Foundation demonstration project for improving palliative care in the intensive care unit. Crit Care Med 2006;399–403.
18. Tilden LB, Williams BR, Tucker RO, MacLennan, Ritchie CS: Surgeons' attitudes and practices in the utilization of palliative and supportive services for patients with a sudden advanced illness. J Pall Med 2009; X:X.
19. National Consensus Project For Quality Palliative Care. Clinical practice guidelines for quality palliative care. 2nd ed. Pittsburgh: National Consensus Project For Quality Palliative Care; 2009. www.nationalconsensusproject.org/Guideline.pdf. Accessed 24 Sept 2009.
20. www.qualityforum.org/publications/reports/palliative.asp. Accessed 24 Sept 2009.
21. Arnold R, Weissman DE. Broaching the topic of a palliative care consultation with patients and families. Fast fact and concept #42. 2nd ed. July 2005. End-of-Life/Palliative Education Resource Center www.eperc.mcw.edu.
22. Baile W, Buckman R. The pocket guide to communication skills in clinical practice including breaking bad news. Cinemedic Distributors. 1998;866-488-8234. Cinemedic@bellnet.ca.
23. Oliver RC, Sturtevant J, Scheetz J, et al. Beneficial effects of a hospital bereavement intervention program after traumatic childhood death. J Trauma. 2001;50:440–8.
24. Linyear AS, Tartaglia A. Family communication coordination: a program to increase organ donation. J Transplant Coord. 1999;9:165–74.
25. Jurkevich GJ, Pierce B, Panenen L, et al. Giving bad news: the family perspective. J Trauma. 2000;48:865–73.
26. www.facs.org/education/tfinterpersonal.html. Accessed 31 January 2010.
27. Prendergast TJ, Claessens MT, Luce JM. A national survey of end-of-life care for critically ill patients. Am J Respir Crit Care Med. 1998;158:1163–7.
28. Dunn GP. Patient assessment in palliative care: how to see the "big picture" and what to do when "there is nothing more we can do". J Am Coll Surg. 2001;193(5):565–73.
29. www.medicare.gov/publications/pubs/pdf/hosplg.pdf. Accessed 31 January 2010.

Chapter 11
Cardiopulmonary Trauma in the Elderly

Jay Menaker and Thomas M. Scalea

Abstract As the baby boom generation age and advances in medicine continue, those over the age of 65 years will increase. As a result, trauma, which was once thought to exclusively affect younger people, will now see an increase in elderly patients. Preexisting medical conditions as well as the older persons inability to compensate after injury lead to higher mortality rates in this patient population. Injuries including rib fractures, flail chest, blunt aortic injuries, sternal fractures, and cardiac contusion require specific age-related considerations and will be the focus of this chapter.

Keywords Elderly • Trauma • Cardiac • Thoracic • Rib fractures • Blunt aortic injury • Flail chest

Introduction

Background

Trauma is the most common cause of death for those under the age of 44. Thus, some consider trauma to be exclusively a disease of the young [1]. However, as the population in the United States (US) ages over the next several decades, the importance of injury in older patients will become more apparent. The elderly, defined as persons aged 65 or greater [2–5] constitute one of the fastest growing segments of the US population. By the year 2030, the number of persons over the age 65 will double relative to the year 2000, representing almost 20% of the nation's total population [6] (Fig. 11.1). This increase is the result of improvement in life expectancy and the aging baby boom generation. The Administration on Aging's Fiscal Year 2009 budget requested 1.381 billion dollars to assist in the long-term needs of these aging baby boomers [7].

J. Menaker (✉)
Department of Surgery, University of Maryland Medical Center,
R. Adams Cowley Shock Trauma Center, Baltimore, MD 21201, USA
e-mail: jmenaker@umm.edu

Thoracic Trauma

Thoracic trauma accounts for 20–25% of all injury related deaths [8, 9] Most of these are a result of motor vehicle collisions (MVCs) and falls [10]. Thoracic trauma represents the second most important factor contributing to death in the elderly trauma victim, behind head injury [11]. The elderly have a significantly higher mortality after blunt chest trauma (BCT) when compared with younger patients with similar injuries [12]. Thus, what may be inconsequential to a younger person can result in significant morbidity and mortality in the elderly. Geriatric patients have an overall higher morbidity than younger patients [12]. Specific complications after thoracic injury may include pain upon inspiration leading to atelectasis, mucus plugging, impaired ventilation, and pneumonia.

The elderly are at risk to the same thoracic injuries as are younger people. Some injuries, including pneumothorax and hemothorax, require essentially identical treatment, and do not require specific age-association considerations. Others including rib fractures, flail chest, blunt aortic injuries, sternal fractures, and cardiac contusion require specific considerations and will be the focus of this chapter.

Physiologic Changes

Understanding the physiologic changes of aging helps explain the increased morbidity and mortality associated with chest trauma in the geriatric population. Elderly patients have a decreased respiratory reserve and thus can decompensate quickly [13]. Decreases in respiratory function in the elderly result from changes in both the chest wall and the lungs [14, 15]. After the age of 30, a 4% per decade decrease in alveolar surface area has a negative effect on gas exchange as well as forced expiratory flow [16]. Alveolar ducts enlarge and the alveoli become flatter and shallower, reducing the area for gas exchange leading to an increase in ventilation perfusion mismatch at baseline.

M.R. Katlic (ed.), *Cardiothoracic Surgery in the Elderly*, DOI 10.1007/978-1-4419-0892-6_11,
© Springer Science+Business Media, LLC 2011

Fig. 11.1 Population growth over time (CDC)

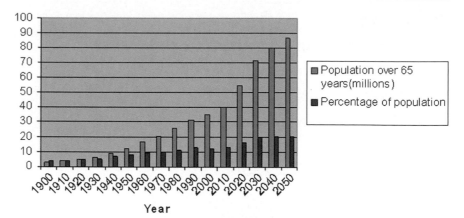

Decreases in chest wall compliance from anatomical changes such as kyphosis and a decline in respiratory muscle strength from muscle fiber atrophy lead to as much as 50% loss in maximal inspiratory and expiratory force [13]. Accessory muscles help to compensate for the decline in respiratory muscle atrophy. Lung elastance also progressively declines causing a collapse of small airways and uneven alveolar ventilation. This results in increased closing volume of the lung.

Additionally, responses to hypoxia and hypercapnia are decreased by 50 and 40%, respectively [13]. Mucociliary function worsens with aging and with fewer cilia per square centimeter, secretion clearance is also impaired. This, in addition to poor dentition, increased oropharyngeal colonization, swallowing dysfunction, and a decreased lower esophageal sphincter tone predispose the elderly to aspiration pneumonia and pulmonary infection [13]. Gram-negative organisms predominate in the oral flora increasing the risk of pulmonary infection from aspiration [16].

Osteopenia of the thoracic cage may increase the rate of pulmonary contusions, rib fractures, and pneumo- and hemo-pneumothoraces as the bony thorax cannot absorb transmitted kinetic energy. Accordingly, flail chest in the elderly correlates with prolonged mechanical ventilation [17]. In those with a flail chest, age has been shown to be the strongest predictor of poor outcome and is directly proportional to mortality [18]. Elderly patients who sustain rib fractures have twice the mortality rate of younger patients with similar injuries [19]. As the number of rib fractures increases, so does the incidence of pneumonia and death [19, 20]. Pain control is critical to allow deep breathing, facilitate clearance of secretions, and prevent as many of pulmonary complications as possible.

Rib Fractures

Young patients with rib fractures and no associated injury have low morbidity and mortality, and are treated with analgesia and ambulation as an outpatient [21, 22]. In the elderly,

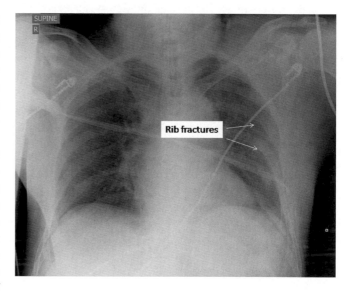

Fig. 11.2 Chest X-ray with rib fractures after trauma

however, rib fractures are a significant cause of morbidity and mortality after trauma (Figs. 11.2 and 11.3). The true incidence of rib fractures after blunt trauma remains unknown. Ziegler and Agarwal reported a 10% overall incidence of rib fractures after trauma [21]; however, this may be an underestimation as many as 50% of rib fractures may be missed on plain X-ray [23]. Other studies have reported the rates of rib fractures after blunt trauma to range from 7 to 21% [9, 24, 25]. Rib fractures have been shown to occur in over two-thirds of all patients who sustain BCT [9]. The elderly have an increased incidence of rib fractures after BCT with higher rates of mortality [12, 20, 24–26] (Fig. 11.4). This increase can be attributed to the elderly having decreased muscle mass and bone density as a result of aging.

The two predominant mechanisms of injury (MOI) causing rib fractures in the elderly are MVCs followed by falls. MVCs have been reported to be the MOI in as many as 75% of injuries causing rib fractures in the elderly [27]. However, most reports suggest that MVCs are the MOI about 50% of the time [19–21, 24, 26]. Falls are typically the second most

Fig. 11.3 Computed tomography of rib fractures after trauma

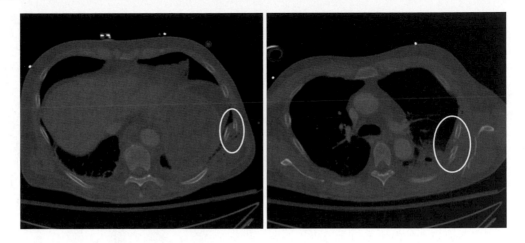

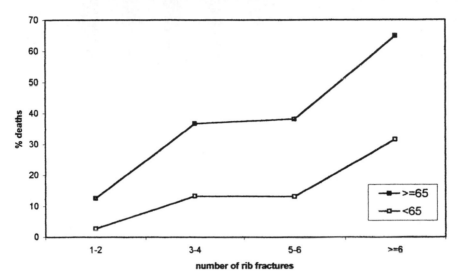

Fig. 11.4 Proportion of deaths by number of rib fractures for each age group (reprinted from Bergeron et al., [20] with permission from Lippincott Williams & Wilkins)

common MOI for rib fractures in the elderly with incidence ranging from 14 to 36% [19–21, 24, 26, 28]. However, one study from Barnea and colleagues demonstrated that falls were the number one cause of rib fractures in the elderly occurring in 53% of cases [28].

A number of studies have focused on the outcome in rib fractures in the elderly [12, 19, 20, 24–26, 29, 30]. Shorr and colleagues did a subset analysis of elderly patients with BCT [12]. Eighty-seven percent of the elderly had rib fractures vs. 73% of the nonelderly. In addition, those over the age of 65 years had a statistically significant increased rate of mortality after BCT. Cameron et al. demonstrated those over 80 years of age had a higher rate of rib fractures when compared with those younger than 80 years of age, also with an increased death rate [24]. In addition, those over the age of 80 with rib fractures had a higher death rate than the same aged cohort without rib fractures.

In 2000, Bulger et al. retrospectively evaluated patients over the age of 65 years with rib fractures compared with

Table 11.1 Outcome measures

Parameter	Age (y)		p value
	≥65	18–64	
Mean ventilator days	4.3 ± 9.2	3.1 ± 9.2	=0.16
Mean ICU days	6.1 ± 10.0	4.0 ± 9.4	<0.05
Mean hospital days	15.2 ± 16.5	11.0 ± 13.1	<0.01
Mortality (%)	22	10	<0.001

ICU intensive care unit
Source: reprinted with permission from Bulger et al. [19]

those younger than 65 [19]. Despite a similar injury severity score (ISS) and chest abbreviated injury score (AIS), the elderly had faired significantly worse in all outcome measures (Table 11.1). These data are consistent with other studies suggesting that ISS may not be a reliable indicator of outcome in the elderly [29, 30]. Additionally, the authors demonstrated a statistically significant increase in mortality rates with each additional rib fracture [19].

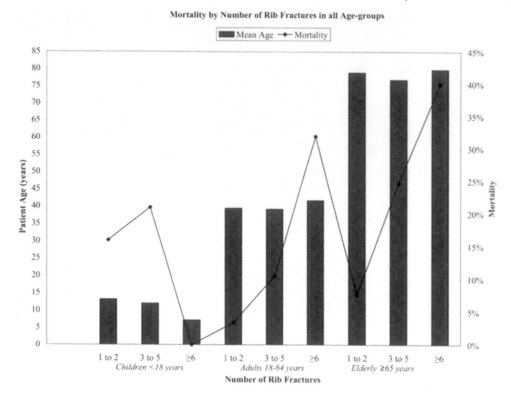

Fig. 11.5 Mortality by number of rib fractures in all-age groups (reprinted with permission from Sharma et al. [25])

Sharma and colleagues demonstrated that those over the age of 65 years had an increased rate of rib fractures as well as mortality rate after BCT [25]. The mortality increased as the numbers of rib fractures increased (Fig. 11.5). The authors showed this twofold increase in mortality in the elderly with rib fractures, despite a lower ISS. Similarly, a 2003 study by Bergeron et al. and a 2004 study by Stawicki et al. reported a lower ISS in the elderly, despite higher rates of both morbidity and mortality [20, 26]. These studies suggest that the elderly patients, even when less severely injured, have minimal abilities to compensate for their injuries.

To demonstrate the impact of rib fractures in the elderly, Barnea and colleagues studied a group of elderly patients with isolated rib fractures [28]. The mean age was 79.9 years and the average number of rib fractures was 2.6. The authors demonstrated an overall morbidity of 38% and mortality of 8%. Increased number of rib fractures, underlying congestive heart failure and diabetes were statistically associated with increased morbidity in the study.

Flail Chest

Flail chest, defined as fractures of three or more consecutive ribs in two or more places, occurs in 5–13% in patients with chest wall trauma [8]. It seems logical that the elderly would be vulnerable to flail chest following trauma because of their decrease muscle mass, decreased bone density, and decreased chest wall compliance. Albaugh and colleagues demonstrated in elderly patients with a flail chest that there was a statistically significant increase in the rate of mortality with increase age (58 vs. 16%, $p=0.002$) [18]. Additionally, the authors showed that for every 10-year increase in age, the likelihood of death increases 132%. For those over the age of 80 years, there was 86% mortality rate for those with a flail chest. Freedland et al. showed that elderly patients with a flail chest had a mortality rate of more than 4 times that of younger persons [31].

Pain Management

Pain control is crucial in the management of rib fractures. It allows for early ambulation, deep breathing, incentive spirometry, clearance of secretions, and prevention of atelectasis. All of these are paramount to prevent complications including pneumonia and respiratory failure. Younger patient's pain is often well controlled with oral narcotics or nonnarcotic medications. However, pain management in the elderly can be a difficult and challenging issue. Many elderly are very sensitive to narcotics and can become somnolent quite easily with only a small dose. Resultant decreased mental status and respiratory drive can occur, sometimes requiring intubation and mechanical ventilation.

Various methods have been used to control pain in elderly patients with rib fractures. Intravenous narcotics and non-narcotics, pleural effusion catheters, rib blocks, and epidural analgesia have been used. Each method has advantages and disadvantages. Intravenous narcotics can be too sedating, while nonnarcotics, such as ketorolec, can be very effective. However, in elderly patients with compromised renal function, nonsteroidals may cause renal failure. Catheter-based analgesia can be very useful for pain control in these patients without causing over sedation; however, preexisting comorbidities such as degenerative spine disease or those requiring the use of aspirin, clopidogrel or warfarin, may preclude its usage. Additionally, injuries such as thoracic vertebral fractures, severe head injury, and upper rib fractures do not allow placement of an epidural catheter. As such, there has been some debate as to the ideal choice of analgesia in the elderly patient with rib fractures [19].

The Eastern Association for the Surgery of Trauma recommends that epidural anesthesia can be provided for persons over the age of 65 years with four or more rib fractures [32]. The use of epidural catheter analgesia in the elderly has been shown to be an independent predictor of decreased mortality and pulmonary complications after chest trauma [19, 33]. The improved outcome in the elderly was felt to offset the increase cost of epidural usage. Additionally, using epidural analgesia has been shown to be cost effective overall. There are savings in both nursing and pharmacy time because of decreased repeated drug administration. Additionally, many institutions do not require intensive care admission for epidural analgesia administrations [33]. A study by Ullman and colleagues demonstrated that the use of epidural analgesia allowed for a statistically decreased length of ICU stay, ventilator days, and total hospital days [34]. Fewer ICU days and total hospital days translates into lower overall costs.

Complications with epidural catheters do occur. Bulger and colleagues demonstrated a 19% complication rate with catheter placement [19]. Most were local infection, transient hypotension, and catheter migration. The authors did not report any epidural hematomas or epidural abscesses as a result of catheter placement. Others have found similar results [35, 36]. Interestingly, the elderly patients who received epidurals had higher rates of pneumonia, ARDS, and ventilator days, but still had a statistically significant lower mortality than those not receiving an epidural [19].

Complications

Pulmonary complications after rib fractures are significantly higher in the elderly than younger people [19] (Fig. 11.6). The incidence of pneumonia in the elderly after rib fractures has varied. Some studies have it being as low as 13–15%,

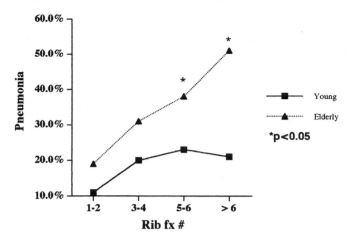

Fig. 11.6 Relationship between pneumonia and number of rib fractures (reprinted with permission from Bulger et al. [19])

while others have it as high as 27–31% [19, 20, 28, 33]. Bulger and colleagues demonstrated that for each additional rib fracture in the elderly, the risk of pneumonia increased by 27% [19]. Additionally, elderly patients with rib fractures have significantly longer ICU and total hospital stays [19].

Blunt Aortic Injury

Early diagnosis of blunt aortic injury (BAI) after trauma requires a high index of suspicion. It has been estimated that lesser than 15% of patients with such an injury survive to emergency department evaluation or die within 30 min of arrival [37]. For those who survive more than 30 min after hospital arrival, 33% die within 6 h and almost 40% die within 24 h without treatment [37]. Often a result of high speed deceleration, BAI commonly occurs after MVCs and falls of significant height. Injuries due to deceleration are believed to occur at points of strain: in the aorta, the isthmus, the point just distal to the left subclavian artery where the ductus arteriosus and thoracic aorta attach [38].

The evaluation modalities for BAI have changed over the past decades. Traditionally, a plain chest roentgenogram (CXR) was used as a screening tool for BAI. Common practice assumed that a widened mediastinum (Fig. 11.7) was suggestive of an aortic injury, while a normal mediastinum ruled out injury. However, many elderly trauma patients have ectatic and tortuous aortas obscuring the normal contour, thus making it difficult to rule out an injury.

Retrograde aortography was then used for definitive diagnosis. It was the most effective modality delineating the extent of injury [37] with a 96% sensitivity and 98% specificity [39, 40]. However, aortography is an invasive procedure and has complication rates of up to 1% depending on the experience level of the operator [41]. In addition,

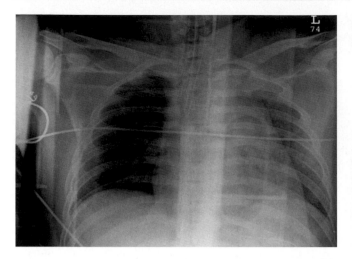

Fig. 11.7 Widened mediastinum on chest X-ray suggestive of a blunt aortic injury

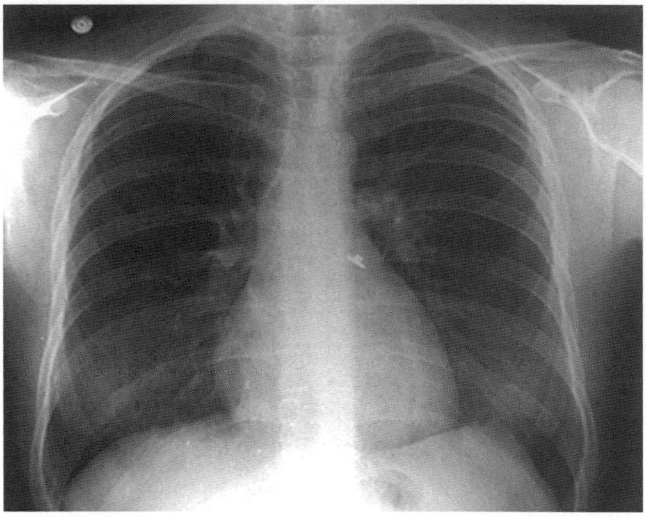

Fig. 11.8 Normal chest X-ray with blunt aortic injury

the intravenous contrast can cause contrast-induced nephropathy (CIN) in patients with underlying renal disease or decreased renal function. This is often a concern in the elderly trauma patient as many have a decreased glomerular filtration rate.

Recently, the notion that a normal CXR ruling out an aortic injury has come into question [42–45]. A 1990 review by Woodring concluded that 7% of BAI will have a normal CXR [42] (Figs. 11.8 and 11.9). The author suggested that the lack of mediastinal hemorrhage or hematoma obscuring the aortic contour explained the normal CXR finding. In a 1997 multicenter trial, Fabian and colleagues also demonstrated that 7% of patients with a BAI had a negative CXR [43]. In the same study, the most common abnormality seen on CXR was a widened mediastinum. More recently, in 2001, Exadaktylos and colleagues demonstrated that 8% of patients with a normal CXR were found to have a BAI [44]. Finally, a 2007 study by Plurad et al. reported a 13.9% incidence of negative CXR in the setting of known BAI [45]. As a result, for the elderly who do in fact have a normal CXR without evidence of an ectatic or tortuous aorta, BAI cannot be safely ruled out.

Currently, computed tomography (CT) is the modality of choice for the diagnosis of BAI (Fig. 11.10). Although early generation CT scanners suffered from poor resolution and low diagnostic accuracy, technological improvement over the past 20 years has now enabled CT to be an effective and rapid mode of diagnosis. Currently, multidetector CT with 2D and 3D reconstructions had yielded sensitivities and specificities of 96.2 and 99.8%, respectively [46]. Although CT represents a less invasive diagnostic modality than aortography with similar results, it still places patients, specifically the elderly, at risk of CIN.

Over the last 10 years, there has been a significant change in the management of BAI. The traditional approach was

immediate surgical repair in the stable BAI or delayed repair for patients with major associated injuries or those with severe comorbidities [47]. However, overall mortalities rates range from 8 to 17%, depending on the surgical technique being used [48]. Additionally, high rates of morbidity including paraplegia, myocardial infarction, stroke result from operative repair [48, 49]. A 1994 study by Camp et al. comparing OR in the young and elderly demonstrated a 163-fold increase likelihood of mortality in the elderly [50]. When excluding all but the "stable" patients, the authors found at least a 40-fold increase in odds of mortality in the elderly. The authors also demonstrated that the elderly had a significantly lower survival rate than that predicted by admission physiologic state and degree of injury. In a multicenter prospective trial comparing "clamp and sew" and various bypass techniques, Fabian colleagues demonstrated that only age was noted to significantly correlate with death [43].

The possibility of nonoperative management for BAI has been suggested by some authors [51–53]. Some BAI are believed to remain stable over time and never rupture [53]. Additionally, Oreskovich et al. suggested that the injured elderly may not be candidate for aggressive treatment including OR, because of their underlying comorbid conditions [30]. Conservative management, with blood pressure and heart rate control, may be a reasonable alternative to surgical repair in this high risk patient population [30, 53]. Camp and colleagues showed a protective effect with conservative, nonsurgical management in the elderly [50].

Recently, there has been an increased utilization of endovascular stent graft (SG) placement for the treatment of BAI (Fig. 11.11). It is a less invasive treatment option that requires only local sedation, causes minimal blood loss, and does not requires an open chest procedure. However, the long-term effects and complications of SG remain unknown. SG was

Fig. 11.9 Computed tomography of blunt aortic injury in a patient with a normal Chest X-ray

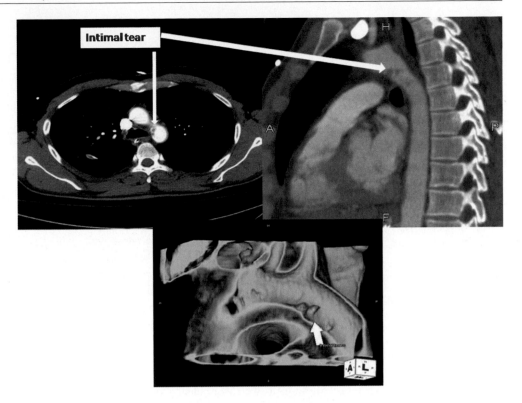

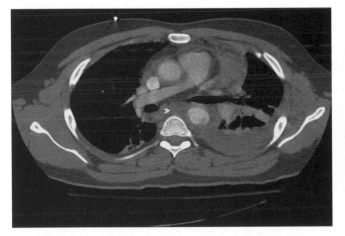

Fig. 11.10 Computed tomography demonstrating blunt aortic injury

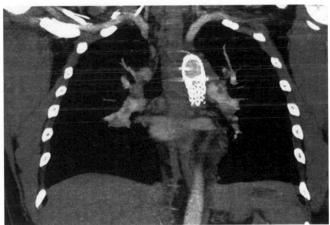

Fig. 11.11 Computed tomography demonstrating stent graft placement for blunt aortic injury

initially recommended for the patients with multiple injuries or those with comorbid diseases, i.e., the elderly [54].

In 2008, Demetriades and colleagues compared results of SG vs. traditional OR [55]. The authors demonstrated that the elderly specifically those over the age of 70 were more likely to have had a SG placed rather than OR. Although there was a statistically significant decrease in mortality in the SG group, age was not a factor in multivariate analysis. That same year, Patel et al. compared open repair vs. endovascular repair in patients older than 75 years of age [56]. The authors demonstrated a reduced early mortality in the SG group as well as a shorter hospital stay. Of note, those in the SG were older and sicker when compared with the OR group. However, long-term results did not show a mortality benefit. Unfortunately, the etiologies of the late deaths are unknown; however, one would have to assume with a mean age of 79 years, underlying comorbid conditions would play a significant role.

Sternal Fractures

The quoted incidence of sternal fractures after trauma varies in the literature and is dependent on the sample population. Recinos et al. demonstrated a 0.33% of sternal fractures in all trauma admissions over a 10-year period [57]. Others have a quoted incidence of 1.36% in blunt trauma, 2.7% in BCT patients, and 5.4% of those with an injury to the thoracic cavity after blunt trauma [9, 58, 59]. In the elderly, the incidence of sternal fractures has been reported to be 5.3% after blunt trauma [60]. Similar to that of rib fractures and flail chest, effective pain control is key to management in the geriatric population.

Cardiac Contusion

Blunt cardiac trauma most frequently occurs after a MVC and results from a direct blow to the chest from the steering wheel or from rapid deceleration [61]. Its diagnosis remains challenging due to nonspecific symptoms as well as no ideal test for diagnosis. Cardiac contusions can result in muscle ischemia, pump failure as well as hemodynamic instability, specifically in the setting on concomitant valvular disruption. Blunt cardiac injury (BCI) must be considered any time a trauma patient has unexplained cardiac dysfunction including heart failure, electrocardiogram (EKG) abnormalities, or complex dysrhythmias [62]. Additionally, hypotension without a clear source in the elderly should prompt evaluation for a cardiac contusion or cardiac dysfunction. The incidence of cardiac contusions after BCT has been reported to be about 4%, regardless of age [9, 59].

The elderly pose additional difficulty in the diagnosis of BCI as many of them have preexisting cardiac dysfunction and underlying arrhythmias. Coronary atherosclerotic disease limiting coronary blood flow, decrease in cardiac output (CO) due to decreased cardiac contraction filling rate and stroke volume cause the elderly lose their ability to respond to a stressful situation such as acute trauma [62]. The CO of an 80-year old is approximately one-half that of a 20-year old person [63].

The diagnosis of BCI is difficult as no single test definitely identifies the injury. The EKG may be normal or show nonspecific abnormalities including diffuse ST elevations or depressions, sinus tachycardia, atrial and ventricular ectopy, and conduction disorders [61]. Cardiac enzymes are often used as a screening to help identify a BCI. Creatinine kinase (CK) is nonspecifically increased in the multitrauma patient because of the skeletal muscle injury. CK-MB, which is thought to be more specific for cardiac injury, had also demonstrated poor correlation in BCI [64, 65]. Some studies have shown that CK-MB is often normal even in the setting of BCI [66, 67]. Additionally, as BCI more often involves the right ventricle [68], which has relatively less muscle mass than the left ventricle, the degree of CK-MB may not correlate with injury [65]. Studies of Troponin I and T have demonstrated high accuracy in the setting of BCI [69, 70]. The authors have suggested that a normal Troponin I or T is a strong indicator of the absence of a cardiac injury.

Echocardiography can provide a direct view of cardiac activity including wall motion and valvular function and has been shown to be an effective tool for diagnosing BCI [71]. A transthoracic echocardiogram (TTE) is noninvasive; however, some patients may not be able to tolerate it because of the chest wall pain, positioning or body habitus. In those situations, a transesophageal echocardiogram (TEE) may be required for evaluation [68]. However, many elderly trauma patients have preexisting wall motion abnormalities and valvular dysfunction complicating the echocardiogram findings and the diagnosis of acute BCI.

Once identified, supportive care with judiciary volume management and inotropes is the mainstay of treatment. Any acute structural lesions should be evaluated for possible operative repair. As the elderly cannot augment CO, they instead increase systemic vascular resistance [72]. This produces a falsely normal blood pressure but may still have badly compromised cardiac performance. Scalea et al. have demonstrated that as many as 50% of those who had "normal" blood pressure in fact had evidence of occult cardiogenic shock and a subsequent poor outcome [73, 74]. Using invasive monitoring, these authors demonstrated significant hemodynamic compromise occurs in elderly patients who were clinically stable after their initial evaluation for blunt trauma [74]. Over a 2-year period, all patients over the age of 65 who were hemodynamically stable after their initial resuscitation had a pulmonary artery catheters inserted. The authors defined patients to be in cardiogenic shock if they had a CO less than 3.5 L/M and/or a mixed venous saturation (MVO$_2$) less than 50%. They demonstrated an increase in survival from 7 to 53% by early optimization of all patients with volume, inotropes, and afterload reduction. The authors concluded that emergent invasive monitoring identifies occult shock early and improves outcome.

Conclusion

The number of persons over the age of 65 years is increasing annually. As a result, the number of geriatric trauma patients is increasing as well. Trauma was once thought to be a disease of the young, but this is no longer the case. Accordingly, clinicians need to be aware of injury patterns and outcomes specifically associated with older age. Although some injuries are managed with similar therapies in the young and the old, some are not. Those over the age of 65 years often have comorbidities that not only predispose them to injury, but also often make it more difficult for them to overcome the injury. Injuries that have minimal effect on the physical being of younger people can have significant morbidity and mortality in the older person. Close attention and aggressive care, often involving a multidisciplinary approach, is needed to decrease the morbidity and mortality after cardio-thoracic trauma in this patient population.

References

1. CDC: 10 Leading Causes of death by age group, United States – 2004. National Center for Injury Prevention and Control. Office of Statistical programming. June 17, 2008.
2. Osler T, Baker SP, Long W. A modification of the injury severity score that both improves accuracy and simplifies scoring. J Trauma. 1997;43:922–6.
3. Champion HR, Copes WS, Buyer D, et al. Major trauma in geriatric patients. Am J Public Health. 1989;79:1278–82.
4. Grossman MD, Miller D, Scaff DW, Arcona S. When is elder old? Effect of preexisting conditions on mortality in geriatric trauma. J Trauma. 2002;52:242–6.
5. Taylor MD, Tracy JK, Meyer W, Pasquale M, Napolitano LM. Trauma in the elderly: intensive care unit resource use and outcome. J Trauma. 2002;53:407–14.
6. US Census Bureau. 65+ in the United States: 2005.
7. U.S. Administration on Aging, Department of Health and Human Services, Washington DC. http://www.aoa.gov. 2008. Accessed 4 Nov 2008.
8. LoCicero 3rd J, Mattox KL. Epidemiology of chest trauma. Surg Clin North Am. 1989;69:15–9.
9. Shorr RM, Crittenden M, Indeck M, et al. Blunt thoracic trauma: analysis of 515 patients. Ann Surg. 1987;206:200–5.
10. Wilson RF, Murray C, Antonenko DR. Non-penetrating thoracic injuries. Surg Clin North Am. 1977;57:17–36.
11. Wang SC, Schneider L. An aging population: fragile, handle with care. Proceedings of the National Highway Traffic Safety Administration. 1999.
12. Shorr RM, Rodriguez A, Indeck MC, et al. Blunt chest trauma in the elderly. J Trauma. 1989;29:234–7.
13. Marik PE. Management of the critically ill geriatric patient. Crit Care Med. 2006;34:176s–82s.
14. DeLorey DS, Babb TG. Progressive mechanical ventilatory constraints with aging. Am J Respir Crit Care Med. 1999;160:169–77.
15. Zeleznik J. Normative aging of the respiratory system. Clin Geriatr Med. 2003;19:1–18.
16. Carpo RO. Aging of the respiratory system. In: Fisherman AP, editor. Pulmonary diseases and disorders. New York: McGraw Hill; 1998. p. 251.
17. Allen JE, Schwab CW. Blunt chest trauma in the elderly. Am Surg. 1985;51:697–700.
18. Albaugh G, Kann B, Puc MM, et al. Age-adjusted outcomes in traumatic flail chest injuries in the elderly. Am Surg. 2000;66:978–81.
19. Bulger E, Arneson MA, Mock CN, et al. Rib fractures in the elderly. J Trauma. 2000;48:1040–7.
20. Bergeron E, Lavoie A, Clas D, et al. Elderly trauma patients with rib fractures are at a greater risk for death and pneumonia. J Trauma. 2003;54:478–85.
21. Ziegler DW, Agarwal NN. The morbidity and mortality of rib fractures. J Trauma. 1994;37:975–9.
22. Lee RB, Bass SM, Morris JA, et al. Three or more rib fractures as an indicator for transfer to a level I trauma center. J Trauma. 1990;30:689–94.
23. Trunkey D. Cervicothoracic trauma. In: Blaisdell F, Trunkey D, editors. Trauma management, vol. 3. New York: Thieme; 1986.
24. Cameron P, Dziukas L, Hadj A, et al. Rib fractures in major trauma. Aust N Z Surg. 1996;66:530–4.
25. Sharma OP, Oswanski MF, Jolly S. Perils of rib fractures. Am Surg. 2008;74:310–4.
26. Stawicki SP, Grossman MD, Hoey BA, et al. Rib fractures in the elderly: a marker of injury severity. J Am Geriatr Soc. 2004;52:805–8.
27. Lotfipour S, Kaku SK, Vaca FE, et al. Factors associated with complications in older adults with isolated blunt chest trauma. West J Emerg Med. 2009;10:79–84.
28. Barnea Y, Kashtan H, Skornick Y, et al. Isolated rib fractures in elderly patients: mortality and morbidity. Can J Surg. 2002;45:43–6.
29. DeMaria EJ, Kenney PR, Merriam MA, et al. Survival after trauma in geriatric patients. Ann Surg. 1987;206:738–43.
30. Oreskovich MR, Howard JD, Copass MK, et al. Geriatric trauma: injury patterns and outcome. J Trauma. 1984;24:565–72.
31. Freedland M, Wilson RF, Bender JS, et al. The management of flail chest injury: factors affecting outcome. J Trauma. 1990;30:1460–8.
32. Simon BJ, Cushman J, Barraco R, et al. Pain management guidelines for blunt thoracic trauma. J Trauma. 2005;59:1256–67.
33. Wisner DH. A stepwise logistic regression analysis of factors affecting morbidity and mortality after thoracic trauma: effect of epidural analgesia. J Trauma. 1990;30:799–804.
34. Ullman DA, Fortune JB, Greenhouse BB, et al. The treatment of patients with multiple rib fractures using continuous thoracic epidural narcotic infusion. Reg Anesth. 1989;14:43–7.
35. Mackersie RC, Karagianes TG, Hoyt DB, et al. Prospective evaluation of epidural and intravenous administration of fentanyl for pain control and restoration of ventilatory function following multiple rib fractures. J Trauma. 1991;31:443–9.
36. Mackersie RC, Shackford SR, Hoyt DB, et al. Continuous epidural fentanyl analgesia: ventilatory function improvement with routine use in treatment of blunt chest trauma. J Trauma. 1987;27:1201–12.
37. Parmley LF, Mattingly TW, Manion WC, et al. Nonpenetrating traumatic injury of the aorta. Circulation. 1958;17:1086–101.
38. Hass G. Types of internal injuries of personnel involved in aircraft accidents. J Aviat Med. 1944;15:77–84.
39. Ahrar K, Smith DC, Bansal RC, et al. Angiography in blunt thoracic trauma. J Trauma. 1997;42:665–9.
40. Johnson MS, Shah H, Harris VJ, et al. Comparison of digital subtraction and cut film arteriography in the evaluation of suspected thoracic aortic injury. J Vasc Interv Radiol. 1997;8:799–807.
41. Fishman JE. Imaging of blunt aortic and great vessel trauma. J Thorac Imaging. 2000;15:97–103.
42. Woodring JH. The normal mediastinum in blunt traumatic rupture of the thoracic aorta and brachiocephalic arteries. J Emerg Med. 1990;8:467–76.
43. Fabian TC, Richardson JD, Croce MA, et al. Prospective study of blunt aortic injury: multicenter trial of the American Association for the Surgery of Trauma. J Trauma. 1997;42:374–83.
44. Exadaktylos AK, Sclabas G, Schmid SW, et al. Do we really need routine computed tomographic scanning in the primary evaluation of blunt chest trauma in patients with "normal" chest radiographs? J Trauma. 2001;51:1173–6.
45. Plurad D, Green D, Demetriades D, et al. The increasing use of chest computed tomography for trauma: is it being overutilized? J Trauma. 2007;62:631–5.

46. Wintermark M, Wicky S, Schnyder P. Imaging of acute traumatic injuries of the thoracic aorta. Eur Radiol. 2002;12:431–42.

47. Nagy K, Fabian T, Rodman G, et al. Guidelines for the diagnosis and management of blunt aortic injury: an EAST practice management guideline work group. J Trauma. 2000;48:1128–43.

48. Jahromi AS, Kazemi K, Safar HA, et al. Traumatic rupture of the thoracic aorta: cohort study and systemic review. J Vasc Surg. 2001;34:1029–34.

49. Von Oppell UO, Dunne TT, De Goot MK, et al. Traumatic aortic rupture: twenty-year metaanalysis of mortality and risk of paraplegia. Ann Thorac Surg. 1994;58:585–93.

50. Camp Jr PC, Rogers FB, Shackford SR, et al. Blunt traumatic thoracic aortic laceration in the elderly: an analysis of outcome. J Trauma. 1994;37:418–23.

51. Hirose H, Gill IS, Malangoni NA. Nonoperative management of traumatic aortic injury. J Trauma. 2006;60:547–601.

52. Aronstam EM, Gomez AC, O'Connell TJ, et al. recent surgical and pharmacologic experience with acute dissecting and traumatic aneurysms. J Thorac Cardiovasc Surg. 1970;59:231–8.

53. Frykberg ER, Vines FS, Alexander RH. The natural history of clinically occult arterial injuries: a prospective evaluation. J Trauma. 1989;29:577–83.

54. Cook J, Salerno C, Krishnadasan B, et al. The effect of changing presentation and management on the outcome of blunt rupture of the thoracic aorta. J Thorac Cardiovasc Surg. 2006;131:594–600.

55. Demetriades D, Velmahos GC, Scalea TM, et al. Operative repair or endovascular stent graft in blunt traumatic thoracic aortic injuries: results of an American Association for the Surgery of Trauma Multicenter Study. J Trauma. 2008;64:561–71.

56. Patel HJ, Williams DM, Upchurch GR, et al. A comparison of open and endovascular descending thoracic aortic repair in patients older than 75 years of age. Ann Thorac Surg. 2008;85:1597–604.

57. Recinos G, Inaba K, Dubose J, et al. Epidemiology of sternal fractures. Am Surg. 2009;75:401–4.

58. Hills MW, Delprado AM, Deane SA. Sternal fractures: associated injuries and management. J Trauma. 1993;35:55–60.

59. Kulshrestha P, Munshi I, Wait R. Profile of chest trauma in a level I trauma center. J Trauma. 2004;57:576–81.

60. Inci I, Ozcelik C, Nizam O, et al. Thoracic in the elderly. Eur J Emerg Med. 1998;5:445–50.

61. Sybrandy KC, Cramer MJ, Burgersdijk C. Diagnosing cardiac contusion: old wisdom and new lights. Heart. 2003;89:485–9.

62. Keough V, Letizia M. Blunt cardiac injury in the elderly trauma patient. Int J Trauma Nurs. 1998;4:38–43.

63. Lakatta EG. Age related alterations in cardiovascular response to adrenergic mediated stress. Fed Proc. 1980;30:3173–7.

64. Frazee RC, Mucha Jr P, Farnell MB, et al. Objective evaluation of blunt cardiac trauma. J Trauma. 1986;26:510–20.

65. Keller KD, Shatney CH. Creatine phosphokinase-MB assays in patients with suspected myocardial contusion: diagnostic test or test of diagnosis? J Trauma. 1988;28:58–63.

66. Potkin RT, Werner JA, Trobaugh GB, et al. Evaluation of non-invasive tests of cardiac damage in suspected cardiac contusion. Circulation. 1982;66:627–31.

67. Mayfield W, Hurley EJ. Blunt cardiac trauma. Am J surg. 1984;148: 162–7.

68. Weiss RL, Brier JA, O'Connor W, et al. The usefulness of transesophageal echocardiography in diagnosing cardiac contusions. Chest. 1996;109:73–7.

69. Adams 3rd JE, Dávila-Román VG, Bessey PQ, et al. Improved detection of cardiac contusion with cardiac troponin I. Am Heart J. 1996;131:308–12.

70. Collins JN, Cole FJ, Weireter LJ, et al. The usefulness of serum troponin levels in evaluating cardiac injury. Am Surg. 2001;67: 821–5.

71. Hiatt JR, Yeatman Jr LA, Child JS. The value of echocardiography in blunt chest trauma. J Trauma. 1988;28:914–22.

72. Oleske DM, Wilson RS, Bernard BA, et al. Epidemiology of injury in people with Alzheimer's disease. J Am Geriatr Soc. 1995;43: 741–6.

73. Scalea TM. Invited commentary (for McMahon et al.: Co-morbidity and trauma in the elderly). World J Surg. 1996;20:116.

74. Scalea TM, Simon HM, Duncan AO, et al. Geriatric blunt multiple trauma: improved survival with early invasive monitoring. J Trauma. 1990;30:129–34.

Chapter 12
Imaging Features of the Normal Aging Chest

Carol C. Wu and Jo-Anne O. Shepard

Abstract As a part of the normal aging process, many changes occur in the lungs, mediastinum, pleura, and thoracic skeleton. Age-related mild pulmonary fibrosis, air trapping, and apical scarring can be seen in the lungs. Tortuous and atherosclerotic vessels and mediastinal lipomatosis are not infrequently seen in elderly patients. With increasing age, diaphragmatic hernia and eventration may become more prominent. Additionally, degenerative changes of the osseous structures can sometimes mimic pulmonary nodules. Familiarity with the imaging appearance of these changes is important to help avoid mistaking these changes as pathologic processes.

Keywords Subpleural reticulation • Tracheal calcification • Apical cap • Airtrapping (f) • Focal fibrosis (f) • Osteophyte (f) • Intraparenchymal lymph node (f) • Lung nodule (f) • Thymus (f) • Mediastinal lipomatosis (f) • Unfolded aorta (f) • Atherosclerosis (f) • Aberrant right subclavian artery (f) • Kommerell diverticulum (f) • Eventration (f) • Diaphragmatic hernia (f) • Costal cartilage calcification (f)

Introduction

Many changes that occur in the lungs, mediastinum, pleura, and thoracic skeleton as part of the normal aging process can be detected on thoracic imaging studies. These changes can sometimes mimic pathologic processes. Familiarity with imaging appearance of the normal aging chest, therefore, is vital for accurate interpretation of the chest radiographs and computed tomography (CT) and can help minimize unnecessary further work-up.

J.-A.O. Shepard (✉)
Department of Radiology, Division of Thoracic Imaging and Intervention, Massachusetts General Hospital, 55 Fruit Street, Founders 202, Boston, MA 02114, USA
e-mail: jshepard@partners.org

Lung

Morphologic Changes

Physiologic and morphologic changes have been identified in the aging lung [1]. Physiological changes occur in the aging lung resulting from loss of elastic recoil in the alveoli and airways [1, 2]. Morphologically, there is an increase in the size of airspaces with dilatation of alveoli and a decrease in gas-exchange surface area and supporting tissue for small airways [1]. Histopathologic studies in animal models have demonstrated increased collagen accumulation and progressive pulmonary fibrosis with aging [3].

In an attempt to establish the "normal" CT appearance in aging lungs, Coplcy et al. have examined the morphology of the lung parenchyma on CT in asymptomatic older patients. Two study groups, an older group above 75 years of age and a younger group below 55 years of age, were scanned with high resolution CT protocol. A subpleural basal reticular pattern was found in the majority (24/40, 60%) of the older group and absent (0/16) in the younger group ($p < 0.0001$) (Fig. 12.1). Small cysts were seen in 25% (10/40) of the older group and in none of the younger group ($p = 0.02$). Bronchial dilatation and wall thickening were also seen significantly more frequently ($p < 0.001$) in the older group (24/40, 60% and 22/40, 55%) than in the younger group (1/16, 6% each), respectively. All of the findings were independent of smoking history, and the majority of patients had normal pulmonary function, likely reflecting the normal spectrum of morphology in the aging lung [4].

Additionally, diffuse calcification of the cartilages of trachea and bronchi is a common appearance in the elderly female (Fig. 12.2). In contrast, abnormal calcium deposition in the airways can be seen in patients with hypercalcemia and patients on warfarin treatment. Cartiaginous calification as a function of aging is of no clinical significance. It should be distinguished from calcifications found in pathologic conditions such as relapsing polychondiritis in which diffuse calcification and smooth thickening is found in the cartilage-bearing

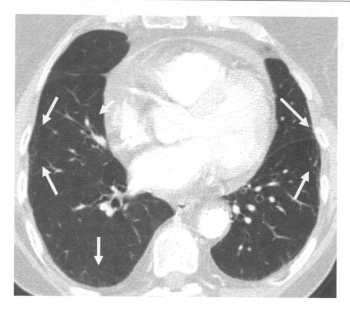

Fig. 12.1 Subtle reticular opacities (*arrows*) are noted in bilateral subpleural lungs

airways or tracheopathia osteochondroplastica in which nodular submucosal cartilaginous deposits are found diffusely throughout the tracheobronchial tree.

Apical Cap

Apical caps are a common feature of advancing age and are usually the result of subpleural scarring not associated with other diseases [5]. Apical subpleural scarring is demonstrated as symmetric smooth or, more often, irregular apical thickening or "apical cap" on chest radiographs. Chest CT images demonstrate symmetric bilateral irregular subpleural apical opacities (Fig. 12.3).

In cases in which the apical opacities are focal or asymmetric, underlying pathology may be suspected. Yousem [6] reviewed 13 cases of pulmonary apical cap (PAC) resected for the exclusion of a clinical diagnosis of lung carcinoma. Radiographically the lesions appeared as spiculated subpleural

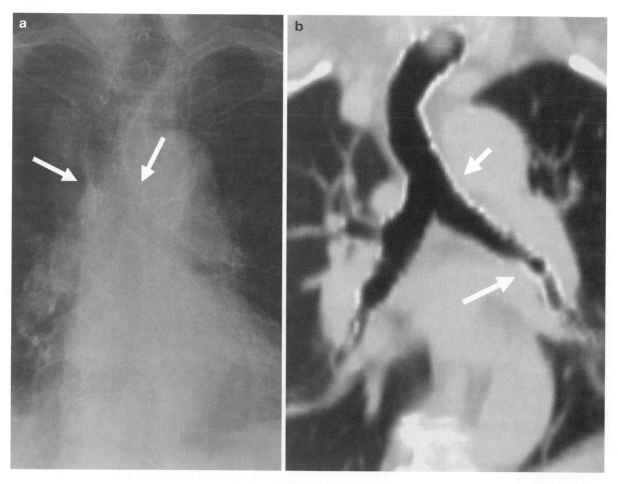

Fig. 12.2 Calcification is noted along the tracheal and bronchial wall (*arrows*) on CXR (**a**) and coronal reformation CT image (**b**)

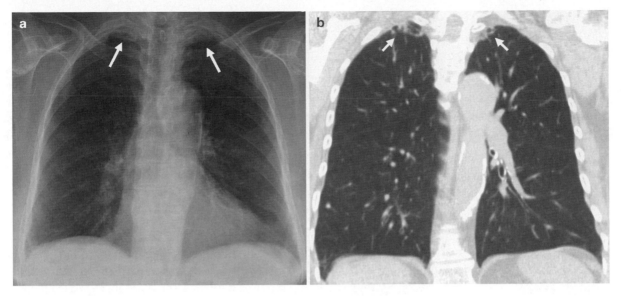

Fig. 12.3 Mild apical reticular opacities (*arrows*) consistent with fibrosis are subtle on CXR (**a**) and better appreciated on coronal reformation CT image (**b**). Note also the atherosclerotic calcification along the wall of the descending aorta

masses ranging from 0.7 to 5.2 cm in diameter. Histologically, these subpleural scars were pyramid shaped with overlying pleural adhesions and hyaline pleural plaques, and were characterized by a dense basophilic fibrosis of the parenchyma with air spaces filled with mature collagen. A chronic ischemic etiology was favored [6]. Apical fibrosis related to ischemic changes can usually be distinguished from other lesions that arise from the lung, pleura, or extra pleural space. These lesions include inflammatory lesion such as tuberculosis, postradiation fibrosis, superior sulcus tumors, posttraumatic subpleural dissection of blood, and mediastinal lipomatosis with subcostal fat extending over the lung apices [5].

Focal Fibrosis

Osteophytes of the spine are a common finding in older patients, and by the age of 50 years, they are found in about 80% of men and 60% of women [7]. Osteophytes are more often found along the right side of the thoracic spine in contact with the lower lobe of the right lung. It is theorized that the pulsations of descending thoracic aorta, which descends on the left side of the spine, prevents the formation of osteophytes [7]. In a retrospective study [8], focal interstitial opacities were present in 45% of patients with osteophytes. In contrast, none were found in patients without osteophytes. Routine chest CT exams commonly demonstrate a focal interstitial opacity adjacent to the right-sided osteophytes (Fig. 12.4). Otake et al. [8] found both reticular and linear patterns on CT images. On prone

images, the interstitial opacities persisted, suggesting that the opacities are irreversible and not just dependent changes [8]. Histologic correlation revealed the adjacent pleura to be white and firm with collapse of the adjacent alveolar spaces. Within the collapsed lung, collagen and elastic fibers were increased consistent with fibrosis [8]. The differential diagnosis includes early interstitial pneumonia, asbestosis or focal organizing pneumonia. However, focal fibrosis is an incidental isolated finding associated with right-sided osteophytes and should not be confused with other disorders.

Air Trapping

Air trapping on CT scans is defined as "decreased attenuation of pulmonary parenchyma, especially during expiration" [9]. On expiratory images, the attenuation of lung parenchyma will normally demonstrate a homogenous increase in attenuation [10]. Air trapping appears as a heterogeneous or a homogeneous increase in lung lucency [11] (Fig. 12.5). Lee et al. [12] assessed the frequency and degree of air trapping on thin-section CT of the lung in relation to age and smoking history in asymptomatic subjects. Thin-section CT was performed prospectively at end inspiration and end expiration in 82 subjects (27 smokers, 55 nonsmokers) without any history of pulmonary diseases or symptoms. The frequency and degree of air trapping were evaluated according to age and smoking status. Air trapping was found in 3/13 (23%) of subjects aged 21–30 years, 7/17 (41%) aged 31–40 years, 9/18 (50%) aged 41–50 years, 11/17 (65%) aged

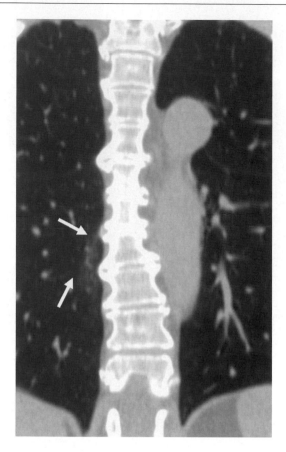

Fig. 12.4 Subtle reticular opacities in the right lower lobe (*arrows*) adjacent to the osteophytes

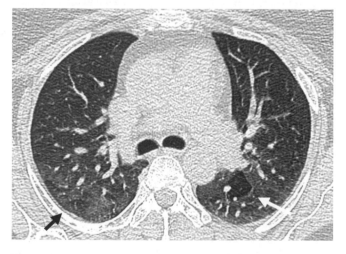

Fig. 12.5 An expiratory image showing subtle hyper-lucent areas (*arrows*) in the lungs consistent with air-trapping

51–60 years, and 13/17 (76%) greater than or equal to 61 years. The frequency of air trapping not only increased with age but also the severity of air trapping had a significant correlation with age and a smoking history of more than 10 pack-years [12].

Benign Intrapulmonary Lymph Nodes/ Perifissural Lymph Nodes (PFNS)

CT scanning has resulted in the frequent detection of small pulmonary nodules, which are often too small to be seen on chest radiographs. The finding of benign intraparenchymal lymph nodes is not an uncommon finding following resection of small peripheral nodules [13, 14]. Bankoff et al. demonstrated that intraparenchymal lymph nodes were found in 18% of their patients who underwent minithoracotomies for evaluation of CT-detected pulmonary nodules. In an autopsy study, Trapnell showed that intraparenchymal lymph nodes were found in 7% (6/92) of their cases. Intraparenchymal lymph nodes are frequently found in patients older than 50 years and are more common in men. They are usually noncalcified, less than 10 mm in diameter, and found in the lower lobes in a subpleural perilymphatic location [15–17] (Fig. 12.6). Intraparenchymal lymph nodes may mimic other nodules such as granulomas or metastases. In a study to determine whether the CT characteristic of benign intrapulmonary lymph nodes and small sarcoma metastases were sufficiently characteristic to allow prospective identification, Sykes et al. [18] found that benign intrapulmonary lymph nodes were statistically more likely to be oval than round, more likely than sarcoma metastases to have a lymphatic distribution, and more likely to be located subpleurally. Although normal lymph nodes are generally ovoid in shape, they may be round in appearance on an axial CT scan if an ovoid nodule were oriented perpendicular to the imaging plane [18]. Coronal and sagittal reformatted images would be helpful to demonstrate the true ovoid shape in such cases. A lymphatic location is a more specific finding. In a pathologic study, Sykes found that 75% (43/57) of benign intrapulmonary lymph nodes were in a lymphatic distribution on CT, and 95% (54/57) were in a lymphatic distribution on pathologic review. Forty-seven percent (27/57) were subpleural, 70% (40/57) were in a septal location, and 31% (17/57) were both septal and subpleural. All but two were located within 2 cm of the pleura. Additionally, 25/57 had a vascular attachment.

Perifissural nodules (PFNs) are frequently seen on CT examinations obtained in older patients who are at high risk for lung cancer. Ahn et al. [19] retrospectively reviewed serial CT images in 128 subjects enrolled in a lung cancer screening trial. Although most PFNs were triangular or oval, round, rectangular and dumbbell shapes were also identified. The mean maximal length was 3.2 mm (range, 1–13 mm). During a 2-year follow up in 71 subjects, 7/159 PFNs increased in size on one scan but were then stable. The authors searched a lung cancer registry 7.5 years after study entry and found 10 lung cancers in 139 of 146 study subjects who underwent complete study follow up.

Fig. 12.6 (**a**) Tiny oval-shaped nodule along the right minor fissure (*arrow*) and (**b**) tiny triangular-shaped nodule along the right major fissure (*arrow*) consistent with intraparenchymal lymph nodes

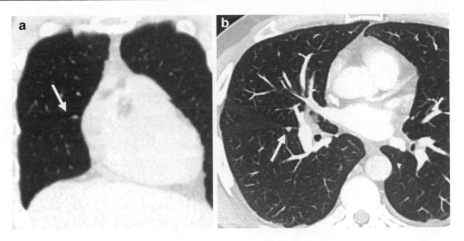

None of these cancers had developed from a PFN, suggesting that the malignant potential of PFNs is low [19]. Small nodules located along the fissures with morphologic characteristics of fissural lymph nodes should be considered benign.

Mediastinum

Thymus

The normal thymus is composed of two lobes that occupy the thyropericardiac space of the anterior mediastinum extending from the level of thyroid gland inferiorly to the base of the heart [20]. From puberty to age 25, the thymus can be identified as a triangular bilobed structure in the anterior mediastinum with flat or concave borders and rarely convex borders. Beginning at puberty, as the thymic gland involutes, atrophied thymic follicles are progressively replaced with fat, causing the attenuation of the thymic tissue to decrease, until about age 60. By age 60, the remaining thymic tissue is negligible or absent [21, 22]. The rate of involution is extremely variable and recognizable thymic tissue can be identified in some subjects even at the age of 40 years. With complete thymic involution, the anterior mediastinal fat may still have CT attenuation higher than subcutaneous fat because of the remaining underlying fibrous skeleton of the thymus [20] (Fig. 12.7).

Mediastinal Lipomatosis

Mediastinal lipomatosis is a benign condition in which there is excessive deposition of unencapsulated fat throughout the mediastinum resulting in mediastinal widening. Mediastinal lipomatosis is associated with obesity, Cushing's syndrome, and steroid treatment. Although lipomatosis may be found in young adults, it is more commonly encountered in the older and obese adult population. Lipomatosis is asymptomatic and requires no treatment.

Mediastinal lipomatosis causes smooth mediastinal widening on chest radiographs, CT, and magnetic resonance imaging (MRI). The excessive fat is deposited throughout the mediastinum, surrounding normal structures without causing compression or obstruction (Fig. 12.8). Excessive fat is commonly more prominent in the superior mediastinum, but is also seen in the paravertebral regions, and the cardiophrenic angles resulting in large paracardiac fat pads (Fig. 12.9). On chest radiographs, the widening in the mediastinum may have a mass-like appearance, mimicking a tumor. However, on CT or MRI, the benign fat can be easily distinguished by its pure fat attenuation and lack of mass effect on adjacent structures. Any stranding of the fat or soft tissue attenuation within the fat is a sign of pathologic process such as hemorrhage or mediastinitis in the acute setting and tumor infiltration, mediastinal fibrosis, or liposarcoma in the chronic setting. Excessive fat may also deposit in the extrapleural space mimicking focal or diffuse pleural thickening on chest radiographs [23–26] (Fig. 12.10).

Aorta and Great Vessels

In normal subjects, the thoracic aorta gradually tapers from its origin to the descending aorta such that the ascending aorta is usually 1 cm greater in diameter than the descending aorta. Aronberg et al. [27] measured the normal diameter of more than 100 adults and found the average diameter

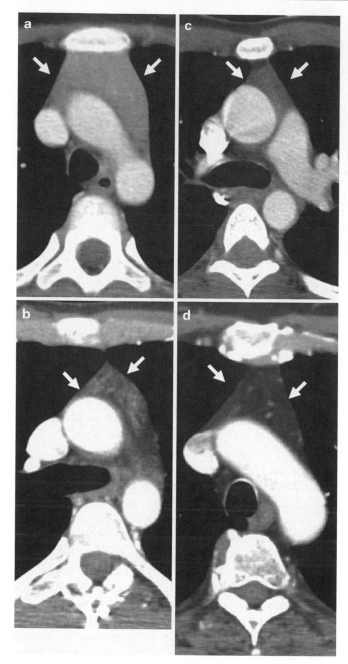

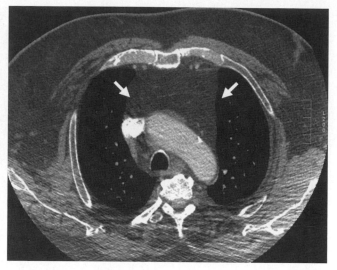

Fig. 12.8 Axial CT shows prominent mediastinal fat (*arrows*) consistent with mediastinal lipomatosis. Significant amount of subcutaneous fat is also present in this obese patient

Fig. 12.7 (**a**) Normal thymus in a 7-year-old child demonstrates convex margin with soft tissue density. (**b**) Normal thymus in a 29-year-old adult has some interspersed fat density and smaller size though still retains a convex margin on the left. (**c**) Normal thymus in another 29-year-old adult consists mostly of fat density but has straight margin. (**d**) Normal thymus in a 73-year-old adult demonstrates complete fatty replacement of the thymic tissue and straight lateral margins

of the proximal ascending aorta is 3.6 cm (range 2.4–4.7 cm), the ascending aorta below the arch is 3.51 cm (range 2.2–4.6 cm), the proximal descending aorta is 2.63 cm (range 1.6–3.7 cm), the middle descending aorta is

2.48 cm (range 1.6–3.7 cm), and the distal descending aorta is 2.42 cm (range 1.4–3.3 cm). Aortic diameters generally increase with advancing age and aortic diameters tend to be greater in men when compared with women [27, 28]. In subjects over 50 years of age, the aorta may appear more prominent or tortuous on chest radiographs without evidence for aneurysm formation. In younger patients, the descending aorta descends in proximity to the thoracic spine in a parallel fashion, while in older normal adults, the aortic arch and descending aorta appear more "unfolded" (Fig. 12.11). Similar changes occur in the right innominate, common carotid and subclavian arteries. With increased age, the arteries may assume a more tortuous appearance. In extreme cases, the vessels may be so tortuous that they cause widening of the superior mediastinum mimicking a mediastinal mass or lymphadenopathy. These findings can be easily clarified by CT correlation or comparison with older chest radiographs to demonstrate long-term stability (Fig. 12.12).

As atherosclerosis develops in older adults and aortic plaques form, focal areas of wall thickening may appear, which is lower in attenuation than the normal aortic wall because of their lipid content [29]. As the atherosclerosis progresses, the plaques calcify. On positron emission tomography (PET) examinations, abnormal fluorodeoxyglucose (FDG) uptake can be detected in atherosclerotic vessels including the aorta and great vessels [30] (Fig. 12.13). The abnormal activity corresponds to inflammatory changes in the atheromatous plaques that can appear as either diffuse or focal uptake in the wall of the

Fig. 12.9 PA and lateral radiographs (**a**, **b**) show prominent paracardiac fat pad (*arrows*), confirmed on CT (**c**)

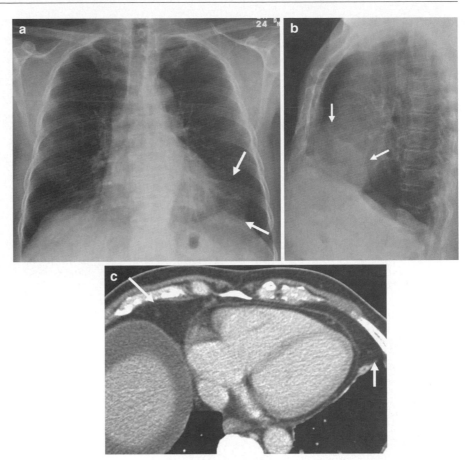

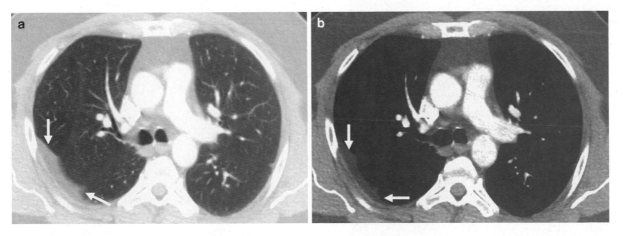

Fig. 12.10 CT images in lung window (**a**) and soft tissue window (**b**). Possible pleural thickening of the right posterolateral thorax (*arrows*) seen in the lung window is of fat density when viewed in the soft tissue window consistent with prominent extra-pleural fat

atherosclerotic artery. Focal uptake may sometimes mimic metastatic lymphadenopathy in PET scans performed for cancer staging. Registration with the concurrent CT examination is important to localize the FDG uptake to the abnormal artery and exclude the presence of lymphadenopathy or other mass.

An aberrant right subclavian artery arising from an otherwise normal left aortic arch is the most common

Fig. 12.11 PA (**a**) and lateral (**b**) chest radiograph show tortuosity or unfolded appearance of the thoracic aorta

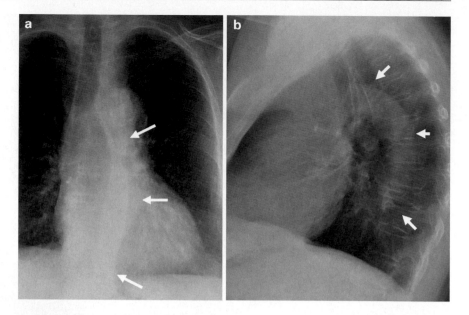

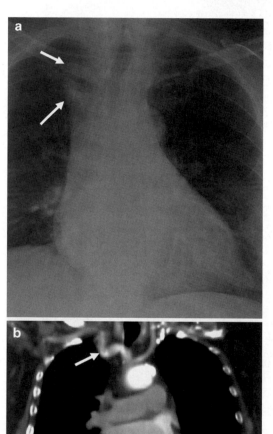

Fig. 12.12 PA chest radiograph (**a**) shows prominent soft tissue in the right paratracheal region (*arrow*) corresponding to a tortuous right subclavian artery on CT (**b**)

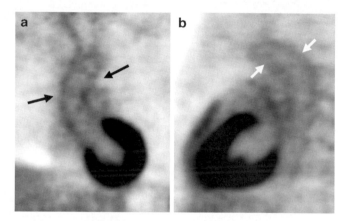

Fig. 12.13 (**a**, **b**) Coronal and sagittal views from a PET study showing FDG uptake along the aortic wall (*arrows*), thought to be due to atherosclerosis. Note the normal uptake by the left ventricular myocardium

congenital abnormality of the aorta occurring in 0.5% of the normal population [31]. The aberrant right subclavian artery arises from the posterior portion of the left-sided aortic arch and crosses the mediastinum posterior to the trachea and esophagus as it courses from left to right. In approximately 60% [28] of cases, there is dilatation of the artery at its origin referred to as a Kommerell diverticulum. The diverticulum can cause compression of the adjacent esophagus resulting in dysphagia. In aging adults, the diverticulum can enlarge, become atherosclerotic, and be a nidus for thrombus formation (Fig. 12.14). In such cases, increased dysphagia or stroke may ensue [32].

Fig. 12.14 Axial (**a**) and coronal (**b**) CT images showing aberrant origin of the right subclavian artery with diverticulum of Kommerell (*short arrow*). The esophagus (*long arrow*) is compressed

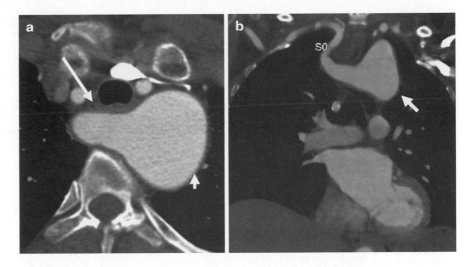

Fig. 12.15 Lateral chest radiograph (**a**) demonstrates a mass-like opacity in the left posterior costophrenic sulcus (*arrow*). Axial CT (**b**, **c**) shows a left posterior diaphragmatic defect (*arrow* in **c**) with herniation of abdominal fat into the left chest cavity (*arrow* in **b**). The patient also has a moderate para-esophageal hiatus hernia (**b**)

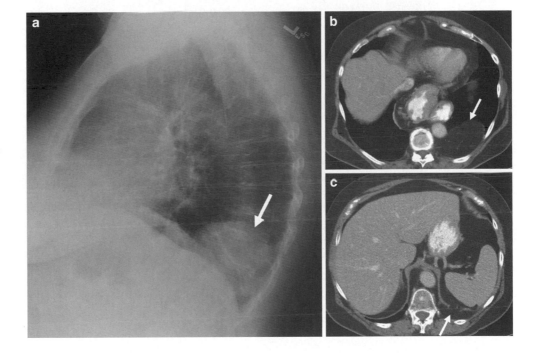

Diaphragm

Age-related changes in the diaphragm have been studied. In a study of 120 subjects evaluated by CT, Caskey et al. [33] failed to identify any change in the thickness of the diaphragm with age. Yet, congenital defects of the diaphragm can become more pronounced with advancing age and in the presence of pulmonary emphysema, especially in men. In this study, none of the patients in their 20s and 30s demonstrated any diaphragmatic defects, whereas 56% of patients in their 60s and 70s were found to have defects. The authors hypothesized that the defects found in older individuals occurred in areas of structural weakness, possibly embryologic in nature [33].

The most common of the diaphragmatic defects, the Bochdalek hernia, is caused by persistence of the embryonic pleuroperitoneal canal. Posterior herniation of abdominal contents such as fat, kidney, and adrenal gland through the defect may simulate an intrathoracic mass (Fig. 12.15). Herniation of intraabdominal fat and viscera may also occur

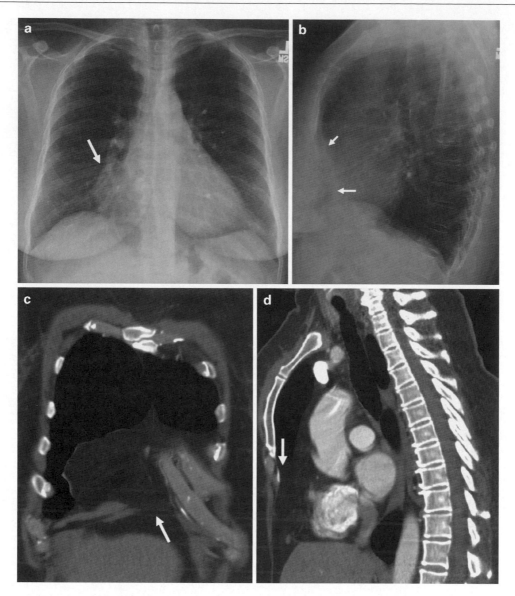

Fig. 12.16 PA and lateral chest radiographs (**a, b**) demonstrate a right para-cardiac opacity (*arrows*). Coronal (**c**) and sagittal (**d**) CT reformation images revealed a defect in the antero-medial aspect of the right hemi-diaphragm (*arrows*) with herniation of abdominal fat and vasculature into the thorax, consistent with Morgagni hernia

through a defect in the anterior costal portion of the diaphragm resulting in a paracardiac Morgagni hernia (Fig. 12.16). These diaphragmatic defects are readily discerned on chest radiographs as an anterior or posterior "mass" contiguous with the diaphragm. CT or MRI evaluation, particularly with sagittal and coronal images, is instrumental in defining the fatty contents and vasculature of the defect and the contiguity with intraabdominal contents [34].

Eventration is a congenital weakness in the muscle of the diaphragm that may occur as a unilateral or bilateral defect. The weakness results in a focal upward bulge in the contour of the diaphragm more commonly in the anterior aspect (Fig. 12.17). In rare cases, the entire extent of the diaphragm may be involved mimicking diaphragmatic paralysis. The distinction of eventration from paralysis can be made by fluoroscopic evaluation of the diaphragm. In the case of paralysis, the diaphragm shows paradoxical motion with a sniff test; the paralyzed hemi-diaphragm will move upward, while the normal contra-lateral hemi-diaphragm will move downward. In eventration, the diaphragm should move downward during the sniff maneuver, as expected with non-paralyzed diaphragm.

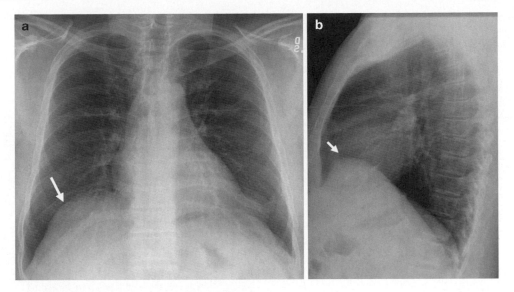

Fig. 12.17 PA (**a**) and lateral (**b**) chest radiograph demonstrate lobulated contour and elevation of the antero-medial aspect of the right hemi-diaphragm, characteristic of eventration

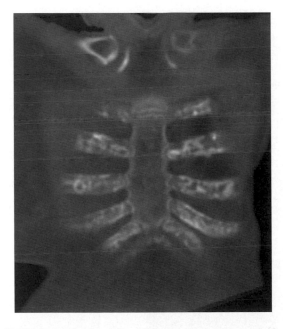

Fig. 12.18 Coronal reformation CT image demonstrates calcification of the costal cartilages

Musculoskeletal

Chest wall compliance demonstrated a significant decrease with increasing age in a study comparing the compliance of the chest wall in subjects aged 24–39 years when compared with those of 55–75 years [35]. Several factors that contribute to decreased chest wall compliance can be demonstrated radiographically. Calcification of the costal cartilages and chondro-sternal junctions increase with advanced age (Fig. 12.18). There are also changes in the shape of the thorax including increased kyphosis relating to osteoporosis and partial or complete vertebral fractures [36, 37]. The increased calcification of the costal cartilages and degenerative osteophytes in the thoracic spine can mimic lung cancers (Figs. 12.19 and 12.20) and, in some instances, can mask significant underlying pathology. For example, the overlying opacities of the head of the clavicle and the first costochondral junction can obscure underlying pathology at the lung apex (Fig. 12.21). The apical location was a common site of missed lung cancers in a retrospective study by Austin et al. [38]. Eighteen radiologists failed to detect 27 potentially resectable bronchogenic carcinomas seen retrospectively on serial chest radiographs. Most of the lung cancers were in an upper lobe ($n=22$ [81%]), particularly the right upper lobe ($n=15$ [56%]) [36]. Shah et al. [39] also found that there was an upper lobe predominance (72%) of missed lung cancers, particularly in the apical or posterior segment of the right upper lobe (38% of cases) or in the apicoposterior segment of the left upper lobe (22% of cases). These three upper zone segments were the sites of missed cancers in 60% of cases in the series of Shah et al. [39] and 59% of cases in the series of Austin et al. Lesions of low conspicuity abound in the upper lung zones, most likely

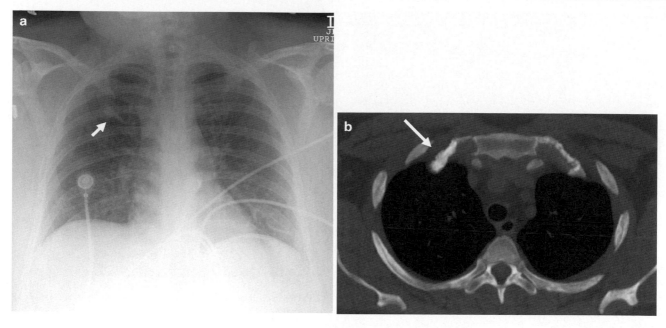

Fig. 12.19 A nodular opacity (*arrow*) was noted on the chest radiograph (**a**), which corresponds to asymmetrically calcified right first costal cartilage on CT (**b**)

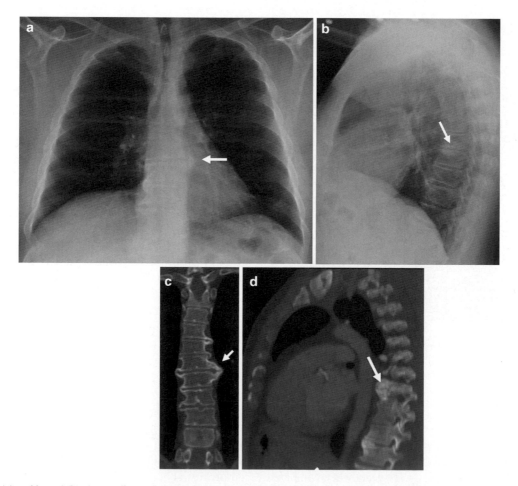

Fig. 12.20 PA (**a**) and lateral (**b**) chest radiograph demonstrate a left paraspinal nodular opacity (*arrow*) which is confirmed to represent bridging osteophytes on coronal (**c**) and sagittal (**d**) reformation CT images

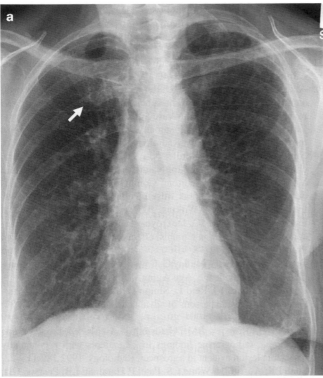

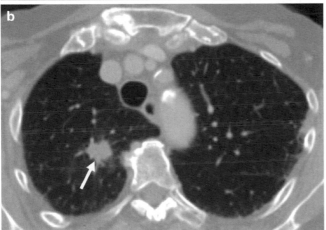

Fig. 12.21 PA chest radiograph (**a**) shows a very subtle opacity in the region of the right first costochondral junction. On CT (**b**), a spiculated nodule, biopsy proven lung cancer, (*arrow*) is found in the right upper lobe at the level of the first costochondral junction

explained by the fact that a clavicle obscured the lesion in 22% of cases [39].

Conclusion

The normal aging process can affect the chest in numerous ways as illustrated in this chapter. By having an understanding of the typical imaging findings frequently seen in elderly patients, one can better distinguish normal aging from pathologic processes and thus avoid common pitfalls and provide appropriate management.

References

1. Janssens JP, Pache JC, Nicod LP. Physiological changes in respiratory function associated with ageing. Eur Respir J. 1999;13:197–205.
2. Gibson GJ, Pride NB, O'Caine C, Quagliato R. Sex and age differences in pulmonary mechanics in normal nonsmoking subjects. J Appl Physiol. 1976;41:20–5.
3. Calabresi C, Arosio B, Galimberti L, Scanziani E, Bergottini R, Annoni G, et al. Natural aging, expression of fibrosis-related genes and collagen deposition in a rat lung. Exp Gerontol. 2007;42:1003–11.
4. Copley SJ, Wells AU, Hawtin KE, Gibson DJ, Hodson JM, Jacques AE, et al. Lung morphology in the elderly: Comparative CT study of subjects over 75 years old versus those under 55 years old. Radiology. 2009;251:566–73.
5. McLoud TC, Isler RJ, Novelline RA, Putman CE, Simeone J, Stark P, et al. The apical cap. AJR Am J Roentgenol. 1981;137:299–306.
6. Yousem SA. Pulmonary apicl cap: a distinctive but poorly recognized lesion in pulmonary surgical pathology. Am J Surg Pathol. 2001;25:679–83.
7. Resnick D, Niwayama G. Degenerative disease of the spine. In: Resnick D, editor. Diagnosis of bone and joint disorders. 3rd ed. Philadelphia: Saunders; 1995. p. 1372–462.
8. Otake S, Takahashi M, Ishigaki T. Focal pulmonary interstitial opacities adjacent to thoracic spine osteophytes. AJR Am J Roentgenol. 2002;179:893–6.
9. Hansell DM, Bankier AA, MacMahon H, McLoud TC, Muller NL, Remy J. Fleischner society: glossary of terms for thoracic imaging. Radiology. 2008;246:697–722.
10. Webb WR, Stern EJ, Kanth N, Gamsu G. Dynamic pulmonary CT: findings in healthy adult men. Radiology. 1993;186:117–24.
11. Stern EJ, Frank MS. Small-airway disease of the lungs: findings at expiratory CT. AJR Am J Roentgenol. 1994;163:37–41.
12. Lee KW, Chung SY, Yang I, Lee Y, Ko EY, Park MJ. Correlation of aging and smoking with air trapping at thin-section CT of the lung in asymptomatic subjects. Radiology. 2000;214:831–6.
13. Bankoff MS, McEniff NJ, Bhadelia RA, Garcia-Moliner M, Daly BD. Prevalence of pathologically proven intrapulmonary lymph nodes and their appearance on CT. AJR Am J Roentgenol. 1996;167:629–30.
14. Trapnell DH. Recognition and incidence of intrapulmonary lymph nodes. Thorax. 1964;19:44–50.
15. Kradin RL, Spirn PW, Mark EJ. Intrapulmonary lymph nodes: clinical, radiologic, and pathologic features. Chest. 1985;87:662–7.
16. Miyake H, Yamada Y, Kawagoe T, Hori Y, Mori H, Yokoyama S, et al. Intrapulmonary lymph nodes: CT and pathologic features. Clin Radiol. 1999;54:640–3.
17. Awai K, Nishioka Y, Tachiyama Y. Intrapulmonary lymph node: findings on high-resolution CT scans. AJR Am J Roentgenol. 1993;161:208–9.
18. Sykes AM, Swensen SJ, Tazelaar HD, Jung SH. Computed tomography of benign intrapulmonary lymph nodes: Retrospective comparison with sarcoma metastases. Mayo Clin Proc. 2002;77:329–33.
19. Ahn MI, Gleeson TG, Chan IH, McWilliams AM, Macdonald SL, Lam S, et al. Perifissural nodules seen at CT screening for lung cancer. Radiology. 2010;254:949–56.

relatively low velocity flow (<2 m/s) and is commonly combined with an estimate of flow area to derive stroke volume (e.g., PW Doppler sample volume is positioned within the left ventricular (LV) outflow tract and combined with an estimate of LV outflow area to measure LV stroke volume).

Color Flow Doppler

Color Doppler is superimposed on the 2D image, with blood velocity at any point on the image assigned a color according to its magnitude and direction. Blood flow towards the ultrasound probe is usually assigned as red, and flow away from the probe is assigned as blue. Blow flow that is turbulent is represented as a mosaic of colors. Since color flow mapping is a form of pulsed wave Doppler, it provides information about velocity and direction of flow within a defined region of interest. The initial echocardiographic assessment of valve stenosis or regurgitation is usually done by positioning a color Doppler sample region over a valve of interest. If abnormal flow pattern are identified, then specific color and spectral Doppler techniques are employed to quantify the degree of valve dysfunction.

Nuclear Myocardial Perfusion Imaging

Since cardiac radionucleotide imaging began in the 1970s, single photon emission computed tomography (SPECT) has become a well established technique for myocardial perfusion imaging (MPI). Numerous studies have validated its role in the detection of coronary artery disease and future risk assessment. With over 10 million studies performed each year alone in the United States, understanding the technique and its implications are paramount to all ordering physicians, including cardiovascular surgeons.

Technique

SPECT-MPI involves injection of radio-isotope tracers (either technecium-99m based or thallium-201 agents) during stress and resting states. These agents are extracted from the bloodstream by viable myocardium in proportion to regional blood flow and decay releasing gamma photon energy. Using a sophisticated system comprising of a detection crystal, collimators, and photomultiplier tubes, the standard nuclear cardiology camera captures and localizes these photoemissions from multiple angles around the body and converts them into an electrical signal. After further processing, the final two dimensional display images are multiple reconstructed slices of the heart representing myocardial

perfusion and regional flow differences. Interpretation of the slices requires comparisons between the resting and stress perfusion images. Areas of the heart with stress induced perfusion defects, but normal resting perfusion are deemed areas of ischemia. Areas of the myocardium with impaired stress and rest perfusion abnormalities are deemed fixed defects, and likely represent infarction especially if the defect is severe. Both semi-quantitative and quantitative analyses have been developed in order to improve reproducibility and to aid in the description of the presence, type, and degree of abnormal findings [1].

MPI is performed in conjunction with either exercise or pharmacological stress to increase coronary blood flow above resting levels. Treadmill exercise using the Bruce protocol to attain at least 85% of age-predicted maximum heart rate is generally preferred as it allows for the concomitant assessment of hemodynamics, functional capacity and symptoms. In the elderly population, co-morbidities and physical ailments frequently preclude treadmill testing or the attainment of target heart rates. Therefore, coronary hyperemia is usually achieved with pharmacological stress agents such as vasodilators (adenosine, regadenoson, or dypridamole) or catecholamines (dobutamine). Finally, SPECT-MPI is performed as a single or two day protocol, depending on patient's body habitus, and generally requires approximately 5 h to complete.

Safety

Stress MPI is, generally, safe and well tolerated. Though infrequent, risks and side effects are related to stress testing and close monitoring is always required. Of more concern recently is ionizing radiation and the potential for significant lifetime exposure with greater risk for malignancy. Substantial differences exist between procedures with use of different radiopharmaceuticals. 99m-Tc rest-stress study averages 10–15 mSv. Doses are much higher for studies using 201Tl (approaching 15–20 mSv) and still higher for dual isotope studies [2]. Great emphasis has been placed on reducing radiation exposure both by increasing awareness, and with new recent hardware and technology advances.

Indications

SPECT-MPI is clinically indicated for a variety of diverse clinical scenarios including the detection of CAD and risk assessment in symptomatic and asymptomatic patients with or without CAD, risk assessment post acute coronary syndromes, preoperative risk assessment of patients undergoing noncardiac surgery, the evaluation of newly diagnosed CHF and the assessment of myocardial viability [3]. Furthermore, over 2 decades of clinical trials have established the prognostic role of SPECT findings in the routine clinical management of subjects with suspected or known CAD. A normal SPECT result generally defines a group with a <1% annual risk of cardiac death and/or nonfatal myocardial infarction, whereas prognosis is progressively poorer the more abnormal the study. Furthermore, quantification of LV ejection fraction has been shown to provide incremental prognostic information to the perfusion and clinical data. In general, post stress LVEF is the best predictor of cardiac death, whereas the amount of ischemia is the best predictor for nonfatal myocardial infarction [4].

Cardiac Computed Tomography (CT)

Traditionally the assessment of coronary artery stenosis has been performed using invasive coronary angiogram (ICA), a technique which provides superior temporal and spatial resolution. However, the risk of ICA is higher in the elderly population with more vascular complications, stroke, myocardial infarctions, and cardiac arrhythmias. Over the last decade, there have been dramatic advances in the performance of cardiac CT. Using state of art technology, scanners can now achieve a high spatial resolution of 0.5 mm and provide a detailed depiction of cardiac structures. In addition, with significantly improved temporal resolution, scanners can now literally "freeze" the coronary arteries to allow for accurate assessment of both the vessel lumen and arterial walls. Performance of MDCT using the intravenous administration of contrast media can noninvasively produce similar high quality angiographic images as ICA but without the potential cardiac, vascular and neurological complications (Fig. 13.1).

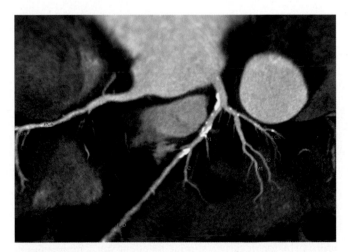

Fig. 13.1 Two dimensional global coronary CT angiogram of a 70 years patient with chest pain. The coronary artery calcium score (CACS) was 556 HU. Notice the severe calcific plaques along the distal LM, proximal and mid LAD. The assessment of luminal stenosis is especially difficult at the level of mid LAD and D2

Although relatively few studies have focused specifically on the elderly; applications of cardiac CT in this population have continued to escalate. Therefore, it is important to be familiar with the strengths and limitations of this relatively new and exciting technology.

Technique

One of the major advantages of CT is the ease with which high quality information is obtained. For optimal image quality, oral and/or IV beta blockers are administrated hours before starting the scan to achieve a heart rate of 60–65 beats per minute. Sublingual NTG is given right before imaging for coronary vasodilation. A low-energy scout film is acquired to ensure the scan volume covers the length of the heart or the structure of interest. CT is performed in inspiratory breathhold after administration of intravenous contrast agent at 4–7 mL/s via an 18-gauge catheter placed in the antecubital vein. The initiation of image acquisition can be done with either bolus tracking or the timing bolus method. The entire CT volume data set for coronary artery visualization can be acquired either in helical (patient table is continuously advanced during the gantry rotation) or step-shoot mode (table intermittently advanced). During the scan, the patient's ECG is continuously recorded. Synchronization of raw CT image data with ECG information enables the reconstruction of axial ECG-gated images. The resulting reconstructed data set is transmitted to an offline workstation where post processing is performed for final review and interpretation. The typical study duration of a 64 slice MDCT scanner is less than 10 s. Newer 320 slices scanner with larger anatomic coverage allow completion of a study within one or two heart beats. This can be very useful in the elderly patient with co-morbidities that prevent them from performing longer breath holds or remaining motionless in a supine position for long periods of time.

Indications

Stenosis detection is currently the leading indication for performing cardiac CT angiography (CTA). Numerous studies have now shown coronary CTA to be highly effective in the evaluation of CAD with an excellent diagnostic accuracy for the detection of significant coronary stenosis when compared to ICA [5]. Furthermore, the diagnostic accuracy of CTA for ruling out the presence of significant CAD has been shown to be very good and can identity patients who would not benefit from ICA [6]. Unlike ICA, coronary CTA further allows the simultaneous assessment of both the lumen and the surrounding arterial wall. It can potentially determine both the type of plaque present and indicate its risk for future plaque rupture and subsequent acute events. Cardiac CT has now extended to cardiovascular surgery patients to assess the patency of coronary artery bypass grafts, or to determine essential anatomy prior to repeat thoracic surgery. Noncoronary indications for cardiac CT include assessment of LV morphology, cardiac chambers sizes, the pericardium, VHD and intra-cardiac masses. The role of cardiac CT for these purposes is usually secondary and mostly performed only when other primary modalities such as echo or MRI cannot provide adequate information.

Limitations

There are potential limitations associated with this new technology, especially in the elderly. A major limitation of CTA is the prevalence of coronary calcification in the elderly which can limit diagnostic accuracy. Calcification causes a blooming artifact which can result in overestimation of stenosis severity and a reduction in diagnostic specificity. One approach to mitigate this would be the performance of a non contrast CT to determine the coronary artery calcium score prior to CTA. If the calcium burden is low, CTA likely will be of diagnostic quality. On the other hand, the presence of high calcium burden should allow the consideration of alternative imaging techniques. There is no well established threshold of calcification for performance of CTA, but a recent large multicenter study used a Housefield unit of 600 as a cutoff for analysis [7]. Contrast related toxicity, another major concern, is much higher in the elderly due to impaired renal function and presence of concomitant comorbidities such as diabetes or HF [8]. The 64 or larger slice scanners fortunately require much lower doses of contrast (usually less than 100 mL per study and comparable to ICA) than the older generation scanners. Finally, although the use of ionizing radiation and its potential long term cancer risk are always concerning, the absolute risk associated with use of radiation is much less in the elderly. Plus, newer imaging protocols have dramatically reduced the amount of total radiation doses that are now delivered (comparable to or lower than ICA).

Cardiac Magnetic Resonance Imaging (CMR)

Cardiac magnetic resonance (CMR) is emerging as the method of choice for the evaluation of a wide range of cardiovascular disorders. Its advancing role is related largely to a variety of hardware and software innovations which allow increasingly rapid and robust data acquisition. Today, CMR has a number of unique advantages over other imaging modalities. First, all imaging is performed without the risks of ionizing radiation and, in many instances, without contrast administration (except for myocardial viability). Second, it provides a view of the entire heart without limitations from inadequate imaging windows or body habitus and can obtain imaging data in any imaging plane prescribed by the scan operator. Next, different CMR pulse sequences enable multiple variant sets of raw data to be gathered from one region – a feature unique to CMR, which provides it with the potential to probe a vast number of biological properties with the same machine (e.g., blood perfusion, contractile function, presence of fat, thrombus, infarction, etc.). These features are also responsible for the increase in the complexity of CMR, since the operator must assess the clinical scenario, select the correct pulse sequences to apply, and then correctly set sequence parameters to achieve optimal image quality.

Indications

CMR is widely considered the gold standard method for the assessment of cardiac morphology [9]. The multifaceted nature of CMR can produce tomographic still images, like CT images, that can accurately and reproducibly assess LV or right ventricular (RV) chamber sizes, wall thickness and mass [9–11]. In addition, CMR is excellent in the evaluation of cardiac or paracardiac masses because of its ability to characterize the composition of abnormal tissue [9, 12–16]. The multifaceted nature of CMR also enables it to be used for functional assessment. Conventional gradient-recalled echo or new steady-state free-precession pulse sequences can be used to construct a cine image, which is a movie of 15–20 frames in which the full cardiac cycle can be seen; each movie frame represents approximately 30–40 ms of the cardiac cycle. These cine images can be acquired in a 5–8 s breath-hold. Newer sequences allow even faster image acquisition, such as three slices in one breath-hold. Figure 13.2 is an example of a complete series of short-axis views throughout the left and right ventricles for the assessment of ventricular function using the steady-state free-precession technique. The high spatial resolution and strong contrast between the myocardium and cavity blood make planimetry of the interface accurate and easily reproducible for assessment of LV and RV function in normal and HF patients [11, 17–21].

CMR can be employed as a noninvasive stress-testing method for the detection and assessment of coronary artery disease. It can be used to assess both inducible wall motion abnormalities (analogous to dobutamine echocardiography) and perfusion reserve (similar to adenosine single photon emission CT). In addition to evaluating the first-pass transit of gadolinium contrast, images can be obtained 10–15 min later, in a pseudoequilibrium phase. In these images, which

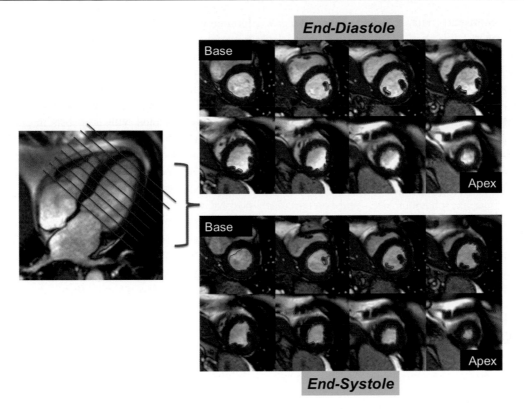

Fig. 13.2 Typical study of ventricular function by CMR. From a 4 chamber long axis view, serial short axis cine images are acquired every 1 cm from base to apex of heart. The left ventricular (LV) endocardial contours are planimetered in both end-diastole and end-systole summed to calculate LV end diastolic volume (LVEDV) and LV end systolic volume (LVESV). The difference between LVEDV and LVESV represents the LV stroke volume. LV ejection fraction (%) can be calculated by dividing the LV stroke volume by the LVEDV and multiplying by 100. The same can be performed for the right ventricle (RV) to ascertain RV end diastolic volume, RV end systolic volume, RV stroke volume, and RV ejection fraction [123]

are usually obtained with a gradient-recalled echo imaging engine and an inversion prepulse modifier, the gadolinium enhancement patterns reflect physiologic processes other than perfusion. This technique, named delayed-enhancement CMR, is useful in the identification of nonviable myocardium, such as where there is acute necrosis or collagenous scarring, which are seen as hyperenhanced or "bright" regions on the images. Delayed-enhancement CMR was first described only 10 years ago [22], but there is already an abundance of validation data in animal models which demonstrate that this method can enable differentiation between reversible and irreversible myocardial injury [22–24]. In addition, evidence of the clinical utility of delayed-enhancement CMR is increasing in both acute and chronic ischemic syndromes [25, 26]. The high spatial resolution provided by delayed-enhancement CMR, along with its ability to directly image both viable and nonviable myocardium [14], make it useful for detecting acute and chronic myocardial infarction and for differentiating ischemic from nonischemic myocardial disorders.

Ischemic Heart Disease

Ischemic Heart Disease Introduction

IHD rises in prevalence and severity with increasing age. Studies employing stress testing or coronary angiography have repeatedly demonstrated age related increases in provocable ischemia, triple vessel and left main disease. Those elderly who present with myocardial infarctions have greater complications, including congestive HF, mitral insufficiency, cardiogenic shock, cardiac rupture, and cardiac death. Despite its prevalence, management of CAD is a continuing challenge in today's burgeoning elderly population as the elderly are commonly undiagnosed or misdiagnosed, presenting with atypical symptoms. Currently, several therapeutic options are available for IHD including medical therapy, percutaneous or surgical revascularization procedures.

Cardiac imaging offers the opportunity to comprehensively evaluate symptomatic or asymptomatic patients with suspected or documented IHD. Cardiac imaging offers needed information to help arrive at the optimal therapy for a patient. First, noninvasive stress testing techniques have been extensively validated for diagnostic accuracy of CAD detection. Although ICA continues to be the accepted gold standard, stress imaging has excellent sensitivities and specificities for the detection of significant disease. Selection of a particular testing modality is frequently based on local expertise, available technology and concomitant patient co-morbidities. Second, imaging parameters are widely used for risk stratification and assessment of long term prognosis. Measurements of cardiac chamber sizes and biventricular ejection fractions, presence of LV hypertrophy, wall motion abnormalities, extent of ischemia, severity of mitral regurgitation, and diastolic function have been found to impact long term survival and therefore clinical decision making. Finally, cardiac imaging techniques provide valuable information on the presence of ischemia and myocardial viability, thereby guiding the appropriate use of aggressive percutaneous or surgical therapies.

Echocardiography

Resting echocardiography is a powerful tool for assessing patients with IHD. It provides valuable information concerning ejection fraction, regional LV wall motion abnormalities, and cardiac morphology including chamber sizes and LV hypertrophy, and RV function. Doppler techniques allow for the assessment of any concomitant valvular abnormalities, intra-cardiac filling pressures and pulmonary artery pressures. In patients with post acute myocardial infarction (AMI), secondary complications can readily be assessed such as LV aneurysms, cardiac thrombi, intra-cardiac shunts and cardiac rupture with resultant pseudo aneurysm (Fig. 13.3).

Several traditional echo parameters have been shown to be closely associated with prognosis in patients with IHD. Elderly patients with LV hypertrophy are at increased risk for both cardiac events such as CHF, unstable angina, arrhythmias, and neurological events such as stroke. Reductions in LV ejection fraction or elevations in LV end systolic volume post MI correlate with increases in mortality [27, 28]. Wall motion score index, reflecting the magnitude of myocardial damage, has been shown to independently predict death or CHF hospitalization [29]. The incidence of mitral regurgitation is high among patients with IHD, and has also been shown to be an independent predictor of cardiovascular mortality and CHF hospitalizations [30]. Finally, diastolic dysfunction, as evidenced by a restrictive filling pattern or enlarged left atrium volumes, has been shown to predict late HF and survival [31]. The increasing use of 3D Echo has provided superior information on LV volumes, LVEF and LV sphericity indices over the recent years, and may predict LV remodeling [32].

Stress echocardiography provides opportunity for risk stratification and the assessment of viability in patients with IHD. Stress echo, is clinically indicated for the detection of CAD and risk assessment in patients with or without chest pain, for risk stratification of patients post ACS or post revascularization, as part of a preoperative evaluation prior to noncardiac surgery, and myocardial viability assessment.

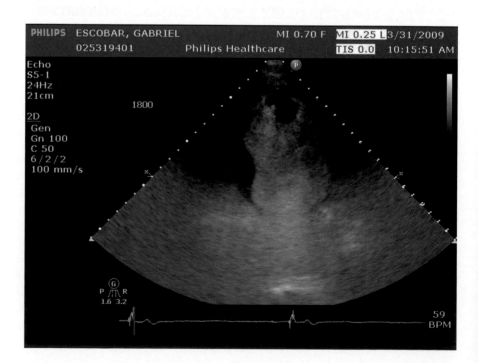

Fig. 13.3 Apical thrombus visualized with intravenous contrast by TTE in a patient with an akinetic apex post LAD infarct

The technique allows assessment of baseline cardiac function and direct evaluation of inducible myocardial ischemia by detecting new or worsening wall motion abnormalities with stress (Fig. 13.4). Studies have shown stress echocardiography to have a similar sensitivity to myocardial perfusion scintigraphy but a higher specificity for the detection of disease [33]. Prognostic parameters of importance in predicting long-term cardiac events in a heterogeneous population are resting LV function, myocardial viability, stress-induced ischemia, vascular extent of wall motion abnormalities, and changes in end-systolic volume and ejection fraction with stress. Patients with normal stress echocardiography have a very low cardiac event rate (0.9%) [34]. Those with increasing abnormalities such as changes in wall motion score index, LV end-systolic volume, and ejection fraction are at increasingly higher risk for death and myocardial infarction and coronary angiography, and subsequent myocardial revascularization may be justified in these patients [35]. In patients with chronic IHD, dobutamine stress echo has a major role in detecting myocardial ischemia and residual viable myocardial tissue. Patients with a substantial amount of dysfunctional but viable or ischemic myocardium have been shown to have a high likelihood of improved function, less adverse remodeling and a better prognosis after subsequent myocardial revascularization [36]. Thus, identifying patients who are high risk for cardiac events allows the appropriate use of invasive procedures for those most likely to benefit.

Recently, myocardial contrast echocardiography (CE) has been used to assess myocardial perfusion and microvascular integrity as indicators of myocardial viability. The extent and severity of perfusion defects have been shown to correlate with perfusion defect size by SPECT imaging LV EF's and the likelihood of functional recovery at follow-up. Large perfusion defects (indicating nonviable tissue) have lower ejection fractions and a low likelihood of regional or global functional recovery over time after acute MI, with an increased risk for the development of adverse LV remodeling [37, 38]. On the other hand, dysfunctional regions with preserved

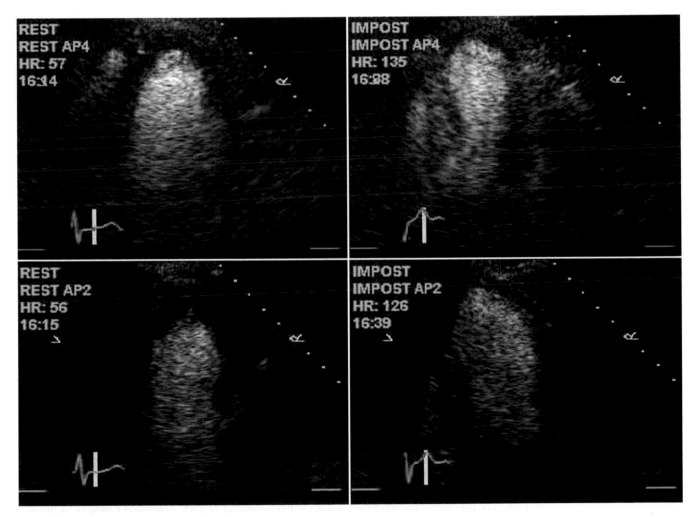

Fig. 13.4 Stress echo demonstrating failure to augment EF with exercise and stress induced wall motion abnormality in the anterior and anteroseptal walls. A proximal LAD lesion was found with invasive angiography

the magnitude of preserved tissue viability. Compared to dobutamine echocardiography, nuclear techniques tend to have a higher sensitivity but lower specificity for prediction of recovery of regional contractile function [51].

Detecting preserved myocardial viability in patients with CAD and significant LV dysfunction using noninvasive imaging techniques prognosticates a patient population at substantial risk of death. This risk has been shown to be significantly reduced by successful revascularization. A recent meta-analysis demonstrated improved survival in individuals with viable myocardium who undergo revascularization as opposed to continued medical therapy [52]. The highest mortality rates were noted in viable patients receiving medical therapy. There was no apparent outcome benefit of revascularization in the absence of demonstrated viability, with a trend toward higher mortality with revascularization. The magnitude of the potential reduction in mortality increased as the severity of LV dysfunction increased. In general, no significant differences exist between nuclear techniques in predicting prognostic benefit with revascularization. A randomized trial comparing viability as demonstrated by FDG PET or Tc-99m sestamibi SPECT showed equivalence by demonstrating no difference between the groups in the proportion of patients sent for revascularization or in 2-year event-free survival [53].

Multislice Computed Tomography and Magnetic Resonance Imaging

Cardiac CT is increasingly used to detect IHD by noninvasively visualizing the coronary arteries with high resolution. The technique allows the direct anatomic assessment of the coronary arteries vessel lumen and arterial wall) rather than relying on their functional consequences. A recent multicenter trial demonstrated on a per-patient basis showed an outstanding sensitivity (95%) and specificity (83%) for the detection of coronary stenosis >50% by invasive angiography in patients with chest pain [54] (Fig. 13.7). Most important, investigations performed with current generations of multidetector CT scanners have consistently reported high negative predictive values that approach 100%. This allows reliable exclusion of significant coronary artery stenosis following a normal or near-normal noninvasive coronary CT angiogram effectively obviating further testing and predicting excellent prognosis [55] (Fig. 13.8). Other useful applications of cardiac CT in IHD are to assess cardiac morphology, LV volumes and ejection fraction, segmental wall motion, patency of coronary artery bypass grafts and coronary stents, LV aneurysms, intracardiac thrombi, and arterial mapping prior to repeat cardiac surgical revascularization. Newer applications include stress MPI for ischemia detection and delayed

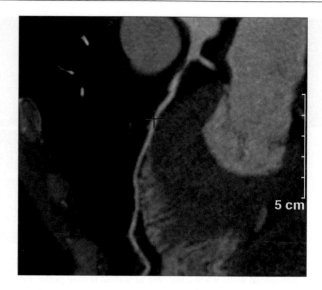

Fig. 13.7 A 70–90% noncalcified stenosis in the proximal LAD detected by cardiac CT in an acute chest pain patient. Invasive angiography demonstrated an 80% stenosis with successful PCI

enhancement imaging for nonviable myocardium. Significant drawbacks to the elderly with Cardiac CT are the use of iodinated contrast dye in those with renal insufficiency and radiation exposure. These are being increasingly addressed with newer generation scanners and imaging protocols. Other limitations include limited lumen visualization in densely calcified or stented segments due to blooming artifact, evaluation of small caliber vessels, excessive image noise in obese patients, and motion artifact from patients unable to remain motionless or perform the 10–15 s breath hold.

Cardiac MR is powerful imaging technique which may provide a comprehensive evaluation of IHD. Apart from providing valuable information on cardiac morphology and regional and global systolic function, its usefulness is further demonstrated by its ability to both detect ischemia and also assess the size and severity of myocardial infarction. Detection of obstructive CAD is best performed by assessing myocardial perfusion reserve with adenosine stress perfusion CMR combined with delayed enhancement imaging. The technique visualizes myocardial hypoperfusion by evaluating the initial first-pass transit of gadolinium through the LV myocardium during vasodilation, and detects myocardial infarction with late gadolinium hyperenhancement. The diagnostic performance has been impressive with a sensitivity of 89% and specificity of 87% for the diagnosis of CAD, with coronary stenosis greater than 70% or left main disease greater than 50% [56] (Fig. 13.9). CMR imaging recently has shown robust prognostication for patients who present with symptoms of ischemia. Patients with neither a reversible perfusion defect nor delayed enhancement have a 98.1% negative annual event rate for death or MI [57]. Contrast enhanced CMR also generates a complete assessment of

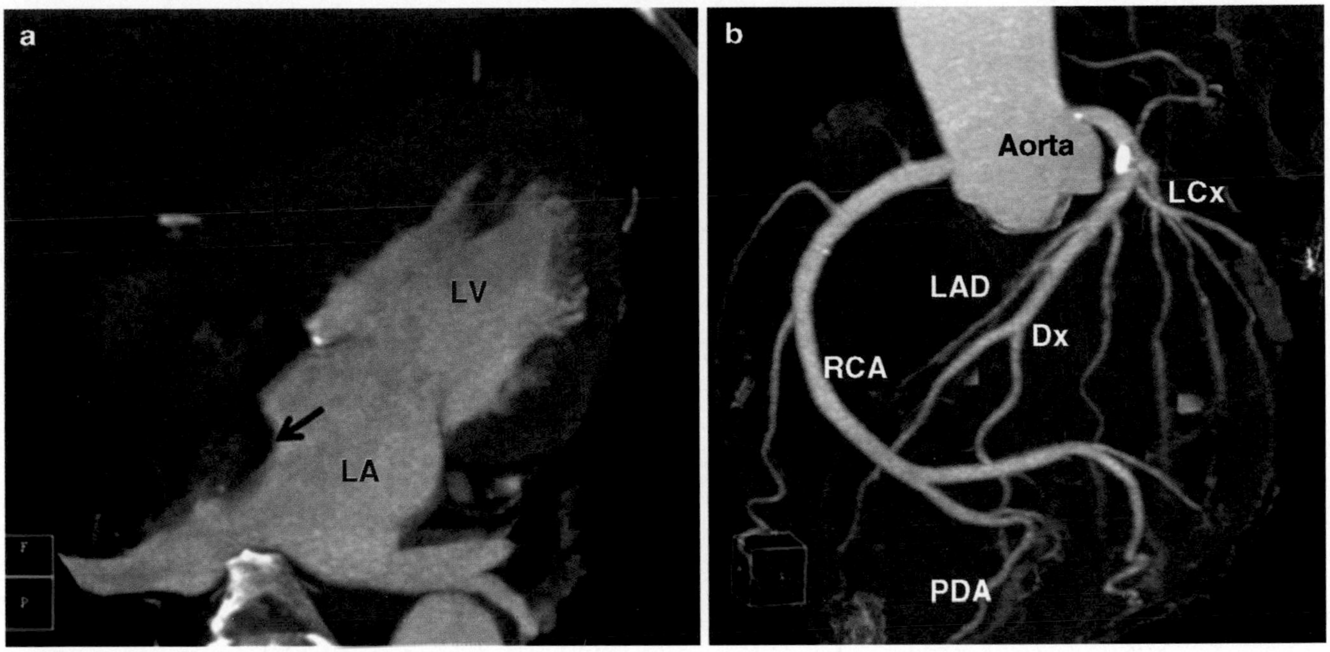

Fig. 13.8 (**a**) Cardiac MDCT of a 68 years woman with chest pain and left atrial myxoma (*arrow*) located in the interatrial septum. (**b**) Pre operative coronary CTA showed non obstructive calcific plaque in the distal LM. Invasive angiogram was avoided

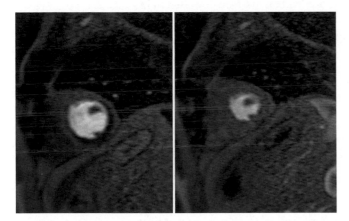

Fig. 13.9 Stress induced perfusion abnormality in the anterior and anteroseptal walls with adenosine stress MRI and first pass perfusion imaging

myocardial viability. With infarction, gadolinium concentrates in the region of the collagenous. The transmural extent of delayed gadolinium enhancement in patients with acute or chronic CAD predicts the improvement in contractile function after coronary revascularization. The likelihood of improvement in regional contractility after revascularization of dysfunctional myocardium decreases progressively as the transmural extent of hyperenhancement before revascularization increases [58]. Further adding contractile reserve assessment with low dose dobutamine, as is performed with echo, has been shown to be additive to the predictive value of late gadolinium hyperenhancement in predicting recovery of

LV function [59]. The importance of identifying viable myocardium is evident from studies that have demonstrated improved survival with revascularization compared to continued medical therapy in patients with viable but dysfunctional myocardium [52]. Finally, CMR has potential uses in the post MI setting other than infarct detection including evaluation of microvascular obstruction, myocardial edema, and thrombus formation (Fig. 13.10).

Congestive Heart Failure

With more than 1 million annual hospital admissions and the leading Medicare billing code, the syndrome of HF is all too prevalent in today's medical landscape [60]. Ever since the CASS trial first demonstrated the benefits of coronary revascularization in ischemic cardiomyopathy, today's cardiac surgeon is frequently operating on patients with reduced ejection fractions [61]. This is likely to increase further given our aging population, more patients surviving myocardial infarctions, and increased patient loads on cardiac transplant lists.

Cardiac imaging has become indispensable for the evaluation of HF and for guiding clinical decision-making. Important clinical information gathered to determine prognosis and guide appropriate medical, device or surgical management include detection and confirmation (systolic or diastolic HF), mechanism of HF (ischemic, valvular, pericardial, infiltrative, other), severity (ejection fraction, morphology, determination

Fig. 13.10 Large apical aneurysm demonstrating transmural infarction on delayed hyperenhancement and evidence of mural thrombus

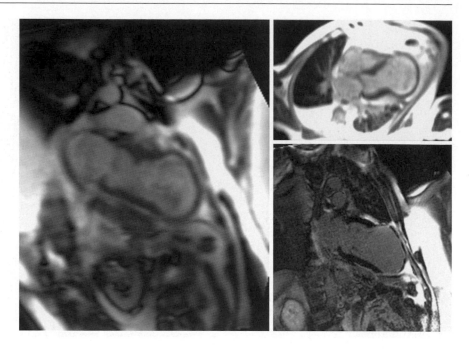

of filling pressures), and concomitant complications (left ventricular hypertroph [LVH], pulmonary hypertension, mitral insufficiency, RV function) [62]. Both inexpensive and ready availability, echocardiography is the generally the most useful initial test for clinical assessment. Apart from evaluating morphology, cardiac function, and presence of valvular disease, it uniquely evaluates diastolic function and provides estimates of intra-cardiac filling pressures. Echo results frequently tailor the use of other imaging procedures to address specific questions. A comprehensive CMR examination takes advantage of varied imaging sequences to help identify and evaluate the underlying etiology of HF by determining cardiac chamber morphology and biventricular function, quantitating volumes, assessing the severity of valvular stenosis and regurgitant insufficiency, and acquiring late gadolinium enhanced images for fibrosis detection [63]. Gadolinium late-enhancement CMR further provides the opportunity to predict functional recovery with revascularization by accurately identifying viable myocardium (ischemic or hibernating) from infarcted or fibrosed myocardium. When evaluating for the presence of IHD in HF, nuclear MPI techniques can identify stress-induced reduction of coronary flow reserve, whereas cardiac CT provides the ability to noninvasively perform accurate coronary angiography.

Assessment of LV Systolic Function

The assessment of LV systolic function, by determining the ejection fraction (LVEF), in patients with HF is essentially due to its significant therapeutic implications. The so called

diastolic CHF or HF with HF with normal EF (HFNEF) is much more prevalent in the elderly, and therapy differs from those with depressed LV function. Virtually all imaging modalities can assess the LV function and dimension, but echo is usually the first test of choice followed by CMR.

Etiology of Systolic Heart Failure

After assessment of LV systolic function by echo, an underlying etiology is generally sought. CAD is the number one cause of depressed LV function accounting for approximately ¾ of cases and determination of coronary anatomy is often mandatory. Patient with CAD and ischemia can present with HF without concomitant angina. Both nuclear imaging using SPECT or PET or stress echo provide indirect evidence of the underlying etiology. The presence of significant reversible/fixed perfusion defect on nuclear stress testing or resting/induced wall motion abnormality on stress echo are markers of CAD. On the other hand, more homogenous tracer uptake or wall motion at rest and with stress usually point to a nonischemic etiology. Although invasive angiography remains the gold standard for establishing ischemic vs. non ischemic etiology of CHF, non invasive coronary CTA with MDCT has been shown to be very useful as well. The absence of significant stenosis with coronary CTA essentially rules out CAD as the cause of depressed LV function [64].

After exclusion of CAD as the cause of CHF, other non ischemic etiologies of HF can be readily assessed with imaging. Presence of hypertension is readily available by history, but echo and MRI can provide the degree of LV hypertrophy

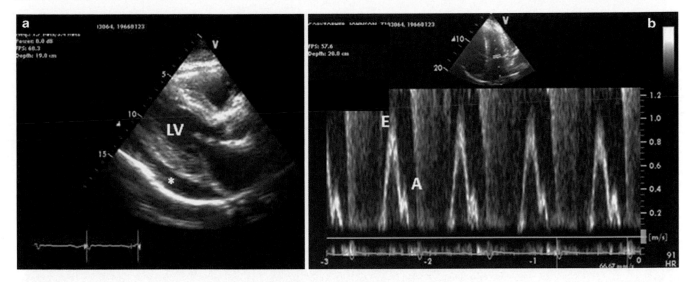

Fig. 13.11 (**a**) Echo images of a patient with cardiac amyloidosis. Noted the biventricular hypertrophy with pericardial effusion. (**b**) Restrictive pattern on mitral inflow

and remodeling. The presence of VHD can be readily evaluated by echo or MRI. Infiltrate cardiomyopathy and pericardial disease are best assessed with combination of echo and cardiac MR or CT (Fig. 13.11).

Nuclear and ECHO for Viability

It is well known that patients with chronic LV dysfunction secondary to CAD often improve their EF after restoration of blood supply, namely the concept of myocardial viability. After determination of coronary anatomy and the presence or absence of ischemia, the evaluation of myocardial viability is essential for prognosis and guiding the need for revascularization vs. continued medical therapy. This information is crucial especially in the elderly as surgical risk increases significantly with age. Pooled observational studies suggest the benefits of revascularization on cardiac outcomes are significantly greater in the presence of ischemia and myocardial viability [51].

Both stress nuclear imaging using SPECT or PET and dobutamine stress echo not only can determine presence of ischemia, but they can also provide information on viability. The diagnosis of myocardial viability with nuclear technique requires myocardial cells with intact cell membranes, (Thallium-201 SPECT imaging), mitochondria (Tc-99m sestamibi or tetrofosmin SPECT imaging), or preserved metabolism (PET with F-18 deoxyglucose) to take up different radioisotope tracers. In general, with stress Thallium-201 or Tc-99m imaging, presence of inducible ischemia (reversible defect) implies a high likelihood for functional improvement

whereas fixed defects of only mild-to-moderate severity using quantitative methods have only an intermediate chance of functional recovery (Fig. 13.12). Nitrate administration has been shown to improve detection of viable myocardium. With PET, evidence of enhanced FDG uptake in segments of decreased blood flow (known as a "mismatch") predicts a high probability of functional improvement following revascularization. For assessment with echo, there should be enough viable cells to respond to inotropic stimulation (contractile reserve assessed by dobutamine echo or MRI) or the presence of microvascular integrity (myocardial CE). With low dose dobutamine infusion, dysfunctional segments with enough viable cells improve in contractility. Similar to radionuclide imaging, the presence of inducible ischemia or a biphasic response with stress echo (improvement of contractility with low dose dobutamine but worsening at higher doses) implies a high likelihood for functional improvement [65].

Clinical studies have shown that the presence of viability by either nuclear imaging or stress echo is an important predictor of probability and magnitude for the regional /global function and symptom improvement after revascularization. Overall, the nuclear technique is more sensitive or has a higher negative predictive value, whereas contractile reserve assessment (dobutamine echo) is more specific or has a higher positive predictive value in predicting recovery [66]. This is probably due to a contractile response to dobutamine which might require greater than 50% viable myocardial cells in a given segment. In comparison, radionuclide MPI can identify segments with fewer viable myocytes and is, therefore, more sensitive among segments with 25–50% viable myocardium [67]. Use of quantitation with radionuclide MPI improves the prediction of viability. A segment with higher counts

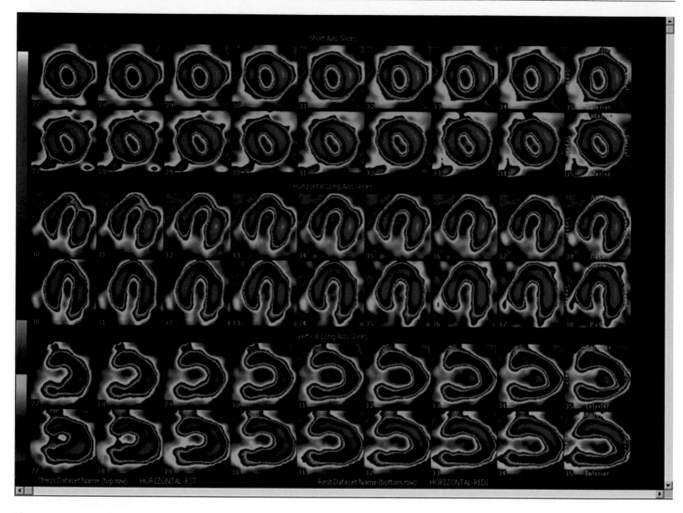

Fig. 13.12 Resting Thallium (*top*) and 4 h redistribution (*bottom*) of the same patient from Fig. 13.3 showing evidence of viability in all three coronaries distribution

is more likely to improve function after revascularization. For either technique, detection of ischemia (reversible perfusion defect or inducible wall motion abnormality) increases significantly the positive predictive value for functional recovery. Other simple negative predictor for functional recovery is an end-diastolic wall thickness ≤6 mm on resting echo.

CMR for Viability

The role of CMR in evaluation of patients with CHF is multifaceted. In patients with ischemic HF, CMR is useful in the assessment of myocardial viability, and for prediction of the likelihood of functional improvement after revascularization. This is performed utilizing a technique called Delayed-enhancement (DE-CMR) which is a relatively simple procedure that can be performed in a single brief examination, requires only a peripheral intravenous catheter, and does not require pharmacologic or physiologic stress (Fig. 13.13) 5-to

CMR Viability Procedure

TIME

- ■ Insert Peripheral IV
- ■ Place Patient In Scanner
- ■ Cine Images
- ■ Inject Gadolinium
- ■ Wait 5-10 Minutes
- ■ Delayed Enhancement Images

Fig. 13.13 Overall sequence of events for performing infarction/viability imaging. *IV* intravenous

10-min after the intravenous administration of gadolinium, delayed enhancement images encompassing the entire heart are obtained using a segmented inversion-recovery gradient echo sequence [26]. Each delayed enhancement image is acquired during an 8- to 10-s breath hold, and the imaging time for the entire examination is generally 45–60 min. Figure 13.14 demonstrates cine and DE-CMR images from a typical patient scan.

Mitral Infl

TD
Lateral A

Fig. 13.16

lateral mitr
both patient
ratio much
diastolic dy

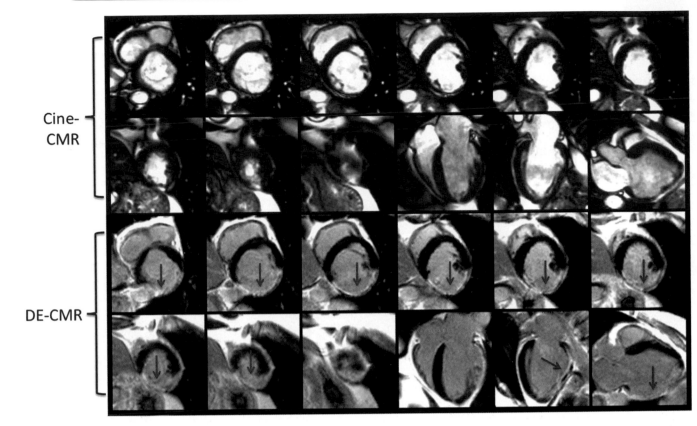

Fig. 13.14 Images from a typical patient scan. Cine and delayed-enhancement images are acquired at 6–8 short-axis locations and at two to three long-axis locations during repeated breath holds. Images are interpreted with the cine images (cine-CMR) immediately adjacent to the delayed-enhancement images (DE-CMR). In this patient example, DE-CMR demonstrates transmural myocardial infarction involving the inferior and inferolateral walls of the left ventricle (*red arrows*). Reprinted with permission from Shah and Dela Cruz [123]

Assessı

Knowled
ating be
A comp
with mi
ing or fl
invasive
can pot
catheter
Noninv
the adn
erative
Mu
early d
(*e′*) or
illary
depres
ratio <
filling

The transmural extent of infarction (TEI), as evident on DE-CMR, has been shown to be a powerful predictor of contractile response to revascularization and medical therapy. DE-CMR-evidenced TEI has been shown to predict response to myocardial revascularization in patients who have established coronary artery disease. This concept was demonstrated by Kim et al. [58], who performed cine and DE-MRI in consecutive patients who had LV dysfunction prior to surgical or percutaneous revascularization. The likelihood of functional improvement was inversely related in a progressive stepwise fashion to TEI. Among all dysfunctional segments, the proportion of segments with improved contractility decreased as TEI increased (*P*<0.001), see Fig. 13.15. When volume of dysfunctional but viable myocardium was calculated on a per-patient basis, this parameter predicted the magnitude of improvement in LV function following revascularization, as measured by mean wall motion score and ejection fraction (*P*<0.001 for both). Similarly, in a patient cohort that had more severe LV dysfunction (mean LVEF, 28±10%), Schvartzman et al. [68] demonstrated an inverse relationship (*P*<0.002) between TEI and postrevascularization functional recovery. These data demonstrate that there is a progressive relationship between the likelihood of contractile response to

revascularization and the TEI, as evidenced by DE-CMR. Thus, use of a single cutoff value on which to base predictions of functional improvement would not have a physiologic basis and would be suboptimal. The ability to grade myocardial viability as a continuum rather than in a binary fashion is one of the greatest strengths of DE-CMR, and highlights an important advantage of DE-CMR over other imaging modalities used to assess viability. Myocardial regions are not interpreted in a binary fashion as viable or nonviable; rather, the transmural extent of viable and infarcted myocardium is directly visualized. Knowledge of infarct transmurality can then be used to predict functional improvement more accurately, and can also be used to understand the underlying physiology of functional response to coronary revascularization.

Diastolic Heart Failure (DHF) or "Heart Failure with Normal Ejection Fraction" (HFNEF)

Diastolic heart failure (DHF) or "heart failure with normal ejection fraction" (HFNEF) is very common in the elderly, and is associated with increased morbidity and mortality.

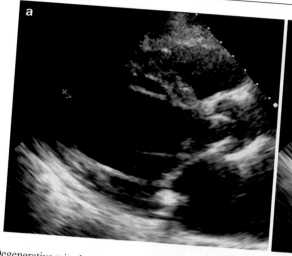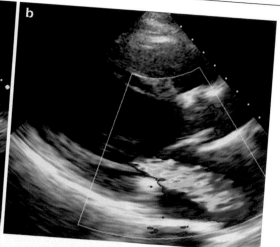

Fig. 13.21 Degenerative mitral valve disease in an 83 years old female. 2D echocardiogram demonstrates mitral annular calcification and mitral leaflet thickening (**a**). Color Doppler imaging reveals degenerative (organic) mitral regurgitation (**b**). *MAC* mitral annular calcification; *LA* left atrium; *LV* left ventricle

Fig. 13.1!
before re
after rev
segments
hypokine

Amon
or near
[69]. F
sion w
diseas
thies.
much
this i
conc
decre
poor
leng
atic

A
DH
DH
mea
dio
ech
inc
for
sui
siz

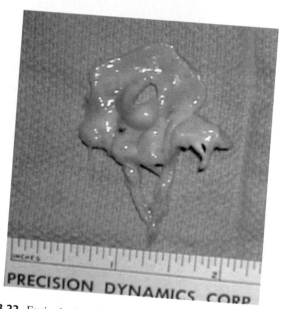

Fig. 13.22 Excised mitral leaflet in a 72 year old male with a history of bacterial endocarditis. The anterior mitral leaflet is shown and appears thickened with a large central perforation

mapping. Although the size of this color jet is proportional to regurgitant volume, care must be taken not to oversimplify the assessment of MR severity. Because the color Doppler map represents flow velocity (not flow volume), the severity of a central MR jet is easily *overestimated* by color Doppler imaging. Likewise, the severity of a very eccentric MR jet that flows along the left atrial wall is easily *underestimated* by color Doppler imaging alone. As such other Doppler imaging tools have been developed. The proximal isoveloc-ity surface area (PISA) method estimates the size of the

regurgitant valve orifice area and flow volume based on the principle of conservation of mass, such that:

$$MR \text{ regurgitant volume (cm}^3) = 2\pi r^2 \times A_{vel}/\text{peak MR velocity(cm/s)},$$

where r is the radius (cm) of the hemisphere converging toward the regurgitant mitral orifice at a defined aliasing velocity (A_{vel}) [87, 92]. This quantification method has proven useful under certain ideal flow conditions, but has limitations when employed to evaluate MR associated with thickened leaflets with irregular coaptation as is common in an elderly population. Another method looks at the width of the origin of the regurgitant color jet. Measurement of this VC zone has been validated by both 2D and 3D techniques to estimate MR severity [93–95]. In an elderly population where degen-erative valve disease is most common, the quantification of MR severity may be best achieved using a comparison of Doppler-derived stroke volumes into and out of the left ven-tricle. In the absence of significant AR, the regurgitant MR volume is equal to the mitral annular diastolic inflow volume minus the LV systolic outflow volume [96, 97]. Using these methods, MR severity can be quantified as mild, moderate, or severe when the effective regurgitant orifice area (EROA) is <0.2, 0.2–0.4 or >0.4 cm² and when the regurgitant volume is <30, 30–60 or >60 mL, respectively [87]. Additional quali-tative evidence such as systolic flow reversal within a pulmo-nary vein, increased early diastolic LV filling velocity and an enlarged left atrium all support a diagnosis of severe MR.

The typical CMR study for evaluating mitral insufficiency involves the performance of a complete set of sequential short-axis (from base to apex) and long-axis (typically standard 2-, 3-, and 4-chamber views) cine images using a steady-state free precession (SSFP) pulse sequence. In addition to providing a gold standard assessment of regional LV and RV function, this data set can be used to planimeter LV and RV volumes in end-diastole and end-systole, thus determining ventricular stroke volume and ejection fraction. All valve coaptation interfaces (A1–P1, A2–P2, and A3–P3) of the mitral valve leaflets are further interrogated with individual cine images by performing sequential long-axis cine slices through each scallop as is shown in Fig. 13.23. This provides insight into mechanism (i.e., prolapse, flail, restricted), and also aids in localization of the abnormality. This information can be crucial for gauging the likelihood of valve repairability. Congenitally abnormal valve leaflets, aberrant papillary muscles or aberrant chordal attachments (parachute mitral valve), leaflet thickening, presence and extent of calcification, leaflet redundancy and prolapse, and commissural fusion are all anatomic descriptions that have been reported by CMR [75]. The phase contrast or velocity-encoded cine CMR pulse sequence is the imaging sequence of choice in quantifying flow and calculating velocities. Protons moving along a magnetic field gradient acquire a phase shift relative to stationary spins [98]. The phase shift is directly proportional to the velocity of the moving protons in a linear gradient. Phase contrast CMR has been shown to be very accurate for assessing antegrade and retrograde flow across semilunar valves and therefore is the technique used for assessing aortic or pulmonic insufficiency [9, 75, 90] (Fig. 13.20). This technique for the mitral valve is more difficult because of significant movement of the mitral annulus during systole. For this reason, quantification of mitral insufficiency volume is obtained by subtracting the aortic forward stroke volume (antegrade flow by phase contrast CMR at the aortic root) from the total LV stroke volume calculated from planimetry of the LV end-diastolic and end-systolic contours (Fig. 13.24). This technique provides accurate calculations in the setting of isolated mitral insufficiency

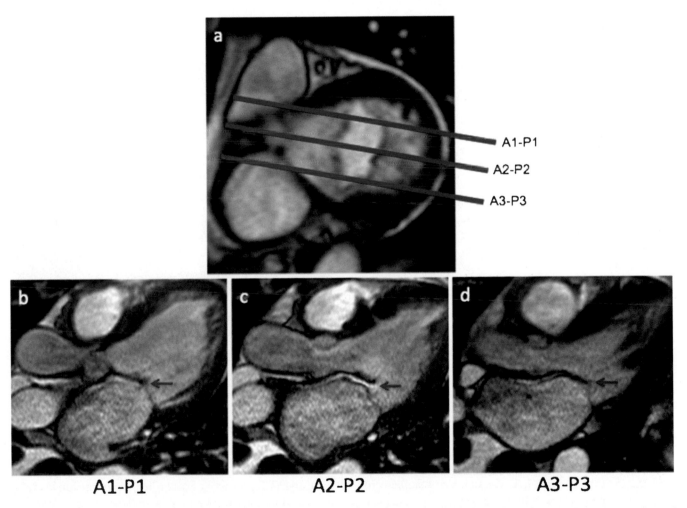

Fig. 13.23 CMR interrogation of the mitral valve. Using a cross-sectional view of the mitral valve as a reference point (**a**), serial long axis views are prescribed through the A1–P1 scallops (**b**), the A2–P2 scallops (**c**), or the A3–P3 scallops (**d**) to produce long axis cine views interrogating the individual scallops and coaptation (*arrow*) points of the mitral valve. In this example there is adequate coaptation (*arrow*) of the A1–P1 scallops (**b**) and the A3–P3 scallops (**d**), but impaired coaptation of the A2–P2 scallops demonstrating a flail P2 scallop (**c**) [123]

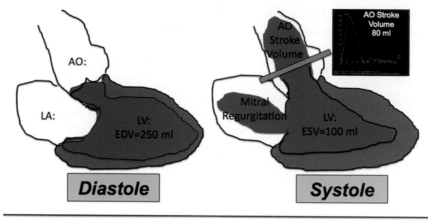

LV STROKE VOLUME (LVSV):	MR VOLUME (MRV):
LVSV = LVEDV – LVESV	MRV = LVSV – Ao Stroke Volume
LVSV = 250 ml – 100 ml	MRV = 150 ml – 80 ml
LVSV = 150 ml	**MRV = 70 ml**

Fig. 13.24 Example of the method used to calculate mitral regurgitant volume, see text for details. *AO* aorta; *LA* left atrium, *LV* left ventricle; *EDV* end diastolic volume; *ESV* end systolic volume; *MR* mitral regurgitation

and also in the setting of coexisting aortic insufficiency, since aortic insufficiency increases both the LV stroke volume *and* aortic forward flow but leaves the difference between the two values unaffected. Numerous validation studies have shown a strong correlation between CMR derived mitral insufficiency quantification and that obtained by echocardiography or cardiac catheterization; additionally regurgitant volumes derived by CMR have also been shown to have low inter-study variability [99–102]. This makes CMR an optimal technique for serial assessment of mitral insufficiency in patients who are managed expectantly.

Novel Valve Imaging Applications

Although 2D echocardiography has been the valve imaging standard for over 25 years, 3D echocardiography technologies are becoming increasing important for the identification and quantification of cardiac valve dysfunction. 3D echocardiography, and in particular live 3D TEE, has undergone significant technological refinement in recent years. Novel applications of 3D color flow have been used to quantify aortic and mitral valve regurgitation, and live 3D TEE is now commonly used to guide surgical mitral valve repair (Fig. 13.25) [95, 103–106]. It is anticipated that these volumetric imaging methods will continue to evolve and provide accurate identification and new insight into the causes of valve dysfunction as well as the development and selection of appropriate therapies for all patients, including the elderly.

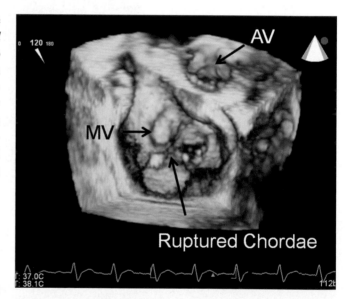

Fig. 13.25 3D Live TEE image of a mitral valve as viewed from the left atrium. In this case severe prolapse of the anterior leaflet is present because of chordae tendinae rupture. *AV* aortic valve; *MV* mitral valve

Prosthetic Valves

The structural and hemodynamic assessment by transthoracic and TEE play an essential role for post operative evaluation and long-term follow-up of prosthetic valve function. The pressure gradient across a normal prosthesis depends upon not only the type, size, and position of the prosthesis but also the flow or cardiac output of the patient. Therefore, an echo Doppler evaluation of the prosthetic valve performed in a hemodynamically stable state (usually 4–6 weeks after surgery) is strongly recommended. The information can serve as baseline reference for future comparison [107].

Patients with prosthetic valve malfunctioning usually present with symptoms of HF and hemolysis can be common as well. There is a wide range of conditions that can lead to prosthetic valve dysfunction. Degeneration of the bioprosthesis ,or the presence of a mass such as pannus, thrombus, or vegetation can interfere with normal leaflet motion resulting in obstruction or regurgitation (Figs. 13.26 and 13.27). Dehiscence of the sewing ring, or a leaflet tear often leads to significant valvular and paravalvular regurgitation or pseudoaneurysm formation (Figs. 13.28 and 13.29). The exact etiology is aided by clinical information such as the age of the valve and the adequacy of anticoagulation, and further refined by important information provided by echocardiography. Although acoustic shadowing caused by the prostheses can hamper structural assessment of the valve, the integration of comprehensive echo/Doppler assessment (chambers size, flow, pressure gradient) often provides the necessary information to determine if a valve is truly stenotic vs. a normal valve with high flow or with the presence of patient prosthesis mismatch (Fig. 13.30). The etiology of stenosis frequently requires visualization of the prosthetic leaflets to evaluate for vegetations, thrombus, pannus or

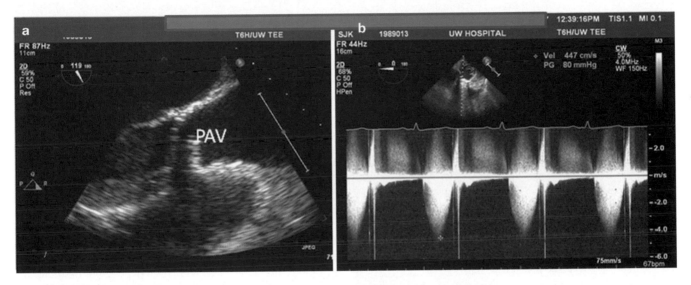

Fig. 13.26 2D TEE (**a**) and Doppler (**b**) of an obstructive aortic valve prosthesis due to pannus formation

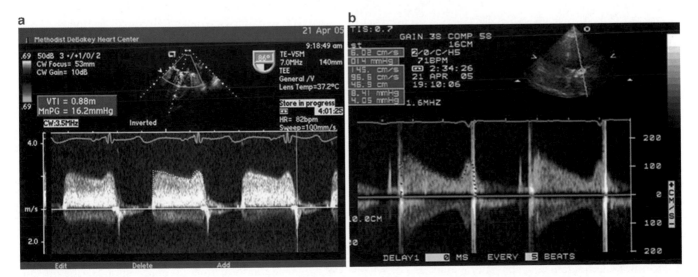

Fig. 13.27 Transmitral Doppler of an obstructive mitral prosthesis due to thrombus before (**a**) and after (**b**) administration of IV thrombolysis

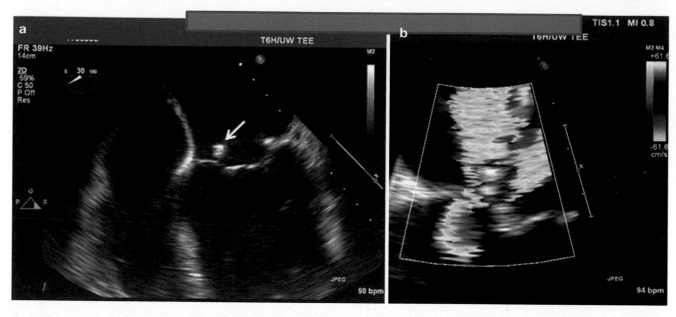

Fig. 13.28 2D TEE (**a**) and color Doppler (**b**) of a mitral valve prosthesis ring dehiscence causing severe paravalvular regurgitation

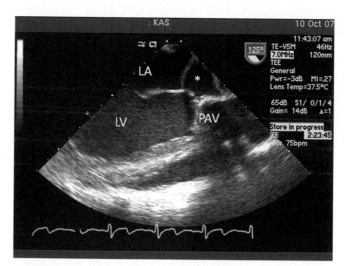

Fig. 13.29 2D TEE of a mechanical PAV complicated by large posterior pseudoaneurysm (*asterisk*) of the intervalvular fibrosa

mal-position of the prosthesis and TEE is often required to make the diagnosis (Fig. 13.31). Similarly, echo and Doppler flow assessment across the prosthesis often provides clues about the presence of prosthetic regurgitation when visualization of the regurgitation jet is hampered. TEE then can be used to confirm the presence and quantify the severity of valvular regurgitation. TEE needs to be performed when transthoracic echocardiogram is technically suboptimal or when suspicious findings on transthoracic echocardiogram are

present. This is especially true during postoperative period in the ICU which the TTE windows are often limited. In general, information obtained by both TTE and TEE are complementary and should frequently be performed together.

In patients with prosthetic valve thrombosis, quantitation of thrombus burden with TEE can help risk-stratify patients undergoing thrombolysis. In an international registry, thrombus area by TEE was an independent predictor of embolization and death. TEE can identify low or high risk groups for thrombolysis irrespective of symptom severity and can guide the medical or surgical management of prosthetic valve thrombosis [108].

MDCT may provide potential benefit in the accurate anatomic assessment of a dysfunctional prosthetic valve (Fig. 13.32). It is probably more useful in assessment of a prosthetic aortic valve due to the limitations of acoustic shadowing with TEE. Cardiac CT has excellent spatial resolution for visualization of all components of the prosthesis and potentially the presence of a thrombus or large vegetation [109]. In addition, like CMR, the ability to assess the surrounding cardiac structures is essential for detecting complications such as abscesses, false aneurysms or fistulas (Fig. 13.33). This is impossible with diagnostic fluoroscopy. Furthermore, the standard cardiac CT protocol allows simultaneous assessment of coronary artery anatomy, which is important for any anticipated surgical management. Therefore, cardiac CT assessment can provide supplemental diagnostic information to guide surgical therapeutic decisions.

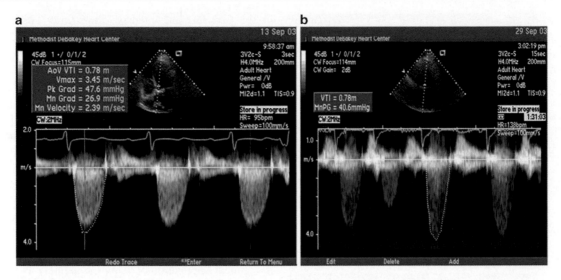

Fig. 13.30 Patient prosthesis mismatch: noted similar gradient across the aortic valve before (**a**) and after (**b**) a mechanical AV replacement due to aortic stenosis

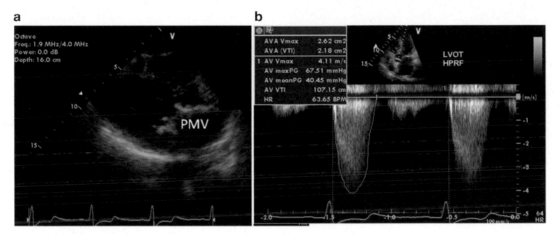

Fig. 13.31 2D echo (**a**) and color Doppler (**b**) of a mitral valve bioprosthesis causing severe LVOT obstruction. Patient presented with exertional syncope

Post Operative Cardiac Imaging

Cardiac surgery and cardiopulmonary bypass result in significant systemic inflammatory reactions which may potentially result in significant physiological changes and end organ dysfunction. Postoperative hemodynamic instability should prompt immediate evaluation, as mechanical complications causing cardiac dysfunction, in particular, have been associated with an increased risk of death and require prompt attention [110]. Along with routine invasive post op hemodynamic monitoring, echocardiography has proven to be indispensable in assessing patients after cardiovascular surgery. Due to its portability, it is routinely used in the ICU for assessing early postoperative cardiac complications, such as occlusion of a coronary artery graft, residual or unexpected valvular disease, prosthetic valve dysfunction, cardiac tamponade, and systolic

anterior motion of the mitral valve with LV outflow tract obstruction [111]. Other imaging modalities are usually non practical due to the frequent presence of renal impairment or supportive devices connected to the patient. Both TTE and TEE are useful in determining left and RV function, wall motion abnormalities, degree of native or prosthetic valve stenosis or incompetence, filling pressures, and for evaluating pericardial effusions. Echocardiography should be performed in all patients with unexplained impairments in cardiac function or hemodynamics following cardiac surgery.

The role of advanced cardiac imaging with CMR or CCT in imaging of the immediate post operative patient is relatively limited since the environment is not ideal for patients with hemodynamic instability, multiple indwelling drainage catheters and temporary pacing wires. However, outside of the immediate post operative window, cardiac CT allows for

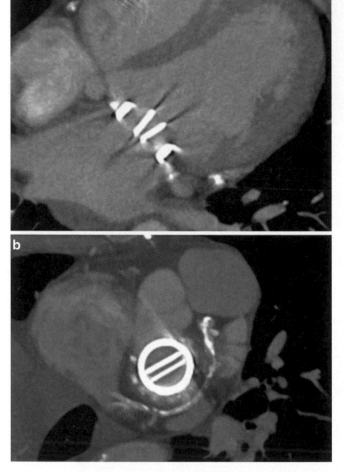

Fig. 13.32 MDCT of a normal functioning mitral mechanical prosthesis. (**a**) Long axis (**b**) short axis

the anatomical assessment of the pericardium, stenosis detection within coronary artery bypass grafts or at graft anastomotic sites, and anatomical mapping prior to a redo sternotomy. CMR, like echo, also allows the opportunity to assess the effects of surgery on various cardiac chambers sizes and their functions, prosthetic valves integrity, the volumetric quantification of paravalvular regurgitation, and pericardial processes such as effusions or constriction (pericardial thickness greater than 4 mm). CMR is safe for all commercially available prosthetic heart valves.

Postoperative LV Function

Assessment of LV function is the most common indication for a postoperative echo in clinically unstable patients with hemodynamic comprise or arrhythmias. However, the assessment of cardiac function using TTE can be quite difficult

in the CV surgical intensive care unit. The presence of bandages, instrumentation and difficulty in positioning the patient make accurate evaluation quite challenging. Before the advent of IV contrast agents, additional semi-invasive procedures such as TEE were often required.

CE using intravenous microbubbles significantly improves endocardial visualization (Fig. 13.34). It has been shown to be accurate, safe, and cost-effective as compared to TEE for evaluating ventricular function in technically difficult studies [112]. Importantly, it also guides patient management by avoiding additional diagnostic procedures and altering drug management in a third of patients. The impact of contrast on management is greater with worsening quality of the nonenhanced study, the highest impact being in intensive care unit patients. Although not formally tested in the elderly, the clinical implication of using CE is likely also to be large, since any unnecessary diagnostic or drug intervention could lead to more complications and worse outcomes in the elderly after CV surgical procedure [113].

Pericardial Effusion and Cardiac Tamponade

Assessment of pericardial effusion and cardiac tamponade is the other common indication for echo in clinically unstable patients after cardiac surgery. Pericardial effusion is a common complication after cardiac surgery occurring in over half of patients. Most of time the effusion does not cause hemodynamic compromise; however, in 0.8–6% of cases the effusion causes cardiac tampondé and can be life threatening [114] (Fig. 13.35). The traditional 2D echocardiographic features of tamponade include large circumferential effusion, RV diastolic collapse, right atrial systolic collapse and an enlarged, plethoric inferior vena cava. Due to pericardial space constraints and ventricular interdependence, there is also exaggerated respiratory variation across the trans-mitral and trans-tricuspid inflows on Doppler examination (Fig. 13.36). Usually these features are present when the effusion is not loculated and there is no pulmonary hypertension or significant left or RV abnormality. Unfortunately, this is frequently not the case in elderly patients after CV surgery in which there often is cardiac dysfunction or the presence of relatively small, loculated effusions which can cause localized increases in intra-pericardial pressure. The detection of these localized effusions by TTE might be difficult due to limited imaging windows. The classical clinical features of pulsus paradoxus and the echocardiographic features of tamponade could be absent in hemodynamically significant effusions in these patients, especially occurring early following cardiac surgery (<72 h). Therefore, if clinical suspicion is high, the diagnosis of tamponade needs to be confirmed with TEE or sometimes with surgical re-exploration. On the other hand, classical

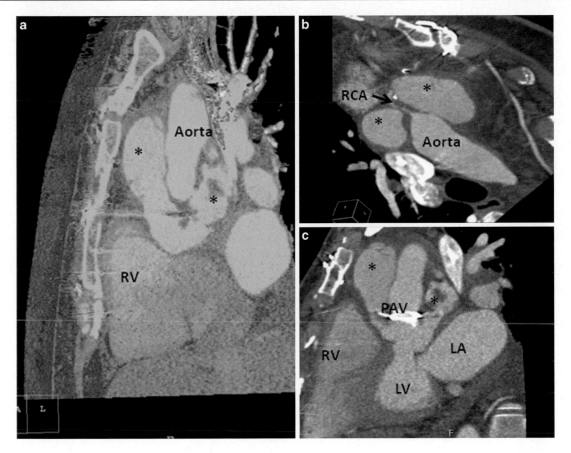

Fig. 13.33 MDCT of a patient undergoing re do AVR for endocarditis of a mechanical PAV complicated by large pseudoaneurysm (*asterisk*). Noted the large pseudoaneurysm surrounded the aortic root circumferentially and extended anteriorly right underneath the sternum (**a**, **c**). In addition, the right coronary artery coursed in the between the pseudoaneurysm (**b**)

clinical and echocardiographic features of tamponade will be usually be present with TTE when tamponade occurs late after cardiac surgery (>72 h) [115]. Cardiac CT also allows reliable examination of the pericardium and could be used to localize loculated effusions in patients without adequate imaging windows and contraindications to TEE.

Pericardial Constriction

Despite an open pericardium, pericardial constriction is an important etiology to consider in patient presenting with HF symptoms after cardiac surgery. Up to a third of cases of constrictive pericarditis occur after cardiac surgery [116]. Echo/Doppler evaluation is crucial in establishing the presence of constrictive physiology. The 2D findings include increased pericardial thickness, abnormal septal bounce, bi-atrial enlargement and dilated or plethoric inferior vena cava and hepatic veins [117]. The Doppler findings reflect ventricular interaction and the dissociation of intracardiac and intrathoracic pressures. It includes elevated early diastolic filling velocity across the right and LV inflow and a prominent E on tissue Doppler. In addition, there are greater respiratory variations with decrease of mitral inflow velocity over 25% and increase on tricuspid velocity in the first cardiac cycle after inspiration. During expiration, the hepatic vein flow reversal increases [118]. However, TTE is neither sensitive nor specific for the evaluation of pericardial thickness. Although TEE could be used to measure the pericardial thickness, the anatomic evaluation of the diseased pericardium usually requires further assessment with high definition images obtained by either cardiac CT or MRI. The advantage of MDCT over echo in the imaging of constrictive pericarditis is based on the ability to rapidly acquire two and three-dimensional reconstruction images. It allows accurate measurement of pericardial thickness, mapping of calcium and its relationship with adjacent structures such as coronaries for surgical planning purposes (Fig. 13.37). Furthermore, contrast administration is not needed to image the pericardium making it an attractive technique in elderly patients. Additionally, CMR can also be useful in establishing the diagnosis of pericardial constriction in the appropriate clinical setting: a pericardial thickness greater than 4 mm on conventional spin echo imaging has been shown to be highly specific for constriction [119] (Fig. 13.38). However, the

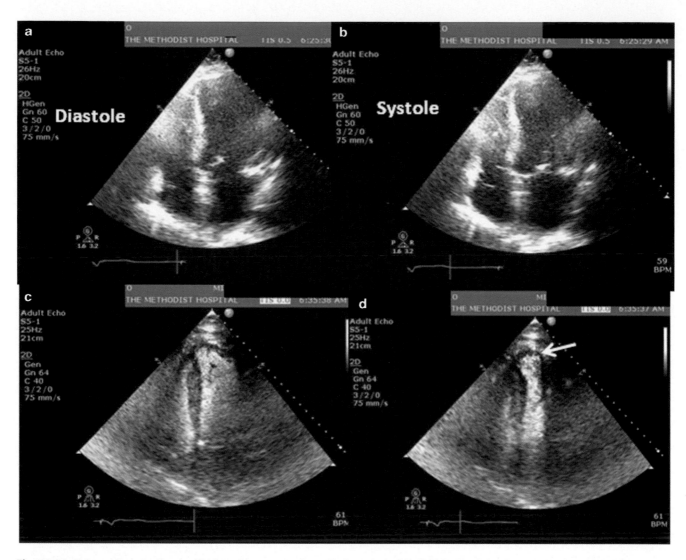

Fig. 13.34 Echo without (*top*) and with (*bottom*) contrast of an elderly patient after CABG. Noted the improved endocardial definition with contrast that allowed detection of apical dyskinesis (*arrow*). (**a**) echo without contrast, diastole; (**b**) echo without contrast, systole; (**c**) echo with contrast, diastole; (**d**) echo with contrast, systole

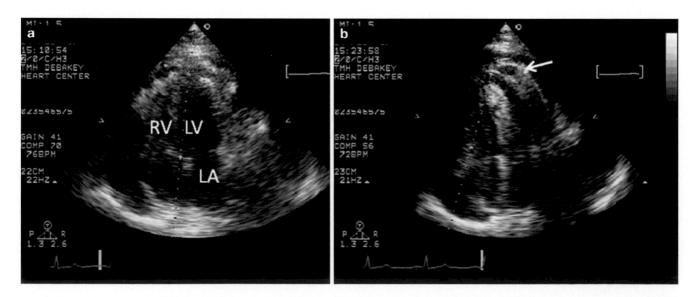

Fig. 13.35 Post CABG echo without (**a**) and with contrast (**b**) of a patient with tamponade. Noted presence of IV contrast in the pericardium (*arrow*) suggestive of myocardial perforation

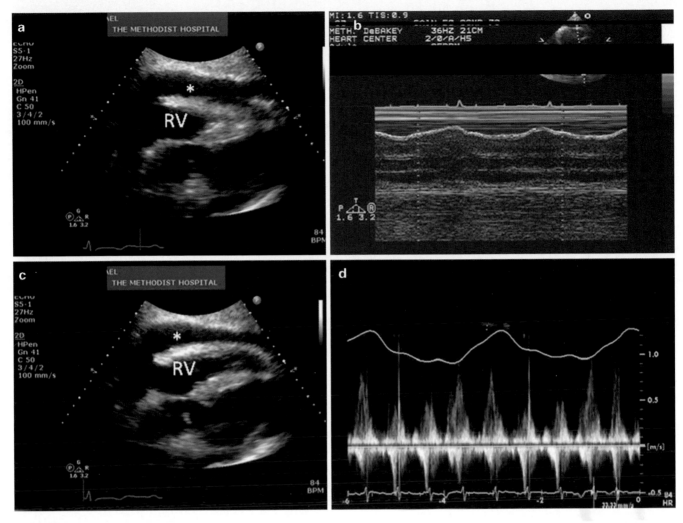

Fig. 13.36 Cardiac tamponade: RV collapse by 2D echo ((**a**) mid diastole and (**b**) end diastole) and M mode (**c**) with significant respiratory variation across the tricuspid inflow (**d**)

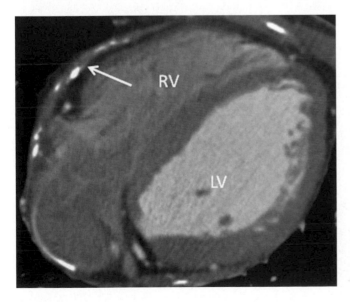

Fig. 13.37 MDCT of a thickened and calcified pericardium

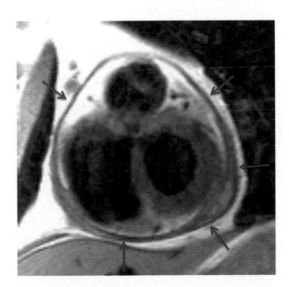

Fig. 13.38 Pericardial constriction. Diffuse thickening of the pericardium (*arrows*) to greater than 4 mm on spin echo CMR imaging. This finding is highly specific for pericardial constriction

absence of pericardial thickening (≥4 mm), does not completely rule out constrictive pericarditis. In difficult cases, the final diagnosis needs to be made in conjunction with clinical, echo Doppler and/or invasive heart catheterization findings.

CT for Assessing Bypass Grafts

Weeks after or during CABG, 5–10% of grafts occlude. In addition, approximately half of venous grafts and one fifth of arterial grafts occlude within 10 years [120]. Invasive catheter-based angiography is the gold standard for the detection of bypass graft disease; but, it carries a much higher procedure related risk when compared to the angiographic assessment of native coronaries. It usually requires larger amount of contrast and a longer procedural duration which can be more detrimental in the elderly population. The larger size of venous grafts with less motion and calcification allow it to be easily assessed by CTA (Fig. 13.39). Artifacts originating from metallic clips, anastomosis indicators, sternal wires may sometimes impair the diagnostic confidence. However, improved temporal resolution and shorter acquisition times of current CT technology can achieve a sensitivity and specificity of 95% or higher for the detection of venous graft occlusion or stenosis [121]. In addition, although arterial grafts are smaller, the diagnosis accuracy of graft occlusion or stenosis by CT is excellent. However, due to

the smaller size, more motion and heavy calcification, the assessment of distal anastomosis sites and native coronary disease progression are not as robust as graft assessment. Therefore, the current clinical application for MDCT remains the assessment of graft disease.

Preoperative Planning for Redo Surgery

With increasing life expectancy and better surgical techniques, it is not unusual that elderly patients require more than one open heart surgery. A redo surgery carries a higher surgical risk (even more so in the elderly) careful preoperative planning is mandatory. Traditionally, selective angiography is used as the gold standard for anatomic evaluation of grafts and native coronary arteries. Besides providing a noninvasive assessment of these structures, MDCT has the advantage of providing the surgeon with information on the relationship of the sternum to the great vessels, existing grafts/conduits, right ventricle, and native coronary arteries. Furthermore, the extent of calcification and atherosclerosis of the aorta can be accurately evaluated. This comprehensive assessment can facilitate surgical planning and may lead to reduced risk of injury to grafts or adjacent cardiac structures during sternotomy and decreased strokes related to cannulation/cross-clamping of a highly calcified and atheromatous aorta.

Findings on MDCTA for high-risk redo surgery are quite common. One study showed that the close proximity (<1 cm)

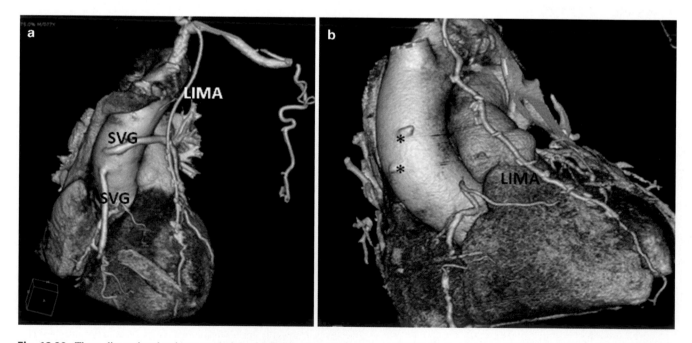

Fig. 13.39 Three dimensional volume rendering of MDCT of two patients post CABG. Patient (**a**) both SVGs and LIMA grafts were patent. Patient (**b**) both SVGs were occluded (*asterisk*) and LIMA graft was patent

of the right ventricle/aorta to the chest wall occurred in 24% of cases and, that in 38% of cases, coronary grafts crossed the midline in close proximity (<1 cm anteroposteriorly) to the sternum. In cases of renal insufficiency or urgent surgery after invasive angiography, administration of additional contrast materials with CTA could be relatively contraindicated. However, a noncontrast CT study can be quite informative in assessing the distance between the right ventricle and the sternum and provide limited but potentially useful information on the ascending aorta and graft location. The routine use of preoperative MDCTA to detect high-risk findings could lead to adoption of preventive surgical strategies in high-risk patients undergoing redo cardiac surgery, and potentially lead to reduced frequency of severe bleeding, graft injuries, and 1-month mortality [122].

References

1. Heller G, Hendel R. Nuclear cardiology: practical applications. New York: McGraw-Hill; 2010.
2. Einstein AJ, Moser KW, Thompson RC, Cerqueira MD, Henzlova MJ. Radiation dose to patients from cardiac diagnostic imaging. Circulation. 2007;116(11):1290–305.
3. Hendel RC, Berman DS, Di Carli MF, et al. ACCF/ASNC/ACR/AHA/ASE/SCCT/SCMR/SNM 2009 appropriate use criteria for cardiac radionuclide imaging: a report of the American College of Cardiology Foundation Appropriate Use Criteria Task Force, the American Society of Nuclear Cardiology, the American College of Radiology, the American Heart Association, the American Society of Echocardiography, the Society of Cardiovascular Computed Tomography, the Society for Cardiovascular Magnetic Resonance, and the Society of Nuclear Medicine. Endorsed by the American College of Emergency Physicians. J Am Coll Cardiol. 2009;53(23):2201–29.
4. Sharir T, Germano G, Kang X, et al. Prediction of myocardial infarction versus cardiac death by gated myocardial perfusion SPECT: risk stratification by the amount of stress-induced ischemia and the poststress ejection fraction. J Nucl Med. 2001;42(6):831–7.
5. Min JK, Shaw LJ, Berman DS. The present state of coronary computed tomography angiography a process in evolution. J Am Coll Cardiol. 2010;55(10):957–65.
6. Bettencourt N, Rocha J, Carvalho M, et al. Multislice computed tomography in the exclusion of coronary artery disease in patients with presurgical valve disease. Circ Cardiovasc Imaging. 2009;2(4):306–13.
7. Miller JM, Rochitte CE, Dewey M, et al. Diagnostic performance of coronary angiography by 64-row CT. N Engl J Med. 2008;359(22):2324–36.
8. Mehran R, Aymong ED, Nikolsky E, et al. A simple risk score for prediction of contrast-induced nephropathy after percutaneous coronary intervention: development and initial validation. J Am Coll Cardiol. 2004;44(7):1393–9.
9. Pennell DJ, Sechtem UP, Higgins CB, et al. Clinical indications for cardiovascular magnetic resonance (CMR): consensus panel report. Eur Heart J. 2004;25(21):1940–65.
10. Semelka RC, Tomei E, Wagner S, et al. Interstudy reproducibility of dimensional and functional measurements between cine magnetic resonance studies in the morphologically abnormal left ventricle. Am Heart J. 1990;119(6):1367–73.
11. Grothues F, Smith GC, Moon JC, et al. Comparison of interstudy reproducibility of cardiovascular magnetic resonance with two-dimensional echocardiography in normal subjects and in patients with heart failure or left ventricular hypertrophy. Am J Cardiol. 2002;90(1):29–34.
12. Grebenc ML, Rosado de Christenson ML, Burke AP, Green CE, Galvin JR. Primary cardiac and pericardial neoplasms: radiologic-pathologic correlation. Radiographics. 2000;20(4):1073–103.
13. Grebenc ML, Rosado-de-Christenson ML, Green CE, Burke AP, Galvin JR. Cardiac myxoma: imaging features in 83 patients. Radiographics. 2002;22(3):673–89.
14. Fuster V, Kim RJ. Frontiers in cardiovascular magnetic resonance. Circulation. 2005;112(1):135–44.
15. Comeau CR, Berke AD, Wolff SD. Ventricular lipoma detection by magnetic resonance imaging. Circulation. 2001;103(10):1485–6.
16. Araoz PA, Mulvagh SL, Tazelaar HD, Julsrud PR, Breen JF. CT and MR imaging of benign primary cardiac neoplasms with echocardiographic correlation. Radiographics. 2000;20(5):1303–19.
17. Otterstad JE, Froeland G, St John SM, Holme I. Accuracy and reproducibility of biplane two-dimensional echocardiographic measurements of left ventricular dimensions and function. Eur Heart J. 1997;18(3):507–13.
18. Helbing WA, Bosch HG, Maliepaard C, et al. Comparison of echocardiographic methods with magnetic resonance imaging for assessment of right ventricular function in children. Am J Cardiol. 1995;76(8):589–94.
19. Grothues F, Moon JC, Bellenger NG, Smith GS, Klein HU, Pennell DJ. Interstudy reproducibility of right ventricular volumes, function, and mass with cardiovascular magnetic resonance. Am Heart J. 2004;147(2):218–23.
20. Bellenger NG, Grothues F, Smith GC, Pennell DJ. Quantification of right and left ventricular function by cardiovascular magnetic resonance. Herz. 2000;25(4):392–9.
21. Barkhausen J, Ruehm SG, Goyen M, Buck T, Laub G, Debatin JF. MR evaluation of ventricular function: true fast imaging with steady-state precession versus fast low-angle shot cine MR imaging: feasibility study. Radiology. 2001;219(1):264–9.
22. Kim RJ, Fieno DS, Parrish TB, et al. Relationship of MRI delayed contrast enhancement to irreversible injury, infarct age, and contractile function. Circulation. 1999;100(19):1992–2002.
23. Rehwald WG, Fieno DS, Chen EL, Kim RJ, Judd RM. Myocardial magnetic resonance imaging contrast agent concentrations after reversible and irreversible ischemic injury. Circulation. 2002;105(2):224–9.
24. Fieno DS, Kim RJ, Chen EL, Lomasney JW, Klocke FJ, Judd RM. Contrast-enhanced magnetic resonance imaging of myocardium at risk: distinction between reversible and irreversible injury throughout infarct healing. J Am Coll Cardiol. 2000;36(6):1985–91.
25. Wu E, Judd RM, Vargas JD, Klocke FJ, Bonow RO, Kim RJ. Visualisation of presence, location, and transmural extent of healed Q-wave and non-Q-wave myocardial infarction. Lancet. 2001;357(9249):21–8.
26. Simonetti OP, Kim RJ, Fieno DS, et al. An improved MR imaging technique for the visualization of myocardial infarction. Radiology. 2001;218(1):215–23.
27. Moller JE, Hillis GS, Oh JK, Reeder GS, Gersh BJ, Pellikka PA. Wall motion score index and ejection fraction for risk stratification after acute myocardial infarction. Am Heart J. 2006;151(2):419–25.
28. White HD, Norris RM, Brown MA, Brandt PW, Whitlock RM, Wild CJ. Left ventricular end-systolic volume as the major determinant of survival after recovery from myocardial infarction. Circulation. 1987;76(1):44–51.
29. Carluccio E, Tommasi S, Bentivoglio M, Buccolieri M, Prosciutti L, Corea L. Usefulness of the severity and extent of wall motion abnormalities as prognostic markers of an adverse outcome after a first myocardial infarction treated with thrombolytic therapy. Am J Cardiol. 2000;85(4):411–5.

30. Bursi F, Enriquez-Sarano M, Jacobsen SJ, Roger VL. Mitral regurgitation after myocardial infarction: a review. Am J Med. 2006;119(2):103–12.

31. Moller JE, Pellikka PA, Hillis GS, Oh JK. Prognostic importance of diastolic function and filling pressure in patients with acute myocardial infarction. Circulation. 2006;114(5):438–44.

32. Li F, Chen YG, Yao GH, et al. Usefulness of left ventricular conic index measured by real-time three-dimensional echocardiography to predict left ventricular remodeling after acute myocardial infarction. Am J Cardiol. 2008;102(11):1433–7.

33. Quinones MA, Verani MS, Haichin RM, Mahmarian JJ, Suarez J, Zoghbi WA. Exercise echocardiography versus 201Tl single-photon emission computed tomography in evaluation of coronary artery disease. Analysis of 292 patients. Circulation. 1992;85(3): 1026–31.

34. Elhendy A, Schinkel AF, Bax JJ, van Domburg RT, Poldermans D. Prognostic value of dobutamine stress echocardiography in patients with normal left ventricular systolic function. J Am Soc Echocardiogr. 2004;17(7):739–43.

35. Sicari R, Pasanisi E, Venneri L, Landi P, Cortigiani L, Picano E. Stress echo results predict mortality: a large-scale multicenter prospective international study. J Am Coll Cardiol. 2003;41(4): 589–95.

36. Rizzello V, Poldermans D, Boersma E, et al. Opposite patterns of left ventricular remodeling after coronary revascularization in patients with ischemic cardiomyopathy: role of myocardial viability. Circulation. 2004;110(16):2383–8.

37. Dijkmans PA, Senior R, Becher H, et al. Myocardial contrast echocardiography evolving as a clinically feasible technique for accurate, rapid, and safe assessment of myocardial perfusion: the evidence so far. J Am Coll Cardiol. 2006;48(11):2168–77.

38. Galiuto L, Garramone B, Scara A, et al. The extent of microvascular damage during myocardial contrast echocardiography is superior to other known indexes of post-infarct reperfusion in predicting left ventricular remodeling: results of the multicenter AMICI study. J Am Coll Cardiol. 2008;51(5):552–9.

39. Khumri TM, Nayyar S, Idupulapati M, et al. Usefulness of myocardial contrast echocardiography in predicting late mortality in patients with anterior wall acute myocardial infarction. Am J Cardiol. 2006;98(9):1150–5.

40. Underwood SR, Anagnostopoulos C, Cerqueira M, et al. Myocardial perfusion scintigraphy: the evidence. Eur J Nucl Med Mol Imaging. 2004;31(2):261–91.

41. Iskandrian AS, Chae SC, Heo J, Stanberry CD, Wasserleben V, Cave V. Independent and incremental prognostic value of exercise single-photon emission computed tomographic (SPECT) thallium imaging in coronary artery disease. J Am Coll Cardiol. 1993;22(3): 665–70.

42. Shaw LJ, Iskandrian AE. Prognostic value of gated myocardial perfusion SPECT. J Nucl Cardiol. 2004;11(2):171–85.

43. Valeti US, Miller TD, Hodge DO, Gibbons RJ. Exercise single-photon emission computed tomography provides effective risk stratification of elderly men and elderly women. Circulation. 2005;111(14):1771–6.

44. Hachamovitch R, Hayes S, Friedman JD, et al. Determinants of risk and its temporal variation in patients with normal stress myocardial perfusion scans: what is the warranty period of a normal scan? J Am Coll Cardiol. 2003;41(8):1329–40.

45. Ladenheim ML, Pollock BH, Rozanski A, et al. Extent and severity of myocardial hypoperfusion as predictors of prognosis in patients with suspected coronary artery disease. J Am Coll Cardiol. 1986;7(3):464–71.

46. Iskander S, Iskandrian AE. Risk assessment using single-photon emission computed tomographic technetium-99m sestamibi imaging. J Am Coll Cardiol. 1998;32(1):57–62.

47. Sharir T, Germano G, Kavanagh PB, et al. Incremental prognostic value of post-stress left ventricular ejection fraction and volume by gated myocardial perfusion single photon emission computed tomography. Circulation. 1999;100(10):1035–42.

48. Mahmarian JJ, Shaw LJ, Filipchuk NG, et al. A multinational study to establish the value of early adenosine technetium-99m sestamibi myocardial perfusion imaging in identifying a low-risk group for early hospital discharge after acute myocardial infarction. J Am Coll Cardiol. 2006;48(12):2448–57.

49. Hachamovitch R, Hayes SW, Friedman JD, Cohen I, Berman DS. Comparison of the short-term survival benefit associated with revascularization compared with medical therapy in patients with no prior coronary artery disease undergoing stress myocardial perfusion single photon emission computed tomography. Circulation. 2003;107(23):2900–7.

50. Shaw LJ, Berman DS, Maron DJ, et al. Optimal medical therapy with or without percutaneous coronary intervention to reduce ischemic burden: results from the Clinical Outcomes Utilizing Revascularization and Aggressive Drug Evaluation (COURAGE) trial nuclear substudy. Circulation. 2008;117(10):1283–91.

51. Schinkel AF, Bax JJ, Poldermans D, Elhendy A, Ferrari R, Rahimtoola SH. Hibernating myocardium: diagnosis and patient outcomes. Curr Probl Cardiol. 2007;32(7):375–410.

52. Allman KC, Shaw LJ, Hachamovitch R, Udelson JE. Myocardial viability testing and impact of revascularization on prognosis in patients with coronary artery disease and left ventricular dysfunction: a meta-analysis. J Am Coll Cardiol. 2002;39(7):1151–8.

53. Siebelink HM, Blanksma PK, Crijns HJ, et al. No difference in cardiac event-free survival between positron emission tomography-guided and single-photon emission computed tomography-guided patient management: a prospective, randomized comparison of patients with suspicion of jeopardized myocardium. J Am Coll Cardiol. 2001;37(1):81–8.

54. Budoff MJ, Dowe D, Jollis JG, et al. Diagnostic performance of 64-multidetector row coronary computed tomographic angiography for evaluation of coronary artery stenosis in individuals without known coronary artery disease: results from the prospective multicenter ACCURACY (Assessment by Coronary Computed Tomographic Angiography of Individuals Undergoing Invasive Coronary Angiography) trial. J Am Coll Cardiol. 2008;52(21): 1724–32.

55. Min JK, Shaw LJ, Devereux RB, et al. Prognostic value of multidetector coronary computed tomographic angiography for prediction of all-cause mortality. J Am Coll Cardiol. 2007;50(12): 1161–70.

56. Klem I, Heitner JF, Shah DJ, et al. Improved detection of coronary artery disease by stress perfusion cardiovascular magnetic resonance with the use of delayed enhancement infarction imaging. J Am Coll Cardiol. 2006;47(8):1630–8.

57. Steel K, Broderick R, Gandla V, et al. Complementary prognostic values of stress myocardial perfusion and late gadolinium enhancement imaging by cardiac magnetic resonance in patients with known or suspected coronary artery disease. Circulation. 2009;120(14):1390–400.

58. Kim RJ, Wu E, Rafael A, et al. The use of contrast-enhanced magnetic resonance imaging to identify reversible myocardial dysfunction. N Engl J Med. 2000;343(20):1445–53.

59. Wellnhofer E, Olariu A, Klein C, et al. Magnetic resonance low-dose dobutamine test is superior to SCAR quantification for the prediction of functional recovery. Circulation. 2004;109(18): 2172–4.

60. Rosamond W, Flegal K, Friday G, et al. Heart disease and stroke statistics – 2007 update: a report from the American Heart Association Statistics Committee and Stroke Statistics Subcommittee. Circulation. 2007;115(5):e69–171.

61. Alderman EL, Fisher LD, Litwin P, et al. Results of coronary artery surgery in patients with poor left ventricular function (CASS). Circulation. 1983;68(4):785–95.

62. Marwick TH, Schwaiger M. The future of cardiovascular imaging in the diagnosis and management of heart failure, part 1: tasks and tools. Circ Cardiovasc Imaging. 2008;1(1):58–69.

63. West AM, Kramer CM. Cardiovascular magnetic resonance imaging of myocardial infarction, viability, and cardiomyopathies. Curr Probl Cardiol. 2010;35(4):176–220.

64. Ghostine S, Caussin C, Habis M, et al. Non-invasive diagnosis of ischaemic heart failure using 64-slice computed tomography. Eur Heart J. 2008;29:2133–40.

65. Underwood SR, Bax JJ, vom Dahl J, et al. Imaging techniques for the assessment of myocardial hibernation. Report of a Study Group of the European Society of Cardiology. Eur Heart J. 2004;25(10):815–36.

66. Bax JJ, Poldermans D, Elhendy A, Boersma E, Rahimtoola SH. Sensitivity, specificity, and predictive accuracies of various noninvasive techniques for detecting hibernating myocardium. Curr Probl Cardiol. 2001;26(2):147–86.

67. Baumgartner H, Porenta G, Lau YK, et al. Assessment of myocardial viability by dobutamine echocardiography, positron emission tomography and thallium-201 SPECT: correlation with histopathology in explanted hearts. J Am Coll Cardiol. 1998;32(6):1701–8.

68. Schvartzman PR, Srichai MB, Grimm RA, et al. Nonstress delayed-enhancement magnetic resonance imaging of the myocardium predicts improvement of function after revascularization for chronic ischemic heart disease with left ventricular dysfunction. Am Heart J. 2003;146(3):535–41.

69. Zile MR, Brutsaert DL. New concepts in diastolic dysfunction and diastolic heart failure: part I: diagnosis, prognosis, and measurements of diastolic function. Circulation. 2002;105(11):1387–93.

70. Nagueh SF, Appleton CP, Gillebert TC, et al. Recommendations for the evaluation of left ventricular diastolic function by echocardiography. Eur J Echocardiogr. 2009;10(2):165–93.

71. Nagueh SF, Middleton KJ, Kopelen HA, Zoghbi WA, Quinones MA. Doppler tissue imaging: a noninvasive technique for evaluation of left ventricular relaxation and estimation of filling pressures. J Am Coll Cardiol. 1997;30(6):1527–33.

72. Nagueh SF. Echocardiographic assessment of left ventricular relaxation and cardiac filling pressures. Curr Heart Fail Rep. 2009;6(3):154–9.

73. Rohde LE, Palombini DV, Polanczyk CA, Goldraich LA, Clausell N. A hemodynamically oriented echocardiography-based strategy in the treatment of congestive heart failure. J Card Fail. 2007;13(8):618–25.

74. Nkomo VT, Gardin JM, Skelton TN, Gottdiener JS, Scott CG, Enriquez-Sarano M. Burden of valvular heart diseases: a population-based study. Lancet. 2006;368(9540):1005–11.

75. Cawley PJ, Maki JH, Otto CM. Cardiovascular magnetic resonance imaging for valvular heart disease: technique and validation. Circulation. 2009;119(3):468–78.

76. Shipton B, Wahba H. Valvular heart disease: review and update. Am Fam Physician. 2001;63(11):2201–8.

77. Bonow RO, Carabello BA, Chatterjee K, et al. focused update incorporated into the ACC/AHA 2006 guidelines for the management of patients with valvular heart disease: a report of the American College of Cardiology/American Heart Association Task Force on Practice Guidelines (Writing Committee to revise the 1998 guidelines for the management of patients with valvular heart disease). Endorsed by the Society of Cardiovascular Anesthesiologists, Society for Cardiovascular Angiography and Interventions, and Society of Thoracic Surgeons. J Am Coll Cardiol. 2008;52(13):e1–142.

78. Mylonakis E, Calderwood SB. Infective endocarditis in adults. N Engl J Med. 2001;345(18):1318–30.

79. Li JS, Sexton DJ, Mick N, et al. Proposed modifications to the Duke criteria for the diagnosis of infective endocarditis. Clin Infect Dis. 2000;30(4):633–8.

80. Sverdlov AL, Taylor K, Elkington AG, Zeitz CJ, Beltrame JF. Images in cardiovascular medicine. Cardiac magnetic resonance imaging identifies the elusive perivalvular abscess. Circulation. 2008;118(1):e1–3.

81. Zoghbi WA, Farmer KL, Soto JG, Nelson JG, Quinones MA. Accurate noninvasive quantification of stenotic aortic valve area by Doppler echocardiography. Circulation. 1986;73(3):452–9.

82. Sondergaard L, Hildebrandt P, Lindvig K, et al. Valve area and cardiac output in aortic stenosis: quantification by magnetic resonance velocity mapping. Am Heart J. 1993;126(5):1156–64.

83. Kilner PJ, Manzara CC, Mohiaddin RH, et al. Magnetic resonance jet velocity mapping in mitral and aortic valve stenosis. Circulation. 1993;87(4):1239–48.

84. Eichenberger AC, Jenni R, von Schulthess GK. Aortic valve pressure gradients in patients with aortic valve stenosis: quantification with velocity-encoded cine MR imaging. Am J Roentgenol. 1993;160(5):971–7.

85. Caruthers SD, Lin SJ, Brown P, et al. Practical value of cardiac magnetic resonance imaging for clinical quantification of aortic valve stenosis: comparison with echocardiography. Circulation. 2003;108(18):2236–43.

86. Sondergaard L, Lindvig K, Hildebrandt P, et al. Quantification of aortic regurgitation by magnetic resonance velocity mapping. Am Heart J. 1993;125(4):1081–90.

87. Zoghbi WA, Enriquez-Sarano M, Foster E, et al. Recommendations for evaluation of the severity of native valvular regurgitation with two-dimensional and Doppler echocardiography. J Am Soc Echocardiogr. 2003;16(7):777–802.

88. Ley S, Eichhorn J, Ley-Zaporozhan J, et al. Evaluation of aortic regurgitation in congenital heart disease: value of MR imaging in comparison to echocardiography. Pediatr Radiol. 2007;37(5):426–36.

89. Honda N, Machida K, Hashimoto M, et al. Aortic regurgitation: quantitation with MR imaging velocity mapping. Radiology. 1993;186(1):189–94.

90. Dulce MC, Mostbeck GH, O'Sullivan M, Cheitlin M, Caputo GR, Higgins CB. Severity of aortic regurgitation: interstudy reproducibility of measurements with velocity-encoded cine MR imaging. Radiology. 1992;185(1):235–40.

91. Chandrashekhar Y, Westaby S, Narula J. Mitral stenosis. Lancet. 2009;374(9697):1271–83.

92. Bargiggia GS, Tronconi L, Sahn DJ, et al. A new method for quantitation of mitral regurgitation based on color flow Doppler imaging of flow convergence proximal to regurgitant orifice. Circulation. 1991;84(4):1481–9.

93. Grayburn PA, Fehske W, Omran H, Brickner ME, Luderitz B. Multiplane transesophageal echocardiographic assessment of mitral regurgitation by Doppler color flow mapping of the vena contracta. Am J Cardiol. 1994;74(9):912–7.

94. Lesniak-Sobelga A, Olszowska M, Pienazek P, Podolec P, Tracz W. Vena contracta width as a simple method of assessing mitral valve regurgitation. Comparison with Doppler quantitative methods. J Heart Valve Dis. 2004;13(4):608–14.

95. Little SH, Pirat B, Kumar R, et al. Three-dimensional color Doppler echocardiography for direct measurement of vena contracta area in mitral regurgitation: in vitro validation and clinical experience. JACC Cardiovasc Imaging. 2008;1(6):695–704.

96. Ascah KJ, Stewart WJ, Jiang L, et al. A Doppler-two-dimensional echocardiographic method for quantitation of mitral regurgitation. Circulation. 1985;72(2):377–83.

97. Quinones MA, Otto CM, Stoddard M, Waggoner A, Zoghbi WA. Recommendations for quantification of Doppler echocardiography: a report from the Doppler Quantification Task Force of the Nomenclature and Standards Committee of the American Society of Echocardiography. J Am Soc Echocardiogr. 2002;15(2):167–84.

98. Masci PG, Dymarkowski S, Bogaert J. Valvular heart disease: what does cardiovascular MRI add? Eur Radiol. 2008;18(2):197–208.

99. Fujita N, Chazouilleres AF, Hartiala JJ, et al. Quantification of mitral regurgitation by velocity-encoded cine nuclear magnetic resonance imaging. J Am Coll Cardiol. 1994;23(4):951–8.

100. Hundley WG, Li HF, Willard JE, et al. Magnetic resonance imaging assessment of the severity of mitral regurgitation. Comparison with invasive techniques. Circulation. 1995;92(5):1151–8.

101. Kizilbash AM, Hundley WG, Willett DL, Franco F, Peshock RM, Grayburn PA. Comparison of quantitative Doppler with magnetic resonance imaging for assessment of the severity of mitral regurgitation. Am J Cardiol. 1998;81(6):792–5.

102. Kon MW, Myerson SG, Moat NE, Pennell DJ. Quantification of regurgitant fraction in mitral regurgitation by cardiovascular magnetic resonance: comparison of techniques. J Heart Valve Dis. 2004;13(4):600–7.

103. Khanna D, Vengala S, Miller AP, et al. Quantification of mitral regurgitation by live three-dimensional transthoracic echocardiographic measurements of vena contracta area. Echocardiography. 2004;21(8):737–43.

104. Ryan LP, Salgo IS, Gorman RC, Gorman III JH. The emerging role of three-dimensional echocardiography in mitral valve repair. Semin Thorac Cardiovasc Surg. 2006;18(2):126–34.

105. Pirat B, Little SH, Igo SR, et al. Direct measurement of proximal isovelocity surface area by real-time three-dimensional color Doppler for quantitation of aortic regurgitant volume: an in vitro validation. J Am Soc Echocardiogr. 2009;22(3):306–13.

106. Sugeng L, Shernan SK, Weinert L, et al. Real-time three-dimensional transesophageal echocardiography in valve disease: comparison with surgical findings and evaluation of prosthetic valves. J Am Soc Echocardiogr. 2008;21(12):1347–54.

107. Zoghbi WA, Chambers JB, Dumesnil JG, et al. Recommendations for evaluation of prosthetic valves with echocardiography and Doppler ultrasound: a report From the American Society of Echocardiography's Guidelines and Standards Committee and the Task Force on Prosthetic Valves, developed in conjunction with the American College of Cardiology Cardiovascular Imaging Committee, Cardiac Imaging Committee of the American Heart Association, the European Association of Echocardiography, a registered branch of the European Society of Cardiology, the Japanese Society of Echocardiography and the Canadian Society of Echocardiography, endorsed by the American College of Cardiology Foundation, American Heart Association, European Association of Echocardiography, a registered branch of the European Society of Cardiology, the Japanese Society of Echocardiography, and Canadian Society of Echocardiography. J Am Soc Echocardiogr. 2009;22(9):975–1014.

108. Tong AT, Roudaut R, Ozkan M, et al. Transesophageal echocardiography improves risk assessment of thrombolysis of prosthetic valve thrombosis: results of the international PRO-TEE registry. J Am Coll Cardiol. 2004;43(1):77–84.

109. Chan J, Marwan M, Schepis T, Ropers D, Du L, Achenbach S. Images in cardiovascular medicine. Cardiac CT assessment of prosthetic aortic valve dysfunction secondary to acute thrombosis and response to thrombolysis. Circulation. 2009;120(19):1933–4.

110. Appelbaum A, Kouchoukos NT, Blackstone EH, Kirklin JW. Early risks of open heart surgery for mitral valve disease. Am J Cardiol. 1976;37(2):201–9.

111. Slama MA, Novara A, Van de PP, et al. Diagnostic and therapeutic implications of transesophageal echocardiography in medical ICU patients with unexplained shock, hypoxemia, or suspected endocarditis. Intensive Care Med. 1996;22(9):916–22.

112. Yong Y, Wu D, Fernandes V, et al. Diagnostic accuracy and cost-effectiveness of contrast echocardiography on evaluation of cardiac function in technically very difficult patients in the intensive care unit. Am J Cardiol. 2002;89(6):711–8.

113. Kurt M, Shaikh KA, Peterson L, et al. Impact of contrast echocardiography on evaluation of ventricular function and clinical management in a large prospective cohort. J Am Coll Cardiol. 2009;53(9):802–10.

114. Pepi M, Muratori M, Barbier P, et al. Pericardial effusion after cardiac surgery: incidence, site, size, and haemodynamic consequences. Br Heart J. 1994;72(4):327–31.

115. Price S, Prout J, Jaggar SI, Gibson DG, Pepper JR. "Tamponade" following cardiac surgery: terminology and echocardiography may both mislead. Eur J Cardiothorac Surg. 2004;26(6):1156–60.

116. Ling LH, Oh JK, Schaff HV, et al. Constrictive pericarditis in the modern era: evolving clinical spectrum and impact on outcome after pericardiectomy. Circulation. 1999;100(13):1380–6.

117. Hoit BD. Imaging the pericardium. Cardiol Clin. 1990;8(4):587–600.

118. Rajagopalan N, Garcia MJ, Rodriguez L, et al. Comparison of new Doppler echocardiographic methods to differentiate constrictive pericardial heart disease and restrictive cardiomyopathy. Am J Cardiol. 2001;87(1):86–94.

119. Masui T, Finck S, Higgins CB. Constrictive pericarditis and restrictive cardiomyopathy: evaluation with MR imaging. Radiology. 1992;182(2):369–73.

120. Goldman S, Zadina K, Moritz T, et al. Long-term patency of saphenous vein and left internal mammary artery grafts after coronary artery bypass surgery: results from a Department of Veterans Affairs Cooperative Study. J Am Coll Cardiol. 2004;44(11):2149–56.

121. Schlosser T, Konorza T, Hunold P, Kuhl H, Schmermund A, Barkhausen J. Noninvasive visualization of coronary artery bypass grafts using 16-detector row computed tomography. J Am Coll Cardiol. 2004;44(6):1224–9.

122. Kamdar AR, Meadows TA, Roselli EE, et al. Multidetector computed tomographic angiography in planning of reoperative cardiothoracic surgery. Ann Thorac Surg. 2008;85(4):1239–45.

123. Shah DJ, Dela Cruz JD. Functional valve assessment: the emerging role of cardiovascular magnetic resonance. Methodist DeBakey Cardiovasc J. 2010;6(1):15–19.

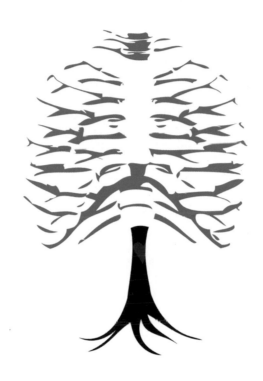

Chapter 14
Invited Commentary

Michael E. Zenilman

As a general surgeon, I have always been jealous of the cardiac surgeons in that the organ they fix is repaired by their operation, and it directly facilitates the postoperative course ("the problem cannot be the heart, we fixed it!"). My patients, on the other hand, are always dependent on that organ to get through the perioperative period. This makes my life that much more interesting.

The heart and lungs age at a predictable rate; not all the organ systems do. Why cardiac function declines along a straight line and the gastrointestinal tract does not is unknown. At the molecular level, many theories have been proposed on the aging process, such as increased DNA damage, impaired repair of damaged DNA by polymerases, and loss of telomerase resulting in shortened telomeres that affect senescence of living cells. The systems that are most directly affected by this process are the cardiac, pulmonary, immune, and neuroendocrine systems. But while the cardiac system is recognized as the most critical one for risk after surgery, we need to understand the aging process of the other critical organ systems since they can directly affect the heart.

The development of cardiac disease is really the result of normal or accelerated aging of the heart and its surrounding systems. Since the heart has been recognized as the most significant risk factor for patients undergoing noncardiac surgery, proactive recognition of its impairment and controlling it with both preventive and interventional measures can keep elective surgery safe. Right now, there are no molecular markers for cardiac disease; the best we have is the nonspecific C-reactive peptide level, a marker of inflammation. But, the molecular and physiologic changes that occur in aging are well established – the development of atherosclerotic plaque due to inflammatory responses, decreased cardiac output and left ventricular hypertrophy due to progressively increased vascular resistance, and the hyposympathetic state due to humoral senescence. In time, a simple blood test will be developed.

The first established way of documenting cardiac risk in noncardiac surgery was the "Goldman Criteria," published in 1977. It focused mostly on cardiac conditions which would affect postoperative cardiac system – e.g., an S3 gallop and jugular venous distention, a nonsinus rhythm, premature ventricular contractions, a recent infarction, or aortic stenosis. In 1999, the criteria were revised to a multisystem list of risk factors, which included active ischemic heart disease, stroke, diabetes, and increased creatinine. These revised criteria amplify the fact that diseases of other systems – renal disease and endocrine – are intimately related to and are part of the equation which predicts cardiac risk. Tuning these organ systems up before surgery decreases risk.

So, in order to decrease cardiac risk, we need to understand the physiology of the heart and its surrounding systems. Yes, perioperative beta blockade is highly effective in preventing perioperative cardiac events in vascular and abdominal surgery, but there is no question that stroke prevention, tight glucose control, and renal protection protect the heart as well.

The multisystem approach to understanding the effect of aging on surgical outcomes is gaining ground, and multiple recent studies are showing that frailty, the condition of weakening and disability (associated) with aging, is likely going to be the most powerful predictor of perioperative mortality. Frailty and its associated disabilities are associated with higher death rates in persons living at home, in patients at hospitals, and in residents of nursing homes. Frailty is associated with cardiac disease. In fact, the best prevention methods for frailty are similar to those of cardiac disease – regular exercise, weight loss, high fiber diet, and smoking cessation. Lifestyle changes have been shown to delay the onset of the disability of frailty by as much as seven years – very similar to the protection in cardiac disease.

The following chapters on physiologic changes are focused on their effect on cardiac disease and cardiothoracic surgery, but these changes are also important for the development of our own frailty as we age and adversely affect the way we respond to all surgical stresses.

So, while the cardiac surgeons still have the advantage of fixing the organ that directly affects the postoperative outcome, frailty is catching up as a predictor of outcome, and it is not reversible.

M.E. Zenilman (✉)
Department of Surgery, Johns Hopkins Medicine,
Bethesda, MD 20814, USA
e-mail: mzenilm1@jhmi.edu

M.R. Katlic (ed.), *Cardiothoracic Surgery in the Elderly*, DOI 10.1007/978-1-4419-0892-6_14,
© Springer Science+Business Media, LLC 2011

Chapter 15
Biology of Aging

Huber R. Warner

Abstract This chapter briefly summarizes what we currently know about some of the biological changes that accompany aging, and then tries to predict which of these may be the most relevant to the onset of age-related cardiac pathology, and the ultimate need for cardiothoracic surgery in older persons. Although cardiovascular diseases are now the major cause of mortality in developed countries, and age is a major risk factor for many of these diseases, it is still not clear just which age-related changes are the most critical in affecting longevity or the risk of dying as a result of cardiovascular pathology.

Keywords Caloric restriction • Oxidative stress • Cell proliferation • Cell death • Insulin-signaling • Telomere function

Introduction

A typical reader could ask why is there a chapter about the biology of aging in this book. While most of the chapters here address very physiological and clinical issues, I have chosen to briefly summarize what we currently know about some of the biological changes that accompany aging, and then try to predict which of these may be the most relevant to the onset of age-related cardiac pathology, and the ultimate need for cardiothoracic surgery in older persons. Although cardiovascular diseases are now the major cause of mortality in developed countries, and age is a major risk factor for many of these diseases, it is still not clear just which age-related changes are the most critical in affecting longevity or the risk of dying as a result of cardiovascular pathology.

The earliest notable milestones in biogerontology include McCay's demonstration that restricting caloric intake increases longevity and delays the onset of age-related diseases in rodents [1], Harman's prediction that the oxygen free radicals that are produced in vivo and damage cellular macromolecules are a major risk factor for aging (the so-called free radical theory of aging) [2], and Hayflick's demonstration that when human fibroblasts are grown in culture, they have a finite life span in terms of the number of times they can divide [3]. These three concepts still provide much of the underpinnings for biogerontolgical research today.

Aging-Related Biological Decline

Extension of Life Span by Caloric Restriction

This is also referred to as dietary restriction, but it is clear that calories are the critical component of the diet that must be reduced to extend longevity [4]. This intervention is reasonably universal, having been shown to be effective in almost every animal species in which it has been adequately tested. Although most studies have been conducted in rodents, primarily rats and mice, nonhuman primates are currently involved in two long-term studies [5, 6], and even humans are being studied in short-term trials [7]. Both species develop physiological responses similar to those seen in calorically restricted (CR) rodents, but mortality data are not yet robust enough in the nonhuman primate studies to unequivocally demonstrate how much average life span can be increased in this species, and no mortality data are available in the short-term human study.

The fundamental observation is that when caloric intake is reduced about 30–40% below what mice or rats with unlimited access to food would consume, the CR animals will live about 30–40% longer than the control animals (Fig. 15.1: compare WT, AL with WT, CR). The CR animals are not sick or malnourished, and in fact the onset of almost every disease associated with aging, e.g., heart disease, cataracts, type 2 diabetes, kidney disease, and cancer, is delayed. In general, restricted animals have lower body temperature, increased physical activity, are more resistant to chemical toxins and

H.R. Warner (✉)
College of Biological Sciences, University of Minnesota, St. Paul, MN 55108, USA
e-mail: warne033@centurylink.net

M.R. Katlic (ed.), *Cardiothoracic Surgery in the Elderly*, DOI 10.1007/978-1-4419-0892-6_15,
© Springer Science+Business Media, LLC 2011

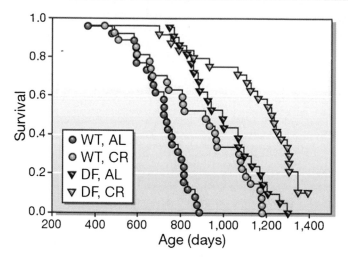

Fig. 15.1 Survival curves of wild type (WT) and dwarf (DF) mice. *AL* mice fed ad libitum; *CR* calorically restricted (From Bartke et al. [48] reprinted by permission from MacMillan)

heat, suffer less oxidative damage to their DNA, proteins and complex lipids, have lower levels of circulating insulin, insulin-like growth factor (IGF), glucose, triglycerides and cholesterol, and more protein turnover and delayed reproduction. The restricted animals are clearly healthier than the control animals, although the ultimate causes of death are fairly similar. Several of the effects listed above can be recognized as potential risk factors for various aspects of heart disease.

In spite of over 70 years of investigation of the CR paradigm, the mechanism of the intervention remains unknown. Sinclair and Howitz [8] have recently provided a comprehensive and up-to-date review proposing how this intervention may work in rodents and invertebrate species. In a major shift from most earlier ideas, they propose that CR represents a stress signal that activates the animal's defense pathways in anticipation of adverse conditions yet to come, e.g., starvation. If correct, this suggests that CR is an active defense response of the organism, evolutionarily designed to promote survival at the expense of growth and reproduction during times of adversity. Thus, energy is perhaps primarily directed to maintain the integrity of the most important components and functions of the cells of the organisms, a process that might be expected to also promote increased longevity.

Several mechanistic corollaries have been discovered so far [9]. CR induces an increase in circulating levels of glucocorticoids such as corticosterone, as do other stresses. Fibroblasts isolated from a variety of long-lived mutants are often more resistant to stresses such as chemicals, heat, and irradiation [10]. CR also induces the expression of certain sirtuin genes [11], and overexpression of these same genes can extend the life span of lower organisms such as nematodes [12]. Compounds that activate sirtuins are also known to extend life span of these same organisms. Sirtuins and their possible roles in aging are described in more detail below under the section "Insulin-Signaling Pathway and Response to Intake of Nutrients."

Oxidative Stress and Macromolecular Damage

As the primary sites of oxygen consumption in eukaryotic cells, mitochondria are also the primary sites for the production of reactive oxygen species (ROS), such as superoxide anion, hydroxyl radicals, and hydrogen peroxide (Fig. 15.2). One of the most enduring theories of aging has been the theory proposed by Harman [2] who proposed that oxygen free radicals are a major risk factor for aging because of their ability to attack bases in DNA [13], oxidize the amino acid side chains of proteins [14], and oxidize the unsaturated fatty acids in complex lipids, thereby producing aldehydic compounds such as malondialdehyde and 4-hydroxynonenal that are capable of interacting nonenzymatically with proteins. These damaged macromolecules must be repaired or eliminated to maintain adequate cellular function and tissue homeostasis.

Some nucleic acid bases are particularly sensitive to oxidation thereby altering their base-pairing properties, in particular guanine and thymine. 8-Oxodeoxyguanosine (8-oxodG) is often used as a measure of DNA oxidation, and the level of this compound in DNA increases with age in spite of the presence of efficient repair systems [15]. If the DNA is not quickly repaired, 8-oxodG in DNA can base pair with adenine instead of cytosine during replication, thus leading to mutations, but faulty repair of this DNA can also lead to mutations. The level of 8-oxodG is usually higher in mitochondrial DNA than in nuclear DNA, because mitochondria are the chief intracellular source of oxygen free radicals. While mutations have not been shown to directly cause aging, depending on where the mutations occurs, such as in an oncogene or tumor suppressor gene, they can lead to cancer. If the DNA damage is heavy, and DNA replication or transcription is blocked by large adducts, cross-linking or fragmentation, the end result may be apoptosis (programmed cell death), and net loss of cells. This result can have direct implications for aging if these cells are not replaced.

While DNA damage is often repaired by simply clipping out the damaged area, and replacing the excised nucleotides in short patches, damaged protein is usually repaired by total degradation of the protein so the undamaged amino acids can be recycled. Large amounts of energy are required to resynthesize these proteins to maintain an adequate supply of essential enzymes and other proteins required for normal cell function with increasing age. This also suggests that cells must maintain robust proteolytic systems to remove specifically damaged proteins that would otherwise accumulate in an old cell. Such proteolytic complexes are found in cells in the form of proteosomes [16]. Cellular proteins are also degraded in the lysosomes in a process known as autophagy [17]. Both of these systems not only provide

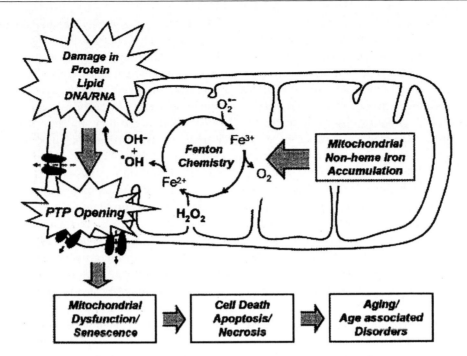

Fig. 15.2 Potential role of mitochondrial iron accumulation in the aging process. Accumulation of iron may increase oxidative stress via Fenton chemistry and the decay of mitochondrial structural components such as proteins, lipids, and nucleic acids. With age, an increase in the susceptibility of the permeability transition pore (PTP) may cause mitochondrial dysfunction and cellular degeneration via apoptosis or necrosis (Reprinted from Seo et al. [75] with permission from Wiley-Blackwell)

cells with a supply of amino acids for synthesis of proteins, but also serves as a quality control role for the proteome of cells. These proteolytic processes also target key regulatory proteins such as transcription factors, cell cycle regulators, tumor suppressors, promoters, etc., so they can have critical roles in maintaining cell function as well. Autophagy declines with age, and CR prevents this decline, suggesting this could be one of many ways by which CR exerts its life-extending effects.

Unsaturated fatty acids are very prone to oxidation by ROS, and longevity negatively correlates with the degree of fatty acid unsaturation of membrane phospholipids. Peroxidation of the double bonds in these side chains produce a variety of end products that can diffuse throughout the cell, modifying proteins and DNA, especially those in the mitochondria near the site of generation of the ROS [18, 19]. Thus, lipid peroxidation not only changes the properties of the membranes themselves, but also can have downstream consequences either near or far from the site of the original damage. For example, some of the end products, such as 4-hydroxy-2-nonenal, are bifunctional and can interact with, and crosslink proteins which inhibits the activity of the proteosomes during their attempt to degrade modified and damaged proteins [20].

Posttranslational Protein Modification

Proteins are also susceptible to nonenzymatic modification through the condensation between the aldehydic groups of free sugars with the amino acid side chains of lysines in proteins in a process known as glycation. These condensation products are Schiff bases which can subsequently rearrange to form a variety of intermediate structures, often with loss of normal function. This property is enhanced in the diabetic individual because of the increased concentration of glucose in their blood. In addition to glycation, proteins are subject to a variety of enzymatic modifications such as glycosylation, phosphorylation, and acetylation, to name a few.

Whereas most enzymatic modifications of cellular proteins are presumably positive modifications that are required for the protein's intended physiological function, a host of other biochemical changes are not. These include biochemical alterations such as glycation, oxidation or deamination of amino acid side chains, and racemization of amino acids from the L form to the D form. Typically, such altered proteins must be completely degraded and replaced through resynthesis. This is an expensive process, as Stadtman [14] has estimated that as many as 50% of proteins in the cell at any one time may have at least one oxidized side chain.

Cell Proliferation and Telomere Function

The mechanistic basis of Hayflick's observation that human cells grown in culture have a limited life span remained a mystery until Harley et al. [21] demonstrated that telomeres shorten each time a cell divides. Telomeres are the structures at the ends of chromosomes containing long noncoding repetitive sequences, and they are synthesized by a special enzyme called telomerase [22]. Telomerase consists of a catalytic protein complexed with a template strand of RNA that determines the repeating sequence of telomeric DNA. Because most somatic cells do not express the gene for the catalytic subunit, as somatic cells continue to divide the length of the telomeric DNA gradually shortens until a lower limit is reached (called the Hayflick limit), at which point proliferation ceases. This nonproliferative state is referred to as cell or replicative senescence. The idea that telomere length is critical to the proliferative potential of cells was strengthened by the observation that transgenically increasing cellular telomerase activity also increases the number of doublings a cell can undergo before reaching the senescent state [23].

Telomeres consist of more than the long noncoding sequence at the 5′ end of each DNA strand. They are complex structures that bind a large number of proteins that are important in the multiple functions of telomeres [24]. These proteins are not only involved in DNA replication, but they also protect the coding sequences near the ends of chromosomes, and prevent the recombination of chromosome ends with each other, or with the double-stranded ends transiently produced during the normal metabolism of DNA. Table 15.1 summarizes some of the roles of these telomere-associated proteins in promoting telomere function.

Telomere length and telomerase activity can impact human health in at least three general ways. One is through the altered phenotype of senescent cells, but adverse effects can also be observed if there is either too much or too little telomerase activity present in the cell. Whereas, fibroblasts normally facilitate the synthesis of the basement membrane that helps to repress the proliferation of cells attached to it, senescent fibroblasts secrete enzymes that degrade this matrix material. This degradation destroys the regulatory properties of the matrix, and Krtolica et al. [25] have shown that senescent cells promote carcinogenesis of nearby preneoplastic cells. Thus, replicative senescence is an example of antagonistic pleiotropy by preventing uncontrolled proliferation of cells in young animals [26], but promoting cancer in the vicinity of senescent cells, a process of increasing relevance as senescent cells accumulate with increasing age.

Table 15.1 Some mammalian age-related pathologies associated with short telomeres

Genotype	Phenotypes	References
Terc or Tert	Dyskeratosis congenita	[65, 66]
Terc, Ku86	Accelerated aging, reduced cancer	[67]
	Heart failure	[68, 69]
wrn	Werner's syndrome	[70]

High telomerase activity is characteristic of germline cells [27], activated lymphocytes [28], and transformed cells [29]. Thus, telomerase activity is associated with the proliferative potential of cells, and is also considered to be a possible local biomarker for cancer. The details of what actually causes telomerase activity to reappear in cancer cells, thus allowing uncontrolled replication, remains to be worked out, but developing cancer drugs that inhibit telomerase is still a sought-after therapeutic intervention.

Even though most cells in an adult organism do not contain telomerase activity, the total absence of telomerase is a serious problem for an organism. The ability to replace damaged cells well into late life depends upon having robust stem cell pools, as the stem cells in these pools divide asymmetrically to produce the needed replacement cells, and telomerase activity is required to maintain the telomere length of the mother stem cell. Humans born with a mutation in either the telomerase catalytic protein or the associated template RNA are defective in telomerase activity, and suffer from a variety of abnormal phenotypes, including abnormal skin pigmentation, premature hair graying, anemia, and bone marrow failure [24]. The latter is not surprising as bone marrow is a well-known source of hematopoetic and mesenchymal stem cells.

If failure to maintain tissue homeostasis contributes to the development of aging phenotypes, then decreased telomerase activity in stem cells is likely to accelerate aging indirectly due to decreased regenerative capacity of the pools [30]. Tomas-Loba et al. [31] provided important evidence for the critical role of telomerase and stem cells in aging by transgenically overexpressing telomerase in mice that were also engineered to be cancer-resistant. This telomerase overexpression delayed the degeneration of both skin and the gastrointestinal tract, and improved neuromuscular coordination and glucose tolerance with aging in these mice. Remarkably, this intervention also increased the median life span, but not the maximum life span, of these mice by 30–40%. These observations strongly implicate telomere maintenance as the main mechanism underlying the antiaging activity of telomerase.

An increasing number of studies have reported a positive association between telomere length in lymphocyte DNA and some independent measure of health. These include all-cause mortality, Alzheimer's disease, psychological stress, parental life span, as well as cardiovascular disease [32]. Neither the mechanistic basis for these associations, nor why these phenotypes correlate with telomere length in lymphocytes is well understood, but they do suggest that environmental factors such as infections that promote lymphocyte expansion may also have an impact on aging phenotypes.

Insulin-Signaling Pathway and Response to Intake of Nutrients

A recent milestone in biogerontology has been the discovery that reducing the activity of the insulin-signaling system also increases longevity. This is the pathway that responds to the binding of IGF-1 to its cell surface receptor. Until the mid-1980s it was widely assumed that aging is not directly regulated by genes, because aging occurs primarily after the reproductive phase of life, and therefore should escape the power of natural selection. However, the isolation of a nematode mutant with a significantly increased life span showed this assumption to be incorrect [33]. The gene mutated was subsequently shown to code for the enzyme phosphatidylinositol 3' kinase (PI3K) an early enzyme in the insulin-signaling pathway [34]. When Kenyon et al. [35] showed that *daf-2* nematode mutants lived twice as long as wild type organisms, and Kimura et al. [36] subsequently showed that the *daf-2* gene codes for an insulin-like receptor, this provided strong evidence that reducing insulin-signaling in nematodes in general might increase longevity. This has subsequently turned out to be true in fruit flies and mice, as well as in nematodes [37].

This signal transduction pathway ultimately induces phosphorylation of a transcription factor known as FOXO in mammals, and reduction in insulin-signaling results in the dephosphorylation and subsequent translocation of the transcription factor FOXO into the nucleus where it activates a series of genes involved in stress responses, e.g., antioxidant enzymes and antibacterial proteins [38, 39]. Because of its ability to regulate the function of this critical transcription factor, the insulin-signaling system also regulates reproduction and lipid metabolism.

Another important regulator of cell growth and proliferation, and even animal size, is a protein kinase called TOR (target of rapamycin) [40]. The mammalian form of TOR, called mTOR, modulates such processes as mRNA translation, ribosome biogenesis, nutrient metabolism, and autophagy. Thus, it indirectly regulates both protein synthesis and protein breakdown. Inhibition of TOR by rapamycin extends life span of nematodes [41] and mice [42], suggesting that it also plays a central role in regulation of longevity. The life span-extending effects of TOR inhibition and CR are not additive, suggesting that CR works at least partially by reducing TOR activity [43, 44]. Deregulation of the mTOR pathway has also been implicated in certain human cancers.

Another recent addition to the longevity regulation scene is the sirtuin family of proteins. A sirtuin is an NAD-dependent protein deacetylase [45]. Like phosphorylation, acetylation is a mechanism for regulating the activity of enzymatic proteins. The name comes from the *sir* genes in lower organisms that regulate gene expression in these organisms.

There are seven sirtuins in mammals, labeled SIRT1 through SIRT7, but SIRT1 is the closest homolog to the original yeast *sir2* gene. Sirtuins are known to deacetylate histones, p53 (a transcription factor and tumor suppressor protein), Ku70 (a protein involved in repair of double strand breaks in DNA), *c-myc* (an oncogene), and a variety of other transcription factors such as FOXO, and nuclear receptors such as PPAR gamma. As mentioned above, CR induces the expression of SIRT1, thereby perhaps contributing to increased longevity [12]. A major breakthrough occurred when Howitz et al. [46] showed that naturally-occurring polyphenolic compounds in plants could activate sirtuins and increase longevity. The best studied of these compounds is resveratrol, a compound found in relative abundance in grapes. Sinclair and Howitz [8] suggest that such polyphenolic sirtuin-activating compounds (STACs) are produced by plants to permit them to respond to various environmental stresses such as drought, nutrient starvation, and UV-light.

A serendipitous finding by Brown-Borg et al. [47] was that dwarf mice live longer than normal mice. As might be predicted, dwarf mice have a defect in either producing or responding to growth hormone, and thus have reduced levels of circulating IGF-1. It doesn't matter whether dwarfism results from a defect in pituitary development, a defect in the growth hormone receptor, or a defect in the growth hormone releasing hormone, all of which result in low circulating levels of IGF-1 [37]. The life span of these long-lived mice can be further extended by CR (Fig. 15.1: compare WT, CR with DF, CR), suggesting that growth hormone deficiency and CR act at least partially by different mechanisms [48].

Other Long-Lived Mouse Mutants

A variety of enzyme deficiencies can also extend life span in mice. Mice that are deficient in the production and/or release of growth hormone into the blood stream are not only dwarf, but also long-lived, when raised in a protected environment [47]. This is apparently due to the reduced activity of the insulin-signaling pathway in these mice. These effects are mimicked in fruit flies and nematodes by mutations that reduce the activity of the insulin-signaling pathway, such as *age-1* (PI3 kinase deficiency) and *daf-2* (an insulin-like receptor) mutants [34, 36]. Mouse life span is also increased by mutations in a protein known as p66[shc]. This protein normally senses oxidative damage [49], and induces programmed cell death of damaged cells [50].

Mice that are deficient in the pregnancy-associated plasma protein A (PAPPA) live about 38% longer than wild type mice [51]. These mice are also dwarf even though dietary intake is normal for their size. They are also resistant to cancer,

Table 15.2 Genetic modifications that increase mouse longevity

Gene	Function/activity	Phenotype of mutant	References
Mutations			
Prop-1	Pituitary development	Dwarf, long-lived	[47, 48]
Pit-1	Pituitary development	Dwarf, long-lived	[71]
GHR/BP	GH receptor	Dwarf, long-lived	[72]
p66^{shc}	Stress response	Long-lived	[50]
MUPA	Regulates appetite	Small, long-lived	[53]
PAPPA	Zn metalloproteinase	Delay thymic atrophy, long-lived, fewer tumors	[51]
Overexpression of genes			
mTERT	Telomerase	Increases median life span of cells in culture	[23]
MCAT	Catalase	Mitochondrial expression increases mouse life span	[73]
klotho	Transmembrane protein, coreceptor for FGF23	Increases mouse life span	[74]

but are not calorically restricted. PAPPA⁻ mice are deficient in a zinc metalloproteinase activity, and resist age-dependent thymic atrophy. Mutations that increase the activity of protective heat shock proteins in nematodes and fruit flies [52], or suppress appetite in mice [53], thereby mimicking caloric restriction, also increase life span of these organisms.

Table 15.2 summarizes some of the mutations or other genetic manipulations that increase mouse longevity. Manipulation of additional genes in yeast, nematodes, and fruit flies also extend longevity, but comparable experiments in mice have not yet been reported.

Cell Death and Turnover

Cell turnover is a natural part of maintaining tissue homeostasis, because damage to a cell may cause it to die by programmed cell death (apoptosis) if the damage is not too severe, or by necrosis if the damage is very severe. Mammalian cells have a stress response gene known as p66^{shc} that sense when the cell is damaged, and induces apoptosis by generating ROS internally [49]. Apoptosis is a proactive process that eliminates damaged cells from an organism, and mice with a mutated p66^{shc} gene are long-lived [50], and more resistant to this oxidative stress-induced apoptosis.

To maintain tissue cell number and function during aging, lost cells must be replaced either by the division of a local cell in a mitotic tissue such as liver, or by recruitment of a cell from a progenitor cell pool in a nonmitotic tissue such as brain. However, the progenitor cell may be already available in the tissue, as in the case of satellite cells in skeletal muscle, and thus not be dependent on recruitment from a distant progenitor pool. Failure to recruit such a replacement cell would result in gradually declining cell number and some tissue atrophy with aging. Although it is not clear whether a declining ability to replace damaged cells is an important factor in normal aging, some believe that it may be [54], and that the mechanism and functional consequences during aging are likely to differ markedly by tissue and cell type [55]. Sharpless and DePinho [30] have argued that "a decline in the regenerative function of stem cells with age contributes to mammalian aging and age-associated disease." This remains to be conclusively demonstrated, however.

A large number of apparently prematurely aging mouse models have been described so far [56], and all are characterized by lower growth rate and smaller adult size than normal mice. One explanation for this could be that cell death is accelerated in these models, and that cell replacement fails to maintain cell number in tissues with increasing age. A good example of a specific age-related-human condition that may be due to an imbalance between cell death and replacement is osteoporosis, where the balance between osteoblasts and osteoclasts is lost due to decreasing osteoblast number after menopause [57].

Figure 15.3 summarizes the events discussed above that may change during aging, and may represent causal events in age-related decline and loss of normal physiological function. Because cell number is dependent on the balance between cell death and cell division, maintaining cellular homeostasis requires tissues both to resist cell loss due to excessive apoptosis, and also to replace lost cells from either a resident or distant progenitor pool. However, it is currently not clear whether cell replacement from stem cell pools eventually becomes limiting with increasing age [55]. Although the frequency of nonproliferating senescent cells in tissues presumably also increases with increasing age [58], there is little evidence to indicate that this creates a problem with increasing age in mammals. More information is needed about these two scenarios to better understand whether maintaining cell number in critical tissues is a problem during mammalian aging, and if it is, in which tissues. One place where this seems most likely to be a problem is in the brain, where a large number of human age-dependent neurodegenerative diseases have now been described, and can be expected to occur with increasing frequency as the human life span continues to increase at a steady rate [59].

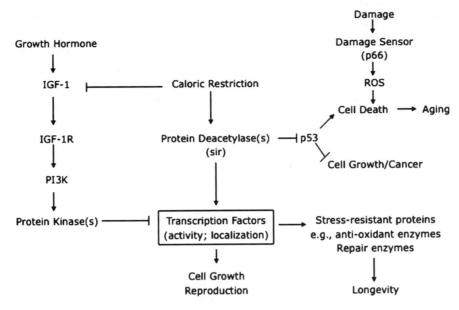

Fig. 15.3   Roles of caloric restriction, insulin-signaling, and oxidative stress in regulating life span

What Could All of This Have To Do with Cardiothoracic Surgery in the Elderly Human?

Human Relevance

As heart disease is the leading cause of death in the United States for both men and women, it is particularly critical to investigate mechanisms for reducing its occurrence, and/or how to repair the damage that promotes cardiovascular aging.

The first question one might ask is whether the results discussed above that were obtained by studying yeast, nematodes, fruit flies, and mice, are even relevant to humans? With regard to general concepts, the answer is probably *yes*, as there is ample evidence that once biology evolves an appropriate pathway or regulatory mechanism to accomplish something such as synthesis or degradation of a particular compound, it tends to conserve that pathway or mechanism during biological evolution. With regard to tissue function, the answer is probably *maybe*. For example, in laboratory mice the chief cause of death is cancer, as many of the laboratory strains were selected for rapid growth and reproduction for use in cancer research.

There is also an important variable with regard to the nature of the adult animal in a species. Because adult fruit flies and nematodes are primarily composed of postmitotic cells, their primary response to macromolecular damage is limited by the activity and fidelity of their repair systems. In contrast, mammals are able to replace severely damaged cells through programmed cell death of the damaged cell, and recruitment of replacement cells from progenitor pools. However, mammalian tissues vary considerably with regard to the latter, so losses in one tissue may be far more critical, e.g., in brain, than is cell loss in a replicative tissue such as liver.

Oxidative Stress

It is likely that oxidative damage contributes to aging in nearly all species studied, but its effects may vary greatly by tissue. In spite of the prediction that oxidative damage is a factor in aging in all species, conclusions drawn from vitamin E clinical trials on human disease incidence are ambiguous, and vitamin E supplementation has rarely extended the longevity of an animal model. In fact, Perez et al. [60] have reported that transgenically altering the levels of specific antioxidant enzymes in mice either up or down has often not supported the free radical theory of aging. Thus, it is clear that we still don't understand the most critical issues with regard to modulating oxidative stress with increasing age.

Cell Replacement

It seems likely that significant oxidative damage may also be occurring in myocytes during normal cardiac metabolism and function, inducing cell death and/or senescence if the damage exceeds some threshold level. The preservation of myocyte number and cardiac mass throughout life is presumed to be critical; this would thus require either activation of resident progenitor cells or recruitment of replacements from a stem cell pool such as bone marrow. Orlic et al. [61] have approached the problem of cell replacement in two ways. In one approach, bone marrow stem cells (BMSC) were injected directly into healthy myocardium adjacent to the damaged area of the left ventricle. In the other approach, cytokines were used to induce BMSC's to enter the blood stream and subsequently traffic to the damaged tissue. In both experiments the BMSC's gave rise to new myocardial cells and blood vessels, thus improving cardiac function and ultimately survival.

As cell number is dependent on the balance between cell death and cell division, maintaining cellular homeostasis not only requires the heart to both resist cell loss due to apoptosis, but also to replace lost cells from either a distant or resident progenitor pool. Increasing age would be expected to increase the rate of cell loss due to continuing oxidative stress, leading eventually to myocyte apoptosis, and/or declining ability to replace lost cells from progenitor pools [62]. These authors propose that continued damage is ultimately responsible for both activation of the cell death program, and development of the senescent phenotype. They also conclude that both maintenance of some telomerase activity to maintain the cell's potential to divide, and attenuation of the production of ROS represent potential intervention targets to delay cardiovascular aging. Increasing age would be expected to increase the rate of cell loss due to continuing oxidative stress leading eventually to apoptosis, and/or decrease the ability to replace lost cells from progenitor pools [63].

Thus, it seems clear that attenuating the low level but chronic generation of ROS to reduce both apoptosis and senescence of myocytes in heart tissue could be one goal of preemptive medicine in older persons. It is well known that acute occlusion of a major coronary artery will lead to myocardial ischemia and the death of myocytes involving both necrotic and apoptotic processes. This is an extreme example of what happens in cardiac tissue in response to oxidative stress, and such infarcts may not readily repair themselves. Whether cell loss is due to such an acute event or to low level chronic damage, the importance of replacing these damaged myocytes implies that maintenance of telomere function in progenitor cells may be a critical factor in the cell replacement part of this process.

Insulin-Signaling

The role of the insulin-signaling pathway in cardiac aging is less clear cut. Torella et al. [64] suggest that IGF-1 overexpression is good for cardiac health, in contrast to the effects it has on the longevity of nematodes, fruit flies, and even mice. They report that IGF-1 potentiates new myocyte formation in the adult heart, decreases myocyte death, inhibits the age-related increase in myocyte size, and in general helps maintain ventricular function and prevent heart failure. Their overall conclusion is that cardiac aging occurs at the cellular level, not the organ level. They also emphasize the overall importance of cardiac stem cells in delaying organ aging and heart dysfunction, implying that maintenance of cardiac cell number is essential for cardiac health.

Caloric Restriction

Human studies of caloric restriction are few, and in general relatively uninformative because of limited power and the short length of human studies [7]. However, it is nonetheless clear that the opposite phenotype, obesity, is a large risk factor for late-life pathologies such as type 2 diabetes and heart disease. Thus, diet in terms of both quantity and quality of food consumed, probably remains one of the best approaches available for reducing the risk to humans of late-life pathology and early death.

References

1. McCay CM, Crowell MF, Maynard LA. The effect of growth upon the length of life span and upon ultimate body size. J Nutr. 1935;10:63–75.
2. Harman D. Aging: a theory based on free radical and radiation chemistry. J Gerontol. 1956;2:298–300.
3. Hayflick L. The limited *in vitro* lifetime of human diploid cell strains. Exp Cell Res. 1965;37:614–35.
4. Weindruch R, Walford RL. The retardation of aging and disease by dietary restriction. Springfield, IL: Charles C. Thomas; 1988.
5. Lane MR, Ingram DK, Roth GS. Nutritional modulation of aging in nonhuman primates. J Nutr Health Aging. 1999;3:69–76.
6. Colman RJ, Anderson RM, Johnson SC, et al. Caloric restriction delays disease onset and mortality in rhesus monkeys. Science. 2009;325:201–4.
7. Heilbronn LK, de Jonge L, Frisard MI, et al. Effect of 6-month calorie restriction on biomarkers of longevity, metabolic adaptation, and oxidative stress in overweight individuals. JAMA. 2006;295:1539–48.
8. Sinclair DA, Howitz KT. Dietary restriction, hormesis, and small molecule mimetics. In: Masoro EJ, Austad SN, editors. Handbook of the biology of aging. 6th ed. New York, NY: Academic Press; 2006. p. 63–104.
9. Masoro EJ. Caloric restriction and aging: an update. Exp Gerontol. 2000;35:299–305.
10. Murakami S, Salmon A, Miller RA. Multiplex stress resistance in cells from long-lived dwarf mice. FASEB J. 2003;17:1565–6.
11. Cohen HY, Miller C, Bitterman KJ, et al. Calorie restriction promotes mammalian survival by inducing the SIRT1 deacetylase. Science. 2004;305:390–2.
12. Tissenbaum HA, Guarente L. Increased dosage of a sir-2 gene extends lifespan in *Caenorhabditis elegans*. Nature. 2001;410:227–30.

13. Campisi J, Vijg J. Does damage to DNA and other macromolecules play a role in aging? If so, how? J Gerontol. 2009;64A:175–8.
14. Stadtman ER. Protein oxidation and aging. Science. 1992;257:1220–4.
15. Hamilton ML, Van Remmen H, Drake JA, et al. Does oxidative damage increase with age? Proc Natl Acad Sci USA. 2001;98:10469–74.
16. Ciechanover A. Proteolysis: from the lysosome to ubiquitin to the proteosome. Nat Rev Mol Cell Biol. 2005;6:79–86.
17. Cuervo AM. Calorie restriction and aging: the ultimate cleansing diet. J Gerontol. 2008;63A:547–9.
18. Pamplona R, Portero-Otin M, Sanz A, et al. Modification of the longevity-related degree of fatty acid unsaturation modulates oxidative damage to proteins and mitochondrial DNA in liver and brain. Exp Gerontol. 2004;39:725–33.
19. Pamplona R. Membrane phospholipids, lipoxidative damage, and molecular integrity: a causal role in aging and longevity. Biochim Biophys Acta. 2008;1777:1249–62.
20. Friguet B, Szweda L. Inhibition of the multicatalytic proteinase (proteosome) by 4-hydroxy-2-nonenal cross-linked protein. FEBS Lett. 1997;405:21–5.
21. Harley CB, Futcher AB, Greider CW. Telomeres shorten during ageing of human fibroblasts. Nature. 1990;345:458–60.
22. Blackburn EH, Greider CW, Henderson E, et al. Recognition and elongation of telomeres by telomerase. Genome. 1989;31:553–60.
23. Bodnar AG, Ouellette M, Frolkis M, et al. Extension of life-span by introduction of telomerase into normal cells. Science. 1998;279:349–52.
24. Blasco MA. Telomere length, stem cells and ageing. Nat Chem Biol. 2007;3:640–7.
25. Krtolica A, Parrinello S, Lockett S, et al. Senescent fibroblasts promote epithelial growth and tumorigenesis: a link between cancer and aging. Proc Natl Acad Sci USA. 2001;98:12072–7.
26. Sedivy J. Telomeres limit cancer growth by inducing senescence: long sought in vivo evidence obtained. Cancer Cell. 2007;11:389–91.
27. Wright WE, Piatyszek MA, Rainey WE, et al. Telomerase activity in human germline and embryonic tissues and cells. Dev Genet. 1996;18:173–9.
28. Liu K, Schoonmaker MM, Levine BL, et al. Constitutive and regulated expression of telomerase reverse transcriptase (hTERT) in human lymphocytes. Proc Natl Acad Sci USA. 1999;96:5147–52.
29. Holt SE, Wright WE, Shay JW. Regulation of telomerase activity in immortal cell lines. Mol Cell Biol. 1996;16:2932–9.
30. Sharpless NE, DePinho RA. How stem cells age and why this makes us old. Nat Rev Mol Cell Biol. 2007;8:703–12.
31. Tomas-Loba A, Flores I, Fernandez-Marcos J, et al. Telomerase reverse transcriptase delays aging in cancer-resistant mice. Cell. 2008;135:609–22.
32. Ogami M, Ikura Y, Ohsawa M, et al. Telomere shortening in human coronary heart disease. Arterioscler Thromb Vasc Biol. 2004;24:546–50.
33. Friedman DB, Johnson TE. A mutation in the age-1 gene in Caenorhabditis elegans lengthens life and reduces hermaphrodite fertility. Genetics. 1988;118:75–86.
34. Morris J, Tissenbaum H, Ruvkun G. A phosphatidylinositol-3 OH kinase family member regulates longevity and diapause in Caenorhabditis elegans. Nature. 1996;382:536–9.
35. Kenyon C, Chang C, Genesch E, et al. A C. elegans mutant that lives twice as long as wild type. Nature. 1993;366:461–4.
36. Kimura D, Tissenbaum HA, Liu Y, Ruvkun G. daf-2, An insulin receptor-like gene that regulates longevity and diapause in Caenorhabditis elegans. Science. 1997;277:942–6.
37. Warner HR. Longevity genes: from primitive organisms to humans. Mech Ageing Dev. 2005;126:235–42.
38. Murphy CT, McCarroll SA, Bargmann CI, et al. Genes that act downstream of DAF-16 to influence the lifespan of Caenorhabditis elegans. Nature. 2003;424:277–84.
39. Wolff S, Dillin A. The trifecta of aging in Caenorhabditis elegans. Exp Gerontol. 2006;41:894–903.
40. Sarbassov DD, Ali SM, Sabatini DA. Growing roles of the mTOR pathway. Curr Opin Cell Biol. 2005;17:596–603.
41. Vellai T, Takacs-Vellai K, Zhang Y, et al. Influence of TOR kinase on lifespan in C. elegans. Nature. 2003;426:620.
42. Harrison DE, Strong R, Sharp ZD, et al. Rapamycin fed late in life extends lifespan in genetically heterogeneous mice. Nature. 2009;460:392–5.
43. Kaeberlein M, Powers R, Steffen K, et al. Regulation of yeast replicative life span by TOR and Sch9 in response to nutrients. Science. 2005;310:1193–6.
44. Stanfel MN, Shamich LS, Kaeberlein M, Kennedy BK. The TOR pathway comes of age. Biochim Biophys Acta. 2009;1790:1067–74.
45. Haigis MC, Guarente LP. Mammalian sirtuins – emerging roles in physiology, aging and calorie restriction. Genes Dev. 2006;20:2913–21.
46. Howitz KT, Bitterman KJ, Cohen HY, et al. Small molecule activators of sirtuins extend Saccharomyces cerevisiae lifespan. Nature. 2003;425:191–6.
47. Brown-Borg HM, Borg KE, Meliska CJ, Bartke A. Dwarf mice and the ageing process. Nature. 1996;384:33.
48. Bartke A, Wright JC, Mattison JA, et al. Extending the life span of long-lived mice. Nature. 2001;414:412.
49. Nemoto S, Finkel T. Redox regulation of forkhead proteins through a p66^{shc}-dependent signaling pathway. Science. 2002;295:2450–2.
50. Migliaccio E, Giorgio M, Mele S, et al. The p66^{shc} adapter protein controls oxidative stress response and life span in mammals. Nature. 1999;402:309–13.
51. Conover CA, Bale LK. Loss of pregnancy-associated plasma protein A extends life span in mice. Aging Cell. 2007;6:727–9.
52. Walker GA, Lithgow GJ. Lifespan extension in C. elegans by a molecular chaperone dependent upon insulin-like signals. Aging Cell. 2003;2:131–9.
53. Mishkin R, Masos T. Transgenic mice over-expressing urokinase-type plasminogen activator in brain exhibit reduced food consumption, body weight and size, and increased longevity. J Gerontol. 1997;52:B118–24.
54. Conboy IM, Rando TA. Aging, stem cells and tissue regeneration: lessons from muscle. Cell Cycle. 2005;4:407–10.
55. Sharpless NE, Schatten G. Stem cell aging. J Gerontol. 2009;64A:202–4.
56. Warner HR. Is cell death and replacement a factor in aging. Mech Ageing Dev. 2007;128:13–6.
57. Jilka RL, Weinstein RS, Parfitt AM, Manolagas SC. Quantifying osteoblast and osteocyte apoptosis: challenges and rewards. J Bone Miner Res. 2007;22:1492–501.
58. Dimri GP, Lee X, Basile G, et al. A novel biomarker identifies senescent human cells in culture and in aging skin in vivo. Proc Natl Acad Sci USA. 1995;92:9363–7.
59. Vaupel JW, Kistowski KG. The remarkable rise in life expectancy and how it will affect medicine. Bundesgesundheitsblatt Gesundheitforschung Gesundheitsschutz. 2005;48:586–92.
60. Perez VI, Bokov A, Van Remmen H, et al. Is the oxidative stress theory of aging dead? Biochim Biophys Acta. 2009;1790:1005–14.
61. Orlic D, Kajstura J, Chimenti S, et al. Bone marrow cells regenerate infracted myocardium. Pediatr Transplant. 2003;7 Suppl 3:86–8.
62. Katsjura J, Rota M, Urbanek K, et al. The telomere-telomerase axis and the heart. Antioxid Redox Signal. 2006;8:2125–41.
63. Kajstura J, Urbanek K, Rota M, et al. Cardiac stem cells and myocardial disease. J Mol Cell Cardiol. 2008;45:505–13.
64. Torella D, Rota M, Nurzynska D, et al. Cardiac stem cell and myocyte aging, heart failure, and insulin-like growth factor-1 overexpression. Circ Res. 2004;94:514–24.
65. Mitchell JR, Wood E, Collins KA. A telomerase component is defective in the human disease dyskeratosis congenita. Nature. 1999;402:551–5.

66. Vulliamy T, Marrone A, Szydlo R, et al. Disease anticipation is associated with progressive telomere shortening in families with dyskeratosis congenita due to mutations in TERC. Nat Genet. 2004;36:447–9.

67. Espejel S, Klatt P, Menissier-de Murcia J, et al. Impact of telomerase ablation on organismal viability, aging and tumorigenesis in mice lacking the DNA repair proteins PARP-1, Ku86, or DNA-PKcs. J Cell Biol. 2004;167:627–38.

68. Oh H, Wang SC, Prahash A, et al. Telomere attrition and Chk2 activation in human heart failure. Proc Natl Acad Sci USA. 2003;100:5378–83.

69. Leri A, Franco S, Zacheo A, et al. Ablation of telomerase and telomere loss leads to cardiac dilation and heart failure associated with p53 upregulation. EMBO J. 2003;22:131–9.

70. Chang S, Multani AS, Cabrera NG, et al. Essential role of limiting telomeres in the pathogenesis of Werner syndrome. Nat Genet. 2004;36:877–82.

71. Miller RA. Kleemeier award lecture: are there genes for aging? J Gerontol. 1999;54A:B297–307.

72. Coschigano KT, Holland AN, Riders ME, et al. Deletion, but not antagonism, of the mouse growth hormone receptor results in severely decreased body weights, insulin, and insulin growth factor I levels and increased life span. Endocrinology. 2003;144: 3799–810.

73. Schriner SE, Linford NJ, Martin GM, et al. Extension of murine life span by overexpression of catalase targeted to mitochondria. Science. 2005;308:1909–11.

74. Kuro-o M. Klotho and aging. Biochim Biophys Acta. 2009;1790: 1049–58.

75. Seo AY, Xu J, Servais S, et al. Mitochondrial iron accumulation with age and functional consequences. Aging Cell. 2008;7: 706–16.

Chapter 16
Hematologic Disorders in the Elderly

Ilene C. Weitz

Abstract Hematologic disorders in the elderly population have become an increasing problem as the general population ages. In the elderly, anemia is associated with increased morbidity and mortality. The etiology of the anemia may be nutritional deficiencies, renal insufficiency, hormone insufficiency, bone marrow dysfunction.

Thrombocytopenia in the elderly patient is associated with a variety of clinical disorders including myelodysplasia and bone marrow failure syndromes, nutritional deficiencies, medications, and immune disorders. Platelet dysfunction is common due to the use of anti-platelet medications, as well as disorders such as myelodysplasia.

While coagulation parameters do not change in the elderly, bleeding complications due to coagulation problems are common in the elderly. Liver failure, the use of anticoagulants, acquired factor inhibitors put elderly patients at risk for bleeding. Thrombosis is common in the elderly. The risk of venous thromboembolism increase with age but is also enhanced by a variety of clinical factors such as surgery, sepsis, hip fractures, cancer, and immobility.

In this chapter we will review the epidemiology, causes, and consequences of anemia in the elderly population. We will discuss platelet disorders, coagulation and thrombotic disorders unique to the elderly.

Keywords Anemia • Elderly • B21 deficiency • Iron deficiency • Anemia of chronic disease • Myelodysplasia • Thrombocytopenia • Immune thrombocytopenia • Thrombosis • Coagulation inhibiots • Heparin induce thrombocytopenia

I.C. Weitz (✉)
Jane Anne Nohl Division of Hematology and Center for Study of Blood Disorders, University of Southern California, Keck School of Medicine, Norris Comprehensive Cancer Center, Los Angeles, CA 90033, USA
e-mail: warne033@centurylink.net

Introduction

Anemia in the Elderly

As average life spans increase, anemia in the elderly population has become a more significant problem. It is now recognized that anemia in this population is common and associated with increased morbidity and mortality.

The accepted criteria, below which anemia is established, has changed over the last 15–20 years. In the past, anemia was defined by the packed cell volume (PCV). However, currently, automated blood analyzers accurately measure hemoglobin (Hgb) levels and calculate the PCV. Therefore, based on the World Health Organization (WHO) criteria uniform definition of anemia, based upon the Hgb is for men a hemoglobin less than 13 g/dL (130 g/L) and for woman a hemoglobin less than 12 g/dL (120 g/L) [1].

The most accurate estimate of anemia in the contemporary US population comes from the National Health and Nutrition Examination (NHANES) III survey of the 39,694 persons selected for this study [2]. Anemia increases significantly with increasing age. In patients aged 50–65, anemia occurs in 4.5% males, 6.5% females, in patients 65–75, anemia occurs in 7.5% in males, 8.5% females (Fig. 16.1). However, in patients over the age of 75, not only does the rate increase significantly, but there is a male predominance, 15% in males compared to 10.3% in females. In octogenarians and nonagenarians the rate continues to increase to 26% in males and 20% in females. Also, there are significant ethnic differences with African Americans having higher rates of anemia (male/female: 27.5/28%) than individuals of Hispanic descent (11.5/9.3%) or Caucasian patients (9.3/8.7%) [3] (Fig. 16.2). In a study of 732 consecutive patients admitted to a geriatric ward, 178 (24%) were found to be anemic with a hemoglobin of 11.5 g/dL or less [4].

Anemia in elderly patients is associated with increased mortality. In a large community-based 10 year study on the impact of anemia in individuals 85 years or older, anemia as defined by WHO criteria, was associated with a significant

M.R. Katlic (ed.), *Cardiothoracic Surgery in the Elderly*, DOI 10.1007/978-1-4419-0892-6_16,
© Springer Science+Business Media, LLC 2011

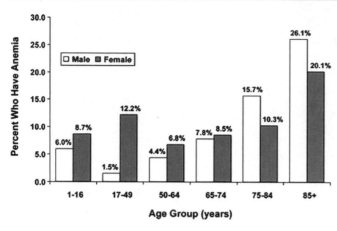

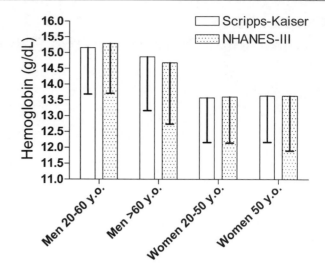

Fig.16.1 Results of the Third National Health and Nutrition Examination Survey. Percentage of persons considered anemic according to age and sex. NHANES III, phases 1 and 2, 1988–1994 (Reprinted from Guralnik et al [2], with permission from the American Society of Hematology)

Fig. 16.2 The mean and 1.65 standard deviations of the hemoglobin values of the white subjects in the Scripps-Kaiser and NHANES-III databases. The bottom of the error bars represents the hemoglobin value below which only 5% of normal values would be predicted to be present (Reprinted from Beutler et al. [3], with permission from the American Society of Hematology.)

increase in mortality in men with a Hgb less than 8.1 g/dL (nL = 13 g/dL) and in women with a Hgb less than 7.5 g/dL (nL = 12 g/dL) [5]. A study of healthy, older patients, age 65–95, found anemia in 8.1% of males and 6.1% females. There was doubling of the mortality rate in anemic patients compared to patients without anemia, 36% of males and 15% of females with anemia died within 5 years compared to 14% in non-anemic men and 9% in non-anemic women. Adjusted for other confounding co morbidities, this represented doubling of the 5 year mortality in male patients (HR 2.2: CI 1.5–2.4) [6]. A study by Culleton demonstrated an increase in all cause mortality in both men and women with anemia [7]. In the prospective Leiden 85 plus study, anemia was associated with more disability, impaired cognitive function and an increased mortality (hazard ratio of 2) in elderly patients greater than 85 years old [8]. Anemia is common in heart failure and is associated with poor outcomes. For patients with congestive heart failure, anemia as a co-morbid condition is associated with a shorter survival [9].

There are multiple causes for anemia in the elderly. In the NHANES III study nutritional deficiencies accounted for 34% of cases. In the other 65% of patients, anemia is due to renal insufficiency, anemia of chronic inflammation (ACI), or a combination of renal insufficiency and ACI [2]. A more recent study noted that nutritional deficiencies accounted for one third of the anemia in the elderly, two thirds of which were due to iron deficiency [10].

Nutritional Deficiencies

Iron deficiency was noted in 16% of elderly patients, with an additional 3.4% having iron deficiency combined with other nutritional deficiencies. The etiology of iron deficiency in the

elderly is always due to blood loss. While dietary issues may on rare occasions play a role in elderly patients, it is not likely to be the sole cause of the iron deficiency state. The etiology of iron deficiency in the elderly includes gastrointestinal blood loss from hiatal hernia, gastro-esophageal reflux disorder (GERD) with gastritis, GI malignancies (gastric, colonic), parasites colonic diverticuli, inflammatory bowel disease, as well as renal losses from renal cell carcinoma [11, 12]. In rare patients with intravascular hemolysis such as PNH, microangiopathic hemolytic anemia or cold agglutinin disease, iron deficiency may occur due to urinary losses.

Early iron deficiency can be diagnosed using measurements for serum ferritin, which indirectly reflects iron stores. In the elderly, a ferritin of less than 45 μg/L suggests iron depletion. A ferritin of less than 20 μg/L is diagnostic of iron deficiency [13]. The serum ferritin may be falsely increased in the setting of inflammation, or renal failure. For patients with significant renal disease, a serum ferritin of <500 μg/L has been used as an indication for iron replacement [14]. As iron deficiency progresses, anemia will develop with an increase in the red cell distribution width (RDW) reflecting red cell populations made at various stages of iron deficiency. A low serum iron and elevated iron binding capacity may be present and finally a microcytic anemia will develop. Soluble serum transferrin receptor assay, and measurements of free erythrocyte protoporphyrin IX may be helpful in patients in whom there is difficulty distinguishing iron deficiency from anemia of chronic inflammation (ACI).

In addition to treating the underlying cause of the iron deficiency anemia, iron replacement should be given. For most patients, oral iron is effective. However, patients using chronic proton pump inhibitor (PPI) therapy, patients with concurrent B12 deficiency, post gastrectomy or post gastric bypass surgery patients, may not have adequate absorbtion of oral iron due to the lack of gastric acid. Ingested iron must be converted from the ferrous form to the ferric form by gastric acid in the stomach. In the duodenum, the iron is converted back to the ferrous form in order to bind to the divalent metal transporter on the luminal surface of the duodenal cell. Poor responses to oral iron may also be due to inadequate dosing or lack of patient compliance due to side effects such as constipation and nausea. Giving stool softeners and laxatives may be helpful. The amount of iron absorbed is inversely correlated with hemoglobin, so as the hemoglobin approaches normalcy, the absorption of oral iron decreases. As a consequence, continued iron replacement for several months after normalization of the hemoglobin is required in order to replace iron stores. If there is no improvement after 3 months of oral therapy, patients should be re-evaluated. If there is no evidence of on-going blood loss with adequate compliance, consideration may be given to intravenous replacement. In patients with risk factors for poor absorption, intravenous iron replacement should be considered. There are several newer intravenous iron preparations which appear to have fewer side effects than iron dextran.

Vitamin B12 (Cobalamine) Deficiency

Vitamin B12 deficiency is rare in young patients. However, in patients over the age of 60, it occurs in occurs in 10–15% of patients. While other recognized causes of B12 malabsorption such as pancreatic insufficiency, terminal ileal disease such as Crohn's disease, radiation enteritis, small bowel lymphoma, nitrous oxide anesthesia do occur in the elderly, pernicious anemia (PA) and food B12 malabsorption (FBM) are the most common causes of B12 deficiency. Women are more commonly affected than males at a ratio of 1.5:1. African American and Hispanic patients with PA may present at an earlier age than Caucasian patients [15]. Low cobalamin levels, even in the absence of clinical findings, were found in 11.8% of elderly patients. In the Leiden 85 study, B12 deficiency occurred in 8% of elderly patients, but was less likely to be associated with anemia than patients who had folate deficiency. Macrocytosis was observed in only 1.8% of patients [16–18]. Patients may present with classic megaloblastic anemia. However, macrocytosis may precede the development of anemia by several months [19]. It is estimated that between 13 and 27% of patients with pernicious anemia may not have significant anemia [19, 20]. Macrocytosis is absent in 7% of anemic patients who have coexisting microcytic processes. Hypersegmentation in neutrophils may be the earliest hematologic finding [21, 22]. Untreated cobalamin deficiency may progress to complete pancytopenia [22]. Atypical presentations of cobalamin deficiency may occur.

In an analysis of 827 Chinese patients in a neurologic department, 19.7% of patients were found to have B12 deficiency, but only 9.8% had evidence of megaloblastic anemia [23]. It is well recognized that folate supplementation can mask the hematologic findings of megaloblastic anemia while the neurologic symptoms progress. On rare occasion, thrombosis with either myocardial infarction, stroke, deep venous thrombosis, or retinal vein thrombosis may be the presentation due to high homocysteine levels [24].

Daily B12 requirements are quite low, 1–2 µg per day, and cobalamin is ubiquitous in animal dietary sources (eggs, meat, and dairy products). With the exception of very strict vegans, B12 deficiency is always do to chronic, poor B12 absorption. Pernicious anemia (PA) is an autoimmune disorder in which antibody mediated destruction of the parietal cells occurs, leading to achlorhydria and loss of intrinsic factor production. In addition, secreted antibodies in gastric fluid may bind to B12 binding site on intrinsic factor blocking B12 binding [25, 26]. Antibodies to parietal cells are found in 90% of patient with PA and are often detectable in other family members, and may be associated with an increased incidence of other immune endocrinopathies such as Hashimoto's thyroiditis, insulin dependent diabetes mellitus, Graves disease, Addison's disease or primary ovarian failure. There also appears to be an increase in antiparietal cell antibodies with increasing age with a fourfold increase in patients in their 80s compared to patients in their 30s [26, 27]. Antibodies to intrinsic factor, while more specific than anti-parietal cell antibodies, are found in only 40–60% of patients.

Atrophic gastritis may also be due to chronic *Helicobactor pylori* infection. This results in low gastric acid-pepsin production. Estimates range from 9 to 30% of gastric hypoacidity as a cause of food B12 malabsorption. Gastric acid is required to release cobalamin from the protein R binder. This results in reduced B12 availability to bind to the intrinsic factor. In elderly patients, low gastric acid production, reflected in elevated serum gastrin levels, has been associated with low B12 levels and low B12 absorption, termed food B12 malabsorption [26–28]. Elderly patients with B12 deficiency should undergo a screening upper endoscopy because of the association of gastric cancer with chronic *H. pylori* infection as well as the high incidence of gastric cancer and carcinoid tumor in patients with PA.

The hallmark laboratory feature of B12 deficiency is a vitamin B12 level of less than 200–250 ng/L. However, 22–30% of these patients may not have evidence of metabolic B12 deficiency as measured by methyl-malonic acid levels nor have evidence of megaloblastic anemia or neurologic impairment. These patients may have transcobalomin I (holocobalamin) deficiency [22]. The sensitivity of the assay used may also affect the number of patients identified with valid B12 deficiency [29]. Cobalamin acts as a cofactor in several important methyl transfer reactions such as conversion of methyl tetra hydrofolate to tetrahydrofolate, which participates in the generation of thymidine from uracil, the conversion homocysteine to methionine and the conversion of methyl malonyl CoA to succinyl CoA. As a result of cobalamin deficiency, these reactions are inhibited with a resulting increase in methyl-malonic acid (MMA), and homocysteine. In addition, as a result of reduced folate polyglutamation, folates tend to leak out of the red blood cells, resulting in a decrease in intracellular RBC folate and an increase in serum folate levels. Carmel recommends using at least two tests, vitamin B12 levels and either MMA or homocysteine levels, to confirm metabolic abnormalities [30]. These levels should be drawn before B12 supplementation starts, because they rapidly normalize with treatment [30]. Unfortunately, the Schilling's test is no longer widely available, making it difficult to confirm the specific diagnosis of PA. Intrinsic factor antibody tests, positive in 40–60% of patients with PA, should be drawn prior to intramuscular B12 replacement [30].

B12 deficiency responds rapidly. to replacement treatment. Carmel recommends initial intramuscular replacement of 1,000 µg. Weekly doses can be given for 4 weeks to replace the stores followed by monthly supplementation [30]. Reticulocyte response occurs about a week after the initial treatment and complete hematologic recovery (normalization of the hemoglobin and MCV) should occur by 8 weeks. In spite of very low hemoglobin values at presentation, transfusions are rarely needed and should be reserved for the patient with cardiac compromise. Daily oral B12 replacement may be more expensive and may be less reliable than intramuscular treatment since it relies on patient compliance.

Folate Deficiency

Folate requirements are much higher and stores are lower than cobalamin deficiency [31]. As a result, anemia due to folate deficiency develops within as little as 2 weeks with inadequate intake [21, 22]. In the Leiden 85 study, folate deficiency had a more profound effect on the development of anemia than did cobalamin deficiency [16]. Fifty percent of the folate in food is lost with cooking. Because of concerns of neural tube defects in the fetus, food and vitamin fortification with folate has significantly reduced the incidence of folate deficiency in the elderly. Nevertheless, elderly patients in countries where folate fortified products are not available, patients with jejunal disease, patients receiving dilantin therapy, patients with bacterial overgrowth, chronic dialysis and alcoholic patients may develop folate deficiency [22]. Alcohol reduces folate absorption and is often coupled with poor dietary intake [22]. Folate is crucial in the generation of

thymidine from uracil, so the lack of folate results in impaired DNA synthesis and macrocytosis and megaloblastosis. Red cell measurements are not widely available so the diagnosis relies on serum levels. Homocysteine levels may also be high in folate deficiency. However, MMA levels are *not* increased unless there is concurrent B12 deficiency. Folate replacement can be given orally and is highly and rapidly effective. The recommended daily dosing, for non-pregnant patients, is 400 µg daily [31].

Anemia of Chronic Inflammation

Aging is an inflammatory process [32]. The prevalence of anemia of chronic inflammation increases with increasing age. Alterations in cytokines with advancing age may contribute to anemia, as well as the "frailty" of older patients [32].The findings of a low serum iron, a low iron binding capacity, an elevated ferritin, a low soluble transferrin receptor suggest the diagnosis of anemia of chronic inflammation. Chronic inflammatory disorders such as diabetes, arthritis, atherosclerosis, and cancer occur more commonly in the elderly,and are associated with the production of inflammatory cytokines such as tumor necrosis factor alpha (TNF) interferon gamma and Interleukin-6 (IL-6). The metabolic syndrome of obesity, hyperlipidemia, and atherosclerosis is associated with increased hepcidin production through increased activation and transcription of the HAMP gene. This may result in the increase in hepcidin production, iron immobilization and the development of anemia of chronic inflammation (ACI) [33]. Hepcidin induces an internalization of the ferroportin receptors on the basolateral membrane of the duodenal cells, as well as on the macrophage cell, resulting in the inability to absorb and mobilize iron. In experimental systems, erythroid colony forming units grow poorly when exposed to serum from patients with chronic inflammation. T cells from patients who did not respond to erythropoietin have been shown to produce increased amounts of interferon gamma and tumor necrosis factor (TNF). This effect can be reversed using antibodies to either TNF alpha or interferon gamma. TNF and gamma interferon induce IL-6 production and can be shown to blunt hypoxia induced erythopoeitin production [34, 35]. Increases in IL-6 levels have been demonstrated in patients over the age of 70, and have been associated with increasing frailty and decreased functionality, anemia and increased mortality [32]. In ACI, hepcidin levels increase in response to increased IL-6. However, measurable increases in hepcidin were not observed in elderly anemic patients [36].

Hormone insufficiency of both estrogen and especially testosterone in older patients may have a role in modulating cytokine production. Both estrogen and especially testosterone appear to suppress NF-kappa B, which may allow an increase in the transcription of IL-6. Androgens have long been associated with an increase in red cell mass observed in men. Androgen deficiency in older males contributes to the increased incidence of anemia seen in the setting of normal bone marrow cellularity. A drop in hemoglobin of 1–2.5 g/dL may occur in patients with prostate cancer treated with androgen ablation. In the Invecchiare in Chianti study (In CHIANTI) of both men and women over the age of 65, there was a linear relationship between testosterone levels and hemoglobin levels. Patients with evidence of lower testosterone levels were at increased risk for developing anemia several years later [34, 37].

When associated with symptoms of anemia, ACI can be treated by erythropoietin supplementation. However, the effect of erythropoietin supplementation in elderly patients with ACI on quality of life and mortality is unknown.

Anemia Due to Renal Insufficiency

Renal dysfunction may be an important cause of anemia in the elderly. The decline in renal function with aging even in healthy elderly patients is well recognized [38, 39]. A study of healthy, non diabetic patients over the age of 60 demonstrated progressive decline in renal function with aging [39]. The presence of anemia was statistically correlated with a progressive decline in renal function at 4 years of follow up [39]. The reduction in renal function may be exacerbated by pre-existing diabetes, hypertension, and medications. As a consequence, erythropoietin (EPO) levels in these patients are significantly less than would be expected. Renal disease associated with diabetic nephropathy can cause a more significant degree of anemia even at relatively normal serum creatinine levels, with more pronounced suppression of EPO production [40]. Significant anemia due to renal insufficiency can be treated with erythropoietin supplementation As mentioned in the section on iron deficiency, iron supplementation with erythropoietin stimulating agents (ESAs) may be indicated in renal failure patients if the serum ferritin is less than 500 µg/L [14].

Bone Marrow Dysfunction and Myelodysplasia

Although hematologic measurements are the same in elderly patients as in younger patients, the ability of the bone marrow to respond to increased demands may be blunted in the elderly patient [41]. There does appear to be a reduction in the reconstituting capacity of hematopoetic stem cells (HSC) from older patients compared to younger patients although

the reason for this is unclear [42]. Stress, such as bleeding or infection, may unmask underlying age associated hematopoetic defects resulting in an impaired bone marrow response. This may be due to a paradoxical reduction in progenitor cells compared to the increase in progenitors seen in younger patients. Clinically this translates into a reduced reticulocyte response to bleeding and an impaired white blood cell response to infection [43]. Epigenetic changes, DNA damage, telomere erosion, increased apoptosis, and alterations in immune function may play a role [42, 44] (Fig. 16.3).

Myelodysplasia (MDS) is a common cause of bone marrow failure in the elderly. The prevalence increases significantly in patients greater than 70 years of age (20/100,000 patients) [41]. The spectrum of presentations is wide, with some patients presenting with isolated anemia, others with pancytopenia. Often, the anemia is macrocytic, with normal B12, MMA and folate levels. Leukopenia and neutropenia are present in 50% of patients with MDS, and thrombocytopenia may be the initial presentation in 25% of patients [41]. Dysplastic changes such as pseudo Pelger–Huet anomaly (bi-lobed neutrophils), or abnormal neutrophil granulation may be seen on peripheral blood smear. However, bone marrow evaluation with cytogenetics or FISH for the characteristic cytogenetic changes (5q- , monosomy 5,7 or 8, deletion /t-11q-, etc.) is the diagnostic test of choice [44]. While the French American British classification still used, the international prognosis staging score (IPSS), has replaced the FAB as the primary mode of classification. IPSS correlates survival with the presence or absence of cytopenias, and bone marrow findings such as the percentage of blasts and the presence or absence of cytogenetic abnormalities. Based on the IPSS, patients with low grade myelodysplasia (IPSS <1) have a considerably longer survival (5.7 years) compared to patients with IPSS Intermediate 1 (3.5 years), intermediate 2 (1.2 years), IPSS 2 (0.4 years) [45]. The IPSS is helpful in deciding on the appropriate therapy for elderly patients with MDS. Patients with low grade MDS may be treated with watchful waiting or ESAs. Patients with higher IPSS may be candidates for more intensive therapy with such as hypo-methylating agents, or histone deacetylase agents.

Thrombocytopenia and Platelet Dysfunction in the Elderly

Thrombocytopenia may be seen in elderly patients for multiple reasons. Many of the same disorders associated with the development of anemia in the elderly such as B12, folate deficiencies or MDS can also be associated with the development of thrombocytopenia. Bone marrow failure due to MDS is the most common cause of chronic thrombocytopenia in the elderly (see previous section). Acute

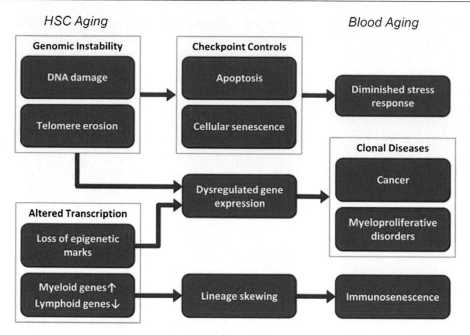

Fig. 16.3 Effect of aging on hematopoetic stem cells and the development of blood disorders. Proposed HSC aging mechanisms and their relationship to blood aging phenotypes. Stem cells accrue DNA damage with age, while the slow cycling of the HSC pool results in telomere erosion. To contain the risk of oncogenesis, cells have defense mechanisms which can sense genomic damage and trigger programmed cell death or permanent cell-cycle arrest (apoptosis and cellular senescence). As the burden of unrepaired damage in the stem cell pool increases, the frequency with which these pathways are activated in HSCs and their downstream progeny rises, and average HSC regenerative potential falls. Although this does not lead to stem cell exhaustion in normal aging, the reserve capacity to meet hematopoietic stress is reduced.

Genomic damage and epigenetic instability can also lead to malignant transformation of HSCs, progenitors or effector cells, manifesting acutely as cancer or chronically as myeloproliferative disorders. Changes in gene expression with age alter the propensity for HSCs to differentiate towards different blood cell lineages, a phenomenon known as "lineage skewing." Lymphoid progenitor numbers are reduced in old age, contributing to a fall in the production of naïve B and T cells. A shift in the peripheral lymphocyte population towards antigen-experienced memory cells and away from naïve cells underwrites the declining response to infection which typifies immunosenescence (Reprinted from Warren and Rossi [42], Copyright 2009, with permission from Elsevier)

thrombocytopenia is often due to infection or medication. Drug induced thrombocytopenia, both immune mediated and marrow suppressive is common [46]. The list of medications inducing thrombocytopenia is extensive. Some of the more frequent drugs are listed in Table 16.1. Of particular importance is heparin induced thrombocytopenia because of the frequency of exposure to heparins in the hospital setting and high risk of thrombosis and the high mortality seen in the disorder (see section on thrombosis).

Immune Thrombocytopenic Purpura

It was previously thought that idiopathic thrombocytopenic purpura (ITP) occurred most often in young female patients with less than 10% of cases occurring in patients over the age of 60 [47]. However, in a recent epidemiologic analysis by Abramson, it is clear that not only does the incidence of ITP increase significantly in patients greater than 60 years of age, but there is a male predominance in the older age population

[48]. Clinically significant fatal bleeding also increases with age [49]. ITP is a disorder characterized by antibody mediated increased platelet clearance as well as and decreased platelet production [50, 51]. Serum thrombopoetin (TPO) levels are not elevated in most cases of ITP. TPO is produced in the liver, binds to the megakaryocyte and platelet, and is removed from the circulation with clearance of the platelet. TPO levels may be low in liver disease and may contribute to the reduction of platelets seen in patients with liver dysfunction. In chronic ITP, significant bleeding usually does not occur until the platelet count drops below 30,000/mcL. Therefore, treatment intervention may not be required if the patient is asymptomatic and has a platelet count of greater than 30,000/mcL. However, if the platelet count falls below 30,000/mcL or the patient has bleeding manifestations intervention may be required. The treatment approach is twofold: first, to acutely increase the platelet count to minimize the bleeding risk using corticosteroids such as prednisone or high dose dexamethasone, anti-RhD or Intravenous immunoglobulin (IvIG). Second is to suppress antibody production using immunologic modulators such as azathioprine,

Table 16.1 Drugs that may commonly cause thrombocytopenia[a]

Drug (brand name)	Number of reports	
	Definite Evidence	Probable Evidence
Abciximab (ReoPro)	6	7
Acetaminophen (Tylenol, Panadol, and others)	3	4
Carbamezapine (Tegretol)	0	10
Chlorpropamide (Diabinese)	0	5
Cimetidine (Tagamet)	1	5
Danazol (Danocrine)	3	4
Diclofenac (Cataflam and Voltaren)	2	3
Efalizumab (Raptiva)	0	6
Eptifibatide (Integrilin)	2	7
Gold (Ridaura, Solganal, and others)	0	11
Hydrochlorothiazide (Aquazide-H, Esidrix, and others)	0	5
Interferon-α (Roferon-A and Intron A)	1	6
Methyldopa (Aldomet)	3	3
Nalidixic Acid (NegGram)	1	5
Quinidine (Quinaglute, Cardioquin, and others)	26	32
Quinine (Quinamm, Quindan, and others)	14	10
Ranitidine (Zantac)	0	5
Rifampin (Rifadin, Rimactane)	5	5
Tirofiban (Aggrestat)	2	6
Trimethoprim/sulfamethoxazole (Bactrim, Septra, and others)	3	12
Vancomycin (Vancoled)	3	4

Source: Reprinted with permission from George and Aster [46]
[a] Data from www.ouhsc.edu/platelets. Drugs were selected for this table because they had five or more published reports of individual patient data or group data with definite or probable evidence for a causal relation to thrombocytopenia

cyclosporine, or rituximab. Splenectomy can induce an unmaintained complete remission in 65% of patients refractory to initial treatment [52].

A new approach in refractory patients is the enhancement megakaryopoesis and platelet production with thrombopoietin receptor agonists, which have recently become available [53, 54]. Achieving a platelet count of 50,000/mcL or greater appears to be associated with a significant reduction in clinical bleeding related episodes [55].

Cardiac bypass may be associated with thrombocytopenia due to mechanical disruption of the platelets [56, 57]. "Late" thrombocytopenia, occurring greater than 5 days post bypass has been associated with prolonged hypothermia [58]. MDS may also be associated with platelet dysfunction as well as thrombocytopenia with significant clinical bleeding manifestations [59]. Medications which purposefully induce platelet dysfunction such as aspirin (ASA), clopedigril, and platelet glycoprotein IIbIIIa antagonists are commonly used in the elderly population.

Coagulation Disorders and Thrombosis

Coagulation parameters are very stable throughout adult life. There do not appear to be any specific alteration of the hemostatic system with aging. However, disorders of coagulation are common in the elderly due to liver dysfunction, anticoagulant therapy, sepsis, and acquired factors inhibitors.

Acquired factor inhibitors, albeit rare, occur with increased frequency in the elderly and may cause massive hemorrhage [60]. These acquired antibody inhibitors may develop after exposure to antibiotics, or vaccines, occur in patients with underlying immune or lymphoproliferative disorders, or may be idiopathic [60, 61]. Patients with inhibitors have markedly abnormal coagulation profiles depending on the nature of the inhibitor. The most frequent acquired inhibitor is against factor VIII. These patients with "acquired" hemophilia, present with profound, life threatening hemorrhage and marked prolongation of the aPTT. Unlike classical hemophilia patients, the inhibitor patients may present with mucosal and skin bleeding, as well as deep tissue and retroperitoneal bleeding. Prompt recognition of the process is crucial for a positive outcome. The treatment goals are: first, control of the hemorrhage using either recombinant Factor VIIa, FEIBA, or porcine factor VIII; second, suppression of antibody production. Corticosteroids and cyclophoshamide as well as rituximab, cyclosporine and azothioprine have been used successfully [61]. A nonrandomized study conducted by the United Kingdom Hemophilia Center Doctors' Organization (UKHCDO) did not find a significant difference among the groups treated with steroid alone, or with a combination of steroids and cytotoxic agents (76 vs. 78%) [62]. Aggarwal et al. treated four patients with autoimmune hemophilia and high-titer inhibitors with rituximab and observed durable complete response in two of them. The other two patients initially responded, then relapsed but responded to second courses of rituximab and prednisone [63]. Rituximab has been successfully used to treat patients with very high-titer acquired factor VIII inhibitors refractory to conventional chemotherapy [64, 65].

Thrombosis in the Elderly

In the elderly, anticoagulation therapy is frequently used to prevent cerebral vascular events in patients with atrial fibrillation, to prevent and treat venous thromboembolism (VTE). However, it is associated with an increased risk of bleeding. The incidence of venous thromboembolism is a phenomenon of aging. In patients aged 19, incidence of VTE is 1 per 100,000 patients. However, starting at age 50 the incidence increases dramatically, with an incidence of 1/1,000 patients,

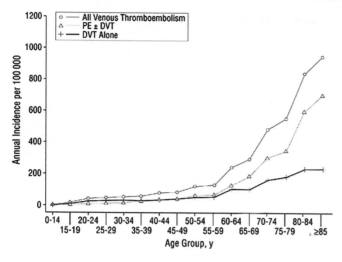

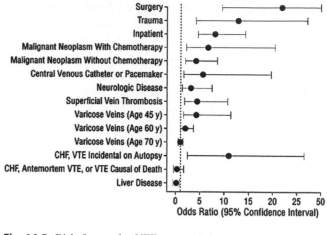

Fig. 16.4 Annual incidence of all venous thromboembolism, deep vein thrombosis (DVT) alone, and pulmonary embolism (PE) with or without deep vein thrombosis (PE (±) DVT) among residents of Olmsted County, Minnesota, from 1966 to 1990, by age (Reprinted with permission from Silverstein et al. [66], Copyright © 1998 American Medical Association. All rights reserved.)

Fig. 16.5 Risk factors for VTE: a population-based case contolled study based case control study (Reprinted with permission from Heit et al. [110], Copyright © 2000 American Medical Association. All rights reserved.)

in patients with cancer the incidence is 1/250 patients, and the risk for patients with cancer getting chemotherapy is 1/100 (Fig. 16.4) [66]. In the elderly, survival after venous thromboembolism is lower than younger patients, and survival after pulmonary embolism is much worse than after deep vein thrombosis alone [67]. The risk of early death among elderly patients with symptomatic pulmonary embolism is 18-fold higher compared to patients with deep vein thrombosis alone [67]. Most patients with underlying congenital hypercoaguable states usually present before the age of 50. However, elderly patients have multiple acquired risk factors for VTE, which predispose them to thrombosis independent of an underlying genetic risk. These include cancer, hip fractures, surgical procedures, hormone replacement therapy (HRT), and congestive heart failure. In a recent prospective analysis of 4486 consecutive patients with deep vein thrombosis (DVT), elderly patients (mean age 78) were more likely to have history of a recent hospitalization (49.2 vs. 44.7% $p=0.03$), congestive heart failure (20.5 vs. 9.9% $p<0.0001$), and recent immobilization (50.5% vs. 39.6% p <0.0001) compared to younger patients (mean age 51) [68]. In this elderly cohort, other comorbidities such as stroke, pneumonia, and chronic obstructive pulmonary disease were common. Elderly patients with DVT were less likely to present with symptoms of leg pain [68]. Less than half of the patients (41%) had received DVT prophylaxis [68, 69]. In view of this, anticoagulation prophylaxis has been strongly recommended for hospitalized elderly patients [68–70] (Fig. 16.5). Patients over the age of 40, with high risk surgeries, such as orthopedic, gynecologic, urogenital, abdominal surgery, cardiothoracic surgery, patients with myocardial

infarction should receive VTE prophylaxis [69]. Patients with cancer, and hip surgeries should be considered for 30 day extended prophylaxis [71, 72]. Low molecular weight heparins, fondiparinux (1A recommendation) as well as unfractionated heparin three times per day subcutaneously (1A recommendation), can be given for prophylaxis [70].

The treatment for patients with VTE should always start with either low molecular weight heparin (LMWH), fondiparinux (FDX) or unfractionated heparin. Vitamin K antagonists (VKA) should not be used acutely to treat the thrombosis as it takes at least 5 day to lower the vitamin K dependent clotting proteins regardless of the dose of VKA used [73]. With the exception of Tinzaparin, which may be used with a creatinine as low as 30 mL/min, patients with renal insufficiency should be treated with unfractionated heparin either intravenously or subcutaneously. Patients can then be transitioned to vitamin K antagonists such as warfarin, for secondary prophylaxis once antithrombotic therapy with heparins or anti Xa treatment has been started [70]. Antithrombotic therapy with heparins should be continued for a minimum of 5 days (even with a therapeutic INR) and until the prothrombin time (PT) INR is 2.5 for 24 h. Patients with active cancer should not be transitioned to warfarin, but continue on low molecular weight heparin as their secondary prophylaxis [70]. Two clinical trials in patients with active cancer receiving chemotherapy demonstrated significant reductions in recurrent events using the low molecular weight heparins, dalteparin (CLOT) or tinzaparin (LITE) compared to VKA [74, 75] The duration of anticoagulationcan be determined by the clinical circumstances associated with the development of the VTE. As per ACCP guidelines, anticoagulants for provoked events should be given for 3 months. Patients with idiopathic DVT or patients with pulmonary embolism should receive at least 6 months of treatment. Patients with persistent risk factors, evidence of residual clot or increased plasma D-Dimers after VKA treatment has stopped should be considered for longer treatment [70].

Because of the narrow therapeutic window, risk of serious bleeding and the need for strict monitoring with VKA, several new oral anticoagulants have been developed. In the recent RE-COVER trial, dabigtran, an oral direct thrombin inhibitor, was given to patients with DVT/PE following initial intravenous heparin or subcutaneous LMWH therapy. In this randomized, double blind, double dummy trial, patients were treated with warfarin or dabigatran for 6 months. There was no evidence of inferiority of the dabigatran, compared to the warfarin, and no evidence of increased bleeding on the dabigatran arm [76]. Unlike warfarin, dabigatran has a wide therapeutic window and does not need monitoring. Recent studies evaluating the role of an oral direct factor Xa inhibitors, Rivaroxiban, and (Apixiban) are quite promising both for treatment and prophylaxis [77–79]. Although approved in Europe and Canada, these medications are still awaiting US Federal Drug Agency (FDA) approval.

Heparin Induced Thrombocytopenia

Heparin use in cardiac and vascular surgery patients is ubiquitous. Therefore, the differential diagnosis of thrombocytopenia in these patients must include consideration of heparin-induced thrombocytopenia (HIT). HIT is the most significant adverse event associated with heparin use. HIT is an immunologic disorder that places patients at a significantly higher risk of developing venous and arterial thrombosis, and is associated with a substantial mortality [80, 81–87]. In contrast to other forms of thrombocytopenia, HIT is not associated with bleeding.

The diagnosis of HIT is based upon clinical findings, including the development of thrombocytopenia and/or thrombosis during or immediately following heparin use [80, 82, 83, 85, 88, 89]. Rapid onset HIT can occur as early as 24 h of heparin treatment in patients who have been exposed to heparin within previous 100 days and have developed HIT antibodies [90]. While the development of thrombocytopenia or an unexplained decrease in the platelet count (>50% of pretreatment baseline) during heparin exposure is the clinical hallmark of this disorder, thrombotic complications develop in 30–70% of HIT patients accounting for much of the morbidity associated with this diagnosis [84, 85, 88, 89]. The death rates due to thrombosis in these retrospective studies are between 40 and 50% [84, 85, 88, 89]. Thrombotic complications may occur even when the platelet count nadir remains

greater than $150 \times 10^9/L$ [88]. Severe thrombocytopenia (platelet count less than 20,000) is rare with HIT. In large clinical studies of HIT, the median platelet count nadir is in the range of $50–60 \times 10^9/L$ [84, 85, 89]. The development of new thrombosis or progression of an existing venous or arterial thrombosis in a patient receiving heparin, particularly if accompanied by a drop in the platelet count is highly suggestive of HIT. The incidence of HIT varies depending upon the patient population, duration and type of heparin utilized, and medical or surgical procedure [81–85, 89–95]. Unlike ITP, where antibody mediated platelet clearance and impaired platelet production reduce the platelet count, HIT is an immunologic disorder in which there is a polyclonal antibody response against neo-antigens expressed on platelet factor 4 (PF4) as a result of heparin binding to this protein. The antibody induces platelet activation by binding to the platelet Fc receptor [96, 97]. Platelet activation is mediated exclusively by IgG antibodies directed against the heparin-PF4 complex [96–98]. The larger heparin molecules, unfractionated heparin, induce larger PF4 bundles which cause greater antibody binding. This may explain the greater incidence of HIT observed with unfractionated heparin as opposed to low molecular weight heparin.

The binding of the heparin-PF4 complex by the Fc domain of the HIT IgG antibodies through the platelet Fc receptors results in platelet activation and vesiculation [99, 100].The activated platelets release membrane microparticles, which express P-selectin capable of to binding monocytes and inducing tissue factor expression, the initiator of the coagulation cascade [101, 102]. However, Heparin-PF4/HIT IgG complexes have also been reported to independently induce tissue factor expression and cytokine release from monocytes and macrophages [103]. Tissue factor generation activates coagulation leading to significant thrombin generation, which in turn activates and aggregates more platelets which worsens the thrombocytopenia. Clinical HIT is similar to disseminated intravascular coagulation, since both syndromes are mediated by excessive thrombin generation resulting in thrombosis and increased platelet consumption [104]. While venous thrombosis predominates over arterial thrombotic events at a rate of 4:1, the targeting of specific thrombotic events in patients with HIT can be explained in part by the clinical circumstances associated with the development of HIT [83]. Patients who develop HIT during treatment of venous thrombosis are most likely to develop new or progressive venous thromboembolism. Antecedent arterial events may precipitate additional arterial thromboses. If HIT is not diagnosed promptly and appropriately treat treated, thrombotic events at multiple sites can occur as seen is patients with disseminated intravascular coagulation [105].

Appropriate platelet monitoring is essential to the early diagnosis of HIT. In heparin naive patients, the platelet count should be monitored every other day beginning 5 days after starting heparin. In patients with previous heparin exposure, the platelets should be monitored with the start of heparin use. A 50% or greater decrease in platelet count from the pre-treatment platelet count should alert the clinician to development of HIT [80, 82, 106]. The development of platelet activating, non-complement fixing IgG antibodies directed against the complex of heparin and platelet factor 4 is the hallmark of this disorder [90, 96, 97, 106]. Confirmation of a clinical suspicion of HIT requires serologic screening for HIT associated heparin/platelet factor 4 (H/PF4) antibodies [90, 96, 97]. Prospective studies of H/PF4 antibody formation indicate that clinical HIT occurs in a minority of patients who form antibodies [107]. Antibody detection can be performed by either the use of functional assays which detect antibodies capable of inducing platelet activation (serotonin release assay), or by a PF4/heparin immunoassay (ELISA). H/PF4 ELISA has significant sensitivity (>90–95%) and specificity (80–90%) [106]. A negative ELISA has a strong negative predictive value of >95%, suggesting an alternate diagnosis for thrombocytopenia. A strongly positive ELISA is also more likely to be associated with a positive functional assay as determined by either a washed platelet C^{14}-serotonin-release assay (SRA) or heparin-induced washed platelet aggregation assay [106]. A positive platelet SRA or platelet aggregation assay has a reported sensitivity of greater than 90% and specificity for clinical HIT of greater than 95% [106]. The combined use of both the PF4/heparin ELISA and a functional assay provide a diagnostic sensitivity approaching 100% for clinical HIT [106].

Prompt recognition of the disorder, immediate cessation of *all forms* of heparin and rapid initiation of a direct thrombin inhibitor such as argatroban, lepirudin or bivalrudin is essential in reducing the morbidity and mortality in HIT. Approximately 50% of patients with HIT presenting with thrombocytopenia alone will develop thrombosis with only discontinuation of heparin [83]. The use of warfarin alone in these patients is *not* protective and warfarin loading after a diagnosis of HIT can result in severe thrombotic complications, such as ischemic limb gangrene [83, 108]. Other thrombotic complications reported in patients with HIT include overt DIC with hypofibrinogenemia, adrenal necrosis, and cutaneous necrosis at the sites of heparin injections [80, 88]. Patients can be transitioned to warfarin after the platelet count has completely recovered, indicating the reduction in thrombin generation. HIT appears to be a unique event in many patients, without recurrence. However, patients within 100 days of diagnosis should not receive any form of heparin therapy [90, 109]. Patients beyond 100 days may receive heparin, if indicated, but should have daily platelet counts monitored. Antibody testing should be closely followed to make sure the patient does not have a recurrence.

As the general population ages, knowledge of the unique hematologic problems seen in the elderly will become increasingly important. Prompt recognition and intervention may result in an improvement in the quality of life and a reduction in mortality in elderly patients.

References

1. World Health Organization. Nutritional anaemias: report of a WHO Scientific Group. Geneva: World Health Organization; 1968.
2. Guralnik JM, Eisenstaedt RS, Ferrucci L, Klein HG, Woodman RC. Prevalence of anemia in persons 65 years and older in the United States: evidence for a high rate of unexplained anemia. Blood. 2004;104:2263–8.
3. Beutler E, Waalen J. The definition of anemia: what is the lower limit of normal of the blood hemoglobin concentration. Blood. 2006;107(5):1747–50.
4. Joosten E, Pelemans W, Hiele M, Noyen J, Verhaeghe R, Boogaerts MA. Prevalence and causes of anaemia in a geriatric population. Gerontology. 1992;38:111–7.
5. Westendorp IGJ, Knook DL RG. The definition of anemia in older patients. JAMA. 1999;281:1714–7.
6. Endres HG, Wedding U, Pittrow D, Thiem U, Trampisch HJ, Diehm C. Prevalence of anemia in elderly patients in primary care: impact on 5 year mortality risk and differences between men and women. Curr Med Res Opin. 2009;25(5):1143–58.
7. Culleton BF, Manns BJ, Zhang J, Tonelli M, Klarenbach S, Hemmelgarn BR. Impact of anemia on hospitalization and mortality in older adults. Blood. 2006;107(10):3841–6.
8. den Elzen WPJ, Willems JM, Westendorp RGJ, de Craen AJM, Assendelft WJJ, Gussekloo J. Effect of anemia and comorbidity on functional status, and mortality in old age: results from the Lieden 85-plus study. CMAJ. 2009;181:151–7.
9. Ezekowitz JA, McAlister FA, Armstromg PW. Anemia is common in heart failure and is associated with poor outcomes: Insight from a cohort of 12,065 patients with new-onset heart failure. Circulation. 2003;107:223–5.
10. Andres E, Federici L, Serraj K. Update of nutrient-deficiency anemia in elderly patients. Eur J Intern Med. 2008;19(7):4888–93.
11. Fleming AF. Iron deficiency in the tropics. Clin Haematol. 1975;11:365–88.
12. Wilson A, Reyes E, Ofam J. Prevalence and outcomes of anemia in inflammatory bowel disease: a systemic review of the literature. Am J Med. 2004;116(s7A):44s–9.
13. Guyatt GH, Patterson C, Ali M, Levine M, Turpie I, Meyer R. Diagnosis of iron deficiency in the elderly. Am J Med. 1990;88:205–9.
14. Grabe DW. Update on clinical practice recommendations and new therapeutic modalities in treating patients with chronic kidney disease. Am J Health Syst Pharm. 2007;13 Suppl 8:S8–14.
15. Carmel R. Prevalence of undiagnosed pernicious anemia in the elderly. Arch Intern Med. 1996;156:1097–100.
16. den Elzen WP, Westendorp RG, Frölich M, de Ruijter W, Assendelft WJ, Gussekloo J. Vitamin B12 and folate and the risk of anemia in old age. Arch Intern Med. 2008;168(20):2238–44.
17. Carmel R, Green R, Jacobsen DW, Rasmussen K, Florea M, Azen C. Serum cobalamin, homocysteine and methylmalonic acid concentrations in a multiethnic elderly population: Ethnic and sex differences in cobalamin and metabolite abnormalities. Am J Clin Nutr. 1999;70:904–10.

18. Carmel R. Macrocytosis, mild anemia, and delay in diagnosis of pernicious anemia. Arch Intern Med. 1979;139(1):47–50.
19. Carmel R. Pernicious anemia: the expected findings of very low serum cobalamin levels, anemia, and macrocytosis are often lacking. Arch Intern Med. 1988;148:1712–4.
20. Chan CW, Liu SY, Kho CS, Lau KH, Chu WR, Ma SK. Diagnostic clues to megaloblastic anaemia without macrocytosis. Int J Lab Hematol. 2007;29:163–71.
21. Herbert V. Experimental nutritional folate deficiency in man. Trans Assoc Am Physicians. 1962;75:307–20.
22. Carmel R. Nutritional Anemias in the Elderly. Semin Hematol. 2008;45(4):225–34.
23. Wang YH, Yan F, Zhang WB, Ye G, Zheng XH, Shao FY. An investigation of vitamin B12 deficiency in elderly inpatients in a neurology department. Neurosci Bull. 2009;25(4):209–15.
24. Barrios M, Alliot C. Venous thrombosis associated with pernicious anaemia. A report of two cases and review. Hematology. 2006;11(2):135–8.
25. Baik HW, Russell RM. Vitamin B12 deficiency in the elderly. Annu Rev Nutr. 1999;19:357–77.
26. Toh BH, van Driel IR, Gleeson P. Pernicious anemia. N Engl J Med. 1997;337(20):1441–8.
27. Strickland RG, Hooper B. The parietal cell heteroantibody in human sera: prevalence in a normal population and relationship to parietal cell autoantibody. Pathology. 1972;4:259–63.
28. Miller A, Furlong D, Burrows BA, Slingland DW. Bound vitamin B12 absorption in patients with low serum B12 levels. Am J Hematol. 1992;40:163–6.
29. Carmel R, Brar S, Agarwal A, Penha PD. Clin Chem. 2000;46(12)2017.
30. Carmel R. How I treat B12 deficiency. Blood. 2008;115(6):2214–21.
31. Panel on Folate, other B Vitamins, and Choline; Institute of medicine. Folate in dietary reference intakes; thiamine, riboflavin, niacin, vitamin B6, folate, vitamin B12, pantothenic acid, biotin, and choline. Washington, DC: National Academy of Science; 1998. p. 196–305.
32. Ershler WB. Biologic interactions of aging anemia: a focus on cytokines. J Am Geriatr Soc. 2003;51:S18–21.
33. Kemna EHJM, Tjalsma H, Willens HL, Swinkels DW. Hepcidin: from discovery to differential diagnosis. Haematologica. 2008;93:90–7.
34. Makipour S, Kanapuru B, Ershler WB. Unexplained anemia in the elderly. Semin Hematol. 2008;45:250–4.
35. Macdougall IC, Cooper AC. Erythropoietin resistance: the role of inflammation and pro-inflammatory cytokines. Nephrol Dial Transplan. 2002;17 Suppl 11:39–43.
36. Gelbart T, Waalen J, Beutler E. Anemia of aging is not associated with increased plasma hepcidin levels. Blood Mol Dis. 2008;41(3):252–4.
37. Ferrucci L, Maggio M, Bandinelli S, Basaria S, Laurentani F, Ble A, et al. Low testosterone levels and the risk of anemia in older men and women. Arch Intern Med. 2006;166:1380–8.
38. Fliser D. Assessment of renal function in elderly patients. Curr Opin Nephrol Hypertens. 2008;17:604–8.
39. Lee YT, Chiu HC, Su HM, Yang JF, Voon WC, Lin TH, et al. Lower hemoglobin concentrations, and subsequent decline in kidney function in an apparently healthy population aged 60 year and older. Clin Chim Acta. 2008;389:25–30.
40. Rarick MU, Espina BM, Colley DT, Chrusoskie A, Gandara S, Feinstein DI. Treatment of a unique anemia in patients with IDDM with epoetin alfa. Treatment of a unique anemia in patients with IDDM with epoetin alfa. Diab Care. 1998;21:423–6.
41. Rothstein G. J Am Geriatr Soc 2003; n51:s22–26.
42. Warren LA, Rossi DJ. Stem cells and aging in the hematopoetic. Mech Ageing Dev. 2009;130:46–53.
43. Buchanan JP, Peters CA, Rasmussen C, Rothstein G. Impaired expression of hematopoetic growth factors: A candidate mechanism for the hematopoetic defect of aging. Exp Gerontol. 1996;31:135–44.
44. Liu Y, Asai T, Nimer SD. Myelodysplasia: battle in the bone marrow. Nat Med. 2010;16(1):30–2.
45. Greenberg P, Cox C, LeBeau MM, et al. International scoring system for evaluating prognosis in myelodysplastic syndromes. Blood. 1998;91:1100.
46. George J, Aster R. Drug-induced thrombocytopenia: pathogenesis, evaluation, and management. Hematology Am Soc Hematol Educ Program. 2009; 153–8.
47. Doan CA, Bouroncel BA, Wiseman DK. Idiopathic and secondary thrombocytopenic purpura: Clinical study and evaluation of 381 cases over a 28 years. Ann Intern Med. 1960;53:861–76.
48. Abrahamson PE, Feudjo-Tepie HSA, Mitrani-Gold FS M, Logie J. The incidence of idiopathic thrombocytopenic purpura among adults: a population-based study and literature review. Eur J Haematol. 2009;83(2):83–9.
49. Cohen YC, Djulbegovic B, Shamai-Lubovitz O, Mozes B. The bleeding risk and natural history of idiopathic thrombocytopenic purpura in patients with persistent low platelet counts. Arch Intern Med. 2000;160:1630–8.
50. Ballen PJ, Segal DM, Stratton JR, et al. Mechanism of response in chronic autoimmune thrombocytopenic purpura. Evidence for impaired platelet production and increased platelet clearance. J Clin Invest. 1987;80:33.
51. Gernsheimer T, Stratton J, Ballem PJ, Slichter SJ. Mechanisms of response to treatment in autoimmune thrombocytopenic purpura. N Engl J Med. 1989;320:974.
52. Kojouri K, Vesely SK, Terrell DR, George JN. Splenectomy for adult patients with idiopathic thrombocytopenic purpura: a systemic review to assess long term platelet responses, prediction of response, and surgical complications. Blood. 2004;104:2623–36.
53. Kuter DJ, Bussel JB, Lyons RM, Pullarkat V, Gernsheimer TB, Senecal FM, et al. Efficacy of romiplostim in patients with chronic immune thrombocytopenic purpura: a double-blind randomised controlled trial. Lancet. 2008;371(9610):395–403.
54. Bussel JB, Provan D, Shamsi T, Cheng G, Psaila B, Kovaleva L, et al. Effect of eltrombopag on platelet counts and bleeding during treatment of chronic idiopathic thrombocytopenic purpura: a randomised, double-blind, placebo-controlled trial. Lancet. 2009;373(9664):641–8.
55. Weitz IC, Sanz M, Henry D, Schipperus M, Godeau B, Gleeson M, et al. Evaluation of bleeding-related episodes in patients with chronic immune thrombocytopenia (ITP) treated with romiplostim in two phase 3 placebo-controlled clinical trials. Washington, DC: American Society of Hematology. 2009: abstr no. 891.
56. Khuri SF, Wolfe JA, Josa M, Axford TC, Szymanski I, Assousa S, et al. Hematologic changes during and after cardiopulmonary bypass and their relationship to bleeding time and nonsurgical blood loss. J Thorac Cardiovasc Surg. 1992;104:94–107.
57. Colman RW. Platelet and neutrophil activation in cardiopulmonary bypass. Ann Thorac Surg. 1990;49:32–4.
58. Ranucci M, Carlucci C, Isgro G, Brozzi S, Boncilli A, Costa E, et al. Hypothermic cardiopulmonary bypass as a determinant of late thrombocytopenia following cardiac operations in pediatric patients. Acta Anaesthesiol Scand. 2009;53:1060–7.
59. Brumitt DR, Barker HF, Pujol-Moix N. A new platelet parameter, the mean platelet component, can demonstrate abnormal platelet function and structure in myelodysplasia. Clin Lab Haematol. 2003;25(1):59–62.
60. Cohen AJ, Kessler CM. Acquired inhibitors. Baillieres Clin Haematol. 1996;9:331–54.
61. Franchini M, Lippi G. Acquired factor VIII inhibitors. Blood. 2008;112(2):250–5.

62. Collins PW, Hirsch S, Baglin TP, et al. Acquired hemophilia A in the United Kingdom: a 2 year national surveillance study by the United Kingdom Center Doctors' Organization. Blood. 2007;109:1870–7.

63. Aggarwal A, Grewal R, Green RJ, et al. Rituximab for autoimmune haemophilia: a proposed treatment algorithm. Haemophilia. 2005;11:13–9.

64. Stasi R, Brunetti M, Stipa E. Amadori S B-cell depletion with rituximab for the treatment of patients with acquired hemophilia. Blood. 2004;103:4424–8.

65. Field JJ, Fenske TS, Blinder MA. Rituximab for the treatment of very high-titre acquired factor VIII inhibitors refractory to conventional chemotherapy. Haemophilia. 2007;13:46–50.

66. Silverstein M, Heit JA, Mohr DN, et al. Trends in incidence of deep venous thrombosis and pulmonary embolism: 25 year population based study. Arch Intern Med. 1998;158:58–593.

67. Heit JA. The epidemiology of venous thromboembolism in the community: implications for prevention and management. J Thromb Thrombolysis. 2006;21(1):23–9.

68. Seddighzadeh PG, Goldhaber SZ A. Deep-vein thrombosis in the elderly. Clin Appl Thromb/Hemost. 2008;14(4):393–8.

69. Bosson JL, Labarere J, Sevestre MA, Belmin J, Beyssier L, Elias A, et al. Deep vein thrombosis in elderly patients hospitalized in subacute care facilities: a multicenter cross-sectional study of risk factors, prophylaxis, and prevalence. Arch Intern Med. 2003; 163(21):2613–8.

70. Geerts WH, Bergqvist D, Pineo GF, Heit JA, Samama CM, Lassen MR, et al. Prevention of venous thromboembolism: American College of Chest Physicians evidence-based clinical practice guidelines (8th edition). Chest. 2008;133(6 Suppl):381S–453.

71. Harrison L, Johnston M, Massicotte MP, Crowther M, Moffat K, Hirsh J. Comparison of 5-mg and 10-mg loading does in initiation of warfarin therapy. Ann Intern Med. 1997;126:133–6.

72. Agnelli G, Bevquist D, Cohen AT, Gallus AS, Gent M, et al. Randomized clinical trial of post operative fonsiparinux versus perioperative dalteparin for the prevention of venous thromboembolism in high risk abdominal surgery. Br J Surg. 2005;92(10): 1212–20.

73. Blanchard E, Ansell J. Extended anticoagulation therapy for the primary and secondary prevention of venous thromboembolism. Drugs. 2005;65(3):303–11.

74. Lee AY, Levine MN, Baker RI, et al. Low-molecularweight heparin versus a coumarin for the prevention of recurrent venous thromboembolism in patients with cancer. N Engl J Med. 2003;349:146–53.

75. Hull RD, Pineo GF, Brant RF, Mah AF, Burke N, Dear R, et al. LITE trial investigators long-term low-molecular-weight heparin versus usual care in proximal-vein thrombosis patients with cancer. Am J Med. 2006;119(12):1062–72.

76. Schulman S, Kearon C, Kakkar AK, Mismetti P, Schellong S, Eriksson H, Baanstra D, Schnee J, Goldhaber SZ, for the RE-COVER Study Group. Dabigatran versus warfarin in the treatment of acute venous thromboembolism. NEJM 2009;361:2342–2352.

77. Eriksson, B.I., Borris, L.C., Friedman, R.J., Haas, S., Huisman, M.V., Kakkar, A.K., Bandel, T.J., Beckmann, H., Muehlhofer, E., Misselwitz, F., Geerts, W. & RECORD1 Study Group. Rivaroxaban versus enoxaparin for thromboprophylaxis after hip arthroplasty. N Engl J Med. 2008;358:2765–75.

78. Kakkar AK, Brenner B, Dahl OE, Eriksson BI, Mouret P, Muntz J, et al. Extended duration rivaroxaban versus short-term enoxaparin for the prevention of venous thromboembolism after total hip arthroplasty: a double-blind, randomized controlled trial. Lancet. 2008;372:31–9.

79. Lassen MR, Ageno W, Borris LC, Lieberman JR, Rosencher N, Bandel TJ, et al. Rivaroxaban versus enoxaparin for thromboprophylaxis after total knee arthroplasty. N Engl J Med. 2008;358: 2776–86.

80. Warkentin TE, Greinacher A. Heparin-induced thrombocytopenia: Recognition, treatment and prevention. Chest. 2004; 126:311S.

81. Kelton JG. The pathophysiology of heparin-induced thrombocytopenia. Biological basis for treatment. Chest. 2005;127:9S.

82. Warkentin TE. New approaches to the diagnosis of heparin-induced thrombocytopenia. Chest. 2005;127:35S.

83. Warkentin TE, Kelton JG. A 14 year study of heparin-induced thrombocytopenia. Am J Med. 1996;101:502.

84. Nand S, Wong W, Yuen B, et al. Heparin-induce thrombocytopenia with thrombosis: incidence, analysis of risk factors, and clinical outcomes in 108 consecutive patients treated at a single institution. Am J Hematol. 1998;56:12.

85. Wallis DE, Workman DL, Lewis BE, et al. Failure of early heparin cessation as treatment for heparin-induced thrombocytopenia. Am J Med. 1999;106:629.

86. Weismann RE, Tobin RW. Arterial embolism occurring during systemic heparin therapy. AMA Arch Surg. 1958;76:219.

87. Rhodes GR, Dixon RH, Silver D. Heparin induced thrombocytopenia with thrombotic and hemorrhagic manifestations. Surg Gynecol Obstet. 1973;136:409.

88. Warkentin TE. Clinical presentation of heparin-induced thrombocytopenia. Semin Hematol. 1998;35(4 suppl 5):9.

89. Warkentin TE. Management of heparin-induced thrombocytopenia: a critical comparison of lepirudin and argatroban. Thromb Res. 2003;110:73.

90. Warkentin TE, Kelton JG. Temporal aspects of heparin-induced thrombocytopenia. N Engl J Med. 2001;344:1286.

91. Hong AP, Cook DJ, Sigouin CS, et al. Central venous catheters and upper extremity deep-vein thrombosis complicating immune heparin-induced thrombocytopenia. Blood. 2003;101:3049.

92. Girolami B, Prandoni P, Stepfani PM, et al. The incidence of heparin-induced thrombocytopenia in hospitalized medical patients treated with subcutaneous unfractionated heparin: a prospective cohort study. Blood. 2003;101:2955.

93. Warkentin TE, Roberts RS, Hirsh J, et al. An improved definition of immune heparin-induced thrombocytopenia in postoperative orthopedic patients. Arch Intern Med. 2003;163:2514.

94. Jackson MR, Gillespie DL, Chang AS, et al. The incidence of heparin-induced antibodies in patients undergoing vascular surgery: A prospective study. J Vasc Surg. 1998;28:439.

95. Lindhoff-Last E, Eichler P, Stein M, et al. A prospective study on the incidence and clinical relevance of heparin-induced antibodies in patients after vascular surgery. Thromb Res. 2000;97:387.

96. Amiral J, Bridey F, Dreyfus M, et al. Platelet factor 4 complexed to heparin is the target for antibodies generated in heparin-induced thrombocytopenia. Thromb Haemost. 1992;68:95.

97. Kelton JG, Smith JW, Warkentin TE, et al. Immunoglobulin G from patients with heparin-induced thrombocytopenia binds to a complex of heparin and platelet factor 4. Blood. 1994;83:3232.

98. Horsewood P, Warkentin TE, Hayward CP, et al. The epitope specificity of heparin-induced thrombocytopenia. Br J Haematol. 1996;95:161.

99. Kelton JG, Sheridan D, Santos A, et al. Heparin-induced thrombocytopenia: laboratory studies. Blood. 1988;72:925.

100. Nieswandt B, Bergmeier W, Schulte V, et al. Expression and function of the mouse collagen receptor glycoprotein VI is strictly dependent on its association with the FcR-gamma chain. J Biol Chem. 2000;275:23998.

101. Warkentin TE, Hayward CP, Boshkov LK, et al. Sera from patients with heparin-induced thrombocytopenia generate platelet-derived microparticles with procoagulant activity: an explanation for the thrombotic complications of heparin-induced thrombocytopenia. Blood. 1994;84:3691.

102. Furie B, Furie BC. P-selectin induction of tissue factor biosynthesis. Haemostasis. 1996;26 suppl 1:60.

103. Pouplard C, Iochmann S, Renard B, et al. Induction of monocytes tissue factor expression by antibodies to heparin-platelet factor 4 complexes developed in heparin-induced thrombocytopenia. Blood. 2001;97(10):3300–2.

104. Liebman HA, Weitz IC. Disseminated intravascular coagulation, Chapter 125. In: Hoffman R, Benz EJ, Shattil SJ, Furie B, Cohen HJ, Silbertein L, McGlave P, editors. Hematology: basic principles and practice. 4th ed. New York, NY: McGraw-Hill; 2004. p. 2169–82.

105. Klein HG, Bell WR. Disseminated intravascular coagulation during heparin therapy. Ann Intern Med. 1974;80:477.

106. Warkentin TE. Platelet count monitoring and laboratory testing for heparin-induced thrombocytopenia. Recommendations of the College of American Pathologists. Arch Pathol Lab Med. 2002;126:1415.

107. Lee DH, Warkentin TE. Frequency of heparin-induced thrombocytopenia. In: Warkentin TE, Greinacher A, editors. Heparin-induced thrombocytopenia. 3rd ed. New York, NY: Marcel Dekker; 2004. p. 107–48.

108. Warkentin TE, Elavathil LJ, Hayward CP, et al. The pathogenesis of venous limb gangrene associated with heparin-induced thrombocytopenia. Ann Intern Med. 1997;127:804.

109. Lubenow N, Kempf R, Eichner A, et al. Heparin-induced thrombocytopenia: temporal pattern of thrombocytopenia in relation to initial use or reexposure to heparin. Chest. 2002;122:37.

110. Heit JA, Silverstein MD, Mohr DN, Petterson TM, O'Fallon WM, Melton III LJ. Risk factors for deep vein thrombosis and pulmonary embolism: a population-based case-control study. Arch Intern Med. 2000;160(6):809.

platelet adhesiveness, and a reduction in thrombolytic activity [5, 6]. Increases in tissue plasminogen activator (tPA), plasminogen activator, fibrinogen, Factors V, VII, VII and IX, proteins S and C and von Willebrand factor all increase with advancing age [7]. Although there are alterations in anticoagulant factors as well, the balance is tipped toward the hemostatic state. Decreased plasminogen tissue activator inhibitor 1 (PAI1) reduces the thrombolytic activity in older adults [6]. In addition to age-associated changes in platelet proclivity to aggregate, the older adult is rendered more prone to thromboembolic events due to changes in the endothelial wall and increases in inflammatory factors such as IL-6, all of which promote hemostasis [6]. Moreover, age-associated changes in venous valves render them less able to coapt which may increase venous pooling and reduce venous return, both of which increase vulnerability of the older patient to VTE. It is also more likely for a person of advanced age to have a history of deep vein thrombosis (DVT) or leg trauma which may further increase their risk of recurrent DVT due to endothelial injury. Comorbidities (malignancies, prior stroke, myelodysplasias) and frailty may also render some surgical patients more immobile post-operatively contributing to blood stasis. These changes significantly augment the risk of older adults for VTE, pulmonary embolism (PE), stroke, coronary events and, rarely, arterial thromboses as well as an increase in prosthetic valve and vascular graft thrombosis [8].

ulcer disease, and diverticulosis are more prevalent. Intracranial hemorrhage (ICH) is also more common in seniors, and is thought to be due to microvasculopathy as well as trauma from falls [10, 11]. Adverse bleeding events can also be associated with metastatic cancer, especially intracranially lesions. Several frequently taken medications in this age group increase the risk of bleeding, including anti-inflammatory drugs (non-steroidal and steroids) and other medications which impact hemostasis including aspirin, thienopyridines, selective serotonin reuptake inhibitors and several herbal substances (garlic, gingko biloba) [12, 13]. Polypharmacy in the older patient also increases the risk of drug-drug interactions, especially with VKA. In fact, much of the elevated bleeding risk in older adults on chronic anticoagulation is due to supratherapeutic levels, often caused by these interactions [10, 11, 14]. As warfarin is bound to plasma protein, those with poor nutrition, synthetic liver dysfunction and/or heart failure may require much lower doses of VKA to achieve therapeutic protimes [14]. Reduction in VKA dose over time occurs as a function of age as is discussed below [15]. In addition, age-related decline in kidney function impacts the dosing of renally cleared anticoagulants, low molecular weight heparins and fondaparinux and creatinine clearance (CrCl) must be calculated in all older patients to accurately measure their kidney function before considering or dosing such medications [1, 16].

Increased Risk of Bleeding in Older Adults

Given that aging is associated with a thrombophilic state, the choice to therapeutically reduce this risk would be evident were it not for the coincident increase in bleeding risk in seniors. Fragility of skin and reduction in subcutaneous fat increases the incidence of bruising and superficial bleeding. Moreover, aging changes and comorbidities commonly seen in older adults may lead to more significant and life altering or deadly bleeding events [9]. In older patients, gastrointestinal (GI) bleeding is more commonly associated with *Helicobacter pylori* infection [10] and gastritis, a history of

Specific Contraindications for Chronic Oral Anticoagulation

Because of the significant elevation in thrombotic risk in older adults, chronic OAT is often recommended [17]. However, given the increase in risk of major bleeding events, falls, ICH and GI bleeding, prescribing OAT is often met with understandable concern. It is important to place this concern in the context of the published absolute and relative contraindications for OAT, noting that many of the most feared risks do not constitute contraindications (Table 17.1) [17].

Table .17.1 Contraindications to chronic oral anticoagulation therapy

Absolute	Relative	No contraindication
Bleeding diathesis	Significant alcohol use (>60 mL/d)	Predisposition to falling
Thrombocytopenia (<50,000/μL)		Perceived inability to adequately control INR status because of age
Untreated or poorly controlled hypertension (consistently>160/90 mmHg)	Conventional NSAID use (without cytoprotection)	Conventional NSAID use with misoprostol or proton pump inhibitor
Noncompliance with medication or INR monitoring	Participation in activities predisposing to trauma	Cyclooxygenase-2 inhibitor-specific NSAID use
		Recent, resolved peptic ulcer disease bleeding (with *Helicobacter pylori* testing and treatment)
		Pervious stroke

Source: Data from Man-Son-Hing [10]

Pharmacologic Changes

Taken together, increased thrombotic risk and elevated bleeding risk in older adults magnifies the importance of vigilant use of anticoagulant medication to keep them in their narrow therapeutic window. This can be challenging, given the issues of a vulnerable substrate, polypharmacy and multimorbidities which can additionally affect the delicate hemostatic balance [14]. Important changes in pharmacokinetics and pharmacodynamics with advancing age impact drug dosing and metabolism must be appreciated to reduce bleeding and thromboembolic complications.

Dosing Considerations

Changes in body composition alter the distribution of fat with aging, and may impact the storage and metabolism of some medications. VKA are highly protein bound, and lower doses may be required in states of poor nutrition, synthetic liver dysfunction, heart failure, or with the use of other highly protein bound drugs such as diltiazem [13, 18]. There are no significant aging alterations in liver metabolism of drugs including cytochrome P450 3A4 enzyme activity. Both the loading and maintenance dose of warfarin decrease as a function of age, regardless of interaction medications (Fig. 17.1). In a study of 107 consecutive OAT patients over 70 years old (mean age 85 years), the typical loading dose of 5 mg daily resulted in supratherapeutic protime international ratio (INR) in 82% of females and 65% of men [19]. The investigators report 4 mg/day load resulted in a significantly higher portion of patients in the therapeutic range more rapidly. These data also highlight that, due to changes in body composition and size, women usually require lower loading and maintenance doses of VKA. Maintenance doses of VKA also decline with age at a rate of 0.4 mg/week/year [18]. This premise argues that older adults need to have their protime monitored in less than monthly intervals to avoid supratherapeutic anticoagulation [14]. In addition to the multitude of drugs that alter the metabolism of VKA, patients must also be wary of excessive intake of vitamin K, which can be found in many liquid nutritional supplements to augment nutrition,

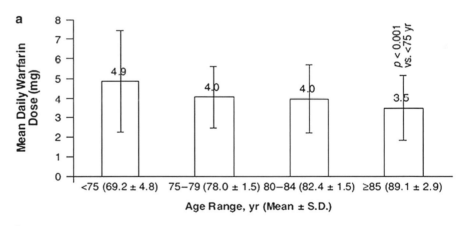

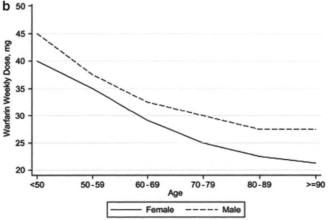

Fig. 17.1 With advancing age, the mean daily (Panel A) dose of warfarin declines and, over time, this translates to a dose decline of approximately 0.4 mg/week/year (Panel B) (Reproduced with permission from ref. [14])

Table 17.2 Medications and supplements commonly prescribed in older adults which impact protime INR

Drugs that increase INR		Drugs that decrease INR	
Antiarrhythmics	**Lipid meds**	**Thyroid replacement**	**Liquid nutritional supplements**
Amiodarone	Gemfibrozil	**GI medications**	Boost®
Propafenone	Lovastatin	Sulcrafate	Ensure®
Quinidine	**Analgesics**	**Neuropsych meds**	Glucerna®
ID medications	Acetominophen	Carbemazepine	Carnation instant breakfast®
Azithromycin	Aspirin	Clozapine	Resource®
Cephalosporins	NSAIDs	Haldoperidol	Equate®
Doxycycline	**Alcohol**	Phenytoin	**Calcium supplements**
Erythromycin	**Endocrine meds**	Trazodone	Viactiv®
Flu vaccine	Methimizole	**ID medications**	**Herbal**
Fluconazole	Sulfonamides	Cyclosporine	St. John's wort
Macrolides	**Neuropsych meds**	Rifampin	Ginseng
Metronidazole	SSRIs	**Spironolactone**	Green tea
Miconazole	Valproate	**Raloxifene**	Coenzyme Q10
Quinolones	Tramadol	**Cholestyramine**	Soy products
Sulfamethoxazole	**Propanolol**		
Tetracycline	**Herbal**		
Tamoxifen	Cassia		
GI medications	Garlic		
Cimetidine	*Gingko biloba*		
Omeptrozole	Feverfew		

in the hospital, rehabilitation, chronic care and home settings (Table 17.2). When chronic OAT is initiated, patient and family education significantly improve the time in therapeutic levels as does frequent monitoring and use of dedicated anticoagulation clinics [20, 21]. It is important to note that approximately 50% of seniors take over-the-counter vitamins, herbals, and supplements but only 49% report their use to their care providers [22]. As many of these substances may interact with VKA, a careful prescription and OTC medication list must be exchanged and monitored to avoid untoward interactions.

Anticoagulants which are primarily cleared renally, such as low molecular weight heparin and fondaparinux, may be contraindicated or must be dose adjusted in older patients with chronic kidney disease, or even age-related kidney dysfunction. As such, calculating the creatinine clearance of candidate patients is important to avoid supratherapeutic levels and resultant dangerous bleeding events [1, 16].

Strategies to Reduce Bleeding Risk

Given the delicate balance between the increased thrombotic and bleeding risks in older patients, strategies to shift the balance to safer anticoagulation should be employed when possible. Pharmacologic anticoagulation-induced bleeding can result in significant morbidity and mortality, especially in older surgical patients. In addition to age-appropriate dosing, frequent monitoring to maintain therapeutic levels, and minimizing interacting and synergistic medications in older

patients, implementation of specific precautions can reduce bleeding risk [4, 14, 20].

Surgical Site

When anticoagulation is clinically indicated postoperatively, either as continuation of ongoing chronic OAT, as a treatment or as VTE prophylaxis, adequate hemostasis of the surgical site must be established first. To reduce surgical site bleeding, anticoagulation with UFH should be initiated, often without a loading bolus. Starting or restarting anticoagulation is dependent on the impact of the bleeding risk (i.e., intracranial bleeding risk with neurosurgery), and the type of surgery. These are addressed in specific sections below. In the setting of cardiac surgery, concurrent aspirin and/or thienopyridines use increase surgical site bleeding [23]. It is important to note that the most vulnerable bleeding sites may not be overtly visible, such as pericardial or anastomotic site bleeding, and careful vigilance for these risks is important.

Gastrointestinal Bleeding

Active GI bleeding is a contraindication to starting or continuing anticoagulation. In contrast, a history of peptic ulcer bleeding increases the risk of GI bleeding on anticoagulation by 13.5-fold, but this risk declines to 1.3%/year if *Helicobacter pylori* is screened and treated [17]. Concomitant use of non-steroidal anti-inflammatory drugs (NSAIDs) significantly increases the risk of GI bleeding to 4.5%/year for those on chronic OAT. If NSAIDs must be used, cotreatment with a proton pump inhibitor or a cytoprotective agent such as misoprostol, reduces the bleeding risk by 50% [10]. Surgical patients being discharged on chronic anticoagulation should be educated on the risk of NSAID use as well as alcohol use, which is a relative contraindication for chronic OAT (Table 17.1).

Intracranial Hemorrhage

The incidence of ICH has been reported to be over threefold higher in those >75 years on chronic OAT (1.8%/year) compared to those <75 years (0.5%/year) [24]. However, retrospective analysis of this study found the majority of older patients with ICH had a supratherapeutic protime international normalized ratio (INR). In older adults with therapeutic INRs, the rate of ICH was similar in older and younger patients [25]. The risk of ICH is also substantially increased by uncontrolled hypertension [11]. Those with systolic blood pressure >160 mmHg and diastolic blood pressure <90 on OAT have a fourfold increased risk of ICH. Other risks for ICH for those on anticoagulation are cerebral angiopathy, intracranial lesions, and concomitant use of high dose aspirin. If aspirin is indicated along with anticoagulation, as with coronary artery disease, low dose aspirin (81 mg) significantly reduced the risk of ICH compared to higher dose aspirin (≥325 mg) [26].

Fall Risk in Older Adults

One of the most commonly cited reason by physicians to not prescribe chronic OAT in older adults is fear of falls [27]. Most falls in older adults tend to be low velocity, resulting in injury and bruising, but rarely in significant bleeding. In the case of OAT for atrial fibrillation, the stroke risk is so elevated in those over 75 years old, that it is estimated that an older patient would have to fall 295 times a year to incur a significant bleeding event serious enough to outweigh the thrombotic protection OAT offers [28]. In the hospital, early ambulation should be encouraged in older patients, but with appropriate precautions, especially in unstable patients. Those who incur long post-operative debilitation should be considered for rehabilitative therapy to increase balance and strength and reduce their fall risk.

The Surgical Patient on Chronic Anticoagulation

Older surgical patients who are on chronic anticoagulation will require differing strategies dependent on their reason for OAT, their risk of thromboembolism/thrombosis, the type of surgery (major vs. minor) they are undergoing as well as the timing of the surgery (elective, urgent or emergent) [1, 29]. Patients who are deemed high risk for acute thrombotic events once OAT is stopped, require "bridging" therapy with a shorter acting anticoagulant (such as unfractionated or low molecular weight heparin) prior to elective surgery. Caution should be used with LMWH if spinal analgesic or anesthesia is proposed due to bleeding risk [30]. If the patient is being treated for an existing VTE (DVT, PE or cardiac mural thrombus), elective surgery that can be safely postponed should be rescheduled until after acute treatment of the clot is completed. Surgical patients who are low risk for immediate thrombotic events may temporarily stop OAT during the surgical period and resume it post-operatively. Finally, some minor surgical procedures are deemed such low risk for bleeding that chronic OAT may be continued throughout the surgical procedure, and in some cases with minor alterations. Table 17.3 summarizes the recommendations for patients on chronic OAT undergoing elective major surgery or surgery associated with a high bleeding risk [1, 29, 30]. Examples of major surgery which carry a high risk of bleeding include coronary artery bypass surgery (CABG) or valve replacement, major vascular surgery (aortic aneurysm repair, peripheral bypass surgery, carotid endarterectomy), intracranial or spinal surgery, major orthopaedic surgery (hip or knee replacement), reconstructive plastic surgery, major cancer surgery, and prostate or bladder surgery. Individual circumstances should be carefully reviewed before an informed decision on modifying OAT is made in the patient undergoing surgery or an invasive procedure.

High Thrombotic Risk Patients

Patients with mechanical mitral valves are at particularly high risk during the perioperative time, as valve thrombosis can occur rapidly and is associated with high mortality (40%) and major morbidity (20%). Those with older mechanical aortic valves such as single tilting disk (Björk–Shiley), and ball-in-cage (Starr Edwards) types are also at higher risk for acute thrombosis and require bridging therapy [1, 29]. Those with a newer model mechanical valve in the aortic position (bileaflet) or bioprosthetic valves in either the aortic or mitral position are deemed low risk, and do not require bridging therapy UNLESS they have additional high risk features for thromboembolism. These high risk features include:

- Chronic atrial fibrillation with MVR
- Prior thromboembolic event
- Known hypercoaguable state

Another tool commonly used for assessing thrombotic risk is the Congestive Heart Failure-Hypertension-Age-Diabetes-Stroke (CHADS$_2$) score [31, 32], which was developed originally for risk stratifying patients with chronic atrial

Table 17.3 Recommendations for those on chronic OAT undergoing elective surgery

Condition for OAT	Thrombotic risk	Stop OAT	Bridging start therapy	Bridging dose	Stop bridge Tx	Resume bridge Tx and OAT	Comment
Mechanical valve							
Mitral – any type or	High risk	If INR 3–4: stop 6 days PTS	Start IV UFH when INR <2	UFH intravenous: Goal aPTT 1.5–2.0 or LMWH Options: Enoxaparin:	UFH: stop 4° PTS or	Adequate hemostatis must be obtained first	Monitor antifactor Xa levels with LMWH 4° after dose (0.5–1.5 U/mL)
Aortic – single-disc (Björk–Shiley) or ball-in-cage (Starr–Edwards) or	High risk	If INR 2–3: stop 5 days PTS	Start LMWH 36° after last warfarin dose	1 mg/kg SC q 12° or 1.5 mg/kg SC q 24°		UFH: resume 6–12° PO Low bleed risk – LMWH 24° PO	
Aortic – bileaflet or tilting disc (Medtronic, CarboMedics) *with high risk features*[a]	High risk	Check INR morning of surgery to ensure <1.5 (1.2 for neurosurgery)		Dalteparin: 120 U/kg SC q 12° or 200 U/kg SC q 24° Tinzaparin: 175 U/kg sc q 24°	LMWH: stop 24° PTS, last dose PTS is ½ dose	High bleed risk – LMWH 48–72° PO Restart OAT night after sursery	LMWH exclusions: wt >150 kg, CrCl <30 mL/min, GI bleed w/i 10 d, H/o HIT, several liver disease, h/o bleeding h/o of ICH, h/o major trauma/ CVA w/i 2 weeks
Aortic – bileaflet or tilting disc *without high risk features*[a]	Low risk[b]	4–6 d PTS, check AM of surgery: INR<1.5	LDLMWH[c] or not required		LDLMWH stop 24° PTS, last dose PTS is ½ dose	Restart OAT 24° PO	
Bioprosthetic valve							
AVR or MVR+ HRF[a]	High risk	5 d PTS	Same as mechanical MVR	Same as mechanical MVR	Same as mechanical MVR	12–24°h PO if adequate hemostasis	
AVR or MVR no HRF[a]	Low risk[b]	5 d PTS	Not required				

VTE therapy		Stop 4 d PTS	UFH when INR<2 or LMWH	UFH if w/i 2 weeks, short surgery, min bleed risk aPTT 1.5–2.5	w/i 2 weeks VTE – stop UFH 6–12° PTS / w/i 2–4 weeks UFH 8–12° PTS	UFH 6° PO without bolus	Do not d/c until INR therapeutic
	Month 1 VTE	Stop 4 d PTS	UFH when INR<2 or LMWH	UFH if w/i 2 weeks, short surgery, min bleed risk aPTT 1.5–2.5	w/i 2 weeks VTE – stop UFH 6–12° PTS / w/i 2–4 weeks UFH 8–12° PTS	UFH 6° PO without bolus	
	Month 2 VTE	5 d PTS	SQ UFH when INR<2	IVC filter if <2 week, major surgery – high bleed risk	UFH 8–12° PTS		Elective surgery should be postponed until at least 1 month, preferably 3 months of Tx
	Month 3 VTE	5 d PTS	or LMWH	Therapeutic dose	LMWH 24° PTS (½ dose)		
Chronic atrial fibrillation	High risk[c] or rheumatic MV	5 d PTS	SC LMWH or IV UFH	IV UFH to aPTT 1.5–2.0 or Therapeutic LMWH	UFH : stop 4° PTS or	Restart OAT PO night	LDMWH can be used if CHADS₂ = 3–4
	Low risk[d]	5 d PTS	LDLMWH or not required	Enoxaparin 30 mg bid, dalteparin 5,000 IU qd	LMWH: stop 24° PTS, last dose PTS is ½ dose	Resume usual OAT dose PO night	
Thrombophilic conditions	High risk	4 d PTS measure INR day 4, if >1.7 give 1 mg vit K SC check INR AM of surgery, if INR>1.3–1.7 give 1 u FFP, INR 1.7–2.0 give 2u FFP	If arterial thrombosis <1 month PTS – IV UFH or LMWH	If art thrombosis <1 month PTS, start IV UFH when INR <2	6°h PTS	IV UFH w/o loading dose 12° PO if w/11 month Tx If high bleed risk, SC UFH or LMW until INR >1.8	
or Prior/current arterial thromboembolism	High risk						
or Cardiac mural thrombus	High risk						

PTS prior to surgery; *PO* post-operatively; *UFH* unfractionated heparin; *LMWH* low molecular weight heparin; *LDLMWH* low dose low molecular weight heparin; *FFP* fresh frozen plasma; *SC* subcutaneous

[a] Atrial fibrillation, left atrial size >5 cm, ejection fraction <35%, >1 prosthetic valve, spontaneous echo contrast or hypercoagulable state

[b] Bridging therapy recommended if pt <3 months post-op from valve replacement

[c] CHADS₂ score (Table 17.4) ≥3 or prior thromboembolism

[d] CHADS₂ score ≤2 (Table 17.4) and no history of prior thromboembolism

fibrillation (Table 17.4). The CHADS$_2$ score assigns points for various thromboembolic risk factors: those with a score of 2 are moderate risk, and those scoring ≥3 are considered high risk. Table 17.5 summarizes anticoagulation recommendations for types of valve replacements, including when to use bridging anticoagulation in the perioperative setting [1, 29, 30]. In the elective surgical setting, and when possible in the semi-urgent setting, vitamin K, especially IV, should *not* be given to those with mechanical valve to expedite correction of anticoagulation due to the high thrombotic risk of the valves [29].

Another setting in which the surgical patient on chronic anticoagulation is at high risk for thrombosis is with a known hypercoagulable disorder. These include deficient levels of Protein C or S, Antithrombin III or factor V Leiden mutation (homozygous) or antiphospholipid antibody syndrome. Certain cancers and myelodysplastic syndromes are also associated with prothrombotic states, and all of these coagulopathies require bridging therapy during the perioperative period [1] (Table 17.3).

Chronic atrial fibrillation is a common condition in older adults, and carries a significantly higher risk of embolic stroke (>8%/year) compared with younger atrial fibrillation patients (1%/year) [9, 33, 34]. A subset of patients on OAT for chronic atrial fibrillation with certain high risk features requires bridging therapy in the perioperative period [1] (Table 17.3). The CHADS$_2$ score is used to evaluate the thromboembolic stroke risk of patients with chronic atrial fibrillation (Table 17.4) [31]. Those with a score of 2 are moderate risk, and those scoring ≥3 are considered high risk. Additional factors that elevate a patient with chronic atrial fibrillation into a high risk category are those with:

- Atrial fibrillation with a mechanical MVR and/or AVR.
- Rheumatic mitral disease with atrial fibrillation
- Previous thromboembolism
- Left ventricular dysfunction
- A hypercoaguable state

Table 17.4 CHADS$_2$ score for stroke risk in patients with non-valvular atrial fibrillation

Clinical parameter	Points
Congestive heart failure (any history)	1
Hypertension (prior history)	1
Age ≥75 years	1
Diabetes mellitus	1
Secondary prevention in patients with a prior ischemic stroke or a transient ischemic attack; most experts also include patients with a systemic embolic event	2

The CHADS$_2$ score estimates the risk of stroke. Patients are considered to be at low risk with a score of 0, at intermediate risk with a score of 1 or 2, and at high risk with a score ≥3. One exception is that most experts would consider patients with a prior ischemic stroke, transient ischemic attack, or systemic embolic event to be at high risk even if they had no other risk factors and therefore a score of 2. However, the majority of these patients usually have other risk factor and a score of at least 3
Source: Data from Gage [31]

Low Thrombotic Risk

Bridging therapy is not required in some patients on chronic OAT as their risk of a thromboembolic event, although high enough to require OAT, is not high enough to pose a significant risk if temporarily stopped for days. These patients include those with chronic atrial fibrillation with CHADS$_2$ score of ≤2 and without prior thromboembolism, those with bioprosthetic valves and those with mechanical bileaflet valves in the aortic position as long as none of these subgroups has additional high risk features listed above. Those

Table 17.5 Summary of anticoagulation recommendations

Valve type	Manufacturer	Bridging therapy	Bridging Therapy	Goal INR	Comments
Mechanical					
Mitral – any type	St. Jude	Yes	VKA	2.5–3.5	Concurrent ASA 81 mg qd if CAD, coronary stent(s)
Aortic – ball-in-cage, older single disc	Björk–Shiley, Starr–Edwards	Yes	VKA	2.5–3.5	
Aortic – bileaflet or newer tilting disc + HRF[a]	St Jude, Medtronics Hall, CarboMedics AVR	Yes	VKA	2.5–3.5	
Aortic – bileaflet or newer tilting disc + no HRF[a]		No	VKA	2.0–3.0[b]	
Bioprosthetic					AVR INR goal 2.5–3.5 for 3 months post implant
Mitral or aortic	Carpentier-Edwards, St. Jude, Medtronic				
With HRF[a]		Yes	VKA + ASA 81qd	2.0–3.0	
No HRF[a]		No	VKAx3 mo,[c] then ASA 81 qd		

[a]HRF-atrial fibrillation, prior thromboembolism, left ventricular dysfunction and hypercoagulable state

[b]INR target 2.5–3.5 for first 3 months post op, then 2.0–3.0

[c]If patient is not OAT candidate, then ASA 325 mg qd indefinitely

with a prior single DVT >12 months prior to surgery without recurrence are also considered low risk [1] (Table 17.3).

Minor Surgical Procedures

Several minor surgical procedures are deemed at such low risk for bleeding, that the thrombotic risk outweighs stopping anticoagulant therapy [1, 30]. Patients taking OAT who are undergoing minor dental (single or multiple tooth extractions or endodontic procedures), or dermatologic procedures (excision of squamous or basal cell carcinomas or removal of malignant or premalignant nevi) should continue OAT throughout the procedure. Similarly, those who are undergoing cataract removal, OAT should not be interrupted for surgery. In contrast, glaucoma surgery has been associated with increased bleeding risk on oral anticoagulation which should be held (with or without bridging dependent of the thrombotic risk level) prior to surgery.

Most minimally invasive procedures can be done with an INR of 1.5. Holding warfarin therapy for 3 days is ideal, however, if necessary, small doses of vitamin K can be given to lower INR more rapidly. Vitamin K should not be given to those with mechanical valves due to the high risk of valve thrombosis [29].

Temporary Reversal of Chronic Anticoagulation for Urgent Surgery

Guidelines for the reversal of anticoagulation depend on the amount of time available before the procedure, and the type of procedure that is being done, and are summarized in Table 17.6 [1, 14, 30]. In semi-urgent procedures that need to be done within 18–24 h, warfarin should be withheld, and vitamin K (2.5–5.0 mg IV) should be administered, and additional blood products will likely not be needed. In urgent situations where reversal of anticoagulation is required in less than one day, warfarin should be withheld, and vitamin K (2.5–5.0 mg po or slow IV) should be given along with fresh frozen plasma (FFP),

prothrombin complex concentrate (PCC), or recombinant factor VIIa. Of these, FFP is usually preferred, but may present volume overload challenges in older adults [30]. Much less data is available for recombinant factor VIIa, and PCC elevates the thrombotic risk more than FFP. It is important to note that the latter three agents will only temporarily reverse VKA, which will continue to be effective until fully metabolized or antagonized with vitamin K. Thus, bleeding risk should be monitored closely when these temporizing agents wear off (12–24 h), and vitamin K should always be given pre-operatively [30]. Emergent surgery in patients on OAT requires the administration of PCC, which does not require blood matching or thawing. The vitamin K-dependent factors in PCC are 25-fold higher than those in FFP, and usually correct the INR in 15 min. The risk of PCC is acute thrombotic events. Vitamin K (5 mg IV slowly infused) should be given with PCC prior to surgery. The dose of PCC is 25–50 units/kg, but in older patients, use of weight-based, initial and desired INR algorithms should be considered [35, 36].

Another clinical scenario in which pharmaceutically induced bleeding may need to be "reversed" is for emergent cardiac surgery after acute myocardial infarction, failed thrombolytics, or percutaneous coronary interventions (PCIs). Optimally, the timing of the surgery should be delayed until short acting fibrinolytics are no longer effective (hours). In the case of glycoprotein IIbIIIa inhibitors, platelet function should be adequate 4 h after stopping tirofiban and eptifibatide infusions. If surgery is more urgent than that time window, or if abciximab (which has a longer half life) is used, platelet transfusion may be necessary along with a reduction in the heparin dose used for the bypass pump [37]. Aspirin and clopidogrel may cause increased bleeding, especially at the surgical site, but their use should not delay surgery [23].

IVC Filters

In patients who have known proximal thrombus, insertion of temporary inferior vena cava filters may reduce the immediate risk of PE in a situation where the bleeding risk is

Table 17.6 Recommendations for VKA reversal for urgent/emergent surgery

Surgical timing	Time frame	Vitamin K	Fresh frozen plasma	Prothrombin complex concentrate	Comment
Semi-urgent	18–24°	2.5–5.0 mg IV[a]	No	No	Check INR prior to surgery
Urgent	<24°	2.5–5.0 mg po[b] or slow IV	4u pre-op, 2u post-op	No	Time for FFP thawing, large volume load
Emergent	<1°	5.0 mg IV slowly	No	25–50 U/kg[c]	

[a]IV vitamin K not recommended with mechanical prosthetic valves due to thrombosis risk
[b]PO vitamin K favored over IV vitamin K in patients with mechanical prosthetic valves due to thrombosis risk
[c]PCC should be used with caution in those with mechanical valves due to thrombosis risk

unacceptably high to continue anticoagulation [1, 16]. An example of this situation is neurosurgery. The filter may then be retrieved when it is safe to resume therapeutic anticoagulation. The use of IVC filters is still debated in many surgical venues and the individualized risk versus benefit ratio should be consider in the older patient.

Specific Surgeries with Recommended Anticoagulation Initiation

Prosthetic Valve Implantation

The surgical correction of valvular heart disease continues to increase in the setting of our growing senior population and increased life expectancy. Mechanical prosthetic heart valves are associated with a variety of complications, including prosthetic valve thrombosis and systemic embolization. The frequency of systemic embolization is about 1% per year in patients on anticoagulation with warfarin, as compared to 4% with no anticoagulation [38].

According to the American College of Cardiology and American Heart Association Guidelines, all patients with mechanical prosthetic valves require anticoagulation with warfarin [29] (Table 17.5). The intensity of recommended OAT varies depending on several factors including the type of valve, the site of valve replacement, underlying risk factors for thrombus formation, and certain clinical settings, such as surgical procedures [30]. Mechanical valves are more thrombogenic as compared to bioprosthetic valves, and the mitral valve site nearly doubles the risk of thromboembolism, as compared to the aortic valve position. The details of dosing and INR goals further depend on other risk factors for thrombus formation including the presence of atrial fibrillation, low left ventricular ejection fraction, and a history of prior thromboembolism. In the setting of thromboembolism, despite antithrombotic therapy, increasing INR goals and/or the addition of aspirin may be necessary [29].

Mechanical Valve Implantation

The risk of mechanical valve thrombosis is at its peak immediate following implantation, even in the setting of anticoagulation, and especially for mitral valves which can have a 5% thrombosis rate within 30 days of implantation (vs. 0.5% for mechanical aortic valves) [38]. Cessation of prior anticoagulation, HIT, and diabetes are risk factors for early thrombosis. Accordingly, as soon as hemostasis has been achieved, UFH or LMWH should be initiated without a bolus as bridging therapy until the INR is therapeutic for two consecutive

days [29, 39]. During this time aPTT should be monitored (goal 1.5–2.5 times control) or anti Factor Xa levels in the case of LMWH use (goal 0.5–1.5 U/mL measured 4 h after dose is given) [40]. Warfarin may be initiated on the day of surgery. The specific recommendations for particular types and placement of valves and goal INR values are listed in Table 17.5.

Bioprosthetic Valve Implantation

Bioprosthetic valves are more commonly used in older adults because of the reduced thrombotic risk which usually doesn't require OAT. Retrospective studies have shown a high thrombotic risk within the first three months of bioprosthetic valves placement, especially in the setting of anticoagulation cessation, valves placed in the mitral position, and in those with a history of thromobembolic events. Thus, several Guidelines recommend OAT for 3 months following bioprosthetic valve implantation in all cases unless there is an absolute contraindication (Table 17.1) [30, 40, 41]. Post-operative anticoagulation with UFH or LMWH is recommended in those who are candidates for VKA as described for mechanical valves until the INR is therapeutic for 2 consecutive days [40]. Long-term anticoagulation is recommended in those with additional risk factors (atrial fibrillation, prior thromboembolism, hypercoagulable state and/or ejection fraction <30%) with INR goal of 2–3. Aspirin is also recommended for all bioprothetic valves at 81 mg a day unless the patient is an OAT candidate who cannot take VKA, in which case aspirin 325 mg a day is recommended.

Cardiac Surgery

Foreign materials within coronary vasculature (stents), in addition to iatrogenic vascular anastamoses, incite inflammatory and thrombotic responses. Additionally, vascular graft sites are at increased risk of thrombosis. Because of this increased risk, all patients with coronary artery disease undergoing CABG are recommended to stay on aspirin (81 mg qd) throughout the surgical period and indefinitely thereafter. If the patient has stopped aspirin prior to surgery, it should be started within 6 hours post-op if hemostasis is secured. Clopdiogrel post-operatively has also been associated with increased graft patency, and is now recommended for 9–12 months post-op from CABG [23, 42]. VKA have not shown added significant benefit in maintaining graft patency when compared to, or in combination with anti-platelet therapy. Because of this, VKA's are not recommended for patients undergoing CABG to maintain graft patency [23]. However, VKA's are recommended for use in addition to aspirin in patients with CABG who have other indications for OAT, including mechanical heart valve replacement or atrial fibrillation.

Vascular Surgery

Older patients undergoing carotid endarterectomy are at significant risk for stroke, and therefore aspirin (81–325 mg) should be initiated prior to surgery and continued indefinitely. Post-operative surgical site bleeding is not uncommon, especially in the setting of combined CABG/CEA and should be monitored closely. Chronic OAT is not recommended after CEA, unless another indication for chronic anticoagulation is met. Similarly, peripheral bypass grafting for claudication are treated with antiplatelet agents such as aspirin rather than OAT.

Surgical Venothromboembolic Prophylaxis

General Issues

DVT affects an estimated 900,000 people in the US each year, resulting in several hundred thousand hospitalizations and about 300,000 deaths from PE [43]. In fact, PE remains one of the most common preventable causes for hospital death in the United States [44]. In the older surgical patient, age over 60 alone places them in the highest risk group for post-surgical DVT, with an incidence of 4–8% and fatal PE incidence of 0.4–1.0% [45]. Multiple age-associated factors contribute to this risk as reviewed above including increased thrombotic factors, endothelial and platelet dysfunction, and venous valve changes. This risk increases further with a prior

history of VTE, history of malignancy, hypercoagulable disorders, immobility, and other comorbidites such as prior stroke. In addition, certain invasive surgical procedures add to thrombotic risk by increasing thrombin generation. Thus, aggressive measures to prevent DVT formation are one of the most important aspects of caring for the older surgical patient.

The guideline recommendations for VTE prophylaxis in surgical patients are described below and have been established by the American College of Chest Physicians in 2008 and are summarized in Table 17.7 [45]. In summary, high risk older surgical patients undergoing a major procedure require both mechanical (when possible) and pharmacological methods of anticoagulation to prevent VTE. Mechanical methods include intermittent pneumatic compression (IPC), graduated compression stockings (GCS), and venous foot pump. Appropriate pharmacological methods include low dose unfractionated heparin (LDUFH) three times a day, weight and procedure based LMWH, or fondaparinux daily in patients with a history of HIT [45]. In some cases, warfarin provides optimal VTE prophylaxis, especially when the risk is prolonged due to immobility or hypercoagulability. All VTE prophylactic measures (medical and mechanical) should ideally be started either before or shortly after surgery and optimally continue until the patient is ambulatory. The pre-operative dose is dependent on the type of surgery where the bleeding risk is low. Early ambulation of the older patient is encouraged as soon as feasible. Aspirin alone does not provide sufficient VTE prophylaxis for any patient group [45].

When considering the medical agent for VTE prophylaxis, several issues arise when caring for the older surgical patient. As renal function declines with age, it is important to calculate the actual creatinine clearance of each older patient to ensure that the agent is dosed adjusted properly or not contraindicated [1, 45]. This is especially important in

Table 17.7 VTE prophylaxis strategies

Type of surgery	DVT prophylaxis medical	Start	Duration of prophylaxis	Non-medical	Comment
General surgery	LDUFH 500 IU SC bid or tid or LMWH[a] or fonda[b]	LDUFH 2° PTS or 4–6° PO LMWH w/i 12–24° PO Fonda 6–24° PO	Ambulatory	ICP+GCS	Monitor platelets with prolonged UFH/LMWH
CABG/valve/thoracic with high bleeding risk	LMWH[a]	LMWH w/i 12–24° PO	Ambulatory	IPC or GCS	Monitor platelets w LMWH IPC/GCS only if high bleed risk
Trauma	LMWH if bleeding risk	When safe	Ambulatory	IPC	IVC if high VTE risk and high bleeding risk
Cancer surgery	Fonda,[b] LMWH	Fonda 6–24° PO LMWH w/i 12–24° PO	28 days	IPC±GCS	Monitor platelets w LMWH

LDUFH: Low dose unfractionated heparin; PTS: prior to surgery; PO: post-operatively; IPC: Intermittent pneumatic compression devices; GCS: graduated compression stockings
[a]LMWH: enoxaparin 30 mg sq q 12°, dalteparin 5,000 IU sq qd
[b]Fonda: fondaparinux 2.5 mg sc qd

women and those with low body weight who can have near normal serum creatinine but significantly impaired renal clearance of drugs. As low molecular weight heparins and fondaparinux are cleared renally, they must be used with caution in older surgical patients. If CrCl is 30 mL/min or less, enoxaparin should be dose adjusted and fondaparinux is contraindicated [1]. Patients given UFH or LMWH must have their platelets monitored regularly for HIT, even with the relatively small doses used for VTE prophylaxis. Another important consideration in agent choice is a patient history of HIT, which requires a non-heparin agent such as fondaparinux. In patients who are at risk for VTE but in whom anticoagulation is not possible (active GI bleed, trauma), mechanical prophylaxis with ICP±GCS should be employed. Certain cancers and chemotherapeutic regimens are associated with hypercoagulability and increased risk of arterial and venous thrombi, and VTE prophylaxis after surgery should continue for 28 days at least [45]. Post-operative VTE has been reported in as many as 40% of patients with known cancers who undergo surgery. If prophylactic anticoagulation is planned, imaging should be performed in tumors with propensity to metastasize to brain and CNS to reduce potential life-threatening bleeds. Lastly, in patients undergoing spinal puncture or epidural catheter placement, LMWH should be used with caution due to the dire consequences of increased bleeding risk.

Perioperative Events Requiring Anticoagulation

New Onset or Recurrent Atrial Fibrillation

Atrial fibrillation is one of the most common cardiovascular conditions in older adults, and is associated with a significantly higher morbidity and mortality in older compared with younger patients [33]. The risk of thrombosis and subsequent cardioembolic stroke is higher in older patients as compared with younger ones [9, 34]. Data from the Framingham Heart Study suggests that risk of stroke increases approximately 1.5% per decade and is as high as 23.5% in patients over 80 years old [34]. Atrial fibrillation is a relatively common post-operative occurrence in older patients, and may be related to directly cardiac manipulation (CABG or valve surgery), volume overload, pain or concurrent infections such as urinary tract infections. In an older post-operative patient with new or recurrent atrial fibrillation, it is reasonable to consider for pulmonary and urinary infections, sepsis, hyperthyroidism, and alcohol withdrawal as etiologies. Most patients who experience atrial fibrillation after cardiac surgery spontaneously convert to sinus rhythm while in the hospital.

Increased bleeding risk associated with cardiac surgery complicates the risk vs. benefit ratio of using IV heparin as a bridge to chronic anticoagulation when new onset atrial fibrillation occurs. The most common concern with early heparin use is significant pericardial effusions and potential tamponade. The current ACC/AHA/ECS recommendation is to initiate VKA, if surgically hemostatic to a target INR of 2.0–3.0 for those with atrial fibrillation lasting ≥48 h, and continue for at least 4 weeks until reevaluation at post-operative follow-up [46]. For cardiac surgery post-op atrial fibrillation lasting >24 h, VKA should be started once hemostasis is secured for 4 weeks with goal INR of 2.0–3.0. Bridging therapy with heparin is not recommended in either setting due to the high risk of bleeding complications [40]. An exception to "bridging" therapy with heparin until INR is therapeutic is in the case of multiple thrombotic risk factors or implantation of a mechanical valve, if bleeding risk is acceptably controlled [30]. These patients must be monitored very closely. In older patients undergoing non-cardiac surgery in whom post-op atrial fibrillation occurs, the decision to initiate heparin depends on the significance of the bleeding risk. If hemostasis is achieved, heparin should be initiated as well as the first dose of VKA, unless an absolute contraindication exists. If the patient is symptomatic or has compromised vitals, cardioversion with direct current should be considered once aPTT is therapeutic if the atrial fibrillation duration is less than 48 h or less without therapeutic anticoagulation. If the patient is stable and asymptomatic in atrial fibrillation, heparin and chronic OAT should be started and continued in a therapeutic range (INR 2.0–3.0) for at least 4 weeks before cardioversion is attempted [46]. Antiarrhythmic drugs such as amiodarone should not be used unless therapeutic anticoagulation is ensured, and either the duration of atrial fibrillation is <48 h or a transesophageal echocardiogram confirms no evidence of a left atrial thrombus. All of these post-op atrial fibrillation recommendations also apply to post-op patients in atrial flutter. If the patient cardioverts in the hospital, spontaneously or with direct current, they should require OAT for 4 weeks as the atrium recovers its full contractile ability [46].

As previously stated, chronic, or even short term anticoagulation in older patients is often met with great fear by prescribers [17]. This is despite the considerable reduction in stroke risk warfarin offers over aspirin (62 as compared to 22%, respectively) in those over 75 years with chronic non-valvular atrial fibrillation [47]. The most commonly cited fear is fall risk followed by the worry of bleeding and creating inconvenience [27]. In a poll of physicians who denied older patients anticoagulation without an absolute or relative indication, the fear of bleeding was overestimated by 670% and the stroke risk was underestimated by 22% [11]. It is important to acknowledge the significantly high stroke risk (>8%/year in octogenarians), appreciate that older adults fear large strokes more than death, and the strategies to reduce bleeding and fall risk previously discussed are all important factors in the decision. Careful warfarin dosing, frequent monitoring and patient education play a key role in reducing bleeding and thrombotic risk of VKAs in older adults [1]. Optimal anticoagulation in older adults with AF also reduces the ischemic stroke related risk of death, dependency, and nursing home placement. The absolute contraindications for OAT are listed in Table 17.1 [10].

Myocardial Infarction

The risk of post-op myocardial infarction and acute coronary syndromes increases with advancing age. Again, the risk of ongoing ischemia/myocardial injury must be weighed against the potential surgical bleeding risk of anticoagulation, usually with heparin. Risk factors associated with post op MI in non-cardiac surgery include age >70 years, abdominal aortic surgery, diabetes, angina, and baseline ST–T wave abnormalities on baseline electrocardiogram [41, 48].

In older post-CABG patients, ischemia and possible graft occlusion within 30 days, is primarily treated with percutenous coronary angioplasty with low pressure balloon inflation. Bare metal stents are preferred if there is reocclusion. Thienopyridines and glycoprotein IIbIIIa inhibitors are used after angioplasty with careful monitoring of bleeding complications [23, 49].

In older patients experiencing an acute coronary syndrome (ACS) after non-cardiac surgery, the therapeutic decision again depends on the bleeding risk of surgery. It should be noted that heparin administration is required in the setting of cardiac catheterization, for sheath management alone, and moreso if PCI is required [49]. Optimal therapy following PCI also may include glycoprotein IIbIIIa inhibitors, thienopyridines, and/or heparin, the risk of which must be weighed against the bleeding risk and the amount of compromise the ischemic injury is causing. Because of the significant risk these additional antiplatelet medications pose, including their use for months after the procedure, some older ACS patients may be more safely managed with aspirin, UFH and beta-blockers as initial therapy.

Left Ventricular Dysfunction

For patients with systolic heart failure in sinus rhythm, data on the utility of anticoagulation to reduce thromboembolic events remains inconclusive. The 2008 American College of Chest Physicians (ACCP) guidelines recommend against routine use of OAT in patients with left ventricular dysfunction due to a nonischemic etiology [14]. However, if patients have a previous history of thromboembolic event or intracardiac thrombus, the 2008 European Society of Cardiology (ESC) heart failure guidelines recommend oral anticoagulant therapy with goal INR 2.0–3.0 [50].

Venothromboembolic Treatment

Anticoagulation

As noted above, DVT/PE is an important cause of morbidity and mortality, especially in hospitalized older patients. The well known triad of risk factors for DVT includes alterations in blood flow or increased stasis, vascular endothelial injury, and variation in blood constituents resulting in hypercoagulability. Because of these basic risk factors, it is inevitable that advanced age will increase the risk of DVT/PE.

In patients with DVT, the primary goals of treatment include preventing clot extension, preventing progression to acute PE, and decreasing the recurrence of thrombosis [16]. Treatment should begin immediately after confirmation of diagnosis, or even before confirmation if clinical suspicion is high. Four options are available for the initial treatment of DVT: (1) body weight-adjusted LMWH administered subcutaneous without monitoring, (2) intravenous UFH with monitoring and dose adjustment, (3) subcutaneous UFH with monitoring and subsequent dose adjustments, and (4) fondaparinux. VKA should be started at the same time as these shorter term anticoagulation strategies. As previously mentioned, the loading dose of warfarin declines with advancing age, and is lower in women than in men.[14, 15, 19] Additionally, the maintenance dose of warfarin also decreases with advancing age, apart from other potential interacting factors (Fig. 17.1). Again, women, those with poor nutrition, heart failure, and vitamin K deficiency also require lower maintenance doses. A starting dose of less than 5 mg in older patients and those at greater risk of bleeding is generally recommended. Heparin can be discontinued when the protime INR is stable and above 2.0 for greater than 48 h [4]. Treatment duration of warfarin for DVT has been studied extensively and ranges from a minimum of three to six months [16]. Table 17.8 summarizes DVT and PE treatment length recommendations in specific patient subgroups.

In patients with DVT who progress to acute PE, the mortality rate is as high as 30% without treatment [51]. As with DVT, anticoagulation with heparin should be started immediately in all patients with confirmed PE, as well as in patients with an intermediate or high clinical probability of PE. The recommended doses of the heparins that are currently approved for the treatment of PE are shown in Table 17.8. Heparin treatment is continued for at least 5–6 days in

Table 17.8 Anticoagulant drugs for the initial treatment of PE

Unfractionated heparin – IV Infusion	80 IU/kg of body weight IV bolus followed by continuous infusion at 18 IU/kg/h	Adjust infusion rate to maintain aPTT between 1.5 and 2.5 times control Monitor platelet count at baseline and q 48° If platelets drop by >50% or a thrombotic event occurs – investigate for HIT
Low molecular weight heparins – subcutaneous injection Enoxaparin	 1 mg/kg every 12 h or 1.5 mg/kg once daily	Not tested or recommended in patients with hypotension or shock Monitor platelet count as above
Tinzaparin	175 U/kg once daily	If creatinine clearance <30 mL/min, reduce dose to 1 mg/kg qd Consider UFH as alternative in patients with renal impairment
Fondaparinux	5 mg – body weight <50 kg 7.5 mg – weight 50–100 kg 10 mg – weight >100 kg Administered once daily	Contraindicated in patients with creatinine clearance <30 mL/min No routine platelet monitoring necessary

Patients with acute PE should also be routinely assessed for treatment with thrombolytic therapy. In patients with acute nonmassive PE, initial treatment with LMWH over IV UFH. In patients with massive PE, in other situations where there is concern about SC absorption, or in patients for whom thrombolytic therapy is being considered or planned, IV UFH is recommended over SC LMWH, SC fondaparinux, or SC UFH
Source: Data from Konstantinides [59]

Table 17.9 Vitamin K antagonists for the long term treatment of VTE

First episode of VTE secondary to a transient (reversible) risk factor
Treatment with a VKA for 3 months (Grade 1A)

First episode of idiopathic, unprovoked VTE
Treatment with a VKA for at least 3 months (Grade 1A)
After 3 months patients should be evaluated for the risk-to-benefit ratio of long-term therapy (Grade 1C)
Patients with a proximal DVT, and in whom risk factors for bleeding are absent and good anticoagulant monitoring is achievable, recommend long-term treatment (Grade 1A)
Patients with a distal DVT, suggest that 3 months of anticoagulant therapy is sufficient rather than indefinite therapy (Grade 2B)

Episode of VTE and cancer
LMWH for the first 3–6 months of anticoagulant therapy (Grade 1A)
Subsequent therapy with VKA or LMWH indefinitely or until cancer is resolved (Grade 1C)

First episode of VTE with documented antiphospholipid antibodies or with two or more thrombophilic conditions (e.g., combined factor V Leiden and prothrombin 20210 gene mutations)
Treatment for 12 months (Grade 1C+)
Indefinite anticoagulant therapy in these patients (Grade 2C)

First episode of VTE with documented deficiency of antithrombin, deficiency of protein C or protein S, or the factor V Leiden or prothrombin 20210 gene mutation, homocysteinemia, or high factor VIII levels (>90th percentile of normal)
Treatment for 6–12 months (Grade 1A)
Indefinite therapy as for patients with idiopathic thrombosis (Grade 2C)

Two or more episodes of objectively documented VTE
Long term treatment (Grade 1A)

In all groups noted above
The dose of VKA should be adjusted to maintain a target INR range, 2.0 and 3.0 for all treatment durations (Grade 1A)
Recommend against high-intensity therapy (INR range, 3.1–4.0) (Grade 1A)
Recommend against low-intensity therapy (INR range, 1.5–1.9) (Grade 1A)
The risk-benefit of continuing such treatment should be reassessed in the individual patient at periodic intervals (Grade 1C)

combination with oral anticoagulation, until the INR is within the therapeutic range (2.0–3.0) for two consecutive days [16]. The recommendations for the long term treatment of PE with OAT are the same as for DVT and are summarized in Table 17.9.

Inferior Vena Cava Filters

Although not a therapy for DVT, inferior vena cava (IVC) filters are indicated in the setting of proximal venous thrombus with an absolute contraindication for anticoagulation. More controversial is the proximal DVT patient with high risk of bleeding, which may be seen in the surgical setting. The most robust long-term follow-up data to date suggests that IVC filters do reduce the risk of PE, but increase incident DVTs and do not affect overall mortality [52, 53]. However, they may offer short term benefit in the certain settings [54].

Specific Anticoagulant Use in Older Patients

Heparins

Unfractionated heparin, and low molecular weight heparin, are very commonly used in initiating and bridging antithrombotic therapy. The heparin preparations work by potentiating the effects of antithrombin, thus resulting in indirect inactivation of thrombin, as well as preventing the conversion of fibrinogen to fibrin. With heparin, the rate of thrombin inhibition is accelerated about 1,000-fold [55]. Specific indications, dosing regimens, and complications are discussed below (Table 17.10).

Table 17.10 Summary of specific anticoagulants

Anticoagulation agent	Dose	Dosing impacted by age	Clearance	Monitor	Therapeutic range	Reversal	Cautions, comments
Unfractionated heparin	IV: 80 U/kg load then 18 U/kg infusion SC: 333 U/kg then 250 U/kg q12°	Yes – may need lower doses	Hepatic	aPTT	1.5–2.5	Protamine sulfate 50mg IV @20mg/min NTE 50mg/10min	HIT, monitor aPTT frequently, aPTT unreliable if prolonged at baseline, skin necrosis
LMWH Enoxaparin	1 mg/kg SC q12° 1.5 mg/kg SC q24°	↓if wt<45 kg Enox qd if CrCl <30 mL/min	Renal	Factor Xa level	0.5–1.0 µg/mL bid dose 1.0–2.0 µg/mL qd dose	Protamine sulfate	May need higher dose w obesity, monitor high risk (mechanical valves, VTE rx)
Dalteparin	100 U/kg SC q12° 200 U/kg SC q24°	Tinza/Dalte best for poor renal fxn	Renal		0.85–1.05 µg/mL	Protamine sulfate	
Tinzaparin	175 IU/kg/24°SC				0.85–1.05 µg/mL	Protamine sulfate	Caution when used around spinal/epidural injections
Direct Thrombin Inhibitors Hirudin	0.4 mg/kg load then 0.15 mg/kg infusion	Reduce dose if CrCl <30 on <60 Avoid if CrCl <30 mL/min	Renal	aPTT	1.5–2.5	None	Possible anaphylaxis in reexposure (Hir) May increase INR Argatroban for *prevention and tx* of HIT
Bivalrudin	0.7 mg/kg load then 1.75 mg/kg/h infusion	No	20% renal			Hemodialysis or hemo-perfusion can remove bivalrudin and agatroban	
Argatroban	2 µg/kg/h infusion	No	Hepatic[a]				
Fondaparinux	5 mg – body wt <50 kg 7.5 mg – wt 50–100 kg 10 mg – wt >100 kg	avoid if CrCl <30 mL/min, caution CrCl 30–50 mL/min	Renal	AntiFactor Xa if fonda used in assay	0.5–1.5 µg/mL	Recombinant factor VIIa	Monitor creatinine and platelets Caution when used around spinal/epidural injections
Warfarin	4–5 mg qd load, less if ♀, heart failure, poor nutrition, low body wt, interact drugs-adjust per INR	Loading and maintenance dose ↓ w age	Cyt P450 3A4	Protime INR	Dependent on indication	Vitamin K, FFP, PCC, Recombinant VIIa	Frequent monitoring to maintain therapeutic index

aPTT activated partial thromboplastin time; *INR* international normalized ratio; *HIT* heparin-induced thrombocytopenia; *LMWH* low molecular weight heparin, *CrCl* creatinine clearance, *FFP* fresh frozen plasma, *PCC* prothrombin complex concentrate

[a] Metabolized by cytochrome P450 3A4

Unfractionated Heparin

One of the major limitations associated with UFH is the necessity to maintain a narrow therapeutic window of adequate anticoagulation, without increasing the bleeding risk. The goal narrow therapeutic window, in combination with a highly variable dose response per individual patient, requires frequent monitoring of the activated partial thromboplastin time (aPTT) with resultant dose adjustments as needed. The goal is for the therapeutic level to be achieved within 24 h. The therapeutic range of aPTT is 1.5–2.5 times the mean of the control value, or the upper limit of the normal aPTT range [55]. In patients who have a prolonged aPTT at baseline, such as those with anticardiolipin antibody or lupus anticoagulant or liver disease, monitoring heparin with aPTT may not be reliable. In these cases, LMWH with Factor Xa monitoring may be a better choice. The aPTT may also be elevated by concurrent administration of warfarin. Because of the risk of heparin-induced thrombocytopenia (HIT), patients on heparin should have their platelet count monitored every 2–3 days at between days 4–14 of heparin therapy. Heparin in contraindicated in patients who have had HIT. There is no specific dosing alterations for older patients, but weight based nomograms should be followed, with vigilant aPTT monitoring. Skin necrosis is a rare complication of heparin. Dosing for full anticoagulation is given in Table 17.10, but dosing for DVT prophylaxis is less (Table 17.7). It should be noted that as of October 2009, the potency of heparin was reduced by 10%. Unfractionated heparin can be reversed by protamine sulfate IV, with full reversal occurring with 1 mg/100 U heparin.

Low Molecular Weight Heparin

Three types of low molecular weight heparins are currently available in the United States: enoxaparin, dalteparin, and tinzaparin [55]. Similar to UFH, LMWHs inactivate factor Xa, but have less effect on thrombin. The anticoagulant properties of LMWH are highly correlated with body weight, and bioavailability is very high making subcutaneous dosing very reliable, convenient, and consistent without the need for frequent monitoring. In situations where adequate anticoagulation must be ensured (mechanical valves, VTE treatment), LMWH should be monitored with Factor Xa levels drawn 4 h after LMWH injection. Because they are renally cleared, LMWH dosing in older patients should be based on the patient's calculated creatinine clearance. Those with CrCl <30 mL/min should receive a lower dose, less frequently (i.e., enoxaparin 30 mg SQ q 24°). In contrast, the dose may need to be adjusted upwards for obese patients. There are several cardiothoracic surgical settings in which LMWH is preferable to UFH for VTE prophylaxis including trauma

patients and cancer surgery. Although still associated with rare skin necrosis, LMWH are less likely to produce HIT than UFH [55]. Protamine sulfate does not completely reverse LMWH, but it is the reversal agent of choice (1 mg/100 anti-Xa units of LMWH), and clinically significant bleeding is not usually seen.

Heparin Induced Thrombocytopenia

Heparin-induced thrombocytopenia (HIT) is an antibody-mediated, adverse effect of heparin. Antibodies are formed against the heparin-platelet factor 4 complex that is strongly associated with venous and arterial thrombosis. HIT usually occurs within five to ten days of initiating therapy, and is a clinicopathologic syndrome classified by HIT antibody formation in addition to an unexplained fall in platelet count (≥50% fall from baseline), skin lesions at heparin injection sites, or acute systemic reaction after IV heparin bolus administration [56].

The risk of HIT antibody formation is especially high in post-operative cardiac surgery patients, even when postoperative anticoagulant prophylaxis with heparin is not administered [56]. Since several other potential causes of thrombocytopenia are often present in these patients, it is difficult to determine whether or not HIT is present. However given the increased risk in these patients, the ACCP guidelines recommend close monitoring of platelets, and excluding a diagnosis of HIT if the platelet count falls by ≥50% (and/or a thrombotic event occurs) between postoperative days 4–day 14 (day of cardiac surgery=day zero) [55, 56].

Thrombosis is the major clinical risk associated with HIT. Treatment is essential to reduce the risk of thrombosis and progression to decompensated disseminated intravascular coagulation http://chestjournal.chestpubs.org/content/126/3_suppl/311S.long - ref-7. The ACCP recommended agents that can be considered for treatment and prevention of HIT associated thrombosis which include DTI (discussed below) and fondaparinux [56].

Direct Thrombin Inhibitors

As described above, the traditional anticoagulants, such as heparin and VKA are indirect inhibitors of thrombin. Although these are commonly used, they are limited by unpredictable anticoagulant response, the need for close monitoring, and complications such as HIT [55, 56]. In the setting of these limitations, emphasis has been placed on developing antithrombotic agents with a more selective mechanism of action aimed at directly inhibiting thrombin. The DTI offer benefits over traditional agents in the treatment and prevention of various thrombotic disorders.

The DTIs interact directly with the thrombin molecule without the need of a cofactor thereby inhibiting both circulating and clot-bound thrombin. Currently approved agents are hirudin, bivalrudin and argatroban. All are approved for the treatment of HIT, but only argatroban is approved for prevention of HIT as well. They offer a more predictable anticoagulant response and have a short half-life, however there is no readily available reversal agent. Recombinant Factor VIIa may help reduce bleeding, but hemodialysis or hemoperfusion are required to remove DTIs (bivalrudin and agatroban only). Hirudin is the only available DTI which is cleared predominantly by the kidneys. Thus, CrCl should be calculated in older adults before administering this agent, which should be dose adjusted if CrCl 30–60 mL/min and avoided if CrCl <30 mL/min. Table 17.10 summarizes the DTIs [55, 57].

Fondaparinux

Fondaparinux is a synthetic analog of the antithrombin-binding sequence found in heparin and low-molecular-weight heparin. Fondaparinux works by binding antithrombin and enhancing its reactivity with factor Xa. Fondaparinux is typically administered once daily subcutaneously and has a plasma half life around seventeen hours [55]. It is renally excreted, and therefore requires dosing adjustments in patients with renal insufficiency, and should be avoided in patients with severely impaired renal function. Like LMWH, CrCl should be calculated in all older patients before considering this agent and should not be used if CrCl <30 mg/min. It does not bind to platelets or platelet factor 4, and therefore heparin-induced thrombocytopenia is unlikely to occur with fondaparinux. One of the limitations of fondaparinux is that it does not interact with protamine sulfate, and is therefore not easily reversible in the setting of uncontrolled bleeding. Recombinant factor VIIa may be effective in the setting of uncontrolled bleeding [58].

Evidence based studies support the use of fondaparinux for the prevention and treatment of venous thromboembolism, and for the treatment of arterial thrombosis. Fondaparinux has been FDA approved for use as venous thromboprophylaxis in high-risk orthopedic patients, or extended DVT prophylaxis following hip fracture surgery, and for patients at risk for thromboembolic complications following abdominal surgery, but not yet for these indications in CT surgery [45, 55].

Fondaparinux has been approved by the FDA for the treatment of acute symptomatic PE and DVT as a bridge to chronic OAT (Table 17.8). The recommended dose for VTE is 5.0, 7.5, or 10 mg SQ once daily for patients weighing <50, 50–100, or >100 kg, respectively. Oral warfarin should be started in addition to initiation of treatment with fondaparinux. Treatment with fondaparinux should be continued for at least five days and until the INR is in the therapeutic range (2.0–3.0) [16].

Combining Agents

Certain clinical scenarios recommend the use of multiple anticoagulant/antiplatelet therapies simultaneously, which must be used with caution in post surgical patients. An example is in a patient with a drug eluting stent less than 1-year old, who is also on anticoagulation for atrial fibrillation or a valve. The risk versus benefit of any elective surgery should be weighed carefully in this scenario, as stopping thienopyridines in such a patient increases the risk of coronary stent thrombosis, and surgical delay may be the safer option in some patients [49]. The risk of stopping anticoagulation/antiplatelet therapy in the higher risk older patient who may have several indications for these medications, must be judged again for the need and urgency of surgery, and the risk of bleeding. These patient-centered decisions often warrant consideration of less invasive mode of therapy when appropriate and available.

Summary

The interface between anticoagulation and surgery is challenging in older patients due to their inherently higher risks of bleeding and thrombosis. These risks are elevated by age-related changes in the coagulation cascade as well as comorbidities and polypharmacy which are common in older patients. Older patients on chronic OAT who undergo surgery are treated differently dependent on their short-term risk of thromboembolism versus their surgical bleeding risk. High risk patients, including those with mechanical mitral valves, bioprosthetic or mechanical aortic and mitral valve, or atrial fibrillation with high risk features, those being treated for VTE, those with cancer, or hypercoagulable states, should be given "bridging" therapy with heparins or fondaparinux with resumption of anticoagulation after the surgery. Older patients on OAT with low risk features may temporarily stop their VKA without bridging for surgery. Anticoagulation should be judiciously administered after valve surgery and for post-operative atrial fibrillation. The risk of VTE post-operatively is also increased in older adults, and aggressive prevention strategies with heparins and fondaparinux as well as mechanical strategies and early ambulation should be employed. Agents which are renally cleared (LMWH, fondaparinux and hirudin) should be used cautiously or avoided in older adults with impaired renal function, and CrCl should always be calculated first. The loading and maintenance doses of warfarin are also reduced, and careful dosing and frequent monitoring significantly reduce the bleeding risk of warfarin in older adults which is often due to supratherapeutic levels. Finally, many physicians' fears to use appropriate anticoagulation in older adults are often unfounded, especially given the high thrombotic risk of older patients.

References

1. Douketis JD, Berger PB, Dunn AS, et al. The perioperative management of antithrombotic therapy. American College of Chest Physicians evidence-based clinical practice guidelines (8th edition). Chest. 2008;133:299–339S.
2. Gurwitz JH, Field TS, Harrold LR. Incidence and preventability of adverse drug events among older persons in the ambulatory setting. JAMA. 2003;289(9):1107–16.
3. Classen DC, Jaser L, Budnitz DS. Adverse drug events among hospitalized Medicare patients: epidemiology and national estimates from a new approach to surveillance. Jt Comm J Qual Patient Saf. 2010;36(1):12–21.
4. Michaels AD, Spinler SA, Leeper B, et al. Medication errors in acute cardiovascular and stroke patients: a scientific statement from the American Heart Association. Circulation. 2010;121(14):1664–82.
5. Franchini M. Hemostasis and aging. Crit Rev Oncol Hematol. 2006;60(2):144–51.
6. Wilkerson WR, Sane DC. Aging and thrombosis. Semin Thromb Hemost. 2002;28(6):555–68.
7. Abatte R, Prisco D, Rostagno C, et al. Age-related changes in the hemostatic system. Int J Clin Lab Res. 1993;23:1–2.
8. Torn M, Bollen WL, van der Meer FJ, et al. Risks of oral anticoagulant therapy with increasing age. Arch Intern Med. 2005;165(13):1527–32.
9. Anonymous. Risk factors for stroke and efficacy of antithrombotic therapy in atrial fibrillation. Analysis of pooled data from five randomized controlled trials. Arch Intern Med. 1994;154:1449–57.
10. Man-Son-Hing M, Laupacis A. Balancing the risks of stroke and upper gastrointestinal tract bleeding in older patients with atrial fibrillation. Arch Intern Med. 2002;162(5):541–50.
11. Hylek EM, Singer DE. Risk factors for intracranial hemorrhage in outpatients taking warfarin. Ann Intern Med. 1994;120:897–902.
12. Nutescu EA, Shapiro NL, Ibrahim S, West P. Warfarin and its interactions with foods, herbs and other dietary supplements. Expert Opin Drug Saf. 2006;5(3):433–51.
13. Hajjar ER, Cafiero AC, Hanlon JT. Polypharmacy in elderly patients. Am J Geriatr Pharmacother. 2007;5(4):345–51.
14. Ansell J, Hirsh J, Poller L, et al. The pharmacology and management of the vitamin K antagonists: the Seventh ACCP Conference on Antithrombotic and Thrombolytic Therapy. Chest. 2004;126:204S–33.
15. Garcia D, Regan S, Crowther M, et al. Warfarin maintenance dosing patterns in clinical practice: implications for safer anticoagulation in the elderly population. Chest. 2005;127:2049–56.
16. Kearon C, Kahn S, Agnelli G, et al. Antithrombotic therapy for venous thromboembolic disease: American College of Chest Physicians evidence based clinical practice guidelines (8th edition). Chest. 2008;133(6 suppl):4545–5455.
17. Man-Son-Hing M, Laupacis A. Anticoagulant-related bleeding in older persons with atrial fibrillation: physicians' fears often unfounded. Arch Intern Med. 2003;163:1580–6.
18. Jacobs LG. Warfarin pharmacology, clinical management, and evaluation of hemorrhagic risk for the elderly. Clin Geriatr Med. 2006;22:17–18i.

19. Siguret V, Gouin I, Debray M. Initiation of warfarin therapy in elderly medical inpatients: a safe and accurate regimen. Am J Med. 2005;118:137–42.
20. Beyth RJ, Quinn L, Landefeld CS. A multicomponent intervention to prevent major bleeding complications in older patients receiving warfarin. A randomized, controlled trial. Ann Intern Med. 2000;133:687–95.
21. Tang EO, Lai CS, Lee KK, et al. Relationship between patients' warfarin knowledge and anticoagulation control. Ann Pharmacother. 2003;37:34–9.
22. Bruno JJ. Ellis JJ.Herbal use among US elderly: 2002 National Health Interview Survey. Ann Pharmacother. 2005 Apr;39(4):643–8.
23. Eagle KA, Guyton RA, Davidoff R, et al. ACC/AHA 2004 guideline update for coronary bypass graft surgery: summary article. J Am Coll Cardiol. 2004;44:1146.
24. Warfarin versus aspirin for prevention of thromboembolism in atrial fibrillation. Stroke Prevention in Atrial Fibrillation II Study. Lancet. 1994;343:687–91.
25. Fang MC, Chang Y, Hylek EM, et al. Advanced age, anticoagulation intensity, and risk for intracranial hemorrhage among patients taking warfarin for atrial fibrillation. Ann Intern Med. 2004;141:745–52.
26. Hart RG, Benavente O, Pearce LA. Increased risk of intracranial hemorrhage when aspirin is combined with warfarin: a meta-analysis and hypothesis. Cerebrovasc Dis. 1999;9:215–7.
27. Bungard TJ, Ghali WA, McAlister FA, et al. Physicians' perceptions of the benefits and risks of warfarin for patients with nonvalvular atrial fibrillation. CMAJ. 2001;165:301–2.
28. Man-Son-Hing M, Nichol G, Lau A, Laupacis A. Choosing antithrombotic therapy for elderly patients with atrial fibrillation who are at risk for falls. Arch Intern Med. 1999;159:677–85.
29. Bonow RO, Carabello BA, Chatterjee K, et al. ACC/AHA 2006 guidelines for the management of patients with valvular heart disease: a report of the American College of Cardiology/American Heart Association Task Force on Practice Guidelines (writing Committee to Revise the 1998 guidelines for the management of patients with valvular heart disease) developed in collaboration with the Society of Cardiovascular Anesthesiologists endorsed by the Society for Cardiovascular Angiography and Interventions and the Society of Thoracic Surgeons. J Am Coll Cardiol. 2006;48(3):e1–148.
30. Thachil J, Gatt A, Martlew V. Management of surgical patients receiving anticoagulation and antiplatelet agents. Br J Surg. 2008;95(12):1437–48.
31. Gage BF, Waterman AD, Shannon W, et al. Validation of clinical classification schemes for predicting stroke: results from the National Registry of Atrial Fibrillation. JAMA. 2001;285:2864.
32. Go AS, Hylek EM, Chang Y, et al. Anticoagulation therapy for stroke prevention in atrial fibrillation: how well do randomized trials translate into clinical practice? JAMA. 2003;290:2685.
33. Go AS. The epidemiology of atrial fibrillation in elderly persons: the tip of the iceberg. Am J Geriatr Cardiol. 2005;1914:56–61.
34. Wolf PA, Abbott RD, Kannel WB. Atrial fibrillation as an independent risk factor for stroke: the Framingham Study. Stroke. 1991;22:983–8.
35. van Aart L, Eijkhout HW, Kamphuis JS, et al. Individualized dosing regimen for prothrombin complex concentrate more effective than standard treatment in the reversal of oral anticoagulant therapy: an open, prospective randomized controlled trial. Thromb Res. 2006;118(3):313–20.
36. Schulman S. Care of patients receiving long-term anticoagulant therapy. N Engl J Med. 2003;349:675.
37. Antman EM, Anbe DT, Armstrong PW, et al. ACC/AHA guidelines for the management of patients with ST-elevation myocardial infarction: a report of the American College of Cardiology/American Heart Association Task Force on Practice Guidelines

(Committee to Revise the 1999 Guidelines for the Management of Patients with Acute Myocardial Infarction). Circulation. 2004;110(9):e82–292.

38. Cannegieter SC, Rosendaal FR, Wintzen AR, et al. Optimal oral anticoagulant therapy in patients with mechanical heart valves. New Engl J Med. 1995;333:11.

39. Allou N, Piednoir P, Berroeta C, et al. Incidence and risk factors of early thromboembolic events after mechanical heart valve replacement in patients treated with intravenous unfractionated heparin. Heart. 2009;95(20):1694–700.

40. Salem DN, O'Gara PT, Madias C, Pauker SG. Valvular and structural heart disease: American College of Chest Physicians evidence-based clinical practice guidelines (8th Edition). Chest. 2008;133:593S.

41. Butchart EG, Gohlke-Barwolf C, Antunes MJ, et al. Recommendations for the management of patients after heart valve surgery. Eur Heart J. 2005;26(22):2463–71.

42. Becker RC, Meade TW, Berger PB, et al. The primary and secondary prevention of coronary artery disease: American College of Chest Physicians evidence-based clinical practice guidelines (8th Edition). Chest. 2008;133:776S.

43. Raskob GE, Silverstein R, Bratzler D, et al. Surveillance for deep vein thrombosis and pulmonary embolism: recommendations from a national workshop. Am J of Prev Med. 2010;38:502.

44. Sandler DA, Martin JF. Autopsy proven pulmonary embolism in hospital patients: are we detecting enough deep vein thrombosis? J R Soc Med. 1989;82:203.

45. Geerts MH, Bergqvist D, Pineo GF, et al. Prevention of venous thromboembolism: ACCP evidence based clinical pracitce guidelines (8th Edition). Chest. 2008;133(6 suppl):3815–4535.

46. Fuster V, Ryden LE, Cannom DS, et al. ACC/AHA/ESC 2006 Guidelines for the Management of Patients with Atrial Fibrillation. A report of the American College of Cardiology/American Heart Association Task Force on Practice Guidelines and the European Society of Cardiology Committee for Practice Guidelines (Writing Committee to Revise the 2001 Guidelines for the Management of Patients With Atrial Fibrillation). J Am Coll Cardiol. 2006;1948:e149–246.

47. Hart RG, Benavente O, McBride R, Pearce LA. Antithrombotic therapy to prevent stroke in patients with atrial fibrillation: a meta-analysis. Ann Intern Med. 1999;131:492–501.

48. McFalls EO, Ward HB, Moritz TE, et al. Predictors and outcomes of a perioperative myocardial infarction following elective vascular surgery in patients with documented coronary artery disease: results of the CARP trial. Eur Heart J. 2008;29(3):394–401.

49. King 3rd SB, Smith Jr SC, Hirshfeld Jr JW, et al. 2007 focused update of the ACC/AHA/SCAI 2005 guideline update for percutaneous coronary intervention: a report of the American College of Cardiology/American Heart Association task force on practice guidelines: 2007 writing group to review new evidence and update the ACC/AHA/SCAI 2005 guideline update for percutaneous coronary intervention, writing on behalf of the 2005 writing committee. Circulation. 2008;117:261.

50. Dickstein K, Cohen-Solal A, Filippatos G, et al. ESC Guidelines for the diagnosis and treatment of acute and chronic heart failure 2008: the Task Force for the Diagnosis and Treatment of Acute and Chronic Heart Failure 2008 of the European Society of Cardiology. Developed in collaboration with the Heart Failure Association of the ESC (HFA) and endorsed by the European Society of Intensive Care Medicine (ESICM). Eur Heart J. 2008;29:2388.

51. Horlander KT, Mannino DM, Leeper KV. Pulmonary embolism mortality in the United States, 1979-1998: an analysis using multiple-cause mortality data. Arch Intern Med. 2003;163:1711.

52. Decousus H, Leizorovicz A, Parent F, et al. A clinical trial of vena caval filters in the prevention of pulmonary embolism in patients with proximal deep-vein thrombosis. Prevention du Risque d'Embolie Pulmonaire par Interruption Cave Study Group. N Engl J Med. 1998;338(7):409–15.

53. PREPIC Study Group. Eight-year follow-up of patients with permanent vena cava filters in the prevention of pulmonary embolism: the PREPIC (Prevention du Risque d'Embolie Pulmonaire par Interruption Cave) randomized study. Circulation. 2005;112(3):416–22.

54. Baglin TP, Brush J, Streiff M. Guidelines on use of vena cava filters. Br J Haematol. 2006;134:590.

55. Hirsh J, Bauer KA, Donati MB, et al. Parenteral anticoagulants: American College of Chest Physicians evidence-based clinical practice guidelines (8th Edition). Chest. 2008;133:141S.

56. Warkentin TE, Greinacher A, Koster A, Lincoff AM. Treatment and prevention of heparin-induced thrombocytopenia: American College of Chest Physicians evidence-based clinical practice guidelines (8th Edition). Chest. 2008;133:340S.

57. Nutescu E, Shapiro N, Chevalier A. New anticoagulant agents: direct thrombin inhibitors. Cardiol Clin. 2008;26(2):169–87.

58. Bijsterveld N, Moons A, Boekholdt S, et al. Ability of recombinant factor VIIa to reverse the anticoagulant effect of the pentasaccharide fondaparinux in healthy volunteers. Circulation. 2002;106:2550–4.

59. Konstantinides S. Clinical practice. Acute pulmonary embolism. New Engl J Med. 2008;359(26):2804–13.

Chapter 18
Medication Usage in Older Cardiothoracic Surgical Patients[1]

Richard A. Marottoli, Sean M. Jeffery, and Roshini C. Pinto-Powell

Abstract Older individuals in general take more medications than other age groups and are more susceptible to potential adverse effects. This chapter reviews the changes that occur with aging and that underlie this increased susceptibility and offers suggestions to minimize adverse effects. Specific medication categories are highlighted that pose particular risk of adverse effects in older cardiothoracic surgery patients. The vast majority of medications can be used safely and effectively in older patients if appropriate precautions are taken in the selection, dosing, and timing of medications, and in the active monitoring of therapeutic effects and side effects.

Keywords Elderly/aging • Cardiothoracic surgery • Medications • Biology of aging • Pharmacokinetics • Polypharmacy • Delirium • Psychoactive medications • Antibiotics • Side effects

As the Baby Boom generation begins reaching age 65 in 2011, we will witness the largest increase in the number of older adults ever. Two-thirds of all people who have ever lived to the age of 65 are alive today [1]. Advances in pharmacotherapy are partially responsible for this increase in longevity and will continue to play a central role in reducing morbidity as this cohort ages. However, medication use in this population is not without potential problems. In older adults medications are often improperly dosed, overprescribed, and poorly monitored for signs of toxicity. Furthermore, changes in pharmacokinetics associated with aging leave little room for error. Older cardiothoracic surgery patients are particularly vulnerable given the nature of the surgery and the underlying conditions. Thus, it is imperative to preoperatively identify potential medication-related problems (MRPs) that can result in postoperative complications. This chapter reviews some of the factors that contribute to MRPs in the elderly, general approaches to prescribing, signs and symptoms to monitor, and highlights of certain drug categories that are commonly used or have substantial potential to cause side effects in older adults.

Biology of Aging

After age 30, organ systems decline in function to some extent with advancing age, but at varying rates, and independently of each other (Table 18.1). In the absence of disease, these declines are not sufficient to impair daily function [2, 3]. However, the reserve capacity of an organ system diminishes with age. Thus, the ability to withstand even a minor insult is decreased, and recovery may be delayed. Appreciating medication-related factors that affect an organ system's reserve capacity is an imperfect science. Understanding the principles of pharmacokinetics will help surgeons to understand how physiologic changes with aging affect response to medications, making it easier to anticipate MRPs [4]. Pharmacokinetics is defined as the delivery of a drug to its site of action. This includes drug absorption, distribution, metabolism, and excretion. These changes are reviewed here in general terms to provide a background for the discussion of individual drug classes (Table 18.2) [5].

Drug Absorption

The amount of oral drug absorption (bioavailability) depends on several factors not related to age, including the presence of food, drug ionization, and dosage formulation [6]. Absorption can occur anywhere along the gastrointestinal tract. Oral drug absorption can also include buccal absorption of orally disintegrating tablets (ODT) for patients with

[1] Portions of this chapter are reprinted with permission from Marottoli RA, Jeffery SM, Pinto-Powell RC. Drug usage in surgical patients: preventing medication related problems. In: Rosenthal RE, Katlic MR, Zenilman ME, editors. Principles and practice of geriatric surgery. 2nd ed. New York: Springer; 2010.

R.A. Marottoli (✉)
Department of Geriatric Medicine, Yale School of Medicine,
VA Connecticut Healthcare System, 950 Campbell Ave, West Haven,
CT 06516, USA
e-mail: richard.marottoli@ynhh.org

M.R. Katlic (ed.), *Cardiothoracic Surgery in the Elderly*, DOI 10.1007/978-1-4419-0892-6_18,
© Springer Science+Business Media, LLC 2011

swallowing difficulties. Some formulations are specifically designed to release medication in response to changes in intestinal pH or osmolality. In general, older adults tend to

have a slight increase in gastric pH. This increase is unlikely to result in altered drug absorption [6, 7]. Achlorhydria, once thought to be a consequence of aging, has diminished as a concern with the identification and treatment of indolent *Helicobacter pylori* infections.

Older adults tend to experience two alterations that can lead to clinically significant changes in the rate of oral drug absorption. First, changes in gastrointestinal blood flow may reduce portal circulation and delay gastric absorption, as seen in some heart failure or cirrhosis patients with substantial hepatic congestion. And second, decreased gastric emptying, resulting from conditions such as Parkinson's disease or diabetes, may also delay the rate of absorption, but not the extent of drug absorbed [7, 8]. Unless therapeutic failure is observed, no changes in dosing are required to overcome delays in gastric absorption.

Oral bioavailability can be substantially altered in the presence of food, so called drug–food interactions. For example, calcium supplementation has variously been reported to reduce the absorption of angiotensin-converting enzyme inhibitors, calcium channel blockers, HMG-CoA reductase inhibitors, and calcium receptor blockers. Conversely, calcium supplementation may increase the effects of α/β-agonists, quinidine, and tocainide. The authors recommend discontinuing most calcium supplementation during the postoperative period to prevent potential chelation interactions with antibiotics. In addition to calcium interactions, many other medications have reduced bioavailability from food. Bisphosphonate bioavailability is exceedingly low when taken with anything other than water. Levodopa absorption is substantially decreased when consumed with a high protein meal [9]. Additionally, certain foods can substantially alter drug levels

Table 18.1 Pharmacokinetic changes with aging

Absorption	Extent not affected
	Rate is reduced or unaltered
	Increased gastric pH
	Unchanged passive diffusion
	Decreased active transport
	Decreased first pass effect
	Decreased GI blood flow with certain diseases (e.g., HF)
Distribution	Decreased total body water
	Decreased lean body mass
	Decreased serum albumin?
	Increased body fat
	↑'d or ↓'d free fraction of highly plasma protein bound drugs
	Higher concentration of water soluble drugs
Metabolism	Decreased liver blood flow
	Decreased liver size
	Decreased enzymatic activity
	Variable decreased and increased $t_{1/2}$ for phase I oxidation drugs
	Decreased clearance and increased $t_{1/2}$ of drugs with high extraction ratio
Excretion	Decreased GFR
	Decreased renal blood flow
	Decreased tubular function
	Decreased clearance and increased $t_{1/2}$ for drugs eliminated primarily by the kidneys

Source: Reprinted with permission from Marottoli RA, Jeffery SM, Pinto-Powell RC. Drug usage in surgical patients: preventing medication related problems. In: Rosenthal RE, Katlic MR, Zenilman ME, editors. Principles and practice of geriatric surgery. 2nd ed. New York: Springer; 2010

Table 18.2 Examples of age-related physiologic changes affecting drug pharmacokinetics

Physiologic change	Direction of change	Drugs affected by this change	Result of change
Serum albumin	↓	Phenytoin, naproxen, valproate, warfarin	Increased free (active) fraction of drug; increased effects
α_1-Acid glycoprotein	↑	Propranolol, antidepressants, lidocaine, methadone, quinidine	Decreased free (active) fraction of drug; decreased effects
Body fat	↑	Fat-soluble drugs (e.g., benzodiazepines)	Increased volume of distribution; increased half-life and potential for accumulation
Lean muscle mass	↓	Digoxin	Decreased volume of distribution; increased concentration; lower loading dose is needed
Body water	↓	Water-soluble drugs (e.g., lithium)	Decreased volume of distribution; increased concentration and effects
Hepatic blood flow	↓	High hepatic extraction ratio drugs (e.g., morphine, meperidine, lidocaine, and isosorbide)	Decreased first-pass metabolism; increased effects
Hepatic metabolism (phase 1: reduction, oxidation, hydroxylation, demethylation)	↓	Diazepam, alprazolam, triazolam, theophylline, quinidine, propranolol, phenytoin, imipramine	Decreased metabolism; increased half-life and concentration
Renal function	↓	Aminoglycosides, digoxin, ciprofloxacin, allopurinol	Decreased clearance; increased effects, toxicity, or both

Source: Reprinted with permission from Marottoli RA, Jeffery SM, Pinto-Powell RC. Drug usage in surgical patients: preventing medication related problems. In: Rosenthal RE, Katlic MR, Zenilman ME, editors. Principles and practice of geriatric surgery. 2nd ed. New York: Springer; 2010

and actions. Patients on warfarin who alter their intake of vitamin K-containing foods risk changes in their international normalized ratio (INR).

Consumption of grapefruit irreversibly inhibits intestinal CYP-450 3A4 isoenzyme activity. This results in presystemic decreases in metabolism leading to increases in therapeutic concentrations that can last for up to 72 h. One of the earliest classes of medications suspected of interacting with grapefruit was the HMG-CoA reductase inhibitors [10]. Such interactions may increase the risk of rhabdomyolysis when dyslipidemia is treated with atorvastatin, lovastatin, or simvastatin. Potential alternative agents are pravastatin, fluvastatin, or rosuvastatin. Grapefruit interactions can result in vasodilation in hypertensive patients receiving the dihydropyridines felodipine, nicardipine, nifedipine, nisoldipine, or nitrendipine. This interaction is not present with amlodipine. Alternately, the efficacy of the angiotensin II type 1 receptor antagonist losartan may be reduced by grapefruit juice. In summary, the rate of absorption may be delayed with aging, but the overall extent of absorption is unlikely to be altered.

Limited information is available about topical drug absorption changes due to aging. Topical administration is gaining popularity as a way to minimize first-pass metabolism, improve medication adherence, and provide more continuous therapeutic drug concentrations. For example, postoperative pain control may include the use of fentanyl or lidocaine patches. Decreases in skin thickness and integrity may alter drug absorption and subsequently peak concentrations. When comparing healthy young volunteers to healthy elderly volunteers receiving transdermal fentanyl patches, older patients demonstrated higher systemic concentrations of fentanyl and correspondingly greater adverse effects resulting in drug discontinuation [11]. An additional concern when administering medications in patch form is the ability to safely remove the patch without damaging the underlying skin. Finally, all patches utilize adhesives that can cause localized skin irritation. The use of presurgical skin disinfectants and body preparations may contribute to heightened skin sensitivity to patch adhesives.

Distribution

The distribution of drugs is altered by the aging process. Total body and intracellular water decrease, as does muscle mass, whereas body fat increases [2, 3]. These changes have important implications for drug distribution that can affect both the half-life of a compound and the concentration of the drug in various tissues (e.g., lipophilic versus hydrophilic saturation). Water-soluble drugs tend to have an increased level per unit dose because of decreased total body and intracellular water. The volume of distribution for lipid-soluble drugs tends to be higher because of increased fat stores, resulting in prolonged and less predictable half-lives. Changes in protein binding can also alter receptor site activity. When medications exhibit substantial protein binding (generally >90%), the potential for protein-binding interactions due to changes in serum albumin becomes more pronounced. For example, in the case of low albumin levels, the relative proportion of free or unbound drug may be increased, enhancing the pharmacologic and toxic properties of the drug. To further illustrate this point consider the highly protein bound drug phenytoin. By convention, when ordering phenytoin levels what is typically reported is the total drug level [12]. In the setting of low albumin, however, the free drug concentration may be high, resulting in toxicity despite a total level in the therapeutic range. In contrast, the carrier protein α1-acid glycoprotein may increase with age, as it does with illness, so drugs that bind to this protein may have a lower proportion unbound; an example is propranolol [13]. Another caveat with drug levels is that normal ranges are often established on young persons; therefore targeting lower therapeutic drug levels may minimize the risk of toxicity. The important exception to this approach is for antibiotic therapy where specific minimum inhibitory concentrations (MIC) are specified. Finally, conformational changes in the ability of albumin to bind drugs may change with age, resulting in reduced affinity of albumin to bind to medications despite a normal albumin level [12].

Metabolism

First-Pass Metabolism and High Hepatic Extraction Ratio Drugs

Liver size and blood flow tend to decrease with age by 20–30%. Drugs that depend on extensive first-pass metabolism may have higher therapeutic levels resulting from decreased hepatic metabolism [9, 14, 15]. For example, it is estimated that morphine exhibits a 33% reduction in clearance in the elderly as a result of decreased first-pass metabolism [15]. Therefore, the effects of morphine may last longer in the elderly. However, this does not constitute a reason to avoid morphine in older patients. Drugs that have high hepatic extraction ratios also exhibit decreased metabolism and potentially increased therapeutic concentrations. Atorvastatin is a high hepatic extraction ratio drug with increased serum concentration (40%) and area under the concentration curve (30%) [15]. Therefore, closer attention to liver function tests and potential dose reduction may be warranted. Similar findings occur with simvastatin and lovastatin.

Delirium is the acute or sub-acute development of an alteration in mental state that fluctuates during the course of the day. Standardized assessment instruments such as the Confusion Assessment Method can be helpful for its detection [47]. Risk factors can be thought of as "predisposing factors," making one vulnerable to developing delirium, and "precipitating factors," which directly or indirectly lead to it. Among the predisposing factors are cognitive impairment, visual impairment, severe illness, and renal insufficiency [48]. Precipitating factors include the use of physical restraints, malnutrition, bladder catheterization, iatrogenic events, and the number and type of medications [49]. Certain medications have been linked to a particular risk of postoperative delirium (e.g., meperidine and benzodiazepines) [50]. The simultaneous addition of three or more medications to a drug regimen in the hospital may also contribute to delirium [49]. This may be due to the sheer volume of new medications overwhelming a vulnerable individual's reserve capacity or to the likelihood of at least one medication being psychoactive when many are prescribed.

Cardiothoracic surgery patients may be at particular risk for developing delirium because of the nature of the procedures, as well as the underlying conditions (with associated comorbidities) necessitating surgery. Although it is difficult to compare across studies because of different patient populations and methods for detecting delirium, a number of risk factors have been identified. These include preoperative (older age, preexisting peripheral/cerebrovascular or renal disease, high comorbidity, cognitive impairment, depression, nutritional deficits), perioperative (complex surgery, long operative time, need for intra-aortic balloon pump, or large volume transfusions), and postoperative (low cardiac output, pneumonia) factors [51–55]. Preoperative prediction rules have been developed to assist in early identification of high-risk patients, including a recent study utilizing separate derivation and validation cohorts that demonstrated a gradient of delirium occurrence of 18–87% based on the presence of preexisting cerebrovascular disease, cognitive impairment, depression, or low albumin [55].

With early identification of at-risk patients and close monitoring for early signs of delirium, a number of strategies may be employed to try to decrease the risk of delirium, including attention to underlying illness and complications. The general prescribing principles outlined above may also be helpful along with specific examples detailed below when discussing individual drug categories. Another factor that is particularly problematic in the hospital setting is the scheduling of medications or treatments at night that require patients to be awakened, sometimes repeatedly. Although it may be necessary for acutely or severely ill patients or during the immediate postoperative period, it is helpful to attempt to minimize the occurrence later in the hospital course. Multifactorial interventions have been shown to reduce the incidence of delirium by 35–40% in medical and post-hip fracture patients [56, 57].

Antipsychotics

Antipsychotics are used to treat hallucinations, delusions, paranoia, and extreme agitation or physical violence [58]. They tend to not be useful for pacing or wandering. Because of potential serious side effects they should not be used to treat insomnia. It is important to look for delirium as the potential cause of a new-onset behavioral disturbance or thought disorder, so the underlying etiology can be determined and treatment of the primary process initiated.

Once a target sign or symptom is identified to gauge the effectiveness of treatment, the choice of agent largely depends on the desired side effect profile. For the most part, neuroleptics are essentially equally effective, so the choice of agent depends on which side effect profile fits the characteristics of the patient or is best tolerated by the patient. "Typical" agents, such as haloperidol (starting dose 0.25–0.5 mg, maximum daily dose 2.0 mg), are inexpensive and are available in oral, intramuscular, and intravenous preparations. The latter parenteral preparations may be particularly helpful in the setting of acute agitation or if the patient is unable to take oral medications. Haloperidol is more likely to produce extrapyramidal side effects, but less likely to cause sedation, orthostasis, and anticholinergic effects than lower potency agents. Among the extrapyramidal effects are Parkinsonian features including tremor, bradykinesia, and masked facies. Although these symptoms may fade over time, they have in the past also been treated with anticholinergic agents such as benztropine and trihexyphenidyl. This approach should be avoided because of the increased potential for delirium with concomitant therapy. A wiser approach might be to decrease the dose or switch to a different agent. Akathisia is manifested as motor restlessness, pacing, or disturbed sleep and may be reported as discomfort or anxiety. A danger is that these features may be misinterpreted as increasing psychosis, with the neuroleptic dose then being increased, resulting in worsened symptoms. As a result, it is often better to decrease the dose as an initial response to such symptoms to see if they are alleviated.

Tardive dyskinesia is a potential serious side effect of neuroleptic use and one of the reasons their use should be limited to the indications described above. Tardive dyskinesia starts as fine movement of the tongue, a facial tic, or lip smacking, but may progress in the extreme to affect speech, eating, and breathing. Furthermore, it may be irreversible. Older adults and women are most likely to develop tardive dyskinesia, and it is more likely to be severe and less likely to be reversible in older adults. It is less clear that treatment duration and type of agent are important contributors to risk [59, 60]. The primary treatment is to taper and discontinue the drug.

"Atypical" agents, such as risperidone (starting dose 0.25–0.5 mg, maximum daily dose 2.5 mg), have been touted as having fewer extrapyramidal side effects, although the risk does increase with increasing dosage. Olanzapine (starting dose 2.5–5 mg, maximum daily dose 20 mg) may be helpful in individuals who have insomnia or poor oral intake in addition to psychosis, although these effects may be problematic with longer term use.

A number of precautions can be taken to minimize the risk or extent of side effects. Once the desired effect is achieved and the target symptom is alleviated, or the inciting event resolves, the drug should be tapered and discontinued. Many of the problems with neuroleptic use result from patients being left on the drug long after the inciting event resolves and after discharge from the hospital. If patients are discharged to a rehabilitation or long-term care facility, it is helpful to indicate a time limit to treatment with these agents, like one would do with a course of antibiotics. If agents are prescribed on an as-needed, or pro re nata (PRN), basis, the indication for use and maximum daily dose should be clearly stated in the orders. The maximum daily doses provided for agents above are guidelines; while they may be exceeded, this should be done cautiously and under close supervision because of the increased risk of side effects.

Of note, recent evidence has raised concern about the limited effectiveness of these agents in controlling behavioral symptoms and the potential risk of other serious adverse effects, such as cardiac and cerebrovascular events and death [61–63]. These effects have been noted in patients with dementia and with long-term use and higher doses, but they may affect the risk–benefit equation in a given patient. They also add to the importance of judiciously using these medications only for the appropriate indications (psychosis and agitation where the health and safety of the patient or caregivers is threatened) and at as low a dose and for as short a duration as is clinically necessary.

Antidepressants

The cardinal features of depression are the "vegetative" or depressive signs and symptoms, including increased or decreased sleep, decreased activity level, fatigue, decreased concentration, increased or decreased appetite or weight, motor slowing or agitation, guilt, suicidality, chronic somatic complaints, and pain [64]. Although standardized instruments, such as the Geriatric Depression Scale, can be useful adjuncts, diagnosis still often relies on the recognition of depressive signs and symptoms [65]. It is important to rule out underlying medical illnesses contributing to depression, such as stroke, myocardial infarction, congestive heart failure, thyroid disorders, uremia,

and certain cancers. Medications may contribute as well, including central-acting antihypertensives and β-blockers, narcotics, neuroleptics, benzodiazepines, antihistamines, and sedative/hypnotics [66].

Once these contributing factors have been ruled out and target signs or symptoms identified, the choice of agent depends in part on the characteristics or features of the patient and the desired side effect profile [64, 67, 68]. There is currently a wide range of therapeutic options to treat depression. While early agents such as tricyclics can be effective, their side effect profiles require much more caution when used in older patients. Tertiary amine tricyclics (e.g., amitriptyline, imipramine, and doxepin) were among the early agents used. Although effective, their side effects are very poorly tolerated by elderly persons and they should be avoided. Their metabolites (secondary amine tricyclics such as nortriptyline and desipramine) are available and are preferred if a tricyclic is to be used. Like the low potency neuroleptics, tricyclics have as potential side effects sedation, orthostasis, and anticholinergic effects. In addition, they have the potential to contribute to arrhythmias. While nortriptyline and desipramine have relatively low arrhythmogenicity, they should be used cautiously in persons with underlying conduction disorders, and PR and QRS intervals should be monitored periodically while on treatment. Desipramine is an activating agent and is preferable for persons who are apathetic, withdrawn, and anhedonic. Nortriptyline is a sedating agent and is preferred in individuals who are anxious or have sleep difficulties as well as depression. Blood levels are available for both agents and can be used to adjust doses depending on effect and side effects (nortriptyline has a therapeutic window – a level beyond the upper limit may lead to less effectiveness and more side effects) [69].

Because of their enhanced safety and tolerablility profiles, selective serotonin and norepinephine reuptake inhibitors (SSRI, SNRI) are the current preferred agents for treating depression in older patients [68, 70]. In general, citalopram/escitalopram, sertraline, and venlafaxine are safe, effective, and well tolerated by older patients and are reasonable initial choices. For patients with certain associated features, other agents may be considered. For patients with poor sleep, poor intake, and anxiety as features of their depression, mirtazapine would be an option. For patients with pain and depression, duloxetine is an alternative. The latter options may minimize the number of medications by treating multiple symptoms with a single agent. Most agents take several weeks to have an effect on mood, but beneficial effects on sleep or appetite may be seen sooner. Potential side effects include gastrointestinal upset, change in sleep, headaches, dizziness, and sexual dysfunction.

Methylphenidate (starting dose 5 mg daily, maximum dose 10 mg twice a day, dosed early), which often exhibits an effect within 24–48 h, may be used as a bridging activating agent for particularly anhedonic or apathetic patients until other agents exert their effect, with its primary side effects being excessive arousal, gastrointestinal upset, and tachycardia [71]. Monoamine oxidase (MAO) inhibitors are used infrequently because of their potential serious interactions with certain medications and tyramine-containing foods. For life-threatening or refractory depression, electroconvulsive therapy can be used safely and effectively in elderly persons [66].

Anxiolytics

Pharmacologic intervention for anxiety is warranted if symptoms are sufficiently severe to interfere with daily coping or enjoyment of life. In general, treatment should be short term: for a grief reaction or as an adjunct to supportive therapy to develop coping strategies. It is important to rule out contributing disorders such as congestive heart failure and chronic obstructive pulmonary disease.

The mainstays of anxiolytic therapy are the benzodiazepines [58, 72]. Given the metabolic changes that occur with aging described above, short-acting agents such as lorazepam (starting dose 0.5 mg/day) and oxazepam (starting dose 7.5 mg/day) are preferred because of their more predictable half-lives and duration of action. All benzodiazepines share potential side effects, including sedation, dizziness, depression, confusion, agitation, and disinhibition. Dependence can develop, and tolerance to their effects often occurs after 2–4 weeks of continuous use. Consequently, it is best to use these agents short term. Because a withdrawal reaction or "rebound" characterized by tremor and agitation can occur after abrupt withdrawal, benzodiazepines should be tapered prior to discontinuing. Buspirone (starting dose 5 mg twice a day) is a non-benzodiazepine anxiolytic that is less likely to cause dependence, sedation, or psychomotor retardation. However, it has a delayed onset of action (several weeks) and lacks the soporific and muscle relaxant effects of benzodiazepines. Its primary side effects are dizziness and nausea. Barbiturates should be avoided because they are less effective and have greater addictive potential than other available agents [72, 73].

Sedative/Hypnotics

Disturbed sleep is a common complaint among older persons, particularly in the hospital [58, 74]. Part of this is due to changes that occur in sleep patterns with aging, including a phase shift (falling asleep and waking up earlier than in prior years) and more disruptions to sleep. Disturbed sleep may manifest as difficulty falling asleep, difficulty staying asleep, or early morning awakening. A variety of medical factors contribute to sleep difficulties, including anxiety, depression,

pain, itching, nocturia, and congestive heart failure. Medications or substances that may contribute include amphetamines, steroids, decongestants, caffeine, and alcohol. A number of other factors may play a role among hospitalized patients, including daytime naps, intravenous lines, catheters, traction, and frequent awakenings for medications or treatments. After establishing by history if sleep is disturbed, the mainstay of treatment should be non-pharmacologic interventions directed at potential contributing factors.

If drug treatment is indicated, there are several potential choices that can be used safely and effectively short term (suggested maximum duration of use is 7–10 days). Among the benzodiazepines, short-acting agents are preferred because they are less likely to cause carryover sedation the following day. Temazepam (starting dose 7.5 mg) has a reasonable duration of action but a delayed onset of action and so must be given approximately 1–2 h before bedtime. Non-benzodiazepine hypnotics, such as zolpidem, zaleplon, and eszopiclone, also appear relatively safe in older persons [75]. If the primary problem is difficulty falling asleep, ramelteon is another option. If persons are depressed and have sleep difficulties, treatment with a sedating antidepressant is preferable to separate treatment with two different medications. Similarly, if someone has a thought disorder and disturbed sleep, a sedating neuroleptic is preferred, but neuroleptics should not be used for sleep alone.

Pain Management

Pain is a common complaint among elderly persons and can have a substantial effect on mood and physical functioning. Adequate treatment is thus important, but caution must be exercised because of the strong potential for adverse effects with many of these agents. Consequently, it is helpful to follow the stepwise approach defined above for assessing the nature and extent of pain, determining its etiology, and starting with lower doses of less potent agents. A variety of instruments are available to help gauge the current severity of pain and the effectiveness of treatment [76, 77].

The first line of therapy often consists of acetaminophen, aspirin, or non-steroidal anti-inflammatory agents (NSAIDs) [77–79]. Although all three possess analgesic and antipyretic properties, acetaminophen lacks the anti-inflammatory properties of the other two classes. Acetaminophen is safe, effective, inexpensive, and well tolerated by older persons. Caution should be exercised in the setting of liver disease or alcohol use, and there may be an increased risk of end-stage renal disease with high-dose long-term use [77, 80]. Caution must also be taken to ensure that patients avoid compound medications that include acetaminophen, which may contribute to their unknowingly exceeding recommended daily limits. Aspirin and non-steroidals can cause gastrointestinal bleeding or renal insufficiency and can interfere with platelet function. A variety of central nervous system (CNS) side effects may also be seen with non-steroidals. Given that these three classes provide roughly equipotent analgesic effects, acetaminophen is a safer initial choice in the absence of inflammation. The most recent guidelines of the American Geriatrics Society recommend acetaminophen rather than non-steroidals for the first-line treatment of pain because of their side effect profiles in older adults [79].

If pain is not controlled with these agents, opioid analgesics are the next line of treatment [77–79]. They are often characterized as mild or strong. Mild opioids, such as codeine and oxycodone, may provide relief alone or in conjunction with the non-opioid analgesics described above. Strong opioids, such as morphine, are used if pain remains unrelieved. All opioids have similar potential side effects, including respiratory depression, constipation, urinary retention, nausea and vomiting, delirium, and myoclonus. The patient should be monitored closely and appropriate dose adjustments made when these side effects appear. Prophylactic bowel regimens are often necessary and should be initiated when the narcotic is started. Tolerance to some of the effects may appear and may be facilitated by continuous, rather than as-needed, administration schedules. For respiratory depression, the opiate antagonist naloxone may be helpful. Meperidine should be avoided in the elderly, as it must be used with caution in patients with renal insufficiency and its metabolite, normeperidine, may cause seizures. Topical analgesics such as capsaicin may be helpful for conditions such as herpes zoster. Non-pharmacologic modalities such as heat, cold, massage, biofeedback, and transcutaneous electrical nerve stimulation (TENS) help in certain situations. Nerve blocks are another potential option for certain types of refractory pain. A recent trial of an interdisciplinary analgesic program in orthopedic patients found that intervention participants had less pain postoperatively and at 6 months and better physical performance [81].

Antihistamines

Histamine H_1 receptor blockers are commonly used for treatment of allergies and allergic reactions; occasionally they are used as sedative/hypnotics. Because of their prominent anticholinergic properties, they should be used cautiously in the elderly. Newer agents with relatively low anticholinergic properties, such as loratadine, are preferred to treat allergy symptoms. Antihistamines such as diphenhydramine should not be used as sleep medications given the availability of safer agents.

Histamine H_2 receptor blockers, used to inhibit gastric acid secretion, can be safely used in elderly persons. All these agents can cause alterations in mental status [82]. The dose

and duration of use should be kept to a minimum and always adjusted for renal function. If used prophylactically during the perioperative period, the dose should be decreased and ultimately discontinued as soon as possible.

Antibiotics

There are two major clinical categories of antibiotic usage among surgical inpatients: perioperative prophylaxis and the treatment of postoperative infections. Surgical site infections account for 11% of nosocomial infections among older patients [83]. Although this chapter does not deal with specific antibiotic recommendations, it addresses the general principles of antibiotic choice, dosing, and specific side effects in the geriatric patient.

As older persons increasingly receive technologic devices (grafts, stents, pacemakers, transplanted organs, and dialysis catheters) to improve and maintain their quality of life, the devices themselves and the medications (immunosuppressive drugs, anticoagulants) that patients may be on as a result need to be taken into consideration when choosing an antibiotic regimen. In the field of cardiothoracic surgery in particular, improving cardiopulmonary bypass technology allows for safer procedures with reduced morbidity and mortality even in older patients. With an ever-expanding array of antibiotics available, the proper choice of antibiotic must take into account possible drug interactions (Table 18.7), the side effect profile of a particular drug, and the appropriate dose in a given patient [84].

The increasing antibiotic resistance noted in several strains of gram-positive bacteria has led to the development of new classes of antibiotics in an effort to combat this problem. All this has improved our ability to successfully care for and treat patients, but has also increased the risk of potential side effects and drug interactions to which patients are exposed. The advent of the electronic medical record, electronic prescribing systems, and electronic prescribing data bases have made the life of a busy clinician easier and have been shown to prevent adverse events [85].

While the maxim of geriatric prescribing, "start low, go slow" is true for most classes of drugs, this practice is not advisable with antibiotic use. This is especially true in the critically ill cardiothoracic surgical patient and may contribute to the problem of antimicrobial resistance. Understanding when pharmacokinetic changes in the elderly are important and call for dose adjustment is imperative [86]. Proper dosing of antibiotics and other drugs in older adults reduces the incidence of ADRs. This is especially important given that the incidence of ADRs increases with advancing age and the effects are more serious in frail elderly patients than in their younger counterparts [87]. Improper dosing is a more frequent cause of error in therapy than is the use of an inappropriate drug [88].

Table 18.7 Selected antibiotics and their drug interactions

Antibiotic	Other drug	Effect
Ampicillin	Anticoagulants	↑ Anticoagulation
Aminoglycosides	Amphotericin B	↑ Nephrotoxicity
	Cyclosporine	↑ Nephrotoxicity
	Loop diuretics	↑ Ototoxicity
	Neuromuscular blockers	↑ Respiratory paralysis
	NSAIDs	↑ Nephrotoxicity
	Vancomycin	↑ Nephrotoxicity
Cefoperazone, cefotetan	Anticoagulants	↑ Anticoagulation
Clindamycin	Muscle relaxants	↑ Frequency of respiratory paralysis
Ciprofloxacin	Antacids/sucralfate/ cations (vitamins, calcium supplements)	↓ Absorption of ciprofloxacin if taken within 2 h
	NSAIDs	↑ Central nervous system (CNS) stimulation/seizures
	Anticoagulants	↑ Anticoagulation
Fluconazole	Tacrolimus	↑ Tacrolimus level with toxicity
	Cyclosporine	↑ Cyclosporine level, nephrotoxicity
	Calcium channel blockers	↑ Calcium channel blocker level
	Anticoagulants	↑ Anticoagulation
	Theophylline	↑ Theophylline level
Metronidazole	Alcohol	Disulfiram-like reaction
	Oral anticoagulants	↑ Anticoagulation
Imipenem– cilastatin	Cyclosporine	↑ Cyclosporine level
Trimethoprim– sulfamethox- azole	Anticoagulants	↑Anticoagulation

Source: Data from Sanford et al. [84]

Table 18.8 Selected antibiotics requiring dose adjustment during renal insufficiency

Antibiotic	Usual dose	Dose for CrCl (10–50 mL/min)	Dose for CrCl (<10 mL/min)
Cefazolin	1–2 g q8 h	1–2 g q12 h	1–2 g q24–48 h
Cefuroxime	0.75–1.50 g q8 h	0.75–1.50 g q12 h	0.75–1.50 g q24 h
Ceftazidime	2 g q8 h	2 g q12–24 h	2 g q24–48 h
Cefotaxime	2 g q8h	2 g q12–24 h	2 g q24 h
Penicillin G	0.5–4.0 million units q4 h	75% of dose	20–50% of dose
Ampicillin	1–2 g q6 h	1–2 g q6–12 h	1–2 g q12–24 h
Pipercillin tazobactam	3.375–4.5 g q6–8 h	2.25 g q6 h	2.25 g q8 h
Piperacillin	3–4 g q4–6 h	3–4 g q6–8 h	3–4 g q8 h
Ticarcillin clavulanate	3.1 g q4 h	3.1 g q8–12 h	2 g q12 h
Aztreonam	2 g q8 h	50–75% of dose	25% of dose
Ertapenem	1 g q24 h	0.5 g q24 h	0.5 g q24 h
Imipenem– cilastatin	0.5 g q6 h	0.25 g q6–12 h	0.125–0.25 g q12 h
Metronidazole	7.5 mg/kg q6 h	7.5 mg/kg q6 h	50% of dose
Vancomycin	1 g q12 h	1 g q24–96 h	1 g q4–7 days
Gentamicin	1.7 mg/kg q8 h	1.7 mg/kg q12–24 h	1.7 mg/kg q48 h
Amikacin	7.5 mg/kg q12 h	7.5 mg/kg q24 h	7.5 mg/kg q48 h
Amphotericin B	0.4–1 mg/kg q24 h	0.4–1 mg/kg q24 h	0.4–1 mg/kg q24 h
Fluconazole	100–400 mg q24 h	50% of dose	50% of dose
Ciprofloxacin (IV)	400 mg q12 h	400 mg q12–24 h	400 mg q18–24 h

CrCl creatinine clearance

Source: Data are from Sanford et al. [91]

Judicious clinical practice requires the prescribing physician to be aware of age-related changes in drug absorption, distribution, metabolism, and elimination. These have been described earlier in this chapter. Of these factors, elimination is the most clinically relevant to antibiotic dosing given the decline in renal function with age. Many disease processes in the elderly, including most notably hypertension and diabetes, contribute to and accelerate this decline [87].

Most clinicians are aware of the need to decrease the dose of certain nephrotoxic antibiotics, such as aminoglycosides, in the setting of frank renal insufficiency or decreased creatinine clearance. However, other commonly used drugs such as quinolones and most cephalosporins need to be dose adjusted for a creatinine clearance of less than 30 mL/min [89]. Table 18.8 lists selected antibiotics requiring dose adjustment [90, 91].

Although aminoglycosides remain important drugs for treating serious infections, alone or in combination with other drugs, the availability of newer agents (quinolones, monobactams, carbapenems) with broad-spectrum coverage and less nephrotoxicity make the use of aminoglycosides less attractive in elderly persons. Risk factors for the development of aminoglycoside-induced nephrotoxicity include diabetes mellitus, dehydration, advanced age, and duration of treatment [92]. In addition to nephrotoxicity, aminoglycosides may cause ototoxicity, particularly in elderly patients if given in high dose or for prolonged periods because ototoxicity is cumulative. Furthermore, the risk of ototoxicity is greater in patients concomitantly taking a loop diuretic [93–95].

Evidence suggests that once-daily dosing of an aminoglycoside is at least as effective as, and less toxic than, conventional dosing regimens of multiple daily dosages as long as trough levels are monitored closely. Several analyses of pooled data from randomized controlled studies in adults found that once-daily aminoglycoside dosing may be associated with less nephrotoxicity and no greater ototoxicity than with conventional dosing [96–99]. However, once-daily aminoglycoside dosing is not appropriate for, or recommended in, any patient with a creatinine clearance less than 30 mL/min.

Table 18.9 Selected antibiotics requiring dose adjustment in the presence of severe hepatic dysfunction

Nafcillin
Cefoperazone
Clindamycin
Erythromycin
Ketoconazole
Isoniazid
Rifampin

Source: Reprinted with permission from Marottoli RA, Jeffery SM, Pinto-Powell RC. Drug usage in surgical patients: preventing medication related problems. In: Rosenthal RE, Katlic MR, Zenilman ME, editors. Principles and practice of geriatric surgery. 2nd ed. New York: Springer; 2010

Although liver size and blood flow tend to decrease with age, in the absence of serious liver disease and subsequent hepatic dysfunction, antibiotic dosages do not need to be adjusted. Drug-induced hepatitis in patients treated with antituberculous agents, especially isoniazid, increases in incidence from 2.8/1,000 in patients <35 years old to 7.7/1,000 in patients ≥55 years old [93, 100]. Therefore, liver function tests must be performed frequently prior to and during the course of antituberculous therapy. Antibiotics that require dose adjustments in patients with hepatic dysfunction include cefoperazone, clindamycin, erythromycin, isoniazid, ketoconazole, nafcillin, and rifampin (Table 18.9).

β-Lactam antibiotics (penicillins, cephalosporins, cephamycins, carbapenems, monobactams) have varying characteristics of absorption, peak concentration, bioavailability, and metabolism. These topics are described in detail in standard texts and are not covered here. In general, bioavailability is relatively poor after oral administration, which has implications for the switch from intravenous to oral preparations, and pharmacokinetics are similar after intramuscular or intravenous administration [90].

Cephalosporins are relatively safe drugs to use in older persons and are recommended as first-line drugs for perioperative prophylaxis in cardiothoracic patients who do not have a β-lactam allergy. Dosages for certain cephalosporins need adjustment for renal insufficiency (Table 18.8). The broad spectrum of activity of ceftriaxone together with its convenient once-daily dosing make it an ideal drug for empiric use in a variety of clinical infections in older adults [101, 102]. It also has both renal and biliary excretion, thus requiring little adjustment for renal insufficiency. A lesser known side effect of ceftriaxone is the formation of biliary sludge with prolonged use [103].

Cefoperazone, a third-generation cephalosporin still in use especially for the treatment of intra-abdominal infections, has primarily biliary excretion and needs no adjustment for renal insufficiency; however, it can cause elevation of the prothrombin time [104]. This side effect is particularly important in the surgical patient. There are three proposed mecha-

nisms of cephalosporin-associated hypoprothrombinemia, two of which involve the *N*-methylthiotetrazole (NMTT) moiety. The most plausible mechanism is NMTT inhibition of vitamin K epoxide reductase in the liver. Patients at increased risk for this adverse event include those with low vitamin K stores, specifically patients who are malnourished with low albumin concentrations and poor food intake. The elderly and patients with liver or renal dysfunction are examples of populations at potential risk. The manufacturer therefore recommends concomitant use of vitamin K once a week during cefoperazone administration, although epidemiologic studies suggest that bleeding complications with antibiotics in general may have more to do with other risk factors than the specific antibiotic [105–108]. It should also be noted that cefoperazone causes a mild disulfiram-like reaction when given within 72 h of alcohol ingestion.

Carbapenems (imipenem cilastatin, meropenem, ertapenem) are a widely used class of drugs especially in the postoperative patient because of their broad spectrum of activity. Their pharmacokinetics are similar to cephalosporins, and renal excretion necessitates dose adjustment for renal insufficiency. The cilastatin component of imipenem cilastatin has no antibacterial activity, but inhibits renal tubular metabolism of imipenem, thereby increasing the urinary concentration of the active drug. Major adverse effects of the carbapenems, especially imipenem cilastatin, are related to the CNS including seizures, somnolence, and confusion [109], particularly in the elderly with a prior history of a CNS lesion, seizure disorder, or renal failure.

Aztreonam is a monobactam that has only aerobic gram-negative bacterial coverage. Its pharmacokinetics are similar to that of the cephalosporins. It is frequently used in patients with renal insufficiency as a substitute for aminoglycosides, although it too needs dose adjustment in such patients. Its use in combination with β-lactam antibiotics for synergy (as with aminoglycosides for enterococcal or pseudomonal infections), however, has not been validated. It lacks cross-reactivity with other β-lactam antibiotics and can be used safely in patients with severe allergy to penicillin or cephalosporins [110, 111].

The fluorinated quinolones have gained wide usage during the past few decades. Compared to the older quinolones (norfloxacin, ciprofloxacin), the third and fourth generation quinolones (ofloxacin, levofloxacin, moxifloxacin) have a broad spectrum of aerobic gram-positive and gram-negative bacterial activity along with the same excellent pharmacokinetic profile. The new generations of quinolones have better gram-positive coverage, especially in vitro activity against *Streptococcus pneumoniae*, than the earlier quinolones (ciprofloxacin). In addition, they are active against intracellular organisms such as *Legionella, Mycoplasma, Chlamydia*, and *Mycobacteria*. They are well absorbed orally, with a high degree of bioavailability that makes them especially useful drugs in the transition from intravenous to oral dosing.

They also have excellent tissue penetration. Care should be taken with the oral administration of these drugs to ensure that they are administered 2 h before or after antacids, sucralfate, or other multivalent metallic cations as their absorption can be severely impaired [112, 113]. Renally eliminated fluoroquinolones (ofloxacin, levofloxacin) need to be dose adjusted when the creatinine clearance is less than 50 mL/min.

With the increased usage of this class of antibiotics, there have been reports of specific side effects in older adults. Certain quinolones can cause QT interval prolongation. They should be avoided in patients with known prolongation of the QT interval, patients with uncorrected hypokalemia or hypomagnesemia, and patients receiving Class I or Class II antiarrhythmic drugs [114]. Elderly patients on corticosteroids, especially in the setting of chronic renal insufficiency, are at risk for Achilles tendon rupture [115]. An important and well-documented drug interaction of quinolones with warfarin is particularly noteworthy in the post-surgical patient. The prothrombin time (PT) and INR need to be closely monitored to prevent bleeding complications [116, 117].

With the current escalating problem of antibiotic resistance and the increase in the numbers of resistant gram-positive infections (Methicillin-resistant *Staphylococcus aureus* and Vancomycin-resistant *Enterococci*), several new antibiotics have been introduced in the past decade as an alternative to Vancomycin. Linezolid and Quinupristin Dalfopristin are two such antibiotics. Linezolid, a fluorinated oxazolidinone active against gram-positive organisms, is a non-selective inhibitor of monoamine oxidase (MAOI). Drug interactions need to be kept in mind when using this antibiotic. Linezolid is on the list of drugs with serotonergic activity that may cause serotonin syndrome – a potentially preventable complex of symptoms that may be fatal if not recognized early. The most common drug combinations associated with serotonin syndrome are MAOIs with selective serotonin reuptake inhibitors (SSRIs). Since SSRIs are frequently used for the treatment of depression, this is an important drug interaction to keep in mind [118–120].

Clostridium difficile-associated diarrhea (CDAD) is a challenge in the care of all hospitalized patients, particularly older ones. Surgical patients comprise 55–75% of all patients with CDAD [121]. Initial treatment regimens remain the same in this population and include oral metronidazole (cheap and effective) or oral vancomycin (expensive and concern for antibiotic resistance). However, there is an increased frequency of treatment failure and CDAD recurrence among elderly persons. A prolonged tapering course of antibiotics, treatment with anion exchange resins, oral lactobacillus or non-pathogenic yeast such as *Saccharomyces boulardii*, and fecal transplants (enema with feces from healthy donors) or combinations of the above may need to be considered in refractory cases. None of these regimens has been proven superior to the others [122].

Summary

A number of factors can potentially influence the risk–benefit equation for drug use in an older population, including age-related physiologic changes in organ system function; increased likelihood of comorbid diseases affecting organ systems that are the intended site of drug action or are responsible for the metabolism or clearance of a drug; and increased likelihood of multiple chronic medications, which may increase the possibility of drug interactions. However, the vast majority of drugs can be used safely and effectively in older cardiothoracic surgical patients if appropriate precautions are taken in the selection, dosing, and timing of drugs and in the active monitoring of effects and side effects.

References

1. Dychtwald K. Age power. How the 21st century will be ruled by the new old. New York: Penguin Putnam; 1999.
2. Shock NW, Watkin DM, Yiengst MJ, Norris AH, Gaffney GW, Gregerman RI, et al. Age differences in the water content of the body as related to basal oxygen consumption in males. J Gerontol. 1963;18:1–8.
3. Forbes GB, Reina JC. Adult lean body mass declines with age: some longitudinal observations. Metabolism. 1970;19:653–63.
4. Gilbaldi M. Revisiting some factors contributing to variability. Ann Pharmacother. 1992;26(7–8):1002–7.
5. Hammerlein A, Derendorf H, Lowenthal D. Pharmacokinetic and pharmacodynamic changes in the elderly. Clin Pharmacokinet. 1998;35:49–64.
6. Pickering G. Frail elderly, nutritional status and drugs. Arch Gerontol Geriatr. 2004;38:174–80.
7. Starner CI, Gray SL, Guay D, Hajjar ER, Handler SM, Hanlon JT. Geriatrics. In: DiPiro JT, Talbert RL, Yee GC, Matzke Gr, Wells BG, Posey LM, editors. Pharmacotherapy: a pathophysiologic approach. 7th ed. New York: McGraw-Hill; 2002. p. 57–66.
8. Turnheim K. Drug dosage in the elderly: is it rational? Drugs Aging. 1998;13:357–9.
9. Robertson DRC, Wood ND, Everest H, Monks K, Waller DG, Renwick AG, et al. The effect of age on the pharmacokinetics of levodopa administered alone and in the presence of carbidopa. Br J Clin Pharmacol. 1989;28:61–9.
10. Bailey DG, Dresser GK. Interactions between grapefruit juice and cardiovascular drugs. Am J Cardiovasc Drugs. 2004;4:281–97.
11. Holdsworth MT, Forman WB, Killilea TA, Nystrom KM, Paul R, Brand SC, Transdermal fentanyl disposition in elderly subjects. Gerontology. 1994;40:32–37.
12. Tozer TN, Winter ME. Phenytoin. In: Burton ME, Shaw LM, Schentag JJ, Evans WE, editors. Applied pharmacokinetics: principles of therapeutic drug monitoring. 4th ed. Philadelphia: Lippincott Williams & Wilkins; 2005. p. 463–88.
13. Paxton JW, Briant RH. Alpha one-acid glycoprotein concentrations and propranolol binding in elderly patients with acute illness. Br J Clin Pharmacol. 1984;1:806–10.
14. Castleden CM, George CF. The effect of ageing on the hepatic clearance of propranolol. Br J Clin Pharmacol. 1979;7:49–54.
15. Tanaka E. In vivo age-related changes in hepatic drug-oxidizing capacity in humans. J Clin Pharm Ther. 1998;23:247–55.

16. Herlinger C, Klotz U. Drug metabolism and drug interactions in the elderly. Best Pract Res Clin Gastroenterol. 2001;15:897–918.

17. Greenblatt DJ, Shader RI, Harmatz JS. Implications of altered drug disposition in the elderly: studies of benzodiazepines. J Clin Pharmacol. 1989;29:866–72.

18. Greenblatt DJ, Harmatz JS, Shader RI. Clinical pharmacokinetics of anxiolytics and hypnotics in the elderly: therapeutic considerations. Part I. Clin Pharmacokinet. 1991;21:165–77.

19. Divoll M, Greenblatt DJ, Ochs HR, Shader RI. Absolute bioavailability of oral and intramuscular diazepam: effects of age and sex. Anesth Analg. 1983;62:1–8.

20. Herman RJ, Wilkinson GR. Disposition of diazepam in young and elderly subjects after acute and chronic dosing. Br J Clin Pharmacol. 1996;42:147–55.

21. Rowe JW, Andres R, Tobin JD, Norris AH, Shock NW. The effect of age on creatinine clearance in men: a cross-sectional and longitudinal study. J Gerontol. 1976;31:155–63.

22. Lindeman RD, Tobin J, Shock NW. Longitudinal studies on the rate of decline in renal function with age. J Am Geriatr Soc. 1985;33:278–85.

23. Bertino Jr JS. Measured versus estimated creatinine clearance in patients with low serum creatinine values. Ann Pharmacother. 1993;27:1439–42.

24. Smythe M, Hoffman J, Kizy K, Dmuchowski C. Estimating creatinine clearance in elderly patients with low serum creatinine concentrations. Am J Hosp Pharm. 1994;51:198–204.

25. Cockcroft DW, Gault MH. Prediction of creatinine clearance from serum creatinine. Nephron. 1976;16:31–41.

26. Sanaka M, Takano K, Shimakura K, Koike Y, Mineshita S. Serum albumin for estimating creatinine clearance in the elderly with muscle atrophy. Nephron. 1996;73:137–44.

27. Levey AS, Bosch JP, Lewis JB, Greene T, Rogers N, Roth D, et al. A more accurate method to estimate glomerular filtration rate from serum creatinine: a new prediction equation. Ann Intern Med. 1999;130:461–70.

28. Lamb EJ, Webb MC, Simpson DE, Coakley AJ, Newman DJ, O'Riordan SE. Estimation of glomerular filtration rate in older patients with chronic renal insufficiency: is the modification of diet in renal disease formula an improvement? J Am Geriatr Soc. 2003;51:1012–7.

29. Reichley RM, Ritchie DJ, Bailey TC. Analysis of various creatinine clearance formulas in predicting gentamicin elimination in patients with low serum creatinine. Pharmacotherapy. 1995;15:625–30.

30. Anonymous. Risk of severe hypoglycemia with glyburide use in elderly patients with renal insufficiency. Veterans Health Administration (VHA) Pharmacy Benefits Management Services (PBM), Medical Advisory Panel (MAP), & Center For Medication Safety (VA Medsafe), July 29, 2009.

31. Gijsen R, Hoeymans N, Schellevis FG, Ruwaard D, Satariano WA, van den Bos GA. Causes and consequences of comorbidity: a review. J Clin Epidemiol. 2001;54:661–74.

32. Hoffman C, Rice D, Sung HY. Persons with chronic conditions: their prevalence and costs. JAMA. 1996;276:1473–9.

33. Field TS, Gurwitz JH, Harrold LR, Rothschild J, Debellis KR, Seger AC, et al. Risk factors for adverse drug events among older adults in the ambulatory setting. J Am Geriatr Soc. 2004;52:1349–54.

34. Safran DG, Neuman P, Schoen C, Montgomery JE, Li W, Wilson IB, et al. Prescription drug coverage and seniors: how well are we closing the gap? Health Aff. 2002;(Suppl web exclusives):W253–68. http://content.healthaffairs.org/cgi/reprint/hlthaff.w2.253v1.pdf. Accessed Feb 2009.

35. Mojtabai R, Olfson M. Medication costs, adherence, and health outcomes among Medicare beneficiaries. Health Aff. 2003;22:220–8.

36. Qato DM, Alexander GC, Conti RM, Johnson M, Schumm P, Lindau ST. Use of prescription and over-the-counter medications and dietary supplements among older adults in the United States. JAMA. 2008;300(24):2867–78.

37. Boyd CM, Darer J, Boult C, Fried LP, Boult L, Wu AW. Clinical practice guidelines and quality of care for older patients with multiple comorbid diseases: implications for pay for performance. JAMA. 2005;294:716–24.

38. Fick DM, Cooper JW, Wade WE, Waller JL, Maclean JR, Beers MH. Updating the Beers criteria for potentially inappropriate medication use in older adults: results of a US consensus panel of experts. Arch Intern Med. 2003;163(22):2716–24.

39. Beyth RJ, Shorr RI. Principles of drug therapy in older patients: rational drug prescribing. Clin Geriatr Med. 2002;18:577–92.

40. Sloan RW. Principles of drug therapy in geriatric patients. Am Fam Physician. 1992;45:2709–18.

41. American Society of Consultant Pharmacists. Top ten dangerous drug interactions in long-term care. http://www.scoup.net/M3Project/topten. Accessed Feb 2009.

42. Jeffery SM. Outpatient geriatric medication reconciliation; 2009.

43. Hanlon JT, Weinberger M, Samsa GP, Schmader KE, Uttech KM, Lewis IK, et al. A randomized, controlled trial of a clinical pharmacist intervention to improve prescribing in elderly outpatients with polypharmacy. Am J Med. 1996;100:428–37.

44. Gillespie U, Alassaad A, Henrohn D, Garmo H, Hammarlund-Udenaes M, Toss H, et al. A comprehensive pharmacist intervention to reduce morbidity in patients 80 years or older: a randomized controlled trial. Arch Intern Med. 2009;169:894–900.

45. Richardson WC, Berwick DM, Bisgard JC, Bristow LR, Buck CR, Cassel CK, et al. The Institute of Medicine Report on Medical Errors: misunderstanding can do harm. Quality of Health Care in America Committee. MedGenMed. 2000; 2(3):E42.

46. Bates DW, Teich JM, Lee J, Segar D, Kuperman GJ, Ma'Luf N, et al. The impact of computerized physician order entry on medication error prevention. J Am Med Inform Assoc. 1999;6(4):313–21.

47. Inouye SK, van Dyck CH, Alessi CA, Balkin S, Siegal AP, Horwitz RI. Clarifying confusion: the confusion assessment method. A new method for detection of delirium. Ann Intern Med. 1990;113:941–8.

48. Inouye SK, Viscoli CM, Horwitz RI, Hurst LD, Tinetti ME. A predictive model for delirium in hospitalized elderly medical patients based on admission characteristics. Ann Intern Med. 1993;119:474–81.

49. Inouye SK, Charpentier PA. Precipitating factors for delirium in hospitalized elderly persons: predictive model and interrelationship with baseline vulnerability. JAMA. 1996;275:852–7.

50. Marcantonio ER, Juarez G, Goldman L, Mangione CM, Ludwig LE, Lind L, et al. The relationship of postoperative delirium with psychoactive medications. JAMA. 1994;272:1518–22.

51. Norkiene I, Ringaitiene D, Misiuriene I, Samalavicius R, Bubulis R, Baublys A, et al. Incidence and precipitating factors of delirium after coronary artery bypass grafting. Scand Cardiovasc J. 2007;41:180–5.

52. Lopenen P, Luther M, Wistbacka JO, Nissinen J, Sintonen H, Huhtala H, et al. Postoperative delirium and health related quality of life after coronary artery bypass grafting. Scand Cardiovasc J. 2008;42:337–44.

53. Tan MC, Felde A, Kuskowski M, Ward H, Kelly RF, Adabag AS, et al. Incidence and predictors of post-cardiotomy delirium. Am J Geriatr Psychiatry. 2008;16:575–83.

54. Katznelson R, Djaiani GN, Borger MA, Friedman Z, Abbey SE, Fedorko L, et al. Preoperative use of statins is associated with reduced early delirium rate after cardiac surgery. Anesthesiology. 2009;110:67–73.

55. Rudolph JL, Jones RN, Levkoff SE, Rockett C, Inouye SK, Sellke FW, et al. Derivation and validation of a preoperative prediction

rule for delirium after cardiac surgery. Circulation. 2009;119: 229–36.

56. Inouye SK, Bogardus ST, Charpentier PA, Leo-Summers L, Acampora D, Holford TR, et al. A multicomponent intervention to prevent delirium in hospitalized older patients. N Engl J Med. 1999;340:669–76.

57. Marcantonio ER, Flacker JM, Wright RJ, Resnick NM. Reducing delirium after hip fracture. J Am Geriatr Soc. 2001;49:516–22.

58. Jenike MA. Psychoactive drugs in the elderly: antipsychotics and anxiolytics. Geriatrics. 1988;43(9):53–65.

59. Task Force on Late Neurological Effects of Antipsychotic Drugs. Tardive dyskinesia: summary of a task force report of the American Psychiatric Association. Am J Psychiatry. 1980;137:1163–72.

60. Smith JM, Baldessarini RJ. Changes in prevalence, severity, and recovery in tardive dyskinesia with age. Arch Gen Psychiatry. 1980;37:1368–73.

61. Schneider LS, Tariot PN, Dagerman KS, Davis SM, Hsiao JK, Ismail MS, et al. Effectiveness of atypical antipsychotic drugs in patients with Alzheimer's disease. N Engl J Med. 2006;335:1525–38.

62. Ray WS, Chung CP, Murray KT, Hall K, Stein CM. Atypical antipsychotic drugs and the risk of sudden cardiac death. N Engl J Med. 2009;360:225–35.

63. Ballard C, Hanney ML, Theodoulou M, Douglas S, McShane R, Kossakowski K, et al. The dementia antipsychotic withdrawal trial (DART-AD): long-term follow-up of a randomized placebo-controlled trial. Lancet Neurol. 2009;8:151–7.

64. Jenike MA. Psychoactive drugs in the elderly: antidepressants. Geriatrics. 1988;43(11):43–57.

65. Yesavage JA, Brink TL, Rose TL, Lum O, Huang V, Adey M, et al. Development and validation of a geriatric depression screening scale: a preliminary report. J Psychiatr Res. 1983;17:37–49.

66. Stimmel GL, Gutierrez MA. Psychiatric disorders. In: Delafuente JC, Stewart RB, editors. Therapeutics in the elderly. 2nd ed. Cincinnati: Harvey Whitney Books; 1995. p. 324–43.

67. Tourigny-Rivard MF. Pharmacotherapy of affective disorders in old age. Can J Psychiatry. 1997;42 Suppl 1:10S–8.

68. Alexopoulos GS, Katz IR, Reynolds CF, Carpenter D, Docherty JP. The expert consensus guideline series: pharmacotherapy of depressive disorders in older patients. Postgrad Med. 2001;Special Report:1–86.

69. Perry PJ, Pfohl BM, Holstad SG. The relationship between antidepressant response and tricyclic antidepressant plasma concentrations: a retrospective analysis of the literature using logistic regression analysis. Clin Pharmacokinet. 1987;13:381–92.

70. Mukai Y, Tampi RR. Treatment of depression in the elderly: a review of the recent literature on the efficacy of single- versus dual-action antidepressants. Clin Ther. 2009;31:945–61.

71. Wallace AE, Kofoed LL, West AN. Double-blind, placebo-controlled trial of methylphenidate in older, depressed, medically ill patients. Am J Psychiatry. 1995;152:929–31.

72. Schneider LS. Overview of generalized anxiety disorder in the elderly. J Clin Psychiatry. 1996;57 Suppl 7:34–45.

73. Shuckit MA. Current therapeutic options in the management of typical anxiety. J Clin Psychiatry. 1981;42(11 Pt 2):15–26.

74. Flamer HE. Sleep problems. Med J Aust. 1995;162:603–7.

75. Vaz Fragoso CA, Gill TM. Sleep complaints in community-living older persons: a multifactorial geriatric syndrome. J Am Geriatr Soc. 2007;55:1853–66.

76. Herr KA, Mobily PR. Pain assessment in the elderly: clinical considerations. J Gerontol Nurs. 1991;17(4):12–9.

77. Ferrell BA. Pain management in elderly people. J Am Geriatr Soc. 1991;39:64–73.

78. Ferrell BA. Pain evaluation and management in the nursing home. Ann Intern Med. 1995;123:681–7.

79. American Geriatrics Society Panel on Pharmacological Management of Persistent Pain in Older Persons. Pharmacological management of persistent pain in older persons. J Am Geriatr Soc. 2009;57:1331–46.

80. Barrett BJ. Acetaminophen and adverse chronic renal outcomes: an appraisal of the epidemiologic evidence. Am J Kidney Dis. 1996;28 Suppl 1:S14–9.

81. Morrison RS, Flanagan S, Fischberg D, Cintron A, Siu AL. A novel interdisciplinary analgesic program reduces pain and improves function in older patients after orthopedic surgery. J Am Geriatr Soc. 2009;57:1–10.

82. Cantu TG, Korek JS. Central nervous system reactions to histamine-2 receptor blockers. Ann Intern Med. 1991;114:1027–34.

83. Kaye KS, Schmader KE, Sawyer R. Surgical site infection in the elderly population. Clin Infect Dis. 2004;39:1835–41.

84. Sanford JP, Gilbert DN, Moellering RC, Sande MA. Anti-infective drug–drug interactions. In: The Sanford guide to antimicrobial therapy. 27th ed. Vienna, VA: Antimicrobial Therapy; 1997. p. 123–6.

85. Smith DH, Perrin N, Feldstein A, Yang X, Kuang D, Simon SR, et al. The impact of prescribing safety alerts for elderly patients in an electronic medical record. Arch Intern Med. 2006;166:1098–104.

86. Bergman SJ, Speil C, Short M, Koirala J. Pharmacokinetic and pharmacodynamic aspects of antibiotic use in high risk populations. Infect Dis Clin North Am. 2007;21:821–46.

87. Gleckman RA. Antibiotic concerns in the elderly. Infect Dis Clin North Am. 1995;9:575–90.

88. Lesar TS, Lomaestro BM, Pohl H. Medication-prescribing errors in a teaching hospital: a 9-year experience. Arch Intern Med. 1997;157:1569–76.

89. Gilbert DN, Bennett WM. Use of antimicrobial agents in renal failure. Infect Dis Clin North Am. 1989;3:517–31.

90. McCue JD. Antimicrobial therapy. Clin Geriatr Med. 1992;8:925–45.

91. Sanford JP, Gilbert DN, Moellering RC, Sande MA. Dosage of antimicrobial drugs in adult patients with renal impairment. In: The Sanford guide to antimicrobial therapy. 27th ed. Vienna, VA: Antimicrobial Therapy; 1997. p. 116–20.

92. Mingeot-Leclercq MP, Tulkens PM. Aminoglycosides: nephrotocicity. Antimicrob Agents Chemother. 1999;43:100–12.

93. Posner JD. Particular problems of antibiotic use in the elderly. Geriatrics. 1982;37(8):49–54.

94. Tablan OC, Reyes MP, Rintelmann WF, Lernov AM. Renal and auditory toxicity of high-dose, prolonged therapy with gentamicin and tobramycin in *Pseudomonas endocarditis*. J Infect Dis. 1984;149:257–63.

95. Moore RD, Smith CR, Lietman PS. Risk factors for the development of auditory toxicity in patients receiving aminoglycosides. J Infect Dis. 1984;149:23–30.

96. Marra F, Partovi N, Jewesson P. Aminoglycoside administration as a single daily dose. Drugs. 1996;52:344–70.

97. Barza M, Ioannidis JPA, Cappelleri JC, Lau J. Single or multiple daily doses of aminoglycosides: a meta-analysis. BMJ. 1996;312:338–45.

98. Hatala R, Dinh T, Cook DJ. Once-daily aminoglycoside dosing in immunocompetent adults: a meta-analysis. Ann Intern Med. 1996;124:717–25.

99. Raveh D, Kopyt M, Hite Y, Rudensky B, Sonnenblick M, Yinnon AM. Risk factors for nephrotoxicity in elderly patients receiving once-daily aminoglycosides. Q J Med. 2002;95:291–7.

100. Van den Brande P, van Steenbergen W, Vervoort G, Demedts M. Aging and hepatotoxicity of isoniazid and rifampin in pulmonary tuberculosis. Am J Respir Crit Care Med. 1995;152:1705–8.

101. Mandell LA, Bergeron MG, Ronald AR, Vega C, Harding G, Saginur R, et al. Once-daily therapy with ceftriaxone compared with daily multiple-dose therapy with cefotaxime for serious

bacterial infections: a randomized, double-blind study. J Infect Dis. 1989;160:433–41.

102. Barriere SL, Flaherty JF. Third-generation cephalosporins: a critical evaluation. Clin Pharm. 1984;3:351–73.

103. Michielsen PP, Fierens H, Van Maercke YM. Drug-induced gallbladder disease: incidence, etiology and management. Drug Saf. 1992;7:32–45.

104. Brogden RN, Carmine A, Heel RC, Morley PA, Speight TM, Avery GS. Cefoperazone: a review of its in vitro antimicrobial activity, pharmacological properties and therapeutic efficacy. Drugs. 1981;22:423–60.

105. Rockoff SD, Blumenfrucht MJ, Irwin RJ, Eng RHK. Vitamin K supplementation during prophylactic use of cefoperazone in urologic surgery. Infection. 1992;20:146–8.

106. Goss TF, Walawander CA, Grasela TH, Meisel S, Katona B, Jaynes K. Prospective evaluation of risk factors for antibiotic-associated bleeding in critically ill patients. Pharmacotherapy. 1992;12:283–91.

107. Grasela TH, Walawander CA, Welage LS, Wing PE, Scarafoni DJ, Caldwell JW, et al. Prospective surveillance of antibiotic-associated coagulopathy in 970 patients. Pharmacotherapy. 1989;9:158–64.

108. Schentag JJ, Welage LS, Williams JS, Wilton JH, Adleman MH, Rigan D, et al. Kinetics and action of N-methylthiotetrazole in volunteers and patients: population-based clinical comparisons of antibiotics with and without this moiety. Am J Surg. 1988;155(5A):40–4.

109. MacGregor RR, Gibson GA, Bland JA. Imipenem pharmacokinetics and body fluid concentrations in patients receiving high-dose treatment for serious infections. Antimicrob Agents Chemother. 1986;29:188–92.

110. Neu HC. Aztreonam activity, pharmacology, and clinical uses. Am J Med. 1990;88(Suppl 3C):2S–6.

111. Fillastre JP, Leroy A, Baudoin C, Humbert G, Swabb EA, Vertucci C, et al. Pharmacokinetics of aztreonam in patients with chronic renal failure. Clin Pharmacokinet. 1985;10:91–100.

112. Davies BI, Maesen FPV. Drug interactions with quinolones. Rev Infect Dis. 1989;11 Suppl 5:S1083–90.

113. Norrby SR, Ljungberg B. Pharmacokinetics of fluorinated 4-quinolones in the aged. Rev Infect Dis. 1989;11 Suppl 5:S1102–6.

114. Stahlmann R, Lode H. Fluoroquinolones in the elderly: safety considerations. Drugs Aging. 2003;20(4):289–302.

115. van der Linden PD, Sturkenboom MC, Herings RM, Leufkens HM, Rowlands S, Stricker BH. Increased risk of Achilles tendon rupture with quinolone antibacterial use, especially in elderly patients taking oral corticosteroids. Arch Intern Med. 2003;163:1801–7.

116. Holbrook AM, Pereira JA, Labiris R, McDonald H, Douketis JD, Crowther M, et al. Systematic overview of warfarin and its drug and food interactions. Arch Intern Med. 2005;165:1095–106.

117. Jones CB, Fugate SE. Levofloxacin and warfarin interaction. Ann Pharmacother. 2002;36:1554–7.

118. Huang V, Gortney JS. Risk of serotonin syndrome with concomitant administration of linezolid and serotonin agonists. Pharmacotherapy. 2006;26:1784–93.

119. Clark DB, Andrus MR, Byrd DC. Drug interactions between linezolid and selective serotonin reuptake inhibitors: case report involving sertraline and review of the literature. Pharmacotherapy. 2006;26:269–76.

120. Taylor JJ, Wilson JW, Estes LL. Linezolid and serotonergic drug interactions: a retrospective survey. Clin Infect Dis. 2006;43:180–7.

121. Jobe BA, Grasley A, Deveney KE, Deveney CW, Sheppard BC. Clostridium difficile colitis: an increasing hospital acquired illness. Am J Surg. 1995;169:480–3.

122. Mylonakis E, Ryan ET, Calderwood SB. Clostridium difficile – associated diarrhea. A review. Arch Intern Med. 2001;161:525–33.

Chapter 19
Wound Healing in the Elderly

Christopher G. Engeland and Praveen K. Gajendrareddy

Abstract Being elderly is a risk factor for delayed wound healing. In aged skin, epidermal turnover is decreased by about 50%. This is accompanied by reductions in vascularization, granulation tissue, collagen, elastin, mast cells and fibroblasts. Age-related changes occur which impact all phases of healing. In general, the elderly have increased rates of infection and wound dehiscence, decreases in wound strength, and slower healing times. This is primarily caused by reductions in re-epithelialization, angiogenesis, macrophage infiltration, and collagen deposition. Paradoxically, wounds heal with less scarring in the aged. It is important to note that healing is delayed but not impaired in the elderly, and the end result of healing, albeit slower, is similar to that of young adults. However, concomitant risk factors for delays or impairments in healing (e.g., disease, medications, malnutrition, immobility, obesity, stress) are more common in the elderly. Each of these risk factors should be tested for, treated, and monitored accordingly prior to surgery to ensure maximal healing. It is not being elderly per se, but being elderly and presenting additional risk factors, that predisposes an individual to impaired healing and poor surgical outcomes.

Keywords Aging • Elderly • Wound healing • Infection • Bacteria • Inflammation • Proliferation • Remodeling • Cytokine • Chemokine • Growth factor • Macrophage • Neutrophil • Fibroblast • Keratinocyte • Epithelial cell • Endothelial cell • Adhesion molecule • Matrix metalloproteinase • Tissue inhibitor of matrix metalloproteinase • Collagen • Elastin • Angiogenesis • Tensile strength • Scarring • Fibrosis • Intrinsic aging • Extrinsic aging • Re-epithelialization • Contraction • Menopause • Estrogen • Testosterone • Phagocytosis • Hormone replacement therapy • Stress • Sex differences • Mucosa • Dermis • Granulation tissue • Myocardium • Heart failure • Cardiac • Infarction • Bone • Fracture • Lung • Fibrosis • Atherosclerotic • Plaque • Ischemia • Hypoxia • Vascular • Oxygen

C.G. Engeland (✉)
University of Illinois at Chicago, College of Dentistry,
801 S Paulina Street, M/C 859, Chicago, IL, USA
e-mail: engeland@uic.edu

Introduction

The world is quickly aging. The elderly (aged ≥65 years) presently comprise the fastest growing population in Western countries and, estimates predict, will make up 20% of the United States population (71.5 million) by 2030 [1]. Moreover, individuals who are 85+ years of age make up the fastest growing segment of the elderly [2].

The treatment of impaired healing costs United States health services more than $9 billion annually [3], much of which has been associated with age-associated delays in wound closure. These delays, in turn, relate to increased risk of infection and medical complications. The elderly have the highest occurrence of wounds of any age group in the United States [2]. Thus, the impact of aging on wound healing is an important issue which severely impacts national health care costs.

In 1916, during World War I, a military surgeon named Lacomte Du Nuoy observed a slower healing rate of open skin wounds in older compared to younger soldiers, which he termed as a "natural delay." Importantly, this was the first report to be published on age-impaired healing [4]. These findings are hard to interpret, however, as his measures were reasonably basic, the soldiers were relatively young (20–40 years), and factors such as wound depth and incidence of infection were not accounted for.

Since then, multiple studies have reported associations between increasing age and poorer healing outcomes in humans [5–7]. In general, however, these studies have not controlled for potentially confounding factors that are more common in older individuals, such as the presence of comorbidity and medication use. Other studies have reported no differences in healing rates between older and younger adults [8–10]. Animal studies, which generally avoid such confounds, have generally found age-associated healing impairments [11–14]. However, animal models have been poor predictors of clinical wound healing [10]. Thus, it remains somewhat unclear in humans if aging per se negatively impacts wound healing [9, 10]. Furthermore, if age-related delays in wound healing do exist, are such effects clinically relevant?

M.R. Katlic (ed.), *Cardiothoracic Surgery in the Elderly*, DOI 10.1007/978-1-4419-0892-6_19,
© Springer Science+Business Media, LLC 2011

The Three Stages of Wound Healing

Wound healing can be divided into three overlapping phases: an inflammatory phase (lasting hours to days), a proliferative phase (days to weeks), and a remodeling phase (weeks to months). These phases are interdependent. Thus, during early inflammation, cytokines and growth factors are released which are essential for the proliferative phase. In turn, elements from the advancing epithelium help to resolve this inflammation. Importantly, the timing and activity of each phase depends upon the resolution of the previous phase. As a result, dysregulation of any phase can impair healing at multiple levels. A dysregulation of inflammation may be particularly important, as this is the earliest phase in the healing cascade. Aging has been shown to affect immune components from every phase of healing.

Inflammatory Phase

The inflammatory phase commences as soon as injury occurs, and is involved in minimizing damage, protecting from infection, debris removal, and initiating the downstream cascade of events necessary for tissue repair [15]. A number of important mediators are released early in the healing process by platelets, white blood cells, and other blood elements in response to injury. These mediators include complement products, kinins, fibrin, and prostaglandins. A provisional matrix is created in the form of a blood clot which helps contain the injury and provides a scaffold for repair.

Cells endogenous to the site of injury are important participants in the early development of inflammation. Following injury, interleukin (IL)-1α (alpha) is released from constitutive stores by endothelial cells. Langerhans cells in the epidermis similarly release inflammatory mediators, and mast cells secrete preformed histamine and tumor necrosis factor (TNF-α). These mediators increase blood flow to the site of injury, and induce the expression of adhesion molecules on endothelial cells (e.g., E-selectin, ICAM) and the release of chemokines from various immune cells (e.g., IL-8 from neutrophils, MCP-1 and MIP-1α from macrophages). Together, these regulate the migration of inflammatory cells from the peripheral circulation into the tissue. Neutrophils appear within minutes and macrophages within hours from the time of injury, followed eventually by lymphocytes. These cells aid in bacterial clearance and the phagocytosis of damaged tissue. They also produce a number of cytokines which further aid in inflammation, and growth factors which aid cells such as fibroblasts, keratinocytes, and endothelial cells in the proliferative phase of healing.

The timeline of inflammation is important and sets the stage for the other healing phases. Normal healing typically involves a strong but short lived inflammatory response which enables quick bacterial clearance from the wound. Too much or too little inflammation will typically retard this process and, in turn, delay re-epithelialization which occurs during the proliferative phase.

Proliferative Phase

This second phase of healing, which entails the rebuilding of damaged structures, involves fibroblasts, epithelial cells and endothelial cells. This phase begins with the proliferation and migration of squamous epithelial cells (keratinocytes) along the wound margin, followed by the proliferation of dermal fibroblasts surrounding the wound. Many of these fibroblasts deposit large amounts of fibronectin which is important for cell migration and adhesion. These fibroblasts also secrete collagen, hyaluronic acid, elastin and other components which make up the extracellular matrix. This new tissue is called granulation tissue. Other fibroblasts migrate to the wound edge, acquire a contractile phenotype and transform into myofibroblasts. These cells play a major role in wound contraction which reduces the area of repair and minimizes reconstructive costs.

Tissue demands for oxygen are highly elevated during wound repair and a strong angiogenic response occurs to meet this need. Endothelial cells migrate to the site of injury, proliferate and form new blood vessels, and nerve sprouting occurs at the leading edge of the wound. The degree of vascularization exceeds what is needed for normal tissue maintenance, and eventually recedes to normal levels once the wound has closed.

As keratinocytes advance and re-epithelialize the wound's surface, they send signals inhibiting further inflammation. Once the wound is covered, the epithelium thickens and secretes structural proteins such as involucrin and keratins to fully restore barrier function (Fig. 19.1).

Remodeling Phase

Similar to changes in vascularization, the connective tissue produced is hypercellular compared to normal tissue. As a result, a remodeling of these cells may continue for a long time after wound closure. The time required for this depends upon the wound's size and depth, the site of injury, etc. Ideally, these extra cells undergo apoptosis (programmed death) and are removed by macrophages. If the cells undergo lysis or necrosis, inflammation will result with additional tissue damage and scarring. Scarring is more likely to occur when there is a higher over-abundance of cells, which may

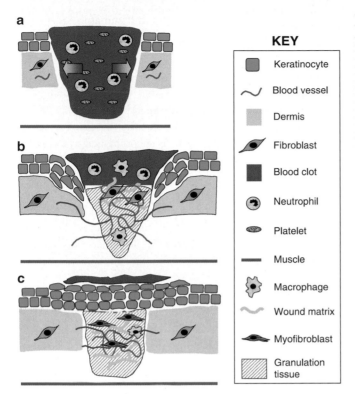

KEY

Keratinocyte

Blood vessel

Dermis

Fibroblast

Blood clot

Neutrophil

Platelet

Muscle

Macrophage

Wound matrix

Myofibroblast

Granulation tissue

Table 19.1 Age related changes in skin

Histological changes
Reduction in epidermal turnover
Reduction in vascularization
Decrease of granulation tissue
Decrease in collagen density
Decrease in elastin content
Reduction in fibroblast numbers
Reduction in mast cells
Decrease in cellular motility

Clinical changes
Atrophy
Drying
Roughness
Altered pigmentation
Sagging
Wrinkling
Tumor formation
Skin becomes thinner (after age 70)

Fig. 19.1 Schematic representation of different stages of wound repair. (**a**) 12–24 h after injury the wounded area is filled with a blood clot. Neutrophils have invaded into the clot. (**b**) At *days 3–7* after injury, the majority of neutrophils have undergone apoptosis. Instead, macrophages are abundant in the wound tissue at this stage of repair. Endothelial cells migrate into the clot; they proliferate and form new blood vessels. Fibroblasts migrate into the wound tissue, where they proliferate and deposit extracellular matrix. The new tissue is called granulation tissue. Keratinocytes proliferate at the wound edge and migrate down the injured dermis and above the provisional matrix. (**c**) 1–2 weeks after injury the wound is completely filled with granulation tissue. Fibroblasts have transformed into myofibroblasts, leading to wound contraction and collagen deposition. The wound is completely covered with a neoepidermis (reprinted from Werner and Grose [96], with permission from the American Physiological Society)

occur due to extended inflammation or as a result of infection. Hence, the avoidance of scarring is dependent upon a quick resolution of the earlier phases of healing.

This remodeling phase involves the synthesis, degradation, reorganization and stabilization (via cross-linking) of collagen. Matrix metalloproteinases (MMPs) and tissue inhibitors of metalloproteinases (TIMPs) are synthesized and control the spatial and temporal aspects of this remodeling.

The Aging Skin

It is well accepted that aging alters skin morphology [8, 13] (Table 19.1). As one ages from 20 to 70 years, epidermal turnover is reduced by about 50% [16]. This is likely due to

an age-related decline in the response of keratinocytes to growth factors, which limits the proliferative capabilities of these cells [17, 18]. In older adult skin there are reductions in vascularization [19], granulation tissue [19], collagen density and production [13, 17, 19], elastin [10, 20], mast cells (<50%) [21], and fibroblast numbers [19] and motility [22, 23].

Many of the deleterious effects of aging on skin pertain to extrinsic aging factors, such as cumulative UV and infra-red exposure, which can result in skin damage over time. In general, extrinsic aging impacts skin morphology more extremely than intrinsic aging [17]. Although these factors are inherently different, at times they offset each other. For instance, photo-aging causes a thinning of the upper dermis, whereas chronological age is associated with a thickening of the lower dermis. As a result, the overall thickness of the epidermis does not appear to change over time [10] until about age 70, at which time it begins to thin [17]. One common effect of intrinsic aging is a drop in elastin content which contributes to the reduced skin elasticity commonly observed in the aged [10].

Clinically, aged skin is characterized by atrophy, drying, roughness, pigment alterations, sagging, wrinkling, and the presence of benign or malignant tumors [13]. The pH of skin remains constant at about 5.5 through adulthood until age 70 and then rises significantly. This increases the susceptibility to infection, as cutaneous acidity inhibits bacterial colonization [24]. As mentioned, a thinning of the skin starts at this same age [10, 17]. Overall, the dermis becomes less dense, less cellular and less vascular with age [10]. In addition, there is a marked reduction in cutaneous blood flow. This affects the ability to adapt to temperature, and likely impacts wound repair due to decreases in oxygen and nutrient transport, and immune cell infiltration [25].

Wound Healing and Aging

Delays in wound closure result in increased incidence of infection and medical complications [13, 26]. Although many studies have reported age-related delays of healing in the elderly (65+ years) [5–7], such findings have been criticized for not controlling for confounding factors which occur more commonly in the aged, such as comorbidity and medication use [8, 10, 14]. Many of these reports are also clinical in nature, so wounds were not standardized and were of dissimilar sizes, shapes and locations. Thus, in humans it remains somewhat unclear if intrinsic aging delays wound healing.

In contrast, animal models typically utilize wounds which are standardized for size, depth, time and location of placement, etc. Such studies have found that aged animals heal 20–60% more slowly than young adult animals [27]. Other studies have more specifically reported that angiogenesis, re-epithelialization and collagen synthesis were delayed in aged mice [11], and macrophages from these mice, though increased in number at the wound site, had decreased phagocytic capabilities (37–43% reduction) compared to young mice [12]. The consensus from animal studies overall is that an age-associated delay, but not an impairment, exists in wound healing [9, 11–14]. Unfortunately, animal models do not seem to be strong predictors of clinical healing [10].

Despite reduced collagen deposition (types I and III) in the wounds of aged mice, the collagen organization has surprisingly been reported to be like normal skin, and exhibits a basket-weave architecture [9]. For determining wound strength, the orientation of collagen fibers may be more important than collagen quantity [28]. Moreover, the final collagen content does not differ between younger and older animals in fully healed wounds [11].

In humans, the functioning of both the innate and acquired immune systems decreases with age (for reviews see [29–31]). Given that local and systemic inflammatory responses are similarly reduced with age [24, 32], a decline in wound healing capabilities in the elderly seems likely.

Human studies indicate that age-related changes in wound healing are qualitative and impact all phases of healing. Such changes include enhanced platelet aggregation [13], increased rates of infection [33], decreases in wound strength and macrophage function, and delays in re-epithelialization, angiogenesis, macrophage infiltration, collagen deposition, and remodeling [10, 13]. In addition, the architecture of collagen fibers (bundles) becomes increasingly disorganized with increasing age. This reduction in, and disorganization of, collagen is thought to be largely responsible for the reduced tensile strength and increased dehiscence rate observed in the surgical wounds of elderly patients [17]. Increased bruising and persistent contact dermatitis are also more common in the elderly [33].

Importantly, many of the differences seen with age do not pertain to cellular defects, but instead to differences in the timing and degree of cellular infiltrate into tissue. In support of this, in vitro studies suggest that cellular responses to cytokines remain unaltered in the aged [34].

In humans there appears to be an early increase in neutrophil infiltration in the aged. This is accompanied by delays in macrophages and lymphocytes with cell numbers peaking at day 84 in the aged, compared to days 7 and 21 for monocytes and lymphocytes in the young, respectively [35]. In addition, several cellular adhesion molecules (CAM) (e.g., intracellular CAM-1, vascular CAM-1) were seemingly delayed and less intently expressed in the aged [35]. Together, these differences might alter the early inflammatory response, thereby affecting the entire healing cascade.

MMPs and TIMPs are involved with the degradation and remodeling of the extracellular matrix in order to aid cell migration. MMP-2 and MMP-9 have been shown to be elevated with age, and TIMPs have been shown to be lower in both acute wounds and in the normal skin of aged humans [36, 37]. This profile of higher MMPs and lower TIMPs may predispose aged skin to tissue breakdown disorders [36] (Fig. 19.2).

Overall it seems that wound closure is delayed, at least to some degree, in the skin of elderly humans. Less is known about the effects of age on wound healing in other tissue types (Table 19.2).

Mucosal Tissue and Aging

Most experimental healing studies involve dermal wounds. Mucosal wounds occur frequently and the healing of mucosa is important in most surgical outcomes. Extrinsic aging (primarily UV exposure) has little to no effect on the mucosa, making these tissues a good model for studying the effects of intrinsic aging. However, little is known about how aging impacts mucosal healing.

Oral wounds occur commonly, and their healing is comparable to wounds in other mucosal tissues with respect to repair rates and susceptibility to infection. Clinical studies have reported that with increasing age there is a greater degree of periodontal breakdown, more inflammation and a slower rate of healing [38]. Using a model of oral mucosal wound healing, Engeland et al. [39] assessed wound closure in younger (18–35 years) and older (50–88 years) human volunteers. A 3.5-mm excisional wound placed ~3 mm from the gingival margin on the hard palate was found to heal slower in older adults. Importantly, this finding occurred regardless of comorbidity or medication use.

Fig. 19.2 Aging is associated with delayed epithelialization resulting from impaired migration and proliferation, excessive inflammation leading to increased levels of proteases (MMPs, elastase) and matrix degradation. Reduced fibroblast production of, and responses to, specific cytokines (e.g., TGF-β1, EGF) results in reduced matrix production, compounding the excessive degradation at the wound site (reprinted with permission from Ashcroft et al. [8].)

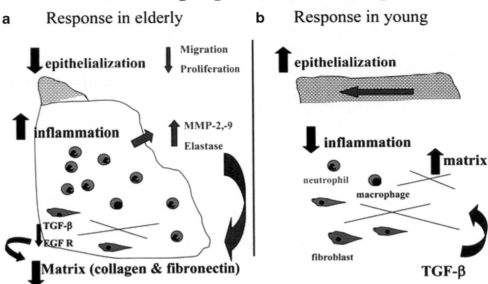

Effects of Ageing on Wound Healing

a   Response in elderly   b   Response in young

Table 19.2 Summary of age related changes in tissues during healing

Tissue	Changes with aging
Skin	Enhanced platelet aggregation
	Decreased/delayed inflammation
	Delayed macrophage infiltration
	Reduced vascularization
	Reduced granulation tissue
	Decreased collagen density/ production
	Lower number of fibroblasts
	Decreased cellular proliferation
	Slower re-epithelialization
Mucosa	Slower re-epithelialization
Myocardium	Impaired angiogenesis
	Increased matrix degradation
Bone	Increased fragility
	Less compressive stiffness
	Increased mineralization and crystallinity
	Decreased osteoprogenitor cells in the marrow
Lungs	Decreased functional capacity
	Decreased proteolytic activity
	Increased collagen accumulation
	Increased fibrosis
Vascular tissues	Decreased angiogenesis
	Decreased survival, migratory capacity and proliferative potential of endothelial progenitor cells
	Endothelial cell dysfunction

As previously mentioned, studies that have assessed aging and healing have been criticized for not accounting for the high rates of comorbidities and medication use in older individuals. In this study, four sets of analyses were performed, which selectively excluded the following individuals: (1) those receiving any type of medication (excluding allergy, birth control, or nutritional supplements such as vitamins); (2) those who presently have or in the past had a serious medical condition (e.g., diabetes, cancer, stroke, heart disease, hypertension, hypothyroidism, arthritis, irritable bowel disease, bacterial meningitis, psychopathological abnormalities such as depression); (3) those who reported to not be in good overall health; and (4) all of the above. After applying any of these exclusion criteria, older individuals still exhibited slower wound closure compared to younger adults (see Figs. 19.3–19.4 for results which exclude individuals taking medication).

Surprisingly, when older individuals taking medication were excluded from the analyses, the age-associated delays in wound healing became significantly stronger (Figs. 19.3–19.4). A common criticism of past studies is that the inclusion of such individuals may exaggerate or even account for age-related healing impairments. However, these findings by Engeland et al. [39] suggest that age impairments in wound healing are not exaggerated by medication use. Furthermore, the deleterious effects of age on wound healing may be stronger than previously suspected.

Observing values obtained 5 days after wounding, wounds were 56% larger in older subjects, and younger individuals were 3.7 times more likely to be considered healed than older individuals. Older women healed the slowest, and their wounds on day 5 were 95% larger than young men (the quickest healing group). Thus, older women appear

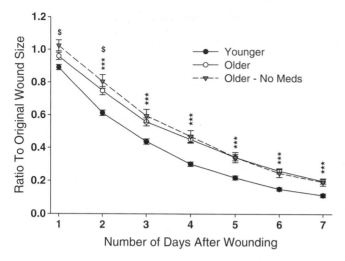

Fig. 19.3 Wound sizes for 7 days after wounding. Compared to younger individuals, older individuals had larger wounds on all days, even when excluding individuals receiving medication (dashed line); young: $n = 104$, older: $n = 92$; older – no meds: $n = 51$. *** $P < 0.001$ (younger vs. older); $ $P < 0.05$ (older – no meds vs. older). Error bars represent SEM (reprinted from [39], Copyright 2006 American Medical Association. All rights reserved)

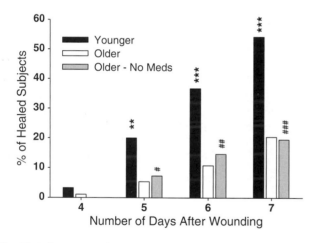

Fig. 19.4 Percentage of subjects considered healed (wounds <10% of original size) on Days 4–7. Compared to the younger group, a lower proportion of the older group were considered healed on Days 5–7, even when excluding individuals receiving medication (gray bars). ** $P < 0.01$, *** $P < 0.001$ (younger vs. older); # $P < 0.05$, ## $P < 0.01$, ### $P < 0.001$ (younger vs. older – no meds) (reprinted from [39], Copyright 2006 American Medical Association. All rights reserved)

to be at the greatest risk for delayed wound closure in mucosal tissues.

Interestingly, women have been found to heal dermal wounds faster than men, but men have a healing advantage in oral mucosal tissues [39]. This highlights the importance of distinguishing between tissue types. Different tissues may undergo similar steps in healing, but the timelines of these steps and the influence of modulating factors, can differ greatly. For instance, stress delays healing in both types of

tissues, but appears to do so by reducing inflammation in dermal tissues and increasing inflammation in mucosal tissues (unpublished observations).

Wound Healing, Menopause and Hormones

Estrogen reduction following menopause has been associated with dryness, atrophy, wrinkling, laxity, and poor healing of the skin [40]. The strength and elasticity of the skin are both reduced due to collagen loss and reduced capillary blood flow [41–44].

Delayed dermal wound healing has been well documented in postmenopausal women [44]. Healing in these women is characterized by increases in neutrophil flux and protease production, decreased phagocytosis, and excessive inflammation [42]. This results in delayed re-epithelialization, reduced collagen deposition and slower healing [44]. In animal studies, ovariectomized mice heal slower than sham operated controls, and exhibit similar healing deficits to those listed above for postmenopausal women [42, 45]. Moreover, these deficits are reversed with estrogen replacement [45].

Interestingly, topical estrogen treatment has been shown to improve the healing of excisional dermal wounds in both elderly men and women (mean ages >70 years) [46]. Specifically, estrogen treatment reduced wound sizes at day 7, increased collagen content at days 7 and 80, and increased wound strength at day 80. A decrease was also noted in neutrophil numbers, with an associated reduction in elastase which may explain the higher observed collagen content [46].

Using the same model of mucosal wound healing as previously described, Engeland et al. [47] identified a small subset of women who were over 50 years old but still premenopausal. The healing patterns of these older premenopausal women were identical to those of young women. Furthermore, these women had faster wound closure when compared to postmenopausal women of the same age (Fig. 19.5). This suggests that aging does not negatively affect wound healing until menopause begins. The delayed healing observed after menopause might be explained by the well-established drop in estrogen levels at this point of time, as estrogen appears beneficial to wound closure rates [40, 46–48]. In support of this notion, postmenopausal women taking hormone replacement therapy (HRT) exhibited a trend for faster wound closure than postmenopausal women of a similar age not taking HRT (Fig. 19.6).

The current literature suggests that age-impaired wound healing in women begins at 35–40 years of age. This conclusion is derived from studies of dermal tissues, which are more vulnerable to factors of extrinsic aging (e.g., UV damage) than mucosal tissues. Although morphological changes

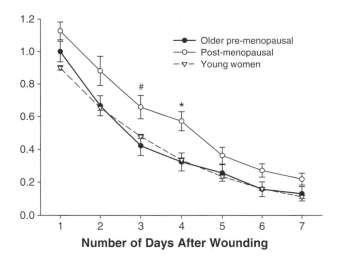

Fig. 19.5 Older women who were premenopausal (50–54 years; $n=6$) showed a pattern of healing similar to that of young women ($n=160$) and dissimilar to that of age-matched (50–55 years) postmenopausal women not taking HRT ($n-13$). This suggests that age is not a negative factor on wound healing in women until menopause begins. * $P<0.05$, # $P<0.10$ Error bars represent SEM (reprinted from Engeland et al. [47], with permission from Elsevier)

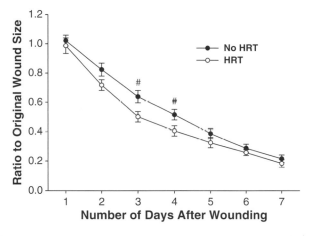

Fig. 19.6 In postmenopausal women, those taking HRT exhibited a trend for faster wound closure compared to those not taking HRT. # $P<0.10$ Error bars represent SEM (reprinted from Engeland et al. [47], with permission from Elsevier)

caused by such factors may affect healing rates, the findings from Engeland et al. [39] suggest that the underlying wound healing mechanism in women remains intact until menopause. Moreover, age may not be a substantial risk factor for delayed wound closure in women until this point of time of a woman's life is reached.

The role of estrogen in wound healing is complicated, and not fully understood but overall estrogen appears to accelerate wound healing (for review see [40]). HRT in women appears beneficial to wound healing rates in different tissue types [44, 47, 49], and studies with ovariectomized animals with HRT support the notion that menopause delays and estrogen benefits dermal wound healing [42, 45].

In men higher testosterone levels relate to slower healing of various tissues [47], and castrating male mice has been shown to speed dermal wound healing [50]. Testosterone in general appears to have an inhibitory effect on both immunity and tissue repair, to the point that being an elderly male is considered a risk factor for delayed dermal healing (for recent reviews see [51, 52]).

Scar Formation and Aging

Paradoxically, following cutaneous surgery, older individuals exhibit less scarring than young adults. In older patients incision lines are less red, the scar is less hypertrophic, and a "normalization" of appearance of the tissue occurs more quickly [17].

Similarly, in aged mice, an improved quality of scarring has been reported both microscopically and macroscopically. This has been associated with reduced levels of transforming growth factor (TGF)-β1 (beta) and a late increase in TGF-β3 [44, 53]. Interestingly, fetal healing, which occurs with little or no inflammation, and without scarring, has reduced levels of TGF-β1 and TGF-β2 isoforms and elevated levels of TGF-β3 [54]. Moreover, applying TGF-β3, or antibodies to TGF-β1 and TGF-β2, to wounds in rodents reduces scar formation [28]. Moreover, the use of HRT in older adults leads to a scarring profile similar to that of young adults [44]. Intriguingly, this TGF-β profile (e.g., the TGF-β1/TGF-β3 ratio) may determine the reduced degree of scarring which occurs in the elderly.

Other mechanistic possibilities for reduced scar formation in the elderly exist. For instance, a decreased proliferative response during the later stages of healing may explain the reduced scar formation commonly observed in the elderly [55]. Another possibility stems from the fact that older individuals, especially women, release more elastin and fibrillin during wound healing [20] which may reduce scar formation. Further exploration of these mechanisms, which may overlap, is obviously needed.

Myocardial Tissue Healing

Healing of the myocardium has unique characteristics that differentiate it from cutaneous wound healing. More than in cutaneous healing, the need for functional recovery in the myocardial tissue determines the quality of healing. This is significant, since the loss of functionality of the myocardium is a major contributor to heart failure following myocardial infarction (MI).

A number of factors such as reperfusion, age [56, 57], estrogen [58, 59], endothelin [60, 61], nitric oxide [62, 63], cytokines [64], TGF-β [65], leukocytes [66], and drugs [67, 68] have been identified as modulators of myocardial healing. Overall, however, the field of myocardial tissue healing is less understood than cutaneous healing.

The cardiac wound, caused mostly due to inadequacies in tissue perfusion, develops in a relatively short duration of time during the ischemic event, and tends to remain ischemic unless reperfused. Rhythmic cardiac contractions can further complicate myocardial healing. The healing process after MI involves four distinguishable phases (reviewed by [69]): cardiomyocyte death, inflammation, formation and remodeling of the granulation tissue, and scar formation.

The death of cardiomyocytes after occlusion of the coronary artery may occur due to cellular apoptosis or necrosis. While apoptosis occurs as early as 6 h after MI, the inability of the neighboring cells to phagocytose the apoptotic cells and their contents may result in necrosis, which happens typically around 12 h to 4 days after infarct formation. The cellular contents released from these cells (i.e., serum glutamine-oxaloacetic transaminase, creatine kinase, troponin T, etc.) can be detected in the general circulation and are often used as early markers of MI. The release of proinflammatory cytokines and the activation of the compliment system mark inflammation after MI. Characteristic of this phase, cellular inflammatory mediators arrive at the site to clear cellular debris.

The formation of granulation tissue is characterized by the deposition of extracellular matrix components and neovascularization. During this stage of healing, the degradation of certain matrix components also occurs, to enable cellular proliferation and migration into the healing tissue. In the healing myocardium the contractile rhythmic stretching of the cardiac tissue influences the remodeling of the granulation tissue and scar formation after MI. Under these influences there appears to be a persistence of cardiac myofibroblasts, while there is a generalized decrease in cellularity by apoptosis during remodeling of the ischemic scar. Importantly, the collagen that was deposited during the earlier phases of healing tends to become completely cross-linked, offering maximal tensile strength to the healing tissue.

Among the various factors associated with myocardial infarcts, age appears to affect both the incidence of MI, and the mortality associated with MI. About 50% of the individuals admitted to hospitals for MI, and 80% of the mortality associated with MI, involve patients 65 years or older. These age-related associations appear to be independent of infarct size [56]. As previously discussed, a number of age-related changes influence healing. These changes, including altered inflammatory responses, dysregulated angiogenic pathways, and increased matrix degradation [9] make older individuals more susceptible to damage from MI and diminish their potential for recovery.

Age has been shown to differentially affect mortality rates in women after MI. Young women who survived hospitalization for MI have a higher mortality rate compared to men. This difference was not observed in older women [70]. This may be related to circulating estrogen levels, as the initiation of HRT after MI has been associated with a greater risk for future cardiac events [71].

Bone Repair and Aging

Aging influences bone healing by increasing the chances of both nonunion and delayed healing. While age and mechanical fixation have significant influences over the healing of fixated fractures, age appears to have the greater influence among the two [72]. As determined by skeletal fragility, the quality of bone decreases with advancing age. While fatigue loading on younger bone inflicts more diffuse damage, older bone suffers microcracks and loses tissue stiffness associated with compression. Such age-related changes may contribute to greater fragility of the bone in older individuals [73]. Increased fragility increases susceptibility for fracture. Additionally, increasing mineralization, crystallinity, and type-b carbonate substitution is associated with decreased elasticity of bone with advancing age [74]. Along with age-associated resorptive changes in bone, these factors can increase the risk of fracture in older individuals. Healing of fractured bone may also be impaired with increasing age, due to the decrease in osteoprogenitor cells in the marrow of older bone [75]. Overall, there is a considerable increase in susceptibility for fractures and delayed fracture healing associated with older age [76].

Lung Fibrosis and Aging

Age associated fibrosis of the lung tissues along with terminal airway closure decrease lung function. Hence, the functional capacity of the lungs decreases with age [77]. Other physiochemical changes associated with aging are known to alter the healing potential of the lung with advancing age. Aging rats showed decreased proteolytic activity of MMPs associated with collagen accumulation in the lung [78]. During healing, extracellular matrix components are laid down in response to injury [79]. An increased deposition of the extracellular matrix or decreased degradation may be associated with age related fibrosis of the lungs. With increasing age, the senescence of the lung epithelial cells, altered regulation of oxidative stress, and changes in matrix composition contribute to an increased susceptibility of the lung to fibrosis following injury.

Angiogenesis and Tissue Oxygenation

Of an estimated 80 million adult Americans who have one or more types of cardiovascular disease, over 38 million are estimated to be 60 years of age or older [80]. Endothelial dysfunction is a key event in atherosclerotic plaque formation, which can be attributed to the majority of cardiovascular disease states. When elderly individuals with clinical atherosclerotic vascular disease were compared with healthy elderly controls and healthy young controls it is seen that age alone, independent of other cardiac risk factors or clinically observed atherosclerosis, is associated with endothelial cell dysfunction [81]. Mechanistically, the endothelial dysfunction translates to impairment in vasodilatation in response to stimuli. In individuals aged 70 years and older, atrial microvessels had a blunted vascular endothelial growth factor (VEGF)-mediated microvascular dilation in comparison to individuals under 70 years of age [82]. The endothelial progenitor cells maintain vascular homeostasis by contributing to regeneration and repair of the vessel wall. In the elderly, endothelial progenitor cells were found to be dysfunctional and exhibited lower survival rates, poorer migratory capacity, and lower proliferative potential [83].

Angiogenesis is a key component of wound healing. Decreased angiogenesis, along with a poor vasodilatory response, can make wounds hypoxic and delay healing. The effects of age and ischemia are additive in the impairment of healing [84]. Hence, it is not surprising that most chronic wounds are seen in the elderly, with these wounds characterized by impaired blood supply and tissue hypoxia. Restoration of adequate blood supply and tissue oxygenation is essential for optimal healing in the elderly.

Clinical Implications

It remains unclear to what degree intrinsic aging impacts wound healing. Few human studies have controlled for confounding factors such as comorbidity and medication use, and factors of extrinsic aging such as cumulative UV exposure likely drive many of the reported findings of age-impaired healing.

Results from mucosal wound healing studies which controlled for medication use and comorbidity, and are not subject to cumulative UV effects, found significantly slower wound closure in men over 50 years of age, and in postmenopausal women [39, 47]. Given these findings, and that vital aspects of both skin morphology and immune function are altered in the elderly, it is almost certain that aging per se impedes some aspects of wound healing (Table 19.3).

Table 19.3 Clinical implications of age related tissue changes

Tissue	Changes with aging
Skin	Delayed healing
	Increased dehiscence
	Reduced tensile strength while healing
	Increased rates of infection
	Reduced skin elasticity
	Decreased scarring
Mucosa	Delayed healing
Myocardium	Greater damage from MI
	Increased mortality associated with MI
Bone	Increased susceptibility to fracture
	Impaired healing
Lungs	Decreased functional capacity
	Increased fibrosis
Vascular tissues	Decreased angiogenesis
	Decreased neovascularization
	Increased tissue hypoxia

The question still remains: Is the degree of impediment which occurs clinically relevant? It is important to note that even if wounds close more slowly in the elderly, healing is essentially normal [19]. New events in healing do not occur, expected events are not absent [32], and the end result is often similar to that of young adults [19]. Moreover, wounds often heal with better esthetics (less scarring) in the aged [17].

The infrequency of wound complications which occur in the elderly, despite delays in wound closure, speaks of the reserve strength found in unwounded skin [7]. Not surprisingly, tissue healing occurs in an overabundant manner. For example, during wound repair, excessive vascularization occurs, and more granulation tissue is created than is needed. After wound closure, this excessive vascularization recedes, and remodeling of the underlying matrix occurs. Even in unwounded skin, the vascularization which exists is about 10 times the amount required for basic nutritional support of the tissue [17]. Thus, our healing capacity is far in excess of what is needed [32]. As a result, surgical operations are routinely and safely performed in elderly patients with normal, albeit slightly slower, recovery times. To date, the contribution of age alone has not been shown to *clinically* impair wound healing.

Importantly, the major increased risk to aged individuals undergoing surgery pertains to other medical complications that affect healing [7]. In addition, the effects of age are interactive with other risk factors for impaired immunity and delayed healing [31, 39]. The risk factors for delayed healing are numerous and include concomitant medical conditions (e.g., diabetes) [2, 85], medication use [19], stress (for recent review see [86]), depression [87], gender (the direction of this disparity varies by tissue type) [39], obesity [88], smoking [89], alcohol [90], nutrition [91, 92], immobility [88], etc.

The presence of any of these risk factors in aged individuals prior to surgery should serve as a red flag to the clinician, and these patients should be given more aggressive postsurgical attention. Importantly, in the presence of such risk factors, medical complications *not* associated with tissue healing are more likely to occur in the elderly [7]. The clinician should take whatever steps necessary to minimize these risks prior to surgery.

The provision of patient education, massage therapy, or relaxation techniques have all been shown to reduce anxiety in surgical patients and improve clinical outcomes [93–95]. This is of particular importance in the elderly who may already have compromised immunity and slower wound healing than younger adults.

The Mini-Nutritional Assessment (MNA) is a good diagnostic tool for identifying nutritional deficits in elderly patients. It was recently reported that total lymphocyte count and MNA scores were lower in patients with delayed wound healing. Moreover, both scores were found to have value in predicting which patients would experience delays in wound healing [92].

Medications which have been shown to inhibit wound healing include anticoagulants, aspirin, phenylbutazone, colchicines, penicillamine and cyclosporine [19]. Corticosteroids can interfere with dermal wound healing at multiple levels, although the effect of a single bolus on mucosal healing (e.g., dental surgery) does not negatively affect wound closure (unpublished observations).

To sum, prior to undergoing surgery, any existing risk factors for delayed healing should be stringently sought out in the elderly. Diseases negatively impact wound healing in the elderly more than in young adults, and pre-existing medical conditions should be treated vigorously prior to surgery to allow for maximal healing [5]. Elderly patients with concomitant risk factors (e.g., diabetes, malnutrition, stress) have a greater susceptibility to chronic infection [19]. Each of these factors should be tested for, monitored, and treated accordingly. It is important to understand that all of these factors occur more commonly in the elderly, and are likely to exacerbate healing.

References

1. US Census Bureau. Interim Projections Consistent With Census 2000. Washington, DC: US Census Bureau; 2004.
2. Pittman J. Effect of aging on wound healing: current concepts. J Wound Ostomy Continence Nurs. 2007;34(4):412–5.
3. Ashcroft GS, Mills SJ. Androgen receptor-mediated inhibition of cutaneous wound healing. J Clin Invest. 2002;110(5):615–24.
4. DuNuoy PL. Cicatrization of wounds. J Exp Med. 1916;24: 461–70.
5. Gerstein AD, Phillips TJ, Rogers GS, Gilchrest BA. Wound healing and aging. Dermatol Clin. 1993;11(4):749–57.
6. Fenske NA, Lober CW. Structural and functional changes of normal aging skin. J Am Acad Dermatol. 1986;15(4 Pt 1):571–85.
7. Goodson III WH, Hunt TK. Wound healing and aging. J Invest Dermatol. 1979;73(1):88–91.
8. Ashcroft GS, Mills SJ, Ashworth JJ. Ageing and wound healing. Biogerontology. 2002;3(6):337–45.
9. Ashcroft GS, Horan MA, Ferguson MW. Aging is associated with reduced deposition of specific extracellular matrix components, an upregulation of angiogenesis, and an altered inflammatory response in a murine incisional wound healing model. J Invest Dermatol. 1997;108(4):430–7.
10. Thomas DR. Age-related changes in wound healing. Drugs Aging. 2001;18(8):607–20.
11. Swift ME, Kleinman HK, DiPietro LA. Impaired wound repair and delayed angiogenesis in aged mice. Lab Invest. 1999;79(12): 1479–87.
12. Swift ME, Burns AL, Gray KL, DiPietro LA. Age-related alterations in the inflammatory response to dermal injury. J Invest Dermatol. 2001;117(5):1027–35.
13. Gosain A, DiPietro LA. Aging and wound healing. World J Surg. 2004;28(3):321–6.
14. Ashcroft GS, Horan MA, Ferguson MW. The effects of ageing on cutaneous wound healing in mammals. J Anat. 1995;187 (Pt 1):1–26.
15. Eming SA, Krieg T, Davidson JM. Inflammation in wound repair: molecular and cellular mechanisms. J Invest Dermatol. 2007;127(3): 514–25.
16. Cerimele D, Celleno L, Serri F. Physiological changes in ageing skin. Br J Dermatol. 1990;122 Suppl 35:13–20.
17. Cook JL, Dzubow LM. Aging of the skin: implications for cutaneous surgery. Arch Dermatol. 1997;133(10):1273–7.
18. Tenchini ML, Savant F, Paini C, Montefusco MC, Donati V, Malcovati M. Autocrine-acting early secreted mitogenic activity: production and responsiveness in cultures of normal human keratinocytes as a function of in vivo and in vitro age. Cell Biol Int. 2001;25(3):197–204.
19. van de Kerkhof PC, Van Bergen B, Spruijt K, Kuiper JP. Age-related changes in wound healing. Clin Exp Dermatol. 1994;19(5):369–74.
20. Ashcroft GS, Kielty CM, Horan MA, Ferguson MW. Age-related changes in the temporal and spatial distributions of fibrillin and elastin mRNAs and proteins in acute cutaneous wounds of healthy humans. J Pathol. 1997;183(1):80–9.
21. Gilchrest BA, Stoff JS, Soter NA. Chronologic aging alters the response to ultraviolet-induced inflammation in human skin. J Invest Dermatol. 1982;79(1):11–5.
22. Pienta KJ, Coffey DS. Characterization of the subtypes of cell motility in ageing human skin fibroblasts. Mech Ageing Dev. 1990;56(2):99–105.
23. Reed MJ, Ferara NS, Vernon RB. Impaired migration, integrin function, and actin cytoskeletal organization in dermal fibroblasts from a subset of aged human donors. Mech Ageing Dev. 2001;122(11):1203–20.
24. Farage MA, Miller KW, Elsner P, Maibach HI. Functional and physiological characteristics of the aging skin. Aging Clin Exp Res. 2008;20(3):195–200.
25. Tsuchida Y. The effect of aging and arteriosclerosis on human skin blood flow. J Dermatol Sci. 1993;5(3):175–81.
26. Robson MC. Wound infection. A failure of wound healing caused by an imbalance of bacteria. Surg Clin North Am. 1997;77(3):637–50.
27. Quirinia A, Viidik A. The influence of age on the healing of normal and ischemic incisional skin wounds. Mech Ageing Dev. 1991;58(2–3):221–32.
28. Shah M, Foreman DM, Ferguson MW. Control of scarring in adult wounds by neutralising antibody to transforming growth factor beta. Lancet. 1992;339(8787):213–4.
29. Plowden J, Renshaw-Hoelscher M, Engleman C, Katz J, Sambhara S. Innate immunity in aging: impact on macrophage function. Aging Cell. 2004;3(4):161–7.

30. Gomez CR, Nomellini V, Faunce DE, Kovacs EJ. Innate immunity and aging. Exp Gerontol. 2008;43(8):718–28.

31. Graham JE, Christian LM, Kiecolt-Glaser JK. Stress, age, and immune function: toward a lifespan approach. J Behav Med. 2006;29(4):389–400.

32. Eaglstein WH. Wound healing and aging. Dermatol Clin. 1986; 4(3):481–4.

33. Lober CW, Fenske NA. Cutaneous aging: effect of intrinsic changes on surgical considerations. South Med J. 1991;84(12):1444–6.

34. Freedland M, Karmiol S, Rodriguez J, Normolle D, Smith Jr D, Garner W. Fibroblast responses to cytokines are maintained during aging. Ann Plast Surg. 1995;35(3):290–6.

35. Ashcroft GS, Horan MA, Ferguson MW. Aging alters the inflammatory and endothelial cell adhesion molecule profiles during human cutaneous wound healing. Lab Invest. 1998;78(1):47–58.

36. Ashcroft GS, Horan MA, Herrick SE, Tarnuzzer RW, Schultz GS, Ferguson MW. Age-related differences in the temporal and spatial regulation of matrix metalloproteinases (MMPs) in normal skin and acute cutaneous wounds of healthy humans. Cell Tissue Res. 1997;290(3):581–91.

37. Ashcroft GS, Herrick SE, Tarnuzzer RW, Horan MA, Schultz GS, Ferguson MW. Human ageing impairs injury-induced in vivo expression of tissue inhibitor of matrix metalloproteinases (TIMP)-1 and -2 proteins and mRNA. J Pathol. 1997;183(2):169–76.

38. Van der V. Effect of age on the periodontium. J Clin Periodontol. 1984;11(5):281–94.

39. Engeland CG, Bosch JA, Cacioppo JT, Marucha PT. Mucosal wound healing: the roles of age and sex. Arch Surg. 2006;141(12): 1193–7.

40. Hall G, Phillips TJ. Estrogen and skin: the effects of estrogen, menopause, and hormone replacement therapy on the skin. J Am Acad Dermatol. 2005;53(4):555–68.

41. Ashcroft GS, Mills SJ, Lei K, Gibbons L, Jeong MJ, Taniguchi M, et al. Estrogen modulates cutaneous wound healing by downregulating macrophage migration inhibitory factor. J Clin Invest. 2003;111(9):1309–18.

42. Ashcroft GS, Ashworth JJ. Potential role of estrogens in wound healing. Am J Clin Dermatol. 2003;4(11):737–43.

43. Raine-Fenning NJ, Brincat MP, Muscat-Baron Y. Skin aging and menopause: implications for treatment. Am J Clin Dermatol. 2003;4(6):371–8.

44. Ashcroft GS, Dodsworth J, van Boxtel E, Tarnuzzer RW, Horan MA, Schultz GS, et al. Estrogen accelerates cutaneous wound healing associated with an increase in TGF-beta1 levels. Nat Med. 1997;3(11):1209–15.

45. Ashcroft GS, Mills SJ, Flanders KC, Lyakh LA, Anzano MA, Gilliver SC, et al. Role of Smad3 in the hormonal modulation of in vivo wound healing responses. Wound Repair Regen. 2003;11(6):468–73.

46. Ashcroft GS, Greenwell-Wild T, Horan MA, Wahl SM, Ferguson MW. Topical estrogen accelerates cutaneous wound healing in aged humans associated with an altered inflammatory response. Am J Pathol. 1999;155(4):1137–46.

47. Engeland CG, Sabzehei B, Marucha PT. Sex hormones and mucosal wound healing. Brain Behav Immun. 2009;23(5):629–35.

48. Kovacs EJ. Aging, traumatic injury, and estrogen treatment. Exp Gerontol. 2005;40(7):549–55.

49. Margolis DJ, Knauss J, Bilker W. Hormone replacement therapy and prevention of pressure ulcers and venous leg ulcers. Lancet. 2002;359(9307):675–7.

50. Gilliver SC, Wu F, Ashcroft GS. Regulatory roles of androgens in cutaneous wound healing. Thromb Haemost. 2003;90(6):978–85.

51. Fimmel S, Zouboulis CC. Influence of physiological androgen levels on wound healing and immune status in men. Aging Male. 2005;8(3–4):166–74.

52. Makrantonaki E, Zouboulis CC. Androgens and ageing of the skin. Curr Opin Endocrinol Diabetes Obes. 2009;16(3):240–5.

53. Ashcroft GS, Horan MA, Ferguson MW. The effects of ageing on wound healing: immunolocalisation of growth factors and their receptors in a murine incisional model. J Anat. 1997;190(Pt 3): 351–65.

54. Wilgus TA. Regenerative healing in fetal skin: a review of the literature. Ostomy Wound Manage. 2007;53(6):16–31.

55. Marcus JR, Tyrone JW, Bonomo S, Xia Y, Mustoe TA. Cellular mechanisms for diminished scarring with aging. Plast Reconstr Surg. 2000;105(5):1591–9.

56. Gillum BS, Graves EJ, Wood E. National hospital discharge survey. Vital Health Stat 13. 1998;133:i–v, 1–51.

57. Maggioni AP, Maseri A, Fresco C, Franzosi MG, Mauri F, Santoro E, et al. Age-related increase in mortality among patients with first myocardial infarctions treated with thrombolysis. The Investigators of the Gruppo Italiano per lo Studio della Sopravvivenza nell'Infarto Miocardico (GISSI-2). N Engl J Med. 1993;329:1442–8.

58. Smith PJ, Ornatsky O, Stewart DJ, Picard P, Dawood F, Wen WH, et al. Effects of estrogen replacement on infarct size, cardiac remodeling, and the endothelin system after myocardial infarction in ovariectomized rats. Circulation. 2000;102:2983–9.

59. Brinckmann M, Kaschina E, Altarche-Xifro W, Curato C, Timm M, Grzesiak A, et al. Estrogen receptor alpha supports cardiomyocytes indirectly through post-infarct cardiac c-kit+ cells. J Mol Cell Cardiol. 2009;47:66–75.

60. Oie E, Vinge LE, Tonnessen T, Grogaard HK, Kjekshus H, Christensen G, et al. Transient, isopeptide-specific induction of myocardial endothelin-1 mRNA in congestive heart failure in rats. Am J Physiol. 1997;273:H1727–36.

61. Sakai S, Miyauchi T, Kobayashi M, Yamaguchi I, Goto K, Sugishita Y. Inhibition of myocardial endothelin pathway improves long-term survival in heart failure. Nature. 1996;384:353–5.

62. Chen Y, Traverse JH, Du R, Hou M, Bache RJ. Nitric oxide modulates myocardial oxygen consumption in the failing heart. Circulation. 2002;106:273–9.

63. Liu YH, Carretero OA, Cingolani OH, Liao TD, Sun Y, Xu J, et al. Role of inducible nitric oxide synthase in cardiac function and remodeling in mice with heart failure due to myocardial infarction. Am J Physiol Heart Circ Physiol. 2005;289:H2616–23.

64. Herskowitz A, Choi S, Ansari AA, Wesselingh S. Cytokine mRNA expression in postischemic/reperfused myocardium. Am J Pathol. 1995;146:419–28.

65. Brown JM, White CW, Terada LS, Grosso MA, Shanley PF, Mulvin DW, et al. Interleukin 1 pretreatment decreases ischemia/reperfusion injury. Proc Natl Acad Sci USA. 1990;87:5026–30.

66. Ashcroft GS, Lei K, Jin W, Longenecker G, Kulkarni AB, Greenwell-Wild T, et al. Secretory leukocyte protease inhibitor mediates non-redundant functions necessary for normal wound healing. Nat Med. 2000;6:1147–53.

67. Wei GC, Sirois MG, Qu R, Liu P, Rouleau JL. Subacute and chronic effects of quinapril on cardiac cytokine expression, remodeling, and function after myocardial infarction in the rat. J Cardiovasc Pharmacol. 2002;39:842–50.

68. Prabhu SD, Chandrasekar B, Murray DR, Freeman GL. beta-adrenergic blockade in developing heart failure: effects on myocardial inflammatory cytokines, nitric oxide, and remodeling. Circulation. 2000;101:2103–9.

69. Blankesteijn WM, Creemers E, Lutgens E, Cleutjens JP, Daemen MJ, Smits JF. Dynamics of cardiac wound healing following myocardial infarction: observations in genetically altered mice. Acta Physiol Scand. 2001;173:75–82.

70. Vaccarino V, Parsons L, Every NR, Barron HV, Krumholz HM. Sex-based differences in early mortality after myocardial infarction. National Registry of Myocardial Infarction 2 Participants. N Engl J Med. 1999;341:217–25.

71. Alexander KP, Newby LK, Hellkamp AS, Harrington RA, Peterson ED, Kopecky S, et al. Initiation of hormone replacement therapy

after acute myocardial infarction is associated with more cardiac events during follow-up. J Am Coll Cardiol. 2001;38:1–7.

72. Strube P, Sentuerk U, Riha T, Kaspar K, Mueller M, Kasper G, et al. Influence of age and mechanical stability on bone defect healing: age reverses mechanical effects. Bone. 2008;42:758–64.

73. Diab T, Sit S, Kim D, Rho J, Vashishth D. Age-dependent fatigue behaviour of human cortical bone. Eur J Morphol. 2005;42:53–9.

74. Akkus O, Adar F, Schaffler MB. Age-related changes in physico-chemical properties of mineral crystals are related to impaired mechanical function of cortical bone. Bone. 2004;34:443–53.

75. Quarto R, Thomas D, Liang CT. Bone progenitor cell deficits and the age-associated decline in bone repair capacity. Calcif Tissue Int. 1995;56:123–9.

76. Bak B, Andreassen TT. The effect of aging on fracture healing in the rat. Calcif Tissue Int. 1989;45:292–7.

77. Ruivo S, Viana P, Martins C, Baeta C. Effects of aging on lung function. A comparison of lung function in healthy adults and the elderly. Rev Port Pneumol. 2009;15:629–53.

78. Calabresi C, Arosio B, Galimberti L, Scanziani E, Bergottini R, Annoni G, et al. Natural aging, expression of fibrosis-related genes and collagen deposition in rat lung. Exp Gerontol. 2007;42:1003–11.

79. Hetzel M, Bachem M, Anders D, Trischler G, Faehling M. Different effects of growth factors on proliferation and matrix production of normal and fibrotic human lung fibroblasts. Lung. 2005;183:225–37.

80. Lloyd-Jones D, Adams R, Carnethon M, De Simone G, Ferguson TB, Flegal K, et al. Heart disease and stroke statistics–2009 update: a report from the American Heart Association Statistics Committee and Stroke Statistics Subcommittee. Circulation. 2009;119:e21–181.

81. Al-Shaer MH, Choueiri NE, Correia ML, Sinkey CA, Barenz TA, Haynes WG. Effects of aging and atherosclerosis on endothelial and vascular smooth muscle function in humans. Int J Cardiol. 2006;109:201–6.

82. Mieno S, Boodhwani M, Clements RT, Ramlawi B, Sodha NR, Li J, et al. Aging is associated with an impaired coronary microvascular response to vascular endothelial growth factor in patients. J Thorac Cardiovasc Surg. 2006;132:1348–55.

83. Heiss C, Keymel S, Niesler U, Ziemann J, Kelm M, Kalka C. Impaired progenitor cell activity in age-related endothelial dysfunction. J Am Coll Cardiol. 2005;45:1441–8.

84. Wu L, Xia YP, Roth SI, Gruskin E, Mustoe TA. Transforming growth factor-beta1 fails to stimulate wound healing and impairs its signal transduction in an aged ischemic ulcer model: importance of oxygen and age. Am J Pathol. 1999;154:301–9.

85. Brem H, Tomic-Canic M, Entero H, Hanflik AM, Wang VM, Fallon JT, et al. The synergism of age and db/db genotype impairs wound healing. Exp Gerontol. 2007;42(6):523–31.

86. Engeland CG, Marucha PT. Wound healing and stress. In: Granstein RD, Luger TA, editors. Neuroimmunology of the skin: basic science to clinical relevance. Berlin: Springer; 2009. p. 233–47.

87. Bosch JA, Engeland CG, Cacioppo JT, Marucha PT. Depressive symptoms predict mucosal wound healing. Psychosom Med. 2007;69(7):597–605.

88. Lowe JR. Skin integrity in critically ill obese patients. Crit Care Nurs Clin North Am. 2009;21(3):311–22, v.

89. Ueng SW, Lee MY, Li AF, Lin SS, Tai CL, Shih CH. Effect of intermittent cigarette smoke inhalation on tibial lengthening: experimental study on rabbits. J Trauma. 1997;42(2):231–8.

90. Radek KA, Ranzer MJ, DiPietro LA. Brewing complications: the effect of acute ethanol exposure on wound healing. J Leukoc Biol. 2009;86(5):1125–34.

91. Thomas DR. The role of nutrition in prevention and healing of pressure ulcers. Clin Geriatr Med. 1997;13(3):497–511.

92. Guo JJ, Yang H, Qian H, Huang L, Guo Z, Tang T. The effects of different nutritional measurements on delayed wound healing after hip fracture in the elderly. J Surg Res. 2010;159:503–8.

93. Holden-Lund C. Effects of relaxation with guided imagery on surgical stress and wound healing. Res Nurs Health. 1988;11(4):235–44.

94. Devine EC. Effects of psychoeducational care for adult surgical patients: a meta-analysis of 191 studies. Patient Educ Couns. 1992;19(2):129–42.

95. Field T, Peck M, Krugman S, Tuchel T, Schanberg S, Kuhn C, et al. Burn injuries benefit from massage therapy. J Burn Care Rehabil. 1998;19(3):241–4.

96. Werner S, Grose R. Regulation of wound healing by growth factors and cytokines. Physiol Rev. 2003;83:835–70.

Chapter 20
Pulmonary Changes in the Elderly

Keenan A. Hawkins and Ravi Kalhan

Abstract There are multiple changes that occur to the respiratory system with aging. In the absence of significant disease, the majority of such changes do not result in any significant impact on lung health. However, such changes do affect physiologic testing and susceptibility to environmental insults which are essential to understand in the context of the patient being considered for thoracic surgery. Normal physiologic changes to the chest wall and supporting structures, airway and lung compliance, alveolar surface area, and pulmonary vasculature all result in a reduction in lung function and may also be associated with reduced exercise capacity. Gas transfer in elderly patients is less efficient than those who are younger, but this seldom is clinically significant. Elderly patients are also more susceptible to infection and a higher mortality associated with such infections due to alterations in host defense mechanisms and the frequency of comorbid conditions.

Keywords Aging • Elderly • Lung function • Compliance • Resistance • Small airways • Senile emphysema • Kyphosis • Respiratory muscles • Spirometry • Vital capacity • Total lung capacity • Residual volume • Closing volume • Diffusing capacity • Maximum oxygen consumption • Host defense • Pneumonia

In 1977, Fletcher and Peto published landmark work which documented that, after attaining peak lung function around age 25, normal aging is associated with loss of lung function [1]. Among non-smokers as well as the majority of smokers, this loss of lung function is not actually associated with the development of obstructive lung disease or significant impairments in gas exchange, and the respiratory system remains capable of carrying out required physiologic functions. Understanding the physiologic changes associated with normal aging, nonetheless, is important within the interpretation of diagnostic testing of lung function. In addition, senescent changes that alter lung host defense may result in increased susceptibility to lung infections.

Structural and Functional Changes of the Respiratory System Associated with Normal Aging

Changes in Chest Wall Mechanics and Respiratory Muscle Performance

Increasing age is associated with substantial decreases in chest wall compliance in both the upper and lower thoracic cavity. In a study of 24–75 year olds, the reduction of chest wall compliance associated with aging was 31% [2]. A variety of factors contribute to reduced chest wall compliance with aging. Changes in the shape of the thoracic cage which occur in association with aging include dorsal kyphosis and increased anterior–posterior diameter (the so-called barrel chest) which may result from vertebral compression fractures. Such findings have been documented with significant frequency in individuals between ages 75 and 93. In a study of 100 chest radiographs in individuals from this age group, 68 had at least moderate kyphosis in the context of vertebral compression fractures [3]. In the same series, calcification at the chondrosternal junctions and degenerative joint disease in the spine were observed frequently and offer additional explanations for reduced chest wall compliance [3].

The altered configuration of the chest wall seen with aging has consequences on respiratory muscle function. Increased anterior–posterior chest diameter and kyphosis collectively lead to worsened diaphragmatic performance [4]. The diaphragm performs optimally with its natural domed configuration during relaxation and any physical alteration which results in "flattening" at rest results in impaired excursion during inspiration. The contractile properties of the diaphragm itself are also altered with aging. The diaphragmatic pressure generated during a maximal sniff was observed to

K.A. Hawkins (✉)
Division of Pulmonary and Critical Care Medicine, Northwestern University Feinberg School of Medicine, Chicago, IL 60611, USA
e-mail: khawkins@nmff.org

13% less in 67–81 year olds compared with 21–40 year olds, and 23% less during bilateral magnetic stimulation of the phrenic nerves [5].

The major respiratory muscles other than the diaphragm are skeletal muscle and skeletal muscle strength decreases with age [6]. Overall strength in the respiratory system is often evaluated via measurement of maximal inspiratory pressure (MIP) which is the pressure at the mouth against a closed valve with maximum inspiration and maximum expiratory pressure (MEP) which is similarly measured during expiration. Notably, MIP incorporates both diaphragmatic and other respiratory muscle strength into a composite measure and is highly correlated with peripheral muscle strength determined by handgrip [7]. In a study of 504 healthy individuals between ages 18 and 82, age was inversely correlated with MIP ($r = -0.24$) [8]. Another correlate of impaired respiratory muscle strength is impaired nutritional status, which is frequent among the elderly. Lean body mass and body weight were both correlated with both MIP and MEP [7]. Post-mortem analysis has documented that there is a correlation between weight and diaphragmatic muscle mass [9]. Suggested mechanisms for loss of respiratory muscle strength with aging include decreased muscle mass as well as decrease number of fast-twitch (type II) muscle fibers, and alternations at the neuromuscular junction including denervation of fast-twitch muscle fibers [4]. Several of the potential chest wall changes that can occur with normal aging are depicted in Fig. 20.1.

Changes in the Airways and Lung Parenchyma

As a part of normal gaining, static elastic recoil pressure of the lung decreases. Peak elastic recoil pressure is achieved in the middle of the third decade of life, and then decreases at a rate of 0.1–0.2 cm H_2O per year [10]. This has been attributed largely to the finding of "senile emphysema" which is an enlargement in the size of airspaces without actual destruction of alveolar walls (a critical distinction from "true" emphysema in which actual alveolar destruction is the principal feature). The most compelling evidence for senile emphysema comes from human data which evaluated airspace size in the context of age in never-smoking subjects 21–93 years old utilizing 16 autopsy specimens and 22 surgical specimens. This study documented that surface area of airspace wall per unit of lung volume ratio (S/V) decreases over the lifespan [11]. The observation of decreased S/V ratio has been validated in the senescence accelerated murine model (SAM mice) In SAM mice, the alveolar ducts increase with aging in a homogenous fashion without alveolar wall destruction, and without cellular infiltration (another important distinction from "true" emphysema) [4]. The mechanism underlying airspace enlargement with aging remains uncertain. An age-associated increase in the ratio of elastin to collagen has been observed in autopsy specimens from individuals who died of non-pulmonary causes [12], but the actual physiologic impact of this change is uncertain. This observation has not been confirmed in SAM mice, although

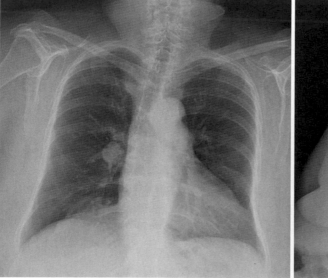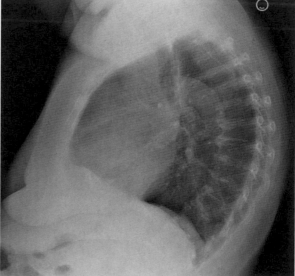

Fig. 20.1 This posteroanterior and lateral chest radiograph from an 86-year-old woman without overt lung disease reveals several changes to the chest wall that can be apparent in the elderly. Notably, disk spaces are reduced indicating likely vertebral compression fractures. In addition, the inspiratory effort is poor which likely is a manifestation of some form of neuromuscular weakness. There is dorsal kyphosis which leads to a barrel configuration of the chest. Finally both hemidiaphragms have a relatively flat appearance compared to what may be seen in individuals of younger age

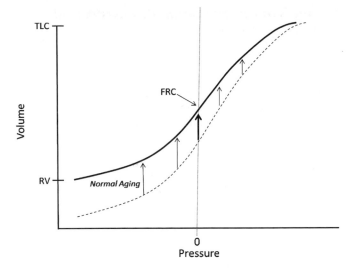

Fig. 20.2 Normal aging results in a shift of the pressure volume curve up and leftward indicating that at any given pressure, lung volumes are increased. The volume of gas in the lung at rest occurs at functional residual capacity (FRC) where the transthoracic pressure is 0 owing to equal and opposite forces between the lung's tendency to collapse (elastic recoil pressure) and the chest wall's tendency to expand. With aging, lung compliance decreases (less elastic recoil pressure). This results in an increase in FRC as well as residual volume (RV) as the forces of increased chest wall resistance do not predominate at lower lung volumes. At higher lung volumes, the reduction in chest wall compliance is likely offset by the increase in lung compliance, and thus, TLC remains constant with normal aging

the elastic fibers from lungs of SAM mice do have reduced recoil pressures [13].

Loss of elasticity and enlargement of the airspaces has an impact on the adjacent small airways (<2 mm diameter airways or terminal bronchioles). Typically terminal bronchioles are "tethered" open by adjacent airspaces which, when enlarged, provide a less robust surrounding support matrix. This fosters a tendency to collapse among the terminal bronchioles which likely results in premature airway closure. In addition, the diameter of bronchioles peaks in the fourth decade of life and then begins to decline [14]. The combined effects of lost elasticity of the lung parenchyma and a tendency of terminal bronchioles to collapse result in an increase in resting lung volumes and diminished flow during forced expiratory maneuvers (see below). The net result of lung parenchyma and chest wall changes with normal aging is a shift of the static pressure–volume curve of the respiratory system up and leftward, indicating increased lung volumes at any given pressure (Fig. 20.2).

Changes in Gas Exchange and Ventilation

The major function of the lung is gas exchange, and it is generally accepted that the alveolar-arterial oxygen gradient widens with aging. The changes in gas exchange with aging

is potentially attributable to several processes including changes in alveolar structure and surface area, change in the pulmonary vasculature, changes in distribution of blood flow, and changes which are a consequence of alterations to the mechanical properties of the lung. Due to the significant amount of reserve acquired throughout the developing years, gas exchange is not meaningfully impacted by loss of alveolar surface area as a normal consequence of aging. Throughout adolescence, the lungs develop an alveolar surface area that is capable of maintaining efficient and effective gas exchange well into adult life. The total reduction in alveolar surface area from 20 to 70 years of age is only 20% ($75–60$ m^2) [15].

Established reference values for arterial blood gases are primarily derived from studies of the normal, healthy young adult. Extrapolation of these values for patients in elderly populations may prove inaccurate. Multiple studies have been performed to investigate the normal age-related changes in arterial blood gas measurements, of which most have failed to demonstrate a clinically significant age-related reduction in PaO$_2$ in the healthy adult despite the increased alveolar-arterial gradient. In addition, the majority of investigations directed toward the normal effects of aging on oxygenation infrequently exclude populations of patients with coexisting morbid conditions [16, 17], making isolation of the effects of normal aging difficult. Arterial carbon dioxide content, specifically in the absence of significant cardiopulmonary disease, has not been documented to undergo any significant age-related changes throughout life.

Changes in the Pulmonary Vasculature

Effects of aging on the pulmonary vasculature result from the age-dependent effects of vascular remodeling and the consequential reduction in pulmonary vascular compliance (or increase in pulmonary vascular resistance). The precise mechanisms responsible for the changes that occur in the pulmonary vascular as a normal result of aging are less well defined in the literature and limited to knowledge gained from investigation in animal models. Studies performed in human populations are limited to those investigating cardiovascular and pulmonary diseases instead of the normal effects of aging with few exceptions. Information derived from a population-based study, the Rochester Epidemiology Project, randomly sampled a general population of 2,042 patients, mean age of 63, and performed assessments of pulmonary artery systolic pressures by echocardiography and followed the changes in pulmonary pressures throughout a duration of 9 years [18]. The studies demonstrated an age-related increase in pulmonary artery pressures independent of elevated left-sided filling pressures. The presence of an increased systolic pulmonary artery systolic pressure was associated with a higher mortality independent of concurrent cardiopulmonary disease (i.e., heart failure, coronary artery disease, hypertension, and chronic obstructive pulmonary disease, and COPD). This finding is consistent with that of earlier studies investigating the normal effects of aging on the pulmonary vasculature [19].

Physiologic Manifestation of Normal Aging in the Lung on Diagnostic Testing

Review of Parameters Obtained in Pulmonary Function Testing

A variety of measurements are made with forced spirometry. The *forced vital capacity (FVC)* is the maximum amount of air exhaled with a maximal forced effort from total lung capacity (TLC). The *forced expiratory volume in 1 s (FEV$_1$)* is the maximal volume of air exhaled in the first second of the FVC maneuver. The *mean forced expiratory flow between 25 and 75% of the FVC (FEF$_{25-75\%}$)*, also termed the maximum mid-expiratory flow, provides a measurement of expiratory flow during the middle phase of the FVC maneuver and provides a measure of small airways obstruction albeit an inconsistent and non-specific one in individual patients [20, 21]. The *FEV$_1$/FVC ratio* can be calculated from the above data and, when low, serves as one of the defining features of obstructive airways disease. A *flow–volume loop* is also constructed as a part of forced spirometry and when analyzed visually can reinforce the presence of airflow obstruction, provide an early indication of airflow obstruction when the FEV$_1$/FVC ratio is not yet reduced, and provide information regarding extrathoracic (upper airway) obstruction. Graphic depictions of information garnered through forced spirometry in the form of a volume—time curve and flow–volume loop are illustrated in Fig. 20.3.

Absolute lung volumes that are measured with pulmonary function testing include *residual volume (RV)*, the volume of gas that remains in the lung after a complete expiration, *functional residual capacity (FRC)*, the volume of gas remaining in the lungs after exhaling a normal tidal breath, and *TLC*, the maximal amount of gas in the lungs after maximal inspiration (Fig. 20.4). Lung volumes are typically measured by either plethysmographic or gas dilution or washout methods. Body plethesymography is considered the optimal method as both ventilated and non-ventilated lung volumes are measured [22].

Changes in Forced Spirometry Associated with Normal Aging

FEV$_1$ and FVC increase into the third decade of life. Lung function then appears to plateau for some period of time until a slow decline in FEV$_1$ commences for the duration of the lifespan [4]. The exact timing of when this decline in lung function occurs in the absence of smoking and other environmental exposures is uncertain. Historically, this decline was thought to commence in the mid-20s, but more recent assessments which evaluate the effects of smoking and other exposures indicate that the plateau in lung function may persist until the mid-30s [23, 24]. The decrease in lung function accelerates with advanced aging with a steady increase in the annual rate of loss of FEV$_1$ [25].

According to the global initiative for obstructive lung disease (GOLD) criteria, a diagnosis of COPD is made when the FEV$_1$/FVC ratio is less than or equal to 0.70 [26]. This may, however, result in overdiagnosis of COPD. According to reference equations published exclusively in a population of healthy, adult, non-smokers from the Cardiovascular Health Study, the FEV$_1$/FVC ratio is normally below 0.70 in men 80 years and older and women 92 years and older [27]. Because of the risk of overdiagnosis, some have advocated that COPD be diagnosed, particularly in the elderly, based on age- and population-appropriate reference equations which identify a "lower limit of normal" for the FEV$_1$/FVC ratio to prevent misclassification of spirometric findings of normal aging as clinical COPD [28–30].

Changes in Lung Volumes Associated with Normal Aging

As outlined above, the elastic recoil pressure of the lung decreases with advanced age, while the chest wall creates increased elastic load. These two concurrent processes appear to counteract each other such that TLC is preserved throughout the normal aging process [31]. Loss of lung elastic recoil pressure combined with reduction in respiratory muscle function and performance results in increased RV in aged individuals. In fact, RV increases by up to 50% over the lifespan and is accompanied by a reduction of 75% in vital capacity (VC) [32]. Normal aging also results in individuals also breathing at higher lung volumes owing largely to the effects of decreased reduced lung parenchymal recoil pressure at lung volumes where the effects of poor chest wall compliance do not predominate resulting in increases in function residual capacity (FRC) [32]. Closing volume increases with normal aging probably due to loss of the

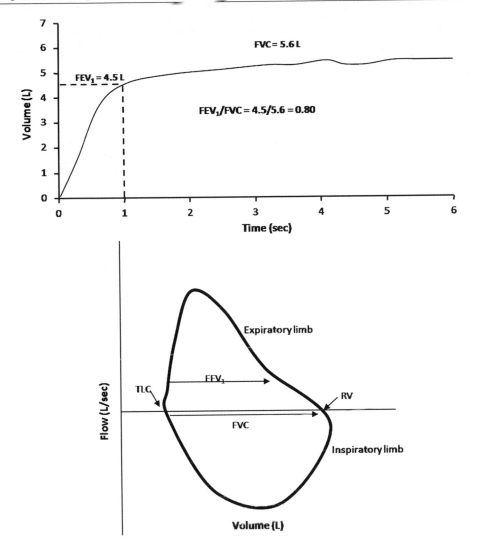

Fig. 20.3 Stereotypical volume–time curve (*top*) and flow–volume loop (*bottom*) in a normal subject. In the volume–time curve, approximately 80% of volume is expired in the first second resulting in a normal forced expiratory volume in 1 s (FEV_1)/FVC ratio of 0.80. The quality of the maneuver is documented by a volume plateau at the termination of the test after 6 s. After inspiration to total lung capacity (TLC), the expiratory limb of the flow–volume loop has a sharp increase in peak expiratory flow rate and then a smooth deceleration in flow over the entire expiration until complete at residual volume (RV). With normal aging, both the FEV_1 and FVC decrease, although, because of loss of elastic recoil pressure, the FEV_1 decrease may be greater than that of FVC. This results in a reduction in the FEV_1/FVC ratio with normal aging

alveolar support structure surrounding small airways. The increase in closing volume may partially explain the increase in alveolar-arterial oxygen gradient observed with normal aging which was described above: when closing volume exceeds FRC (which likely occurs between ages 45 and 65), tidal breathing occurs without significant portions of the lung contributing to ventilation. This results in ventilation–perfusion mismatch (in this case an increase in low V/Q lung zones), although direct measurement of ventilation–perfusion relationships has not documented that such increases are clinically significant [33].

Changes in Measurements of Gas Transfer Associated with Normal Aging

Several of the changes described earlier in this chapter result in reduction in alveolar gas transfer including loss of alveolar surface area, increased pulmonary vascular resistance and resultant reduction in capillary blood volume, and alterations of ventilation–perfusion relationships result in reduction in alveolar gas transfer. Diffusion capacity of carbon monoxide (D_LCO) as measured in pulmonary function tests, therefore, decreases with normal aging, although

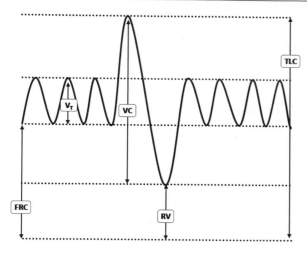

Fig. 20.4 Tidal volume (V_T): The volume air inhaled and exhaled with normal breathing; functional residual capacity (FRC): the volume of gas remaining in the lung after exhaling a normal tidal breath; residual volume (RV): the volume of gas that remains in the lung after a complete expiration; total lung capacity (TLC): the volume of gas in the lung after maximal inspiration; vital capacity (VC): the difference between TLC and RV, or the maximum volume of air available to be exchanged by the lung

Table 20.1 Manifestations of normal aging on pulmonary diagnostic testing

Vital capacity (VC)	Decreased
Forced expiratory volume in 1 s (FEV$_1$)	Decreased
FEV$_1$/VC	Decreased
Total lung capacity (TLC)	Unchanged
Functional residual capacity	Increased
Residual volume	Increased
Diffusion capacity of carbon monoxide (D$_L$CO)	Decreased
Maximal oxygen consumption (VO$_{2\,max}$)	Decreased
Alveolar-arterial (A–a) oxygen gradient	Increased
Pulmonary arterial systolic pressure	Increased

aging is not a significant contributor to pathologic reductions in this parameter.

Alterations in Exercise Capacity Associated with Normal Aging

Although there is no evidence that the normal changes in structure and function of the lung have a meaningful impact on normal daily activities, it is conceivable that during periods of increased physiologic demands (such as surgery), they may have a greater impact. The most precise measure available to determine exercise capacity is maximum oxygen consumption (VO$_{2\,max}$) although its measurement is heavily confounded by degree of fitness. Some attempts have been made to isolate these effects independent of aging. A study of individuals who were well-conditioned athletes all over the age of 62 determined performed VO$_{2\,max}$ measurements separated by 6 years. Consistent with the expected findings the participants did not have significant changes in TLC or D$_L$CO, but did have a reduction in FVC, FEV$_1$ and an increase in RV. VO$_{2\,max}$ was reduced by 11% over the 6-year period with greater reductions in those who were older at the baseline examination indicating that normal aging is associated, to some extent, with maximal exercise capacity [34]. The changes that occur with normal aging on diagnostic testing are summarized in Table 20.1.

Changes in Lung Host Defense Mechanisms Associated with Normal Aging and Vulnerability to Respiratory Infections

The risk of developing pulmonary infections is increased in elderly patients. The incidence of health care-associated pneumonia is higher in elderly populations and it increased in both institutionalized patients as well as those living at home. Alterations in immune function that occur with aging are likely contributors to this finding. The mortality associated with the development of pneumonia in patients of advanced age is also significantly higher than younger patients with rates approaching up to 40% [35]. There are multiple factors responsible for the higher mortality of pneumonia in the elderly including the absence of usual signs and symptoms resulting in a delay in diagnosis as well as the frequent presence of multiple comorbid conditions which complicate the presentation and management of these infections (i.e., swallowing dysfunction, depressed levels of alertness, and cardiac disease). In addition, there are changes in the immune response to infection that result diminished defense mechanisms against infection. While cellular mechanisms of immunity are not felt to be quantitatively affected by advanced age, it is thought that there is a qualitative defect in humoral defense mechanisms, particularly with respect to adaptive immunity, that likely play a role in creating greater susceptibility to infection [36]. Other factors that may contribute to the increased incidence of pneumonia in the elderly include but are not limited to frequent prior courses of antibiotics leading to the emergence of resistant pathogens, alterations in nutritional status, frequent use immunosuppressive therapies such as corticosteroids, and waning humoral and cell-mediated immunity to vaccinations to influenza and pneumococcal pneumonia. Postural and structural changes to the airways and contour of the chest, normally associated with aging, such as the aforementioned kyphosis, costovertebral and rib cartilage calcifications, and vertebral compression fractures also may disrupt effectiveness of cough and other bronchial clearance regimens.

References

1. Fletcher C, Peto R. The natural history of chronic airflow obstruction. Br Med J. 1977;1:1645–8.
2. Estenne M, Yernault JC, De Troyer A. Rib cage and diaphragm-abdomen compliance in humans: effects of age and posture. J Appl Physiol. 1985;59:1842–8.
3. Edge JR, Millard FJ, Reid L, Simon G. The radiographic appearances of the chest in persons of advanced age. Br J Radiol. 1964;37:769–74.
4. Janssens JP, Pache JC, Nicod LP. Physiological changes in respiratory function associated with ageing. Eur Respir J. 1999;13:197–205.
5. Polkey MI, Harris ML, Hughes PD, et al. The contractile properties of the elderly human diaphragm. Am J Respir Crit Care Med. 1997;155:1560–4.
6. Bassey EJ, Harries UJ. Normal values for handgrip strength in 920 men and women aged over 65 years, and longitudinal changes over 4 years in 620 survivors. Clin Sci (Lond). 1993;84:331–7.
7. Enright PL, Kronmal RA, Manolio TA, Schenker MB, Hyatt RE. Respiratory muscle strength in the elderly. Correlates and reference values. Cardiovascular Health Study Research Group. Am J Respir Crit Care Med. 1994;149:430–8.
8. Hautmann H, Hefele S, Schotten K, Huber RM. Maximal inspiratory mouth pressures (PIMAX) in healthy subjects–what is the lower limit of normal? Respir Med. 2000;94:689–93.
9. Arora NS, Rochester DF. Effect of body weight and muscularity on human diaphragm muscle mass, thickness, and area. J Appl Physiol. 1982;52:64–70.
10. Turner JM, Mead J, Wohl ME. Elasticity of human lungs in relation to age. J Appl Physiol. 1968;25:664–71.
11. Gillooly M, Lamb D. Airspace size in lungs of lifelong non-smokers: effect of age and sex. Thorax. 1993;48:39–43.
12. Pierce JA. Age related changes in the fibrous proteins of the lungs. Arch Environ Health. 1963;6:50–4.
13. Kurozumi M, Matsushita T, Hosokawa M, Takeda T. Age-related changes in lung structure and function in the senescence-accelerated mouse (SAM): SAM-P/1 as a new murine model of senile hyperinflation of lung. Am J Respir Crit Care Med. 1994;149:776–82.
14. Niewoehner DE, Kleinerman J. Morphologic basis of pulmonary resistance in the human lung and effects of aging. J Appl Physiol. 1974;36:412–8.
15. Wahba WM. Influence of aging on lung function–clinical significance of changes from age twenty. Anesth Analg. 1983;62:764–76.
16. Sorbini CA, Grassi V, Solinas E, Muiesan G. Arterial oxygen tension in relation to age in healthy subjects. Respiration. 1968;25:3–13.
17. Blom H, Mulder M, Verweij W. Arterial oxygen tension and saturation in hospital patients: effect of age and activity. Br Med J. 1988;297:720–1.
18. Lam CS, Borlaug BA, Kane GC, Enders FT, Rodeheffer RJ, Redfield MM. Age-associated increases in pulmonary artery systolic pressure in the general population. Circulation. 2009;119:2663–70.
19. Davidson Jr WR, Fee EC. Influence of aging on pulmonary hemodynamics in a population free of coronary artery disease. Am J Cardiol. 1990;65:1454–8.
20. Pellegrino R, Viegi G, Brusasco V, et al. Interpretative strategies for lung function tests. Eur Respir J. 2005;26:948–68.
21. Miller MR, Hankinson J, Brusasco V, et al. Standardisation of spirometry. Eur Respir J. 2005;26:319–38.
22. Wanger J, Clausen JL, Coates A, et al. Standardisation of the measurement of lung volumes. Eur Respir J. 2005;26:511–22.
23. Kerstjens HA, Rijcken B, Schouten JP, Postma DS. Decline of FEV1 by age and smoking status: facts, figures, and fallacies. Thorax. 1997;52:820–7.
24. Kalhan R, Arynchyn A, Colangelo LA, Dransfield MT, Gerald LB, Smith LJ. Lung function in young adults predicts airflow obstruction 20 years later. Am J Med. 2010;123:468.e1–7.
25. Burrows B, Lebowitz MD, Camilli AE, Knudson RJ. Longitudinal changes in forced expiratory volume in one second in adults. Methodologic considerations and findings in healthy nonsmokers. Am Rev Respir Dis. 1986;133:974–80.
26. Rabe KF, Hurd S, Anzueto A, et al. Global strategy for the diagnosis, management, and prevention of chronic obstructive pulmonary disease: GOLD executive summary. Am J Respir Crit Care Med. 2007;176:532–55.
27. Enright PL, Kronmal RA, Higgins M, Schenker M, Haponik EF. Spirometry reference values for women and men 65 to 85 years of age. Cardiovascular health study. Am Rev Respir Dis. 1993;147:125–33.
28. Schermer TRJ, Smeele IJM, Thoonen BPA, et al. Current clinical guideline definitions of airflow obstruction and COPD overdiagnosis in primary care. Eur Respir J. 2008;32:945–52.
29. Vaz Fragoso CA, Concato J, McAvay G, et al. The ratio of FEV1 to FVC as a basis for establishing chronic obstructive pulmonary disease. Am J Respir Crit Care Med. 2010;181:446–51.
30. Carlos AVF, John C, Gail M, et al. Defining chronic obstructive pulmonary disease in older persons. Respir Med. 2009;103:1468–76.
31. Janssens JP. Aging of the respiratory system: impact on pulmonary function tests and adaptation to exertion. Clin Chest Med. 2005;26:469–84, vi–vii.
32. Crapo RO. The aging lung. In: Mahler DA, editor. Pulmonary disease in the elderly patient. New York: Marcel Dekker; 1993. p. 1–21.
33. Cardus J, Burgos F, Diaz O, et al. Increase in pulmonary ventilation-perfusion inequality with age in healthy individuals. Am J Respir Crit Care Med. 1997;156:648–53.
34. McClaran SR, Babcock MA, Pegelow DF, Reddan WG, Dempsey JA. Longitudinal effects of aging on lung function at rest and exercise in healthy active fit elderly adults. J Appl Physiol. 1995;78:1957–68.
35. Loeb M, McGeer A, McArthur M, Walter S, Simor AE. Risk factors for pneumonia and other lower respiratory tract infections in elderly residents of long-term care facilities. Arch Intern Med. 1999;159:2058–64.
36. Kirkwood TB, Ritter MA. The interface between ageing and health in man. Age Ageing. 1997;26 Suppl 4:9–14.

Chapter 21
Cardiac Changes in the Elderly

Wilbert S. Aronow and William H. Frishman

Abstract Cardiovascular function in elderly persons is significantly affected by the aging process itself and by those acquired diseases of the cardiovascular system that are more prevalent with age. Some of the cardiovascular disorders that are more prevalent in elderly persons include hypertension, left ventricular hypertrophy, left atrial enlargement, abnormal LVEF, atrial fibrillation, CHF (especially with a normal LVEF), coronary artery disease, ischemic and thromboembolic stroke, peripheral arterial disease, extracranial carotid arterial disease, aortic stenosis, aortic regurgitation, mitral regurgitation, mitral annular calcium, hypertrophic cardiomyopathy, and pacemaker rhythm. These physiologic and pathologic changes of the aging cardiovascular system must be taken into consideration during the clinical assessment and management of elderly patients who need to undergo surgical procedures and general anesthesia.

Keywords Cardiovascular aging • Vascular stiffness • Left ventricular ejection fraction • Congestive heart failure • Atrial fibrillation • Coronary artery disease • Stroke • Peripheral arterial disease • Aortic valvular disease • Mitral valvular disease • Conduction defects

Age-related changes in the cardiovascular system, overt and occult cardiovascular disease, and reduced physical activity affect cardiovascular function in the elderly. With aging, there is a loss of myocytes in both the left and right ventricles with a progressive increase in myocyte cell volume per nucleus in both ventricles [1], and an inability to regenerate new myocytes [2]. There is also a progressive reduction in the number of pacemaker cells in the sinus node, with only 10% of the number of cells present at age 20 remaining at age 75 [3]. Wall thickening and dilatation are structural changes that occur within large elastic arteries during aging [4].

W.S. Aronow (✉)
New York College of Medicine, Macy Pavillion, Room 138,
Valhalla, NY 10595, USA
e-mail: wsaronow@aol.com

Afterload

Resistance to the ejection of blood by the left ventricle is called afterload. There are two components to afterload: peripheral vascular resistance and characteristic aortic impedance. Peripheral vascular resistance is the steady-state component and provides opposition to steady blood flow. Characteristic aortic impedance is the dynamic component and opposes pulsatile blood flow. Peripheral vascular resistance is measured by dividing the mean arterial pressure by the cardiac output; it is inversely proportional to the cross-sectional area of the peripheral vascular beds. Characteristic aortic impedance is measured as the time variation in mean arterial pressure/flow through the aorta; it is inversely proportional to the arterial compliance (the distensibility of the arterial wall). An indirect measurement of afterload is the pulse wave velocity, which measures the propagation speed of pressure waves traveling from proximal to distal arterial segments; it increases as arteries become less compliant.

With aging, the large elastic arteries become dilated with a reduction in compliance [5]. Progressive thickening of the aortic media and intima are associated with aortic enlargement [6]. There is an age-associated increase in arterial stiffness resulting from changes in the arterial media, such as thickening of the smooth muscle layers, increased fragmentation of elastin, an increase in the amount and characteristics of collagen, and increased calcification [7]. These structural changes are associated with a reduction in aortic distensibility due to increased aortic stiffness with an increase in pulse wave velocity [8]. The structural changes in the arterial wall are independent of coexisting atherosclerosis. Avolio et al. [8] showed an increase in pulse wave velocity with age in farmers from Guanzhou Province in southern China despite a low prevalence of atherosclerosis in this population. The age-associated increase in stiffness and decrease in distensibility of large elastic arteries are not found in distal arteries [9].

The increase in arterial wall thickening and decrease in endothelial function with aging [10] are associated with an increase in arterial stiffness and a decrease in compliance.

M.R. Katlic (ed.), *Cardiothoracic Surgery in the Elderly*, DOI 10.1007/978-1-4419-0892-6_21,
© Springer Science+Business Media, LLC 2011

Table 21.1 Age-associated structural changes in arterial media that increase vascular stiffness

Increased collagen content
Covalent cross-linking of collagen
Calcification
Decreased elastin content
Elastin fracture

Age-associated structural changes in the arterial media that increase vascular stiffness include increased collagen content, covalent cross-linking of the collagen, decreased elastin content, elastin fracture, and calcification (Table 21.1) [11, 12].

Impedance spectral patterns have shown an age-related increase in characteristic aortic impedance and peripheral vascular resistance [13]. The reduction in arterial compliance contributes more to the age-related increase in afterload than does the loss of peripheral vascular beds [13]. Peripheral vascular resistance was not age related in healthy persons screened for occult coronary artery disease in the Baltimore Longitudinal Study of Aging [14], but increased with age in persons not screened for occult coronary artery disease [15]. Arterial stiffening appearing as an increase in pulse wave velocity is associated with degeneration of the vascular media independent of atherosclerosis. Arterial stiffening causes earlier occurrence of wave reflection from peripheral sites to the ascending aorta during left ventricular ejection. Therefore, aortic and carotid phasic pressures increase to a greater magnitude at a later time during left ventricular ejection, causing an increase in systolic and pulse pressures and a delayed peak in the aortic pressure pulse contour.

Circulating levels of catecholamines increase with age, especially with stress, although β-adrenergic vasodilation of vascular smooth muscle decreases [16]. α-Adrenergic vasoconstriction of vascular smooth muscle does not change with age [17]. The impaired vasodilator response to β-adrenergic stimulation with age is most important during exercise and contributes to the increased afterload associated with aging.

Increased afterload causes an increase in blood pressure. With aging, there is an increase in systolic blood pressure and a widened pulse pressure. A slight decrease in diastolic blood pressure occurs after the sixth decade [18]. The increase in systolic blood pressure is due to interactions of aging, cardiovascular disease, and life style factors, such as dietary sodium intake, body weight, and level of physical activity. An age-associated increase in the index of aortic stiffening was not found in normotensive persons on a low sodium chloride diet [19]. The increase in carotid augmentation index (an index of aortic stiffening) in highly trained elderly men was half of that expected on the basis of age alone [20]. The prevalence of abnormal aortic stiffness increases steeply in the community

with advancing age, especially in the presence of diabetes mellitus and obesity [21].

As aortic compliance decreases with aging, the transfer of kinetic energy from the blood ejected during left ventricular systole to potential energy stored in the elasticity of the aortic wall decreased. Consequently, return of the potential energy stored in the elasticity of the aortic wall back to the kinetic energy of blood flow during diastole also decreased. Therefore, the left ventricle must eject its stroke volume into a less compliant aorta with greater pressure and force to achieve adequate cardiac output. The increased pulse wave velocity also causes the pressure in the aorta to increase and peak later during systole, contributing to the increased systolic blood pressure and widened pulse pressure.

Posterior left ventricular wall thickness increased with increasing age in normotensive men and women screened for occult coronary artery disease in the Baltimore Longitudinal Study of Aging [5]. Data from persons in this study suggested that the increase in left ventricular wall thickness associated with aging is mediated by an increase in systolic blood pressure [22]. Aging is also associated with an increase in the prevalence of hypertension and cardiovascular disease and, therefore, with the left ventricular hypertrophy seen by echocardiography.

Age-associated left ventricular hypertrophy is caused by an increase in the volume but not in the number of cardiac myocytes. Fibroblasts undergo hyperplasia, and collagen is deposited in the myocardial interstitium. Increased afterload results in an increase in left ventricular systolic stress and the addition of sarcomeres, in parallel, which causes increased left ventricular wall thickness with a normal or reduced left ventricular chamber size and an increased relative wall thickness.

In the Framingham Heart Study, echocardiographic left ventricular hypertrophy was observed in 33% of men and 49% of women older than 70 years [23]. In our elderly population, echocardiographic left ventricular hypertrophy was found in 226 of 554 men (41%) with a mean age of 80 and in 539 of 1,243 women (43%) with a mean age of 82 [24].

In our elderly population systolic or diastolic hypertension was present in 255 of 664 men (38%) with a mean age of 80 and in 651 of 1,488 women (44%) with a mean age of 82 [25]. In another study of our elderly population, systolic or diastolic hypertension occurred in 108 of 215 Blacks (50%) with a mean age of 81, in 411 of 1,140 Whites (36%) with a mean age of 82, and in 19 of 54 Hispanics (35%) with a mean age 81 [26]. Echocardiographically diagnosed left ventricular hypertrophy occurred in 66 of 92 hypertensive Blacks (72%), in 194 of 346 hypertensive Whites (56%), and in 8 of 15 hypertensive Hispanics (53%) [26]. However, it was observed in only 2 of our 88 elderly persons (2%) without hypertension or overt cardiac disease [27].

Regular aerobic endurance exercise attenuates age-related reductions in central arterial compliance and restores levels in previously sedentary healthy middle-aged and elderly men [28]. Regular aerobic endurance exercise also can prevent the age-associated loss in endothelium-dependent vasodilation and restore levels in previously sedentary middle-aged and elderly healthy men [29]. These are mechanisms by which regular aerobic endurance exercise contributes to a decreased risk of cardiovascular disease in the elderly [28, 29].

Preload

Preload is the filling volume of the left ventricle. Preload is determined by many factors that influence blood return to the heart and by the mechanical properties of the heart during diastolic filling of the left ventricle.

Resting left ventricular end-diastolic volume, measured by radionuclide ventriculography using multiple gated pool acquisition imaging or by echocardiography, is not age related in healthy persons, indicating that the resting preload does not change with age [5, 10, 14, 30]. Although resting preload does not change with age, left ventricular early diastolic filling decreases with age.

Passive filling of the left ventricle occurs during the rapid filling and diastasis phases of early diastole. With age, left ventricular stiffness increased, left ventricular compliance decreased, left ventricular wall thickness increased, left ventricular relaxation impaired, and left ventricular early diastolic filling decreased. This may result in hypotension if preload is reduced. An age-related increase in systolic blood pressure also reduces left ventricular early diastolic filling, leading to hypotension if preload is reduced. Left ventricular filling during early diastole decreased 50% from age 20 to 80 [5, 31, 32].

Despite the reduction in early diastolic filling of the left ventricle with age, preload is maintained because left atrial contraction becomes more vigorous to increase late diastolic filling of the left ventricle [5, 30–36]. Augmentation of late diastolic filling of the left ventricle prevents a decrease in left ventricular end-diastolic volume. The ratio of late diastolic Doppler peak transmitral velocity (peak atrial, or A wave, velocity) to early diastolic Doppler peak transmitral velocity (peak rapid filling, or E wave, velocity) increases from approximately 0.6 at 30 years of age to 1.2 at 70 years of age [37]. A reduction in the E/A wave ratio with age reflects a reduction in left ventricular compliance. An age-related increase in left atrial size resulting from increased wall stress due to increased left atrial pressure counteracts the effects of decreased left ventricular compliance with age.

In our older population, 619 of 1,797 older persons (34%) had echocardiographic left atrial enlargement [24].

Age was the most powerful independent variable for left ventricular filling in healthy persons in the Framingham Heart Study [38]. Age was inversely associated with the E wave (peak early diastolic filling velocity) and was directly associated with the A wave (peak late diastolic filling velocity). Other independent variables that contribute to a lesser degree to left ventricular filling were heart rate, PR interval measured from the electrocardiogram (ECG), gender, left ventricular systolic function, and systolic blood pressure. Increasing the heart rate reduces peak early diastolic filling and increases peak late diastolic filling velocity. The PR interval on the ECG is inversely associated with peak early diastolic filling velocity. Women have slightly higher peak early diastolic filling velocities than men. Left ventricular systolic function is directly associated with peak early diastolic filling velocity. Increasing the systolic blood pressure increases the peak late diastolic filling velocity [38, 39]. Age-associated abnormalities in Doppler measures of myocardial filling and relaxation are only partially minimized by lifelong endurance training [40].

A decrease in preload is not well tolerated in elderly persons. Reduced intravascular volume, reduced venous return to the heart, vasodilation by drugs or disease states, and use of drugs such as nitrates or diuretics reduce preload and may cause reduced cardiac output and hypotension in older persons. Decreased compliance of the left ventricle and decreased cardiac and vascular responsiveness to β-adrenergic stimulation [41] cause elderly persons to be highly dependent on the Frank–Starling mechanism to increase cardiac output. Elderly persons are more susceptible to developing orthostatic hypotension [42–44]. Impaired baroreceptor reflex sensitivity [45], decreased cardiac responsiveness to β-adrenergic stimulation [41], loss of arterial compliance, decreased venous return due to increased venous distensibility, impaired compensatory mechanisms for maintenance of fluid volume and electrolyte balance, increased incidence of common precipitating diseases and disorders, and the use of multiple drugs contribute to orthostatic hypotension. Older persons are also more susceptible to developing postprandial hypotension [41–44].

Marked reductions in postprandial systolic blood pressure in elderly persons may predispose them to symptomatic hypotension and to falls, syncope, angina pectoris, and transient cerebral ischemic attacks [46–50]. At 29-month follow-up, a marked decrease in postprandial systolic blood pressure in elderly persons was associated with an increased incidence of falls, syncope, new coronary events, new stroke, and total mortality [50]. Whether therapeutic interventions to prevent a marked reduction in postprandial systolic blood pressure in elderly persons can reduce the incidence of falls, syncope, new coronary events, new stroke, and total mortality at long-term follow-up must be investigated.

Because left atrial contraction can contribute up to 50% of left ventricular filling in a poorly compliant left ventricle, the development of atrial fibrillation may result in a marked reduction in cardiac output because of loss of the left atrial contribution to left ventricular late diastolic filling. A rapid ventricular rate associated with atrial fibrillation also reduces the time for diastolic filling of the left ventricle, resulting in a marked decrease in cardiac output.

The incidence of atrial fibrillation also increased with age [51, 52]. In 2,101 elderly persons in a nursing home, the prevalence of chronic atrial fibrillation was 5% in persons aged 60–70, 13–14% in persons aged 71–90, and 22% in persons 91 years and older [52]. Atrial fibrillation in elderly persons is associated with an increased incidence of new thromboembolic stroke [51, 52] and new coronary events [53, 54].

Cardiac output increases during exercise in healthy elderly persons owing to an increase in venous return to the heart, increasing the diastolic filling of the left ventricle and allowing an increased stroke volume to be ejected during exercise [55]. This is the Frank–Starling mechanism. The maximal heart rate response to exercise decreased with age in healthy persons in the Baltimore Longitudinal Study of Aging [14], whereas exercise stroke volume increased with age to maintain the exercise cardiac output [14]. The increase in exercise stroke volume resulted from an increase in left ventricular end-diastolic volume (preload) via the Frank–Starling mechanism. In contrast, healthy nonelderly persons achieved an increase in exercise cardiac output primarily by an increase in heart rate. Exercise stroke volume increased in nonelderly healthy persons owing to a slight increase in the left ventricular end-diastolic volume and a large decrease in the left ventricular end-systolic volume. The exercise-induced increase in heart rate and reduction in left ventricular end-systolic volume in nonelderly persons are probably mediated by β-adrenergic stimulation. The increase in left ventricular end-diastolic volume during exercise in healthy older persons suggests that the age-associated reduction in resting early diastolic filling of the left ventricle does not persist during exercise.

Contractility

The intrinsic ability of the heart to generate force does not change with age in healthy persons, although the duration of contraction and relaxation is prolonged in senescent animals [56, 57]. Prolongation of the left ventricular ejection time [58] and the preejection period [59] with age in healthy persons indicates that prolongation of contraction occurs

with age. Prolongation of the duration of contraction in senescent animals is associated with increased muscle stiffness and prolongation of the action potential duration [60]. These age-related changes are associated with cellular changes in the excitation–contraction coupling mechanism [61] and are an adaptive response to preserve contractile function in response to an age-induced increase in afterload.

There is no reduction in resting left ventricular ejection fraction (LVEF) or circumferential fiber shortening in old persons with no evidence of heart disease [5, 14, 30, 62, 63]. However, systolic function with exercise decreases with age. In the Baltimore Longitudinal Study of Aging, old persons showed less exercise-induced increase in LVEF than did younger persons because of an age-related increase in left ventricular end-systolic volume [14]. However, the absolute values of LVEF at maximal exercise in healthy old persons rarely decrease from basal values [14]. Age-associated reductions in maximal heart rate and left ventricular contractility during maximal exercise are manifestations of decreased β-adrenergic responsiveness, with aging partially offset by exercise-induced dilation of the left ventricle [64].

Diastolic Function

Aging is associated with prolongation of the isovolumic relaxation time, reduced early diastolic filling of the left ventricle, and augmented late diastolic filling of the left ventricle [31, 34, 37]. Normal aging changes that affect the left ventricular diastolic function include increased systolic blood pressure, increased left ventricular wall thickness, decreased left ventricular early diastolic filling, prolonged left ventricular diastolic relaxation, increased left atrial size, and increased left ventricular late diastolic filling [65].

With aging occurs slowing of the rate at which calcium is sequestered by the sarcoplasmic reticulum following myocardial excitation, which causes reduced relaxation of the left ventricle [52, 61, 66]. Accumulation of calcium at the onset of diastole may reduce left ventricular diastolic relaxation and early diastolic filling [67]. Reduced oxidative phosphorylation and cumulative mitochondrial peroxidation occurring with age may also reduce the left ventricular diastolic function [68, 69].

Increased left ventricular stiffness with age due to increased interstitial fibrosis and cross-linking of collagen in the heart impairs left ventricular diastolic relaxation and filling [1, 70–72]. Myocardial ischemia in the absence of coronary artery disease caused by decreases in capillary density and coronary reserve with age may further decrease left ventricular diastolic function in elderly persons [1, 73].

In addition to a reduction in left ventricular diastolic relaxation and early diastolic filling caused by age, elderly persons are more likely to have left ventricular diastolic dysfunction because they have an increased prevalence of hypertension, myocardial ischemia due to coronary artery disease, and left ventricular hypertrophy due to hypertension, coronary artery disease, valvular aortic stenosis, hypertrophic cardiomyopathy, and other cardiac disorders. The increased stiffness of the left ventricle and prolonged left ventricular relaxation time decrease left ventricular early diastolic filling and cause higher left ventricular end-diastolic pressures at rest and during exercise in elderly persons [74, 75].

In patients with congestive heart failure (CHF) associated with left ventricular systolic dysfunction, the LVEF is less than 50%. There is a reduced amount of myocardial fiber shortening, the stroke volume is reduced, the left ventricle is dilated, and the patient is symptomatic.

With CHF due to left ventricular diastolic dysfunction with normal left ventricular systolic function, the LVEF is normal. Kitzman et al. [76] demonstrated that during exercise, persons with CHF and normal left ventricular systolic function but abnormal left ventricular diastolic function were unable to increase stroke volume normally, even in the presence of increased left ventricular filling pressure. Myocardial hypertrophy, ischemia, or fibrosis causes slow or incomplete left ventricular filling at normal left atrial pressures. The left atrial pressure increases to augment left ventricular filling, resulting in pulmonary and systemic venous congestion. The development of atrial fibrillation may also cause a reduction in cardiac output and the development of pulmonary and systemic venous congestion because of loss of the left atrial contribution to left ventricular late diastolic filling and decreased diastolic filling time due to a rapid ventricular rate.

In a prospective study of 2,535 persons older than 60 years (mean 82 years), CHF developed in 677 (27%) [77]. In a prospective study of 1,160 men and 2,464 women older than 60 years, with a mean age of 81, CHF developed in 29% of elderly men and in 26% of elderly women [78]. Elderly persons are more likely than nonelderly persons to develop CHF because of abnormal left ventricular diastolic dysfunction with normal left ventricular systolic function. Table 21.2 shows that the prevalence of normal LVEF in older persons with CHF ranges from 34 to 52% [77, 79–84]. The prevalence of normal LVEF with CHF is also higher in elderly women than in elderly men [77, 80–84].

A normal LVEF was present in older persons with CHF in 44% of 55 African-American men versus 58% of 110 African-American women, in 46% of 24 Hispanic men versus 56% of 34 Hispanic women, in 35% of 148 White men versus 57% of 303 White women, and in 38% of 227 older men versus 57% of 447 older women [84]. Table 21.3 shows

Table 21.2 Prevalence of normal left ventricular ejection fraction (LVEF) in elderly patients with congestive heart failure (CHF)

Study	Results for patients with CHF and normal LVEF
Wong et al. [79]	41% of 54 Persons, mean age 80
Aronow et al. [80]	47% of 247 Persons, mean age 82
Cardiovascular Health Study [81]	59% of 186 Persons, mean age 73
Framingham Heart Study [82]	51% of 73 Persons, mean age 73
Pernenkil et al. [83]	34% of 501 Persons, mean age 81
Aronow et al. [77]	50% of 572 Persons, mean age 82
Aronow et al. [84]	51% of 674 Persons, mean age 81

Source: Reprinted with permission from Aronow WS, Frishman WH. Physiologic changes in cardiac function with aging. In: Rosenthal RE, Katlic MR, Zenilman ME, editors. Principles and practice of geriatric surgery. 2nd edition. New York: Springer; 2010

Table 21.3 Association of CHF with normal LVEF with gender and age in 572 elderly patients

Age (years)	Normal LVEF
60–69	22% of 18 Men and 37% of 38 women
70–79	33% of 54 Men and 44% of 79 women
80–89	41% of 86 Men and 59% of 219 women
≥90	47% of 19 Men and 73% of 59 women
All ages	37% of 177 Men and 56% of 395 women with CHF

Source: Data from Aronow et al. [77]

the prevalence of a normal LVEF in 572 older persons with CHF in men and women of different age groups [77]. In the community, advancing age and female gender are associated with increases in vascular and ventricular systolic and diastolic stiffness even in the absence of cardiovascular disease [85]. This contributes to the increased prevalence of CHF with a normal LVEF in elderly persons, especially in elderly women.

LVEF should be measured in all patients with CHF in order that appropriate therapy may be given [86–90]. For example, digoxin should not be used to treat persons with CHF and normal LVEF if sinus rhythm is present [65, 91–95]. By increasing contractility through increasing intracellular calcium ion concentration, digoxin may increase left ventricular stiffness, increasing left ventricular filling pressure, and adversely affecting CHF due to left ventricular diastolic dysfunction. Patients with CHF due to abnormal LVEF tolerate higher doses of diuretics than do patients with CHF and normal LVEF. Patients with CHF due to left ventricular diastolic dysfunction with normal LVEF need high left ventricular filling pressures to maintain an adequate stroke volume and cardiac output and cannot tolerate intravascular depletion. These patients should be treated with a low salt diet with cautious use of diuretics, rather than with large doses of diuretics. Patients with abnormal LVEF should not be treated with calcium channel blockers [96, 97].

Cardiovascular Response to Exercise

The maximal oxygen consumption (VO$_2$max) is the best overall measurement of cardiovascular fitness [98]. VO$_2$max is the product of cardiac output and systemic arteriovenous oxygen difference at peak exercise. Maximal cardiac output – the heart rate multiplied by the stroke volume at peak exercise – is a more direct measurement of cardiovascular reserve than is VO$_2$max [98]. VO$_2$max decreased with age [99, 100]. The degree of decrease of VO$_2$max with age is affected by physical conditioning, subclinical coronary artery disease, smoking, and body weight. Table 21.4 lists the cardiovascular responses to exercise in healthy elderly persons and clinical implications.

In the Baltimore Longitudinal Study of Aging, older male athletes had a higher peak exercise VO$_2$max than older sedentary men [101]. The greater peak exercise VO$_2$max in older male athletes than in older sedentary men was achieved by a higher cardiac index and a greater systemic arteriovenous oxygen difference. The higher peak exercise cardiac index in older male athletes than in older sedentary men was due to a higher stroke volume index with similar maximal heart rates. Long-term endurance training also is associated with enhanced ventricular diastolic filling indices [102]. Older age is associated with a decreased exercise efficiency and an increase in the oxygen cost of exercise, which contributes to a decreased exercise capacity. These age-related changes are reversed with exercise training [103].

A decrease in maximal systemic arteriovenous oxygen difference occurs with age [104]. The decrease in muscle mass with age may play a major role in the reduction in systemic arteriovenous oxygen difference at peak exercise and in VO$_2$max [105].

Fleg et al. [106] also investigated the effect of age on peak upright cycle exercise in healthy sedentary men and women aged 22–86 in the Baltimore Longitudinal Study of Aging. Peak cycle work rate was reduced with age in both men and women but was greater in men than in women at any age. Both men and women had peak exercise reductions in heart rate, cardiac index, and LVEF and increases in the left ventricular end-diastolic volume index and end-systolic volume index with age. Peak exercise stroke volume index did not vary with age in men or women. The exercise-induced reduction in left ventricular end-systolic volume index and the increases in cardiac index, stroke volume index, and LVEF from rest were greater in elderly men than in elderly women.

Age-Related Changes in Cardiovascular Function

Table 21.5 lists some age-related changes in cardiovascular function in healthy elderly persons and clinical implications. Contractility at rest does not change with age, but the duration of left ventricular contraction and relaxation is prolonged. Age-associated decreases in maximal heart rate and left ventricular contractility during maximal exercise are manifestations of reduced β-adrenergic responsiveness with age partially offset by exercise-induced dilation of the left ventricle.

Decreased arterial compliance contributes more to the age-related increase in afterload than does the loss of peripheral vascular beds. The impaired vasodilator response to β-adrenergic stimulation with age is most important during exercise and contributes to the increased afterload associated with age. Resting preload does not change with age. Left ventricular early diastolic filling decreased with age. Augmentation of late diastolic filling of the left ventricle prevents a reduction in left ventricular end-diastolic volume with age. The maximal heart rate response to exercise decreased with age. Exercise stroke volume increased with age to maintain the exercise cardiac output, resulting from an increase in preload by the Frank–Starling mechanism.

Table 21.4 Cardiovascular responses to exercise in healthy elderly persons

Maximal heart rate decreased with age

Exercise stroke volume increased with age to maintain cardiac output

Increased exercise stroke volume with age results primarily from increase in left ventricular end-diastolic volume by Frank–Starling mechanism

Decrease in muscle mass with age plays role in age-associated decreases in systemic arteriovenous oxygen difference and in VO$_2$max at peak exercise

Left ventricular end-diastolic and end-systolic volumes increased during peak exercise with age

Peak exercise LVEF reduced with age

Exercise-induced decrease in the left ventricular end-systolic volume index and increases in the cardiac index, stroke volume index, and LVEF from rest are greater in elderly men than in elderly women

Table 21.5 Some age-related changes in cardiovascular function in healthy elderly persons

Contractility at rest does not change with age

Duration of left ventricular contraction and relaxation prolonged with age

Decrease in arterial compliance contributes more to age-related increase in afterload than does loss of peripheral vascular beds

Resting preload does not change with age

Left ventricular early diastolic filling decreased with age

Augmentation of late diastolic filling of the left ventricle prevents a reduction in left ventricular end-diastolic volume with age

Cardiovascular responses to exercise with age are noted in Table 21.4

Age-associated reductions in maximal heart rate and left ventricular contractility during maximal exercise are manifestations of decreased β-adrenergic responsiveness with age partially offset by exercise-induced dilation of the left ventricle

Aging selectively impairs endothelium-dependent function

VO$_2$max and the systemic arteriovenous oxygen difference at peak exercise decreased with age. Aging also selectively impairs endothelium-dependent function [107].

In addition to age-related changes in cardiovascular function and deconditioning due to a sedentary life style, elderly persons also have a higher prevalence and incidence of cardiovascular disorders that impair cardiovascular performance than do nonelderly persons. Elderly persons are more likely than nonelderly persons to develop CHF secondary to abnormal left ventricular diastolic dysfunction with normal left ventricular systolic function. There is also an age-related increase in pulmonary artery systolic pressure [108].

Treatment of Congestive Heart Failure

The LVEF should be measured in all persons with CHF in order for appropriate therapy to be given [86–90]. For example, digoxin should not be used to treat persons with CHF and normal LVEF if a sinus rhythm is present [65, 91–95]. Large doses of diuretics and nitrates should also be used cautiously in persons with CHF and a normal LVEF [97].

Calcium channel blockers such as diltiazem, nifedipine, and verapamil exacerbate CHF in persons with CHF associated with abnormal LVEF [109]. Diltiazem increased mortality in patients with pulmonary congestion associated with abnormal LVEF after myocardial infarction [110]. The Multicenter Diltiazem Postinfarction Trial showed, in persons with a LVEF less than 40%, that late CHF at follow-up increased in patients randomized to diltiazem (21%) versus those randomized to placebo (12%) [111]. Prospective studies have demonstrated that the vasoselective calcium channel blockers amlodipine [112] and felodipine [113] did not significantly affect survival compared with placebo in

patients with CHF associated with abnormal LVEF. There was a significantly higher incidence of pulmonary edema in the persons treated with amlodipine (15%) than in those treated with placebo (10%) [112]. The American College of Cardiology Foundation (ACCF)/American Heart Association (AHA) guidelines recommend that calcium channel blockers should not be given to persons with CHF associated with abnormal LVEF [96].

Abnormal Left Ventricular Ejection Fraction

Table 21.6 shows the ACCF/AHA Class I recommendations for treating patients with current or prior symptoms of CHF with reduced LVEF [96]. Elderly persons with CHF associated with abnormal LVEF should be treated with a low sodium diet and with diuretics plus an angiotensin-converting enzyme (ACE) inhibitor [114, 115] plus a β-blocker such as metoprolol CR/XL [116], carvedilol [117], bisoprolol [118], or nebivolol [119]. An angiotensin receptor blocker should be used if the patient is intolerant to an ACE inhibitor because of cough or angioneurotic edema [120]. Regular physical activity such as walking should be encouraged in patients with mild to moderate HF to improve functional status and to decrease symptoms. Patients with CHF who are dyspneic at rest at a low work level may benefit from a formal cardiac rehabilitation program [120].

An implantable cardioverter-defibrillator and cardiac resynchronization therapy should be used according to ACC/AHA guidelines [96, 121–123]. Statins should also be used in these patients to reduce appropriate cardioverter-defibrillator shocks and mortality [124, 125]. An aldosterone antagonist such as spironolactone [126] or eplerenone [127] should be used according to ACC/AHA guidelines [96].

Table 21.6 Class I recommendations for treating patients with current or prior symptoms of heart failure with reduced LVEF

Treat underlying and precipitating causes of heart failure

Use diuretics and salt restriction in persons with fluid retention

Use angiotensin-converting enzyme (ACE) inhibitors

Use β-blockers

Use angiotensin II receptor blockers if intolerant to ACE inhibitors because of cough or angioneurotic edema

Avoid or withdraw nonsteroidal anti-inflammatory drugs, most antiarrhythmic drugs, and calcium channel blockers

Recommend exercise training

Implant cardioverter-defibrillator in persons with a history of cardiac arrest, ventricular fibrillation, or hemodynamically unstable ventricular tachycardia

Implant cardioverter-defibrillator in persons with ischemic heart disease ≥40 days post myocardial infarction or nonischemic cardiomyopathy, a LVEF ≥30%, New York Heart Association Class II or III symptoms on optimal medical therapy, and an expectation of survival of ≥1 year

Use cardiac resynchronization therapy in persons with a LVEF ≥35%, New York Heart Association Class III or IV symptoms despite optimal therapy, and a QRS duration >120 ms with or without a cardioverter-defibrillator

Add an aldosterone antagonist in selected patients with moderately severe to severe symptoms of heart failure who can be carefully monitored for renal function and potassium concentration (serum creatinine should be ≥2.5 mg/dL in men and ≥2.0 mg/dL in women; serum potassium should be <5.0 mEq/L)

Use hydralazine plus nitrates in patients self-described as African-Americans with moderate to severe symptoms on optimal therapy with ACE inhibitors, β-blockers, and diuretics

Source: Adapted from Jessup et al. [96], Copyright Elsevier 2009, with permission from the American College of Cardiology

Table 21.7 shows the ACC/AHA Class IIa recommendations for treating patients with current or prior symptoms of CHF with reduced LVEF [96]. Isosorbide dinitrate plus hydralazine was very effective in treating Blacks with CHF in the African-American Heart failure trial [128, 129] and is now recommend in Blacks with a Class I indication as stated in Table 21.6. The serum digoxin level should be maintained between 0.5 and 0.8 ng/mL to avoid an increase in mortality [97, 130, 131].

Normal Left Ventricular Ejection Fraction

Table 21.8 shows the therapy for elderly persons with CHF associated with a normal LVEF. β-Blockers [119, 132], ACE inhibitors [133, 134], and angiotensin receptor blockers [135] are efficacious in the treatment of these patients.

In elderly persons with CHF associated with a normal LVEF, pulmonary congestion is reduced by a low sodium diet, diuretics, and nitrates. Sinus rhythm is maintained to increase the left ventricular filling time. The ventricular rate is slowed below 90 beats/min by a β-blocker to increase left ventricular filling time. Myocardial ischemia should be decreased and is best achieved by giving a β-blocker. Elevated systolic blood pressure decreased by diuretics and an ACE inhibitor. The left ventricular mass is reduced by an ACE inhibitor. Left ventricular relaxation should be improved by ACE inhibitors or β-blockers.

Cardiovascular Disease

In addition to age-related changes in cardiovascular function and deconditioning due to a sedentary life style, old persons also have a higher prevalence and incidence of cardiovascular disorders, which impair cardiovascular performance, than nonelderly persons. Table 21.9 lists the prevalence of some cardiovascular disorders in an elderly population in a long-term health care facility [78, 136, 137].

Aortic Valve Disease

Valvular aortic stenosis in elderly persons is usually due to stiffening, scarring, and calcification of aortic valve leaflets.

Table 21.7 Class IIa recommendations for treating persons with current or prior symptoms of heart failure with decreased LVEF

Angiotensin II receptor blockers may be used instead of ACE inhibitors if patients are already taking them for other reasons

Hydralazine plus nitrates may be used if symptoms of heart failure persist despite ACE inhibitors and β-blockers

Implant cardioverter-defibrillator in patients with LVEF of 30–35% of any origin with New York Heart Association Class II or III symptoms on optimal medical therapy with a life expectancy of >1 year

Digoxin can be used in patients with persistent symptoms to reduce hospitalization for heart failure

Source: Adapted from Jessup et al. [96], Copyright Elsevier 2009, with permission from the American College of Cardiology

Table 21.8 Therapy of patients with heart failure and normal LVEF

Treat underlying and precipitating causes of heart failure

Avoid use of inappropriate drugs such as nonsteroidal anti-inflammatory drugs

Treat hypertension, especially systolic hypertension, hyperlipidemia, myocardial ischemia, and anemia

Treat with cautious use of diuretics

Treat with β-blockers

Treat with ACE inhibitor or angiotensin receptor blocker if patient cannot tolerate ACE inhibitor because of cough, angioneurotic edema, rash, or altered taste sensation

Add isosorbide dinitrate plus hydralazine if heart failure persists

Avoid digoxin if sinus rhythm is present

Exercise training as an adjunctive approach to improve clinical status in ambulatory patients

Control ventricular rate in patients with atrial fibrillation

Source: Data from Hunt SA, Abraham WT, Feldman AM, et al. ACC/AHA 2005 guideline update for the diagnosis and management of chronic heart failure in the adult-summary article. J Am Coll Cardiol. 2005;46:1116–43

Table 21.9 Prevalence of cardiovascular disorders in elderly persons in a long-term health care facility

Cardiovascular disorder	Mean age (years)	Prevalence Number	%
Coronary artery disease [78]	81	1,521/3,624	42
Thromboembolic stroke [78]	81	1,131/3,624	31
Peripheral arterial disease [78]	81	1,011/3,624	28
40–100% Extracranial carotid arterial disease [136]	81	281/1,846	19
Congestive heart failure [78]	81	978/3,624	27
Hypertension [78]	81	2,136/3,624	59
Aortic stenosis [137]	81	463/2,805	17
Mitral annular calcium [137]	81	1,321/2,805	47
≥1+ Mitral regurgitation [137]	81	928/2,805	33
≥1+ Aortic regurgitation [137]	81	824/2,805	29
Rheumatic mitral stenosis [137]	81	37/2,805	1
Hypertrophic cardiomyopathy [137]	81	108/2,805	4
Idiopathic dilated cardiomyopathy [137]	81	29/2,805	1
Atrial fibrillation [78]	81	495/3,624	14
Pacemaker rhythm [78]	81	186/3,624	5
Abnormal left ventricular ejection fraction [137]	81	687/2,805	24
Left ventricular hypertrophy [137]	81	1,224/2,805	44
Left atrial enlargement [137]	81	987/2,805	35

Source: Reprinted with permission from Aronow WS, Frishman WH. Physiologic changes in cardiac function with aging. In: Rosenthal RE, Katlic MR, Zenilman ME, editors. Principles and practice of geriatric surgery. 2nd edition. New York: Springer; 2010

Calcific deposits in the aortic valve are common and may lead to valvular aortic stenosis [24, 138–140]. Calcific deposits in the aortic valve were present in 22 of 40 necropsied patients (55%) aged 90–103 [139]. Aortic cuspal calcium was present in 295 of 752 men (36%), with a mean age of 80, and in 672 of 1,663 women (40%), with a mean age of 82 [140].

Calcific valvular aortic stenosis was present at autopsy in 18% of 366 octogenarians [141]. Valvular aortic stenosis was diagnosed by continuous-wave Doppler echocardiography in 463 of 2,805 old persons (17%) with a mean age of 81 [78]. Severe aortic stenosis was present in 2% of these 2,805 old persons [78]. Severe aortic stenosis was also diagnosed in 3% of 501 persons aged 75–86 in the Helsinki Ageing Study [142].

Aortic valve calcium, mitral annular calcium, and coronary artery disease in older persons have similar predisposing factors for atherosclerosis [140, 142–148]. Elderly persons with extracranial carotid arterial disease [143] and with peripheral arterial disease [144] have an increased prevalence of aortic stenosis. Older patients with aortic stenosis [149, 150] and valvular aortic sclerosis [151, 152] have an increased incidence of new coronary events.

The prevalence of aortic regurgitation also increases with age [24, 153, 154]. Aortic regurgitation was diagnosed by pulsed Doppler recordings of the aortic valve in 526 of 1,797 elderly persons (29%) with a mean age of 81 [78]. Severe or moderate aortic regurgitation was diagnosed by pulsed Doppler recordings of the aortic valve in 74 of 450 elderly persons with a mean age of 82 [155]. Margonato et al. [153] linked the increased prevalence of aortic regurgitation with age to aortic valve thickening.

Mitral Valvular Disease

Two degenerative aging processes – mitral annular calcification and mucoid (or myxomatous) degeneration of the mitral valve leaflets and chordae tendineae – can cause significant mitral valvular dysfunction [156–158]. Mitral annular calcification was diagnosed by two-dimensional echocardiography in 36% of 924 elderly men and in 52% of 1,881 elderly women, with a mean age of 81 [78]. Mitral annular calcium was present in 11 of 57 persons (19%) 62–70 years of age, in 53 of 158 persons (34%) 71–80 years of age, in 190 of 301 persons (63%) 81–90 years of age, in 75 of 85 persons (88%) 91–100 years of age, and in 3 of 3 persons (100%) 101–103 years of age [159].

Breakdown of lipid deposits on the ventricular surface of the posterior mitral leaflet at or below the mitral annulus and on the aortic surfaces of the aortic valve cusps is probably responsible for the calcification [160]. Elderly men and women with mitral annular calcium have a higher prevalence of coronary artery disease [161–163], peripheral arterial disease [163, 164], extracranial carotid arterial disease [163, 165, 166], and aortic atherosclerotic disease [163] than elderly men and women without mitral annular calcium.

Conduction Defects

The increased prevalence of conduction defects in elderly persons is due to age-related degeneration of the conduction system and the development of cardiovascular disease. Aging is associated with regional conduction slowing, anatomically determined conduction delay at the crista, and structural changes including areas of low voltage [167]. Impairment of sinus node function and an increase in atrial refractoriness occur with aging, predisposing to atrial fibrillation [167]. Table 21.10 lists the prevalence of conduction defects in 1,153 elderly persons, with a mean age of 82 [168]. At 45-month follow-up, elderly persons with second-degree atrioventricular block, left bundle branch block, intraventricular conduction defect, and pacer rhythm had an increased incidence of new coronary events [168]. At 45-month follow-up, elderly persons with first-degree atrioventricular block, left anterior fascicular block, or right bundle branch block did not have an increased incidence of new coronary events [168].

Conclusions

Cardiovascular function in elderly persons is significantly affected by the aging process itself and by those acquired diseases of the cardiovascular system that are more prevalent with age. These physiologic and pathologic changes of the aging cardiovascular system must be taken into consideration during the clinical assessment and management of elderly patients who need to undergo surgical procedures and general anesthesia.

Table 21.10 Prevalence of conduction defects in 1,153 elderly persons

Defect	Prevalence (%)
First-degree atrioventricular block	6
Left anterior fascicular block	8
Right bundle branch block	10
Left bundle branch block	4
Intraventricular conduction defect	3
Second-degree atrioventricular block	1
Pacemaker rhythm	4

Source: Adapted with permission from Aronow [168], with permission from S. Karger AG, Basel

References

1. Olivetti G, Melissari M, Capasso JM, Anversa P. Cardiomyopathy of the aging human heart: myocyte loss and reactive cellular hypertrophy. Circ Res. 1991;68:1560–8.
2. Bolli R, Anversa P. Stem cells and cardiac aging. In: Leri A, Anversa P, Frishman WH, editors. Cardiovascular regeneration and stem cell therapy. Oxford, UK: Blackwell/Futura; 2007. p. 171–81.
3. Davies MJ. The pathological basis of arrhythmias. Geriatr Cardiovasc Med. 1988;1:181–3.
4. Lakatta EG. Cardiovascular regulatory mechanisms in advanced age. Physiol Rev. 1993;73:13.
5. Gerstenblith G, Fredericksen J, Yin FCP, Fortuin NJ, Lakatta EG, Weisfeldt ML, et al. Echocardiographic assessment of a normal adult aging population. Circulation. 1977;56:273–8.
6. Safar M. Aging and its effects on the cardiovascular system. Drugs. 1990;39 Suppl 1:1–8.
7. Yin FCP. The aging vasculature and its effects on the heart. In: Weisfeldt ML, editor. The aging heart: its function and response to stress. New York: Raven; 1980. p. 137–214.
8. Avolio AP, Fa-Quan D, Wei-Qiang L, et al. Effects of aging on arterial distensibility in populations with high and low prevalence of hypertension: comparison between urban and rural communities in China. Circulation. 1985;71:202–10.
9. Boutouyrie P, Laurent S, Benetos A, Girerd XJ, Hoeks AP, Safar ME. Opposing effects of ageing on distal and proximal large arteries in hypertensives. J Hypertens. 1992;10:587–91.
10. Celermajer DS, Sorenson KE, Spiegelhalter DJ, Georgakopoulos D, Robinson J, Deanfield JE. Aging is associated with endothelial dysfunction in healthy men years before the age-related decline in women. J Am Coll Cardiol. 1994;24:471–6.
11. Lakatta EG, Levy D. Arterial and cardiac aging: major shareholders in cardiovascular disease enterprises. Part I: aging arteries a "set up" for vascular disease. Circulation. 2003;107:139–46.
12. Lakatta EG. Arterial and cardiac aging: major shareholders in cardiovascular disease enterprises. Part III: cellular and molecular clues to heart and arterial aging. Circulation. 2003;107:490–7.
13. Nichols WW, O'Rourke MF, Avolio AP, et al. Effects of age on ventricular-vascular coupling. Am J Cardiol. 1985;55:1179–84.
14. Rodeheffer RJ, Gerstenblith G, Becker LC, Fleg JL, Weisfeldt ML, Lakatta EG. Exercise cardiac output is maintained with advancing age in healthy human subjects: cardiac dilatation and increased stroke volume compensate for a diminished heart rate. Circulation. 1984;69:203–13.
15. Brandfonbrener M, Landowne M, Shock NW. Changes in cardiac output with age. Circulation. 1955;12:557–66.
16. Pan HY, Hoffman BB, Pershe RA, Blaschke TF. Decline in beta-adrenergic receptor-mediated vascular relaxation with aging in man. J Pharmacol Exp Ther. 1986;239:802–7.
17. Buhler F, Kowski W, Van Brumeler P. Plasma catecholamines and cardiac, renal and peripheral vascular adrenoceptor mediated response in different age groups in normal and hypertensive subjects. Clin Exp Hypertens. 1980;2:409–26.
18. Landahl S, Bengtsson C, Sigurdsson JA, Svanborg A, Svardsudd K. Age-related change in blood pressure. Hypertension. 1986;8:1044–9.
19. Avolio AP, Clyde KM, Beard TC, Cooke HM, Ho KK, O'Rourke MF. Improved arterial distensibility in normotensive subjects on a low salt diet. Arteriosclerosis. 1986;6:166–9.
20. Vaitkevicius PV, Fleg JL, Engel JH, et al. Effects of age and aerobic capacity on arterial stiffness in healthy adults. Circulation. 1993;88:1456–62.
21. Mitchell GF, Guo C-Y, Benjamin EJ, et al. Cross-sectional correlates of increased aortic stiffness in the community. The Framingham heart study. Circulation. 2007;115:2628–36.
22. Lima JAC, Gerstenblith G, Weiss JL, et al. Systolic blood pressure, not age mediates the age-related increase in left ventricular wall thickness within a normotensive population [abstract]. J Am Coll Cardiol. 1988;11:81A.
23. Levy D, Anderson KM, Savage DD, Kannel WB, Christiansen JC, Castelli WP. Echocardiographically detected left ventricular hypertrophy: prevalence and risk factors. The Framingham heart study. Ann Intern Med. 1988;108:7–13.
24. Aronow WS, Ahn C, Kronzon I. Prevalence of echocardiographic findings in 554 men and in 1243 women aged >60 years in a long-term health care facility. Am J Cardiol. 1997;79:379–80.
25. Aronow WS, Ahn C. Risk factors for new coronary events in a large cohort of very elderly patients with and without coronary artery disease. Am J Cardiol. 1996;77:864–6.
26. Aronow WS, Kronzon I. Prevalence of coronary risk factors in elderly Blacks and Whites. J Am Geriatr Soc. 1991;39:567–70.
27. Aronow WS, Koenigsberg M, Schwartz KS. Usefulness of echocardiographic left ventricular hypertrophy in predicting new coronary events and atherothrombotic brain infarction in patients over 62 years of age. Am J Cardiol. 1988;61:1130–2.
28. Tanaka H, Dinenno FA, Monahan KD, Clevenger CM, DeSouza CA, Seals DR. Aging, habitual exercise, and dynamic arterial compliance. Circulation. 2000;102:1270–5.
29. DeSouza CA, Shapiro LF, Clevenger CM, et al. Regular aerobic exercise prevents and restores age-related declines in endothelium-dependent vasodilation in healthy men. Circulation. 2000;102:1351–7.
30. Gardin JM, Henry WL, Savage DD, Ware JH, Burn C, Borer JS. Echocardiographic measurements in normal subjects: evaluation of an adult population without clinically apparent heart disease. J Clin Ultrasound. 1979;7:439–47.
31. Bryg RJ, Williams GA, Labovitz AJ. Effect of aging on left ventricular diastolic filling in normal subjects. Am J Cardiol. 1987;59:971–4.
32. Iskandrian AS, Aakki A. Age related changes in left ventricular diastolic performance. Am Heart J. 1986;112:75–8.
33. Spirito P, Maron BJ. Influence of aging on doppler echocardiographic indices of left ventricular diastolic function. Br Heart J. 1988;59:672–9.
34. Miyatake K, Okamoto J, Kinoshita N, et al. Augmentation of atrial contribution to left ventricular flow with aging as assessed by intracardiac Doppler flowmetry. Am J Cardiol. 1984;53:587–9.
35. Sartori MP, Quinones MA, Kuo LC, Taube J, Goldberg AP, Lakatta EG. Relation of Doppler-derived left ventricular filling parameters to age and radius/thickness ratio in normal and pathologic states. Am J Cardiol. 1987;59:1179–82.
36. Fleg JL, Shapiro EP, O'Connor F, Taube J, Goldberg AP, Lakatta EG. Left ventricular diastolic filling performance in older male athletes. JAMA. 1995;273:1371–5.
37. Gardin JM, Rohan MK, Davidson DM, et al. Doppler transmitral flow velocity parameters: relationship between age, body surface area, blood pressure and gender in normal subjects. Am J Noninvasive Cardiol. 1987;1:3–10.
38. Benjamin EG, Levy D, Anderson KM, et al. Determination of Doppler indexes of left ventricular diastolic function in normal subjects (the Framingham heart study). Am J Cardiol. 1992;70:508–15.
39. Villari B, Hess OM, Kaufmann P, Krogmann ON, Grimm J, Krayenbuehl HP. Effect of aortic valve stenosis (pressure overload) and regurgitation (volume overload) on left ventricular systolic and diastolic function. Am J Cardiol. 1992;69:927–34.
40. Prasad A, Popovic ZB, Arbab-Zadeh A, et al. The effects of aging and physical activity on Doppler measures of diastolic function. Am J Cardiol. 2007;99:1629–36.
41. Lakatta EG. Age-related alterations in the cardiovascular response to adrenergic mediated stress. Fed Proc. 1980;39:3173–7.

42. Robbins AS, Rubenstein LZ. Postural hypotension in the elderly. J Am Geriatr Soc. 1984;32:769–74.

43. Aronow WS, Lee NH, Sales FF, Etienne F. Prevalence of postural hypotension in elderly patients in a long-term health care facility. Am J Cardiol. 1988;62:336.

44. Lipsitz LA, Jonsson PV, Marks BL, Parker JA, Royal HD, Wei JY. Reduced supine cardiac volumes and diastolic filling rates in elderly patients with chronic medical conditions: implications for postural blood pressure homeostasis. J Am Geriatr Soc. 1990;38:103–7.

45. Gribbin B, Pickering TG, Sleight P, Peto R. Effect of age and high blood pressure on baroreflex sensitivity in man. Circ Res. 1971;29:424–31.

46. Lipsitz LA, Nyquist Jr RP, Wei JY, Rowe JW. Postprandial reduction in blood pressure in the elderly. N Engl J Med. 1983;309:81–3.

47. Vaitkevicius PV, Esserwein DM, Maynard AK, O'Connor FC, Fleg JL. Frequency and importance of postprandial blood pressure reduction of elderly nursing-home patients. Ann Intern Med. 1991;115:865–70.

48. Aronow WS, Ahn C. Postprandial hypotension in 499 elderly persons in a long-term health care facility. J Am Geriatr Soc. 1994;42:930–2.

49. Kamata T, Yokota T, Furukawa T, Tsukagoshi H. Cerebral ischemic attack caused by postprandial hypotension. Stroke. 1994;25:511–3.

50. Aronow WS, Ahn C. Association of postprandial hypotension with incidence of falls, syncope, coronary events, stroke, and total mortality at 29-month follow-up in 499 older nursing home residents. J Am Geriatr Soc. 1997;45:1051–3.

51. Wolf PA, Abbott RD, Kannel WB. Atrial fibrillation as an independent risk factor for stroke: the Framingham study. Stroke. 1991;22:983–8.

52. Aronow WS, Ahn C, Gutstein H. Prevalence of atrial fibrillation and association of atrial fibrillation with prior and new thromboembolic stroke in elderly patients. J Am Geriatr Soc. 1996;44:521–3.

53. Kannel WB, Abbott RD, Savage DD, McNamara PM. Epidemiologic features of chronic atrial fibrillation: the Framingham study. N Engl J Med. 1982;306:1018–22.

54. Aronow WS, Ahn C, Mercando AD, Epstein S. Correlation of atrial fibrillation, paroxysmal supraventricular tachycardia, and sinus rhythm with incidences of new coronary events in 1359 patients, mean age 81 years, with heart disease. Am J Cardiol. 1995;75:182–4.

55. Poliner LR, Dehmer GJ, Lewis SE, Parkey RW, Blomqvist CG, Willerson JT. Left ventricular performance in normal subjects: a comparison of the responses to exercise in the upright and supine positions. Circulation. 1980;62:528–34.

56. Fraticelli A, Josephson R, Danziger R, Lakatta E, Spurgeon H. Morphological and contractile characteristics of rat cardiac myocytes from maturation to senescence. Am J Physiol. 1989;257:H259–65.

57. Capasso JM, Malhotra A, Remly RM. Effects of age on mechanical and electrical performance of rat myocardium. Am J Physiol. 1983;245:H72–81.

58. Willems JL, Roelandt H, DeGeest H, Kesteloot H, Joossens JV. The left ventricular ejection time in elderly subjects. Circulation. 1970;42:37–42.

59. Shaw DJ, Rothbaum DA, Angell CS, Shock NW. The effect of age and blood pressure upon the systolic time intervals in males aged 20–89 years. J Gerontol. 1973;28:133–9.

60. Lakatta EG. Do hypertension and aging have similar effects on the myocardium? Circulation. 1987;75(Suppl I):69–77.

61. Lakatta EG, Yin FCP. Myocardial aging: functional alterations and related cellular mechanisms. Am J Physiol. 1982;242:H927–41.

62. Port S, Cobb FR, Coleman RE, Jones RH. Effect of age on the response of the left ventricular ejection fraction to exercise. N Engl J Med. 1980;303:1133–7.

63. Aronow WS, Stein PD, Sabbah HN, Koenigsberg M. Resting left ventricular ejection fraction in elderly patients without evidence of heart disease. Am J Cardiol. 1989;63:368–9.

64. Fleg JL, Schulman S, O'Connor F, et al. Effect of acute β-adrenergic receptor blockade on age-associated changes in cardiovascular performance during dynamic exercise. Circulation. 1994;90:2333–41.

65. Tresch DD, McGough MF. Heart failure with normal systolic function: a common disorder in older people. J Am Geriatr Soc. 1995;43:1035–42.

66. Morgan JP, Morgan KG. Calcium and cardiovascular function: intracellular calcium levels during contraction and relaxation of mammalian cardiac and vascular smooth muscle as detected with aequorin. Am J Med. 1984;77(Suppl 5A):33–46.

67. Wei JY, Spurgeon HA, Lakatta EG. Excitation-contraction in rat myocardium: alterations with adult aging. Am J Physiol. 1984;246:H784–91.

68. Bandy B, Davison AJ. Mitochondrial mutations may increase oxidative stress: implications for carcinogenesis and aging? Free Radic Biol Med. 1990;8:523–39.

69. Corral-Debrinski M, Stepien G, Shoffner JM, Lott MT, Kanter K, Wallace DC. Hypoxemia is associated with mitochondrial DNA damage and gene induction: implications for cardiac disease. JAMA. 1991;266:1812–6.

70. Lie JT, Hammond PI. Pathology of the senescent heart: anatomic observations on 237 autopsy studies of patients 90 to 105 years old. Mayo Clin Proc. 1988;63:552–64.

71. Schaub MC. The aging of collagen in the heart muscle. Gerontologia. 1964;10:38–41.

72. Verzar F. The stages and consequences of aging collagen. Gerontologia. 1969;15:233–9.

73. Hachamovitch R, Wicker P, Capasso JM, Anversa P. Alterations of coronary blood flow and reserve with aging in Fischer 344 rats. Am J Physiol. 1989;256:H66–73.

74. Ogawa T, Spina R, Martin III WH, et al. Effects of aging, sex and physical training on cardiovascular responses to exercise. Circulation. 1992;86:494–503.

75. Manning WJ, Shannon RP, Santinga JA, et al. Reversal of changes in left ventricular diastolic filling associated with normal aging using diltiazem. Am J Cardiol. 1991;67:894–6.

76. Kitzman DW, Higginbotham MB, Cobb FR, Sheikh KH, Sullivan M. Exercise intolerance in patients with heart failure and preserved left ventricular systolic function: failure of the Frank-Starling mechanism. J Am Coll Cardiol. 1991;17:1065–72.

77. Aronow WS, Ahn C, Kronzon I. Normal left ventricular ejection fraction in older persons with congestive heart failure. Chest. 1998;113:867–9.

78. Aronow WS, Ahn C, Gutstein H. Prevalence and incidence of cardiovascular disease in 1160 older men and 2464 older women in a long-term health care facility. J Gerontol: Med Sci. 2002;57A:M45–6.

79. Wong WF, Gold S, Fukuyama O, Blanchette PL. Diastolic dysfunction in elderly patients with congestive heart failure. Am J Cardiol. 1989;63:1526–8.

80. Aronow WS, Ahn C, Kronzon I. Prognosis of congestive heart failure in elderly patients with normal versus abnormal left ventricular systolic function associated with coronary artery disease. Am J Cardiol. 1990;66:1257–9.

81. Kitzman DW, Gardin JM, Arnold A, et al. Heart failure with preserved systolic LV function in the elderly: clinical and echocardiographic correlates from the Cardiovascular Health Study [abstract]. Circulation. 1996;94(Suppl I):I-433.

82. Vasan RS, Benjamin EJ, Evans JC, et al. Prevalence and clinical correlates of diastolic heart failure: Framingham heart study [abstract]. Circulation. 1995;92(Suppl I):666.

83. Pernenkil R, Vinson JM, Shah AS, Beckham V, Wittenberg C, Rich MW. Course and prognosis in patients ≥70 years of age with congestive heart failure and normal versus abnormal left ventricular ejection fraction. Am J Cardiol. 1997;79:216–9.

84. Aronow WS, Ahn C, Kronzon I. Comparison of incidences of congestive heart failure in older African-Americans, Hispanics, and whites. Am J Cardiol. 1999;84:611–2.

85. Redfield MM, Jacobsen SJ, Borlaug BA, et al. Age-and gender-related ventricular-vascular stiffening. A community-based study. Circulation. 2005;112:2254–62.

86. Konstam MA, Dracup K, Baker DW, et al. Heart failure: management of patients with left-ventricular systolic dysfunction. Quick Reference Guide for Clinicians, No. 11, AHCPR Publication No. 94-0613. Rockville, MD: Agency for Health Care Policy and Research; 1–21 June 1994.

87. Aronow WS. Echocardiography should be performed in all elderly patients with congestive heart failure. J Am Geriatr Soc. 1994;42:1300–2.

88. Williams Jr JF, Bristow MR, Fowler MB, et al. Guidelines for the evaluation and management of heart failure. Report of the American College of Cardiology/American Heart Association Task Force on Practice Guidelines (Committee on Evaluation and Management of Heart Failure). J Am Coll Cardiol. 1995;26:1376–98.

89. American Medical Directors Association. Heart failure. Clinical practice guideline. Columbia, MD: American Medical Directors Association; 1996. p. 1–8.

90. Aronow WS. Commentary on American Geriatrics Society Clinical Practice Guidelines from AHCPR Guidelines on Heart Failure: evaluation and treatment of patients with left ventricular systolic dysfunction. J Am Geriatr Soc. 1998;46:525–9.

91. Aronow WS. Digoxin or angiotensin converting enzyme inhibitors for congestive heart failure in geriatric patients: which is the preferred treatment? Drugs Aging. 1991;1:98–103.

92. Rich MW, McSherry F, Williford WO, Yusuf S. Effect of age on mortality, hospitalizations and response to digoxin in patients with heart failure: the DIG Study. J Am Coll Cardiol. 2001;38:806–13.

93. Ahmed A, Aronow WS, Fleg JL. Predictors of mortality and hospitalization in women with heart failure in the Digitalis Investigation Group trial. Am J Ther. 2006;13:325–31.

94. Ahmed A, Rich MW, Fleg JL, et al. Effects of digoxin on morbidity and mortality in diastolic heart failure. The Ancillary Digitalis Investigation Group trial. Circulation. 2006;114:397–403.

95. Ahmed A, Zile MR, Rich MW, et al. Hospitalizations due to unstable angina pectoris in diastolic and systolic heart failure. Am J Cardiol. 2007;99:460–4.

96. Jessup M, Abraham WT, Casey DE, et al. 2009 Focused update: ACCF/AHA guidelines for the diagnosis and management of heart ailure in adults. A report of the American College of Cardiology Foundation/American Heart Association Task Force on Practice Guidelines Developed in collaboration with the International Society for Heart and Lung Transplantation. J Am Coll Cardiol. 2009;53:1343–82.

97. Aronow WS. Epidemiology, pathophysiology, prognosis, and treatment of systolic and diastolic heart failure. Cardiol Rev. 2006;14:108–24.

98. Fleg JL. Alterations in cardiovascular structure and function with advancing age. Am J Cardiol. 1986;57:33C–44.

99. Dehn MM, Bruce RA. Longitudinal variations in maximal oxygen intake with age and activity. J Appl Physiol. 1972;33:805–7.

100. Heath GW, Hagberg JM, Ehsani AA. A physiological comparison of young and older endurance athletes. J Appl Physiol. 1981;51:634–40.

101. Fleg JL, Schulman SP, O'Connor FC, et al. Cardiovascular responses to exhaustive upright cycle exercise in highly trained older men. J Appl Physiol. 1994;77:1500–6.

102. Forman DE, Manning WJ, Hauser R, Gervino EV, Evans WJ, Wei JY. Enhanced left ventricular diastolic filling associated with long-term endurance training. J Gerontol. 1992;47:M56–8.

103. Woo JS, Derleth C, Stratton JR, Levy WC. The influence of age, gender, and training on exercise efficiency. J Am Coll Cardiol. 2006;47:1049–57.

104. Julius S, Amery A, Whitlock LS, Conway J. Influence of age on the hemodynamic response to exercise. Circulation. 1967;36:222–30.

105. Fleg JL, Lakatta EG. Role of muscle loss in the age-associated reduction in VO_{2max}. J Appl Physiol. 1988;65:1147–51.

106. Fleg JL, O'Connor F, Gerstenblith G, et al. Impact of age on the cardiovascular response to dynamic upright exercise in healthy men and women. J Appl Physiol. 1995;78:890–900.

107. Chauhan A, More RS, Mullins PA, Taylor G, Petch C, Schofield PM. Aging-associated endothelial dysfunction in humans is reversed by L-arginine. J Am Coll Cardiol. 1996;28:1796–804.

108. Lam CSP, Borlaug BA, Kane GC, Enders FT, Rodeheffer RJ. Age-associated increases in pulmonary artery systolic pressure in the general population. Circulation. 2009;119:2663–70.

109. Elkayam U, Amin J, Mehra A, Vasquez J, Weber L, Rahimtoola SH. A prospective, randomized, double-blind, crossover study to compare the efficacy and safety of chronic nifedipine therapy with that of isosorbide dinitrate and their combination in the treatment of chronic congestive heart failure. Circulation. 1990;82:1954–61.

110. Multicenter Diltiazem Postinfarction Trial Research Group. The effect of diltiazem on mortality and reinfarction after myocardial infarction. N Engl J Med. 1988;319:385–92.

111. Goldstein RE, Boccuzzi SJ, Cruess D, Nattel S. Diltiazem increases late-onset congestive heart failure in postinfarction patients with early reduction in ejection fraction. Circulation. 1991;83:52–60.

112. Packer M, O'Connor CM, Ghali JK, et al. Effect of amlodipine on morbidity and mortality in severe chronic heart failure. N Engl J Med. 1996;335:1107–14.

113. Cohn JN, Ziesche SM, Loss LE, et al. Effect of the calcium antagonist felodipine as supplementary vasodilator therapy in patients with chronic heart failure treated with enalapril. V-HeFT III. Circulation. 1997;96:856–63.

114. Garg R, Yusuf S, Collaborative Group on ACE Inhibitor Trials. Overview of randomized trials of angiotensin-converting enzyme inhibitory on mortality and morbidity in patients with heart failure. JAMA. 1995;273:1450–6.

115. Pitt B, Segal R, Martinez FA, et al. Randomised trial of losartan versus captopril in patients over 65 with heart failure (Evaluation of Losartan in the Elderly Study, ELITE). Lancet. 1997;349:747–52.

116. MERIT-HF Study Group. Effect of metoprolol CR/XL in chronic heart failure: Metoprolol CR/XL Randomised Intervention Trial in Congestive Heart Failure (MERIT-HF). Lancet. 1999;353:2001–7.

117. Packer M, Coats AJS, Fowler MB, et al. Effect of carvedilol on survival in chronic heart failure. N Engl J Med. 2001;344:651–8.

118. CIBIS-II Investigators and Committees. The Cardiac Insufficiency Bisoprolol Study II (CIBIS-II): a randomised trial. Lancet. 1999;353:9–13.

119. Flather MD, Shibata MC, Coats AJS, et al. Randomized trial to determine the effect of nebivolol on mortality and cardiovascular hospital admission in elderly patients with heart failure (SENIORS). Eur Heart J. 2005;26:215–25.

120. Granger CB, McMurray JJV, Yusuf S, et al. Effects of candesartan in patients with chronic heart failure and reduced left-ventricular systolic function intolerant to angiotensin-converting-enzyme inhibitors: the CHARM-Alternative trial. Lancet. 2003;362:772–6.

121. Bardy GH, Lee KL, Mark DB, et al. Amiodarone or an implantable cardioverter-defibrillator for congestive heart failure. N Engl J Med. 2005;352:225–37.

122. Aronow WS. CRT plus ICD in congestive heart failure. Use of cardiac resynchronization therapy and an implantable cardioverter-

defibrillator in heart failure patients with abnormal left ventricular dysfunction. Geriatrics. 2005;60(2):24–8.

123. Cleland JGF, Daubert J-C, Erdmann E, et al. The effect of cardiac resynchronization on morbidity and mortality in heart failure. N Engl J Med. 2005;352:1539–49.

124. Lai HM, Aronow WS, Kruger A, et al. Effect of beta blockers, angiotensin-converting enzyme inhibitors or angiotensin receptor blockers, and statins on mortality in patients with implantable cardioverter-defibrillators. Am J Cardiol. 2008;102:77–8.

125. Desai H, Aronow WS, Tsai FS, et al. Statins reduce appropriate cardioverter-defibrillator shocks and mortality in patients with heart failure and combined cardiac resynchronization and implantable cardioverter-defibrillator therapy. J Cardiovasc Pharmacol Ther. 2009;14(3):176–9.

126. Pitt B, Zannad F, Remme WJ, et al. The effect of spironolactone on morbidity and mortality in patients with severe heart failure. N Engl J Med. 1999;341:709–17.

127. Pitt B, Remme W, Zannad F, et al. Eplerenone, a selective aldosterone blocker, in patients with left ventricular dysfunction after myocardial infarction. N Engl J Med. 2003;348:1309–21.

128. Taylor AL, Ziesche S, Yancy C, et al. Combination of isosorbide dinitrate and hydralazine in blacks with heart failure. N Engl J Med. 2004;351:2049–57.

129. Aronow WS. Race, drugs, and heart failure. Geriatrics. 2005; 60(7):8–9.

130. Rathore SS, Curtis JP, Wang Y, Bristow MR, Krumholz HM. Association of serum digoxin concentration and outcomes in patients with heart failure. JAMA. 2003;289:871–8.

131. Ahmed A, Aban IB, Weaver MT, et al. Serum digoxin concentration and outcomes in women with heart failure: a bi-directional effect and a possible effect modification by ejection fraction. Eur J Heart Fail. 2006;8:409–41.

132. Aronow WS, Ahn C, Kronzon I. Effect of propranolol versus no propranolol on total mortality plus nonfatal myocardial infarction in older patients with prior myocardial infarction, congestive heart failure, and left ventricular ejection fraction ≥40% treated with diuretics plus angiotensin-converting-enzyme inhibitors. Am J Cardiol. 1997;80:207–9.

133. Aronow WS, Kronzon I. Effect of enalapril on congestive heart failure treated with diuretics in elderly patients with prior myocardial infarction and normal left ventricular ejection fraction. Am J Cardiol. 1993;71:602–4.

134. Cleland JG, Tendera M, Adamus J, et al. The perindopril in elderly people with chronic heart failure (PEP-CHF) study. Eur Heart J. 2006;27:2257–9.

135. Yusuf S, Pfeffer MA, Swedberg K, et al. Effects of candesartan in patients with chronic heart failure and preserved left-ventricular ejection fraction: the CHARM-Preserved trial. Lancet. 2003;362: 777–81.

136. Aronow WS, Ahn C, Schoenfeld MR, Gutstein H. Association of extracranial carotid arterial disease and chronic atrial fibrillation with the incidence of new thromboembolic stroke in 1,846 older persons. Am J Cardiol. 1999;83:1403–4.

137. Aronow WS, Ahn C, Kronzon I. Comparison of echocardiographic abnormalities in African-American, Hispanic, and white men and women aged >60 years. Am J Cardiol. 2001;87:1131–3.

138. Roberts WC, Perloff JK, Costantino T. Severe valvular aortic stenosis in patients over 65 years of age. Am J Cardiol. 1971;27: 497–506.

139. Waller BF, Roberts WC. Cardiovascular disease in the very elderly: an analysis of 40 necropsy patients aged 90 years or over. Am J Cardiol. 1983;51:403–21.

140. Aronow WS, Schwartz KS, Koenigsberg M. Correlation of serum lipids, calcium, and phosphorus, diabetes mellitus and history of systemic hypertension with presence or absence of calcified or thickened aortic cusps or root in elderly patients. Am J Cardiol. 1987;59:998–9.

141. Shirani J, Yousefi J, Roberts WC. Major cardiac findings at necropsy in 366 American octogenarians. Am J Cardiol. 1995;75: 151–6.

142. Lindroos M, Kupari M, Heikkila J, et al. Prevalence of aortic valve abnormalities in the elderly: an echocardiographic study of a random population sample. J Am Coll Cardiol. 1993;21:1220–5.

143. Aronow WS, Kronzon I, Schoenfeld MR. Prevalence of extracranial carotid arterial disease and of valvular aortic stenosis and their association in the elderly. Am J Cardiol. 1995;75:304–5.

144. Aronow WS, Ahn C, Kronzon I. Association of valvular aortic stenosis with symptomatic peripheral arterial disease in older persons. Am J Cardiol. 2001;88:1046–7.

145. Nassimiha D, Aronow WS, Ahn C, Goldman ME. Rate of progression of valvular aortic stenosis in persons ≥60 years. Am J Cardiol. 2001;87:807–9.

146. Nassimiha D, Aronow WS, Ahn C, Goldman ME. Association of coronary risk factors with progression of valvular aortic stenosis in older persons. Am J Cardiol. 2001;87:1313–4.

147. Palta S, Pai AM, Gill KS, Pai RG. New insights into the progression of aortic stenosis. Implications for secondary prevention. Circulation. 2000;101:2497–502.

148. Aronow WS, Schwartz KS, Koenigsberg M. Correlation of serum lipids, calcium and phosphorus, diabetes mellitus, aortic valve stenosis and history of systemic hypertension with presence or absence of mitral anular calcium in persons older than 62 years in a long-term health care facility. Am J Cardiol. 1987;59: 381–2.

149. Aronow WS, Ahn C, Shirani J, Kronzon I. Comparison of frequency of new coronary events in older persons with mild, moderate, and severe valvular aortic stenosis with those without aortic stenosis. Am J Cardiol. 1998;81:647–9.

150. Livanainen AM, Lindroos M, Tilvis R, Heikkila J, Kupari M. Natural history of aortic valve stenosis of varying severity in the elderly. Am J Cardiol. 1996;78:97–101.

151. Otto CM, Lind BK, Kitzman DW, Gersh BJ, Siscovick DS. Association of aortic-valve sclerosis with cardiovascular mortality and morbidity in the elderly. N Engl J Med. 1999;341:142–7.

152. Aronow WS, Shirani J, Kronzon I. Comparison of frequency of new coronary events in older subjects with and without valvular aortic sclerosis. Am J Cardiol. 1999;83:599–600.

153. Margonato A, Cianflone D, Carlino M, Conversano A, Nitti C, Chierchia S. Frequence and significance of aortic valve thickening in older asymptomatic patients and its relation to aortic regurgitation. Am J Cardiol. 1989;64:1061–2.

154. Akasaka T, Yoshikawa J, Yoshida K, et al. Age-related valvular regurgitation: a study by pulsed Doppler echocardiography. Circulation. 1987;76:262–5.

155. Aronow WS, Kronzon I. Correlation of prevalence and severity of aortic regurgitation detected by pulsed Doppler echocardiography with the murmur of aortic regurgitation in elderly patients in a long-term health care facility. Am J Cardiol. 1989;63:128–9.

156. Sell S, Scully RE. Aging changes in the aortic and mitral valves. Am J Pathol. 1965;46:345–65.

157. Pomerance A, Darby AJ, Hodkinson HM. Valvular calcification in the elderly: possible pathogenic factors. J Gerontol. 1978;33:672–6.

158. Roberts WC. The senile cardiac calcification syndrome. Am J Cardiol. 1986;58:572–4.

159. Aronow WS, Schwartz KS, Koenigsberg M. Correlation of atrial fibrillation with presence of absence of mitral annular calcium in 604 persons older than 60 years. Am J Cardiol. 1987;59: 1213–4.

160. Roberts WC, Perloff JK. Mitral valvular disease: a clinicopathologic survey of the conditions causing the mitral valve to function abnormally. Ann Intern Med. 1972;77:939–75.

161. Aronow WS, Ahm C, Kronzon I. Association of mitral annular calcium and of aortic cuspal calcium with coronary artery disease in older patients. Am J Cardiol. 1999;84:1084–5.

162. Adler Y, Herz I, Vaturi M, et al. Mitral annular calcium detected by transthoracic echocardiography is a marker for high prevalence and severity of coronary artery disease in patients undergoing coronary angiography. Am J Cardiol. 1998;82:1183–6.

163. Tolstrup K, Roldan CA, Qualls CR, Crawford MH. Aortic valve sclerosis, mitral annular calcium, and aortic root sclerosis as markers of atherosclerosis in men. Am J Cardiol. 2002;89:1030–4.

164. Aronow WS, Ahn C, Kronzon I. Association of mitral annular calcium with symptomatic peripheral arterial disease in older persons. Am J Cardiol. 2001;88:333–4.

165. Antonini-Canterin F, Capanna M, Manfroni A, Brieda M, Grandis U, Sbaraglia F, et al. Association between mitral annular calcium and carotid artery stenosis and role of age and gender. Am J Cardiol. 2001;88:581–3.

166. Seo Y, Ishimitsu T, Ishizu T, et al. Relationship between mitral annular calcification and severity of carotid atherosclerosis in patients with symptomatic ischemic cerebrovascular disease. J Cardiol. 2005;46:17–24.

167. Kistler PM, Sanders P, Fynn SP, et al. Electrophysiologic and electroanatomic changes in the human atrium associated with aging. J Am Coll Cardiol. 2004;44:109–16.

168. Aronow WS. Correlation of arrhythmias and conduction defects on the resting electrocardiogram with new cardiac events in 1,153 elderly patients. Am J Noninvasive Cardiol. 1991;75:182–4.

Chapter 22
Renal Changes in the Elderly

Carlos G. Musso and Dimitrios G. Oreopoulos

Abstract After the age of 30 many structural and functional changes appear gradually in the kidney. These changes can lead to what has been referred to as *nephrogeriatric giants*, six conditions present in the majority of the old people: senile hypofiltration (progressive reduction in glomerular filtration), renal vascular changes (atheromatosis and dysautonomy of the renal vessels), tubular dysfunction (reduction of several functions of the renal tubules), tubular frailty (tubular susceptibility to develop necrosis, and delayed recovery), medullary hypotonicity (reduced medulla tonicity), and obstructive uropathy. These changes explain the appearance of several disorders such as renal failure, ischemic nephropathy, hypo or hyperkalemia, sodium depletion, hyponatremia, dehydration, and urosepsis in the elderly.

Keywords Nephrogeriatric giants • Senile hypofiltration • Renal vascular changes • Tubular dysfunction • Tubular frailty • Medulla hypotonicity • Urinary obstruction • Renal failure • Ischemic nephropathy • Dyskalemia • Sodium depletion • Hyponatremia • Dehydration • Urosepsis

Introduction

More than 50% of aged kidneys are normal in appearance, while approximately 14% display cortical scars scattered across their surface [1]. The weight of the kidney slowly decreases from 400 g in the third decade to less than 300 g in the ninth decade of life and its length diminishes by 2 cm during this period. The renal cortex loses more mass than the medulla, while the latter shows an increase in its interstitial tissue; this is accompanied by fibrosis and increase of fat content at the level of the renal sinus, a constant finding is the presence of cysts along the distal nephron. Tubular cells undergo fatty degeneration with age, showing an irregular thickening of their basal membrane. Microdissection shows that the diverticula that arise from the distal and convoluted tubules become more frequent with age [2, 3].

After the age of 30 renal functional capacity gradually decreases due either to a progressive loss of functioning nephrons alone or a decrease in the number of energy-producing mitochondria, lower concentration of adenosine triphosphatase activity and other enzymes, or decreased tubular cell transport capacity [4, 5].

The structural and functional changes of the aged kidney can lead to what has been referred to as *nephrogeriatric giants*, six conditions present in the majority of the old people and characterized by profound changes in renal physiology [6]: These changes are (1) decrease in glomerular filtration rate (GFR) (senile hypofiltration), (2) renal vascular changes, (3) tubular dysfunction, (4) hypotonicity of the medulla, (5) tubular "frailty," and (6) obstructive uropathy. Below we will describe these entities and their clinical consequences in detail (Table 22.1).

Decrease in GFR (Senile Hypofiltration)

Glomerular sclerosis begins at approximately 30 years of age, and the "obsolete" glomeruli vary between 1 and 30% in persons aged 50 or older [7]. The glomerular tuft appears partially or totally hyalinized, and this is the basis of the glomerulosclerosis, which leads to a reduction in the effective filtration surface in the elderly glomeruli [8, 9]. At the same time, the mesangium increases to nearly 12% by the age of 70 [2]. Microangiographic examination shows obliteration particularly of juxtamedullar nephrons, but not of those sited more peripherally, with the formation of a direct channel between afferent and efferent arterioles of the former (phenomenon called *aglomerular circulation*) (Fig. 22.1). Presumably this change contributes to the maintenance of medullary blood flow, and perhaps contributes to medullary

C.G. Musso (✉)
Department of Nephrology, Hospital Italiano de Buenos Aires, Gascon 450, C1181 Ciudad de Buenos Aires, Argentina
e-mail: carlos.musso@hospitalitaliano.org.ar

M.R. Katlic (ed.), *Cardiothoracic Surgery in the Elderly*, DOI 10.1007/978-1-4419-0892-6_22,
© Springer Science+Business Media, LLC 2011

Table 22.1 Nephrogeriatric giants and their potential clinical consequences

Nephrogeriatric giant	Potential clinical consequences
Senile hypofiltration	Drug dose toxicity
	Saline load (pulmonary congestion)
	Water load (hyponatremia)
Renal vascular changes	Atheroembolia
	Ischemic nephropathy
	Secondary hypertension
Tubular dysfunction	Hyperkalemia
	Hypokalemia
	Sodium loss (hypotension, hyponatremia)
Tubular frailty	Acute renal failure
	Chronic renal failure
Medulla hypotonicity	Water loss (dehydration)
	Nocturia
Obstructive uropathy	Acute renal failure
	Chronic renal failure
	Urosepsis

hypotonicity in the aged [10] (Fig. 22.2). Because of all these changes, aging is accompanied by a decrease of GFR), renal plasma flow (RPF), and renal blood flow (RBF) [11]. The GFR evaluation with ^{51}Cr EDTA confirms that the elderly have lower GFRs than the young [12]. At the third decade of life, creatinine clearance (Ccr) peaks at approximately 140 mL/min/1.73 m^2, and from then on, it progressively declines at a rate of 8 mL/min/1.73 m^2 per decade [12]. The fall in Ccr is accompanied by a concomitant decrease in creatinine production (senile sarcopenia), and consequently serum creatinine does not increase with the progressive decrease in GFR with age [13] (Fig. 22.2). In daily clinical practice, to estimate the Ccr in the elderly the equation of Cockcroft and Gault (CG) (Ccr = (140 − age) × (body weight) /72 × serum creatinine; in women, it is 15% lower) is quite useful [14] (Table 22.2; Fig. 22.3).

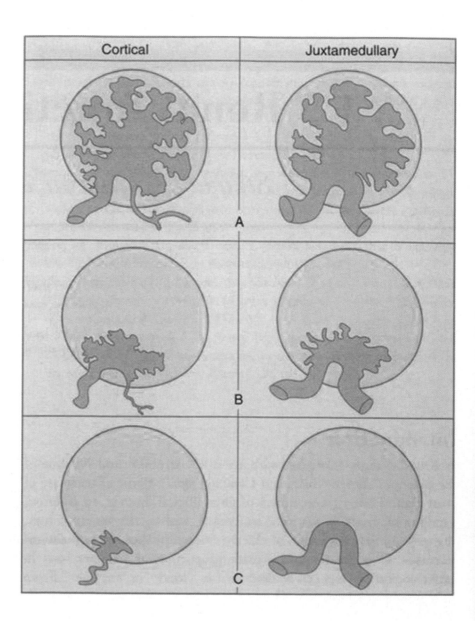

Fig. 22.1 Cortical and juxtamedullary glomerulosclerosis and aglomerular circulation. (Reprinted from McLachlan [52], by permission of Oxford University Press. Data from Takazakura et al. [53])

Fig. 22.2 Creatinine clearance reduction and serum creatinine stability in aging (Reprinted from Kampmann et al. [54], with permission from Wiley)

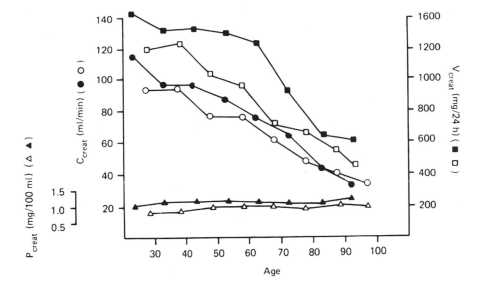

Table 22.2 Senile hypofiltration: its mechanisms

Senile hypofiltration
Glomerulosclerosis
Mesangial expansion
Aglomerular circulation

Table 22.3 Senile renal vascular changes: its mechanisms

Renal vascular changes
Renal atherosclerosis
Vascular dysautonomy
Arteriole subendotelial hyalinosis
Aglomerular circulation

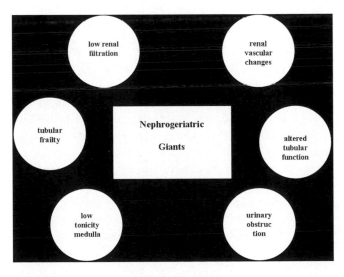

Fig. 22.3 Nephrogeriatric giants' mechanisms

Clinical Consequences

- A serum creatinine concentration of 1 mg/dL reflects a Ccr of 120 mL/min in a 20-year-old person and 50 mL/min in a 80-year-old one [12].
- It should be remembered that because of the senile decrease in Ccr, the dose of prescribed drugs must be corrected to the measured or estimated GFR and not serum creatinine [15]. Estimation of Ccr by the CG formula is adequate for adjustment in dose of prescribed drug.
- The *senile decrease in GFR* together with diastolic cardiac failure secondary to the normal aging (called *presbicardia*) predispose healthy old people to pulmonary congestion after they receive a saline load [6].

Renal Vascular Changes

In apparently normal aged individuals, prearterioles, from which afferent arterioles arise, show subendothelial deposition of hyaline and collagen fibers that produce intimal thickening [7]. In small arteries the intima is thickened due to proliferation of the elastic tissue. This is associated with atrophy of the media. Another characteristic of the aging kidney is the formation of anastomosis among afferent and efferent arterioles following obliteration of the glomeruli [16]. Besides, there is a defect in the autonomic renal vascular reflex in the elderly that normally protects the kidney from hypotensive and hypertensive states in the young people (see tubular frailty) [6] (Table 22.3).

Clinical Consequences

In the presence of the changes mentioned above, the elderly are predisposed to develop the following pathological entities:

- Ischemic nephropathy: An important cause of chronic kidney disease in the elderly patient with essential hypertension [17, 18].
- Atheroembolic disease: It occurs when plaque material breaks free from the diseased vessel and enters the distal microcirculation. This intra-renal atheroemboli may lead to an acute kidney injury (AKI) from which the patient rarely recovers [19].
- Renovascular disease: Reversible renal failure may develop after the use of angiotensin-converting enzyme (ACE) inhibitors in patients with unequal-sized kidneys on ultrasound. It is important to make this diagnosis, because even in end-stage renal disease (ESRD), angioplasty of the stenosed renal artery may restore some renal function [18, 19].

Tubular Dysfunction

Renal tubules undergo fatty degeneration with age and show an irregular thickening of their basal membrane. Microdissection shows diverticuli arising from the distal and convoluted tubules [16]. Also there are increasing zones of tubular atrophy and fibrosis, which may relate to the defects in concentration and dilution that are part of the normal renal aging process [2, 3].

Sodium

Probably hypernatremia and hyponatremia are the most common and better known disturbances in aged individuals. In spite of the lower sodium tubular load, 24-h urinary sodium output and fractional excretion of sodium are significantly greater in old and very old people compared to the young [20, 21]. This suggests that the renal tubule of the elderly is unable to conserve sodium adequately. As a result, in a setting of sodium deprivation, the mean half time for a reduction of sodium excretion is around 18 h in persons under 30 years, reaching around 31 h in persons over 60 years, apparently mediated by the concomitant reduction in GFR [22]. As GFR declines with age and the amount of filtered sodium is lower than in young subjects, an aged person takes longer to eliminate any salt load given to them [23]. However, when sodium is restricted to 50 mmol per day, the period required to achieve equilibrium is 5 days in the young

and 9 days in the elderly. As a result of these slow adaptations, both hypernatremia and hyponatremia are frequent in geriatric patients [24, 25]. Under normal conditions, the old are not salt depleted because any renal sodium losses are matched by salt contained in the diet. The inability of the aged kidney to conserve sodium may explain the tendency in old people to develop volume depletion in case of diminished sodium intake (<50 mmol/24 h) [26, 27]. The diminished capacity to reabsorb sodium by the ascending limb of Henle's loop in healthy elderly persons [28, 29] has two direct important consequences: First, the amount of sodium arriving at more distal segments of the nephron (distal convoluted and collecting tubules) increases; and at the same time, the capacity to concentrate in the medullary interstitium is diminished, causing elderly subjects to exhibit both increased sodium excretion and inability to maximally concentrate the urine [30]. Kirkland et al. found greater urinary elimination of water and electrolytes during the night in the elderly, which can, at least in part, explain the nocturia observed in 70% of elderly persons [31]. Basal plasma concentrations of renin and aldosterone and the response to stimuli such as walking and salt restriction are also diminished in old age [20]. Thus, a dual effect of low aldosterone secretion and a relative insensitivity of the distal nephron to the hormone could account for diminished sodium reabsorption at this site [32].

Potassium

Total body potassium content is lower in the old than in the young and the correlation with age is linear [33]. As 85% of potassium is deposited in muscle, and muscular mass diminishes with age, this may largely account for the fall in total body potassium, with other factors such as poor intake also playing some role [34]. Under normal conditions, plasma potassium is normal in the elderly, but when patients are placed on diuretics, the elderly develop hypokalemia more rapidly than do the young [31]. On the other hand, the total renal excretion of potassium is significantly lower in the aged population than in the young. A clinical consequence of this tendency to lower excretion of potassium by the aging kidney is the vulnerability of elderly persons to hyperkalemia [35–37] (Table 22.4).

Table 22.4 Senile tubule-interstitial changes: its mechanisms

Tubule-interstitial changes
Tubular diverticuli
Tubular atrophy
Tubular fat degeneration
Reduced sodium reabsorption
Reduced potassium secretion
Interstitial fibrosis
Medulla hypotonicity

Clinical Consequences

- It has been suggested that diverticuli in the senile distal and convoluted tubules may serve as reservoirs for recurrent urinary tract infection in the old [16].
- When normotensive old patients are salt restricted or when they become ill and lose their appetite, they may develop salt and volume depletion and even acute renal failure (ARF) [26].
- The reduced capability of the aging kidney to excrete potassium explains the vulnerability of the elderly to hyperkalemia. This electrolyte disturbance is particularly frequent when elderly individuals are treated (either alone or in combination) with non-steroidal anti-inflammatory drugs (NSAIDs), ACE inhibitors, and beta-blockers or potassium-sparing diuretics [36].

Medullary Hypotonicity

Senescence reduces the capacity of the kidney to concentrate the urine. The maximum urinary concentration remains constant until about the third decade and then falls by about 30 mosmol/kg per decade. The decrease in the concentrating ability correlates with the fall in GFR with age. The relative increase in medullary blood flow (because of aglomerular circulation described above) also may contribute to the impairment of renal concentration capacity. The defect in sodium chloride reabsorption in the ascending limb of Henle's loop and in distal urea reabsorption are both important mechanisms for the development of a **hypotonic** medulla, which **leads to the inadequate** water reabsorption **and to the** decrease in the capacity to concentrate urine detected in the aged [29, 38]. The decrease in responsiveness of tubular epithelium of the collecting tubules to antidiuretic hormone (ADH) is another mechanism for the impairment of the urine concentrating ability. Also this may explain why plasma vasopressin levels are higher in the elderly compared to the adult person [36, 39]. Furthermore, when healthy active elderly volunteers were water restricted for 24 h, their threshold for thirst was increased and water intake was reduced compared with a control group of younger subjects [40]. Dryness of the mouth, a decrease in taste, alteration in mental capacity or cortical cerebral dysfunction, and a reduction in the sensitivity of both osmoreceptors and baroreceptors all may contribute to this increased threshold for thirst. Finally, concentration of angiotensin, a powerful generator of thirst, is lower in the elderly [36]. Total body water is diminished with age, comprising only 54% of total body weight compared to 65% in young, probably because old people have a greater proportion of body weight as fat than the young. The decrease in total body water seems to be due predominantly to a decrease in the intracellular compartment [20, 36, 41]. Urinary dilution capability also is decreased. Thus, there is a minimum urine concentration of only 92 mOsmol/kg in the elderly compared to 52 mOsmol/kg in the young [42, 43]. Maximum free water clearance also is reduced in the elderly from 16.2 mL/min to 5.9 mL/min. Again, the functional impairment of the diluting segment of the thick ascending limb, described above, seems to account for the decrease in the capacity to dilute urine observed in the aged [27] (Table 22.4).

Clinical Consequences

- Alterations in the senile loop of Henle induce a lower urine dilution capability in the elderly, which predisposes them to hyponatremia in a setting of free water load [34].
- In the elderly the characteristic reduced ability to concentrate urine contributes to the trend to develop nocturia and dehydration in settings such as hot weather, febrile syndromes, or delirium, as well as characteristic low serum urea levels in healthy oldest old [23, 34].

Tubular Frailty

In the elderly, renal tubular cells may develop acute tubular necrosis (ATN) rapidly, and they on the contrary recover slowly. Because of this, AKI is frequent in the elderly [6, 44]. Among the various causes of AKI, the most common are [44, 45]:

1. *Prerenal*: Loss of fluids (diarrhea, diuretics), inadequate fluid intake, loss of blood (hemorrhage), shock (cardiogenic and septicemic).
2. *Renal*: ATN due to the persistent prerenal causes and/or to nephrotoxins; rapidly progressive damage due to collagen disorders, such as Goodpasture's syndrome and Henoch–Schonlein purpura; arterial or venous thrombosis; acute interstitial nephritis (drug toxicity).
3. *Postrenal (Obstructive)*: Stones, clots, tumors, strictures, prostatic hypertrophy. Prerenal and postrenal causes of AKI are of particular importance in the elderly since their early identification and treatment may prevent the development of established ATN.

Finally, it must be noted that continuation of treatment with ACEs, ARBs, or NSAIDs in febrile-dehydrated elderly patients has a serious effect on the aged kidney [45] (Table 22.4).

Clinical Consequences

- The incidence of AKI in the elderly is higher than in the young, because of the frequency of systemic illnesses, polypharmacy (especially NSAIDs, ACEs, and ARBs), and because of the renal aging process itself [46]. In a particular individual AKI is often multifactorial, i.e., inadequate fluid replacement before surgery, followed by dehydration, hypotension, infection, or inappropriate antibiotics (particularly aminoglycosides) [44, 45].
- The kidneys in the elderly are particularly susceptible to the toxic effect of drugs and other chemical agents for the following reasons: (a) they have a rich blood supply; (b) drugs are concentrated in the hypertonic medulla; (c) drug accumulation is associated with impaired renal function; (d) hypersensitivity reaction with vasculitis is common in the kidney; and (e) concomitant inhibition of hepatic enzymes (present in elderly persons) increases drug toxicity [47].

Obstructive Uropathy

Prostatic hypertrophy occurs to the same degree in almost all aging males, but in a proportion of them it provides a slow obstruction to urinary outflow that gradually decreases kidney function. Often this is not recognized until it is too late, largely because the patient becomes polyuric rather than oliguric [48]. Other causes of urinary tract obstruction are uterine prolapse, stones, strictures, and neurogenic bladder due to diabetes mellitus and posterior column dysfunction [49] (Table 22.5).

Clinical Consequences

- By the time urinary obstruction is diagnosed, irreversible damage may have taken place, so that even with the relief of obstruction, renal function recovers only partially [48].
- Urinary tract infection is the most common infection in the elderly and is especially prevalent in debilitated,

institutionalized old individuals. The pathogenesis is strongly related to obstructive uropathy. Moreover, the incidence of bacteriuria increases with advancing age since several non-obstructive mechanisms predispose the aged to urinary infection such as vaginal and urethral atrophy, puddling related to bed rest, and bladder catheterization [50, 51].

Conclusions

The aging kidney becomes less efficient in coping with stressful situations such as overload or deprivation. If one does not pay attention to this, one may expose the elderly to ARF or congestive cardiac failure. In the elderly, drug abuse, dehydration, renal artery stenosis, and urinary outflow obstruction are frequent important but often asymptomatic complications. With clinical experience, the physician can avoid these complications and thus prevent renal failure.

References

1. Zhou X, Laszik Z, Silva F. Anatomical changes in the aging kidney. In: Macías Núñez JF, Cameron S, Oreopoulos D, editors. The aging kidney in health and disease. New York: Springer; 2008. p. 40–54.
2. Baert L, Steg A. Is the diverticulum of the distal and collecting tubules a preliminary stage of the simple cyst in the adult? J Urol. 1977;118:707–10.
3. Macías Nuñez JF. The normal ageing kidney-morphology and physiology. Rev Clin Gerontol. 2008;18:175–97.
4. Musso C, Fainstein I, Kaplan R, Galinsky D, Macías Nuñez JF. The patient with acid base and electrolytes disorders. In: Macias JF, Guillén Llera F, Rivera Casado JM, editors. Geriatrics since the beginning. Barcelone: Glosa; 2001. p. 245–52.
5. Beauchene RE, Fanestil DD, Barrows CH. The effect of age on active transport and sodium-potassium-activated ATPase activity in renal tissue of rats. J Gerontol. 1965;20:306–10.
6. Musso CG. Geriatric nephrology and the "nephrogeriatric giants". Int Urol Nephrol. 2002;34:255–6.
7. McLachlan MSF, Guthrie JC, Anderson CK, Fulker MJ. Vascular and glomerular changes in the ageing kidney. J Pathol. 1977;121:65–77.
8. Rosen H. Renal disease of the elderly. Med Clin North Am. 1976;60:1105.
9. Goyal VK. Changes with age in the human kidney. Exp Gerontol. 1982;17:321–31.
10. Takazakura E, Sawabu N, Handa A, et al. Intrarenal vascular changes with age and disease. Kidney Int. 1972;2:224–30.
11. Cohen MP, Ku L. Age-related changes in sulfation of basement membrane glycosaminoglycans. Exp Gerontol. 1983;18:447–50.
12. Rowe JW, Andres R, Tobin JD, et al. The effect of age on creatinin clearance in man: a cross-sectional and longitudinal study. J Gerontol. 1976;31:155–63.
13. Swedko P, Clark H, Paramsothy K, Akbari A. Serum creatinine is an inadequate screening test for renal failure in the elderly patients. Arch Intern Med. 2003;163:356–60.
14. Cockcroft DW, Gault MH. Prediction of creatinine clearance from serum creatinine. Nephron. 1976;16:31–41.

Table 22.5 Senile urinary obstruction: its mechanisms

Uro-obstruction
Prostatic hyperplasia
Prostate carcinoma
Renal lithiasis
Uterine prolapse
Urethral strictures
Neurogenic bladder

15. Musso C, Enz P. Pharmacokinetics in the elderly. Rev Arg Farm Clin. 1996;3:101–5.

16. Darmady EM, Offer J, Woodhouse MA. The parameters of the ageing kidney. J Pathol. 1973;109:195–207.

17. Ritz E, Fliser D. Clinical relevance of albuminuria in hypertensive patients. Clin Investig. 1992;70:s114–9.

18. Weir MR. Hypertensive nephropathy: is a more physiologic approach to blood pressure control an important concern for the preservation of renal function? Am J Med. 1992;93:s27–37.

19. Meyrier A. Renal vascular lesions in the elderly: nephrosclerosis or atheromatous renal disease? Nephrol Dial Transplant. 1996;11 Suppl 9:45–52.

20. Musso CG, Macías Nuñez JF. Renal handling of water and electrolytes in the old and old-old healthy aged. In: Macías Núñez JF, Cameron S, Oreopoulos D, editors. The aging kidney in health and disease. New York: Springer; 2008. p. 141–54.

21. Musso CG, Macías Núñez JF, Musso Musso, et al. Fractional excretion of sodium in old-old people on a low sodium diet. FASEB. 2000;14:A659.

22. Meyer BR. Renal function in ageing. J Am Geriatr Soc. 1989;37:791–800.

23. Fish LC, Murphy DJ, Elahi D, Minaker KL. Renal sodium excretion in normal aging: decreased excretion rates lead to delayed sodium excretion in normal aging. Geriatr Nephrol Urol. 1994;4:145–51.

24. Solomon LR, Lye M. Hypernatremia in the elderly patient. Gerontology. 1990;36:171–9.

25. Roberts MM, Robinson AG. Hyponatremia in the elderly: diagnosis and management. Geriatr Nephrol Urol. 1993;3:43–50.

26. Macias JF, Garcia-Iglesias C, Tabernero JM, et al. Renal management of sodium under indomethacin and aldosterone in the elderly. Age Ageing. 1980;9:165–72.

27. Macias JF, Garcia-Iglesias C, Bondia A, et al. Renal handling of sodium in old people: a functional study. Age Ageing. 1978;7:178–81.

28. De Santo N, Anastasio P, Coppola S, et al. Age-related changes in renal reserve and renal tubular function in healthy humans. Child Nephrol Urol. 1991;11:33–40.

29. Musso CG, Fainstein I, Kaplan R, Macías Núñez JF. Tubular renal function in the oldest old. Rev Esp Geriatr Gerontol. 2004;39(5):314–9.

30. Fulop T, Worum I, Csongor J, et al. Body composition in elderly people. Gerontology. 1985;31:6–14.

31. Kirkland JL, Lye M, Levy DW, Banerjee AK. Patterns of urine flow and electrolyte secretion in healthy elderly people. Br Med J (Clin Res Ed). 1983;285:1665–7.

32. Heim JM, Gottmann K, Weil J, et al. Effects of a bolus of atrial natriuretic factor in young and elderly volunteers. Eur J Clin Invest. 1989;19:265–71.

33. Cox JR, Shalaby WA. Potassium change with age. Gerontologie. 1981;27:340–4.

34. Lye M. Distribution of body potassium in healthy elderly subjects. Gerontologie. 1981;27:286–92.

35. Musso CG, Miguel R, Algranati L, Farias Edos R. Renal potassium excretion: comparison between chronic renal disease patients and old people. Int Urol Nephrol. 2005;37(1):167–70.

36. Andreucci V, Russo D, Cianciaruso B, Andreucci M. Some sodium, potassium and water changes in the elderly and their treatment. Nephrol Dial Transplant. 1996;11 Suppl 9:9–17.

37. Eiam-Ong S, Sabatini S. Effect of ageing and potassium depletion on renal collecting tubule k-controlling ATPases. Nephrology. 2002;7:87–91.

38. Rowe JW, Shock NW, De Fronzo RA. The influence of age on the renal response to water deprivation in man. Nephron. 1976;17:270–8.

39. Bengele HH, Mathias RS, Perkins JH, Alexander EA. Urinary concentrating defect in the aged rat. Clin J Physiol. 1981;240:147–50.

40. Phillips PA, Rolls BJ, Ledingham DM, et al. Reduced thirst after water deprivation in healthy elderly men. N Engl J Med. 1984;311:753–9.

41. Shannon RP, Minaker KL, Rowe JW. Aging and water balance in humans. Semin Nephrol. 1984;4:346–53.

42. Dontas AS, Marketos S, Papanayioutou P. Mechanisms of renal tubular defects in old age. Postgrad Med J. 1972;48:295–303.

43. De Toro Casado R, Macías Núñez JF. Physiologic characteristics of the renal ageing: clinical consequences. Ann Med Interna. 1995;12:157–9.

44. Macías Núñez JF, López Novoa JM, Martínez Maldonado M. Acute renal failure in the aged. Semin Nephrol. 1996;16:330–8.

45. Musso CG, Macías Núñez JF. The aged kidney: morphology and function. Main nephropathie. In: Salgado A, Guillén F, Ruipérez I, editors. Geriatrics handbook. Barcelon: Masson; 2002. p. 399–412.

46. Kafetz K. Renal impairment in the elderly: a review. J R Soc Med. 1983;76:398–401.

47. Evans DB. Drugs and the kidney. Br J Hosp Med. 1980;24:244–51.

48. Sacks SH, Aparicio SAJR, Bevan A, et al. Late renal failure due to prostatic out flow obstruction: a preventable disease. Br Med J. 1989;298:180–9.

49. Alivizatos G, Skolarikos A. Obstructive uropathy and benign prostatic hyperplasia. In: Macías Núñez JF, Cameron S, Oreopoulos D, editors. The aging kidney in health and disease. New York: Springer; 2008. p. 257–72.

50. Rodríguez Pascual C, Olcoz Chiva M. Infectious diseases in geriatric patients. In: Salgado A, Guillén F, Ruipérez I, editors. Geriatrics handbook. Barcelona: Masson; 2002. p. 542–8.

51. Nicolle LE. Urinary tract infection in the elderly. J Antimicrob Chemother. 1994;33:99–109.

52. McLachlan M. Anatomic structural and vascular changes in the ageing kidney. In: Macías-Núñez JF, Cameron JS, editors. Renal functional and disease in the elderly. London: Butterworths; 1987. p. 3–26.

53. Takazakura E, Sawabu N, Handa A, Takada A, Shinoda A, Takeuchi J. Intrarenal vascular change with age and disease. Kidney Int. 1972;2:224–30.

54. Kampmann J, Siersbaek-Nielsen K, Kristensen M, Hansen JM. Rapid evaluation of creatrinine clearance. Acta Med Scand. 1974;196(6):517–20.

Chapter 23
Gastrointestinal and Liver Changes in the Elderly[1]

Vadim Sherman, John A. Primomo, and F. Charles Brunicardi

Abstract Within the gastrointestinal tract, a number of subtle changes occur with aging. An understanding of these expected changes will help the clinician decide whether the clinical presentation is expected, or due to a pathological process. The foregut undergoes some significant alterations in physiology which lead to clinically significant phenomenon in the elderly. These include an increased risk of aspiration and malnutrition. Age-related changes in the colon include a significantly increased incidence of diverticular disease, constipation, and colitis.

The hepatobiliary system also undergoes normal physiological alteration with age. Overall, there is little clinical impairment of liver function. Similarly, the gallbladder continues to function in a normal fashion, although there is an increased incidence of gallstones. With regard to the pancreas, the data is not clear as to whether age related changes are the determinant of alterations in pancreatic function.

Keywords Esophagus • Stomach • Small bowel • Colon • Liver • Biliary system • Pancreas • Elderly • Physiology • Age-related changes • Aging

Introduction

As we know, a number of physiological changes occur with aging. Although not as dramatic and sometimes significant as changes with other vital organs such as the heart and brain, the gastrointestinal tract does undergo subtle alterations in function. A knowledge and understanding of these alterations helps the clinician decide whether the clinical presentation is consistent with the patient's physiology, or whether it is a pathological process. Furthermore, an appreciation of

gastrointestinal changes with aging also affords the clinician the opportunity to expect and prevent certain conditions which are more likely to occur.

The Esophagus

Anatomy

The word esophagus originates from the Greek words of Oisen, meaning to carry, and Phagein, meaning to eat. Throughout its serpiginous 25–30 cm course, the esophagus is subdivided into cervical, thoracic, and abdominal portions. Blood supply is from the inferior thyroid, the bronchial, the left gastric, and the paired phrenic arteries. Though it begins as a midline structure, the esophagus deviates to the left of the trachea as it passes the thoracic inlet. It then courses to the right and distal to the carina, it passes again to the left under the mainstem bronchus, finally entering the abdominal cavity through the esophageal hiatus. During its course the esophagus is narrowed at three distinct areas: the cricopharyngeus muscle, the left mainstem bronchus, and the diaphragmatic hiatus.

Unlike the remainder of the intestinal tract, the esophagus is composed of only two layers: the mucosa and the muscularis propria, thereby lacking an outer serosal layer. Distal to the cricopharyngeal muscle the esophagus has two concentric muscle bundles, an inner circular and outer longitudinal layer. The upper third of musculature is striated, whereas the lower two thirds is composed of smooth muscle. The complex muscular construction of the esophagus includes an upper and lower esophageal sphincter (LES) that provide crucial functionality (Fig. 23.1). The upper esophageal sphincter (UES) is characterized by the end of the pharyngeal constrictor muscles. The cricopharyngeus muscle is solely responsible for maintaining the UES. The space between the thyropharngeus muscle and the cricopharyngeus muscle marks an area of weakening which contributes to the formation of Zenkers diverticulm. The LES is maintained by the diaphragmatic crura, the phrenoesophageal membrane, and

---

[1] Portions of this chapter are reprinted with permission from Sherman and Brunicardi [1].

V. Sherman (✉)
Michael E. DeBakey Surgery Department,
Baylor College of Medicine, Houston, TX 77030, USA
e-mail: vsherman@bcm.tmc.edu

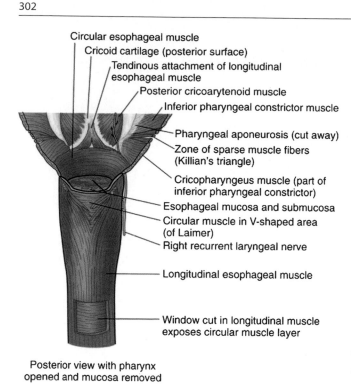

Circular esophageal muscle
Cricoid cartilage (posterior surface)
Tendinous attachment of longitudinal
esophageal muscle
Posterior cricoarytenoid muscle
Inferior pharyngeal constrictor muscle
Pharyngeal aponeurosis (cut away)
Zone of sparse muscle fibers
(Killian's triangle)
Cricopharyngeus muscle (part of
inferior pharyngeal constrictor)
Esophageal mucosa and submucosa
Circular muscle in V-shaped area
(of Laimer)
Right recurrent laryngeal nerve
Longitudinal esophageal muscle
Window cut in longitudinal muscle
exposes circular muscle layer

Posterior view with pharynx
opened and mucosa removed

Fig. 23.1 Muscles of the esophagus (reprinted from Townsend: Sabiston Textbook of Surgery, 18th ed. Copyright © 2007 Saunders, An Imprint of Elsevier)

the 1–2 cm of intrabdominal esophagus. It is recognized endoscopically by the Z-line and the transition to the rugal folds of the stomach. Externally it is recognized when the circular muscle fibers of the esophagus join the oblique fibers of the stomach.

Physiology

Swallowing is comprised of three distinct, yet highly coordinated phases: oral, pharyngeal and esophageal. The oropharyngeal phase takes only 1.5 s but involves six events. These include elevation of the tongue, posterior movement of the tongue, elevation of the soft palate, elevation of the hyoid, elevation of the larynx, and tilting of the epiglottis. The UES will then relax, while posterior pharyngeal constrictors push a food bolus into the esophagus. Utilization of the pressure differential between the positive pressure of the cervical esophagus, and the negative intrathoracic pressure helps mobilize the food bolus into the thoracic esophagus. This is followed by a postrelaxation contraction that initiates peristalsis and prevents reflux into the pharynx. The UES returns to a resting pressure of 60 mmHg as the peristaltic wave propagates into the midesophagus.

The food bolus is brought distally by esophageal peristalsis. Three types of esophageal contractions occur: primary,

secondary, and tertiary. Primary contractions are voluntary and progress at a rate of 2–4 cm/s, generating an intraluminal pressure of 40–80 mmHg. Subsequent swallows will experience peristalsis in a similar fashion, with esophageal relaxation occurring to help maintain coordinated movement. Secondary peristalsis also involves progressive contractions. However, these are usually involuntary, and stimulated by distention or irritation of the esophagus. Tertiary contractions represent uncoordinated contractions of the esophageal smooth muscle and are nonprogressive and nonperistaltic, occurring with both voluntary and involuntary swallow.

The last phase of bolus progression occurs at the LES and requires vagal-mediated relaxation of the LES. This occurs around 1.5–2.5 s after pharyngeal swallowing and lasts for 4–6 s, followed by a postrelaxation contraction to restore the barrier to reflux.

Age Related Changes in the Phrenoesophageal Swallow Mechanism

Age related alterations include an overall slowing that begins at the oropharyngeal swallow mechanism. Patients older than 65 demonstrate significantly attenuated laryngeal and pharyngeal events related to slowed laryngeal vestibule closure, maximal hyolaryngeal excursion, and delayed UES opening. This results in a food bolus spending a greater time adjacent to the airway, causing increased pooling in the pharyngeal recess and a resultant increase risk of aspiration (Fig. 23.2). The resultant airway penetration happens more often and with greater consequences in the elderly [2, 3]. The swallowing mechanism in the elderly is also more sensitive to alterations and disturbances, resulting in an inability to compensate. One such circumstance is placement of a nasogastric tube (NGT). One study demonstrated airway aspiration occurred more frequently when a NGT was placed in patients over 70 [2].

In addition to a mechanical slowing, recent attention has been placed on the central and peripheral neurophysiologic alterations accompanying swallowing [4, 5]. The use of MRIs has demonstrated that slower swallowing is associated with an increase in periventriculiar white matter hyperintensities (PVH's) in the cerebral white matter tracts of normal adults [6]. As one ages, there is an increase in the frequency and degree of PVHs. In addition to the decrease in cerebral blood flow and cerebral atrophy, an increase in PVHs may contribute to a central neurophysiologic alteration in swallowing among the elderly. Alterations in the peripheral nervous system occur as well, and may be related to sarcopenia of the head and neck muscles. Sarcopenia refers to the reduction in muscle mass and cross-sectional areas of muscle, as a result of decreasing number and size of muscle fibers [7–10].

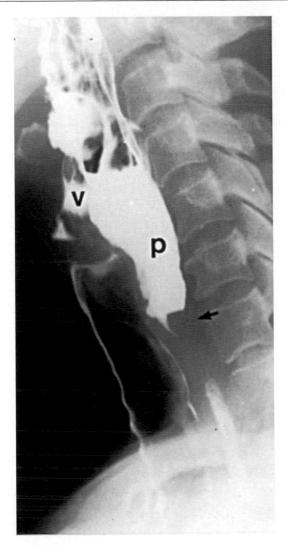

Fig. 23.2 Lateral film from a barium esophagogram in an elderly patient with oropharyngeal dysphagia and cricopharyngeal dysfunction. The film demonstrates a prominent indentation by the cricopharyngeus muscle (*arrow*). Dilatation of the piriform sinuses (*p*) is present, and aspiration of barium into the laryngeal vestibule (*v*) and trachea is well demonstrated (reprinted from Feldman: Sleisenger & Fordtran's Gastrointestinal and Liver Disease, 8th ed. Copyright © 2006 Saunders, An Imprint of Elsevier)

Studies have shown that with aging comes a reduction in tongue musculature, as well as an increase in fatty and connective tissue in the blood vessels of the tongue. Another study demonstrated a replacement of fast (type II) laryngeal muscle fibers with slow (Type I) muscle fibers.

Age Related Changes in Esophageal Contraction

Studies on age related changes of esophageal peristalsis have been conducted since the 1960s. Early studies with

debilitated patients, including those with neurologic disorders and diabetes, claimed that elderly patients had more nonpropulsive contractions, tertiary contractions, esophageal dilation, and delayed esophageal emptying [11, 12]. Reevaluation in 1974 by Hollis and Castel found a decrease in peristaltic amplitude, but no significant change in the speed, duration or incidence of dysmotiltiy in healthy men over 80. More recent data continue to be contradictory, with some supporting normal transit time in the elderly, and others supporting slowed transit time, mostly across the LES.

Evaluation by Richter et al. [13] found that contractile duration remained stable, however distal esophageal amplitude increased significantly each decade until a plateau at age 60. In contrast, Ren et al. [14] and Aly and Abdel-Aty's [15] showed that esophageal transit time was longer with an increased duration across the LES. A recent manometric study evaluating this finding showed a significant decrease in peristaltic wave amplitude, a decrease in LES and UES pressures, and an increased number of failed contractions [16]. In support of this conclusion, a recent Japanese study demonstrated an increasing number of failed peristalsis and synchronous contractions in the elderly, mostly observed with more viscous substances [16–18].

Studies utilizing impedance manometry along with intraesophageal balloon distention, allowing for biomechanical and visceral sensation assessment in the elderly, have demonstrated a significantly larger esophageal lumen. Compliance of the smooth muscle was impaired, whereas no appreciable difference in the striated muscle was noted [19]. Few Studies have evaluated secondary peristalsis, however, Ren et al. demonstrated that this was absent or significantly impaired in healthy elderly individuals (>74) compared to healthy controls (aged 35) [14].

Given the differing patient selection, methods, techniques, and technology of each study, it is difficult to compare them. What can be extrapolated is that patients over the age of 90 have associated comorbidities, which predispose to esophageal motility disorders, making it difficult to distinguish whether age or the associated disease process is causing the alteration. Healthy individuals between 80 and 90 years of age demonstrate esophageal muscle weakness, and associated decrease in the number of enteric neurons, however, the swallow function remains relatively intact. The clinical relevance of observed decreases in the amplitude of peristaltic pressures and increase in nonpropulsive repetitive contractions [18] remains controversial.

Ultimately these changes work in concert with the phrenoesophageal age related changes to alter the swallowing function of the elderly, and may explain the increase in airway aspiration and dysphagia in the elderly. As demonstrated, the above physiologic changes involve both mechanical and neurological components. The mechanical alterations of decreased UES pressure, reduced opening, and delayed relaxation following deglutination [20–22] are complex and poorly defined. Likely, there is an additive effect of age related sarcopenia, central and peripheral neurologic alterations, and decreased esophageal motility, all contributing to the overall slowing of the swallowing mechanism, and possibly placing these patients at increased risk of airway aspiration.

The Stomach

Anatomy

The stomach is a highly distensible organ bound proximally by the LES and distally by the pylorus. It is composed of a series of regions that are difficult to distinguish by gross examination. The uppermost aspect of the stomach is the cardia and connects to the esophagus. Laterally and superiorly, the fundus is attached to the spleen via short gastric vessels. The main portion of the stomach is called the body, and it transitions to the antrum as the stomach makes an angular directional change around the angularis incisura. The stomach is extremely well vascularized, due to blood supply from the left and right gastric arteries supplying the lesser curvature, and left and right gastroepiploic arteries along the greater curvature. Additional supply comes from the inferior phrenic and short gastric arteries. The significant cross connections between these vessels allow the stomach to remain well vascularized even in the face of ligation of three out of four main vessels. Innervation of the stomach is through the left and right vagal trunks, which provide parasympathetic innervation and are involved in both motility and acid secretion.

Physiology

The purpose of the stomach is to initiate digestion of the food bolus, and propulse it into the duodenum for additional digestion and absorption. The stomach accomplishes this through chemical and mechanical digestion. The chemical digestion is secondary to gastric acid degradation. Gastric acid secretion from the parietal cell is stimulated by acetylcholine, histamine, and gastrin. Acetylcholine is released directly from the vagus nerve and parasympathetic ganglion cells. The vagus also innervates G cells which produce gastrin. Gastrin subsequently acts directly on parietal cells to increase acid secretion, and acts indirectly by stimulating the secretion of histamine. Histamine is the most important positive regulator of gastric acid secretion. The acid secretion occurs through three intertwined phases: cephalic, gastric, and intestinal. The cephalic phase begins with thought, sight, smell, or taste of food. When the food bolus enters the gastric lumen, the direct interaction with the microvilli of antral cells leads to gastrin release and the gastric phase. The intestinal phase occurs following the movement of partially digested products into the duodenum. This phase proceeds as long as remnants of food remain within the stomach.

Gastric motility is enabled through both extrinsic controls, such as the parasympathetic and sympathetic nerves, and intrinsic neural mechanisms. Similar to the esophagus, a series of coordinated peristaltic waves act to not only propel the food, but to also grind it in the antrum, thereby mechanically digesting it. During a fasting state, the stomach is mechanically active, exhibiting a series of slow waves and electrical spikes known as the myoelectric migrating complex (MMC). The MMC is likely independent of vagal stimulation as the mechanism remains intact even following vagal denervation. Once food enters the stomach, the resting tone decreases in what is known as receptive relaxation and gastric accommodation, a vagally-mediated action. The food is then propelled against the pylorus in vigorous and short contractions that act to grind the food before it is transported into the duodenum. Emptying of gastric contents occurs according to highly coordinated neuro-hormonal mechanisms. These can be influenced by internal gastric temperature, properties of the food, and psycho-motor influences such as fear and anxiety. Receptors within the duodenum and small bowel are also involved in the feedback loops of gastric emptying.

Gastric Acid Secretion and the Elderly

Recent studies demonstrate that healthy individuals over 90 without atrophic gastritis maintain the ability to secrete acid [23]. Haruma et al. [24] showed that H pylori status was more important than age in determining which patients had hypochlorhydria. H pylori positive patients have an increased number of inflammatory cytokines and a higher incidence of atrophic gastritis, both of which inhibit parietal cells. Recent studies from Japan, evaluating the long term effects of H-pylori, concluded that H-pylori infection, not age, caused atrophic gastritis and intestinal metaplasia [25].

The resultant atrophic gastritis, observed in 50–80% of patients over 80, [26] may cause two problems: bacterial overgrowth and gastric malabsorption. The prevalence of small bowel bacterial overgrowth is around 15.6% in the elderly [27]. This incidence is associated with lower body weights, lower body mass index, lower plasma albumin levels, and a higher degree of diarrhea. The prevalence of gastric malabsorption plays an important role in vitamin B12 absorption.

Kaptan et al. [28] showed that 40% of Vitamin B12 levels returned to normal following treatment of H-pylori. Overall the hypochlorhydria seen in the elderly has been demonstrated to be secondary to H-pylori infection. The recognition and treatment of atrophic gastritis in this patient population is crucial, because the consequences of bacterial overgrowth and gastric malabsorption contribute to malnutrition in the elderly.

Aging and Gastric Emptying

The effective role of aging on gastric emptying remains controversial. The work of Madsen et al. [29, 30] evaluated gastric transit time in healthy individuals over the age of 80 utilizing gamma camera technique. They found no difference in gastric transit time, or frequency of postprandial antral contractions in the healthy elderly population. However, other studies have demonstrated that radiolabeled solids and liquids emptied slower in older patients, even though the change was minimal. One study, using electrogastography and 13C-acetate breath test, comparing active and inactive healthy elderly subjects, showed a decrease in postprandial peristalsis and contractile gastric force within the inactive group [31]. Another report concluded that lipid had a delaying effect on gastric emptying which could be reversed in the elderly by the administration of lipase [32]. In addition, rodent models have shown an age related neurodegeneration of the enteric nervous system along the gastrointestinal tract [33, 34]. The clinical relevance of these minor changes is questionable.

Aging and Gastric Carcinogenesis

The effect of aging on the stomach begins at the cellular level. Studies comparing young and old rodents showed that gastric epithelial cells in older rodents remain in a state of hyperproliferation [35]. This may be related to the finding that less gastric cells undergo apoptosis in older generations [36]. In addition, dietary stimuli have differing affects on the younger and older rodent populations. Holt et al. [37] showed that caloric restriction in older rodents resulted in significantly less apoptotic regulation compared to matched younger rodents. This state of cellular hyperproliferation and decreased apoptosis, along with increased exposures to carcinogens may help explain the increased incidence of gastric cancers later in life. In addition, recent attention has been turned to the increased incidence of mutations of the APC, DCC, and p 53 tumor suppressor genes found in the gastric mucosa of the elderly [38].

The Small Bowel

Anatomy

The small bowel is comprised of the duodenum, jejunum, and ileum. The duodenum begins at the pylorus, and transitions to the jejunum at the ligament of Treitz, as it passes through the mesocolon. There is no obvious demarcation between the jejunum and ileum, however there are some differences that can be appreciated by gross inspection. The jejunum is a larger caliber and thicker than the ileum. Also, arterial arcades within the jejunal mesentery usually number one or two, whereas the blood supply to the ileum may consist of four to five separate arcades.

Physiology

The principle role of the small intestine is the absorption of nutrients, water, and electrolytes. In addition to its length (approximately 300 cm), the small intestine is also invested with an immense amount of surface area secondary to microvilli. Following the initiation of digestion within the stomach, ingested food undergoes additional digestion within the proximal small bowel, secondary to secretion of digestive enzymes into the small bowel lumen. Brush border enzymes also populate the lining of the small bowel, allowing carbohydrates to be digested to their simplest molecular states. The brush border is also responsible for the direct absorption of nutrients from the intestinal lumen into the blood supply. The physiological function of the small intestine has been heavily studied from a histological basis, with little attention focused on the gross physiology. Similar to the esophagus and stomach, motility of the small intestine is mediated via neural and hormonal mechanisms.

Small Bowel Changes with Aging

The small bowel maintains its architecture in the elderly. No alterations at the surface area, villous height, depth, crypt-to-villous ratio, brush border, enterocytes or Brunner glands occur [39]. In addition, the small bowel appears to maintain the ability to absorb nutrients. When patients with renal failure or bacterial overgrowth are excluded from evaluation, elderly subjects show minimal reduction in small bowel absorption [40]. With regard to fat absorption, there are conflicting reports. Some studies show no correlation between aging and 72 h fecal fat excretion. Others demonstrate that fat absorption takes longer in the elderly with consequent postprandial satiety occurring.

The Large Intestine

Anatomy

The transition of the terminal ileum into the cecum marks the beginning of the colon. The ileocecal valve, a semicircular thickening, maintains a unidirectional flow of contents into the colon. At the most inferior end of the cecum lies the appendix, a small tubular shaped organ. The cecum is differentiated from the remainder of the colon in that it has a spherical shape, as opposed to a tubular one. Although distensible, the cecum's shape makes it prone to ischemia and perforation in times of colonic dilatation. Following the cecum, the colon continues as the ascending, then transverse, then descending colon. The partitions are based on fixed positions of the colon at the hepatic and splenic flexures. Both the ascending and descending colon lie in the right and left paracolic gutters respectively, making the colon both a peritoneal and retroperitoneal organ. At the pelvic brim, the descending colon transitions into the sigmoid colon, so named due to its curvaceous course. In contrast to the small intestine, the outer muscular layer of the colon is organized into three distinct muscular bands known as taeniae. At the junction of the sigmoid and rectum, these muscular bands converge to form the outermost layer of the rectum, thereby permitting gross identification. The rectum occupies the pelvic basin and persists for approximately 10–15 cm, before joining with the exterior as the anus.

Physiology

The function of the colon is to reclaim the necessary intestinal constituents back to the body, and then eliminate wastes through stool formation and defacation. Although the small bowel functions to absorb the majority of nutrients, the colon functions to recover the remainder, along with a significant amount of water and electrolytes. In addition to the mucosa, these functions are carried out by an expansive array of microflora that symbiotically exist within the lining and lumen of the colon. The colon receives approximately 1,500 mL of fluid per day, yet stool contains only 10% of this total, indicating a very efficient fluid reabsorption. In addition, sodium is efficiently reabsorbed via cellular active transport mechanisms. The fuel for these mechanisms is derived from colonic bacteria, that produce it from breakdown of dietary fiber. Lack of dietary fiber therefore leads to decreased sodium and water reabsorption and subsequent diarrhea. The colon is also active in recovering any bile acids that are not reabsorbed in the terminal ileum. Bile acids are absorbed passively across the colonic mucosa. However, once capacity is exceeded, colonic flora act to deconjugate the bile acids which interfere with sodium and water reabsorption and result in diarrhea.

The colon may be functionally subdivided into three portions: the right, left, and rectum. The right colon contains the most metabolically active colonic flora and therefore acts as the fermentation chamber of the colon. The left side is involved with absorption of water as stool passes through. Lastly, the rectum is involved in storage and expulsion of stool. Motility of the colon is related to these functional arrangements, in that the right colon experiences antiperistaltic waves to accommodate the retrograde flow into the cecum. The left colon, on the contrary, is involved in forward-propulsive peristalsis aimed at moving the stool bolus forward. A number of factors can increase the colonic transit time, including gender, meal intake, nicotine, and intestinal disease states. An appropriate amount of colonic transit time is necessary to have regular bowel movements. The factors which determine continence are difficult to elucidate. On the one hand, a rectum can become filled with stool, and remain filled with no voluntary contraction of the external sphincter. However, a rectum affected by radiation proctitis, with intact sphincter tone, may empty upon entry of any stool from the sigmoid. The mechanisms are not fully understood, however, and are likely due to an interplay of voluntary, involuntary and sensory innervation.

Age Related Changes in the Colon

One of the most apparent changes in the colon of elderly patients is diverticular disease. Diverticulosis is characterized by the presence of false diverticulae within the colonic wall. The outpouchings of mucosa form between the taenie and may lead to significant complications such as lower gastrointestinal bleeding and perforation. Necropsy-based studies do implicate aging as a primary risk factor for diverticular disease [41]. Separate historical studies confirmed similar results of diverticular disease and aging. There was a prevalence of approximately 13% up to 54 years of age, compared to 40–50% in those over 75 [42, 43]. Much focus has been placed on the role of diet, implicating Western diets lacking in fiber as a primary reason for the development of diverticular disease. A study from Singapore indicates an increase in the prevalence of diverticulosis, possibly due to increased Western influence in local diet [44]. Although most patients will remain asymptomatic, the 10–25% that experience a complication do so at an average age of 62 [45]. In addition to diet, colonic motility has also been implicated in the pathogenesis of diverticulosis. Intraluminal pressure measurements in patients with symptomatic disease have demonstrated abnormal motor and propulsive activities within the affected regions [46].

Table 23.1 Common associations with constipation in the elderly

Nongastrointestinal medical conditions
  Endocrine and metabolic disorders
    Diabetes mellitus
    Hypothyroidsim
    Hyperparathyroidism
    Chronic renal disease
  Electrolyte disturbances
    Hypercalcemia
    Hypokalemia
    Hypermagnesemia
  Neurologic disorders
    Parkinson disease
    Multiple sclerosis
    Autonomic neuropathy
    Spinal cord lesions
    Dementia
  Myopathic disorders
    Amyloidosis
    Scleroderma
  Other
    Depression
    General disability
Medications
  Analgesics (opiates, tramadol, NSAIDs)
  Anticholinergic agents
  Calcium channel blockers
  Tricyclic antidepressants
  Antiparkinsonian drugs (dopaminergic agents)
  Antacids (calcium and aluminum)
  Calcium supplements
  Bile acid binders
  Iron supplements
  Antihistamines
  Diuretics (furosemide, hydrochlorothiazide)
  Iron supplements
  Antipsychotics (phenothiazine derivatives)
  Anticonvulsants

Source: Bouras and Tangalos [117]

Constipation is another entity that is subject to intestinal motility (Table 23.1). The prevalence of constipation increases with age: from 4.5% in those 65–74 years old to 10.2% in those 75 years and older. Motility of the intestinal tract is determined by neuro-hormonal mechanisms. The innervation is dependent on both extrinsic and intrinsic sources. Extrinsic innervation includes parasympathetic preganglionic fibers and postganglionic sympathetic fibers. There is no definitive evidence of age-related changes of the extrinsic innervation of the intestinal tract. Intrinsic nerves, which regulate the action of smooth muscle cells within the colon, have been implicated in age-related alteration. Human studies have demonstrated that there exists an age-related loss of inhibitory nerve input to the circular smooth muscle of the colon [47, 48]. This decrease of inhibitory input may play a central role in the development of constipation in the elderly by preventing the normal colonic relaxation or decreasing the normal inhibition of nonpropogating colonic contractions. Lastly, appropriate relaxation of smooth muscle is dependent on adequate smooth muscle number and function. There is little evidence implicating myopathy as an age-related reason for abnormal intestinal motility. In any case, studies have demonstrated an age-related decrease in left sided transit of colonic material, specifically in the recto-sigmoid region [49]. The cause of constipation in the elderly is likely due to a superimposition of chronic disease, such as diabetes mellitus, opiate use, polypharmacy, and dietary changes to subtle physiological changes. In many patients, the exact cause remains unclear.

Fecal incontinence also appears to increase with age. Although it is infrequently brought to the attention of physicians and caregivers, the incidence is estimated to be up to 18% in those aged 65 or older [50]. Similar to constipation and colonic motility, it is unclear whether fecal incontinence in the elderly is subject to changes in the anal sphincter or by secondary diseases that affect sphincter function. Studies have demonstrated that anal canal and sphincter pressures decrease with age, however, an overwhelming majority of patients with fecal incontinence are also found to have concurrent neurological diseases, diabetes, prior trauma, or cognitive impairment [51]. Anal manometry helps to determine the level of sphincter tone, anal canal pressure and maximal squeeze pressure. Moreover, patients with fecal incontinence must be investigated to rule out overflow incontinence, which occurs secondary to rectal impaction or loss of sphincter tone. In these patients, evacuation of the rectal vault will usually improve fecal incontinence.

Elderly patients are also at an increased risk of various forms of colitis. Epidemiological studies of inflammatory bowel disease patients, including ulcerative colitis and Crohn's colitis, have determined that there is a bimodal distribution amongst age groups. The peaks in incidence occure between ages 15 and 30, and 55 and 80. The etiology of each has yet to be determined; however ,a number of factors have been implicated including family history, exposure to antigens, and possible infectious etiologies. Other significant colitis presentations in the elderly include inflammatory, infectious and ischemic colitis. NSAID use may independently lead to inflammatory colitis, or may exacerbate ulcerative colitis, or Crohn's colitis. NSAIDs are well known causal agents of ulcers and other complications in the foregut, but they may also lead to ulceration, bleeding, perforation, or stricture within the colon [52, 53]. NSAID-induced inflammatory colitis in the elderly may present as acute or chornic inflammation. The most common presentation of infectious colitis in the elderly population is secondary to *C. difficile*. This spore-producing bacteria can survive in an inactive form for significant amounts of time in hospitals, nursing homes, and extended care facilities. The bacteria is normally present within the colonic flora; however, the growth of the active organism is usually suppressed by other bacteria of the colon. Administration of antibiotics may suppress the colonic flora that inhibit the proliferation of *C. difficile*, thereby predisposing to *C. difficile* toxin-induced diarrhea and possible colitis. Although possible at any age, the elderly are predisposed to *C. difficile* colitis due to antibiotic use, concomitant medical conditions, and living arrangements within medical facilities. Ischemic colitis results from inadequate blood supply to the colon. Factors that predispose a patient to ischemic colitis include vascular, cardiogenic or coagulopathic states happen to occur in the elderly with increased frequency [54]. Considering the increased incidence of diabetes and hypertension among the elderly, ischemic colitis is significantly more prevalent in this population. The condition is less likely to result from large vessel disease or thrombosis, but is more likely to occur from transient hypotension or dehydration, which may result from an episode of illness or malnutrition [55].

The Liver and Hepatobiliary System

Liver Anatomy

The liver is the largest solid organ in the body, extending from the level of the nipples to slightly below the costal margin. The horizontal axis spans the right hemidiaphragm and a portion of the left hemidiaphragm. Liver anatomy is determined

according to the Couinaud nomenclature, rather than historic classifications based on external topography (Fig. 23.3). The gross anatomical landmarks include the ligamentum teres (round ligament of the liver), which appears to divide the liver into a small left and larger right lobe. However, the anatomic classification divides the left and right lobe of the liver based on Cantlie's line, which represents the plane of the middle hepatic vein, and the primary bifurcation of the portal vein. Cantlie's line can also be visualized as the plane extending from the gallbladder fossa to the inferior vena cava. The liver receives dual vascularization from the portal and systemic vasculature. The portal vein, hepatic artery, and biliary ductal system generally run in parallel, each bifurcating just before entry into the hilum and sending major branches to each hepatic lobe. Couinaud's functional anatomical classification divides the liver into eight segments according to the anatomic relation of portal vein and hepatic vein branches [56]. This results in a functional and anatomical collection of eight subsegments.

Liver Physiology

The liver is vital to a number of processes aimed at maintaining health and homeostasis. The functions of the liver include detoxification, protein synthesis, bile acid synthesis, storage of substances, and metabolism of proteins, carbohydrates and lipids. Toxins, both internally produced and externally acquired, are filtered from the blood through the action of the liver.

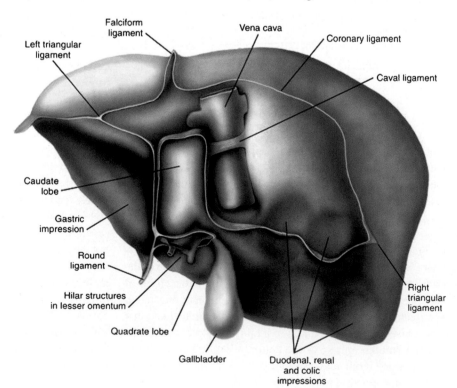

Fig. 23.3 Posterior view of the liver. The shape of the liver is determined by molding against adjacent organs (reprinted from Feldman: Sleisenger & Fordtran's Gastrointestinal and Liver Disease, 8th ed. Copyright © 2006 Saunders, An Imprint of Elsevier)

Toxins are cleared through a series of enzymatic reactions that render the toxins water or fat-soluble, thereby allowing for their secretion in urine or bile. Furthermore, the liver produces the bile that acts as a vehicle of export for various offending agents.

In addition to toxins, bile also transports bilirubin, cholesterol, bile salts, and phospholipids to the intestinal tract for excretion. Moreover, bile acids are required in the digestion of fats, thereby facilitating their absorption. Approximately 500–1,000 mL of bile is secreted per day. Nearly all of the bile acids that are excreted into the intestines are reclaimed by hepatocytes, thereby preventing their loss into the systemic circulation. The hepatocytes reconjugate the extracted product into the formation of new bile, thereby completing the circuit. This is referred to as the enterohepatic circulation of bile acids. The rate of new bile acid formation is therefore dependent on the rate of intestinal reabsorption and hepatocyte extraction. At the level of hepatocytes, bile is formed by the oxidation of cholesterol. Dietary intake and availability of lipoprotein carriers also affect cholesterol metabolism. Although insoluble in water, cholesterol remains soluble in bile if the relative concentrations of bile salts and phospholipids are maintained within certain limits. Supersaturation and crystallization of cholesterol can occur, which can be a prelude to gallstone formation.

The liver is also a central point in the metabolism of carbohydrates. The liver manages the surplus or deficit of metabolic fuels by engaging in storage or distribution of glucose. Both the liver and muscle are capable of glucose storage, however, only the liver is involved in the conversion of glycogen to glucose for systemic use. Other catabolic functions of the liver include gluconeogenesis and ketogenesis. Anabolic functions of the liver include glycogenesis and synthesis of plasma proteins, such as albumin, transferrin, haptoglobin, and numerous coagulation factors.

Age Related Changes in Hepatic Function

As a person ages, the liver undergoes "brown atrophy," which is caused by accumulation of pigmented lipofuscin granules in hepatocytes and Kupffer cells. These granules are thought to be the depository of residues, predominantly exogenous dietary contaminants, that the liver cannot metabolize. The pertinent morphologic and physiologic changes are summarized in Table 23.2. On an average, liver weight is decreased 6.5% in males and 14.3% in females [57]. The absolute number of hepatic lobules remains constant, but they undergo a decrease in the size of each lobule. Consequently, the number of hepatocytes decreases, yet each hepatocyte assumes an increased volume. Postmortem liver tissue analysis in subjects over 60 years old demonstrates decreased microsomal

Table 23.2 Morphologic and physiologic changes observed in the liver of elderly persons

Parameter	Change with age	Functional impact
Organ size (absolute and relative)	↓	None
Hepatocyte number	↓	None
Cell volume, ploidy, organelle constituents	↑	None
Hepatic blood flow	↓	min↓
Liver function tests	No change	None
Metabolic function	No significant change?	None

↑ increased; ↓ decreased; ? not proven or consistent
Source: adapted with permission from Sherman and Brunicardi [1]

enzyme activity, and a decreased hepatic concentration of smooth endoplasmic reticulum [58]. Furthermore, the number of mitochondria per hepatocyte decreases with [59]. Although these are not very significant changes on their own, when coupled with a decreased hepatic blood flow, this may account for a reduced capacity for metabolism of certain drugs and toxins. Hepatic blood flow, measured with dye clearance tests, shows a corresponding decrease with age at an estimated 0.3–1.5% decline per year. Reduced blood flow is attributed to the diminution of hepatic parenchymal mass with aging. As a result of this decline, individuals aged 65 years have 40–45% less total hepatic blood flow than they had at age 25 [60].

Examination of human and rat hepatocytes has provided insight into mechanisms of impaired drug metabolism by the aging liver. Hepatocytes isolated from young and old rats and humans demonstrated no difference in rates of oxidative phase I drug metabolism and phase II conjugation reactions [61]. In contrast, in vivo rates of oxidative phase I drug metabolism was impaired in older rats, yet glucuronidation was preserved [62]. A possible explanation for these observations is that older animals experience a degree of hypoxia. The decreased oxygen delivery may be a result of the creation of a diffusion barrier secondary to pseudocapillarization of hepatic sinusoids. The sinusoids of older rats has been found to have thicker endothelium, and increased deposition of type IV collagen. Therefore, the pseudocapillarization and subsequent relative hypoxia in older rats may have implications for elderly humans. That is, this finding may impact drug therapy in the elderly, specifically those drugs whose clearance involves undergoing oxidative metabolism [63].

Despite the aforementioned changes the liver undergoes with normal aging, the result is little to no significant clinical impairment. Several studies have documented that standard liver function tests (LFTs) do not vary significantly with increasing age alone [64, 65]. Therefore, presence of abnormal liver chemistries in the elderly should not be considered normal, and investigation of possible hepatobiliary disease should be undertaken. Regardless, standard

LFTs – including serum bilirubin, aminotransferases, and alkaline phosphatase – do not reflect the true dynamic function of the liver. To this end, other study techniques have been used to assess liver function. Prior studies investigating hepatic clearance or retention in the elderly have been controversial and conflicting, requiring control for multiple comorbid diseases, medications, and decreased hepatic blood flow [64–66]. To date, the most definitive study is that of Kampmann and associates, which demonstrated no significant variation in retention of anionic dyes in 43 carefully selected patients aged 50–88 years, when compared with younger persons [67].

Studies in old rats have demonstrated that although hepatic regeneration following hepatectomy is slower, these livers will eventually achieve their original volume [68]. In humans, clinical data has also demonstrated the longevity of aging livers through results garnered from liver transplants. Five patients whose transplanted livers were from donor patients over 80 years old, experienced similar clinical outcomes to the group ($n=35$) that received livers from patients under 80 years old [69]. In terms of function, synthesis of most hepatic proteins remains intact with some impaired catabolism. Also, the activities of certain hepatic enzymes necessary for cholesterol metabolism are thought to be affected by the aging process. These age-related changes in hepatic enzyme activity may well be contributing factors in the pathogenesis of gallstone formation in the elderly.

Biliary Anatomy

After being secreted by the hepatocyte, bile drains along canaliculi that form into progressively larger intrahepatic ducts. These continue to coalesce within each lobe to form the right and left lobar ducts, which then exit the hilum and join to form the common hepatic duct (CHD). The CHD, in its course to the intestine, becomes the common bile duct (CBD) once it joins with the cystic duct from the gallbladder. The gallbladder is a pear-shaped, blind-ended, organ lying on the inferior surface of the liver that receives and drains bile through the cystic duct. The CBD then courses towards the second portion of the duodenum, where it empties into the ampulla of Vater within the duodenal wall. Shortly before entering the duodenum, the CBD also joins with the pancreatic duct, although variations to this anatomy are common. The sphincter of Oddi is a complex muscular structure surrounding the distal portions of the CBD, main pancreatic duct, and ampulla of Vater that is separate from the duodenal musculature. This sphincter coordinates appropriate release of biliary and pancreatic secretions during a meal, while preventing harmful reflux of duodenal contents into the CBD.

Biliary Physiology

The purpose of the gallbladder is to store and concentrate bile during the fasting state. Following ingestion of a meal, the secretion of gastrointestinal hormones such as secretin, gastrin, and CCK results in the release of bile from the gallbladder into the intestinal tract. Although the gallbladder generally holds only 40–50 mL of bile, its remarkable absorptive capacity allows it to accommodate the 500–1,000 mL of bile produced by the liver each day [56]. The mucosa of the gallbladder performs this function by absorbing significantly more sodium and water than cholesterol and calcium. As the concentration of calcium increases in bile, it also affects the solubility of cholesterol. In turn, the increased concentrations of cholesterol and calcium may result in precipitation and creation of gallstones.

Between meals, the gallbladder passively fills with bile that is continuously produced by the liver. With the sphincter of Oddi contracted, the pressure within the CBD increases above that of the gallbladder lumen, thereby facilitating passive movement of bile into the cystic duct. Periodically, a small amount of bile (10–30%) is released from the gallbladder. This process of partial emptying and filling seems to be coordinated with late phase II and phase III activity of the MMC, which is associated with increases in plasma concentrations of the hormone motilin [66]. The turnover of gallbladder bile during fasting may serve as a mechanism to prevent or expel cholesterol crystals prior to macroscopic stone formation.

Following a meal of fatty acids or amino acids, vagal stimulation and CCK result in contraction of the gallbladder and the release of approximately 50–70% of the stored bile. The presence of intraluminal gastric acid, fatty acids, and certain amino acids triggers the release of CCK from epithelial cells in the proximal intestine, primarily in the duodenum. In addition to the release of bile from the gallbladder, CCK also impacts the contraction and relaxation of the sphincter of Oddi. This coordinated reflex allows flow of bile and pancreatic juice into the duodenum to aid in the digestive process. At physiologic levels, CCK seems to influence vagal cholinergic innervation of the gallbladder by means of CCK-A receptors on postganglionic neurons [70]. This neurohumoral interaction may provide control of basal gallbladder smooth muscle tone, and coordination of postprandial gallbladder contraction.

Biliary Function in the Elderly

Similar to the liver, the gallbladder undergoes minor changes with aging. There is little effect on size, contractility, or absorptive capacity (Table 23.3). The effect of a decreased

Table 23.3 Morphologic and physiologic changes observed in the biliary system of elderly persons

Parameter	Change with age
Bile duct size	↑
Gallbladder contractility	No change
Gallbladder absorptive capacity	No change
Cholecystokinin plasma levels	↑
Gallbladder cholecystokinin sensitivity	↓
Cholelithiasis incidence	↑
Bile cholesterol saturation	↑

↑ increased; ↓ decreased; ? not proven or consistent
Source: adapted with permission from Sherman and Brunicardi [1]

Table 23.4 Prevalence of gallstones at autopsy in women in various countries

Age (years)	Prevalence of gallstones (%)			
	UK [118]	USA [75]	Sweden [76]	Chile [77]
10–19	–	0	–	7.2
20–29	6.8	4.2	14.3	25.1
30–39	–	8.6	16.7	26.4
40–49	9.7	12.1	15.0	46.5
50–59	28.0	23.3	27.6	55.6
60–69	31.5	27.5	40.0	65.3
70–79	33.6	30.6	52.7	63.7
80–89	42.6	34.9	51.9	77.1
90+	42.7	44.4	58.4	–

Sources: data from Bateson [15], Lieber [76], Lindström [77], and Marinovic et al. [78]
The table illustrates the geographic variation of gallstone disease and increasing prevalence with advancing age. This table is reprinted with permission from Sherman and Brunicardi [1]

responsiveness to CCK may not have clinical significance. Khalil and colleagues demonstrated that gallbladder sensitivity to CCK decreases with age, but fasting and fat-stimulated plasma levels of CCK are significantly higher in older individuals. These physiologic alterations appear to offset each other functionally, as the rate of gallbladder emptying in the elderly is similar to that of younger individuals [71]. The age-related increase in serum concentration of pancreatic polypeptide may also depress gallbladder emptying, however the data to date is conflicting and further studies are needed to clarify the role of this hormone in hepatobiliary function in the elderly [72].

The most significant age-related change involving the hepatobiliary system involves the CBD. Namely, the duct increases in size, in a similar fashion to the pancreatic duct. One study by Nagase and associates used intravenous cholangiography to measure the CBD size in 84 healthy Japanese persons and documented a mean diameter of 9.2 mm at age 70, compared to 6.8 mm at age 20 [73]. Other studies have confirmed the upper normal size of the CBD as 10 mm in patients over 75 years old, and 14 mm post cholecystectomy [74]. The distal portion of the CBD and the sphincter of Oddi become progressively narrower with age, possibly predisposing to stone impaction, nevertheless, biliary obstruction in older adults is usually due to malignancy rather than to choledocholithiasis. The most common malignancy is adenocarcinoma of the pancreas, but may be caused by other malignancies such as ampullary, gallbladder, bile duct, duodenal, and metastatic cancers. Benign strictures can result from cholangitis or common duct injuries. Primary sclerosing cholangitis is rare in those older than 65 years of age.

Gallstone Pathogenesis

Epidemiological studies have shown that cholesterol gallstones occur infrequently in adolescence, and the presence increases linearly with age (Table 23.4) [75–79]. The incidence of gallstones increases approximately 1–3% per year [80].

Recent studies have even indicated that the incidence of gallstones in females approaches 50% by age 70 [81]. In fact, the most common abdominal operation performed in the geriatric population is cholecystectomy, with the total number of cases performed annually for nonfederal inpatients 65 years of age and over approximating 161,000 [79]. Furthermore, the risk of complications from gallstone disease is increased in elderly patients, with an increased incidence of CBD obstruction, perforation, and gangrene [82].

Gallstones are classified according to their cholesterol content as either cholesterol stones or pigment stones. Pigment stones are further classified as black or brown. In the United States, gallstones are most commonly composed of cholesterol (70–80%) with pigment stones accounting for the remaining 20–30% [56].

Cholesterol Gallstone Pathogenesis

Three independent but mutually inclusive processes appear to be necessary for gallstone formation: (1) cholesterol supersaturation; (2) nucleation (also known as crystallization); and (3) stone growth. Excess biliary cholesterol can result from hypersecretion of cholesterol with a normal bile acid pool, or with normal cholesterol secretion in conjunction with a diminished bile acid pool. Therefore, cholesterol supersaturation can be produced by decreased activity of cholesterol 7-α-hydroxylase (decreasing the conversion of hepatic cholesterol to bile acids), overactivity of HMG-CoA reductase (the rate-controlling enzyme in the synthesis of cholesterol), or terminal ileal disease or resection (interrupting the enterohepatic conservation of bile acids).

Cholesterol supersaturation alone is a common finding in normal patients free of biliary pathology [83, 84]. Nucleation, or the precipitation of supersaturated bile cholesterol into solid cholesterol monohydrate crystals, usually occurs due to a combination of depressed biliary kinetics and procrystallizing protein action on the bile. Nucleation time, the rate at which cholesterol crystals form, is decreased from approximately 15 days in control patients free of biliary disease, to 3 days in patients with gallstones [85]. Concentration of bile within the gallbladder causes the formation of large, cholesterol-rich multilamellar vesicles that can precipitate cholesterol crystals. Also, concentration of calcium salts within the gallbladder leading to saturation may serve as a nidus for nucleation.

Lastly, the gallstone attains clinical significance when its size grows to the point at which it causes an obstruction of the biliary system. Macroscopic stone formation from cholesterol crystals results from progressive enlargement of individual crystals with deposition of insoluble material onto its outer surface or by fusion of crystals into a larger conglomerate. However, patients may also present with typical biliary disease symptoms, without expected radiological findings such as definitive stones. This biliary "sludge," also known as biliary microlithiasis, is a precipitation of cholesterol crystals and calcium bilirubinate granules in bile with a high mucin content, not infrequently observed in states of prolonged bowel rest or with use of total parenteral nutrition (TPN). Nevertheless, the pathogenesis of cholesterol gallstones is clearly multifactorial (Table 23.5).

The subtle age-related changes of the liver and biliary system, namely gallbladder mucosal function and contractility, play key roles in lithogenesis. Gallbladder hypomotility, with infrequent or incomplete emptying of the gallbladder contents, may predispose to bile stasis and crystal formation. As previously discussed, gallbladder kinetics are decreased in the elderly population, thereby increasing the risk of development of cholelithiasis. It is also important to consider other mechanisms that predispose to cholelithiasis, that may be present within a comorbid illness in the elderly patient.

Table 23.5 Factors contributing to cholesterol gallstone formation

Cholesterol supersaturation
Cholesterol hypersecretion
Diminished bile acid pool
Ileal disease or resection
Nucleation
Mucin glycoproteins
Pronucleating substances: phospholipase C, fibronectin
Nucleation-inhibiting substances: apolipoprotein A1
Calcium concentration
Gallbladder dysmotility
Altered cholecystokinin (CCK) plasma levels or receptors
Neurohumoral influences: CCK somatostatin, estrogen
Vagolysis, mechanical or functional

Source: adapted with permission from Sherman and Brunicardi [1]

For instance, the elderly patient may require TPN, which further delays gallbladder emptying. Another notable condition that may predispose a patient to gallstone formation is rapid weight loss, which may be due to poor dietary intake or chronic illness [86].

Pigment Gallstone Pathogenesis

Pigment stones are formed by the precipitation of bilirubin in bile, which, like cholesterol, is insoluble in water. Bilirubin becomes soluble within the liver, where it is conjugated, although a small percentage (3%) remains unconjugated. In healthy patients, this is inconsequential. Hyperparathyroidism may predispose a patient to pigment stones by increasing the level of ionized calcium. Pigment stones may also occur secondary to an increase in unbound bilirubinate. This is due to chronic hemolysis (cirrhosis or sickle cell disease), or increased synthesis of unconjugated bilirubin as a result of increased activity of β-glucuronidase (which converts conjugated bilirubin to unconjugated) [87]. When an increase in insoluble bilirubin comes into contact with insoluble calcium, a black pigment stone of solid consistency forms. Brown pigment stones are more common in Asian populations and are associated with chronic biliary tract infections or bile stasis. They are almost always associated with colonization of bile by *E. coli*, *Bacteroides* or *Clostridium* [88]. The stones are much more fragile than cholesterol or black pigment stones, crumbling readily when manipulated. Brown pigment stones are usually found in the bile ducts where β-glucuronidase produced by bacteria hydrolyzes conjugated bilirubin to the free form, a hydrophobic solute that readily combines with calcium to produce a nidus for gallstone formation.

Lithogenic Factors in the Elderly

A multitude of factors is responsible for the increased incidence of gallstones in the elderly. Ahlberg and associates demonstrated age-associated changes of biliary cholesterol saturation and bile acid kinetics in a group of nonobese, normolipidemic subjects known to be gallstone-free [89]. Specifically, this investigation was able to show a direct correlation between advancing age and increasing cholesterol saturation of bile, presumably due to an increased rate of hepatic cholesterol secretion (Fig. 23.4). Additionally, bile acid synthesis and pool sizes were noted to decrease with advancing age (Fig. 23.5). Each of these changes contributes to the enhanced lithogenicity of bile in the elderly. In terms of whether changes in hepatocyte enzyme activity for HMG-CoA reductase and 7-α-reductase influence lithogenicity, results have been inconclusive [89, 90].

To explore whether aging increases cholesterol supersaturation of bile and gallstone prevalence, Wang studied age-related changes in hepatic and biliary lipid metabolism in gallstone-susceptible and resistant mice of varying ages [81]. The rats were fed a lithogenic diet for 8 weeks ,and then evaluated for gallstone prevalence, gallbladder size, biliary lipid secretion, and HMG-CoA reductase activity.

These outcomes were all increased in the gallstone-susceptible mice. Furthermore, increasing age augmented biliary secretion and intestinal absorption of cholesterol, reduced hepatic synthesis and biliary secretion of bile salts, and decreased biliary contractility, all of which increased susceptibility to cholesterol gallstones in susceptible mice. The research concluded that aging was an independent risk factor for cholesterol gallstone formation.

Furthermore, gallbladder stasis may play an active role in the formation of gallstones. Factors that may lead to gallbladder dysmotility in older patients include increasing saturation of bile with cholesterol, and altered sensitivity of the gallbladder smooth muscle to CCK. Reviews of CCK receptor stimulants, motilin agonists, and procholinergic agents provide encouragement for emerging pharmacotherapy as treatment options for gallbladder hypomotility [85, 91].

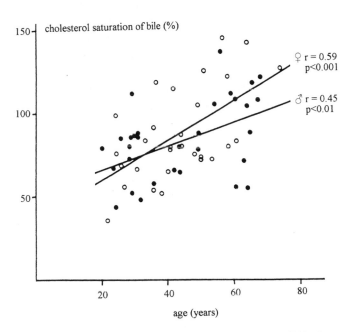

Fig. 23.4 Relation between age and cholesterol saturation of bile. Open symbols denote women, and closed circles denote men (from Einarsson et al. [116]. © Massachusetts Medical Society, with permission)

Pancreas

Anatomy

The pancreas is a retroperitoneal organ in the upper abdomen, posterior to the stomach. During the fourth week of gestation, two buds develop from the duodenum, a hepatic diverticulum and a dorsal bud. The anterior bud develops into the liver and biliary system, while the dorsal bud eventually forms the body and tail of the pancreas. During the 32nd week of gestation, the hepatic diverticulum gives rise to the ventral bud, which ultimately forms the uncinate process. It then

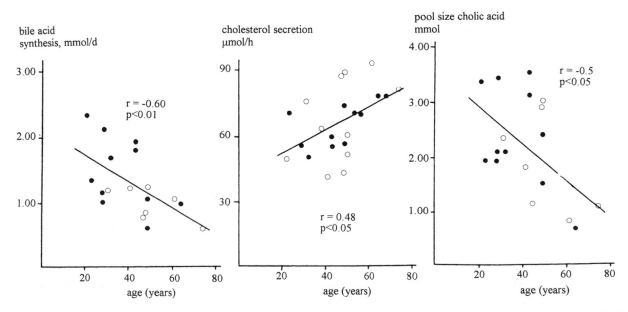

Fig. 23.5 Relation between age and hepatic cholesterol secretion, total bile acid synthesis, and size of the cholic acid pool. Open circles denote women, and closed circles denote men (from Einarsson et al. [116]. © Massachusetts Medical Society, with permission)

rotates 180° clockwise around the duodenum, and fuses with the dorsal pancreatic bud to form the mature pancreas. The main pancreatic duct of Wirsung, formed by fusion of the ventral duct and the distal portion of the dorsal pancreatic duct, drains most of the pancreas into the duodenum at the ampulla of Vater. The diameter of the main pancreatic duct is 2.0–3.5 mm in healthy young adults [92]. The CBD joins with the main pancreatic duct at the ampulla of Vater and empties through the greater duodenal papilla. The proximal ductal system of the dorsal bud persists as the accessory pancreatic duct of Santorini, draining the superior portion of the pancreatic head via the lesser papilla into the duodenum proximal to the greater papilla.

Physiology

The pancreas has dual functions, both exocrine and endocrine. The exocrine activity is geared towards facilitating digestion, neutralizing gastric acid, and regulating intraintestinal pH. Pancreatic endocrine activity is vital for glucose homeostasis. Because of the great functional reserve of this organ, 90% of pancreatic function can be lost before signs of insufficiency become clinically evident [93].

Exocrine Function

The exocrine pancreas accounts for approximately 85% of the total mass and produces 500 mL of secretions per day. The acinar cells of the pancreas secrete enzymes responsible for digestion, and centroacinar cells and the ductal system direct the exocrine secretions to the duodenum, modifying the electrolyte concentration and water content of the pancreatic fluid as it passes. The acinar cells are innervated by the sympathetic and parasympathetic nervous systems. The parasympathetic system increases secretions, whereas the sympathetic system inhibits them [94]. The enzymes produced by the acinar cells include amylase (isoamylase type P), lipase, trypsinogen, chymotrypsinogen, procarboxypeptidases A and B, deoxyribonuclease, ribonuclease, proelastase, and trypsin inhibitor.

Similar to gastric acid secretion, pancreatic juices are secreted in a cephalic, gastric, and intestinal phase. The cephalic phase accounts for 10–15% of meal-stimulated pancreatic secretion, and may be mediated by direct stimulation and increased gastric acid secretion in the stomach, which indirectly stimulates pancreatic secretion due to duodenal acidification and secretin release. The gastric phase also accounts for 10–15% of meal-stimulated pancreatic secretion, and is due to gastric distention brought on by the ingested meal. The increase in gastric acid leads to duodenal

acidification, which triggers the release of secretin. This, in turn, leads to pancreatic secretions aimed at raising the pH. Pancreatic secretions are alkaline, and have a pH that varies from 7.6 to 9.0, depending on the rate of bicarbonate secretion from the ductal epithelium. This alkaline pH is necessary to maintain the inactive proteolytic enzymes, and transport them to the appropriate acidic milieu of the duodenum where they undergo activation. Secretin is the major stimulant for pancreatic electrolyte and water secretion, with CCK, gastrin, and peripherally released acetylcholine acting as weaker stimulants. Lastly, the intestinal phase is secondary to food and gastric contents entering the proximal intestine, which again increases secretin release. Dietary fats and proteins in the duodenum also stimulate the release of CCK, which then stimulates acinar secretion. The intestinal phase is the most important determinant of pancreatic secretion.

In addition to the water and electrolyte secretions, the exocrine pancreas secretes major proteolytic enzymes, such as trypsin. It is initially secreted in an inactive form, but activated within the duodenum by increasing acidity and enterokinase, a hormone produced by duodenal mucosa. Only amylase is secreted directly from the acinus in an active form. The other enzymes are initially secreted as inactive proenzymes, requiring trypsin and the acidic environment of the duodenum for activation. Inappropriate early activation of enzymatic action can result in autodigestion of the pancreatic substance, as may be seen in acute pancreatitis. The protein, fat and carbohydrate constituents of diet alter the absolute amount and ratio of enzymes secreted. Regulation of enzyme secretion is primarily through the hormone CCK and acetylcholine. Secretin, vasoactive intestinal peptide (VIP), and pancreatic islet hormones weakly stimulate acinar secretion [93].

Endocrine Function

The main physiologic function of the endocrine pancreas is the regulation of energy through the hormonal regulation of carbohydrate metabolism. This is achieved via the islets of Langerhans, clusters of specialized endocrine cells which are scattered throughout the exocrine tissue. Most islets contain approximately 3,000–4,000 cells, consisting of four major cell types: alpha cells which secrete glucagon, beta cells which secrete insulin, delta cells which secrete somatostatin, and PP or F cells which secrete pancreatic polypeptide.

The predominant and most studied pancreatic hormone is insulin. Insulin secretion occurs in response to elevated blood glucose levels, and is suppressed by hypoglycemia. Insulin secretion is greater in response to orally administered glucose than intravenous glucose, even when serum glucose levels are equal. Insulin secretion occurs in two phases, the first being the release of stored insulin. The second phase is longer and related to the sustained release of newly produced insulin. Type I diabetes results from a combination of genetic, environmental and autoimmune factors ,which lead to selective destruction of β-cells. The endocrine tissue of the pancreas has excellent reserve, thereby requiring destruction of at least 80% of the tissue before clinical manifestations are evident.

Insulin binds to specific membrane-associated glycoprotein receptors that effect an increase in membrane-bound glucose transporters (GLUT-1 to GLUT-5), thereby facilitating glucose transport from the blood into cells. Skeletal muscle accounts for the majority of insulin-mediated glucose uptake, and impaired insulin action at the level of the muscle is the cause of insulin resistance in type II diabetes [95]. In the liver, insulin facilitates glycogen deposition, while inhibiting gluconeogenesis and glycogenolysis, resulting in a net increase in glucose uptake. Insulin also promotes lipogenesis and protein synthesis. As part of the insulin resistance syndrome, malfunction of insulin at the level of the liver can lead to abnormal lipid accumulation in hepatocytes, leading to nonalcoholic steatohepatitis (NASH) [96].

Glucagon's purpose is to counteract the effects of insulin and increase the concentration of blood glucose. Similar to insulin, glucose is the primary regulator of glucagon secretion, although with glucagon, it causes an inhibitory effect. Furthermore, insulin and somatostatin also serve as negative regulators of glucagon secretion. Secretion is stimulated by hypoglycemia, acetylcholine, and generalized stressed states such as occur with infection, trauma, or inflammation. Glucagon promotes an elevation of blood glucose levels, with mobilization of intracellular fuels by hepatic glycogenolysis, gluconeogenesis, ketogenesis, and lipolysis. It is the provision of metabolic fuels during times of stress, that resulted in glucagon being grouped with epinephrine, cortisol, and growth hormone as stress hormones.

Endocrine release of somatostatin occurs during a meal, in response to intraluminal fat. However, its exact role in the pancreas remains unclear, but it has been shown to inhibit the release of almost all peptide hormones, and to inhibit gastric, pancreatic, and biliary secretion. Some researchers have suggested that somatostatin may regulate adjacent islet cell functions, but this has not been proven in vivo. The potent inhibitory effects of somatostatin and octreotide, a long-acting synthetic analogue, have been used to treat a variety of endocrine and exocrine disorders.

Pancreatic polypeptide's (PP) most important roles may be as a mediator of the hepatic response to insulin. It has been demonstrated that abnormal glucose homeostasis associated with PP deficiency in patients with chronic pancreatitis is due to impaired suppression of hepatic glucose production by insulin [97]. This relative hepatic resistance to insulin is a consequence of diminished insulin receptor concentration, rather than altered receptor affinity, and can be ameliorated by administration of PP [98]. This mechanism of glucose metabolism has been further clarified by studies suggesting that hepatic insulin resistance in chronic pancreatitis is due to impaired transcription of the insulin receptor gene. Additionally, PP increases hepatic insulin-binding sites perhaps by upregulating insulin receptor gene expression [99]. PP is known to inhibit pancreatic exocrine secretion, choleresis, and motilin release [100]. PP release is augmented by cholinergic stimulation, with the normal postprandial rise in PP levels being ablated by vagotomy, antrectomy, or both [93].

PP is part of the polypeptide-fold family of peptide hormones, along with the central nervous system peptide, neuropeptide Y and peptide tyrosine-tyrosine (PYY). Each of these is believed to play an important role in the regulation of appetite. PP was the first of these hormones to be isolated, from an impure insulin extraction. PP functions as a component of the "ileal brake" since it acts in various ways to slow the transit of food through the gut. It delays gastric emptying, attenuates pancreatic exocrine secretion, and inhibits gallbladder contraction [101]. The role of PP in obesity is undergoing increasing investigation. Preliminary data suggest that PP reduced postprandial secretion is associated with obesity, whereas elevated postprandial levels of PP are found in patients with anorexia nervosa [102].

Pancreatic Anatomy in the Elderly

The pancreas undergoes an aging process resulting in minimal amounts of atrophy, fatty infiltration, and fibrosis. One of the main age-related changes occurs with ductal anatomy, specifically an increase in the caliber of the main pancreatic duct and ectasia of branched ducts. One review by Kreel and Sandin of in situ retrograde pancreatography at necropsy in 120 subjects older than 30 years revealed the main pancreatic duct width to increase with age at a rate of 8% per decade[103]. Regardless, the pancreatic duct was not found to be more than 3 mm, which if detected, should be considered a pathologic finding and not solely age-related [104]. Acinar atrophy, an increased amount of intralobular fibrosis and fatty infiltration, and calcified pancreatic ductal calculi seem to be common findings in the pancreas over the age of 70 [105]. Because of the increasing frequency of intercurrent disease states and degrees of malnutrition in the elderly, the proportion of these morphologic changes that are due to age alone vs. pathology has yet to be determined. In summary, the morphologic changes of the aging pancreas can be considerable, requiring clinicians to take caution when interpreting ERCP and computed tomography (CT) findings in the elderly (Table 23.6).

Table 23.6 Morphologic and physiologic changes observed in the aging pancreas

Parameter	Change
Organ size	↓
Ductal size	↑
Acinar glands	↓
Pancreatic lithiasis	↑
Exocrine function	No change
Glucose tolerance	↓
Glucagon levels	↑ ?
Pancreatic polypeptide levels	↑

↑ increased; ↓ decreased; ? not proven or consistent
Source: adapted with permission from Sherman and Brunicardi [1]

Aging of the Exocrine Pancreas

Conflicting data exists as to the change in pancreatic exocrine function with aging. For instance, Laugier determined that patients over 65 years of age demonstrated a decrease in the volume and bicarbonate output of pancreatic secretion, and the concentrations of pancreatic protein and lipase in response to stimulation from secretin and CCK stimulation [106]. In contrast, Gullo and associates failed to show any decrease in bicarbonate, trypsone or lipase in response to continuous stimulation in elderly patients when compared to younger controls [107]. Regardless of the contrasting results, the clinical significance of age-related changes in exocrine function is limited to a decrease of 10–30%. Therefore, the presence of steatorrhea in the elderly patient must be considered outside of expected aging, and in the greater scope of other pathologies such as intraductal papillary mucinous neoplasms, or pancreatic carcinoma [108].

Insulin Resistance in the Elderly

It has long been recognized that persons over 60 years of age more commonly exhibit dysfunction of glucose regulatory mechanisms in response to a glucose challenge. Minimal morphologic alteration occurs in the aging endocrine pancreas, but a number of functional tests suggest progressive impairment of glucose tolerance in the elderly [109]. Clinical studies show an age-related increase in fasting blood glucose levels of about 1–2 mg/dL per decade, which may be less marked in lean, physically active individuals [110]. The prevalence of diabetes over the past decade has increased enormously, largely due to a concomitant rise in the prevalence of obesity. As the aging population continues to grow and their life expectancy increases, so too does the rate of diabetes. Currently, about 20% of patients over 65 years suffer from diabetes [111].

Type II diabetes results from a multifactorial, progressive disease state and decompensation. The spectrum begins with glucose intolerance and progresses to frank diabetes, once the β-cell can no longer compensate for peripheral hormone resistance. Numerous changes associated with aging may contribute to this. Proposed mechanisms include altered insulin metabolism (depressed secretion, increased clearance, or diminished prohormone activation), increased resistance of peripheral tissues to insulin (receptor aberration, altered postreceptor pathways, or altered glucose transporter), and loss of hepatic sensitivity to insulin, causing reduced glycogenesis, increased glucagon levels, and an age-associated increase in adipose tissue [112]. Studies which have specifically examined age-related effects on β-cell function have demonstrated variable results. This may be due to the small magnitude of the age effect, different techniques of measurement and the presence of confounding factors such as obesity.

Current theories involving aging and insulin secretion highlight the interplay between a decreased β-cell secretory function, and failure of peripheral glucose uptake mechanisms. The number and affinity of insulin receptors are similar across the spectrum of age groups. Therefore, in the absence of other risk factors, insulin resistance in the elderly is also due to impairments at the postreceptor level and β-cell dysfunction. A number of age-related effects on β-cells is known, such as decreased sensitivity to incretins and impaired compensation to insulin resistance, thereby predisposing older people to develop impaired glucose tolerance and diabetes [113]. Future studies aimed at delineating β-cell function may shed additional light on the subject.

Glucagon

Little is known about glucagon metabolism and actions in the elderly. Berger and associates reported that fasting plasma glucagon levels are significantly higher after age 30, when compared to those of a younger cohort [110]. However, after age 30, plasma glucagon levels did not significantly increase with advancing age. These findings are compared with those from the more recent work of Simonson and DeFronzo, who showed no correlation between advancing age and glucagon levels in 111 subjects aged 21–75 years [114]. Additionally, this study demonstrated no difference in glucagon concentrations or clearance in young and old subjects receiving glucagon infusion, but hepatic sensitivity to the hormone appeared to be enhanced in the older age groups. Although the mechanism for this effect is not known, heightened hepatic sensitivity to glucagon in the elderly may be one of several factors contributing to progressive glucose intolerance of aging. Although some follow up studies have confirmed no age-related changes in glucagon concentrations, other studies have shown reduced and elevated glucagon levels in the elderly [115].

References

1. Sherman V, Brunicardi FC. Hepatobiliary and pancreatic function: physiologic changes. In: Rosenthal RE, Katlic MR, Zenilman ME, editors. Principles and practice of geriatric surgery, 2e. New York: Springer; 2010.

2. Robbins JA, Hamilton JW, Lof GL, Kempster G. Oropharyngeal swallowing in normal adults of different ages. Gastroenterology. 1992;103:823–9.

3. Robbins JA, Coyle J, Rosenbek J, et al. Differentiation of normal and abnormal airway protection during swallowing using penetration aspiration scale. Dysphagia. 1999;14:228–32.

4. Welford AT. Reaction time, speed of performance, and age. Ann NY Acad Sci. 1988;515:1–17.

5. Birren IE, Woods AM, Williams MV. Speed of behavior as an indicator of age changes and the integrity of the nervous system. Brain function in old age. Berlin: Springer; 1979. p. 10–44.

6. Levine R, Robbins JA, Maser A. Periventricular white matter changes and oropharyngeal swallowing in normal individuals. Dysphagia. 1992;7:142–7.

7. Brown M, Hasser EM. Differential effects of reduced muscle use (hindlimb unweighting) on skeletal muscle with aging. Aging (Milano). 1996;8:99–105.

8. Carlson BM. Factors influencing the repair and adaptation of muscles in aged individuals: satellite cells and innervation. J Gerontol. 1995;50:96–100.

9. Lexell J. Human aging, muscle mass, and fiber type composition. J Gerontol. 1995;50:11–6.

10. Lexell J, Taylor CC, Sjostrom M. What is the cause of ageing atrophy? Total number, size and proportion of different fiber types studied in whole vastus lateralis muscle from 15 to 83–year old men. J Neurol Sci. 1988;84:275–94.

11. Zboralske FF, Amberg JR, Soergel KH. Presbyesophagus: cineradiographic manifestations. Radiology. 1964;82:463–7.

12. Soergel KH, Zboralske FF, Amberg JR. Presbyesophagus: esophageal motility in nonagenarians. J Clin Invest. 1964;43:1472–9.

13. Richter JE, Wu WC, Johns DN, et al. Esophageal manometry in 95 healthy adult volunteers. Variability of pressures with age and frequency of "abnormal" contractions. Dig Dis Sci. 1987;32:583–92.

14. Ren J, Shaker R, Kusano M, et al. Effect of aging on the secondary esophageal peristalsis: presbyesophagus revisited. Am J Physiol. 1995;268:G772–9.

15. Aly YA, Abdel-Aty H. Normal oesophageal transit time on digital radiography. Clin Radiol. 1999;54:545–9.

16. Grande L, Lacima G, Ros E, et al. Deterioration of esophageal motility with age: a manometric study of 79 healthy subjects. Am J Gastroenterol. 1999;94:1795–801.

17. Nishimura N, Hongo M, Yamada M, et al. Effect of aging on the esophageal motor functions. J Smooth Muscle Res. 1996;32:43–50.

18. Ferriolli E, Dantas RO, Oliveira RB, Braga FJ. The influence of ageing on oesophageal motility after ingestion of liquids with different viscosities. Eur J Gastroenterol Hepatol. 1996;8:793–8.

19. Rao SS, Mudipalli RS, Mujica VR, Patel RS, Zimmerman B. Effects of gender and age on esophageal biomechanical properties and sensation. Am J Gastroenterol. 2003;98:1688–95.

20. Fulp SR, Dalton CB, Castell JA, Castell DO. Aging-related alterations in human upper esophageal sphincter function. Am J Gastroenterol. 1990;85:1569–72.

21. Wilson JA, Pryde A, Macintyre CC. The effects of age, sex, and smoking on normal pharyngoesophageal motility. Am J Gastroenterol. 1990;85:686–91.

22. Shaker R, Ren J, Podvrsan B. Effect of aging and bolus variables on pharyngeal and upper esophageal sphincter motor function. Am J Physiol. 1993;264:G427–32.

23. Hurvitz A, Brady DA, Schaal E, et al. Gastric acidity in older adults. JAMA. 1997;278:659–62.

24. Haruma K, Kamada T, Kawaguchi H, et al. Effect of age and Helicobacter pylori infection on gastric acid secretion. J Gastroenterol Hepatol. 2000;15:277–83.

25. Asaka M, Sugiyama T, Nobuta A, et al. Atrophic gastritis and intestinal metaplasia in Japan: results of a large multicenter study. Helicobacter. 2001;6:294–9.

26. Pilotto A, Salles N. Helicobacter pylori infection in geriatrics. Helicobacter. 2002;7:56–62.

27. Parlesak A, Klein B, Schecher K, et al. Prevalence of small bowel bacterial overgrowth and its association with nutrition intake in nonhospitalized older adults. J Am Geriatr Soc. 2003;51:768–73.

28. Kaptan K, Beyan C, Ural A, et al. Helicobacter pylori: is it a novel causative agent in vitamin B_{12} deficiency? Arch Intern Med. 2000;160:1349–53.

29. Madsen JL, Graff J. Effects of aging on gastrointestinal motor function. Age Aging. 2004;33:154–59.

30. Madsen JL. Effects of gender, age, and body mass index on gastrointestinal transit times. Dig Dis Sci. 1992;37:1548–53.

31. Shimamoto C, Hirata I, Hiraike Y. Evaluation of gastric motor activity in the elderly by electrogastrography and the ^{13}C-acetate breath test. Gerontology. 2002;48:381–6.

32. Nakae Y, Onouchi H, Kagaya M, et al. Effects of aging and gastric lipolysis on gastric emptying of lipid in liquid meal. J Gastroenterol. 1999;34:445–9.

33. Phillips RJ, Powley TL. As the gut ages: timetables for aging of innervation vary by organ in the Fisher 344 rat. J Comp Neurol. 2001;434:358–77.

34. El-Salhy M, Sandstrom O, Holmlund F. Age-induced changes in the enteric nervous system in the mouse. Mech Aging Dev. 1999;107:93–103.

35. Atillasoy E, Holt PR. Gastrointestinal proliferation and aging. J Gerontol. 1993;48:B43–9.

36. Ferriolli E, Dantas RO, Oliveira RB, et al. The influence of aging on oesophageal motility after ingestion of liquids with different viscosities. Eur J Gastroenterol Hepatol. 1996;8:793–8.

37. Holt PR, Moss SF, Heydari AR, Richardson A. Diet restriction increases apoptosis in the gut of aging rats. J Gerontol A Biol Sci Med Sci. 1998;53:B168–72.

38. Majumdar AP. Regulation of gastrointestinal mucosal growth during aging. J Physiol Pharmacol. 2003;54(S4):143–54.

39. Corazza GR, Frazzoni M, Gatto MR, et al. Aging and small-bowel mucosa: a morphometric study. Gerontology. 1986;32:60–5.

40. Woudstra T, Thomson ABR. Nutrient absorption and intestinal adaptation with aging. Best Pract Res Clin Gastroenterol. 2002;16:1–15.

41. Commane DM, Arasaradnam RP, Mills S, et al. Diet, ageing and genetic factors in the pathogenesis of diverticular disease. World J Gastroenterol. 2009;15(20):2479–88.

42. Eide TJ, Stalsberg H. Diverticular disease of the large intestine in Northern Norway. Gut. 1979;20:609–15.

43. Parks TG. The clinical significance of diverticular disease of the colon. Practitioner. 1982;226:643–8.

44. Lee YS. Diverticular disease of the large bowel in Singapore. An autopsy survey. Dis Colon Rectum. 1986;29:330–5.

45. Parks TG. Natural history of diverticular disease of the colon. Clin Gastroenterol. 1975;4:53–69.

46. Heise CP. Epidemiology and pathogenesis of diverticular disease. J Gastrointest Surg. 2008;12:1309–11.

47. Koch TR, Carney JA, Go VLW, Szurszewski JH. Inhibitory neuropeptides and intrinsic inhibitory innervation of descending human colon. Dig Dis Sci. 1991;36(6):712–8.

48. Wester T, O-Briain DS, Buri P. Notable postnatal alterations in the myenteric plexus of normal human bowel. Gut. 1999;44(5):666–74.

49. Eastwood HDH. Bowel transit studies in the elderly: radio-opaque markers in the investigation of constipation. Gerontol Clin. 1972; 14:154–9.

50. Johanson JF, Lafferty J. Epidemiology of fecal incontinence: the silent affliction. Am J Gastroenterol. 1996;91(1):33–6.

51. McHugh SM, Diamant NE. Effect of age, gender, and parity on anal canal pressures: contribution of impaired anal sphincter function to fecal incontinence. Dig Dis Sci. 1987;32(7):726–36.

52. Hawkey CJ. NSAIDs, coxibs and the intestine. J Cardiovasc Pharmacol. 2006;47:S72–5.

53. Faucheron JL. Toxicity of non-steroidal anti-inflammatory drugs in the large bowel. Eur J Gastroenterol Hepatol. 1999;11:389–92.

54. Sreenarasimhaiah J. Diagnosis and management of intestinal ischaemic disorders. Br Med J. 2003;326:1372–6.

55. Laurell H, Hansson LE, Gunnarson U. Acute abdominal pain among elderly patients. Gerontology. 2006;52:339–44.

56. Klein AS, Lillemoe KD, Yeo CJ, Pitt HA. Liver, biliary tract, and pancreas. In: O'Leary JP, editor. The physiologic basis of surgery. 2nd ed. Baltimore: Williams & Wilkins; 1996. p. 441–78.

57. Popper H. Aging and the liver. Prog Liver Dis. 1986;8:659–83.

58. Schmucker DL, Jones AL. Hepatic fine structure in young and aging rats treated with oxandrolone: a morphometric study. J Lipid Res. 1975;16(2):143–50.

59. Tauchi H, Sato T. Age changes in size and number of mitochondria of human hepatic cells. J Gerontol. 1968;23(4):454–61.

60. Thompson EN, Williams R. Effect of age on liver function with particular reference to Bromsulphalein excretion. Gut. 1965;6: 266–9.

61. Williams D, Woodhouse K. Age related changes in NADPH cytochrome c reductase activity in mouse skin and liver microsomes. Arch Gerontol Geriatr. 1995;21(2):191–7.

62. Le Couteur DG, McLean AJ. The aging liver: drug clearance and an oxygen diffusion barrier hypothesis. Clin Pharmacokinet. 1998;34(5):359–73.

63. Junaidi O, Di Bisceglie AM. Aging liver and hepatitis. Clin Geriatr Med. 2007;23(4):889–903.

64. Kampmann JP, Sinding J, Møller-Jørgensen I. Effect of age on liver function. Geriatrics. 1975;30:91–5.

65. Koff RS, Garvey AJ, Burney SW, et al. Absence of an age effect on sulfobromophthalein retention in healthy men. Gastroenterology. 1973;65:300–2.

66. Qvist N. Motor activity of the gallbladder and gastrointestinal tract as determinants of enterohepatic circulation: a scintigraphic and manometric study. Dan Med Bull. 1995;42:426–40.

67. Rafsky HA, Newman B. Liver function tests in the aged (the serum cholesterol partition, Bromsulphalein, cephalinflocculation and oral and intravenous hippuric acid tests). Am J Dig Dis. 1943;10: 66–9.

68. Sawada N, Ishikawa T. Reduction of potential for replicative but not unscheduled DNA synthesis in hepatocytes isolated from aged as compared to young rats. Cancer Res. 1998;48(6):1618–22.

69. Zapletal C, Faust D, Wullstein C, et al. Does the liver ever age? Results of liver transplantation with donors above 80 years of age. Transplant Proc. 2005;37(2):1182–5.

70. Gadacz TR. Biliary anatomy and physiology. In: Greenfield LJ, editor. Surgery: scientific principles and practice. Philadelphia: Lippincott; 1993. p. 925–36.

71. Khalil T, Walker JP, Wiener I, et al. Effect of aging on gallbladder contraction and release of cholecystokinin-33 in humans. Surgery. 1985;98:423–9.

72. Rajan M, Wali JP, Sharma MP, et al. Ultrasonographic assessment of gall bladder kinetics in the elderly. Indian J Gastroenterol. 2000;19(4):158–60.

73. Nagase M, Hikasa Y, Soloway RD, et al. Surgical significance of dilatation of the common bile duct: with special reference to choledocholithiasis. Jpn J Surg. 1980;10:296–301.

74. Kaim A, Steinke K, Frank M, et al. Diameter of the common bile duct in the elderly patient: measurement by ultrasound. Eur Radiol. 1998;8(8):1413–5.

75. Lieber MM. The incidence of gallstones and their correlation with other diseases. Ann Surg. 1952;135:394–405.

76. Lindström CG. Frequency of gallstone disease in a well-defined Swedish population. Scand J Gastroenterol. 1977;12:341–6.

77. Marinovic I, Guerra C, Larach G. Incidencia de litiasis biliar en material de autopsias y analisis de composicion de los calculos. Rev Med Chil. 1972;100:1320–7.

78. Heaton KW. The epidemiology of gallstones and suggested aetiology. Clin Gastroenterol. 1973;2:67–83.

79. National Center for Health Statistics. National Hospital Discharge Survey: Annual Summary, 1994. Series 13: Data from the National Health Care Survey, No. 128. DHHS Publ No. (PHS) 97-1789. Hyattsville, MD: National Center for Health Statistics, May 1997.

80. Attili AF, Capocaccia R, Carulli N, et al. Factors associated with gallstone disease in the MICOL experience. Multicenter Italian study on epidemiology of cholelithiasis. Hepatology. 1997;26(4): 809–18.

81. Wang DQ. Aging per se is an independent risk factor for cholesterol gallstone formation in gallstone susceptible mice. J Lipid Res. 2002;43(11):1950–9.

82. Reiss R, Deutsch AA. Emergency abdominal procedures in patients above 70. J Gerontol. 1985;40:154–8.

83. Tang WH. Serum and bile lipid levels in patients with and without gallstones. J Gastroenterol. 1996;31:823–7.

84. Holan KR, Holzbach RT, Hermann RE, et al. Nucleation time: a key factor in the pathogenesis of cholesterol gallstone disease. Gastroenterology. 1979;77:611–7.

85. Portincasa P, Stolk MFJ, van Erpecum KJ, et al. Cholesterol gallstone formation in man and potential treatments of the gallbladder motility defect. Scand J Gastroenterol. 1995;30 Suppl 212:63–78.

86. Festi D, Colecchia A, Larocca A. Review: low caloric intake and gall-bladder motor function. Aliment Pharmacol Ther. 2000;14 Suppl 2:51–3.

87. Carey MC. Pathogenesis of gallstones. Am J Surg. 1993;165(4): 410–9.

88. Lambou-Gianoukos S, Heller SJ. Lithogenesis and bile metabolism. Surg Clin North Am. 2008;88(6):1175–94.

89. Ahlberg J, Angelin B, Einarsson K. Hepatic 3-hydroxy-3-methylglutaryl coenzyme A reductase activity and biliary lipid composition in man: relation to cholesterol gallstone disease and effects of cholic acid and chenodeoxycholic acid treatment. J Lipid Res. 1981;22:410–22.

90. Bowen JC, Brenner HI, Ferrante WA, Maule WF. Gallstone disease: pathophysiology, epidemiology, natural history, and treatment options. Med Clin North Am. 1992;76:1143–57.

91. Patankar R, Ozmen MM, Bailey IS, Johnson CD. Gallbladder motility, gallstones, and the surgeon. Dig Dis Sci. 1995;40: 2323–35.

92. Anderson DK, Brunicardi FC. Pancreatic anatomy and physiology. In: Greenfield LJ, editor. Surgery: scientific principles and practice. Philadelphia: Lippincott; 1993. p. 775–91.

93. DiMagno EP, Vay LWG, Summerskill WHJ. Relations between pancreatic enzyme outputs and malabsorption in severe pancreatic insufficiency. N Engl J Med. 1973;288:813–5.

94. Havel PJ, Taborsky GJ. The contribution of the autonomic nervous system to changes of glucagon and insulin secretion during hypoglycemic stress. Endocr Rev. 1989;10(3):332–50.

95. Lara-Castro C, Garvey WT. Intracellular lipid accumulation in liver and muscle and the insulin resistance syndrome. Endocrinol Metab Clin North Am. 2008;37(4):841–56.

96. Viljanen AP, Lautamäki R, Järvisalo M, et al. Effect of weight loss on liver free fatty acid uptake and hepatic insulin resistance. J Clin Endocrinol Metab. 2009;94(1):50–5.

97. Brunicardi FC, Chaiken RL, Ryan AS, et al. Pancreatic polypeptide administration improves abnormal glucose metabolism in patients with chronic pancreatitis. J Clin Endocrinol Metab. 1996;81:3566–72.

98. Seymour NE, Volpert AR, Lee EL, et al. Alterations in hepatocyte insulin binding in chronic pancreatitis: Effects of pancreatic polypeptide. Am J Surg. 1995;169:105–10.

99. Spector SA, Frattini JC, Zdankiewicz PD, et al. Insulin receptor gene expression in chronic pancreatitis: the effect of pancreatic polypeptide. In: Surgical Forum. Proceedings for the 52nd Annual Sessions of the Owen H. Wangensteen Surgical Forum; 1997 Oct 12–17; Chicago. Lawrence: Allen Press; 1997. p. 168–71.

100. Brunicardi FC, Druck P, Sun YS, et al. Regulation of pancreatic polypeptide secretion in the isolated perfused human pancreas. Am J Surg. 1988;155:63–9.

101. Kojima S, Ueno N, Asakawa A, et al. A role for pancreatic polypeptide in feeding and body weight regulation. Peptides. 2007;28:459–63.

102. Jayasena CN. Role of gut hormones in obesity. Endocrinol Metab Clin North Am. 2008;37(3):769–87.

103. Kreel L, Sandin B. Changes in pancreatic morphology associated with aging. Gut. 1973;14:962–70.

104. Glaser J, Stienecker K. Pancreas and aging: a study using ultrasonography. Gerontology. 2000;46(2):93–6.

105. Nagai H, Ohtsubo K. Pancreatic lithiasis in the aged. Gastroenterology. 1984;86:331–8.

106. Laugier R, Sarles H. The pancreas. Clin Gastroenterol. 1985;14:749–56.

107. Gullo L, Ventrucci M, Naldoni P, Pezzilli R. Aging and exocrine pancreatic function. J Am Geriatr Soc. 1986;34:790–2.

108. Walsh RM. Innovations in treating the elderly who have biliary and pancreatic disease. Clin Geriatr Med. 2006;22(3):545–8.

109. Taylor R, Agius L. The biochemistry of diabetes. Biochem J. 1988;250:625–40.

110. Berger D, Crowther RC, Floyd Jr JC, et al. Effect of age on fasting plasma levels of pancreatic hormones in man. J Clin Endocrinol Metab. 1978;47:1183–9.

111. Mazza AD. Insulin resistance syndrome and glucose dysregulation in the elderly. Clin Geriatr Med. 2008;24(3):437–54.

112. Timiras PS. The endocrine pancreas and carbohydrate metabolism. In: Timiras PS, editor. Physiological basis of aging and geriatrics. 2nd ed. Boca Raton: CRC Press; 1994. p. 191–7.

113. Chang AM, Halter JB. Aging and insulin secretion. Am J Physiol Endocrinol Metab. 2003;284(1):E7–12.

114. Simonson DC, DeFronzo RA. Glucagon physiology and aging: evidence for enhanced hepatic sensitivity. Diabetologia. 1983;25:1–7.

115. Pagano G, Marena S, Scaglione L, et al. Insulin resistance shows selective metabolic and hormonal targets in the elderly. Eur J Clin Invest. 1996;26(8):650–6.

116. Einarsson K et al. Influence of age on secretion of cholesterol and synthesis of bile acids by the liver. N Engl J Med. 1985;313:277–82.

117. Bouras EP, Tangalos EG. Chronic constipation in the elderly. Gastroenterol Clin N Am. 2009;38:463–80.

118. Bateson MC. Gallbladder disease and cholecystectomy rate are independently variable. Lancet. 1984;2:621–4.

Chapter 24
Neurologic and Cognitive Changes in the Elderly

J. Riley McCarten

Abstract Neurologic changes, particularly cognitive changes, are common disease-related conditions in older adults. Cognitive impairment, most often caused by Alzheimer's disease, is easily overlooked. Patients typically look normal and may not recognize deficits. Families may attribute symptoms of dementia to normal aging. Such patients are at increased risk for peri-operative complications, specifically, delirium. Establishing a baseline, preoperative mental status is essential for managing the often difficult recovery from major surgery. Knowing that a patient is demented and at increased risk for delirium prepares the patient, family, and healthcare team, and may even provide a contraindication for surgery. Inquiring about changes typical of memory and cognitive disorders, such as repeating, misplacing, relying more on notes and calendars, forgetting names of familiar persons, forgetting medications, and getting lost driving may suggest an underlying dementia. Simple bedside testing focusing on the patient's ability to learn and remember new information and to follow instructions is key to the mental status examination. Additional neurologic evaluation, including visual fields, extraocular movements, speech, facial symmetry, gait, and drift testing are simple, high yield, reproducible, and readily identify deficits, efficiently enhancing your neurologic assessment.

Keywords Neurologic • Cognition • Cognitive • Dementia • Alzheimer's • Delirium • Memory • Mental status • Visual fields • Extraocular movements • Speech • Gait

Introduction

Changes are often observed in the central and peripheral nervous system of older adults. Most of these, however, are not a natural part of aging, but rather are the result of age-related disease affecting the nervous system, either directly or indirectly. Both central and peripheral nervous systems are tremendously dynamic and capable of maintaining good function throughout life. In the peripheral nervous system, common problems, such as peripheral neuropathy, are the result of associated disease, such as diabetes. Limitation in motor function may be related to problems with bones, joints, and connective tissue. Healthy nerves and muscles work well into late life. Similarly, a healthy brain functions well, even in late life. If one compares the nervous system to other organ systems, it is most like blood; responding rapidly to changes in the environment, and with a high turnover of its constituent proteins. Though neurons have a low rate of turnover, their cell membranes are constantly being remodeled.

While the integrity of the motor and sensory pathways of the peripheral nervous system may influence rehabilitation, it is impairment in brain function, and specifically, cognitive function, that is most likely to manifest as problems in surgical practice. Cognitive impairment is common in older adults [1, 2], affecting as many as 1/3 of persons age 70 and older. The incidence may be higher in persons with cardiovascular disease as vascular risk factors increase the likelihood of Alzheimer's disease (AD) [3–5]. Certainly, the risk of delirium is highest in those that already have impaired brain function [6], and delirium may even accelerate the rate of decline in AD [7].

It cannot be overstated that older adults with cognitive impairment, including many persons who have moderately severe dementia, may look normal. They interact appropriately, attend to conversations, give plausible – though typically inaccurate – histories, and may deny or minimize any cognitive problems. Families also may not report concerns, chalking up cognitive deficits to old age, reluctant to speak in front of the patient, or simply denying the problem. Without cognitive testing, a physician cannot know the integrity of a patient's mental status. Fortunately, some simple bedside tests can provide important clues to the presence of cognitive impairment. Prior to an operation when a patient is at baseline, the important questions are: Can the patient learn and remember new information? Can he/she follow complex instructions? If the answers are yes, the patient is reasonably

J.R. McCarten (✉)
Department of Neurology, University of Minnesota
Medical School, VA Medical Center, One Veterans Drive,
Minneapolis, MN 55417, USA
e-mail: mccar034@umn.edu

M.R. Katlic (ed.), *Cardiothoracic Surgery in the Elderly*, DOI 10.1007/978-1-4419-0892-6_24,
© Springer Science+Business Media, LLC 2011

cognitively intact, and the physician can give that patient advice – and write him or her a prescription. If the answers are no, it is unreasonable of the physician to make that patient responsible for the physician's advice and directions. Such patients are not noncompliant. They do not have the option of complying because of brain disease.

Given that sometimes dramatic postoperative cognitive changes in patients are observed by families, alerting the patient and family to an increased likelihood of such changes in a vulnerable patient prepares them, and may protect the physician and staff from angry reproaches. Trying to establish a pre-existing dementia after surgery may be difficult, and even seen by the family as an attempt to shift blame. Simple baseline cognitive screening may prepare the clinical team, patient and family for the often challenging recovery of the cognitively impaired patient. In some cases it may even provide a strong relative contraindication to surgical intervention.

A Brief History of Dementia

The origin of the distinction between AD and senile dementia is beautifully reviewed by Amaducci et al. [8]. Briefly the syndrome of "senile dementia" first came to light in the medical literature in Germany in the mid 1800s. In 1892, microscopic senile plaques, now called amyloid plaques, were first described and, in 1907, were correlated with dementia in older adults. In the same year, Alois Alzheimer described the case of Frau D, a woman in her 50s who developed dementia. Using Nissl's then new staining methods, Alzheimer was the first to report neurofibrillay tangles in the brain of a demented person. He also observed abundant senile plaques. His rivals, using the new staining methods, later identified neurofibrillary tangles in their cases of senile dementia (Fig. 24.1). It was known, therefore, from near the time of Alzheimer's first report, that both his case of a middle aged woman with

dementia, and the cases of senile dementia both had the hallmark plaques and tangles that define AD neuropathologically. The head of Alzheimer's department in Munich, Kraepelin, a prominent and powerful neuroscientist of his day, believed that Alzheimer's case represented a distinct disease entity. Alzheimer was persuaded, and "presenile dementia," or AD, was born. In fact, numerous subsequent series revealed that senile vs. presenile dementia could not be distinguished either clinically or neuropathologically. Still, because of this early distinction, AD was defined as a rare disease of midlife, while senile dementia was tacitly acccepted as reflecting the inexorable march of time, a normal process of aging.

An interesting aside is that, in the early 1900s, when senile and presenile dementia were defined, the most common cause of dementia was syphilis. Because neuropsyphilis is associated with vascular infiltration of meningeal vessels, it was imperative that any publication on dementia in the preantibiotic era carefully address the brain's blood vessels. Apparently, neither Alzheimer nor his rivals in the senile dementia camp believed that cerebrovascular disease, apart from syphilitic vasculitis, was a significant contributor to dementia.

In the late 1960s, Tomlinson et al. published a series of manuscripts, including two seminal works, "Observations on the Brains of Non-Demented Old People" [9], and "Observations on the Brains of Demented Old People" [10]. They concluded that the clinical distinctions between demented and nondemented older adults rested upon the quantity of pathology, most specifically, plaques, tangles, and cerebrovascular disease. In their demented cohort, 50% had the pathology of AD, 8–18% had mixed AD and cerebrovascular (CVD) pathology, and 12–15% had predominantly CVD. Among females, 15/16 had AD changes, while only 10/34 males had AD changes. They concluded further, that "Arteriosclerotic dementia is almost certainly overdiagnosed clinically." Given the advances in treating cerebrovascular disease since the 1950s and 1960s – better control

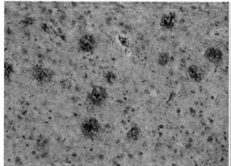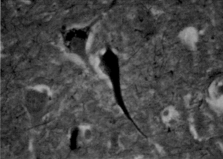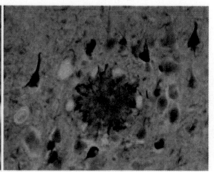

Fig. 24.1 Senile (amyloid) plaques (*left*), a neurofibrillary tangle (NFT; *middle*), and a plaque with surrounding intraneuronal NFTs and normal appearing neurons (*right*). Note difference in magnification. Plaques are relatively large, extracellular structures. NFTs are intraneuronal, though they may be extruded after the neuron dies. Plaques and NFTs are the pathological hallmarks of Alzheimer's disease (AD)

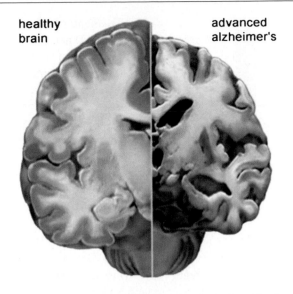

healthy brain   **advanced alzheimer's**

Fig. 24.2 Coronal section of healthy brain vs. brain with advanced AD. Note the marked atrophy of mesial temporal lobe (hippocampus) in AD (*arrows*). Cell loss is a late feature of AD. The gross anatomy of the brain in early AD may not be distinguishable from healthy brain. © 2010 Alzheimer's Association. www.alz.org. All rights reserved. Image credit: Jannis Productions. Stacy Jannis. Reprinted with permission

Table 24.1 Medications with moderate to high CNS anticholinergic effects commonly used in the elderly

Common indications for medications	Common medications with CNS[a] anticholinergic effects
Peri-operative adjuncts (multiple indications)	Atropine, hydroxyzine, hyoscyamine, scopolamine
Sedation, sleep	Diphenydramine, amitryptiline, nortriptyline, doxepin
Bladder urgency	Oxybutynin, hyoscyamine
Nausea, diarrhea, irritable bowel	Chlorpromazine, scopolamine, dicyclomine, hyoscyamine
Agitation; psychotic disorders	Olanzapine, chlorpromazine, clozapine, thioridazine
Depression, anxiety	Paroxetine, amitryptiline, nortriptyline, doxepin
Allergies, pruritis	Diphenhydramine, hydroxyzine, doxepin
Chronic pain	Amitryptiline, nortriptyline

Anticholinergic drugs impair memory and cognition, as well as drying secretions, blocking smooth muscle contractions (bladder and bowel), and blocking vagally mediated slowing of the heart. Illness, other stressors, and concomitant medications may increase the brain's permeability to drugs, including anticholinergic drugs with typically low CNS penetrance, e.g., tolterodine and ranitidine
[a]*CNS* central nervous system
Source: Data from Chew et al. [39]

of hypertension, hyperlipidemia, and diabetes, and less smoking – the relative contribution of CVD to dementia has decreased, while that of AD has increased. Equally important, the authors reported that brain weight and ventricular size did not vary greatly between healthy older adults and younger age groups, and cerebral atrophy was slight or absent in the healthy elderly (Fig. 24.2). It should be noted that the commonly seen age-related "atrophy" seen on neuroimaging often is not evident to the pathologist examining the fixated brain. True atrophy on neuroimaging is more likely if the volume loss is focal in nature, e.g., the mesial temporal lobe in AD [11], or the cerebellar vermis in alcoholism.

The Rediscovery of Alzheimer's Disease and the Cholinergic Hypothesis

Despite the reports of Tomlinson et al. in the late 1960s, for many years AD was still largely considered a rare disease of mid-life, distinct from the "normal" brain aging of senile dementia. The situation began to change, beginning in the mid 1970s and into the early 1980s, because of several discoveries: (1) Anticholinergic medications were found to impair memory [12] (Table 24.1); (2) Choline acetyl transferase (CAT), the enzyme responsible for generating acetylcholine (ACh), is deficient in the brains of persons with AD [13]; (3) The basal forebrain nuclei sends projections throughout the neocortex and to the hippocampus, providing virtually all of the brain's ACh [14]; and (4) The basal

forebrain nuclei degenerate in AD [15]. The excitement over these discoveries was obvious to neurologists, since the situation appears directly analogous to Parkinson's disease (PD). Like PD, AD is a slowly progressive degenerative brain disease. The differences between PD and AD were simple: (1) Instead of dopamine (DA), the deficient neurotransmitter is ACh; (2) Instead of a pool of neurons in the substantia nigra, the pool of neurons is in the basal forebrain; (3) Instead of motor symptoms, there are memory and cognitive symptoms; and, most importantly, (4) Instead of good treatment, there was no treatment. By the early 1980s, L-DOPA therapy had revolutionized the treatment of PD, and new ways to better replace deficient DA were moving the field forward. It stood to reason that the same strategy to replete a diminished neurotransmitter – in this case, ACh – would have a similar magnitude of benefit to the symptoms of AD. The early and mid 1980s saw an explosion of interest in AD in anticipation of good treatments based on this cholinergic hypothesis (Fig. 24.3).

While the cholinergic hypothesis indeed may be valid, effectively increasing the level of ACh in the brain is much more difficult than increasing the level of DA. The CAT enzyme is not a rate-limiting step in ACh synthesis, and precursor loading with choline, unlike with L-DOPA, is not an effective strategy to increase ACh neurotransmitter levels. Direct stimulation of ACh receptors, unlike DA receptors, also provides little benefit. Blocking ACh esterase with cholinesterase inhibitors (CIs; e.g., donepezil – Aricept®, galantamine – Razadyne®, and rivastigmine – Exelon®) does prolong the effect of ACh in the synapse, but the effects are

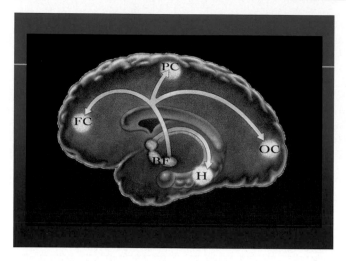

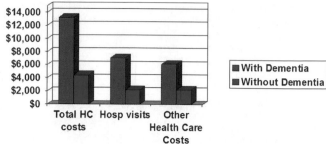

Fig. 24.4 Healthcare costs among older adults with comparable healthcare problems except for dementia. Dementia as a co-morbidity triples healthcare costs. Most of the excess cost is in hospitalizations. Most of the remainder is in long term care costs. From the Alzheimer's Association [41]. www.alz.org.

Fig. 24.3 The cholinergic hypothesis of AD: Cholinergic neurons in the basal forebrain (BF) project to frontal (FC), parietal (PC), and occipital cortex (OC), as well as to the hippocampus (H), providing virtually all of the acetylcholine (ACh) for the brain. ACh is crucial for memory and cognitive function and is deficient in AD. Neurons in the BF degenerate and die in AD. Adapted from McNeil [40]

modest and analogous to a third or fourth line treatment in PD. In contrast to DA levels, which remain fairly constant in the brain throughout the circadian cycle, ACh levels change significantly during waking, non-REM and REM sleep. This makes ACh levels, unlike DA levels, a moving target, and may explain in part the limited effect of cholinergic treatment strategies.

Alzheimer's Disease and Dementia Today

While the cholinergic hypothesis did not lead to a major treatment advance, once we began looking for AD in anticipation of effective treatments, it became evident that the disease affects millions of people and costs billions of dollars. Indeed, the estimates for 2010 are that 5.3 million people in the United States have at least the early symptoms of AD [16], with care costs of $172 billion, including $123 billion for Medicare and Medicaid [17]. Healthcare costs for persons with AD are three times that of comparable older adults without AD (Fig. 24.4) [18]. While rare before the age of 65, the incidence of AD basically doubles every 5 years thereafter [19]. With the rapidly growing population of older adults, a huge growth in AD and related dementia is inevitable. It has become clear that, despite early failures, we must find ways to address this disease.

Much has been learned about AD and, indeed, it is one of the most active areas of scientific research. The dominant hypothesis in AD research today is the beta-amyloid hypothesis which states that AD is the result of the accumulation of beta amyloid (Aβ [A-beta]), causing neuronal dysfunction and eventually cell death [20]. Aβ is the cleavage product of the amyloid precursor protein (APP), one of the most abundant of brain proteins (Fig. 24.5). All of the nearly 200 known mutations which cause familial AD (FAD), all autosomal dominant disorders, involve point mutations on either the APP protein in or near the Aβ portion of the molecule, or in the protein presenilin, the key molecule in the gamma secretase complex which generates of Aβ from APP (Fig. 24.6) [21]. Persons with Down's syndrome, in which trisomy 21 yields three copies of the gene for APP, invariably develop the plaques and tangles of AD [22]. Of the three ApoE alleles, ApoE 4 is associated with decreased clearance of Aβ and significantly increases the risk of developing AD [23]. There are no other proven genetic risk factors for AD that do not directly involve the production and/or clearance of Aβ. Still, effective pharmacological therapy has been elusive.

There are, of course, other forms of dementia, but AD deserves special attention. Not only is it the most common cause of dementia in older adults, it is the easiest to overlook. Unlike dementia associated with cerebrovascular disease or parkinsonian syndromes – the other most common etiologies of dementia (Fig. 24.7) – with AD there typically are no other indicators of brain disease. AD also reflects a fundamental characteristic of the brain:healthy brain cells adapt and survive, sick brain cells malfunction and die. Dementia is the result of sick brain cells. The determination of brain health, even after serious injury, depends primarily upon the number of healthy neurons remaining. All physicians have seen dramatic brain injuries due to stroke, trauma, infection, or tumors from which patients make amazing recoveries after treatment. Given enough time to accommodate the insult, the brain even learns to function remarkably well in the face of otherwise lethal toxins, whether endogenous or exogenous. All of these injuries are extrinsic to the brain. When the lesion involves the brain's cellular machinery, however, recovery is compromised. If the disorder spreads across the brain, dementia is inevitable.

Fig. 24.5 Processing of the transmembrane amyloid precursor protein (APP). α alpha secretase; β beta secretase; γ gamma secretase; *aa* amino acid; *sAPP* soluble APP (fragment); *CTF* C-terminal fragment. Aβ and p3 are cleavage products. Aβ is believed to play a pivotal role in the pathogenesis of AD (courtesy of Dr. Sylvain Lesne, Department of Neuroscience, University of Minnesota, Minneapolis MN)

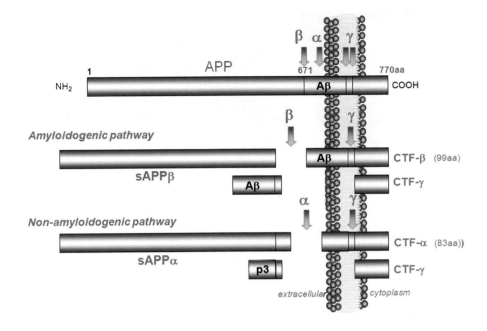

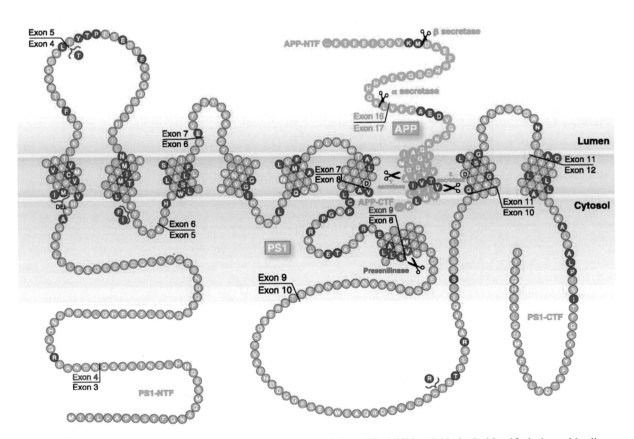

Fig. 24.6 Presenilin, the APP and the genetics of Familial AD. Each circle is an amino acid. The *red circles* indicate point mutations associated with a known kindred with Familial Alzheimer's Disease (FAD). The *blue* strand is the presenilin molecule, a key component in the γ (gamma) secretase complex. The green strand is the Aβ [A-beta] part of the APP. Additional kindreds identified since this diagram was made also have point mutations in one of these two molecules. The presenilin molecule creates a pore in the membrane – not evident in this two dimensional representation – surrounding APP at the cleavage site (reprinted with permission from Hardy and Selkoe [21])

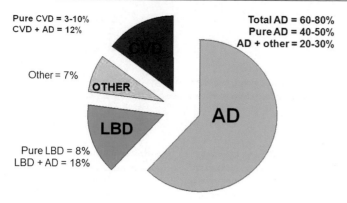

Pure CVD = 3-10%
CVD + AD = 12%

Total AD = 60-80%
Pure AD = 40-50%
AD + other = 20-30%

Other = 7%

Pure LBD = 8%
LBD + AD = 18%

Fig. 24.7 Neuropathologically confirmed etiologies of dementia in older adults. *AD* Alzheimer's disease; *CVD* cerebrovascular disease; *LBD* Lewy body disease (courtesy of Dr. David S. Knopman, Department of Neurology, Mayo Clinic, Rochester, MN)

Most forms of dementia in older adults lack a clear premorbid biomarker. Diagnostic criteria, such as outlined by the DSM-IV [24], provide guides to reasonably good premorbid diagnostic accuracy, particularly in the later stages of disease. Identifying dementia in its early, even incipient stages, is important to identify those patients at increased risk for delirium in the hospital setting. Diagnosis naturally is less accurate the more ambiguous the clinical findings, which is the case in the early stages of most progressive dementias. Agreement amongst several experts – a consensus diagnosis – is the gold standard for defining cognitive impairment in older adults. The Geriatric Research, Education and Clinical Center (GRECC) at the Minneapolis VA Healthcare System operationalized the published criteria for various types of cognitive impairment, and attempted to apply them rigorously to patients evaluated in a dementia clinic, and reviewed in a consensus diagnosis conference. The results (Table 24.2) reveal not only the numerous etiologies that must be considered, but also the preponderance of neurodegenerative diseases in general, and AD or incipient AD, as reflected in the diagnosis of mild cognitive impairment (MCI), in particular. While these results are skewed by the nature of the population – referral based, predominantly Caucasian and male – they accurately reflect the effort that is involved in correctly diagnosing cognitive impairment in older adults.

The Clinical Evaluation of Cognitive Impairment in Older Adults

Arriving at a specific diagnosis for cognitive impairment in older adults is most often the purview of a dementia specialist. Recognizing the symptoms of cognitive impairment and gauging the severity, are reasonable and necessary skills for every physician. The broad etiologies of brain disease – degenerative, vascular, infectious, traumatic, neoplastic, toxic/metabolic (T/M) – also should be familiar to every physician, as this determines to large extent the relative urgency of the evaluation. Failure to recognize baseline cognitive impairment in an older patient often leads to the emergent evaluation of a potentially unstable patient postoperatively for a disease that could have been evaluated electively prior to surgery.

The History

The first question the physician should ask any older adult seen in the office setting is, "Did you come with anyone?" Often, a family member is in the waiting room, assuming, or at least hoping, that the doctor will identify a cognitive problem. The patient often will deny or minimize a cognitive problem, and genuinely may not recognize it in themselves. When family members are available, it is important for the physician to establish full control over the interview and examination from the outset. Family members often are reticent to discuss concerns about the patient's cognition in front of the patient, but practically and ethically the patient should be present. Not only does the patient have a right to know what is discussed, but the patient's full involvement in the process is necessary to building the trust essential for therapy, particularly surgery. A patient may be demented, but they know whom they trust. Treat cognitive disorders in a matter-of-fact manner. They are common in older adults, and it is not only reasonable, but essential that the physician inquire about them.

In the interview, do not let the patient sit across from family members. The nonverbal communication between them will compromise the history provided by the family, which already may be difficult to elicit. Give the patient his/her chance, but if the history seems overly long, tangential or confusing, do not waste time with a potentially unreliable historian. With the patient's permission, direct questions to the family. If the patient interrupts, remind him/her that they have had their chance, and re-direct the interview.

For family that does not live with the patient, the first question is, "How often do you see your [mother, father, etc.]?" Clearly establish their familiarity with the patient in the recent past. A given family member may be present only because of the potential for major surgery, and otherwise may have had little recent contact with the patient. Someone who knows the patient well is the necessary informant. When asking if the patient has any problems with thinking or memory, do not dismiss a response such as, "No more than anyone his/her age." Age is a risk factor, not a cause of cognitive decline. Clarify the question by asking when the

Table 24.2 Compilation of diagnoses generated in the Minneapolis VA Healthcare System Geriatric Research, Education and Clinical Center (GRECC) Memory Loss Clinic through consensus diagnosis using published criteria

Consensus diagnosis – all cases

Etiologies of cognitive impairment (CI)	Primary etiology			Secondary etiology(s)
	Number of patients	% of total	% with secondary causes	Frequency as secondary cause
Neurodegenerative disease	342	83.4	17.8	9
Mild cognitive impairment	55	13.4	12.7	4
Possible	13	3.2	23.1	4
Probable	41	10.0	7.3	0
Alzheimer's disease	249	60.7	17.4	4
Possible	52	12.7	21.2	3
Probable	196	47.8	16.3	1
Frontotemporal dementia	15	3.7	20.0	1
Possible	7	1.7	42.9	1
Probable	6	1.5	0.0	0
Pick-like	2	0.5	0.0	0
Primary prog. aphasia/language variant	5	1.2	0.0	0
With motor neuron disease (ALS)	0	0.0	–	0
Diffuse Lewy body disease	14	3.4	35.7	0
Possible	8	2.0	37.5	0
Probable	6	1.5	33.3	0
Parkinson's disease	3	0.7	66.7	0
Progressive supranuclear palsy	1	0.2	0.0	0
Multiple system atrophy	3	0.7	33.3	0
Corticobasal degeneration	2	0.5	0.0	0
Huntington's disease	0	0.0	–	0
Vascular disease	10	2.4	70.0	16
Possible	1	0.2	0.0	13
Probable	9	2.2	77.8	3
Psychiatric disorder	14	3.4	93.3	28
Depression	12	2.9	100.0	21
Anxiety	1	0.2	0.0	8
Psychotic disorder	0	0.0	–	0
Other psychiatric disorder	1	0.2	100.0	4
Sleep disorder	1	0.2	100.0	25
Obstructive sleep apnea	1	0.2	100.0	21
Other sleep disorder	0	0.0	–	8
Toxic/metabolic conditions	7	1.7	42.9	24
Alcohol	0	0.0	–	9
Possible	0	0.0	–	8
Probable	0	0.0	–	1
Korsakoff's (B1/thiamine deficiency)	0	0.0	–	0
Drugs/medications	5	1.2	60.0	11
Thyroid disease	0	0.0	–	0
Other toxic/metabolic	2	0.5	0.0	4
B12/folic acid deficiency	0	0.0	–	2
Infection	0	0.0	–	0
HIV	0	0.0	–	0
Creutzfeldt-Jacob disease	0	0.0	–	0
Postinfectious	0	0.0	–	0
Other infections	0	0.0	–	0
Trauma	5	1.2	40.0	3
Traumatic brain injury	5	1.2	40.0	2
Subdural hematoma	0	0.0	–	0
NPH	1	0.2	0.0	3
Neoplasm	0	0.0	–	0
Other (DEM-NEC)	0	0.0	–	–
Etiology unknown (DEM-NOS)	19	4.6	36.8	–
No cognitive impairment	11	2.7		
Total	410	100.0		

Note the preponderance of neurodegenerative etiologies in general, and Alzheimer's disease specifically. Mild Cognitive Impairment is included as a neurodegenerative disorder only when the consensus is that the patient is likely to progress to full blown neurodegenerative dementia. Degenerative dementias when present are felt most often to be exclusively responsible for the dementia syndrome. Other dementia etiologies are more often secondary, not primary, causes

patient's thinking and memory was last completely normal for him/her – 100%, no problems. If a cognitive problem is present, be aware that families tend to report when things got bad. The question is not when they got bad, but when they started. Onset and course are the key to establishing a neurological diagnosis. The further back the onset of symptoms can be pushed, the more likely it is a degenerative brain disease. Symptoms that began insidiously, have been apparent for at least 6 months and preferably longer, and have been only gradually progressive, are almost invariably due to a degenerative dementia. In contrast, sudden onset and improving or static symptoms characterize a stroke or head injury; somewhat less acute but progressive symptoms (hours–days, rarely weeks) may suggest infection; sub-acute onset and progression (weeks–months) may indicate a slowly growing mass lesion, typically accompanied by headache and/or focal neurological deficits; and a fluctuating course is most commonly seen in toxic and metabolic conditions.

When investigating the syndrome of memory loss, much like investigating any other chief complaint, there are specific questions that need to be addressed. Open ended questions, particularly when patient and family are together, may lead to a replay of a disagreement that does little to clarify the situation. More constructive are simple, direct questions that typify the nature of most dementing illnesses: Does the patient repeat? Misplace? Rely more on notes and calendars? Struggle with names of people he/she should know? While patients may be aware of some of these problems, almost no one is aware that they repeat themselves. Families, however, often find the constant repetition of questions exhausting and frustrating. Other simple questions relate to trouble finding words (language), getting lost driving (visuospatial memory and orientation), and having trouble keeping track of the day (temporal orientation). Surprisingly, even when many or all of these symptoms are endorsed, the family assumes that the patient is competent to manage a complex regimen of medications, and also to handle financial affairs. If the family does not endorse any concerns, if may be useful to ask if the patient could live independently. Not infrequently a patient would not be left alone even overnight, despite the denial of any problems by the family. For a cognitively intact individual, in the absence of incapacitating physical ailments, independent living should be possible regardless of age.

The prior neurological and psychiatric histories are of particular importance in the past medical history when investigating possible cognitive impairment. Simply asking if the patient has ever had a serious head injury, stroke, seizure, or other known nervous system disease is usually adequate to address the neurological history. Similarly, simply asking if a patient has ever seen a psychiatrist, or been treated for depression or other nervous/mental disorder is adequate for the psychiatric history.

Medications commonly cause or, more often, aggravate cognitive dysfunction in older adults. In addition to medications with anticholinergic activity, many other medications should be avoided [25]. In particular medications with central nervous system (CNS) effects, and particularly anxiolytics and sedative/hypnotics, may contribute to cognitive dysfunction – and also often an increase risk for falls. Most sedating medications share features of alcohol: If someone is sleepy, they will hasten sleep onset. If someone is wide-awake, they will produce cognitive and motoric impairment. Be aware, however, that – just like alcohol – the brain has tremendous capacity to develop tolerance to, and also dependence on, medications. Even medications typically to be avoided in older adults, such as benzodiazepines, are best left alone if the patient has been on a stable dose for many years. Eliminating drugs from a list of those to avoid does not substitute for clinical judgment [26].

Other important features to consider in the history of possible cognitive impairment are family and social histories. Often, older adults may be familiar with, or misinformed about, dementia. It is important to know the patient's and families' expectations. A patient's level of education and occupation also are important to factor into an evaluation of cognition. Well-educated, formerly high functioning individuals – such as physicians – may pass easily for being cognitively intact in the face of significant impairment. Conversely, someone with very little education and limited occupational skills may be difficult to distinguish from someone who has an evolving dementia.

The Examination

The first and foremost purpose of the neurological examination is localization. If there is a lesion, where is it? Without a locus, the differential diagnosis is moot. For example, if a patient were to complain of "weakness" in a hand, it may relate to: a lesion in the premotor or motor cortex or anywhere along the course of the upper motor neuron; a nerve root or peripheral motor nerve injury; dysfunction at the neuromuscular junction; disease of the muscle; impairment in the sensory apparatus or nerves leading to the spinal cord; impaired sensory input to the thalamus or to projections from thalamus to parietal lobe; or in either basal ganglia or cerebellar extrapyramidal systems. The differential diagnosis of the weakness depends entirely on the location of the lesion.

To localize a lesion, neurologists consider the nervous system in a very deliberate manner. The neurological examination has five basic elements, each building on the foregoing part. The five parts, in order, are: I. Mental Status; II. Cranial Nerves: III. Motor (III.A. Deep tendon reflexes [DTRs]); IV. Sensory; and V. Coordination/Station/Gait. The mental status considers the cerebral hemispheres, and particularly the cortex of the brain. The cranial nerves add a consideration of the brainstem. The motor examination adds the spinal cord and efferent nerves. The sensory examination adds a consideration of afferent nerves projecting to cord, thalamus and, ultimately, to the parietal cortex. Finally, coordination, station and gait testing add a consideration of basal ganglia and cerebellum. It is important to know the relative integrity of the mental status in order to evaluate the rest of the neurological examination. A decreased level of alertness, attentiveness, cooperation or cognitive ability will flavor the rest of the examination findings, potentially limiting what can be tested. Cranial nerves, and particularly vision and hearing, also obviously may influence other examination findings. Except in rare circumstances, such as a sensory level on the trunk suggesting a spinal cord lesion, motor findings are always considered before sensory findings because motor findings are "harder" and less influenced by the patient's subjective report. DTRs naturally are considered after the motor signs. If weakness is found, the next logical question is: What are the reflexes? An increased reflex indicates an upper motor neuron (UMN) lesion, while a decreased reflex goes with a lower motor neuron (LMN) lesion. When sensory symptoms are reported, ask the patient to outline the area of numbness. Distal, symmetrical numbness is consistent with a peripheral polyneuropathy, such as in diabetes. Reflexes should be decreased distally in that setting. Focal numbness that conforms to a dermatome suggests a peripheral root or nerve lesion, while less distinct but compelling focal numbness, particularly of a densely innervated structure, such as the hand or face, may indicate a central lesion. The complaint of an entire limb being numb, particularly in the absence of compelling motor signs, is of questionable localizing value. Finally, coordination, station and gait (C/S/G) testing are considered last, because they require integrated nervous system function. The basal ganglia and cerebellum work through the motor system to augment motor function. In turn the motor system relies on sensory feedback to work properly. C/S/G testing relies also on cognitive function and to some extent on vision, hearing, and the ability to communicate. In sum, the neurological examination is designed to build a picture of the nervous system. Considered in order, that picture emerges to reveal localized deficits. Considered out of order, the exam is often uninterruptible. The admittance exam that includes, "neuro grossly normal," "neuro non-focal," or "neuro grossly non-focal," is of little value to the physician trying to decide if the patient has suffered a new neurological deficit.

The Mental Status Exam

Neurologists and psychiatrists consider the mental status examination from different viewpoints. The neurologist is a mechanic, asking "How is the vehicle running?" The psychiatrist is a driving evaluator, trying to answer "How's my driving?" While there is overlap – just as a poorly operating vehicle can make a one look like an impaired driver, or an impaired driver can make a vehicle appear to malfunction – the neurologist's approach is concrete, always with an eye to localization.

Level of Consciousness

First off is the question of level of consciousness (LOC). Alertness is a function of the reticular activating system (RAS). Acutely, a decreased LOC is due most often to global suppression of the cerebral hemispheres, such as with medications or global hypoxia. With an intact RAS, one functioning cerebral hemisphere is adequate for an alert state, as is evident even after a large unilateral hemisphere stroke. Even with both hemispheres impaired, however, an intact RAS eventually will generate an alert state, if only manifest by spontaneous eye opening. A persistent vegetative state – "The lights are on but nobody's home" – reflects the re-established sleep/wake cycle of a patient with severe injury to both cerebral hemispheres. When the LOC is decreased, a behavioral description of the minimum stimulus needed to provoke an arousal should be documented. Descriptors such as "lethargic," "stuporous," and "obtunded" are open to interpretation, while statements such as, "opens eyes to [loud voice, gentle touch, moderate pressure on the nail bed]," "localizes and fends off painful stimulation," or "withdraws appropriately to pain" offer examination findings that can be retested and monitored.

Attention

If a patient is alert, the next mental status feature is attentiveness. Attention reflects the integrity of the connections between the thalamus and the cortex – the thalamocortical circuits. It is easy to believe that a person who is alert and interactive is attentive. Still, the degree to which attention can be impaired in a normal appearing patient may be stunning. A physician on rounds may feel as though he/she has had a normal conversation with a patient, only to be called shortly thereafter because of a disruptive outburst, or other confused behavior by the patient. Impaired and fluctuating attention is the hallmark of delirium. Much of delirium is "quiet delirium," however, and may go unnoticed. Even in these cases, the morbidity of delirium is high [27]. The physician should test any patient in whom delirium is a risk, i.e., any older perioperative patient, by asking the patient to perform a task requiring attention. Relatively difficult tasks include serial seven subtractions – "Count backwards from 100 by 7s" – and months in reverse – "Recite the months of the year in reverse order." If a patient stumbles with these tasks, try easier tasks, such as, "Do a countdown from 20," or "Recite the months of the year." Try to identify and document the maximum level of attention the patient is able to sustain, even if simply counting to 10. While delirium is characterized by fluctuation, intact attention, even if for relatively brief intervals, is a good sign, while fluctuations only between bad and worse are ominous. The Intensive Care Unit nurse potentially is invaluable as an observer of evolving delirium. Cultivating a care team with nursing staff empowered to assess for the presence of delirium will serve the surgeon well. Again, the physician should not underestimate the degree to which a delirious patient may appear normal.

Memory

The next feature of the mental status examination, given that a patient is alert and attentive, is memory. The brain structures most critical for memory are the hippocampi, deep in the mesial temporal lobes. Though part of the brain cortex, the hippocampus is not neocortex, but rather much more primitive archicortex, consistent with its location near the midline. The evolving brain was not reinvented, but rather added features that gradually mushroomed over the primitive brainstem. Memory understandably is a primitive function, following naturally after alertness and attentiveness in its value to survival. The blood supply to the hippocampus is quite variable, with the main branches usually from the posterior circulation, but also anterior circulation branches directly off the internal carotid artery. Consequently, memory loss is rarely a prominent or even evident feature of stroke; posterior circulation strokes often causing other devastating injuries if the hippocampus is involved, and anterior circulation strokes typically occurring distal to branches to the hippocampus.

Because different disciplines and persons, such as psychology vs. neurology vs. family members, may use different terms, it is important to be clear what is meant by "memory." Memory function is divided in various ways. Immediate memory, sometimes called attention span or "short term memory," is the ability to recall what was just registered, such as being able to repeat back a phone number or a short list. This is more accurately a test of attention and not truly an assessment of hippocampal function and the ability to learn. Semantic memory – the conscious recollection of factual information independent of context and personal relevance, such as remembering the names of objects – and

procedural memory – the "unconscious memory" of how to do something, like riding a bike – also are not dependent primarily on the hippocampal formation, but rather neocortical (semantic memory) and extrapyramidal systems (procedural memory). Episodic memory is the conscious memory of personal events and can be divided into remote and recent memory. Remote memory is the ability to recall memories from the distant past and can be divided into personal memories, such as related to family, high school, and occupation, and nonpersonal memories, such as Presidents and major events in history. Remote memories are more "hard wired" than recent memories, and may remain relatively intact long after recent memory function has begun to decline. Recent memory – also often called "short term memory" – is the ability to recall what happened in the recent past – typically minutes to hours ago. A practical example would be to recall what one was doing before being interrupted by a phone call. It is recent memory that is most clearly dependent on hippocampal function, is most critical for new learning, and is most important to test in older adults.

Recent memory is the function impaired first and foremost in AD, and is almost invariably involved to some degree in other degenerative dementias. It is most important because the ability to learn and remember new information is key to recovery and independent living. Patients having suffered devastating neurological injuries may be able to live independently if they are able to learn. Conversely, the most physically fit patient always will be dependent without the ability to learn and remember.

Testing Recent Memory

The key to testing recent memory is to provide an adequate interference task – the mental challenge the patient has between registration and recall. The time interval is much less important. Consequently, an adequately difficult interference task, even if as brief as 10 s, may suffice to identify impairment in recent memory. The tests of attention described above are not only good interference tasks, but expedite the evaluation. By giving the patient something to remember – typically, three unrelated words – and then testing attention, the examiner integrates testing these two critical aspects of the mental status. Recent memory is so important that it is reasonable to check it multiple times during a given evaluation. Start the exam by saying, "I'm going to start with a short quiz. I'm going to say three words. Say them after me and try to remember them" (Table 24.3). Then have the patient do the interference (attention) task. Then ask "What were the three words?" If the words are not recalled, give first letter or category cues and, if necessary, multiple choice. Prompted recall is better than no recall. Still, if words are not

Table 24.3 Five alternate word lists used in the Minneapolis VA Healthcare System GRECC Memory Loss Clinic

Baby	Daughter	Village	Kitchen	Captain
Garden	River	Heaven	Nation	Season
Leader	Table	Finger	Picture	Mountain

The lists are matched for the frequency with which the words occur in the English language

spontaneously recalled, make sure that the patient repeats them a second time and ask for them later in the exam or interview. If they are not recalled a second time, again make sure that they are repeated and test a third time. Patients who don't recall the first time may have not clearly understood the intention of the test. If not recalled a second time, it becomes more concerning. If not recalled a third time, there is very likely a problem. As with any other part of the examination, the physician should seek to convince himself or herself that there either is or is not a problem. A failure of recent memory has profound implications.

Neocortical Function

The remaining mental status domains are basically language (dominant, usually left, temporoparietal cortex), visuospatial (nondominant, usually right temporoparietal cortex), and executive (frontal lobe) function. While all are eventually involved in AD, the symptoms are usually mild in the early stages and may not be evident at the bedside. Sudden difficulty with speech or language is usually obvious and, of course, concerning for an acute stroke. Neurologists are careful to distinguish deficits in speech, manifest by dysarthria, e.g., slurring, (motor function, usually brainstem or cerebellar dependent and posterior circulation), from language, characterized by difficulty finding words, use of wrong words, and/or difficulty with understanding words (expression and comprehension, neocortically dependent, anterior circulation). Persons with language deficits at least intermittently speak without dysarthria, such as the "automatic language" of a well-articulated expletive [28], whereas those with true dysarthria are unable to speak clearly under any circumstances. Sudden changes in visuospatial or executive function, however, may be more difficult to recognize and characterize, often looking like acute confusion. An inability to recognize faces, common objects or surroundings in a patient who is able to see and converse may suggest an acute nondominant hemisphere stroke. Peculiar, inappropriate behavior, such as a loss of concern, immodesty and a blunted affect, may suggest an acute frontal lobe stroke. Persons with frontal lobe (executive) dysfunction also have difficulty organizing or sequencing information, or shifting from one topic to another, often without any insight into their deficits. Typically, cortical strokes involving language, visuospatial, and/or executive function have other neurological findings which help distinguish them from delirium.

Bedside Mental Status Examinations

Several brief mental status examinations for use at the bedside or in the office have been published [29]. The utility of these exams is that they provide structure, are typically quick and easy to administer, and yield a single number to estimate global cognitive function. None can, by themselves, either make or rule out a diagnosis of dementia, though poor performance on any is usually indicative of significant cognitive problems. All should be administered rigorously to minimize variability and enhance reliability. Because they are generally scripted and straight-forward, virtually any member of the clinical team can be taught to administer the simpler bedside tests.

The most widely used bedside test of cognitive function is the mini-mental state exam (MMSE [30]), a 30 point test of orientation (5 temporal, 5 spatial points), three word registration (3 points), attention/concentration (5 points), three word recall (3 points), language (8 points) and visuospatial function (1 point). The MMSE is cited in over 5,000 journal articles and is a common primary or secondary outcome in numerous clinical studies. Most clinicians have a general idea of the meaning of the MMSE score: 30 points reflects no errors; above 26 indicates either intact cognition or only mild impairment; 20–26 typically reflects at least mild and sometimes moderate cognitive difficulties; 10–20 indicates moderate difficulties; and below 10 is usually indicative of marked cognitive deficits. The test is too simple, however, to be a diagnostic tool. In the clinical setting, there are no strict cut-offs, particularly at the upper end of the MMSE scale, that assure that a patient is cognitively intact. Intelligent, well-educated persons may score perfectly on the MMSE despite significant cognitive deficits. The MMSE is not sensitive in particular to frontal lobe (executive) dysfunction, as the structure of the test removes the need for the patient to plan and organize responses – executive functions. Unfortunately, by the time a patient's behavior typically prompts an MMSE, deficits are unambiguous (Figs. 24.8 and 24.9). In AD, the decline on the MMSE is usually insidious and independent of age [31], gender and education [32], potentially contributing to the lack of recognition early in the disease as patients, families and clinicians are inclined to attribute subtle deficits to "normal" aging.

In choosing from the many alternatives to the MMSE, both the content and the length of the test are cardinal considerations. Orientation generally is not a sensitive indicator of cognitive dysfunction. At baseline, by the time a patient is

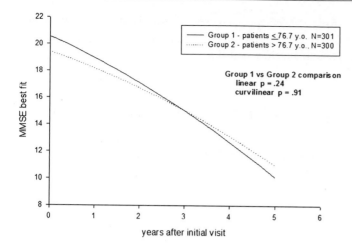

Fig. 24.8 Rate of decline on the MMSE in 601 patients with a diagnosis of Alzheimer's disease followed at the Minneapolis VA Healthcare System GRECC. Note that the average MMSE is about 20 when patients are initially diagnosed. There is no significant effect of age on rate of decline. Older patients tend to be identified later in the disease course. *MMSE* mini-mental state exam

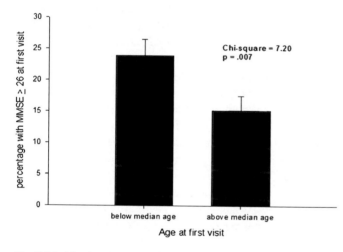

Fig. 24.9 Numbers/percentages of patients diagnosed with AD at a MMSE≥26 (mild dementia) at the Minneapolis VA Healthcare System GRECC. Total patients followed=601. Median age=76.7 years old. Note that the older cohort is significantly less likely to be identified at an early stage of AD

disoriented, cognitive symptoms are pronounced. In an acute care setting, if a disoriented patient – such as someone emerging from anesthesia – can be readily re-oriented and retains that information, there is no cause for concern. The important issues for the patient are the abilities to learn and remember new information and to follow instructions. A combination of three-word recall and the clock-drawing task (CDT [33]), the Mini-Cog™ [34, 35] assesses recent memory as well as language (ability to follow complex instructions), visuospatial and executive (planning and organization) skills in the CDT interference task. There are numerous methods to score clock drawing [36, 37], and tracking

performance (saving the drawing) may be a useful indicator of recovery. The Mini-Cog™ itself scores clock drawing simply as correct (2 points: All 12 numbers in the correct order and direction, and two hands pointing to the correct numbers) or incorrect (0 points). The 3 word registration (0 points), clock draw (2 points), and delayed recall (3 points) generate a 5 point score where 5 is best. Alternate versions of the word list and clock times allow the test to be administered serially. While the clock times of 11:10, 1:45 and 8:20 are of basically equivalent difficulty, word lists which appear to be of equal difficulty are not [38]. Matching lists for the frequency with which words appear in the language should minimize this problem (Table 24.3).

As noted previously, recent memory is so important that it should be tested multiple times if there is any doubt as to its integrity. Patients who struggle with free recall but improve with cues or multiple choice are less impaired than those who do not improve with these aids. Patients who volunteer incorrect responses, either spontaneously or to a cue, or select a foil from a multiple choice list, are more likely to be impaired. The physician must be aware that neither the three words nor the cues nor multiple choices are tests that can be made up on the fly; having two or three word lists memorized as well as the cues and multiple choices used for each list will make the job easier.

The Remainder of the Neurological Examination

A detailed review of the neurological examination is beyond the scope of this text. Several simple tests, however, can be performed by any practitioner and are outlined here. The rationale, specific test procedure and normal and abnormal finding for each test are defined.

Cranial Nerves (CN)

Visual Fields (VF; CN II)

Rationale: An extensive amount of tissue, from the retina to the occipital lobes, is traversed in the course of the VFs, and everything is arranged in quadrants VFs may be abnormal in structural brain lesions involving optic tracts (postchiasmatic), optic radiations (temporal and parietal lobes), and occipital lobes.
Procedure: While standing/seated face to face with patient, say, "Look at me. Which hand moves?" Right and left eyes are tested simultaneously, unless there is a known history of serious eye problems. Hold each hand squarely and symmetrically in upper or lower quadrants, approximately 12 in. to each side and almost flush with patient's face. Left and

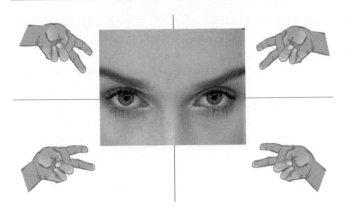

Fig. 24.10 Testing visual fields: Hold each hand clearly in the upper or lower quadrants and nearly flush with the patient's face. Test both upper and both lower quadrants simultaneously (double simultaneous stimulation)

right are tested simultaneously, first upper then lower quadrants (double simultaneous stimulation, or DSS) with a quick flick of the fingers of each hand (Fig. 24.10).

Normal: Patient responds "Both," or the equivalent. If the patient can see both stimuli simultaneously, there is no need to test left and right independently. Be aware of physical features (droopy lids, heavy brows) that may interfere with the assessment of upper quadrants.

Abnormal: (1) Patient reports seeing only one hand move. If this is a consistent finding, test each eye and each quadrant separately to distinguish monocular vs. binocular problem and an absolute VF cut vs. extinction. Extinction – seeing one hand move only when there is no competition from the opposite, homologous quadrant – is a more subtle but still significant VF deficit. (2) Patient does not see hands move unless they are positioned closer to the center of vision, suggesting a constricted field and likely an ocular problem, e.g., glaucoma.

Comment: Patients with dementia or delirium tend to perseverate and/or become distracted. When testing VFs, keep the instructions simple. The initial response may be the only reliable response. A newly documented VF deficit should be addressed electively prior to surgery or, postoperatively, in urgent fashion to rule-out a newly acquired structural lesion.

Visual Acuity (VA; CN II)

Rationale: Diminished visual acuity (VA) is a source of excess disability.

Procedure: Give the patient a card/paper with small print (preferably a standard card with graduated print as used in an eye clinic) and ask him/her to read. Always test best-corrected vision (i.e., with glasses when needed). Alternate covering each eye while the patient reads. Intact near VA assures integrity of central vision. Problems with distant vision are refractive errors.

Normal: Patient reads small print held at approximately 14 in.

Abnormal: The patient unable to read small print (VA < 14/28) needs further evaluation unless he or she has known eye disease and is followed for it.

Comment: Test VA after VFs to avoid potential confusion from a left VF deficit, in which the patient may miss items on the left of the page. This is particularly a problem if patients are asked to read numbers.

Extraocular Movements (EOMs; CNs III, IV, VI)

Rationale: Normal EOMs require input from extensive regions of brain, including frontal and parietal cortex, several brainstem nuclei, basal ganglia and cerebellum. At least subtle abnormalities in smooth pursuit eye movements are present in most brain diseases. EOMs are abnormal in some structural lesions, as a side-effect of drugs, and most prominently in the degenerative brain disease progressive supranuclear palsy (PSP).

Procedure: Holding a finger 3 ft away, ask the patient to "Follow my finger with your eyes." Move finger to extremes of gaze in all directions. Do not hold finger too close to eyes, as older adults have difficulty converging, and smooth pursuit movements may appear impaired as a result.

Normal: Patient follows finger with full and conjugate voluntary gaze and no nystagmus. (Very mild, symmetrical nystagmus at extremes of horizontal gaze is "physiological nystagmus" and within normal limits.)

Abnormal: Patient has (new) dysconjugate gaze, lacks full ROM other than mildly limited up gaze, or has significant nystagmus. A decrease in smoothness of pursuit movements also is abnormal, though very nonspecific and difficult to quantify for the exam.

Facial Symmetry (CN VII)

Rationale: Lateralized facial weakness may indicate a brain structural lesion (Central VIIth).

Procedure: Tell the patient "Show me your teeth," and "Close your eyes tight." Also observe symmetry of palpebral fissures and nasolabial folds at rest.

Normal: Symmetrical.

Abnormal: Asymmetrical.

Hearing (CN VIII)

Rationale: Diminished hearing is a source of excess disability.

Procedure: While standing two feet from the patient and while the patient is looking away, ask, in a low voice, his or her middle name.

Normal: Patient responds with a middle name or other statement to reflect that the question was heard and understood.

Abnormal: Patient does not hear adequately based on examiner's assessment of response.

Speech (CNs V, VII, IX, X; See Also CN XII Below)

Rationale: Speech may be abnormal in bilateral corticobulbar (pseudobulbar) lesions, bulbar (lower brainstem), basal ganglia and cerebellar disorders and some lateralized structural lesions.

Procedure: Assess speech quality during interview.

Normal: Speech clear, normal volume.

Abnormal: Hypophonia (diminished volume), dysphonia (hoarseness), nasal speech, or dysarthria (slurred speech, not 100% intelligible).

Cervical Rotation (CN XI; Sternocleidomastoid Muscles)

Rationale: Limited head movement is a source of excess disability (particularly with driving).

Procedure: Tell the patient and/or demonstrate, "Turn your head as far as you can to the right; now the left."

Normal: Full range of motion (90°) to right and left.

Abnormal: Significant limitation cervical in range of motion.

Tongue (CN XII)

Rationale: The tongue reveals fasiculations and atrophy in motor neuron disease; a change in appearance in nutritional deficiencies; and deviation in structural lesions.

Procedure: Look at the tongue.

Normal: Tongue is normal in appearance.

Abnormal: Atrophy, fasiculations, deviation, or macroglossia.

Motor

Strength

Rationale: Lateralized weakness suggests a structural lesion. Proximal weakness is typical of myopathies. Distal weakness is typical of neuropathies. Weakness is a source of excess disability.

Proximal Extremity Strength

Procedure for upper extremities (UEs): Drift: Ask the patient to extend arms with palms up at shoulder level, shoulder width apart, eyes closed.

Normal: Patient holds for 10 s without significant movement of arms/hands. (Tremor may be present, but should be discounted in interpretation of drift.)

Abnormal: One arm pronates. The weak arm also may drift downward, but it must pronate to be consistent with a corticospinal tract lesion. An arm that drifts laterally to 45° may suggest ipsilateral cerebellar dysfunction. An arm that drifts upward is rare but suggestive of a proprioceptive deficit.

Procedure for lower extremities (LEs): Ask the patient to cross arms over chest and stand up.

Normal: Patient stands easily without pushing off.

Abnormal: The patient: (1) Struggles but stands without pushing off; (2) Must push off to stand; (3) Needs assistance to stand; (4) Cannot stand.

Comment: The subsequent assessment of gait determines lateralized vs. generalized weakness.

Distal Extremity Strength

Procedure for UEs: Ask patient to squeeze examiner's fingers "as hard as you can."

Normal: Symmetrical grip from which examiner cannot pull away.

Abnormal: Asymmetrical or generalized weakness of grip from which examiner can pull away.

Procedure for LEs: Ask patient to walk on tiptoes and on heels. If patient has difficulty because of gait instability, allow patient to hold examiner's hands.

Normal: Patient is able to walk on tiptoes and on heels.

Abnormal: Patient cannot walk on tiptoes or heels; note if weakness is lateralized.

Bulk

Rationale: Fasiculations (small, local contractions of muscles seen under the skin) indicate an irritated LMN and are seen in motor neuron disease (amyotrophic lateral sclerosis, ALS). LMN lesions (ALS, root, ganglia, peripheral nerve) are associated with marked atrophy, with loss of about 90% of bulk. Upper motor neuron lesions have the more modest atrophy of disuse, about 25% loss of bulk.

Procedure: Visually inspect muscle groups of shoulders, forearms, calves. If it is inconvenient to visibly inspect, palpate muscles to assess bulk.

Normal: Normal and symmetrical bulk.

Abnormal: Diffuse, focal, or lateralized atrophy and/or fasiculations.

Tone

Rationale: Muscle tone is increased in: basal ganglia disorders (rigid); UMN lesions (spastic); in more advanced dementia, and also with anxiety, i.e., paratonia or gegenhalten – an increased resistance that becomes less prominent when the patient is distracted. When paratonia is prominent, other abnormalities of tone are difficult to assess. Tone is decreased diffusely in cerebellar disorders. In severe peripheral nerve injuries, such as an avulsion of nerve roots, tone is very decreased.

Procedure: Passively move each arm at elbow and wrist.

Normal: Very mild resistance.

Abnormal: (1) Diffuse or lateralized hypertonia. If the increase in tone is the same throughout the range of motion, tone is rigid. Rigidity may or may not have associated cogwheeling, which likely reflects underlying tremor. If tone changes with the degree and/or speed of passive movement, tone is spastic. More marked UE spasticity is characterized by flexion at the wrist and elbow and decreased fine motor control of the hand. Variable changes suggest paratonia, which may overlie rigidity or spasticity; (2) Diffuse or lateralized hypotonia. This is uncommonly identified. If diffuse, such patients typically have a pendular patellar reflex.

Comment: It is important to check strength before tone and tone before DTRs. If weakness is identified, particularly lateralized weakness, a change in tone and reflexes may be anticipated and should be sought. Spastic tone from an UMN lesion should be associated with increased DTRs.

Deep Tendon Reflexes (DTRs)

Rationale: DTRs are asymmetrical in lateralized UMN (increased DTRs) or LMN (decreased DTRs) lesions. DTRs are reduced symmetrically in peripheral polyneuropathy.

Procedure: Tap on tendon while palpating and/or observing corresponding muscle.

Normal: Ankle jerk (AJ; Achilles reflex; S1–2), knee jerk (KJ; patellar reflex; L3–4) brachioradialis (C5–6), biceps (C5–6), and triceps (C7–8) are present and symmetrical.

Abnormal: Absence or asymmetry of DTR. Symmetrical diffuse decrease of DTRs in a patient with an otherwise normal motor examination are likely not clinically significant. Absent AJs suggest peripheral neuropathy. Present AJs are not expected in peripheral neuropathy, such as in long-standing diabetics, and actually may represent a hyperactive reflex.

Plantar Reflex

Rationale: The plantar reflex is used universally as a test of UMN integrity.

Procedure: Scrape from lateral sole to base of great toe with any tool capable of mild irritation.

Normal: Toes flex symmetrically. No movement is equivocal, but if symmetrical, is considered normal.

Abnormal: Great toe extends, other toes may fan. If clearly asymmetrical with toes on one side flexing (normal), the contralateral side is abnormal.

Comment: Almost any noxious stimuli on or near the foot may provoke an involuntary extensor (positive) plantar reflex. Involuntary flexion at the ankle, knee and hip – a triple flexion response – is a more dramatic sign of UMN compromise. Tapping the top of the great toe with a pin may clarify withdrawal from a positive plantar reflex. The appropriate withdrawal response to the pin is to flex the toe. The involuntary extensor response actually pulls the toe into the pin.

Sensory

Rationale: Sensory disturbances are found most commonly in association with peripheral neuropathy from diabetes mellitus (DM), peripheral vascular disease (PVD), or alcohol abuse, and also are a prominent feature of B12 deficiency.

Position

Procedure: Position (proprioception): Have patient stand with feet together and eyes closed for 5 s (Romberg). If not evident, ask patient, "Do you feel a little more unsteady [normal], or a lot more unsteady [positive Romberg]?"

Normal: Negative Romberg.

Abnormal: Positive Romberg: Patient unable to maintain balance and/or reports significant increase in unsteadiness.

Light Touch

Procedure: Light touch: Ask patient, "Do you have any numbness?" If yes, have patient specify where. Touch backs of toes, then backs of fingers, and ask, "Does this feel about the same?"

Normal: Patient denies numbness; reports feet/hands feel the same to touch.

Abnormal: Patient endorses numbness in an anatomical distribution, for e.g., consistent with a peripheral neuropathy, or in a dermatomal pattern consistent with a peripheral nerve or root lesion; more diffuse/less distinct lateralized numbness may suggest a CNS lesion and is usually associated with corresponding motor and DTRs changes.

Coordination, Station and Gait

Gait

Rationale: A normal gait requires integrated motor, sensory, cerebellar and basal ganglia function. Apart from the mental status, nothing reveals more about the integrity of the nervous system than the patient's gait. While the character of an abnormal gait may be difficult to define and may require a specialist, a normal gait is easy to identify and may be an invaluable piece of documentation.

Procedure: Tell the patient, "Take a fast walk down the hall [to bring out abnormalities]." Then, "Come on back [to observe turns.]" Note base, stride, posture, arm-swing, turns (stability).

Normal: Walks normally 30 ft down the hallway and returns.

Abnormal: Hemiplegic (affected leg is stiff and circducts when moving forward; arm swing decreased on affected side); Neuropathic (steppage gait with foot slap); Parkinsonian (flexed posture, reduced stride length and arm swing, but narrow base and symmetrical stride); Ataxic (variable base and stride with tendency to cross step; staggers. Ataxia is specific to cerebellar lesions); Choreiform (abrupt, unpredictable jerky movements of limbs and trunk during walking that the patient may incorporate into gait); Magnetic (feet appear to stick to the floor and patient must make deliberate, conscious effort with each step; a gait "apraxia," the inability to perform a learned motor skill).

Comment: The gait is always abnormal in untreated PD and often abnormal in other neurodegenerative diseases, including dementia with Lewy bodies (DLB), PSP, multiple system atrophy (MSA), corticobasal degeneration (CBD), Huntington's disease (HD), and some frontotemporal dementias (FTDs). Gait abnormalities are seen also post-CVA or traumatic brain injury (TBI), in normal pressure hydrocephalus (NPH), and in cerebellar or T/M disorders. Gait disorders due to pain (antalgic) or joint (orthopedic) disease are common in older adults, but not an indicator of nervous system disease.

Postural Stability

Rationale: Postural stability is impaired in basal ganglia disorders and is a major contributor to falls.

Procedure: While the patient is standing with feet together, stand behind him/her and say, "I'm going to bump you. Keep your balance." Apply a quick tug on both shoulders, pulling patient backwards. (Use caution with low back injuries, as a patient's sudden need to catch self may exacerbate pain and spasm.)

Normal: Patient maintains balance. Patient may take one step backwards to catch self, but does not fall.

Abnormal: Patient falls backwards without being able to catch self and stop. (Examiner catches patient.)

Comment: It is a good time to test hearing while standing behind the patient.

Coordination

Rationale: Coordination is abnormal in some frontal and parietal cortical lesions (CBD; possibly FTD; decreased fine motor post-CVA), and in basal ganglia and cerebellar disorders.

Procedure 1: Rapid alternating movements: Tell patient to "Do this as fast as you can." Demonstrate rapidly turning hand over and back, patting hand on lap or in other hand; demonstrate rapid heel tapping on the floor. Do right and left separately, as the hand and foot movement often will look symmetrical when tested together. Look for rate, range, and rhythm.

Normal: Alternating hand movements and heel tapping is at least 2 Hz (ten rhythmic movements in 5 s).

Abnormal: Slowed and/or arrhythmic tapping or either hand or foot.

Procedure 2: Finger-to-nose testing: After patient has maintained drift posture for 10 s, say, "Make a pointer with the first finger on your right hand [or touch the finger and say 'with this finger'] and touch the tip of your nose. Now do it with the left hand." Remind the patient to keep eyes closed.

Normal: Touches tip of nose – may have two practice trials if needed.

Abnormal: Misses nose after two trials.

Comment: If a patient consistently misses to the same spot, e.g., touching the same spot on the cheek repeatedly, this is an embellishment (i.e., a deliberate effort to mislead the examiner) and not true dysmetria.

Involuntary, Uncontrolled, or Diminished Movements

Rationale: The character of a movement abnormality may suggest a specific disorder.

Procedure: Observe patient for: bradykinesia (generalized slowness or paucity of movement; seen in PD, DLB, PSP), tremor (PD, DLB, T/M), dysmetria (difficulty with directed hand movements, over- or under-shooting, often with shaky, uncoordinated appearance, as though hand/wrist are weighted down; seen in cerebellar or possibly cortical disorders), choreoathetosis (chorea is quick, involuntary movements, athetosis is more writhing in appearance; both affect groups of muscles; seen in HD), dystonia (involuntary, sustained contraction of muscles, producing unusual postures of limb or trunk; seen in CBD, PSP), myoclonus (quick, usually random twitches of isolated muscles; seen in Creutzfelt-Jacob disease, CJD; late in AD; T/M encephalopathies); stereotyped movements (e.g., tics; also seen in FTD; complex partial seizures). In general, adverse drug effects should always be considered when a movement disorder appears.

Summary and Conclusions

Cognitive changes in the elderly are common and are the result of brain disease. AD (Fig. 24.11), the most common cause of dementia in older adults, is insidiously progressive, is associated with few, if any, other neurological symptoms or signs, and is easily overlooked. Demented patients are more prone to delirium and can be anticipated to have more difficulty recovering from major surgery. Simple bedside tests focusing on learning and memory may identify unrecognized cognitive problems, and help to identify patients most at risk for delirium. In addition to mental status testing, several simple bedside tests may help to identify significant neurological problems. High yield examination procedures include assessing visual fields, extraocular movements, speech, drift, finger-to-nose, grip, and, if at all possible, gait. As opposed to an assessment such as "neuro non-focal," the statement of a few specific findings may be invaluable. "Recent memory 3/3, readily recites months in reverse [mental status], VFF, EOMI, face symmetrical, speech articulate [cranial nerves], gait normal [motor, sensory, basal ganglia cerebellar], drift negative [upper extremity motor; cerebellar; sensory], postural reflexes intact [basal ganglia], finger to nose normal [cerebellar hemispheres]" conveys useful information that can be used to document a patient's baseline function and monitor recovery.

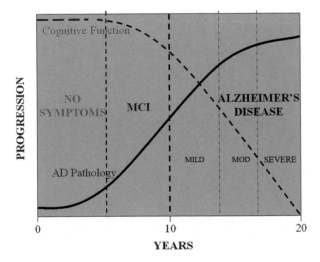

Fig. 24.11 Hypothetical progression of AD. AD pathology may begin even decades prior to onset of symptoms. A prodromal phase of insidious cognitive loss (MCI) typically precedes the appearance of full blown symptoms of dementia, by which time the pathology is well-established. The correlation of pathology and dementia severity is poor, other than to note that wide-spread, severe pathology is almost invariably associated with advanced clinical dementia. *MCI* mild cognitive impairment

References

1. Plassman BL, Langa KM, Fisher GG, Heeringa SG, Weir DR, Ofstedal MB, et al. Prevalence of cognitive impairment without dementia in the United States. Ann Intern Med. 2008;148(6): 427–34.
2. Plassman BL, Langa KM, Fisher GG, Heeringa SG, Weir DR, Ofstedal MB, et al. Prevalence of dementia in the United States: the aging, demographics, and memory study. Neuroepidemiology. 2007;29(1–2):125–32.
3. de Toledo Ferraz Alves TC, Ferreira LK, Wajngarten M, Busatto GF. Cardiac disorders as risk factors for Alzheimer's disease. J Alzheimers Dis. 2010;20(3):749–63.
4. Carlsson CM. Type 2 diabetes mellitus, dyslipidemia, and Alzheimer's disease. J Alzheimers Dis. 2010;20(3):711–22.
5. Rocchi A, Orsucci D, Tognoni G, Ceravolo R, Siciliano G. The role of vascular factors in late-onset sporadic Alzheimer's disease. Genetic and molecular aspects. Curr Alzheimer Res. 2009;6(3): 224–37.
6. Lee HB, DeLoatch CJ, Cho S, Rosenberg P, Mears SC, Sieber FE. Detection and management of pre-existing cognitive impairment and associated behavioral symptoms in the Intensive Care Unit. Crit Care Clin. 2008;24(4):723–36, viii.
7. Fong TG, Jones RN, Shi P, Marcantonio ER, Yap L, Rudolph JL, et al. Delirium accelerates cognitive decline in Alzheimer disease. Neurology. 2009;72(18):1570–5.
8. Amaducci LA, Rocca WA, Schoenberg BS. Origin of the distinction between Alzheimer's disease and senile dementia: how history can clarify nosology. Neurology. 1986;36(11):1497–9.
9. Tomlinson BE, Blessed G, Roth M. Observations on the brains of non-demented old people. J Neurol Sci. 1968;7(2):331–56.
10. Tomlinson BE, Blessed G, Roth M. Observations on the brains of demented old people. J Neurol Sci. 1970;11(3):205–42.
11. Davis PC, Gearing M, Gray L, Mirra SS, Morris JC, Edland SD, et al. The CERAD experience, part VIII: neuroimaging-neuropathology correlates of temporal lobe changes in Alzheimer's disease. Neurology. 1995;45(1):178–9.
12. Drachman DA, Leavitt J. Human memory and the cholinergic system. A relationship to aging? Arch Neurol. 1974;30(2):113–21.
13. Davies P, Maloney AJ. Selective loss of central cholinergic neurons in Alzheimer's disease. Lancet. 1976;2(8000):1403.
14. Johnston MV, McKinney M, Coyle JT. Evidence for a cholinergic projection to neocortex from neurons in basal forebrain. Proc Natl Acad Sci U S A. 1979;76(10):5392–6.
15. Whitehouse PJ, Price DL, Clark AW, Coyle JT, DeLong MR. Alzheimer disease: evidence for selective loss of cholinergic neurons in the nucleus basalis. Ann Neurol. 1981;10(2):122–6.
16. Hebert LE, Scherr PA, Bienias JL, Bennett DA, Evans DA. Alzheimer disease in the US population: prevalence estimates using the 2000 census. Arch Neurol. 2003;60(8):1119–22.
17. The Lewin Group for the Alzheimer's Association. Alzheimer's disease facts and figures 2010: total payments for healthcare, long term care and hospice. Alzheimer's Dementia. 2010;6:34.
18. Alzheimer Association. Alzheimer's disease and chronic health conditions: the real challenge for 21st century medicare. Alzheimer's disease facts and figures. Washington: Alzheimer Association; 2008.
19. Hendrie HC, Ogunniyi A, Hall KS, Baiyewu O, Unverzagt FW, Gureje O, et al. Incidence of dementia and Alzheimer disease in 2 communities: Yoruba residing in Ibadan, Nigeria, and African Americans residing in Indianapolis, Indiana. JAMA. 2001;285(6):739–47.
20. Selkoe DJ. Soluble oligomers of the amyloid beta-protein impair synaptic plasticity and behavior. Behav Brain Res. 2008;192(1): 106–13.

21. Hardy J, Selkoe DJ. The amyloid hypothesis of Alzheimer's disease: progress and problems on the road to therapeutics. Science. 2002;297(5580):353–6.

22. Ringman JM, Rao PN, Lu PH, Cederbaum S. Mosaicism for trisomy 21 in a patient with young-onset dementia: a case report and brief literature review. Arch Neurol. 2008;65(3):412–5.

23. Kim J, Basak JM, Holtzman DM. The role of apolipoprotein E in Alzheimer's disease. Neuron. 2009;63(3):287–303.

24. American Psychiatric Association. Diagnostic and statistical manual of mental disorders, fourth edition (DSM-IV). Washington: American Psychiatric Association; 1994.

25. Starner CI, Norman SA, Reynolds RG, Gleason PP. Effect of a retrospective drug utilization review on potentially inappropriate prescribing in the elderly. Am J Geriatr Pharmacother. 2009;7(1):11–9.

26. Steinman MA, Rosenthal GE, Landefeld CS, Bertenthal D, Kaboli PJ. Agreement between drugs-to-avoid criteria and expert assessments of problematic prescribing. Arch Intern Med. 2009;169(14):1326–32.

27. Fong TG, Tulebaev SR, Inouye SK. Delirium in elderly adults: diagnosis, prevention and treatment. Nat Rev Neurol. 2009;5(4):210–20.

28. Van Lancker D, Cummings JL. Expletives: neurolinguistic and neurobehavioral perspectives on swearing. Brain Res Brain Res Rev. 1999;31(1):83–104.

29. Brodaty H, Low LF, Gibson L, Burns K. What is the best dementia screening instrument for general practitioners to use? Am J Geriatr Psychiatry. 2006;14(5):391–400.

30. Folstein MF, Folstein SE, McHugh PR. "Mini-mental state." A practical method for grading the cognitive state of patients for the clinician. J Psychiatr Res. 1975;12(3):189–98.

31. McCarten JR, Hemmy LS, Rottunda SJ, Kuskowski MA. Patient age influences recognition of Alzheimer's disease. J Gerontol A Biol Sci Med Sci. 2008;63(6):625–8.

32. Wilkosz PA, Seltman HJ, Devlin B, Weamer EA, Lopez OL, DeKosky ST, et al. Trajectories of cognitive decline in Alzheimer's disease. Int Psychogeriatr. 2010;22(2):281–90.

33. Tuokko H, Hadjistavropoulos T, Miller JA, Beattie BL. The Clock Test: a sensitive measure to differentiate normal elderly from those with Alzheimer disease. J Am Geriatr Soc. 1992;40(6):579–84.

34. Borson S, Scanlan J, Brush M, Vitaliano P, Dokmak A. The mini-cog: a cognitive "vital signs" measure for dementia screening in multilingual elderly. Int J Geriatr Psychiatry. 2000;15(11):1021–7.

35. Borson S, Scanlan JM, Chen P, Ganguli M. The Mini-Cog as a screen for dementia: validation in a population-based sample. J Am Geriatr Soc. 2003;51(10):1451–4.

36. Mendez MF, Ala T, Underwood KL. Development of scoring criteria for the clock drawing task in Alzheimer's disease. J Am Geriatr Soc. 1992;40(11):1095–9.

37. Nolan KA, Mohs RC. Screening for dementia in family practice. In: Richter RW, Blass JP, editors. Alzheimer's disease: a guide to practical management, part II. St. Louis: Mosby; 1994. p. 81–95.

38. McCarten JR, Anderson P, Kuskowski MA, Borson S. Analysis of the equivalency of different versions of the Mini-CogTM. Alzheimer's Dementia. 4(4), T443. 7-15-2008. Abstract.

39. Chew ML, Mulsant BH, Pollock BG, Lehman ME, Greenspan A, Mahmoud RA, et al. Anticholinergic activity of 107 medications commonly used by older adults. J Am Geriatr Soc. 2008;56(7): 1333–41.

40. McNeil. Alzheimer's disease: unraveling the mystery. National Institute of Health; 1995, p. 1–48.

41. Alzheimer's Association. Alzheimer's disease and chronic health conditions: the real challenge for 21st century medicare. Chicago: Alzheimer's Association; 2003.

Chapter 25
Hormonal Changes During and After Cardiac Surgery

Marcello Maggio, Chiara Cattabiani, and Gian Paolo Ceda

Abstract Aging is associated with changes in serum concentrations of various hormones, including growth hormone, insulin-like growth factor-1 (IGF-1), testosterone, estrogens, dehydroepiandrosterone, cortisol, and thyroid hormones. Studies suggest that these hormonal alterations may be responsible for some of the physiologic changes seen with aging and also play a path physiological role in many age-related medical conditions. The overall result of the hormonal changes is an imbalance between catabolic hormones that increase and anabolic hormones that decrease. In this age-related hormonal context, a surgical stress, especially cardiovascular surgery, may usually lead to a more profound catabolic status than in young adult subjects. This peculiar vulnerable status observed in older population after surgery has been recently defined as *acute postoperative frailty*. The correct interpretation of the hormonal response to surgical stress is extremely important and may contribute to identify new interesting therapeutic target to improve poor clinical and functional outcomes in older patients undergoing cardiac surgery.

Keywords Hormonal changes • Elderly • Frailty • CABG • Oxidative stress • Inflammation • Testosterone • Estradiol • DHEA • Cortisol • IGF-1 • Thyroid • Anabolic deficiency • Anemia • Therapeutic target • Adaptive response

Endocrine Changes During Aging

Aging process is characterized by an imbalance between catabolic and anabolic hormones.

In particular, anabolic hormones such as testosterone, estradiol (E2), insulin-like growth factor-1 (IGF-1), and dehydroepiandrosterone sulphate (DHEAS) dramatically decrease with age, while serum cortisol levels decrease less or are substantially stable, thyroid-stimulating hormone (TSH) increase or decrease according to iodine intake with increase in free thyroxine (FT4) and decrease in free triiodothyronine (FT3) [1].

These hormonal alterations can be part of physiological changes occurring with age [2], but they are also involved in the development of frailty defined as state of vulnerability to stressors and difficulty in maintaining homeostasis, because of the decreased physiological reserves. Hormonal changes may also play a path-physiological role in many age-related conditions, such as sarcopenia [3], chronic heart failure [4] and other cardiovascular disease [5–7], and rheumatoid arthritis [8, 9].

The alteration in one single hormone has been associated with specific symptoms and clinical signs defined as andropause or more appropriately late onset hypogonadism (LOH), menopause, somatopause, and adrenopause.

Changes in Pituitary-Gonadal Function During Aging in Men and Women

The condition of lower testosterone levels associated with aging is called LOH. The decline in serum testosterone concentration is mainly due to decreased production rates in older men, as a result of abnormalities at all levels of the hypothalamic-pituitary-testicular axis [10, 11]. There is an increase in serum luteinizing hormone (LH) and follicle-stimulating hormone (FSH) levels with age with a parallel reduced response of testosterone to LH and human chorionic gonadotropin. Moreover, the circadian rhythm of testosterone secretion is generally lost in older men [12].

Changes in testosterone levels in men have been associated with adverse clinical outcomes including the development of metabolic syndrome and diabetes [13, 14], cardiovascular disease [15, 16], sarcopenia [17], osteoporosis [18], anemia [19], decline in cognitive function [20], and depression [21]. Recently, low levels of bioavailable testosterone were independently associated with worse frailty status [22], whereas other studies failed to find any association between total or free testosterone levels and frail phenotype [23, 24].

The relationship between testosterone levels and mortality is still debated with some studies showing that lower levels

M. Maggio (✉)
Department of Internal Medicine and Biomedical Sciences,
Section of Geriatrics, University of Parma, Parma 43100, Italy
e-mail: marcellomaggio2001@yahoo.it

M.R. Katlic (ed.), *Cardiothoracic Surgery in the Elderly*, DOI 10.1007/978-1-4419-0892-6_25,
© Springer Science+Business Media, LLC 2011

Fig. 25.1 Sequential mechanisms of pathophysiological events after cardiac surgery

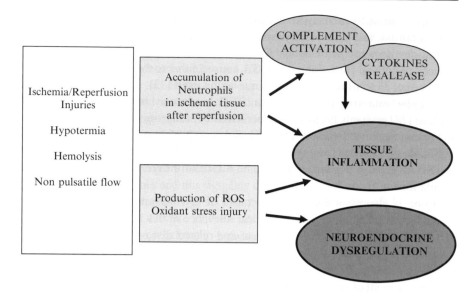

CABG, whereas the trend toward TNF-α increase in early hours reached statistical significance only 48 h after on-pump CABG [81]. None or minor differences in the kinetic of IL-6 were observed during on-pump and off-pump CABG [82, 83].

Similarly to TNF-α and IL-6, the myocardium and the lungs are major sources of IL-8 during CPB. A randomized study showed increased plasma levels of IL-8 in on-pump CABG patients from 1 to 24 postoperative hours, whereas no relevant changes were detected over time in off-pump CABG [84]. Another study showed no significant difference in the time course of IL-8 between on-pump and off-pump CABG [81].

IL-10, a cytokine with antiinflammatory properties have a rapid and significant increase in on-pump CABG, just after reperfusion and returns to baseline levels within 2–4 h after surgery. By contrast, no statistically significant changes in IL-10 levels are observed in off-pump CABG [85].

An increase in oxidative stress occurs in patients undergoing CABG with CBP (on-pump). During reperfusion, the oxygen supply in tissue is restored and the ROS are more produced causing changes in biological molecules. Off-pump procedures are associated with significantly lower levels of markers of oxidative stress during the first 24 h after surgery [86]. Even if the burst of oxidative stress that occurs during CABG has been related to myocardial ischemia-reperfusion due to cardioplegic arrest, a separate contribution of CBP to oxidative stress has also been shown [81].

In conclusion, both on-pump and off-pump CABG elicit systemic inflammatory activation. Consistent biological differences are limited to some markers of inflammation, hemostasis, and oxidative stress for the time span between the final steps of the surgical procedure and the early hours of the postoperative course. The surgical trauma, due to the unavoidable tissue injury produced by the surgical access itself, is important as the CPB in terms of inflammatory and oxidative activation. CPB might amplify the decreased neutrophil

apoptosis observed in all surgical stresses prolonging the survival of activated neutrophils and, consequently, amplifying the inflammatory response [83].

Therefore, as shown in Fig. 25.1, hormonal dysregulation occurring especially after on-pump CABG is only the final step of other phenomena associated with surgical procedure and including the complement activation and the inflammatory response.

We now list some of the most important hormonal changes occurring after CABG describing observational and, whereas available, intervention studies.

Changes in Thyroid Hormones After CABG

CABG with CPB is associated with thyroid changes consistent with "euthyroid sick syndrome." Similar changes have been observed in patients undergoing general surgical procedures. Euthyroid sick syndrome, or non-thyroidal illness syndrome (NTIS), is characterized by marked decrease in circulating triiodothyronine (T3) levels with the onset of illness or fasting [87].

Observational Studies

As already observed in the severely burned patients and critically ill patients, CBP induces the euthyroid sick syndrome, which is characterized by depression of T3 and free T3 concentrations with a concomitant increase in reverse T3 levels in the presence of normal levels of TSH [88].

As summarized in Table 25.1, several studies have analyzed the modifications in thyroid hormones after CABG. Marked decreases in serum total T3 and T4 levels occur

Table 25.1 Changes in thyroid hormones during and after CABG

References	Population	Period of observation	Results
Holland et al. [88]	14 Subjects Age 41–70	−1, +8 h, +24 h	Total T3 and free T3 were significantly depressed up to 24 h after CABG TSH, T4 and free T4 levels remained within normal range at all sampling time
Cerillo et al. [90]	40 Subjects Age 64.4 ± 9	Preoperatively, at 0, 12, 48, 120 h postoperatively, and at 6-month follow up	Non thyroidal illness was observed in all patients FT3 was still reduced by postoperative day 5 At 6 month follow up 87% of patients had normal thyroid profile, 4.5% developed overt hypothyroidism
Spratt et al. [89]	59 Subjects 7 Females 52 males Age 63.7 ± 1.7 years	Preoperatively, +1, +6, +12, +18, +24, +36 h	FT3 decreased markedly and remained low for all study period. TSH remained within the normal range
Spratt et al. [79]	17 Males Age 42–75 years (59 ± 1.8)	−1, preoperatively, 0, +1, +2, +3, +4, +5, +6 days, at 2 weeks, 4 weeks, 5 weeks	Marked decrease in serum total T3 and T4 occurring with surgery T3 levels remained below baseline through 4 wk after discharge and recovery was evident by the 2nd postoperative day Recovery of T4 occurred through 6 days
Velissaris et al. [91]	52 Subjects Age <75 years (62 ± 8 years)	−1, 0, +24 h	TSH and FT4 remained within normal range, whereas FT3 levels at 24 h after surgery were significantly lower than baseline values
Bettendorf et al. [92]	40 Children 24 Males, 16 females Age <18 years	Preoperatively, +2, +24, +72 h	During early postoperative period lowered thyroxine and triiodothyronine plasma levels, and correlate with the subsequent intensive care course. Triiodothyronine concentrations are decreased during dopamine

during and after surgery. Serum T3 levels remained significantly below the baseline levels for 6 days during hospitalization through 4 weeks after hospital discharge. A trend toward recovery is evident by the second postoperative day. Recovery of serum T4 levels occurred more rapidly in the first 6 days after surgery [89]. No significant modification in TSH levels was observed.

Changes in the components of thyroid gland condition are considered as a transient and completely reversible phenomenon and persist several days after CABG surgery. In a recent study, Cerillo et al. assessed thyroid function in 40 patients undergoing uncomplicated CABG at 0, 12, 48, and 120 h after surgery and following these patients during 6-month follow-up period. Typical NTIS was observed in all patients with free T3 concentrations still reduced by postoperative day 5. During the 6-month follow-up period, in most of the patients (87.5%) thyroid function returned to normal [90].

Other studies listed in Table 25.1 have analyzed thyroid function after CBP. All studies showed a significant decline in total and free T3, normal TSH concentration and serum T4 levels in normal range or low, in both sexes and in both older [91] and younger population [92].

Changes in thyroid function after CABG were examined by Cerillo et al. in adults and in 40 old subjects (mean age 64.4 ± 9 years) during the 6-month follow-up period. The typical changes of non-thyroidal illness were observed in all patients [90].

Spratt et al. have studied 59 subjects (mean age 63.7 ± 1.7 years) for 36 h after CBP and demonstrated a decline in T3 levels while TSH concentration remained in normal range [89]. Vellissaris analyzed 52 patients undergoing primary elective CABG (age <75 years, 62 ± 8 years) for 24 h after surgery. In the first postoperative hours, there was a significant decline in FT3 levels, but not in TSH and FT4 values [92].

Intervention Studies Using T3 in CABG

A few studies have analyzed the effects of T3 administration in patients undergoing CABG surgery or heart transplant, both of which have NTIS, with contrasting results. Some authors have reported an improvement in cardiac function [93, 94], whereas others suggested for NTIS a role of adaptive response of the organism to counteract catabolism [95].

To evaluate whether non-thyroidal illness syndrome is a physiologic response to the early stages of major illness, Spratt et al. performed a prospective randomized placebo-controlled study evaluating the effects of T3 treatment on cardiac function, protein metabolism, different hormonal axes, and iron response. T3 was infused for 24 h after surgery but the correction of T3 levels during early stages of NTIS in acute illness had minimal and transient effects in cardiac function without any significant effects on protein metabolism, endocrine balance, or iron response to acute illness [95].

The lack of discernable benefits indicates that T3 therapy should not be recommended in CABG patients.

Adrenal Hormones and CABG

Changes in Cortisol and ACTH Levels After Cardiac Surgery

The hypothalamic-pituitary-adrenal system is one of the main components of endocrine stress response after surgical stress [96]. The changes in glucocorticoid secretion is one of the best studied perioperative phenomena. Changes in HPA

Table 25.3 Changes in hypothalamus pituitary gonadal axis after CABG

References	Population	Period of observation	Results
Spratt et al. [79]	17 males Age 42–75 years (59 ± 1.8)	Preoperatively, 0, and 1st, 2nd, 3rd, 4th, 5th, 6th day, at 2nd, 4th, 5th week	Gonadotrophins but not testosterone decreased during surgery Decrease in serum testosterone was evident on the 1st day after surgery and persisted for 2 weeks Low LH levels persisted for 6 days The duration of FSH suppression was longer than LH A trend toward increasing of LH, FSH, Te was evident by the 5th day Increase in serum E1 and E2 levels Decline in SHBG levels since 2nd day after surgery
Aono et al. [101]	25 Males Middle age	Preoperatively, 0, +1, +2 days	Testosterone decreased during surgery LH increased during surgery and reached the maximum levels 30 min after the beginning Shortly after the end of surgery, LH returned to its preoperative level, while testosterone continued to fall A decline in LH levels was observed on the 2nd postoperative day, when plasma testosterone showed the most marked decrease FSH levels were not influenced by surgical stress
Spratt et al. [117]	20 Postmenopausal women	Admission, day 5	Two patterns of changes in sex steroids Admission serum levels of androstenedione, Estrone (E1), Estradiol (E2) were higher compared with healthy controls. Androstenedione and E1 then decreased toward normal by day 5 in parallel with cortisol In contrast, admission serum DHEA and DHEAS were not elevated and testosterone levels were lower than controls Testosterone and DHEA continued to decrease by day 5, in parallel with gonadotrophin levels
Spratt et al. [119]	14 Subjects 11 Males 3 Females Age 42–69 years	Preoperatively, 0, 1st, 2nd, 3rd, 4th postoperative day	Testosterone levels decreased on 1st postoperative day In contrast, estrogens were stable or increased The postoperative increase in serum E1 and E2 may be different Maximum serum E1 and E2 was in 2nd postoperative day and then declined E1 and E2 rising go on in 3rd and 4th postoperative days The mean increase in E2 was not statistically significant Androstenedione increased at the end on the 1st or in 2nd day and decreased to baseline in the 4th day
Maggio et al. [108]	19 subjects 12 males, 7 females Age 62–80 years (70.1 ± 6.1 years)	Preoperatively, on the day of procedure and 1st, 2nd, 3rd, 4th and 30th day after CABG	In men, significant drop in Testosterone (Te) levels during the first 4 days after surgery In women Te increased significantly already on the 1st day after surgery, and declined progressively thereafter remaining statistically higher for the 4 day follow up E2 increased in both sexes reaching significance on the 2nd day in men and on 3rd day in women In both sexes decline in SHBG levels but statistically significant only in men and during the first 3 post surgical days

production of DHEA/DHEAS, secondary to ACTH stimulation, and then to an increase conversion from DHEAS to testosterone [115, 116].

Serum levels of estrone (E1) and estradiol (E2) rise in both men and postmenopausal women [108, 117] after CABG. The causes of the elevated serum estrogen levels could be different. Some studies suggest that the increase in estrogen levels is the consequence of general adrenal activation with increasing supply of androgen precursors available for estrogen production [118]. By contrast, recent data indicate that the increased serum estrogen concentrations reported in acute illness are primarily caused by increased peripheral aromatization rates due to an increased expression of aromatase in both men and women [119]. The increased circulating cortisol or cytokine concentrations during critical illness may potentially contribute to an increase in aromatase expression. Glucocorticoids stimulate aromatase activity in vitro [120, 121], although in vivo studies have not confirmed this effect. Tumor necrosis factor- α, IL-1, IL-6, and IL-10 are all elevated in acute illness and have been demonstrated to increase aromatase activity in vitro [121, 122].

The clinical effects of elevated estrogen levels in critical illness remain to be interpreted. Estrogens are known to promote arterial vasodilatation and coronary flow [123], to enhance myocardial function after trauma/hemorrhage, and may have beneficial effects against hypoxic tissue damage by enhancing the production of several hepatic proteins, including factors in coagulation cascade and acute phase proteins [124, 125].

Changes in serum estrogen levels following coronary artery bypass graft surgery undergo significant individual variation. Spratt et al. tested three representative models [119]: in the first model, estrone (E1) markedly increased the second day after surgery and further rose in third and fourth postoperative day. Estradiol (E2) levels increased until the third postoperative day, and then did not change or decreased. In the second model, plasma E1 and E2 concentrations increased in the second postoperative day, then decreased. Finally, the third model showed no significant change in E2 levels [119].

These different changes in serum E1 from baseline to postoperative day 2 were highly correlated with the change in serum ASD levels [119]. Percent conversion of ASD to E1 via aromatization increased strikingly postoperatively. These data suggest that the increased adrenal androgen precursor availability may contribute to increased E1 production, even if increased aromatization rates are the primary mechanism. Recovery of reproductive axis was prolonged, requiring at least 4 weeks after surgery. In particular, recovery of FSH values was more prolonged than LH and testosterone values, suggesting that FSH secretion is more susceptible to suppression by illness than LH. The elevated estrogen response to surgery was less protracted with estrone returning to baseline levels by the fifth postoperative day [109].

This divergence of the time courses of hypogonadotropic hypogonadism and elevated estrogen observed in men suggest that the two responses are distinct, suggesting a different regulating mechanism [119]. Sex hormone binding globulin (SHBG) levels were also affected by cardiovascular surgery including CABG. SHBG is a major carrier of sex hormones in humans and is produced by the liver. The SHBG levels changes with age with a significant increase commonly observed in aging male, and scant and contradictory data available in women [126, 127].

There is increasing evidence of a protective role of SHBG on the risk of metabolic syndrome and type 2 diabetes. Low SHBG levels are an independent correlate of metabolic syndrome and an independent risk factor for diabetes also in elderly population [128–131]. Two different studies performed in 19 older participants and in 14 adult subjects undergoing CABG showed that SHBG levels declined significantly after cardiac surgery. This decline is more profound in men than in women, occurs by the first postoperative day or by third postoperative day depending on the study with a return to the preoperative levels 30 days after the surgical procedure [108, 119]. The mechanism underlying this decline might be related to the increased inflammation associated with cardiac surgery with inhibition of secretion of SHBG production from the liver.

Changes in GH-IGF-1 Levels After Cardiac Surgery

Table 25.4 summarizes the data concerning the response in GH-IGF-1 axis after cardiac surgery. In young patients, the stress response is characterized by an elevation of growth hormone secretion, which is not followed by the corresponding increment in IGF-1 and IGF-binding Protein-3 (IGFBP-3) concentrations. Plasma levels of IGF-1 decreased

Table 25.4 Changes in GH-IGF-1 axis after CABG

References	Population	Period of observation	Results
Balcells et al. [32]	23 children Age ≤18 years	Preoperatively, and on 1st, 2nd, 7th postoperative day.	IGF-1 levels were low and remained low throughout the study period. Not significant decline in IGFBP-3 The IGFBP-1 was initially high but then declined toward normal values Urinary GH concentrations were high from days 1–7
Wallin et al. [133]	20 subjects: 17 men, 3 women Age 44–81 years	Preoperatively, at 1st post operative day, and at discharge (7th)	During CABG a rapid decrease in total IGF-1 occurred GH secretion was stimulated by surgery When extracorporeal circulation stopped, there was a prompt rise in IGFBP-1 levels
Maggio et al. [108]	19 subjects 12 males 7 females Age 70.1 ± 6.1 years	Preoperative day, 0, 1st, 2nd, 3rd, 4th and 30th postoperative day	60% decline in IGF-1 levels in both sexes during the first 4 days after CABG
Cavaliere et al. [136]	24 subjects Age 41–80	Preoperative, at 2nd and 5th day after surgery	66% of patients presented an increase of IGF-1 levels after surgery 34% of patients showed unchanged or decreased levels

during CABG and remained low during the first week after surgery [108, 132, 133]. Immediately after cessation of ECC, there is also a prompt rise in another IGF-binding protein, IGFBP-1, with a progressive return to baseline values during postoperative period [133].

All these postsurgical changes in GH-IGF-1 axis, namely the increase in GH with no increase or decrease in IGF-1 levels, suggest a state of GH resistance associated with cardiac surgery [134, 135].

In older population, the decline in IGF-1 levels is even more profound. One study reports a significant decrease of about 60% in serum IGF-1 levels in both sexes during the first 4 days after on pump CABG [108] contributing to catabolic/anabolic imbalance observed in this particular age group [3, 4].

Different mechanisms may explain the postsurgical decline of IGF-1. The IGF levels are strictly related to energy intake, and IGF-1 levels have been proposed as an index of acute malnutrition in critically ill patients. Cavaliere et al. have demonstrated a significant relationship between low IGF-1 levels and worse nutritional index after coronary revascularization [136]. Moreover, the IGF-1 concentration is influenced by circulating levels of IGF-binding proteins-1 (IGFBP-1) and IGFBP-3. Animal studies have shown that hypoxia, occurring during CPB, is a potent stimulus for the secretion of these proteins [134]. Finally, during CBP, the rise in inflammatory cytokines levels with inhibitory effects on the production of IGF-1 by the liver has been proposed as one of the main facilitating factors of the development of acquired GH resistance [135].

The Significance of Hormonal Changes in Young vs. Older Population

All the hormonal changes previously described occurring after cardiac surgery are such important in adult and older patients. However, since the functional reserve and homeostatic mechanisms are already altered in older individuals, where there is also a higher prevalence of subclinical and clinical endocrine dysfunction, the impact in this population deserves further attention

The difficulty in maintaining homeostasis in the face of perturbations due to decreased physiologic reserves induces the development of a state of vulnerability to stressor, defined "frailty" [137].

Recent studies suggest that although single hormonal derangement is not frequently associated with frailty, there is a strong relationship between the parallel changes in multiple hormonal axes, typical of the elderly, and the so-called accelerated aging. Neuroendocrine dysregulation has been shown an important determinant of the clinical development of frailty [24, 48, 64, 138, 139].

This state of vulnerability of older subjects may contribute to the higher incidence of complications observed in elderly after acute illness or a type surgical stress as CABG.

For example, thyroid function changes during aging. Also in subjects with normal thyroid function, TSH levels were slightly lower at older than in younger ages; in parallel, FT3 levels were lower and FT4 levels were higher. These concomitant divergent changes may suggest that in humans the hepatic 5′ deiodinase activity declines with age, with consequence of a decreased peripheral T4 degradation [140]. Moreover, there is an age-dependent increase in the prevalence of antithyroid antibodies. All these age-related modifications in thyroid function facilitate in older population the development of euthyroid sick syndrome after critical illness or surgical stress.

Also adrenal function is also affected by age, with decrease in DHEAS concentration and relative increase of cortisol level in both sexes [64]. The higher cortisol/DHEAS ratio observed in older individuals may contribute to increased vulnerability of these subjects after CABG [107, 141].

Testosterone levels exhibit a progressive decline in men with age with smaller changes in women. Since the testosterone levels in men are generally already low, a state of "relative hypogonadism" with total testosterone levels below 200 ng/mL, occurring after surgical stress and during critical illness testosterone levels in older men, is more profound than in younger population [108] with potential consequences on frailty and mortality [29, 142, 143].

In contrast, serum levels of estrone and estradiol do not change or more likely rise in both men and postmenopausal women after CABG. This increment in circulating levels of E2 is likely explained by an increment in biological conversion from DHEA and DHEAS and by an enhanced aromatization of androgens to estrogens [108, 119].

Finally, IGF-1 serum levels decline over the life span [144]. In older persons, lower IGF-1 levels are associated with an increased risk of disability and all-cause and cardiovascular mortality [145]. Studies conducted in younger adults have observed either an increase [136] or decrease in IGF-1 levels immediately after cardiac surgery in both men and women [132, 133].

Despite the potential specific importance of the postsurgical hormonal dysregulation in older individuals, only few studies have focused on the hormonal changes occurring in the older population [89, 90, 98, 104, 108].

Maggio et al. examined the acute endocrine response occurring in older individuals (12 men and 7 women) with lower ventricular function and undergoing on pump CABG. In this group of patients, a dramatic drop in testosterone levels below 200 ng/ml in old men and a decline of about 60% in IGF-1 were observed in both sexes during the first 4 days after CABG. Serum cortisol levels significantly increased in both men and women with DHEAS increased progressively but became statistically significant only in the third day after surgery, while in women DHEAS increased fourfold on the first postoperative day and remained higher for the first 4 postsurgical days [108].

Spratt et al. [89] and Cerillo et al. [90] have evaluated changes in thyroid function after CBP in older subjects. In both of these studies, euthyroid sick syndrome occurred as in younger individuals. Roth-Isigkeit et al. showed in very older population (>70 years), a transient increase in ACTH levels after surgery. Cortisol levels rose and remained higher than the baseline values during the study period [98, 104].

Until now, no study has tested possible differences in endocrine changes in older and younger individuals.

Duration of Hormonal Changes and Recovery to Baseline

All these hormonal changes following CABG gradually recover to baseline after the end of the surgical procedure and probably the end of oxidative stress consequent to the cell damage. The duration of changes depends from the hormone studied with each single hormone showing a specific trajectory.

Thyroid Hormones

A marked decrease in total T3 and T4 concentration with T3 levels remaining below baseline levels through 5 weeks after surgery but with a trend toward recovery by the second postoperative day.

Recovery of serum T4 levels occurs more rapidly occurring in the first 6 days after surgery with no significant modification in TSH levels [89]. NTIS is generally observed in all patients with reduced free T3 concentrations by postoperative day 5. This condition is considered as a transient and completely reversible phenomenon and is persistent several days after CABG surgery.

Generally after 6 months, most of patients (87.5%) have a return to normal thyroid function [90].

Adrenal Hormones

The changes in HPA axis is one of the best studied per operative phenomena.

Pre and intraoperatively, there was no evidence of significant change in plasma cortisol or ACTH levels. These parameters are significantly increased between 6 and 8 h after surgery compared with preoperative values. ACTH levels recover to baseline concentrations during the first or second postoperative day. Plasma cortisol levels remain high and significantly elevated over the first four postsurgical follow up days. All changes in Cortisol, DHEA, DHEAS, and Cort/DHEA molar ratio return to baseline levels after 30 days, since the surgical procedure [108].

Sex Hormones

CABG has been demonstrated to produce modifications in sex hormone concentrations.

A decline in testosterone levels occurs in the first four days after CABG. A marked decrease in testosterone concentrations is evident in men on the first day after surgery [108, 119] and low serum testosterone levels persist for 2 weeks following surgery [119] and then gradually returned to baseline values (30 days) [108]. The amplitude of the decline is different from study to study [108, 119].

In women, testosterone levels increase significantly already on the first day after surgery and decline progressively thereafter. However, testosterone remains statistically higher than the baseline for the first 4 days after surgery and recovers to baseline values in the first month after CABG [108].

Estradiol levels increase after surgery in both sexes. In men, this increase is significant on postoperative day 2, in women on day 3, and persist during hospitalization period. One month after surgical procedure, estradiol levels return to baseline values in both men and women [79, 108].

LH decreases profoundly during surgery and low LH levels persist throughout hospitalization (5 days after surgery) [108].

A trend toward increasing serum levels of LH and FSH is evident by the fifth postoperative day [119].

Decrease in serum SHBG levels is evident by the second postoperative day, but it is statistically significant only in men and return to baseline levels 30 days after surgery.

GH-IGF-1 Axis

In both men and women, serum GH levels increase in the first postoperative hours and are still higher during the postsurgical period, although the magnitude of increment is modest and not statistically significant. In contrast, IGF serum levels decrease quickly after surgery and remain significantly lower than baseline over the first 4 days after CABG. Within a month, these changes recover to baseline levels [108, 133].

Possible Clinical Implications of Postsurgical Endocrine Changes: Adaptive Phenomenon or Therapeutic Targets?

The significance of the hormonal changes occurring after surgery is uncertain. There is no agreement to consider these endocrine changes a physiological or adaptive mechanism useful for recovery during the postoperative period [146].

In favor of this hypothesis is the non-thyroidal illness, which is a transient and completely reversible phenomenon, and is considered a protective mechanism from the catabolic postsurgical state [87]. In fact, when T3 replacement is performed in adult undergoing CBP, no significant improvement in cardiac function, protein metabolism, and iron response is achieved [95].

Conversely, other authors suggest that postsurgical hormonal modifications are not only the surrogate of the other concurring phenomena including oxidative stress and proinflammatory state but may also worsen the metabolic, functional, and cognitive function of individuals during the postoperative period.

For example, the dramatic decline in testosterone and IGF-1 observed in older men might have in this specific population important clinical and functional consequences. Theoretically, through anabolic, antiinflammatory properties, testosterone replacement therapy during surgery could improve rehabilitative and functional outcomes [78, 147]. Another potential beneficial effect of testosterone treatment is on hemopoiesis [19, 148]. Since anemia (due to inflammation, hem dilution, malnutrition, bleeding) is a frequent clinical complication after surgery, testosterone might help to counteract the development of anemia especially in older population where testosterone levels before the surgical procedure are already low.

Similarly, the decline in IGF-1 levels occurring in both men and women after surgery have important clinical consequences, since IGF-1 is a modulator of catabolic/anabolic equilibrium and vascular function, and a good nutritional marker especially in older population. Epidemiological studies in general population have shown that low IGF-1 levels are associated with an increased risk in ischemic heart disease and stroke [145, 149, 150].

Therefore, for testosterone (at least in men) and IGF-1 (in both sexes), the hypothesis that these hormonal responses are an adaptive mechanism is unlikely. More credit deserves the alternative theory that these modifications can worsen the impact of surgical stress and might eventually represent potential therapeutic targets in the specific setting of older frail individuals [147, 151].

In both sexes, serum DHEA and DHEAS levels increased from the first postoperative day and then progressively decline. The increase in DHEA, due to an increase of the serum levels

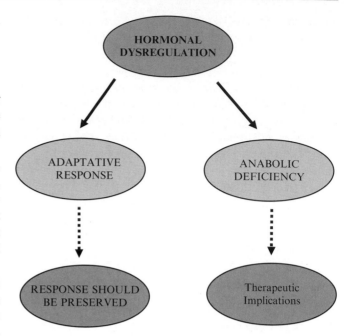

Fig. 25.2 Interpretation and possible therapeutic implications of endocrine changes after cardiac surgery in older patients

of the stimulating adrenocorticotrophic hormone, seems to be advantageous in critical illness and during CPB.

Finally, the increased estrogen levels after CABG found in several studies [79, 108, 119] argue against the use of estrogens prior to surgery in men and postmenopausal women undergoing CBP, a treatment advocated by some researchers [152, 153]. (Fig. 25.2)

References

1. Lamberts SW, van den Beld AW, van der Lely AJ. Endocrinology of aging. Science. 1997;278(5337):419–24.
2. Ceda GP, Dall'Aglio E, Maggio M, Lauretani F, Bandinelli S, Falzoi C, et al. Clinical implications of the reduced activity of GH-IGF-I axis in older men. J Endocrinol Invest. 2005;28(11 Suppl Proceedings):96–100.
3. Roubenoff R, Parise H, Payette HA, Abad LW, D'Agostino R, Jacques PF, et al. Cytokines, insulin-like growth factor-1, sarcopenia and mortality in very old community-dwelling men and women: the Framingham heart study. Am J Med. 2003;115:429–35.
4. Ceda GP, Dall'Aglio E, Salimbeni I, Rocci A, Mazzoni S, Corradi F, et al. Pituitary function in chronic heart failure in the elderly. J Endocrinol Invest. 2002;25(10 suppl):24–8. Review.
5. Muller M, van der Schouw YT, Thijssen JHH, Grobbee DE. Endogenous sex hormones and cardiovascular disease in men. J Clin Endocrinol Metab. 2003;88(11):5076–86. Review.
6. Saccà L, Cittadini A, Fazio S. Growth hormone and the heart. Endocr Rev. 1994;15(5):555–73.
7. Vasan RS, Sullivan LM, D'Agostino RB, Roubenoff R, Harris T, Sawyer DB, et al. Serum insulin like growth factor I and risk for heart failure in elderly individuals without a previous myocardial infarction: the Framingham Heart Study. Ann Intern Med. 2003;139(8):642–8.

8. Ferrucci L, Guralnik JM. Inflammation, hormones, and body composition at a crossroad. Am J Med. 2003;115(6):501–2.

9. Tengstrand B, Carlstrom K, Hafstrom I. Bioavailable testosterone in men with rheumatoid arthritis – high frequency of hypogonadism. Rheumatology (Oxford). 2002;41(3):285–9.

10. Ishimaru T, Pages L, Horton R. Altered metabolism of androgens in elderly men with benign prostatic hyperplasia. J Clin Endocrinol Metab. 1977;45(4):695–701.

11. Mulligan T, Iranmanesh A, Johnson ML, Straume M, Veldhuis JD. Aging alters feed-forward and feedback linkages between LH and testosterone in healthy men. Am J Physiol. 1997;273(4, Pt2): R1407–13.

12. Chahal HS, Drake WM. The endocrine system and ageing. J Pathol. 2007;211(2):173–80. Review.

13. Laaksonen DE, Niskanen L, Punnonen K, Nyyssonen K, Tuomainen T-P, Valkonen V-P, et al. Testosterone and sex hormone binding globulin predict the metabolic syndrome and diabetes in middle aged men. Diab Care. 2004;27(5):1036–41.

14. Rodriguez A, Muller DC, Metter EJ, Maggio M, Harman SM, Blackman MR, et al. Aging, androgens, and the metabolic syndrome in a longitudinal study of aging. J Clin Endocrinol Metab. 2007;92(9):3568–72.

15. Hak AE, Witteman JC, de Jong FH, Geerlings MI, Hofman A, Pols HA. Low levels of endogenous androgens increased risk of atherosclerosis in elderly menthe Rotterdam study. J Clin Endocrinol Metab. 2002;87(8):3632–9.

16. Muller M, van den Beld AW, Bots ML, Grobbee MI, Lamberts SW, van der Schouw YT. Endogenous sex hormones and progression of carotid atherosclerosis in elderly men. Circulation. 2004;109(17):2074–9.

17. Doherty TJ. Invited review: aging and sarcopenia. J Appl Physiol. 2003;95(4):1717–27.

18. Fink HA, Ewing SK, Ensrud KE, Barrett-Connor E, Taylor BC, Cauley JA, et al. Association of testosterone and estradiol deficiency with osteoporosis and rapid bone loss in older men. J Clin Endocrinol Metab. 2006;91(10):3908–15.

19. Ferrucci L, Maggio M, Bandinelli S, Basaria S, Lauretani F, Ble A, et al. Low testosterone levels and the risk of anemia in older men and women. Arch Intern Med. 2006;166(13):1380–8.

20. Yeap BB, Almeida OP, Hyde Z, Chubb SA, Hankey GJ, Jamrozik K, et al. Higher serum free testosterone is associated with better cognitive function in older men, whilst total testosterone is not. Clin Endocrinol. 2008;68(3):404–12.

21. Shores M, Sloan KL, Matsumoto AM, Moceri VM, Felker B, Kivlahan DR. Increased incidence of diagnosed depressive illness in hypogonadal older men. Arch Gen Psychiatry. 2004;61(2): 162–7.

22. Cawthon PM, Ensrud KE, Laughlin GA, Cauley JA, Dam TT, Barrett-Connor E, et al. Sex hormones and frailty in older men: the osteoporotic fractures in men (MrOS) study. J Clin Endocrinol Metab. 2009;94(10):3806–15.

23. Mohr BA, Bhasin S, Kupelian V, Araujo AB, O'Donnel AB, McKinlay JB. Testosterone, sex hormone-binding globulin and frailty in older men. J Am Geriatr Soc. 2007;55(4):548–55.

24. Cappola AR, Xue QL, Fried LP. Multiple hormonal deficiencies in anabolic hormones are found in frail older women: the Women's Health and Aging studies. J Gerontol A Biol Sci Med Sci. 2009;64(2):243–8.

25. Shores MM, Matsumoto AM, Sloan KL, Kivlahan DR. Low serum testosterone and mortality in male veterans. Arch Intern Med. 2006;166(15):1660–5.

26. Khaw KT, Dowsett M, Folkerd E, Bingham S, Wareham N, Lube R, et al. Endogenous testosterone and mortality due to all causes, cardiovascular disease, and cancer in men: European prospective investigation into cancer Norfolk (EPIC-Norfolk) prospective population study. Circulation. 2007;116(23):2694–701.

27. Laughlin GA, Barrett-Connors E, Bergstrom J. Low serum testosterone and mortality in older men. J Clin Endocrinol Metab. 2008;93(1):68–75.

28. Smith GD, Ben-Shlomo Y, Beswick A, Yarnell J, Lightman S, Elwood P. Cortisol, testosterone, and coronary heart disease: prospective evidence from the Caerphilly Study. Circulation. 2005; 112(3):332–40.

29. Araujo A, Kupelian V, Page ST, Handelsman DJ, Bremner J, McKinlay JB. Sex steroids and all-cause and cause-specific mortality in men. Arch Intern Med. 2007;167(12):1252–60.

30. Maggio M, Lauretani F, Ceda GP, Bandinelli S, Ling SM, Metter JE, et al. Relationship between low levels of anabolic hormones and 6-years mortality in older men: the Aging in the Chianti Area (InCHIANTI) Study. Arch Intern Med. 2007;167(20):2249–54.

31. Johnson SR. Menopause and hormone replacement therapy. Med Clin North Am. 1998;82(2):297–320. Review.

32. Speroff L, Symons J, Kempfert N, Femhrt Study Investigators. The effect of varying low-dose combinations of norethindrone acetate and ethinyl estradiol (FEMHRT) on the frequency and intensity of vasomotor symptoms. Menopause. 2000;7(6):383–90.

33. Nordin BE, Wishart JM, Clifton PM, McArthur R, Scopacasa F, Need AG, et al. A longitudinal study of bone-related biochemical changes at the menopause. Clin Endocrinol (Oxford). 2004;61(1):123–30.

34. Shaywitz SE, Shaywitz BA, Pugh KR, Fulbright RK, Skudlarski P, Mencl WE, et al. Effect of estrogen on brain activation patterns in postmenopausal women during working memory tasks. J Am Med Assoc. 1999;281(13):1197–202.

35. Hendrix SL, Cochrane BB, Nygaard IE, Handa VL, Barnabei VM, Iglesia C, et al. Effects of estrogen with or without progestin on urinary incontinence. JAMA. 2005;293(8):935–48.

36. Khan AS, Sane DC, Wannenburg T, Sonntag WE. Growth hormone, insulin like growth factor-I and the aging cardiovascular system. Cardiovasc Res. 2002;54(1):25–35. Review.

37. Lieberman SA, Mitchell AM, Marcus R, Hintz RL. Hoffman AR the insulin like growth factor I generation test: resistance to growth hormone with aging and estrogen replacement therapy. Horm Metab Res. 1994;26(5):229–33.

38. Hameed M, Harridge SDR, Goldspink G. Sarcopenia and Hypertrophy: a role for insulin like growth factor-1 in aged muscle? Exerc Sport Sci Rev. 2002;30(1):15–9. Review.

39. Fryburg DA. Insulin like growth factor I exert growth hormone- and insulin like actions on human muscle protein metabolism. Am J Physiol. 1994;267(2 Pt 1):E331–6.

40. Sandhu M, Heald A, Gibson J, Cruickshank JK, Dunger DB, Wareham NJ. Circulating concentrations of insulin like growth factor-I and development of glucose intolerance: a prospective observational study. Lancet. 2002;359(9319):1740–5.

41. Puglielli L. Aging of brain, neurotrophin signalling, and Alzheimer disease: is IGF1-R the common culprit? Neurobiol Aging. 2008;29(6):795–811.

42. Wilder RL. Hormones and autoimmunity: animal models of arthritis. Baillières Clin Rheumatol. 1996;10(2):259–71. Review.

43. Bayes-Genis A, Conover CA, Schwartz RS. The insulin like growth factor axis: a review of atherosclerosis and restenosis. Circ Res. 2000;86(2):125–30. Review.

44. Conti E, Carrozza C, Capoluongo E, Volpe M, Crea F, Zuppi C, et al. Insulin like growth factor- 1 as a vascular protective factor. Circulation. 2004;110(15):2260–5. Review.

45. Baserga R. The insulin like growth factor 1 receptor: a key to tumor growth? Cancer Res. 1995;55(2):249–52.

46. Fürstenberger G, Senn HJ. Insulin like growth factors and cancer. Lancet Oncol. 2002;3(5):298–302. Review.

47. Samani A, Yakar S, LeRoith D, Brodt P. The role of IGF system in cancer growth and metastasis: overview and recent insights. Endocr Rev. 2007;28(1):20–47. Review.

48. Leng SX, Cappola AR, Andersen RE, Blackman MR, Koenig K, Blair M, et al. Serum levels of insulin like growth factor-I (IGF-I) and dehydroepiandrosterone sulfate (DHEA-S) and their relationships with serum interleukin-6 in the geriatric syndrome of frailty. Aging Clin Exp Res. 2004;16(2):153–7.

49. Puts MT, Visser M, Twisk JW, Deeg DJ, Lips P. Endocrine and inflammatory markers as predictors of frailty. Clin Endocrinol (Oxford). 2005;63(4):403–11.

50. Brugts MP, van den Beld AW, Hofland LJ, van der Wansem K, van Koetsveld PM, Frystyk J, et al. Low circulating insulin like growth factor-I bioactivity in elderly men is associated with increased mortality. J Clin Endocrinol Metab. 2008;93(7):2515–22.

51. Cappola AR, Xue QL, Ferrucci L, Guralnik JM, Volpato S, Fried L. Insulin like growth factor I and Interleukin-6 contribute synergistically to disability and mortality in older women. J Clin Endocrinol Metab. 2003;88(5):2019–25.

52. Friedrich N, Haring R, Nauck M, Lüderimann J, Rosskopf D, Spilcke-Liss E, et al. Mortality and serum insulin like growth factor-I and IGF binding protein 3 concentrations. J Clin Endocrinol Metab. 2009;94(5):1732–9.

53. Roubenoff R, Parise H, Payette HA, Abad LW, D'Agostino R, Jacques PF, et al. Cytokines, insulin like growth factor 1, sarcopenia and mortality in very old community-dwelling men and women: the Framingham Heart Study. Am J Med. 2003;115(6):429–35.

54. Arai Y, Takayama M, Gondo Y, Inagaki H, Yamamura K, Nakazawa S, et al. Adipose endocrine function, insulin like growth factor-1 axis and exceptional survival beyond 100 years of age. J Gerontol A Biol Sci Med Sci. 2008;63A(11):1209–18.

55. Laughlin GA, Barrett-Connor E, Criqui MH, Kritz-Silverstein D. The prospective association of serum insulin like growth factor-I (IGF-I) and IGF-binding protein-1 levels with all cause and cardiovascular disease mortality in older adults: The Rancho Bernardo Study. J Clin Endocrinol Metab. 2004;89(1):114–20.

56. Saydah S, Graubard B, Ballard-Barbash R, Berrigan D. Insulin like growth factors and subsequent risk of mortality in the United States. Am J Epidemiol. 2007;166(5):518–26.

57. Yamaguchi H, Komamura K, Choraku M, Hirono A, Takamori N, Tamura K, et al. Impact of serum insulin like growth factor-1 on early prognosis in acute myocardial infarction. Intern Med. 2008;47(9):819–25.

58. Andreassen M, Kistorp C, Raymond I, Hildebrandt P, Gustafsson F, Kristensen LØ, et al. Growth Horm IGF Res. 2009;19(6):489–90.

59. Hu D, Pawlikowska L, Kanaya A, Hsueh WC, Colbert L, Newman AB, et al. Health, Aging and Body Composition Study. Serum insulin like growth factor-1, binding protein 1 and 2 and mortality in older adults: the health, aging, and body composition study. J Am Geriatr Soc. 2009;57(7):1213–8.

60. Kaplan R, McGinn AP, Pollak MN, Kuller L, Strickler HD, Rohan TE, et al. Total insulin like growth factor-I and insulin like growth factor binding protein levels, functional status, and mortality in older adults. J Am Geriatr Soc. 2008;56(4):652–60.

61. Raynaud Simon A, Lafort S, Berr C, Dartigues JF, Baulieu EE, Le Bouc Y. Plasma insulin like growth factor I levels in the elderly: relation to plasma dehydroepiandrosterone sulfate levels, nutritional status, health and mortality. Gerontology. 2001;47(4):198–206.

62. Major JM, Laughlin GA, Kritz-Silvestein D, Wingard DL, Barrett-Connor E. Insulin like growth factor I and cancer mortality in older men. J Clin Endocrinol Metab. 2010;95(3):1054–9.

63. Orentreich N, Brind JL, Rizer RL, Vogelman JH. Age changes and sex differences in serum dehydroepiandrosterone sulfate concentrations throughout adulthood. J Clin Endocrinol Metab. 1984;59(3):551–5.

64. Valenti G. Aging as an allostatic condition of hormones secretion: summing up the endocrine data from the InCHIANTI study. Acta Biomed. 2010;81 Suppl 1:9–14.

65. Parker Jr CR, Mixon RL, Brissie RM, Grizzle WE. Aging alters zonation in adrenal cortex of men. J Clin Endocrinol Metab. 1997;82(11):3898–901.

66. Yen SS, Laughling GA. Aging and the adrenal cortex. Exp Gerontol. 1998;33(7–8):897–910. Review.

67. Baulieu EE. Dehydroepiandrosterone (DHEA): a fountain of youth? J Clin Endocrinol Metab. 1996;8(9):3147–51.

68. Trivedi DP, Khaw KT. Dehydroepiandrosterone sulfate and mortality in elderly men and women. J Clin Endocrinol Metab. 2001;86(9):4171–7.

69. Barrett-Connor E, Khaw KT, Yen SS. A prospective study of dehydroepiandrosterone sulfate, mortality, and cardiovascular disease. N Engl J Med. 1986;315(24):1519–24.

70. Mazat L, Lafont S, Berr C, Debuire B, Tessier JF, Dartigues JF, et al. Prospective measurements of dehydroepiandrosterone sulfate in a cohort of elderly subjects: relationship to gender, subjective health, smoking habits, and 10-yr mortality. Proc Natl Acad Sci USA. 2001;98(14):8145–50.

71. Barrett-Connor E, Khaw KT. Absence of an inverse relation of dehydroepiandrosterone sulfate with cardiovascular mortality in postmenopausal women. N Engl J Med. 1987;317(11):711.

72. Barrett-Connor E, Edelstein SL. A prospective study of dehydroepiandrosterone sulfate and cognitive function in an older population: the Rancho Bernardo Study. J Am Geriatr Soc. 1994;42(4):420–3.

73. Mariotti S, Franceschi C, Cossarizza A, Pinchera A. The aging thyroid. Endocr Rev. 1995;16(6):686–715.

74. Sawin CT, Geller A, Kaplan MM, Bacharach P, Wilson PW, Hershman JM. Low serum thyreotropin (thyroid stimulating hormone) in older person without hyperthyroidism. Arch Intern Med. 1991;151(1):165–8.

75. Greenspan SL, Klinbanski A, Rowe JW, Elahi D. Age related alterations in pulsatile secretion of TSH: role of dopaminergic regulation. Am J Physiol. 1991;260(3 Pt 1):E486–91.

76. Ferrari E, Cravello L, Muzzoni B, Casarotti D, Paltro M, Solerte SB, et al. Age-related changes of hypothalamic-pituitary-adrenal axis: pathophysiological correlates. Eur J Endocrinol. 2001;144(4):319–29.

77. Kudielka BM, Schmidt-Reinwald AK, Hellhammer DH, Kirschbaum C. Psychological and endocrine responses to psychosocial stress and dexamethasone/corticotropin-releasing hormone in healthy postmenopausal women and young controls: the impact of age and a two week estradiol treatment. Neuroendocrinology. 1999;70(6):422–30.

78. Ferrucci L, Maggio M, Ceda GP, Beghi C, Valenti G, De Cicco G. Acute postoperative frailty. J Am Coll Surg. 2006;203(1):134–5.

79. Spratt DI, Kramer RS, Morton JR, Lucas F, Becker K, Longcope C. Characterization of a prospective human model for study of the reproductive hormone response to major illness. Am J Physiol Endocrinol Metab. 2008;295(1):E63–9.

CABG and Oxidative Stress

80. Biglioli P, Cannata A, Alamanni F, Naliato M, Porqueddu M, Zanobini M, et al. Biological effects of off-pump vs. on-pump coronary artery surgery: focus on inflammation, hemostasis and oxidative stress. Eur J Cardiothorac Surg. 2003;24(2):260–9.

81. Matata BM, Sosnowski AW, Galinanes M. Off-pump bypass graft operation significantly reduces oxidative stress and inflammation. Ann Thorac Surg. 2000;69(3):785–91.

82. Schulze C, Conrad N, Schutz A, Egi K, Reichenspurner H, Reichart B, et al. Reduced expression of systemic proinflammatory cytokines after off pump versus conventional coronary artery bypass grafting. Thorac Cardiovasc Surg. 2000;48(6):364–9.

83. Chello M, Mastroroberto P, Quirino A, Cuda G, Perticone F, Cirillo F, et al. Inhibition of neutrophil apoptosis after coronary bypass operation with cardiopulmonary bypass. Ann Thorac Surg. 2002; 73(1):123–30.

84. Ascione R, Lloyd CT, Underwood MJ, Lotto AA, Pitsis AA, Angelini GD. Inflammatory response after coronary revascularization with or without cardiopulmonary bypass. Ann Thorac Surg. 2000;69(4):1198–204.

85. Wan S, Izzat MB, Lee TW, Wan IY, Tang NL, Yim AP. Avoiding cardiopulmonary bypass in multivessel CABG reduces cytokine response and myocardial injury. Ann Thorac Surg. 1999;68(1):52–6.

86. Gerritsen WBM, van Boven WJ, Driessen AH, Haas FJ, Aarts LP. Off-pump versus on-pump coronary artery bypasses grafting: oxidative stress and renal function. Eur J Cardiothorac Surg. 2001;20(5):923–9.

CABG and Thyroid Function

87. Langton JE, Brent GA. Nonthyroidal illness syndrome: evaluation of thyroid function in sick patients. Endocrinol Metab North Am. 2002;31(1):159–72.

88. Holland FW, Brown Jr PS, Weintraub BD, Clark RE. Cardiopulmonary bypass and thyroid function: a "euthyroid sick syndrome". Ann Thorac Surg. 1991;52(1):46–50.

89. Spratt DI, Frohnauer M, Cyr-Alves H, Kramer RS, Lucas FL, Morton JR, et al. Physiological effects of nonthyroidal illness syndrome in patients after cardiac surgery. Am J Physiol Endicrinol Metab. 2007;293(1):E310–5.

90. Cerillo AG, Storti S, Mariani M, Kallush E, Bevilacqua S, Parri MS, et al. The non-thyroidal illness syndrome after coronary artery bypass grafting: a 6-month follow-up study. Clin Chem Lab Med. 2005;43(3):289–93.

91. Velissaris T, Tang AT, Wood PJ, Hett DA, Ohri SK. Thyroid function during coronary surgery with or without cardiopulmonary bypass. Eur J Cardiothorac Surg. 2009;36(1):148–54.

92. Bettendorf M, Schmidt KG, Grulich-Henn J, Ulmer HE, Heinrich UE. Triiodothyronine treatment in children after cardiac surgery: a double blind, randomised, placebo-controlled study. Lancet. 2000;356(9229):529–34.

93. Novitzky D. Novel actions of thyroid hormone: the role of triiodothyronine in cardiac transplantation. Thyroid. 1996;6(5):531–6.

94. Rosendale JD, Kauffman HM, McBride MA, Chabalewski FL, Zaroff JG, Garrity ER, et al. Hormonal resuscitation yields more transplanted hearts, with improved early function. Transplantation. 2003;75(8):1336–41.

95. Gardner DF, Kaplan MM, Stanley CA, Utiger RD. Effect of triiodothyronine replacement on the metabolic and pituitary responses to starvation. N Engl J Med. 1979;300(11):579–84.

CABG and Adrenal Function

96. Weissman C. The metabolic response to stress: an overview and update. Anesthesiology. 1990;73(2):308–27.

97. Weiskopf M, Braunstein GD, Bateman TM, Sowers JR, Conklin CM, Matloff JM, et al. Adrenal function following coronary bypass surgery. Am Heart J. 1985;110(1 Pt):71–6.

98. Roth-Isigkeit AK, Dibbelt L, Schmucker P. Blood levels of corticosteroid-binding globulin, total cortisol and unbound cortisol in patients undergoing coronary artery bypass grafting surgery with cardiopulmonary bypass. Steroids. 2000;65(9):513–20.

99. Vogeser M, Felbinger TW, Kilger E, Röll W, Fraunberger P, Jacob K. Corticosteroid-binding globulin and free cortisol in the early postoperative period after cardiac surgery. Clin Biochem. 1999;32(3):213–6.

100. Chernow B, Alexander RH, Smallridge RC, Thomson WR, Cook D, Beardsley D, et al. Hormonal responses to graded surgical stress. Arch Intern Med. 1987;147(7):1273–87.

101. Lanuza DM. Postoperative circadian rhythms and cortisol stress response to two types of cardiac surgery. Am J Crit Care. 1995;4(3):212–20.

102. McIntosh TK, Lothrop DA, Lee A, Jackson BT, Nabseth D, Egdahl RH. Circadian rhythm of cortisol altered in postsurgical patients. J Clin Endocrinol Metab. 1981;53(1):117–22.

103. Span LF, Hermus AR, Bartelink AK, Hoitsma AJ, Gimbrere JSF, Smals AG, et al. Adrenocortical function: an indicator of severity of disease and survival in chronic critically ill patients. Intensive Care Med. 1992;18(2):93–6.

104. Roth-Isigkeit A, Schmucker P. Postoperative dissociation of blood levels of cortisol and adrenocorticotropin after coronary artery bypass grafting surgery. Steroids. 1997;62(11):695–9.

105. Späth-Schwalbe E, Born J, Schrezenmeier H, Bornstein ST, Stromeyer P, Drechsler S, et al. Interleukin-6 stimulates the hypothalamus-pituitary adrenocortical axis in man. J Clin Endocrinol Metab. 1994;79(4):1212–4.

106. Vogeser M, Felginger TW, Röll W, Jacob K. Cortisol metabolism in the postoperative period after cardiac surgery. Clin Endocrinol Diabetes. 1999;107(8):539–46.

107. Straub RH, Lehle K, Herfarth H, Weber M, Falk W, Preuner J, et al. Dehydroepiandrosterone in relation to other adrenal hormones during an acute inflammatory stressful disease state compared with chronic inflammatory disease: a role of interleukin-6 and tumor necrosis factor. Eur J Endocrinol. 2002;146(3):365–74.

108. Maggio M, Ceda GP, De Cicco G, Cattadori E, Visioli S, Ablondi F, et al. Acute changes in circulating hormones in older patients with impaired ventricular function undergoing on pump coronary artery bypass grafting. J Endocrinol Invest. 2005;8:711–9.

CABG and Sex Hormones

109. Canbaz S, Ege T, Sunar H, Cikirikcioglu M, Acipayam M, Duran E. The effects of cardiopulmonary bypass on androgen hormones in coronary artery bypass surgery. J Intern Med Res. 2002;30(1):9–14.

110. Aono T, Kurachi K, Mizutani S, Hamanaka Y, Uozumi T, Nakasima A, et al. Influence of major surgical stress on plasma levels of testosterone, luteinizing hormone and follicle-stimulating hormone in male patients. J Clin Endocrinol Metab. 1972;35(4):535–42.

111. Finkelstein JS, O'Dea LS, Whitcomb RW, Crowley Jr WF. Sex steroid control of gonadotropic secretion in the human male. II. Effects of estradiol administration in normal and gonadotropin releasing hormone deficient men. J Clin Endocrinol Metab. 1991;73(3):621–8.

112. Matsumoto AM. Andropause: clinical implications of the decline in serum testosterone levels with aging in men. J Gerontol A Biol Sci Med Sci. 2002;57(2):M76–99. Review.

113. Dong Q, Salva A, Sottas CM, Niu E, Holmes M, Hardy MP. Rapid glucocorticoid mediation of suppressed testosterone biosynthesis in male mice subjected to immobilization stress. J Androl. 2004;25(6):973–81.

114. Mauduit C, Gasnier F, Rey C, Chauvin MA, Stocco DM, Louisot P, et al. TNF alpha inhibits leyding cell steroidogenesis through a decrease in steroidogenic acute regulatory protein expression. Endocrinology. 1998;139(6):2863–8.

115. Mortola JF, Yen SS. The effects of oral dehydroepiandrosterone on endocrine metabolic parameters in postmenopausal women. J Clin Endocrinol Metab. 1990;71(3):696–704.

116. Laughlin GA, Barrett-Connor E, Kritz-Silverstein D, von Muhlen D. Hysterectomy, oophorectomy, and endogenous sex hormone levels in older women: the Rancho Bernardo Study. J Clin Endocrinol Metab. 2000;85(2):645–51.

117. Spratt DI, Longcope C, Cox PM, Bigos ST, Wilbur-Welling C. Differential changes in serum concentrations of androgens and estrogens (in relation with cortisol) in postmenopausal women with acute illness. J Clin Endocrinol Metab. 1993;76(6):1542–7.

118. Christeff N, Benassayag C, Carli-Vielle C, Carli A, Nunez EA. Elevated estrogen and reduced testosterone levels in the serum of male septic shock patients. J Steroid Biochem. 1988;29(4):435–40.

119. Spratt DI, Morton JR, Kramer RS, Mayo SW, Longcope C, Vary CP. Increases in serum estrogen levels during major illness are caused by increased peripheral aromatization. Am J Physiol Endocrinol Metab. 2006;291(3):E631–8.

120. Iida S, Moriwaki K, Fujii H, Gomi M, Tsugawa M, Nakamura Y, et al. Quantitative comparison of aromatase induction by dexamethasone in fibroblasts from a patient with familiar cortisol resistance and patient with cortisol hyperreactive syndrome. J Clin Endocrinol Metab. 1991;73(1):192–6.

121. Lueprasitsakul P, Longcope C. Aromatase activity in human adipose tissue stromal cells; the effect of fetal bovine serum fractions on dexamethasone-stimulated aromatization. J Steroid Biochem Mol Biol. 1991;39(3):353–7.

122. Simpson ER, Clyne C, Rubin G, Boon WC, Robertson K, Britt K, et al. Aromatase – a brief overview. Annu Rev Physiol. 2002;64:93–127. Review.

123. Wild RA, Reis SE. Estrogens, progestins, selective estrogen receptor modulators, and the arterial tree. Am J Obstet Gynecol. 2001;184(5):1031–9.

124. Clemente C, Russo F, Caruso MG, Giangrande M, Fanizza G, DiLeo A. Ceruloplasmin serum level in post-menopausal women treated with oral estrogens administered at different time. Horm Metab Res. 1992;24(4):191–3.

125. Tuck CH, Holleran S, Berglund L. Hormonal regulation of lipoprotein(a) levels: effects of estrogen replacement therapy on lipoprotein(a) and acute phase reactants in postmenopausal women. Artheroscler Thromb Vasc Biol. 1997;17(9):1822–9.

Sex Hormone Binding Globulin and Cardiac Surgery

126. Anderson DC. Sex hormone binding globulin. Clin Endocrinol. 1974;3(1):69–86. Review.

127. Maggio M, Lauretani F, Basaria S, Ceda GP, Bandinelli S, Metter EJ, et al. Sex hormone binding globulin levels across the adult lifespan in women – the role of body mass index and fasting insulin. J Endocrinol Invest. 2008;31(7):597–601.

128. Maggio M, Lauretani F, Ceda GP, Bandinelli S, Basaria S, Paolisso G, et al. Association of hormonal dysregulation with metabolic syndrome in older women: data from the InCHIANTI study. Am J Physiol Endocrinol Metab. 2007;292(1):E353–8.

129. Maggio M, Lauretani F, Ceda GP, Bandinelli S, Basaria S, Ble A, et al. Association between hormones and metabolic syndrome in older Italian men. J Am Geriatr Soc. 2006;54(12):1832–8.

130. Perry JR, Weedon MN, Langenberg C, Jackson AU, Lyssenko V, Sparsø T, Thorleifsson G, Grallert H, Ferrucci L, Maggio M, Paolisso G, Walker M, Palmer CN, Payne F, Young E, Herder C, Narisu N, Morken MA, Bonnycastle LL, Owen KR, Shields B, Knight B, Bennett A, Groves CJ, Ruokonen A, Jarvelin MR, Pearson E, Pascoe L, Ferrannini E, Bornstein SR, Stringham HM, Scott LJ, Kuusisto J, Nilsson P, Neptin M, Gjesing AP, Pisinger C, Lauritzen T, Sandbaek A, Sampson M; MAGIC, Zeggini E, Lindgren CM, Steinthorsdottir V, Thorsteinsdottir U, Hansen T, Schwarz P, Illig T, Laakso M, Stefansson K, Morris AD, Groop L, Pedersen O, Boehnke M, Barroso I, Wareham NJ, Hattersley AT, McCarthy MI, Frayling TM. Genetic evidence that raised sex hormone binding globulin (SHBG) levels reduce the risk of type 2 diabetes. Hum Mol Genet. 2010;19(3):535–44.

131. Ding EL, Song Y, Manson JE, Hunter DJ, Lee CC, Rifai N, et al. Sex hormone-binding globulin and risk of type 2 diabetes in women and men. N Engl J Med. 2009;361(12):1152–63.

CABG and GH/IGF-1 Axis

132. Balcells J, Moreno A, Audì L, Roqueta J, Iglesias J, Carrascosa A. Growth Hormone/Insulin like growth factors axis in children undergoing cardiac surgery. Crit Care Med. 2001;29(6):1234–8.

133. Wallin M, Barr G, öWall A, Lindahl SG, Brismar K. The influence of glucose-insulin-potassium (GIK) on GH/IGF-I/IGFBP-1 axis during elective coronary artery bypass surgery. J Cardiothorac Vasc Anesth 2003;17(4):470–7.

134. Lang CH, Nystrom GJ, Frost RA. Regulation of IGF binding protein-1 in hep G2 cell by cytokines and reactive oxygen species. Am J Physiol. 1999;276(3 Pt 1):G719–27.

135. Lang CH, Hong-Brown L, Frost RA. Cytokine inhibition of JAK-STAT signaling: a new mechanism of growth hormone resistance. Pediatr Nephrol. 2005;20(3):306–12.

136. Cavaliere F, Guarnieri S, Varano C, Di Francesco P, Possati GF, Schiavello R. Somatomedin C plasma levels after coronary revascularization. J Cardiovasc Surg (Torino). 1992;33(6):761–4.

137. Butcher SK, Lord JM. Stress responses and innate immunity: aging as a contributory factor. Aging Cell. 2004;3(4):151–60.

138. Fried LP, Ferrucci L, Darer J, Williamson JD, Anderson G. Untangling the concepts of disability, frailty, and comorbility: implications for improved targeting and care. J Gerontol A Biol Sci Med Sci. 2004;59(3):255–63.

139. Maggio M, Cappola AR, Ceda GP, Basaria S, Chia CW, Valenti G, et al. The hormonal pathway of frailty in older men. J Endocrinol Invest. 2005;28(11 Suppl Proceedings):15–9. Review.

140. Ceresini G, Lauretani F, Maggio M, Ceda GP, Morganti S, Usberti E, et al. Evaluation of thyroid function over the life span and of the relationship between hyperthyroidism and cognitive impairment in the elderly. Results from the InCHIANTI study. J Am Geriatr Soc. 2009;57(1):89–93.

141. Voznesensky M, Walsh S, Dauser D, Brindisi J, Kenny AM. The association between dehydroepiandrosterone and frailty in older men and women. Age Ageing. 2009;38(4):401–6.

142. Cawthon PM, Ensrud KE, Laughlin GA, Cauley GA, Dam TT, Barrett-Connor E, et al. Osteoporotic fractures in Men (MrOS) Research Group. Sex hormones and frailty in older men: the osteoporotic fractures and frailty in older men (MrOS) study. J Clin Endocrinol Metab. 2009;94(10):3806–15.

143. Shores MM, Matsumoto AM, Sloan KL, Kivlahan DR. Low serum testosterone and mortality in male veterans. Arch Intern Med. 2006;166(15):1660–5.

144. Maggio M, Ble A, Ceda GP, Metter EJ. Decline in insulin-like growth factor-I levels across adult life span in two large population studies. J Gerontol A Biol Sci Med Sci. 2006;61(2):182–3.

145. Juul A, Scheike T, Davidsen MJ, Gyllenborg T, Jorgensen JO. Low insulin like growth factor I is associated with an increased risk of ischemic heart disease: a population based case-control study. Circulation. 2002;106(8):939–44.

146. Vanhorebeek I, Langouche L, Van den Berghe G. Endocrine aspects of acute and prolonged critical illness. Nat Clin Pract Endocrinol Metab. 2006;2(1):20–31. Review.

147. Spratt DI. Altered gonadal steroidogenesis in critical illness: is treatment with anabolic steroids indicated ? Best Pract Res Clin Endocrinol Metab. 2001;15(4):479–94.

148. Coviello AD, Kaplan B, Lakshman KM, Chen T, Singh AB, Bhasin S. Effects of graded doses of testosterone on erythropoiesis in healthy young and older men. J Clin Endocrinol Metab. 2008; 93:914–9.
149. Denti L, Scoditti U, Tonelli C, Saccavini M, Caminiti C, Valcavi R, et al. The poor outcome of ischemic stroke in very old people: a cohort study of its determinants. J Am Geriatr Soc. 2010; 58(1):12–7.
150. Denti L, Annoni V, Cattadori E, Salvagnini MA, Visioli S, Merli MF, et al. Insulin-like growth factor 1 as a predictor of ischemic stroke outcome in the elderly. Am J Med. 2004;117(5):312–7.
151. Wolfe RR. Optimal nutrition, exercise, and hormonal therapy promote muscle anabolism in the elderly. J Am Coll Surg. 2006;202(1):176–80.
152. Wei M, Kuukasjarvi P, Kaukinen S, Laurikka J, Pehkonen E, Laine S, et al. Anti-inflammatory effects of 17 beta estradiol pretreatment in men after coronary artery surgery. J Cardiothorac Vasc Anesth. 2001;15(4):455–9.
153. Nussmeier NA, Marino MR, Vaughn WK. Hormone replacement therapy is associated with improved survival in women undergoing coronary artery bypass grafting. J Cardiothorac Surg. 2002; 124(6):1225–9.

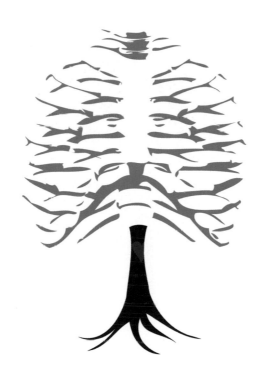

Part IX
Cardiac Surgery

Chapter 26
Invited Commentary

William A. Baumgartner

It is a real pleasure to write a commentary on the Cardiac Surgery section of this comprehensive book which outlines, discusses, and reviews the surgical care of elderly patients with cardiothoracic disease. In this section on Cardiac Surgery, Dr. Katlic has secured recognized experts in the important topics of Adult Cardiac Surgery. A good friend and colleague of mine once told me that pediatric patients were not little adults. Similarly, the elderly patient has unique and different physiology, psychology, and functional aspects, clearly distinct from the younger adult. My training and practice of cardiac surgery have spanned over three and a half decades – amazing, as I don't think of myself as approaching the definition of elderly! As a resident, an "older patient" was someone in their mid to late 60s. As junior faculty, "older" referred to someone in his or her 70s. At the end of my clinical practice, we routinely operated on patients in their 80s and some in their 90s.

One of the real benefits of having a geriatric practice during this particular time period was the opportunity to get to know the members of the "world's greatest generation"(according to Tom Brokaw). It was a real honor to be able to care for and know the men and women who survived the Great Depression and World War II. Although they almost universally had the will of a lion and the enthusiasm of a young adult, they often did not have the reserve to tolerate a complicated operation. Although we recognized early on that these patients were different from their younger cohort, we were unable to provide them with definite reasons why they were at increased risk other than their increased age alone. For example, we realized that these older patients had a tendency to bleed more, have more neurocognitive problems, were more likely to develop infections, and often needed rehabilitation.

Recently, the field of geriatrics has evolved yielding very interesting insights into the elderly patient. The word "frailty"

has become a medical term associated with a significant impact on the elderly patient. As our population ages, more patients will require cardiac surgical procedures. Currently, our ability to access risk is challenging and is primarily based on associated morbidities. Frailty provides one method of measuring physiological reserve in this group of older patients. It has been shown that a patient who is considered frail is more likely to sustain a postoperative fall, develop delirium, and progress to disability. Although the definition of frailty continues to evolve, one particular hallmark of this significant risk factor is the disregulation of homeostatic systems at both the molecular and physiological levels. This can be manifested as decreased muscle mass, variation of cortisol levels, and clotting studies as well as certain biomarkers.

At our own institution, Dr. Martin Makary and his associates prospectively looked at a group of surgical patients of age 65 years or older, who were being evaluated for elective surgery. Frailty was based on a validated scoring system characterized by decline in five domains including weight loss, weakness, exhaustion, low physical activity, and slowed walking speed. Weight loss was measured as greater than ten pounds in the past year. Weakness was assessed by a hand-held dynamometer. Exhaustion and low physical activity were analyzed by questionnaire. Slowed walking speed was measured by which the speed a patient could walk fifteen feet. The Hopkins group found that frailty had a significant influence on surgical outcomes following major surgical procedures compared to minor procedures. One of their conclusions is as follows: "As the phenotype becomes better studied, patients may benefit from interventions to reduce risk, such as, preoperative conditioning, nutrition, or even pharmacological therapy. At a minimum, providers will be alerted to special needs and risks of older surgical patients." They concluded that frailty is common in older surgical patients and is independently associated with a greater risk of postoperative complications, increased length of stay, and being discharged to an assisted or skilled nursing facility. This paper is to be published in the Journal of American College of Surgeons, 2010. Continued investigation into better defining the inherent risk of the elderly population will

W.A. Baumgartner (✉)
Department of Surgery, Division of Cardiac Surgery,
The Johns Hopkins Hospital, 600 North Wolfe Street, Baltimore,
MD 21205, USA
e-mail: wbaumgar@jhmi.edu

M.R. Katlic (ed.), *Cardiothoracic Surgery in the Elderly*, DOI 10.1007/978-1-4419-0892-6_26,
© Springer Science+Business Media, LLC 2011

provide cardiac surgeons advanced information to be able to counsel their patients and their family members. It may also lead to deliberate preoperative, intraoperative, and postoperative interventions to reduce the risk of postoperative complications in patients who are designated as most susceptible to injury.

This section and the book as a whole will be a very important resource for cardiothoracic surgeons, anesthesiologists, intensivists, residents, and nurses who take care of geriatric patients. It has become clear with investigational research that the geriatric patient is not just an older adult. Understanding the current state of the care of patients undergoing a variety of cardiac surgical operations, as described in this section, will improve the quality of care given to our older patients with cardiovascular disease, which will clearly be needed as the sizable baby boomer generation becomes elderly.

Chapter 27
Preoperative Evaluation and Preparation in the Elderly Cardiac Surgery Patient

Joseph C. Cleveland Jr.

Abstract The physiologic response of the elderly patient to cardiac surgical procedures differs substantially from their younger peers. Indeed, traditional preoperative assessment and tools which seek to estimate peri-operative risk for mortality and complications focus almost exclusively on mortality alone. Important considerations for geriatric patients who elect to undergo cardiac operations include functional mobility, quality of life, and maintenance of their independent status. The purpose of this chapter will be to review the current status of preoperative preparation and evaluation of the geriatric cardiac surgery patient. We will attempt to emphasize strategies which highlight some of the unique risk factors that are operant in the elderly patient undergoing cardiac surgery. Attention will also be directed to evaluation of risk in a manner other than evaluating traditional organ system risks. This chapter will focus on nutritional evaluation, screening for delirium, and disability before cardiac surgery, as these three entities are unique to the elderly population who undergo cardiac surgery. Lastly, emphasis on advanced directives, and the designation of a single person who will be responsible for important medical and or end-of life decisions for this group of patients will be discussed.

Keywords Preoperative evaluation • Peri-operative risk • Functional mobility • Quality of life • Nutritional evaluation • Delirium screening • Cardiac surgery

Introduction

Cardiovascular disease is the leading cause of morbidity and mortality in the aging United States population. In 2006, over 7,000,000 cardiovascular procedures were performed in the United States, over 50% of these procedures were performed in patients ≥65 years of age, and the total cost for cardiovascular disease in 2010 is estimated at over \$500 billion dollars [1]. Indeed, the Society of Thoracic Surgeons Adult Cardiac Database documented a significant increase in the age of patients undergoing coronary artery bypass during the decade of 1990–1999 [2].

The physiologic response of the elderly patient to cardiac surgical procedures differs substantially from their younger peers. Indeed, traditional preoperative assessment and tools which seek to estimate peri-operative risk for mortality and complications focus almost exclusively on mortality alone. Important considerations for geriatric patients who elect to undergo cardiac operations include functional mobility, quality of life, and maintenance of their independent status. A more holistic approach to the unique risk factors of geriatric patients has been difficult to quantify. The purpose of this chapter will be to review the current status of preoperative preparation and evaluation of the geriatric cardiac surgery patient. For the purpose of this discussion, we will attempt to emphasize strategies which highlight some of the unique risk factors that are operant in the elderly patient undergoing cardiac surgery. Attention will also be directed to evaluation of risk in a manner other than evaluating traditional organ system risks. This chapter will focus on nutritional evaluation, screening for delirium, and disability before cardiac surgery, as these three entities are unique to the elderly population who undergo cardiac surgery. Lastly, emphasis on advanced directives, and the designation of a single person who will be responsible for important medical and or end-of life decisions for this group of patients will be discussed.

Nutritional Evaluation

The elderly are at risk for malnutrition for a variety of reasons. Commonly cited reasons which promote malnutrition include: alterations in taste/smell with age; appetite reduction secondary to co-existing medical disorders and medications; loss of dentition, limited income; and reduced access to protein calories. The prevalence of malnutrition in elders

J.C. Cleveland Jr. (✉)
Department of Surgery, University of Colorado Health Sciences Center, 12631 East 17th Avenue, Aurora, CO 80045, USA
e-mail: joseph.cleveland@ucdenver.edu

M.R. Katlic (ed.), *Cardiothoracic Surgery in the Elderly*, DOI 10.1007/978-1-4419-0892-6_27,
© Springer Science+Business Media, LLC 2011

ranges from 1% in community-healthy elders to 37% in institutionalized patients. Clearly, a spectrum exists and a screening tool to identify the higher risk elders is desirable. The Mini Nutritional Assessment (MNA) was developed and validated as a screening tool for malnutrition [3]. (Fig. 27.1) The full MNA is an 18 item questionnaire which utilizes BMI, mid-arm and calf circumference, and a questionnaire regarding dietary intake, a global assessment, and a self assessment. The MNA-SF is an abbreviated version of the MNA, and comprises 6 of the 18 items. A MNA-SF score of 12 or greater or MNA score of 24 or greater, in general, documents a patient who is not at risk for malnutrition. A MNA score between 17 and 24 or a MNA-SF score between 8 and 11 predicts that the patient is at risk for malnutrition; and an MNA score of below 17 or MNA-SF score below 7 indicates the patient is suffering from malnutrition. Unfortunately, situations exist which preclude optimization of an elderly patient's nutritional status because of urgency of surgical procedure (i.e., L main coronary artery disease, valvular endocarditis). However, if one has the opportunity to identify and correct these nutritional deficiencies, then aggressive nutritional correction should ensue.

Protein intake has emerged as a critical factor in promoting functional capacity and preventing chronic wasting and some features of the frailty syndrome. These benefits extend beyond assisting community based elders, but recent data have emerged to support the recovery of hospitalized elderly patients to recover from surgery, trauma, and disease [4]. Unfortunately, as is often the case, the recommended daily allowance (RDA) of protein established by the USDA, of 0.8 g protein/kg/day, was empirically based upon data gathered in young males. Data exist supporting the need for greater protein intake in the elderly to avoid negative nitrogen balance [5], and therefore the optimal RDA for protein intake in elderly males and females remains unknown. Recent investigations, however, do support increasing the intake of protein above the current RDA in elders to increase muscle anabolism. In fact, a single serving of 113 g of high quality lean beef (90% lean ground beef patty) was observed to increase muscle protein synthesis by 50% in healthy young and elderly patients [6]. It seems almost intuitive that preoperative screening for malnutrition should also emphasize adequate daily protein intake, to prevent muscle catabolism and loss of functional capacity after cardiac surgery. Based upon these available data, it would seem reasonable to emphasize that patients undergoing cardiac surgery should receive daily high quality protein –rich foods such as lean ground beef. Attention to maintenance of positive protein balance should extend throughout the perioperative and postoperative recovery period.

Hormonal replacement therapy merits strong consideration for elderly males undergoing cardiac surgery. Alterations in anabolic and catabolic hormones including cortisol, dehydroepiandrosterone, luteinizing hormone, estradiol, testosterone, sex hormone binding globulin, and insulin-like growth factor-1 were observed following coronary artery bypass grafting surgery in elderly males and females [7]. A substantial decrease in serum testosterone levels and insulin growth factor-1 was most pronounced in elderly males undergoing operation. Of interest, an elevation in several cytokines, such as IL-6, which may lead to sarcopenia after operation has been independently observed, and is postulated to promote this drop in testosterone. Based upon these observations, testosterone replacement in males undergoing cardiac surgery seems strongly worthy of consideration. However, at the present time, data are lacking which demonstrate a positive effect on outcomes with hormonal replacement (Table 27.1).

Assessment of Risk for Delirium

A vast body of literature exists which describes a variety of post-operative cognitive changes following cardiac surgery. Rather than focusing on these changes, attention will be directed towards screening patients for high risk of developing delirium. Delirium is a clinical syndrome in which an acute disruption of attention and cognition occurs. It often waxes and wanes – and it may have a very abrupt onset. Unfortunately, cardiac surgery remains one of the most common procedures which incites delirium in elderly patients. While the exact mechanisms promoting the development of delirium remain unknown, several accepted tents regarding this clinical syndrome exist. Most noteworthy is the universal observation that the development of postoperative delirium is associated with increased morbidity and mortality [8]. Established preoperative risk factors for delirium include: history of alcohol abuse, pre-existing cognitive dysfunction, pre-existing physical impairment, type of surgery, and metabolic abnormalities. Screening for cognitive evaluation before cardiac surgery is paramount, and simple tests such as the Mini-Cog Test (combined three item recall with a clock draw test) is reliable and easily administered. Identifying patients with pre-existing cognitive dysfunction should trigger consultation with a geriatrics team, who can assist in the post-operative management of these patients to either reduce the likelihood of delirium, or assist in the management of delirium.

The mechanisms underlying why cardiac surgery should provoke delirium remain uncharacterized. However, a differential elaboration of chemokines in the serum of patients who developed delirium versus those who did not following cardiac surgery has been reported, and clearly warrants

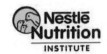

Mini Nutritional Assessment
MNA®

Last name:		First name:	
Sex:	Age:	Weight, kg:	Height, cm:	Date:

Complete the screen by filling in the boxes with the appropriate numbers. Total the numbers for the final screening score.

Screening

A Has food intake declined over the past 3 months due to loss of appetite, digestive problems, chewing or swallowing difficulties?
0 = severe decrease in food intake
1 = moderate decrease in food intake
2 = no decrease in food intake ☐

B Weight loss during the last 3 months
0 = weight loss greater than 3 kg (6.6 lbs)
1 = does not know
2 = weight loss between 1 and 3 kg (2.2 and 6.6 lbs)
3 = no weight loss ☐

C Mobility
0 = bed or chair bound
1 = able to get out of bed / chair but does not go out
2 = goes out ☐

D Has suffered psychological stress or acute disease in the past 3 months?
0 = yes   2 = no ☐

E Neuropsychological problems
0 = severe dementia or depression
1 = mild dementia
2 = no psychological problems ☐

F1 Body Mass Index (BMI) (weight in kg) / (height in m²)
0 = BMI less than 19
1 = BMI 19 to less than 21
2 = BMI 21 to less than 23
3 = BMI 23 or greater ☐

IF BMI IS NOT AVAILABLE, REPLACE QUESTION F1 WITH QUESTION F2.
DO NOT ANSWER QUESTION F2 IF QUESTION F1 IS ALREADY COMPLETED.

F2 Calf circumference (CC) in cm
0 = CC less than 31
3 = CC 31 or greater ☐

Screening score ☐☐
(max. 14 points)

12-14 points: Normal nutritional status
8-11 points: At risk of malnutrition
0-7 points: Malnourished

For a more in-depth assessment, complete the full MNA® which is available at **www.mna-elderly.com**

Ref.   Vellas B, Villars H, Abellan G, et al. *Overview of the MNA® - Its History and Challenges*. J Nutr Health Aging 2006;10:456-465.
            Rubenstein LZ, Harker JO, Salva A, Guigoz Y, Vellas B. *Screening for Undernutrition in Geriatric Practice: Developing the Short-Form Mini Nutritional Assessment (MNA-SF)*. J. Geront 2001;56A: M366-377.
            Guigoz Y. *The Mini-Nutritional Assessment (MNA®) Review of the Literature - What does it tell us?* J Nutr Health Aging 2006; 10:466-487.
            ® Société des Produits Nestlé, S.A., Vevey, Switzerland, Trademark Owners
            © Nestlé, 1994, Revision 2009. N67200 12/99 10M
            For more information: www.mna-elderly.com

Fig. 27.1 The Mini Nutritional Assessment [13–15]; ®Société des Produits Nestlé, S.A., Vevey, Switzerland, Trademark Owners. ©Nestlé, 1994, Revision 2009. N67200 12/99 10M. For more information: www.mna-elderly.com)

Table 27.1 Nutritional evaluation

| Nutritional screening with MNA |
| Encourage protein intake (1 lean meat serving/day) |
| Consider hormonal replacement (testosterone for males) |

Table 27.2 Risk factors for delirium

| History of alcohol abuse |
| Pre-existing cognitive dysfunction |
| Type of surgery (cardiac is strong risk factor) |
| Pre-existing physical impairment |
| Metabolic abnormalities |

further investigation [9]. Clinical data regarding anti-inflammatory strategies have largely proven inconsistent in preventing delirium, and therefore remain unproven for preventing delirium.

The number of medications taken daily by elderly patients is substantial. It is not uncommon to evaluate a patient for a cardiac operation who takes 20–30 pills daily. While polypharmacy is often used as a surrogate for co-morbidities, it remains vitally important to thoroughly review each patient's medication list (including herbal and over-the-counter, OTC) medications prior to undertaking cardiac surgical operations. Particular attention should be directed towards benzodiazepine and other sedative type medications. Strong consideration should be given to trimming the medication list, as drug-drug interactions can precipitate delirium. Many elders remain on anticoagulants – in particular Coumadin and Plavix – for relatively non-specific indications. Dialog with both patients and their treating physicians should include a reassessment of the necessity of these particular medications. As mentioned previously, many elderly patients will often self-initiate OTC medications or herbal supplements (saw palmetto, ginseng, etc.). Elderly patients should be specifically asked about the use of OTC or herbal supplements, as certain supplements (ginseng, garlic, and gingko) can promote bleeding at the time of cardiac surgery.

While it remains difficult to develop a specific pre-operative strategy to prevent delirium, simple screening for delirium risk can target those patients where early intervention in the peri-operative period may prevent or ameliorate the delirium syndrome (Table 27.2).

Assessment of Disability

Disability refers to loss of ability to perform activities of daily living (ADL). A very practical and clinically easily administered screening tool for disability is the Katz index for disability [10]. This index assigns one point for independence in each of 6 of the ADL (bathing, toileting, dressing,

transferring, feeding, and continence). Patients are scored from 0 to 6 with 6 representing independence in all these domains, and 0 representing complete dependence in these domains. While the Katz index represents a simple screening tool for evaluation of disability, strong debate still exists in the geriatric literature whether disability can be independently assessed as a risk factor for poor outcomes. Many believe that there is a strong synergy that exists between disability, frailty, and comorbidity towards promoting poor outcomes after surgical procedures. Recent data which address this complex interaction provide a very robust evaluation of these three syndromes in predicting outcomes. Robinson and colleagues prospectively evaluated 110 patients aged >65 undergoing major general, thoracic, cardiac, vascular, and urological operations. In this very comprehensive evaluation, the strongest predictor of adverse post-operative outcome was any functional dependence as assessed by the Katz screening tool. Other variables which predicted poor outcome include impaired cognition, recent falls, low albumin (<3.3), anemia, functional dependence, and increased comorbidities [11]. Quantification of disability seems much more rigorous to screen patients than the age old "eyeball test." Intuitively, while disability may relate to other geriatric syndromes, it seems that loss of independence in any of the six domains of the ADL would predict a very poor outcome after cardiac surgery. Hence, appropriate identification of patients who may not be appropriate candidates for open operations is desirable, to either avoid or appropriately counsel patients regarding very high risk cardiac operations.

Advance Directives/Medical Proxy

The traditional cardiac surgical approach to the care of elderly patients raises several potential conflicts,regarding the boundaries of strong personal commitment and desire to provide aggressive care, by surgeons juxtaposed with patients' desire to retain autonomy – particularly with end-of-life decisions. On the one hand, it is quite frustrating for an individual surgeon to perform a highly complex, technically difficult operation, only to have the outcome be withdrawal of care if the desired outcome is not achieved. Conversely, it is impossible to ignore the observations from two multiinstitutional studies, indicating that elders often received ICU resuscitative care despite patient preferences for comfort care [12]. Unfortunately, two very important decisions are often overlooked in the preoperative evaluation of elderly patients. (1) If a designated procedure does produce complications or a suboptimal outcome, then how aggressive does the patient wish to remain regarding future and further care? (2) If for some reason the patient is unable to provide medical decision making after a cardiac surgical procedure, then who will make those decisions? A follow-up question for the second question would also inquire as to whether the designated medical decision maker has had a thorough conversation with the patient, to ensure that indeed the patient's wishes are known and followed, if a complication occurs that precludes the patient from participating in these decisions. Certainly patient and surgeon do not approach a cardiac operation anticipating complications or poor outcomes; however, a discussion during the preoperative visit to establish what the patient's wishes regarding aggressiveness of care following their operation is crucial. This discussion should also include some specific known circumstances – such as whether death is preferable to partial dependence or full dependence. Many elderly patients fear losing independence more than dying, and the surgeon can thus properly understand each patient's preferences. It is useful to estimate prognosis of various operations and complications for patient counseling. For example, mediastinal bleeding after cardiac surgery, which requires reoperation, will have a low likelihood of permanent adverse outcomes. Conversely, a perioperative cerebrovascular accident (CVA) which results in a dense hemiparesis and aphasia, is likely to strongly and negatively influence the patient's duration and quality of life. It is advisable that these preoperative discussions be conducted with both patient and their surrogate present – to avoid any miscommunication or misperceptions of the patient's wishes.

Conclusion

The preoperative evaluation and preparation of the elderly cardiac surgical patient demands a thoughtful and thorough consideration of concepts that differs from our traditional "organ based" physiological assessment of risk/benefit. Clearly, the surgeon who is asked to intervene on a nonagenarian assumes a greater responsibility for ensuring that optimal outcomes will be achieved. As with many cardiac surgical procedures, the benefit of restoration to an active and vigorous existence often occurs. Indeed, the vast majority of elders who undergo either valvular or coronary surgery return to full independence, and have improvement in their health related quality of life. Attention to detail and evaluation of nutrition, cognition, functional dependence, and understanding patients' wishes regarding aggressiveness of care are fundamental geriatric principles which should be included in the preoperative evaluation of the geriatric cardiac surgery patient.

References

1. Lloyd-Jones D, Adams RJ, Brown TM, et al. Heart disease and stroke statistics – 2010 update: a report from the American Heart Association. Circulation. 2010;121:e1–170.
2. Ferguson Jr TB, Hammill BG, Peterson ED, Delong ER, Grover FL. A decade of change – risk profiles and outcomes for isolated coronary artery bypass grafting procedures, 1990–1999: a report from the STS national database committee and the duke clinical research institute. Ann Thoracic Surg. 2002;73:480–90.
3. Guigoz Y, Lauque S, Vellas BJ. Identifying the elderly at risk for malnutrition The Mini Nutritional Assessment. Clin Geriatr Med. 2002;18:737–57.
4. Schurch MA, Rizzoli R, Slosman D, Vadas L, Vergnaud P, Bonjour JP. Protein supplements increase serum insulin – like growth factor -1 levels and attenuate proximal femur bone loss in patients with recent hip fracture: a randomized, double-blind, placebo controlled trial. Ann Intern Med. 1998;128:801–9.
5. Campbell WW, Crim MC, Dallal GE, Young VR, Evans WJ. Increased protein requirements in elderly people: new data and retrospective assessments. Am J Clin Nutr. 1994;60:501–9.
6. Symons TB, Sheffield-Moore M, Wolfe RR, Paddon-Jones D. A moderate serving of high-quality protein maximally stimulates skeletal muscle protein synthesis in young and elderly subjects. J Am Diet Assoc. 2009;109:1582–6.
7. Maggio M, Ceda GP, De Cicco G, et al. Acute changes in circulating hormones in older patients with impaired ventricular function undergoing on-pump coronary artery bypass grafting. J Endocrinol Invest. 2005;28:711–19.
8. Marcantonio ER, Goldman L, Mangione CM, et al. A clinical prediction rule for delirium after noncardiac surgery. JAMA. 1994;271:134 9.
9. Rudolph JL, Ramlawi B, Kuchel GA, et al. Chemokines are associated with delirium after cardiac surgery. J Gerontol. 2008;63A: 184–89.
10. Katz S, Downs TD, Cash HR, et al. Progress in development of the index of ADL. Gerontologist. 1970;10:20–30.
11. Robinson TN, Eiseman B, Wallace JI, et al. Redefining geriatric preoperative assessment using frailty, disability, and co-morbidity. Ann Surg. 2009;250:449–55.
12. Phillips RS, Hamel MB, Covinsky KE, Lynn J. Findings from SUPPORT and HELP: an introduction. J Am Geriatr Soc. 2000;48 (5 Suppl):S1–5.
13. Vellas B, Villars H, Abellan G, et al. Overview of the MNA® – its history and challenges. J Nutr Health Aging. 2006;10:456–65.
14. Rubenstein LZ, Harker JO, Salva A, Guigoz Y, Vellas B. Screening for undernutrition in geriatric practice: developing the short-form Mini Nutritional Assessment (MNA-SF). J Gerontol. 2001;56A: M366–377.
15. Guigoz Y. The mini-nutritional assessment (MNA®) review of the literature – What does it tell us? J Nutr Health Aging. 2006;10:466–87.

Chapter 28
Cardiac Anesthesia in the Elderly

Eric W. Nelson and James H. Abernathy III

Abstract Elderly patients have more comorbidities and are increasingly undergoing more complex procedures. Despite the ever aging population, expected mortality continues to decline. This is based in part on our increased understanding of the complex physiology of the elderly and improved medications and monitoring techniques now in use to mitigate adverse outcomes.

Keywords Transesophageal echocardiogram • Epiaortic ultrasound • Postoperative cognitive dysfunction • Diastolic dysfunction • Cerebral oximetry • Anesthetic management • Pulmonary artery catheter • Benzodiazepines • Acid–base management

The elderly patient provides a unique set of challenges to the anesthesiologist. These challenges are amplified during cardiac surgery as the patients themselves have many comorbidities and the surgeries are complicated. In this chapter, we will outline the anesthetic considerations for the elderly patient undergoing cardiac surgery starting from the preoperative holding area, to the operating room, and finally postoperatively in the intensive care unit (ICU).

Preoperative Considerations

Neurological

One of the first things the anesthesiologist notices about a patient when we meet them in the holding area is their neurological status. By age 65, 10–15% of patients have cognitive dysfunction, and by age 80, 50% of the population has some form of dementia [1]. This plays an important role when dealing with consent and a patients' understanding of

J.H. Abernathy III (✉)
Department of Anesthesia and Perioperative Medicine, Division of Cardiothoracic Anesthesiology, Medical University of South Carolina, 25 Courtenay Dr., Suite 4200, MSC 240, Charleston, SC 29425, USA
e-mail: abernatj@musc.edu

the anesthetic process and postop ICU stay. Benzodiazepines can have an exaggerated sedative effect on a patient with pre-existing dementia. Benzodiazepines have also been found to increase the risk of postop delirium in patients even if they receive them prior to admission to the surgical ICU [2].

The elderly patients have a higher incidence for stroke when compared with younger patients. This increased incidence is most likely from age-related risk factors such as hypertension, peripheral vascular disease, cardiac disease, smoking, prior stroke, and use of aspirin and anticoagulants[3–7]. The biggest risk factor for perioperative stroke is a prior stroke. In fact, one study placed the risk at 5–10 times more common in patients with a history of stroke [8]. The majority of these perioperative strokes are attributed to thrombotic or embolic events [7]. It is therefore imperative for the anesthesiologist to be diligent in examining preoperative studies such as echocardiograms, carotid ultrasounds, and computed tomography scans to assess risk for an embolic event and take the necessary precautions to decrease this risk such as keeping mean arterial pressure higher or changing aortic cannulation sites if plaque is noted in the ascending aorta.

Despite the numerous neurological changes the aging brain undergoes, it is important to keep in mind that cerebral autoregulation is preserved. The elderly patients have an increased incidence of hypertension, which results in a shift of the cerebral autoregulatory curve to the right. This shift causes the lower limit of autoregulation of cerebral perfusion pressure to be higher than in a patient without hypertension, which could lead to cerebral hypoperfusion at a higher mean arterial pressure than in the normal population.

Cardiovascular

The numerous changes the cardiovascular system undergoes as patients age is also important to take into consideration during the preoperative period, so that the anesthesiologist will be able to properly plan an anesthetic. One important consideration is diastolic dysfunction (Fig. 28.1). Elderly patients have a higher rate of diastolic dysfunction, even with

M.R. Katlic (ed.), *Cardiothoracic Surgery in the Elderly*, DOI 10.1007/978-1-4419-0892-6_28,
© Springer Science+Business Media, LLC 2011

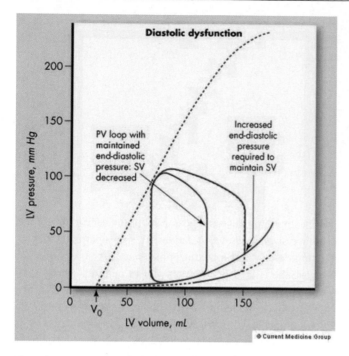

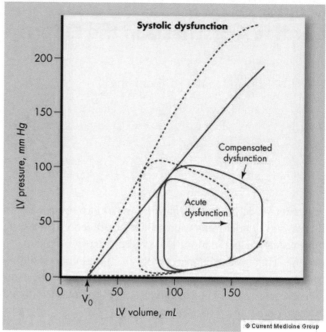

Fig. 28.1 Diastolic dysfunction: Effect of decreased left ventricular compliance. At a given end-diastolic pressure, the end-diastolic volume is reduced and stroke volume falls as well (reprinted with permission from Reves et al. [59])

Fig. 28.2 Systolic dysfunction: With negative inotropy, the end-systolic pressure–volume point is shifted to the right and down. Stroke volume is reduced with compensation utilizing preload reserve, and stroke volume is restored at the expense of ejection fraction (reprinted with permission from Reves et al. [59])

preserved systolic function, than the normal population [9, 10]. Because of the stiffening of the ventricle as one ages, there is a progressive decline in ventricular filling during the early diastole and a decrease in the early diastolic filling rate. Thus, the aging heart is increasingly dependent upon atrial filling and contraction to maintain adequate ventricular filling. A slow sinus rhythm is preferred. Given that by age 80, 10% of the population has atrial fibrillation this may be difficult to achieve [11]. The other implication of diastolic dysfunction for the anesthesiologist is an increase in difficulty in weaning from bypass [12]. Even in the preoperative period, one must begin to think about which vasopressors and other methods will have to be employed to successfully separate from bypass at the end of the procedure.

Although diastolic dysfunction occurs in the elderly without systolic dysfunction, systolic dysfunction also occurs at an increasing rate in the aging population. There is an age-related decrease in systolic function, especially in those with hypertension (Fig. 28.2). The decrease in systolic function is often masked because cardiac output is maintained at rest via prolonged myocardial contraction [13]. However, the physiologic stress of surgery, rapidly unmasks this age-related decline in contractile reserve. In a study by Turner, when phenylephrine was used to acutely increase systemic vascular resistance (SVR), in turn increasing left ventricular wall stress, an age-related decrease in contractile reserve was noted [14].

Blood vessels also undergo numerous changes as the body progresses in age. There is a progressive decrease in vascular

compliance leading to an increase in systolic blood pressure. The increase in afterload places a greater burden on the heart often leading to ventricular concentric hypertrophy. Systolic blood pressure increases without a concomitant rise in diastolic blood pressure creating an increased pulse pressure predisposing the elderly patient to a myocardial oxygen supply and demand mismatch.

As patients age, parasympathetic innervation to the myocardium decreases. Despite this decrease in parasympathetic activity, sympathetic outflow and vascular response to sympathetic stimulation are maintained [15].

Pulmonary

One of the biggest concerns of the anesthesiologist is the airway. When it comes to evaluating the airway of the elderly patient, keeping in mind the effects the aging process has on the musculoskeletal system is important. First, osteoarthritis is a common problem in the elderly. Arthritis of the cervical spine and limited neck extension often manifest as difficulty in successfully placing an endotracheal tube via standard direct laryngoscopy. There is also a gradual decrease in muscle mass over time. This decrease results in hypotonia of the hypopharyngeal and genioglossal muscles of the upper airway. This hypotonia may manifest as upper airway obstruction, which not only would cause difficulty in bag mask ventilation, but also ventilation by an awake patient lying supine. The decrease in muscle mass not only affects the upper airway, but also the muscles of respiration as well. Decreased strength of the respiratory muscles contributes to easy fatigability, which can complicate weaning from mechanical ventilation [16]. The aging pulmonary system is also subjected to a decrease in chest wall compliance and a decrease in elastic recoil, both of which act to increase the work of breathing.

Elderly patients have a decreased response to hypercarbia and hypoxemia as well. This is caused by a decreased sensitivity to carbon dioxide. Because opioids reduce the respiratory response to hypoxemia and hypercarbia, it is imperative that they be used judiciously and only with proper monitoring in the preoperative period [16]. Benzodiazepines also produce respiratory depression, which may be exaggerated in the elderly patient secondary to the increased potency of these agents [17].

Renal

The steady decline in renal function, 10% per decade after the age of 50, experienced by the elderly, has an important effect on the pharmacokinetics and pharmacodynamics for the medications anesthesiologists choose [18]. Not only anesthetics but also many of the other medications used by anesthesiologists during cardiac surgery are cleared by the kidneys. This decline in renal function makes it imperative to take measures to protect the kidneys as much as possible during the perioperative period. A preoperative evaluation of renal function will allow the anesthesiologist to properly formulate a plan for appropriate medication choices and renal protection; from keeping the patient well hydrated, to giving mannitol prior to bypass, to using a dopaminergic agent such as fenoldopam [19].

Endocrine

Nearly 1 out of every 5 persons over the age of 60 is a diabetic [20]. By the year 2025, two-thirds of the adult diabetic population will be composed of those over 60 years of age [21]. Preoperatively, these patients must have their blood sugars checked, especially after being allowed nothing by mouth (NPO) for an extended period of time to prevent hypo or hyperglycemia. It is also important to have an intraoperative plan in place to manage blood sugars not only in the diabetic, but also in the non-diabetic elderly population as hyperglycemia has been found to be a cause of perioperative morbidity. The latest studies have suggested that moderately tight glucose control with a blood sugar of less than 180 mg, rather than intensive glucose control of 81–108 mg, is the safest glucose management strategy for patients [22].

Fluid Balance

Almost all patients presenting for surgery have a fluid deficit secondary to their NPO status. This fluid deficit tends to be more pronounced in the elderly. The elderly patients have a decreased thirst mechanism, which leads them to be somewhat dehydrated at baseline [23]. They also have a diminished capacity to conserve water and salt secondary to decreased renal function [24]. Coupled with being NPO for 8 h or greater can lead to a large deficit in intravascular volume, which causes a much greater degree of hypotension with the decrease in SVR seen with many of our induction agents.

Induction of Anesthesia

Monitors

Standard monitoring of cardiac surgical patient includes invasive blood pressure, pulse oximetry, ECG, central venous pressure, temperature, and capnography. An arterial line is started prior to induction of anesthesia so variations in blood pressure may be detected and swiftly remedied. The radial artery is superficial and easily accessed by most practitioners. There is also collateral circulation to the hand which is easily checked and typically adequate. However, due to the distal position of the radial artery, there is often a discrepancy in blood pressure between the pressure tracing and the aortic pressure when coming off bypass (Fig. 28.3). This discrepancy

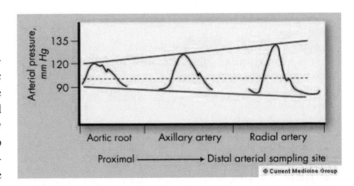

Fig. 28.3 Arterial pressure: Arterial line waveforms as the sampling site is moved more peripherally from the heart (reprinted with permission from Reves et al. [59])

is more apparent in patients with decreased vascular compliance such as the elderly population.

A central line and CVP monitoring are also standard for cardiac surgery. A large bore central venous catheter will allow infusion of vasoactive drugs and also large amounts of fluids quickly should the need arise. Although CVP does not give direct left-sided filling pressures, in patients who have good left ventricular function it can be used as an estimate of left-sided filling pressures.

Pulmonary artery catheters allow monitoring of not only pulmonary artery pressures and inference of left ventricular filling pressures, but also continuous monitoring of SVO_2, blood temperature, cardiac output, and some also have the ability to temporarily pace the heart. Despite all this usefulness, controversy continues to exist regarding their risk/benefit ratio [25, 26]. Clinical indications along with absolute and relative contraindications are listed in Table 28.1.

Temperature is also a very important monitor for cardiac surgery, but especially in the elderly. Temperature is typically measured at numerous sites to approximate the patient's

Table 28.1 Clinical use of the pulmonary artery catheter

Diagnosis
Differentiation among causes of shock
  Cardiogenic
  Hypovolemic
  Distributive (sepsis)
  Obstructive (massive pulmonary embolism)
Differentiation between mechanisms of pulmonary edema
  Cardiogenic
  Noncardiogenic
Evaluation of pulmonary hypertension
Diagnosis of pericardial tamponade
Diagnosis of left-to-right intracardiac shunt
Diagnosis of lymphangitic spread of tumor and fat embolism (case
  reports based on blood aspirated from wedge position)

Therapy
Management of perioperative patient with unstable cardiac status
Management of complicated myocardial infarction
Management of patients following cardiac surgery
Management of severe preeclampsia
Guide to pharmacologic therapy
  Vasopressors
  Inotropes
  Vasodilators (for patients with pulmonary hypertension)
Guide to nonpharmacologic therapy
  Fluid management
Gastrointestinal bleed
Traumatic exsanguination
Burns
Renal failure
Sepsis
Heart failure
Decompensated cirrhosis
Ventilator management (assessment of best PEEP for O_2 delivery)

(continued)

Table 28.1 (continued)

Complications of central venous catheterization
Immediate
  Bleeding
  Arterial puncture
  Arrhythmia
  Air embolism
  Thoracic duct injury (with left SC or left IJ approach)
  Catheter malposition
  Pneumothorax or hemothorax

Delayed
  Infection
  Venous thrombosis, pulmonary emboli
  Catheter migration
  Catheter embolization
  Myocardial perforation
  Nerve injury

Contraindications
Absolute
  Tricuspid or pulmonary valve stenosis
  Prosthetic tricuspid or pulmonary valve
  Right atrial or right ventricular mass
  Cyanotic heart disease
  Latex allergy
  Previous pneumonectomy
Relative
  Severe arrhythmias
  Anticoagulation
  Proposed pneumonectomy
  Attempted floatation during cardiopulmonary bypass

core temperature. Blood temperature can be measured when a PAC is utilized. We also measure temperature via the bladder or rectum and the esophagus. Hypothermia has been found to lead to ischemia, arrhythmias, coagulopathy, increased risk of postop wound infection, impaired drug metabolism, and shivering; all of which may lead to complications in both the operating room and postoperatively in the ICU.

Urine output is measured with a foley catheter during cardiac surgery. This allows the anesthesiologist to assess volume status via urine output. Kidney function can also be assessed by the amount of urine the patient produces. It is also a good way to assess a post cardiopulmonary bypass (CPB) coagulopathy as the urine will begin to turn pink or red if a coagulopathy exists or if hemolysis is present.

One of the newer monitors that has come into vogue in the past few years is the cerebral oximeter. This monitor measures intravascular regional hemoglobin oxygen saturation via transcranial near infrared spectroscopy and is meant to be used as an estimate of cerebral perfusion and cerebral blood flow. As determined by studies in awake patients, [27] a decline in the oxygen supply-demand balance is reflected as a decline in cerebral oximetry. Studies have found a decline of 20% from baseline or an absolute value of 50 or less are clinically important [28, 29]. A recent study from England has shown interventions to correct decreased cerebral oximetry by increasing oxygen delivery via increasing cardiac output, blood pressure, and hemoglobin; reduce neurological injury, major organ morbidity, mortality, and duration of hospital stay [30].

The BIS monitor is another commonly used monitor by anesthesiologists during cardiac surgery. This monitor has proved especially useful during rewarming and separation from bypass as these are two of the most common times of patient awareness. A BIS number less than 60 is associated with general anesthesia and thus a low risk of awareness [31].

Intraoperative transesophageal echocardiography (TEE) has become an invaluable tool to anesthesiologists and surgeons during cardiac surgery, especially surgery involving the valves and aorta. A comprehensive TEE exam allows the anesthesiologist to confirm and refine the preoperative diagnosis, detect new or unsuspected pathology, adjust the anesthetic and surgical plan, and assess results of the surgical intervention. Unique and critical information is able to be obtained in the TEE exam that was not available previously in the operating room [32]. In fact, the American Society of Anesthesiologists and American Society of Echocardiography recommend the use of TEE in all open heart and thoracic aortic surgical procedures and should be considered in coronary artery bypass graft surgery as well [33]. Studies have found that TEE influences cardiac surgical decisions in almost 10% of cases [34].

Epiaortic ultrasound is an ultrasound modality, which allows better detection of artheromatous disease in the aorta than either TEE or direct palpation. Cerebral embolism risk from aortic artheroma has been repeatedly described throughout the history of cardiac surgery [35]. One study showed a 25% risk of stroke in patients with mobile atheromatous plaque in the aortic arch compared with 2% rate in those with limited disease [36]. This modality may be employed as a way to avoid atheromas during cannulation, cross clamp, and vein graft placement. A study by Rosenberger found that the overall stroke rate in patients in whom epiaortic ultrasound was used was lower when compared with all patients undergoing surgical procedures. The use of epiaortic ultrasound was also found to influence surgical decision making in greater than 4% of cardiac surgical patients [37]

Drugs

Sedative Hypnotics

The induction of anesthesia for cardiac surgery is at times the most stressful part of the procedure for the anesthesiologist. Abrupt changes in coronary perfusion pressure, preload or contractility can lead to a patient's demise. It is especially important to remember that the elderly patient is more dependent on sympathetically mediated vasoconstriction to control their SVR; thus any inhibition of the sympathetic nervous system, as often occurs with anesthetic drugs, will have a more profound hypotensive effect on these patients when compared with younger patients. It is also important to remember that the elderly patient has a decreased central volume of distribution, decreased systemic clearance, and decreased intercompartmental clearance of drugs [17]. The elderly cardiac patient requires judicious, slow dosing of anesthetic drugs to prevent untoward effects (Tables 28.2 and 28.3).

There are many anesthetic drugs available for use in cardiac surgery. A study by Tuman et al. demonstrated no difference in outcome, based on the anesthetic drug chosen for cardiac surgery [38, 39]. With this in mind, some of the more commonly used drugs for induction and maintenance will be addressed.

Propofol is one of the most common drugs used for induction of anesthesia. It may be used in the elderly patient for induction for cardiac surgery; however, one must beware of

Table 28.2 Hemodynamic goals for induction of anesthesia

	Preload	HR	Afterload
Aortic stenosis	Full	Avoid extremes	Elevated
Aortic regurgitation	Full	Increased	Decreased
Mitral stenosis	Full	Slow	Decreased
Mitral regurgitation	Balanced	Fast	Decreased
Ischemia	Balanced	Slow	Decreased

Table 28.3 Hemodynamic effects of induction agents

	SVR	HR	Stroke volume	PVR
Propofol	Decreased	Decreased	Decreased	Decreased
Etomidate	Decreased	Increased	Decreased	Increased
Midazolam	Decreased	Unchanged	Decreased	Unchanged
Thiopental	Increased	Increased	Decreased	Unchanged
Opiates	Decreased	Decreased	Unchanged	Unchanged

the drop in blood pressure caused by a decreased SVR, preload, and contractility associated with propofol. These effects are more pronounced in elderly patients as propofol impairs the already decreased baroreceptor response. Despite these cardiovascular changes, they can be diminished if propofol is given slowly over a long period of time [40].

Thiopental is another commonly used induction agent. Like propofol, thiopental causes a decrease in blood pressure through peripheral venodilation and a decrease in contractility. When compared with propofol, thiopental also causes an increase in heart rate, which may be deleterious in patients with impaired coronary arteries as this will increase myocardial oxygen consumption. Thiopental also causes a decrease in cardiac output and blood pressure in hypovolemic patients; however, these decreases are typically not as pronounced as that seen with propofol [41–43].

Etomidate is yet another sedative hypnotic used for induction of anesthesia. Etomidate is structurally unrelated to all other induction medications. Unlike other induction agents, etomidate has very little effect on the cardiovascular system. It does cause a mild decline in blood pressure secondary to decreased SVR; however, it does not appear to have any depressant effects on the myocardium. This may be the drug of choice for induction in a patient with low intravascular volume, coronary artery disease, or decreased ventricular function. Despite these advantages, etomidate does cause a high incidence of nausea and vomiting and also pain on injection. A single bolus dose also has been found to cause widespread adrenal inhibition in critically ill patients, which is reversible in 48 h [44]. Considering cortisol levels peak 24 h after CPB, steroid supplementation may be required in patients who are induced with etomidate.

Benzodiazepines are also used for anesthesia induction. Midazolam has a quick onset and is short acting compared with alprazolam and diazepam, which makes it a better choice in the elderly population. Midazolam causes a dose-related decrease in SVR. In spite of this, midazolam has been safely used for induction even in patients with severe aortic stenosis [45]. It must be kept in mind that induction with high dose midazolam will take longer than with propofol or thiopental [46]; however, the amnesic properties of midazolam are more reliable thus making it a good choice for cardiac surgery. There has been found to be an increased incidence of postoperative delirium in elderly patients who receive benzodiazepines, even when they are given prior to admission to the ICU [2]. The elimination half life of benzodiazepines is also increased by CPB, hence the anesthesiologist must be judicious in dosing these medications [47].

Dexmedetomidine is a novel alpha2-adrenergic agonist. It is able to produce sedation and analgesia without respiratory depression. This medication has been found to lower the requirements of other anesthetic agents, and at high enough doses can be used as a complete anesthetic. Side effects include decreases in heart rate and cardiac output, which is more pronounced at higher doses thus making it a less than ideal choice as the sole anesthetic for cardiac surgery. Despite this, studies have shown that dexmedetomidine does no influence hemodynamics after surgery. May be its most important attribute is how it can reduce postoperative delirium after cardiac surgery [48, 49].

Opiates

High-dose opiate anesthesia has been a mainstay of cardiac anesthesia for decades. With the exception of meperidine, all opiates produce some degree of bradycardia, which is beneficial to the patient with coronary artery disease. The most commonly used opiates used in cardiac anesthesia will be discussed here.

Fentanyl and its analogs, sufentanyl, remifentanyl, alfentanyl, have been in use in cardiac anesthesia since the late 1970s [50]. These synthetic narcotics lack cardiovascular depression, which is especially important during induction. They also have the advantage of being highly lipid soluble; have a more rapid onset of action, increased anesthetic potency, absence of histamine release, and independence of renal function for drug clearance. Opiate drugs have amnesic properties; therefore, it is important to use a concurrent sedative hypnotic agent. Side effects of these medications, like all narcotics, include pruritis, constipation, urinary retention, and nausea.

Morphine is a naturally occurring opiate that has been coming back into vogue in cardiac anesthesia. Morphine was the first opiate used in high doses for cardiac anesthesia; however, it had fallen out of favor due to the fact that it causes histamine release, which leads to hypotension. It also may cause muscle rigidity at high doses, which may impair ventilation immediately after induction. However, a recent study by Murphy et al. demonstrated that morphine provided superior postop recovery in patients who had received it intraoperatively when compared with those who received fentanyl. Patients who received morphine had lower pain scores, required less analgesics, and had fewer febrile reactions [21]. This is most likely due to both the longer duration of action and the antiinflammatory affects of morphine when compared with that of the fentanyl group of opiates.

Muscle Relaxants

The choice of muscle relaxant in cardiac anesthesia for the elderly patient is an important one as many of these drugs effect more than just the nicotinic receptors on skeletal muscles. One must also remember that the elderly have a smaller volume of distribution and typically have less muscle mass; therefore, the dose of all muscle relaxants should be reduced in this group of patients.

Succinylcholine is the only depolarizing muscle relaxant still in use. This drug is typically reserved when a rapid sequence intubation is required as it tends to cause an increase in heart rate. This drug is also not optimal in the elderly population as they typically have decreased renal function, and succinylcholine causes an increase in potassium. This increase (0.5 mMol) usually is not enough to make the patient hyperkalemic; however, it should be kept in mind that these patients may have decreased excretion of potassium due to their renal function.

The other muscle relaxants used in cardiac anesthesia are nondepolarizing muscle relaxants. Pancuronium is an older muscle relaxant not used very often in adult cardiac anesthesia secondary to undesirable tachycardia. It is also important to keep in mind that it is very long acting and is cleared mainly by the kidneys, making it a suboptimal choice. Vecuronium is commonly used in cardiac surgery and is well suited for the elderly patient. It is intermediate acting without muscarinic affects and is excreted through the bile and kidney. Rocuronium has a similar side effect profile to vecuronium. It should be kept in mind that rocuronium is shorter acting so more frequent redosing is necessary. Cisatracurium is unlike vecuronium, rocuronium, or pancuronium in that it is not cleared by the kidneys at all. It is cleared in the blood by the Hoffman Reaction. Because it does not depend on renal or hepatic excretion, it is the muscle relaxant of choice in patients with hepatic or renal failure. Its side effect profile is similar to those of vecuronium and rocuronium.

Volatile Anesthetics

All volatile anesthetics are able to produce amnesia, some degree of analgesia, and some degree of muscle paralysis making them ideally suited as a sole anesthetic. However, the volatile anesthetics also produce decreases in blood pressure from arterial vasodilatation and depression of myocardial contractility at their general anesthetic doses. It is important to keep in mind that volatile anesthetics have a greater myocardial depressant effect on diseased myocardium so when used on patients undergoing cardiac surgery the circulatory effects will be much more profound. Volatile anesthetics also affect the pacemaker cells in the heart, at times causing a junctional rhythm, which may not be tolerated in the cardiac surgical patient. These effects are dose dependent; therefore, the volatile anesthetics are typically used in lower doses than that which is required for general anesthesia and combined with an opiate for pain control and a muscle relaxant for paralysis.

Although any of the commonly used volatile anesthetics can be used in cardiac surgery, desflurane should be used with caution as it may cause tachycardia. Both isoflurane and sevoflurane are appropriate to use; however, isoflurane has the benefit of being able to be run with lower fresh gas flows in the ventilator, which preserves moisture and prevents heat loss through the airway.

It is important to keep in mind that all volatile anesthetics possess vasodilatory and cardiac depressant effects. These are typically not well tolerated in the elderly cardiac patient at higher doses. For this reason, the volatile anesthetic is typically used at a lower dose and supplemented with a narcotic. A high-dose narcotic anesthetic has the benefit of not only providing potent analgesia and blunting the sympathetic response to surgery, but also may decrease heart rate via its vagotonic effect, which is beneficial in ischemic and stenotic heart lesions.

Maintenance of Anesthesia

Prebypass

After induction of anesthesia and placement of lines and monitors, the patient is turned over to the surgeon for their cardiac procedure. It is at this time baseline labs are checked. A baseline ACT is checked to help assess anticoagulation for bypass and a baseline ABG is also checked. Any electrolyte abnormalities are corrected and glucose is also managed. It is important to keep in mind that the elderly patients have a higher incidence of diabetes [51] making them more prone to hyperglycemia than the younger population. Much has been studied regarding perioperative glucose control. Hyperglycemia increases risk after myocardial infarction, stroke, and cardiac surgery [52, 53]. Therefore, glucose control is important in this surgical population; however, overly aggressive glucose control in diabetic patients increases hypoglycemia risk, which carries severe consequences if not detected and treated early [54].

Acid–base management is also important. It has long been debated whether alpha-stat or pH stat acid–base management is superior. Alpha-stat management helps to maintain normal cerebral auto regulation via the coupling of cerebral metabolism to CBF. Alpha-stat monitoring allows adequate cerebral perfusion while avoiding an increased cerebral perfusion that is seen with pH stat monitoring [55]. Any increase in blood flow above what is necessary for cerebral metabolism increases the risk for emboli. Alpha-stat monitoring has also been found to improve neurocognitive outcomes in bypass surgery [56].

The goal of anesthesia maintenance at this time is to keep the patient hemodynamically stable to provide organ protection. This is accomplished typically through the use of a volatile anesthetic and narcotic technique, or via total intravenous anesthesia (TIVA). The inhaled, volatile anesthetics are preferred agents in cardiac surgery because of the anti-ischemic preconditioning that they provide. Recent studies have shown desflurane and sevoflurane reduce postoperative mortality and incidence of myocardial infarction following cardiac surgery and also decrease postoperative cardiac troponin release, the need for inotrope support, mechanical ventilation time, time spent in the ICU, and overall hospital stay [57].

Both infusions and boluses of vasoactive drugs are utilized to achieve the desired blood pressure and heart rate in the prebypass period. Short acting drugs, which are easily titratable, are preferred such as phenylephrine, ephedrine (an indirect acting cholinergic), nitroglycerin, and esmolol.

Bypass

During the bypass period, careful monitoring of the mean arterial pressure is imperative for both end organ and cerebral protection. It is also important to make sure that an adequate anesthetic depth is achieved to prevent awareness and to keep the patient comfortable. Titrating a volatile anesthetic or a sedative hypnotic infusion to a BIS of less than 50 will ensure that the patient is at an appropriate level of anesthesia. Muscle relaxants are also given during the bypass period to ensure the patient does not move or have subclinical shivering, which could increase oxygen consumption during a time when oxygen delivery may be impaired.

Blood gasses are serially monitored and adjusted once again with alpha-stat interpretation to achieve a neutral acid–base balance. Blood sugars are also checked and an insulin infusion is adjusted accordingly. Patients often become insulin resistant and hypoglycemic while hypothermic and on CPB so the insulin requirements are greatly increased during this time. Close glucose monitoring is especially important when rewarming begins as a rebound effect is often seen and a precipitous drop in glucose may occur. Our practice is often to decrease the insulin dose by half at the start of rewarming to avoid hypoglycemia. Further adjustments to the insulin infusion are then made based on glucose measurements.

Separation from Bypass

Weaning and separation from bypass takes a coordinated effort between surgery, anesthesia, perfusion, and nursing. The condition of the patient preoperatively oftentimes dictates how they will separate from bypass. Patients with diastolic dysfunction typically require higher inotropic support [12]. The elderly patient with hypertension also has a higher

Table 28.4 Separation from bypass checklist

Adequate anesthesia and paralysis
Stable rhythm, preferable sinus with synchronized atrial contraction
Normothermia
Potassium, calcium, and other electrolytes within normal range
Serum glucose within normal range
Normal acid–base status
Acceptable hematocrit
Normal SVR
No evidence of intracardiac air by TEE
Inotropes, vasopressors, and vasodilators available

risk of systolic dysfunction [13], which would increase the need for inotropic support of the heart when separating from bypass.

The anesthesiologist has a checklist in his or her head for separation from bypass to ensure that weaning and separation from bypass will be successful (Table 28.4).

Post Bypass

Once the patient is successfully weaned from bypass, heparin is reversed and labs are evaluated to check for coagulopathy and assess that the patient's blood gas, electrolytes, and glucose are all optimized. It is imperative for the anesthesiologist to remain vigilant during this time as hemodynamics may abruptly change with chest closure.

New anesthetic techniques take advantage of short acting sedative hypnotics such as propofol and dexmedetomidine postoperatively so that excessive sedation does not hinder extubation. These drugs provide the benefits of rendering patients comfortable while intubated, and also being easily titratable and having a short half life.

Postoperative Period

After the elderly cardiac surgical patient is stable and extubated, it is important to keep in mind the higher incidence of postoperative central nervous system dysfunction this population has. Delirium is the most common form of cognitive impairment in hospitalized patients with positive predictors including age greater than 70, preexisting cognitive impairment, a history of delirium, comorbidities, cardiac surgery, and poor functional status. This patient population is inherently more at risk for delirium and other forms of postoperative cognitive dysfunction because of the positive predictors they possess. For this reason it is prudent as anesthesiologists to avoid drugs such as benzodiazepines and anticholinergics, which have been found to contribute to postoperative cognitive dysfunction to reduce the already high risk as much as possible [57].

The elderly cardiac surgical patient presents many challenges to the anesthesiologist all the way from the preoperative visit until they are discharged from the hospital. Tailoring anesthetic technique to this unique population helps to not only guide them safely through the perioperative period, but also contribute to overall patient safety and satisfaction. Despite the increasing age of cardiac surgical patients and the increased morbidity and mortality associated with this aging, operative mortality has not substantially increased. This can be attributed to multiple factors including improved surgical techniques, dedicated cardiac anesthesiologists, better CPB machines, improved pharmacologic interventions, and better anesthetic techniques and technology [58].

References

1. Keefover RW. Aging and cognition. Neurol Clin. 1998;16(3):635–48.
2. Pandharipande P, Cotton BA, Shintani A, Thompson J, Pun BT, Morris Jr JA, et al. Prevalence and risk factors for development of delirium in surgical and trauma intensive care unit patients. J Trauma. 2008;65(1):34–41.
3. Larsen SF, Zaric D, Boysen G. Postoperative cerebrovascular accidents in general surgery. Acta Anaesthesiol Scand. 1988;32(8):698–701.
4. Parikh S, Cohen JR. Perioperative stroke after general surgical procedures. NY State J Med. 1993;93(3):211–5.
5. Kim J, Gelb AW. Predicting perioperative stroke. J Neurosurg Anesthesiol. 1995;7(3):211–5.
6. Kam PC, Calcroft RM. Peri-operative stroke in general surgical patients. Anesthesia. 1997;52(9):879–83.
7. Limburg M, Wijdicks EF, Li H. Ischemic stroke after surgical procedures: clinical features, neuroimaging, and risk factors. Neurology. 1998;50(4):895–901.
8. Landercasper J, Merz BJ, Cogbill TH, et al. Perioperative stroke risk in 173 consecutive patients with a past history of stroke. Arch Surg. 1990;125:986–9.
9. Zile MR, Brustsaert DL. New concepts in diastolic dysfunction and diastolic heart failure: part II: Causal mechanisms and treatment. Circulation. 2002;105:1503.
10. Vasan R, Larson M, Benjamin E, et al. Congestive heart failure in subjects with normal versus reduced left ventricular ejection fraction: prevalence and mortality in a population-based cohort. J Am Coll Cardiol. 1999;33:1948–55.
11. Ebert TJ, Rooke GA. Alterations in circulatory function. In: Silverstein JH, Rooke GA, Reves JG, McLeskey CH, editors. Geriatric anesthesiology. 2nd ed. New York: Springer; 2008. p. 137–48.
12. Groban L, Dolinski SY. Transesophageal echocardiographic evaluation of diastolic function. Chest. 2005;128(5):3652–63.
13. Vinch CS, Aurigemma GP, Simon HU, et al. Analysis of left ventricular systolic function using midwall mechanics in patients >60 years of age with hypertensive heart disease and heart failure. Am J Cardiol. 2005;19:59–64.
14. Turner MJ, Cm M, Spina RJ, et al. Effects of age and gender on cardiovascular responses to phenylephrine. J Gerontol Med Sci. 1999;54A:M17–24.
15. Brodde O-E, Leineweber K. Autonomic receptor systems in the failing and aging human heart: similarities and differences. Eur J Pharmacol. 2004;500:167–76.
16. Carti-Ceba R, Spring J, Gajic O, Warner D. The aging respiratory system: anesthetic strategies to minimize perioperative pulmonary complications. In: Silverstein JH, Rooke GA, Reves JG, McLeskey CH, editors. Geriatric anesthesiology. 2nd ed. New York: Springer; 2008. p. 149–64.
17. McEvoy MD, Reves JG. Intravenous hypnotic anesthetics. In: Silverstien JH, Rooke GA, Reves JG, McLeskey CH, editors. Geriatric anesthesiology. 2nd ed. New York: Springer; 2008. p. 229–45.
18. Epstein M. Aging and the kidney. J Am Soc Nephrol. 1996;7:1106–22.
19. Cogliati AA, Vellutini R, Nardini A, Urovi S, Hamdan M, Landoni G, et al. Fenoldopam infusion for renal protection in high-risk cardiac surgery patients: a randomized clinical study. J Cardiothorac Vasc Anesth. 2009;23(1):128.
20. Jack Jr L, Boseman L, Vinicor F. Aging Americans and diabetes. A public health and clinical response. Geriatrics. 2004;59:14–7.
21. King H, Aubert RE, Herman WH. Global burden of diabetes, 1995-2025: prevalence, numerical estimates, and projections. Diabetes Care. 1998;21:1414–31.
22. Finfer S, Chittock DR, et al. Intesnsive versus conventional glucose control in critically ill patients. N Engl J Med. 2009;360(13):1283–97.
23. Phillips PA, Rolls BY, Ledingham JG, Forsling ML, Morton JJ, Crowe MJ. Reduced thirst after water deprivation in healthy elderly men. N Engl J Med. 1984;311:753–9.
24. Weidmann P, Demyttenaere-Bursztein S, Maxwell MH, DeLima J. Effect of againg on plasma rennin and aldosterone in normal man. Kidney Int. 1975;8:325–33.
25. Robin ED. Defenders of the pulmonary artery catheter. Chest. 1988;93:1059.
26. Dalen JE, Bone RC. Is it time to pull the pulmonary artery catheter? JAMA. 1996;276:916.
27. Roberts KW, Crnkowic AP, Linneman LJ. Near-infrared spectroscopy detects critical cerebral hypoxia during carotid endarterectomy in awake patients. Anesthesiology. 1998;89(3A):A934.
28. Cho H, Nemoto E, Yonas H. Cerebral monitoring by means of oximetry and somatosensory evoked potential during carotid endarterectomy. J Neurosurg. 1998;89:533.
29. Monk TG, Reno KA, Olsen BS, et al. Postoperative cognitive dysfunction is associated with cerebral oxygen desaturations. Anesthesiology. 2000;93:A167.
30. Vohra HA, Modi A, Ohri SK. Does use of intra-operative cerebral regional oxygen saturation monitoring during cardiac surgery lead to improved clinical outcomes? Interact Cardiovasc Thorac Surg. 2009;9(2):318–22.
31. Myles PS, Leslie K, McNeil J, et al. Bispectral index monitoring to prevent awareness during anaesthesia: the B-Aware randomized controlled trial. Lancet. 2004;363:1757.
32. Kahn RA, Shernan SK, Konstadt SN. Intraoperative echocardiography. In: Kaplan JA, Reich DL, Lake CL, Konstadt SN, editors. Kaplan's cardiac anesthesia. 5th ed. Philadelphia: Saunders Elsevier; 2006. p. 437–88.
33. Thys DM, et al. Practice guidelines for perioperative transesophageal echocardiography. Anesthesiology 2010;112(1).
34. Eltzschig HK, Rosenberger P, Loffler M, Fox JA, Aranki SF, Shernan SK. Impact of intraoperative transesophageal echocardiography on surgical decisions in 12, 566 patients undergoing cardiac surgery. Ann Thorac Surg. 2008;85(3):845–52.
35. Hartman GS, Yao FS, Bruefach 3rd M, et al. Severity of aortic atheromatous disease diagnosed by transesophageal echocardiography predicts stroke and other outcomes associated with coronary artery surgery: a prospective study. Anesth Analg. 1996;83:701.
36. Katz ES, Tunick PA, Rusinek H, et al. Protruding aortic atheromas predict stroke in elderly patients undergoing cardiopulmonary bypass: experience with intraoperative transesophagela echocardiography. J Am Coll Cardiol. 1992;20:70.
37. Rosenberger P, Shernan SK, Loffler M, Shekar PS, Tuli FJA, JK NM, et al. The influence of epiaortic ultrasonography on intraoperative

surgical management in 6051 cardiac surgical patients. Ann Thorac Surg. 2008;85(2):548–53.

38. Tuman KJ, McCarthy RJ, Spiess BD, Ivankovich AD. Comparison of anesthetic techniques in patients undergoing heart valve replacement. J Cardiothorac Anesth. 1990;4(2):159–67.

39. Tuman KJ, McCarthy RJ, Spiess BD, DaValle M, Dabir R, Ivankovich AD. Does choice of anesthetic agent significantly affect outcome after coronary artery surgery? Anesthesiology. 1989;70(2):189–98.

40. Schnider TW, Minto CF, Gumbus PL, et al. The influence of method of administration and covariates on the pharmacokinetics of propofol in adult volunteers. Anesthesiology. 1998;88(5):1170–82.

41. Ball C, Westhorpe R. The history of intravenous anaesthesia: the barbiturates. Part 1. Anaesth Intensive Care. 2001;19(2):97.

42. Ball C, Westhorpe R. The history of intravenous anaesthesia: the barbiturates. Part 2. Anaesth Intensive Care. 2001;29(3):219.

43. Ball C, Westhorpe R. The history of intravenous anaesthesia: the barbiturates. Part 3. Anaesth Intesive Care. 2001;29(4):323.

44. Vinclair M, Broux C, Faure P, Brun J, Genty C, Jaquot C, et al. Duration of adrenal inhibition following a single dose of etomidate in critically ill patients. Intesive Care Med. 2008;34(4):714–9.

45. Reves JG, Fragen RJ, Vinik HR, et al. Midazolam: pharmacology and uses. Anesthesiology. 1985;62:310.

46. Harper KW, Collier PS, Dundee JW, et al. Age and nature of operation influence the pharmacokinetics of midazolam. Br J Anesth. 1985;57:866.

47. Ishikawa S, Kugawa S, Neya K, Suzuki Y, Kawasaki A, Hayama T, et al. Hemodynamic effects of dexmedetomidine in patients after cardiac surgery. Minerva Chir. 2006;61(3):215–9.

48. Maldonado JR, Wysong A, van der Starre PJ, Block T, Miller C, Reitz BA. Dexmedetomidine and the reduction of postoperative delirium after cardiac surgery. Psychosomatics. 2009;50(3):206–17.

49. Stanley TH, Webster LR. Anesthetic requirements and cardiovascular effects of fentayl-oxygen and fentanyl-diazempam-oxygen anesthesia in man. Anesth Analg. 1978;57:411.

50. Murphy GS, Szokol JW, Marymont JH, et al. Morphine-based cardiac anesthesia provides superior early recovery compared with fentanyl in elective cardiac surgery patients. Anesth Analg. 2009;109(2):311–9.

51. Ouattara A, Lecomte P, LeManach Y, et al. Poor intraoperative blood glucose control is associated with a worsened hospital outcome after cardiac surgery in diabetic patients. Anesthesiology. 2005;103:4.

52. Egi M, Bellomo R, Stachowski E, et al. Variability of blood glucose concentration and short-term mortality in critically ill patients. Anesthesiology. 2006;105:2.

53. van den Berghe G, Wouters P, Weekers F, et al. Intensive insulin therapy in the surgical intensive care unit. N Engl J Med. 2001;345:1359.

54. Nauphal M, El-Khatib M, Taha S, Haroun-bizri S, Alameddine M, Baraka A. Effect of alpha-stat vs. pH-stat strategies on cerebral oximetry during moderate hypothermic cardiopulmonary bypass. Eur J Anaesthesiol. 2007;24(1):15–9.

55. Patel RL, Turtle MR, Chambers DJ, et al. Alpha-stat acid-base regulation during cardiopulmonary bypass improves neuropsychologic outcome in patients undergoing coronary artery bypass grafting. J Thorac Cardiovasc Surg. 1996;111:1267.

56. Landoni G, Fochi O, Tritapep L, Garracino F, Belloni I, Bignami E, et al. Cardiac protection by volatile anesthetics. A review. Minerva Anestesiol. 2009;75(5):269–73.

57. Culley DJ, Monk TG, Crosby G. Postoperative central nervous system dysfuncion. In: Silverstein JH, Rooke GA, Reves JG, McLeskey CH, editors. Geriatric anesthesiology. 2nd ed. New York: Springer; 2008. p. 123–36.

58. Abernathy JH. Cardiac procedures. In: Silverstien JH, Rooke GA, Reves JG, McLeskey CH, editors. Geriatric anesthesiology. 2nd ed. New York: Springer; 2008. p. 229–45.

59. Reves JH, Reeves S, Abernathy JH, editors. Atlas of cardiothoracic anesthesia. 2nd ed. New York: Current Medicine Group, Springer; 2009.

Chapter 29
Postoperative and Critical Care in the Elderly Cardiac Surgery Patient

Christopher J. Barreiro, Kerry J. Stewart, and Glenn Whitman

Abstract As the population of our country continues to age, the number of elderly patients requiring cardiac surgery is inevitably going to rise. The limited functional and physiological reserve of the elderly provides additional challenges in the perioperative care of these patients. However, there is still much benefit and quality of life to be gained by providing expert cardiac surgical care to the elderly. To do this effectively, close attention must be paid to their preoperative, intraoperative, and postoperative care. In addition, aggressive postoperative cardiac rehabilitation is necessary to achieve our goal of returning our elderly patients to a normal life expectancy with reasonable quality of life.

Keywords Coronary artery bypass grafting • Off-pump coronary artery bypass • Aortic stenosis • Aortic valve replacement • Acute renal failure • Glomerular filtration rate • Carotid endarterectomy • Forced expiratory volume • Forced vital capacity • Mediastinitis • Cardiac rehabilitation

Introduction

The average age of cardiac surgery patients continues to increase as the population of the United States ages. Over the next 25 years, the population aged above 65 will grow at a rate 5 times than that of those under 65. The population aged above 85 will grow even more rapidly, making it the fastest growing segment of the population. In fact, between 2000 and 2050, the elderly population over 65-years-old will more than double [1]. Although the indications for surgery do not necessarily change based on a patient's age, the elderly patients have a lower functional reserve and a higher prevalence of comorbidities. Therefore, greater attention to their

preoperative risk stratification and postoperative care is required.

Clearly, the goal of surgery for all patients, including the elderly, is to return them to a normal life expectancy with a reasonable quality of life when compared with their peers. In fact, major improvements in surgical and anesthetic techniques, cardiopulmonary bypass (CPB), and postoperative critical care management have resulted in improved survival and decreased morbidity for elderly patients undergoing cardiac surgery [2]. Nevertheless, the inevitable loss of reserve in each organ system that accompanies the aging process creates an increased vulnerability to postoperative complications. Elderly patients have a higher risk for neurologic impairment including not only stroke, but also postoperative delirium, depression, and subtle neurocognitive deficits. A higher prevalence of obstructive pulmonary disease and general decline in pulmonary function result in longer ventilator dependence and increased length of stay. A slow but steady decline in renal glomerular filtration rate, as we age, results in higher rates of renal insufficiency, and therefore difficulty in managing electrolytes and fluid status postoperatively. Suboptimal nutrition and osteoporosis lead to increased rates of sternal dehiscence and wound complications. All of these factors necessitate a more intense approach to risk factor assessment and management in the elderly, both pre- and postoperatively.

The importance of age as a risk factor in cardiac surgical outcomes cannot be underestimated. The Society of Thoracic Surgery Risk Calculator can provide a concrete example of this: consider a theoretical male patient of medium height and weight, with hypertension, diabetes, and a previous history of a myocardial infarction. He has stable angina, known three vessel disease and normal left ventricular function. If this patient presents for first time, elective, isolated coronary artery bypass grafting at age 50, his risk of mortality is 0.3%. If this same patient were to present for surgery at age 65, his mortality risk doubles to 0.6%, and increases by a factor of 5–1.5% at age 80. The overall risk of morbidity or mortality in this 50-year-old patient almost doubles from 5.8 to 11.2% as his age increases to 80. The individual risk of renal failure

C.J. Barreiro (✉)
Division of Cardiothoracic Surgery, Johns Hopkins Hospital,
600 N Wolfe Street, Blalock 618, Baltimore, MD 21287, USA
e-mail: cbarrei1@jhmi.edu

M.R. Katlic (ed.), *Cardiothoracic Surgery in the Elderly*, DOI 10.1007/978-1-4419-0892-6_29,
© Springer Science+Business Media, LLC 2011

Table 29.1 The impact of age on the incidence of postoperative complications following coronary artery bypass in a low risk, idealized patient, based on the Society of Thoracic Surgery Risk Calculator

Age (years)	50 (%)	65 (%)	80 (%)
Risk of mortality	0.3	0.6	1.5
Morbidity or mortality	5.8	7.3	11.2
Renal failure	0.8	1.3	2.5
Permanent stroke	0.4	0.7	1.2

Table 29.2 Independent predictors of mortality for patients following CABG

Age	Gender
Prior CABG	Vascular disease
COPD	History of CHF
Shock or emergency procedure	Impaired ejection fraction
Renal insufficiency	Preoperative MI

and stroke also triples in this theoretical patient (see Table 29.1) [3]. These are quite impressive statistics when you consider that the only variable is the patient's age. However, despite the physiologic challenges posed by the elderly, there is good evidence that the current practice of cardiac surgery allows them to experience a meaningful improvement in functional capacity and quality of life postoperatively.

Operation-Specific Risk Factors

Cardiovascular disease is the leading cause of death in the US. As the population continues to age, the prevalence of elderly patients with symptomatic coronary artery disease requiring bypass is also increasing. Historically, studies have shown the morbidity and mortality of elderly patients undergoing cardiac surgery to be significantly higher when compared with their younger counterparts. Independent predictors of mortality for patients of any age following coronary artery bypass grafting (CABG) are shown in Table 29.2: age, gender, prior CABG, vascular disease, COPD, history of CHF, shock or emergency procedure, impaired left ventricular ejection fraction (LVEF), renal insufficiency, and preoperative MI. The National Cardiovascular Network (NCN) revascularization database is a collaboration of 22 US high volume centers. A recent report from this database reviewed 64,467 patients undergoing CABG alone, and compared patients <80 (n=60,161) with those ≥80-years old (n=4,306) [2]. Both groups had a similar preoperative LVEF. However, the patients aged ≥80-years had more extensive coronary artery disease, a higher frequency of preoperative shock, left ventricular assist device placement, and surgery under emergency circumstances. The elderly patients had a significantly

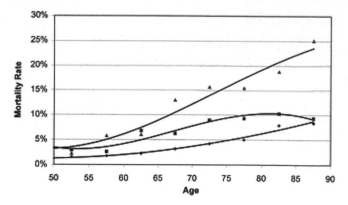

Fig. 29.1 Observed in-hospital mortality after cardiac surgery among all patients. *Diamond*=CABG; *solid square*=CABG/AVR; *triangle*=CABG/MVR. *AVR* aortic valve replacement; *CABG* coronary artery bypass grafting; *MVR* mitral valve repair or replacement (reprinted from Alexander et al. [2], Copyright Elsevier 2000, with permission from the American College of Cardiology)

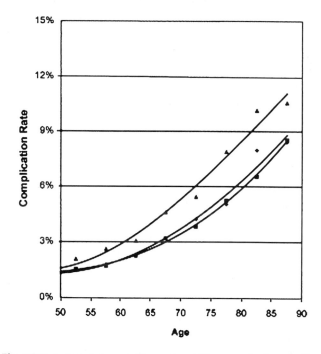

Fig. 29.2 In-hospital mortality, postoperative neurologic complications and postoperative renal failure after CABG by age. *Diamond*=mortality; *square*=renal failure; *triangle*=neurologic events (reprinted from Alexander et al. [2], Copyright Elsevier 2000, with permission from the American College of Cardiology)

higher operative mortality at 8.1% vs. 3% in the younger patients (see Fig. 29.1). Postoperative renal failure and neurologic complications were also twice as high in the patients ≥80-years old (see Fig. 29.2).

Another study evaluating predictors of mortality and outcomes following CABG in the elderly analyzed 3,683 patients at a single institution in the UK over a 5-year period. Risk factors for operative mortality were female gender, severe angina, prolonged CPB time, preoperative arrhythmias, and renal impairment. The elderly group, ≥75-years old, comprised 18% of the cohort (659) and had a 1-year mortality of 9% compared with 4% in the 60–74 age group [4]. However, this mortality in the elderly group dropped from 15%, in the first year of the study, to 7%, in the last year of the study, while the mortality rate remained relatively stable in the younger population. The authors attributed the 50% drop in mortality to improved CPB management and more experience in the postoperative care of these elderly patients.

One of the goals of cardiac surgery has been to minimize the morbidity and mortality in all patients, but most notably the elderly, as they are most at risk. Out of this effort sprang "off pump" coronary bypass surgery. Off-pump coronary artery bypass (OPCAB) avoids hypothermia, CPB, aortic cannulation, and in some cases even eliminates significant manipulation of the aorta. All of these features have significant theoretical advantages for the elderly. In fact, many studies report lower incidences of morbidities such as postoperative renal failure and stroke with OPCAB when compared with conventional CABG [5]. However, long-term clinical outcomes with OPCAB in the elderly show trends toward lower survival and higher rates of repeat revascularization [6]. Yet another obvious way to continue to improve survival is through earlier intervention in the elderly patients prior to acute deterioration of symptoms and left ventricular impairment.

The surgical treatment of elderly patients with valvular heart disease will inevitably come under new scrutiny as well, with the advent of percutaneous valve implantation techniques. Aortic valve stenosis (AS) is the most commonly acquired heart valve lesion in the elderly, with a prevalence of 2% in Americans over 65-years old, caused by degenerative changes with complex calcification of the native leaflets and annulus. Aortic valve replacement (AVR) in the elderly has been demonstrated to have excellent functional outcomes with satisfactory long-term survival rates. A review of 247 patients >70-years old undergoing AVR at Johns Hopkins Hospital demonstrated a 6.1% operative mortality, with a 1-year actuarial survival of 89.5% [7]. Some of the most commonly quoted risk factors for operative mortality with valvular heart disease as seen in Table 29.3 are as follows: older age, reduced ejection fraction, NYHA functional class, pulmonary hypertension, respiratory dysfunction, peripheral vascular disease, urgent surgery, renal dysfunction and

previous cardiac surgery [8]. Long-term survival has been shown to be detrimentally influenced by aortic valve regurgitation, postoperative renal failure, stroke, and intra-aortic balloon pump usage [9].

Combining valve surgery with coronary revascularization leads to additional mortality risk. The 345 octogenarians in the NCN revascularization database undergoing combined CABG/AVR had a mortality rate of 10.1% vs. 7.9% for those <80-years old [2]. Interestingly, the addition of an AVR appears to increase mortality by the same increment regardless of age category, whereas MVR adds increasingly to operative mortality risk with advancing age (see Fig. 29.1). Those patients ≥80-years old undergoing combined CABG/MVR ($n=92$) had a mortality of 19.6% (11.5% higher than CABG alone), whereas in the group <80-years old, the mortality was 12.2% (9.2% higher than a CABG alone). Despite their increased age, aggressive surgical treatment is still warranted in the symptomatic, elderly patient, at least until more data are available on newer less invasive percutaneous techniques.

Renal Insufficiency

Acute renal insufficiency is a serious complication of cardiac surgery and is associated with significant morbidity and mortality when renal replacement therapy becomes necessary. Acute renal failure (ARF) requiring dialysis occurs in 1–5% of patients following cardiac surgery and is dependent on many preoperative, intraoperative, and postoperative factors. The mortality of ARF requiring dialysis following cardiac surgery is upwards of 50% in some studies [10]. Some of the most significant risk factors for postoperative ARF include preoperative renal insufficiency, diabetes, prolonged CPB time, postoperative hypotension, and age [11].

As we age, many structural and functional changes occur to our kidneys, which lead to diminished nephron reserve and a reduced capacity of renal autoregulation. Chronic diseases such as hypertension, diabetes, and cardiovascular disease also become more prevalent in the elderly, which promotes renal damage. Anatomic changes to the kidneys with age include a decrease in volume and weight due to glomerulosclerosis and tubulointerstitial fibrosis. These structural changes that occur with advancing age result in functional alterations and a concomitant decrease in glomerular filtration rate (GFR) (see Fig. 29.3) [12]. The Cockcroft-Gault equation is a simplified estimation of GFR based on the patient's age, weight, gender, and creatinine:

$$GFR = \frac{(140 - age) \times (wgt \text{ in kg}) \times (0.85 \text{ for females})}{72 \times creatinine}.$$

Table 29.3 Risk factors for operative mortality with valvular heart disease

Age	Reduced ejection fraction
NYHA functional class	Pulmonary hypertension
Respiratory dysfunction	Peripheral vascular disease
Urgent surgery	Renal dysfunction
Reoperative cardiac surgery	

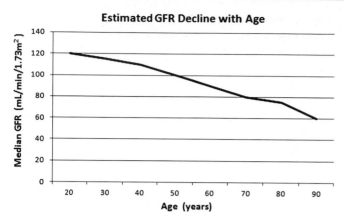

Fig. 29.3 Estimated GFR vs. age

The significant impact of age on GFR can be observed with this formula. Roughly speaking, for every year of life you lose 1 cc of glomerular filtration. For example, a 40-year old, 75 kg male patient with a creatinine of 1.0 mg/dL has a GFR of 104 mL/min. Using the Cockcroft-Gault equation, this same patient 40 years later, at 80 years of age, would have a GFR of only 62 mL/min. In addition to this loss of glomerular filtration, there is also a decrease in the autoregulatory vascular defense and an increase in renal tubular fragility [13]. All of these factors combine to make the elderly patient less capable of withstanding the acute nephrotoxic insults incurred in the perioperative period.

The detrimental effects on kidney function specific to CPB can be attributed to renal hypoperfusion, nonpulsatile flow, hypothermia, and stimulation of the systemic inflammatory response. Bypass in and of itself is associated with a mild decrease in GFR, filtration fraction, and renal vascular resistance, and at the same time increases the fractional excretion of sodium and free water clearance. There is also a concomitant release of renin, aldosterone, angiotensin II, and vasopressin. In an effort to minimize the hormonal and physiological chaos that is detrimental to kidney function, off-pump surgery has been proposed as a means of minimizing this renal insult. Unfortunately, studies have failed to demonstrate a reduction in renal morbidity with off-pump when compared with conventional on-pump cardiac surgery [14].

The Society of Thoracic Surgery database defines postoperative ARF as a rise in the serum creatinine to greater than 2.0 mg/dL associated with at least a doubling of the patient's preoperative creatinine, not as a need for renal replacement therapy. Perhaps an even more sensitive way of defining postoperative renal dysfunction would involve estimation of postoperative GFR, a more accurate assessment of renal function. Preoperatively, once the GFR falls below 60 mL/min, there is a significant increase in the risk of postoperative renal dysfunction. To reduce these risks preoperatively, all potentially nephrotoxic medications should be discontinued and the patient should be adequately hydrated. Perioperatively,

hemodynamics should be optimized to avoid any periods of hypotension. Ischemic acute tubular necrosis (ATN) most often results from hypotension and a low cardiac output state, and is the most common etiology of postoperative ARF. It is often due to hypovolemia or the use of vasoconstricting alpha agents, which overwhelm the ability of the kidney to auto-regulate GFR and maintain perfusion and filtration. Postoperative volume administration must be aggressive to maintain adequate intravascular volume, to ensure an appropriate cardiac output and renal perfusion. However, it must simultaneously be judicious, so as to avoid jeopardizing pulmonary function. As patients age, the tipping point is even narrower.

Postoperative renal insufficiency and failure, as is the case in all instances of renal dysfunction, can be categorized as nonoliguric or oliguric. Nonoliguric renal failure creates a more easily negotiated balance regarding volume overload and electrolyte homeostasis. In this situation, it is paramount to avoid further insults to the kidneys while awaiting spontaneous recovery of function. In oliguric renal failure, high-dose diuretics are often used to try to convert to a nonoliguric phase with the hope of minimizing the impact of fluid retention and volume overload on pulmonary function and tissue edema. However, in this situation, renal replacement therapy often becomes necessary as a result of hypervolemia, hyperkalemia, uremia, and metabolic acidosis. Correction of electrolytes can be achieved with either intermittent hemodialysis or with continuous venovenous hemodialysis, which is frequently used as a result of the commonly associated hemodynamic instability in this patient population. However, renal replacement therapy is not benign, and its use is associated with a close to 50% mortality in this postoperative population. In fact, in our population, renal replacement therapy in octogenarians was required in over 4% of patients, 2–3 times that seen in a typical population of open heart surgery patients viewed as a whole, and was associated with a mortality of over 60% [15].

Gastrointestinal Complications

Gastrointestinal (GI) complications occur in 0.5–4% of postoperative cardiac surgery patients and cause significant morbidity and mortality [16]. Complications include GI bleeding, mesenteric ischemia, pancreatitis, cholecystitis, perforated ulcers, as well as ileus/obstruction. The pathophysiologic mechanism for many of these complications is vasoconstriction and hypoperfusion of the splanchnic bed in the perioperative period. Contributing factors include hemodilution and nonpulsatile flow, which are usually unavoidable during CPB, but postoperative low cardiac output and the use of vasopressors must be viewed as significant contributors as well. Decreased visceral and mucosal perfusion of the GI tract leads to bacterial translocation, sepsis, and multiorgan failure. Older age has been shown in many studies to be an independent predictor of GI complications after cardiac surgery [16–18].

In addition to age, other independent risk factors for GI complications include renal failure, prolonged CPB time, and urgent/emergent operative status. Patients developing GI complications postoperatively have been shown to require additional procedures, have a higher incidence of postoperative arrhythmias, and are more likely to develop neurologic, pulmonary, renal, and sternal wound complications [19]. These patients predictably spend more time in the ICU, have prolonged ventilator times and overall length of hospitalization. The development of any GI complication significantly increases operative mortality up to fivefold in some studies [16].

Identifying the risks preoperatively for postoperative GI complications is important to sensitize the practitioner and allow for early recognition of the complications, and earlier intervention, with the hope of minimizing the associated morbidity and mortality. When patients exhibit signs and symptoms of an acute intraabdominal process such as abdominal pain/tenderness or gross/occult GI bleeding, suspicion and a search for the etiology should be immediate. However, frequently the presentation is subtle, with the first hint of a problem being an elevated white blood cell count or slightly abnormal liver function tests (LFTs). A serum amylase/lipase or random lactate level can be extremely helpful in this setting. Successful treatment hinges on early identification of the underlying etiology as postoperative cardiac patients, particularly the elderly, are usually too fragile to withstand the stress of prolonged intestinal ischemia, sepsis, or bleeding. The importance of serial abdominal exams should not be underestimated, and should be associated with timely laboratory evaluations, abdominal imaging with ultrasound or computed tomography, as well as endoscopy in the case of GI bleeding or possible colonic ischemia. The key to therapy is early diagnosis.

Neurologic Impairment

Neurologic complications following cardiac surgery are extremely common in the elderly and result in prolonged length of hospital stay and subsequent rehabilitation. The spectrum of neurologic sequelae ranges from stroke, which is seen in up to 6% of patients undergoing CAB, to much more prevalent, subtle neurocognitive changes [20, 21]. These include mild deficits in memory, attention, concentration, and language, and can be seen in 60–70% of patients undergoing cardiac surgery. The three main etiologic factors involved are cerebral embolization, hypoperfusion,

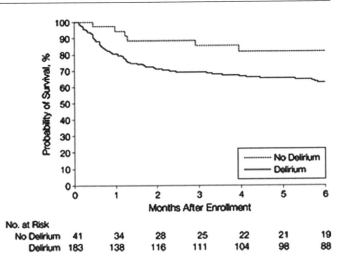

Fig. 29.4 Kaplan-Meyer analysis of delirium in the intensive care unit and 6-month survival (reprinted with permission from Ely et al. [22]. Copyright 2004 American Medical Association. All rights reserved)

and generalized perioperative inflammation. Also commonly seen in the elderly is the postoperative delirium, a transient but global impairment in cognitive function, which occurs in up to 80% of the ICU population [22]. It is a major postoperative morbidity factor, associated with a significant increase in mortality and length of stay (see Fig. 29.4). Delirium is a persistent problem in the ICU, without a clearly defined therapy or a well understood etiology, except for being multifactorial. Inciting events and risk factors other than age include preoperative organic brain disease, metabolic derangements, alcohol withdrawal, low cardiac output, hypoxia, sepsis, and medications.

Preoperative predictors of neurologic sequelae after cardiac surgery include the following: advanced age, prior neurologic events, hypertension, diabetes, and peripheral/carotid vascular disease [23, 24]. These risk factors identify individuals with widespread cerebrovascular disease, impaired cerebral blood flow, or increased susceptibility to thromboembolic events. Studies have also identified intraoperative predictors for perioperative neurologic events. These independent risk factors include the following: the presence of significant aortic arch atherosclerosis, longer duration of CPB, and CAB with concomitant carotid endarterectomy (CEA) [25]. The issue of performing a concomitant CAB/CEA in patients with significant (>70%) internal carotid artery (ICA) stenosis has been debated in the literature, and the benefits remain unclear. However, it is important to identify those patients with significant carotid disease through appropriate screening so that operative decisions can be made with regards to a concomitant, vs. staged, CAB and CEA. A retrospective analysis of 1,421 consecutive CAB patients at Johns Hopkins Hospital was performed to identify the potential merits of preoperative carotid screening. The study reinforced the notion that significant carotid stenosis

patient found that despite the higher prevalence of comorbidities at the start of cardiac rehabilitation, age was not a factor in the extent of physiological and risk factor improvements that accrued through participation in a cardiac rehabilitation program [53].

A review by Stewart et al. highlights the scientific and clinical evidence for cardiac rehabilitation in patients who have undergone percutaneous revascularization, heart transplant, and heart valve surgery [54]. Across these diagnoses, regardless of age, there is considerable benefit of cardiac rehabilitation and supervised exercise training for increasing functional capacity, favorably modifying disease-related risk factors, decreasing symptoms, detecting signs and symptoms of disease before they become serious complications, and improving quality of life. The available evidence for this component of cardiovascular disease management, albeit not perfect, still warrants its more widespread application.

In 2007, the American Heart Association and the American Association of Cardiovascular and Pulmonary Rehabilitation recommended that cardiac rehabilitation programs provide several important core components consisting of baseline patient assessment, nutritional counseling, risk factor management (lipids, hypertension, weight, diabetes, and smoking), psychosocial management, physical activity counseling, and exercise training [46]. The American Heart Association also recommends these cardiac rehabilitation components for the elderly [48]. Although secondary prevention therapies such as pharmacological management of atherosclerosis risk factors and depression are provided by clinicians in their offices, cardiac rehabilitation is often the most advantageous setting for bringing many of these core components together in a comprehensive approach to provide exercise training, patient education, behavioral counseling, and psychosocial support. Studies of efficacy and effectiveness of cardiac rehabilitation document reductions in mortality and improvements in clinical and behavioral outcomes beyond the improvements in morbidity and mortality already available through revascularization and optimal pharmacotherapy. Yet cardiac rehabilitation, like many preventive measures, is underutilized [55].

Unfortunately, it is estimated that only 10–40% of eligible patients participate in cardiac rehabilitation programs [56, 57]. These rates of participation are even less for older patients, a group with the highest prevalence of cardiovascular disease [58, 59]. Medicare provides payment for cardiac rehabilitation for the diagnoses of myocardial infarction, coronary artery bypass surgery, stable angina, and more recently, percutaneous revascularization, heart transplant, and heart valve surgery. Thus, cardiac rehabilitation services are generally available for the Medicare population who has undergone cardiac revascularization procedures. Insurance coverage by other third-party payers varies considerably throughout the US, although most payers generally follow Medicare policy. One review found that the lower rates of

participation in older patients was primarily due to less aggressive rates of referrals from physicians rather than lack of benefit accruing to the older patients [60]. This problem is even worse for women who have a decreased likelihood of receiving a physician referral to cardiac rehabilitation after revascularization, despite being matched for age and undergoing the same procedure [61]. Thus, there is the need for education initiatives of all healthcare providers on the comprehensive nature and benefits of cardiac rehabilitation in the secondary prevention of cardiovascular disease, with a particular emphasis on women.

A review of all components of cardiac rehabilitation and secondary prevention (such as smoking cessation, behavioral counseling, and pharmacotherapy) is beyond the scope of this section. To some extent, the scope is also limited by the studies on cardiac rehabilitation, which uses supervised exercise training as the primary treatment modality. Although not fully evaluated in large-scale trials, a comprehensive approach to cardiac rehabilitation should be more than just exercise training, and presumably would produce greater improvements in health and functional status for patients than is evident in the literature [62]. A structured exercise program may be novel to older individuals, or in some instances, an activity in which they have not participated in for many years. Furthermore, for older persons with coronary heart disease, the clinical manifestations represent the effects of the disease superimposed on the physiological effects of age, which too often leads to decreases in exercise capacity and overall physical activity. Nevertheless, there is considerable evidence that exercise training by itself produces substantial physiological benefits, improves risk factors, reduces mortality, and increases aerobic capacity, muscle strength, and functional performance.

Contemporary cardiac rehabilitation programs are also experienced in addressing the educational deficiencies of older patients including the special needs of those with cardiac pacemakers and implanted defibrillators, chronic heart failure, diabetes, peripheral arterial disease, and other comorbidities. In recent years, there is also increased recognition of the importance of resistance training for individuals with and without cardiovascular disease. The American Heart Association recently updated its Scientific Advisory on "Resistance Exercise in Individuals with and without Cardiovascular Disease," which noted that after appropriate screening, resistance training is an effective method for improving muscular strength and endurance, preventing and managing a variety of chronic medical conditions, modifying cardiac risk factors, enhancing psychosocial well-being, and increasing functional capacity [63]. This latter benefit is of particular importance for older patients, many of whom are slower to recover from surgical procedures and have reduced functional capacity before surgery. A key benefit of resistance exercise training is an increase in muscle mass and strength, and improved flexibility and balance, all of which reduces the risk of falls. Though weight machines are most commonly used in cardiac rehabilitation programs, alternative modes of resistance training are calisthenics, isometrics, and use of elastic stretch bands. These modalities are commonly used when the older patient lacks the initial strength or has orthopedic limitations that preclude use of weight machines.

Most activities requiring lifting and straining, such as weight training, have a large static component. In such activities, there is increased peripheral vascular resistance, with an expected increase in blood pressure but much less of an increase in heart rate or cardiac output compared with aerobic exercise. Nevertheless, brief periods of moderate resistive exercise appear safe and may pose less of a cardiac burden than aerobic exercises of similar effort. In fact, studies show that cardiac patients who were required to carry or lift weights or to perform isometric exercise after a myocardial infarction had fewer ischemic electrocardiographic changes and arrhythmias during resistance exercise than during aerobic exercises. There is no evidence that short term increases in blood pressure during resistance training is of concern, even in older patients, who commonly have higher baseline blood levels secondary to greater arterial stiffness. Gradual involvement in resistance training may, therefore, be beneficial and desirable, especially for older patients for whom preventing or reversing sarcopenia is of great concern.

Exercise prescription for increasing functional capacity and enhancing recovery from open heart surgery has been a core component of cardiac rehabilitation for decades [64, 65]. The expected outcomes are similar to those for younger persons, though the levels of functional capacity are less in the older patient and achieving positive benefits may require longer program participation. The specific methods for prescribing exercise for cardiac patients have been published and generally do not require significant modification for the older patient [48, 64, 65]. The main need for modification depends primarily on existing comorbidities that might limit mobility. After open heart surgery, light stretching and calisthenics are used to maintain flexibility and range of motion of the upper torso. However, heavier forms of resistance training should be avoided until there is sufficient healing of the sternum, as determined by physical examination by the surgeon. Participation in lower body exercise can be undertaken sooner, in addition to aerobic exercise such as walking or cycling.

References

1. US Department of Commerce, Bureau of the Census. http://www.census.gov/main/www/cen2000.html.
2. Alexander KP, Anstrom KJ, Muhlbaier LH, et al. Outcomes of cardiac surgery in patients age ≥ 80 years: results from the cardiovascular network. J Am Coll Cardiol. 2000;35:731–8.
3. Online STS Risk Calculator. http://209.220.160.181/STSWebRisk Calc261/de.aspx.
4. Naughton C, Feneck RO, Roxburgh J. Early and late predictors of mortality following on-pump coronary artery bypass graft surgery in the elderly as compared to a younger population. Eur J Cardiothorac Surg. 2009;36:621–7.
5. Yan L, Zheng Z, Hu S. Early and long-term outcomes in the elderly: comparison between off-pump and on-pump techniques in 1191 patients undergoing coronary artery bypass grafting. J Thorac Cardiovasc Surg. 2008;136:657–64.
6. Racz MJ, Hannan EL, Isom OW, et al. A comparison of short and long-term outcomes after off-pump and on-pump coronary artery bypass graft surgery with sternotomy. J Am Coll Cardiol. 2004;43: 557–64.
7. Tseng EE, Lee CA, Cameron DE, et al. Aortic valve replacement in the elderly. Risk factors and long-term results. Ann Surg. 1997;225:793–802.
8. Kolh P, Kerzmann A, Honore C, et al. Aortic valve surgery in octogenarians: predictive factors for operative and long term results. Eur J Cardiothorac Surg. 2007;31:600–6.
9. Melby SJ, Zierer A, Kaiser SP, et al. Aortic valve replacement in octogenarians: risk factors for early and late mortality. Ann Thorac Surg. 2007;83:1651–7.
10. Ostermann ME, Taube D, Morgan CJ, et al. Acute renal failure following cardiopulmonary bypass: a changing picture. Intensive Care Med. 2000;26:565–71.
11. Suen WS, Mok CK, Chiu SW, et al. Risk factors for development of acute renal failure requiring dialysis in patients undergoing cardiac surgery. Angiology. 1998;49:789–800.
12. National Kidney Foundation: KDOQI Guidelines. http://www.kidney.org/PROFESSIONALS/kdoqi/guidelines_ckd/p4_class_g1.htm.
13. Fliser D, Ritz E, Franek E. Renal reserve in the elderly. Semin Nephrol. 1995;15:463–7.
14. Chukwuemeka A, Weisel A, Maganti M, et al. Renal dysfunction in high-risk patients after on-pump and off-pump coronary artery bypass surgery: a propensity score analysis. Ann Thorac Surg. 2005;80:2148–54.
15. Wijeysundera DN, Karkouti K, Dupuis JY, et al. Derivation and validation of a simplified predictive index for renal replacement therapy after cardiac surgery. JAMA. 2007;297:1801–9.
16. Rodriguez F, Nguyen TC, Galanko JA, Morton J. Gastrointestinal complications after coronary artery bypass grafting: a national study of morbidity and mortality predictors. J Am Coll Surg. 2007;205:741–47.
17. Filsoufi F, Rahmanian PB, Castillo JG, Scurlock C, Legnani PE, Adams DH. Predictors and outcome of gastrointestinal complications in patients undergoing cardiac surgery. Ann of Surg. 2007;246:323–29.
18. Recht MH, Smith JM, Woods SE, Engel AM, Hiratzka LF. Predictors and outcomes of gastrointestinal complications in patients undergoing coronary artery bypass graft surgery: a prospective, nested case-control study. J Am Coll Surg. 2004;198: 742–47.
19. Roach GW, Kanchuger M, Mangano CM, et al. Adverse cerebral outcomes after coronary bypass surgery. N Engl J Med. 1996;335:1857–63.
20. Redmond JM, Greene PS, Goldsborough MA, et al. Neurologic injury in cardiac surgical patients with a history of stroke. Ann Thorac Surg. 1996;61:42–7.
21. Hogue CW, Murphy SF, Schechtman KB, et al. Risk factors for early or delayed stroke after cardiac surgery. Circulation. 1999;100: 642–7.
22. Ely EW, Shintani A, Truman B, et al. Delirium as a predictor of mortality in mechanically ventilated patients in the intensive care unit. JAMA. 2004;291:1753–62.

23. Bucerius J, Gummert JF, Borger MA, et al. Stroke after cardiac surgery: a risk factor analysis of 16, 184 consecutive adult patients. Ann Thorac Surg. 2003;75:472–8.

24. Cernaianu AC, Vassilidze TV, Flum DR, et al. Predictors of stroke after cardiac surgery. J Card Surg. 1995;10:334–9.

25. Durand DJ, Perler BA, Roseborough GS, et al. Mandatory versus selective preoperative carotid screening: a retrospective analysis. Ann Thorac Surg. 2004;78:159–66.

26. Vohra HA, Modi A, Ohri SK. Does use of intra-operative cerebral regional oxygen saturation monitoring during cardiac surgery lead to improved clinical outcomes? Interact Cardiovasc Thorac Surg. 2009;9:318–22.

27. Edmonds HL. Multi-modality neurophysiologic monitoring for cardiac surgery. Heart Surg Forum. 2002;5:225–8.

28. Selnes OA, Grega MA, Borowicz LM, et al. Cognitive changes with coronary artery disease: a prospective study of coronary artery bypass graft patients and nonsurgical controls. Ann Thorac Surg. 2003;75:1377.

29. Selnes OA, Grega MA, Bailey MM, et al. Do management strategies for coronary artery disease influence 6-year cognitive outcomes? Ann Thorac Surg. 2009;88:445–54.

30. Breuer AC, Furlan AJ, Hanson MR, et al. Central nervous system complications of coronary artery bypass graft surgery: prospective analysis of 421 patients. Stroke. 1983;14:682.

31. Grocott HP, Croughwell ND, Amory DW, et al. Cerebral emboli and S100β during cardiac surgery. Ann Thorac Surg. 1998;65:1645.

32. Kannel WB, Hubert H, Lew EA. Vital capacity as a predictor of cardiovascular disease: the Framingham Study. Am Heart J. 1983;105:311–5.

33. Knudson RJ. Aging of the respiratory system. Curr Pulmonol. 1989;10:1–24.

34. Griffith KA, Sherill DL, Siegel EM, et al. Predictors of loss of lung function in the elderly. Am J Respir Crit Care Med. 2001;163:61–8.

35. Liptay MJ, Basu S, Hoaglin MC, et al. Diffusion lung capacity for carbon monoxide (DLCO) is an independent prognostic factor for long-term survival after curative lung resection for cancer. J Surg Oncol. 2009;100:703–7.

36. Yavas S, Yagar S, Mavioglu L, et al. Tracheostomy: how and when should it be done in cardiovascular surgery ICU? J Card Surg. 2009;24:11–8.

37. Rahmanian PB, Adams DH, Castillo JG, et al. Tracheostomy is not a risk factor for deep sternal wound infection after cardiac surgery. Ann Thorac Surg. 2007;84:1984–92.

38. Karra R, McDermott L, Connelly S, et al. Risk factors for 1-year mortality after postoperative mediastinitis. J Thorac Cardiovasc Surg. 2006;132:537–43.

39. Reeves BC, Murphy GJ. Increased mortality, morbidity, and cost associated with red blood cell transfusion after cardiac surgery. Curr Opin Cardiol. 2008;23:607–12.

40. Choong CK, Gerrard C, Goldsmith KA, et al. Delayed re-exploration for bleeding after coronary artery bypass surgery results in adverse outcomes. Eur J Cardiothorac Surg. 2007;31:834–8.

41. Lepelletier D, Poupelin L, Corvec S, et al. Risk factors for mortality in patients with mediastinitis after cardiac surgery. Arch Cardiovasc Dis. 2009;102:119–25.

42. Braxton JH, Marrin CA, McGrath PD, et al. 10-year follow-up of patients with and without mediastinitis. Semin Thorac Cardiovasc Surg. 2004;16:70–6.

43. Cabbabe EB, Cabbabe SW. Immediate versus delayed one-stage sternal debridement and pectoralis muscle flap reconstruction of deep sternal wound infections. Plast Reconstr Surg. 2009;123:1490–4.

44. Robicsek F, Cook JW, Rizzoni W. Sternoplasty for incomplete sternum separation. J Thorac Cardiovasc Surg. 1998;116:361–2.

45. Schimmer C, Reents W, Berneder S, et al. Prevention of sternal dehiscence and infection in high risk patients: a prospective randomized multicenter trial. Ann Thorac Surg. 2008;86:1897–904.

46. Balady GJ, Williams MA, Ades PA, et al. Core components of cardiac rehabilitation/secondary prevention programs: 2007 update. Circulation. 2007;115:2675–82.

47. Lloyd-Jones D, Adams R, Carnethon M, et al. Heart disease and stroke statistics–2009 update: a report from the American Heart Association Statistics Committee and Stroke Statistics Subcommittee. Circulation. 2009;119:e21–181.

48. Williams MA, Fleg JL, Ades PA, et al. Secondary prevention of coronary heart disease in the elderly (with emphasis on patients > or =75 years of age): an American Heart Association scientific statement from the Council on Clinical Cardiology Subcommittee on Exercise, Cardiac Rehabilitation, and Prevention. Circulation. 2002;105:1735–43.

49. Peterson ED, Cowper PA, Jollis JG, et al. Outcomes of coronary artery bypass graft surgery in 24, 461 patients aged 80 years or older. Circulation. 1995;92:II85–91.

50. Barzilay JI, Kronmal RA, Bittner V, et al. Coronary artery disease and coronary artery bypass grafting in diabetic patients aged > or = 65 years (report from the Coronary Artery Surgery Study [CASS] Registry). Am J Cardiol. 1994;74:334–9.

51. O'Keefe Jr JH, Sutton MB, McCallister BD, et al. Coronary angioplasty versus bypass surgery in patients > 70 years old matched for ventricular function. J Am Coll Cardiol. 1994;24:425–30.

52. Edwards FH, Carey JS, Grover FL, et al. Impact of gender on coronary bypass operative mortality. Ann Thorac Surg. 1998;66:125–31.

53. Maniar S, Sanderson BK, Bittner V. Comparison of baseline characteristics and outcomes in younger and older patients completing cardiac rehabilitation. J Cardiopulm Rehabil Prev. 2009;29:220–9.

54. Stewart KJ, Badenhop D, Brubaker PH, et al. Cardiac rehabilitation following percutaneous revascularization, heart transplant, heart valve surgery, and for chronic heart failure. Chest. 2003;123:2104–11.

55. Bittner V, Sanderson B. Cardiac rehabilitation as secondary prevention center. Coron Artery Dis. 2006;17:211–8.

56. Thomas RJ, Miller NH, Lamendola C, et al. National survey on gender differences in cardiac rehabilitation programs. J Cardiopulm Rehabil. 1996;16:402–12.

57. Wenger NK, Froelicher ES, Smith LK, et al. Cardiac rehabilitation as secondary prevention. Agency for Health Care Policy and Research and National Heart, Lung, and Blood Institute. Clin Pract Guide Quick Ref Guide Clin. 1995;17:1–23.

58. Lavie CJ, Milani RV. Cardiac rehabilitation and preventive cardiology in the elderly. Cardiol Clin. 1999;17:233–42.

59. Ades PA. Cardiac rehabilitation in older coronary patients. J Am Geriatr Soc. 1999;47:98–105.

60. Pasquali SK, Alexander KP, Peterson ED. Cardiac rehabilitation in the elderly. Am Heart J. 2001;142:748–55.

61. Caulin-Glaser T, Blum M, Schmeizl R, et al. Gender differences in referral to cardiac rehabilitation programs after revascularization. J Cardiopulm Rehabil. 2001;21:24–30.

62. Thomas RJ, King M, Lui K, et al. AACVPR/ACC/AHA 2007 performance measures on cardiac rehabilitation for referral to and delivery of cardiac rehabilitation/secondary prevention services. J Am Coll Cardiol. 2007;50:1400–33.

63. Williams MA, Haskell WL, Ades PA, et al. Resistance exercise in individuals with and without cardiovascular disease: 2007 update. Circulation. 2007;116:572–84.

64. American Association of Cardiovascular & Pulmonary Rehabilitation. Guidelines for cardiac rehabilitation and secondary prevention programs. 4th ed. Champaign: Human Kinetics; 2004.

65. American Association of Cardiovascular & Pulmonary Rehabilitation. AACVPR cardiac rehabilitation resource manual: promoting health and preventing disease. Chicago: Human Kinetics; 2006.

Chapter 30
Surgery for Ischemic Coronary Disease in the Elderly[1]

Margarita T. Camacho and Melissa L. Wong

Abstract As the elderly population grows each year, so does the number of these patients referred for cardiac intervention. The morbidity and mortality associated with these procedures have substantially decreased since the 1980s, but judicious patient selection and optimization can lower perioperative risks even further. The older the patient, the more likely the presence of multiple chronic noncardiac diseases, increased tissue fragility, and limited organ reserves for stressful events. Systematic assessment of cognitive and other functions, when possible, will help predict the operative risk and guide for the optimization of the preoperative elderly patient. During the process of deciding whether to offer cardiac surgical intervention to elderly patients, the relief of symptoms and improved quality of life should assume more importance than the issue of increased life expectancy. Comorbidities and concerns raised by the patient and family should be acknowledged and factored into the decision-making process. The overall goal is to select the least morbid and most effective procedure that is currently available.

Keywords Elderly • Ischemic coronary disease • Comorbidities • Mortality and morbidity risk • Optimization • Quality of life

As the elderly population rises steadily each year, so does the number of patients referred for cardiac surgical procedures. The US Census Bureau predicted that the population would contain approximately 7.4 billion people above the age of 80 by 2008, when compared with 6.2 billion in 2000 [2]. Recent data reported that elderly patients aged above 70 with no functional limitations can be expected to live 14.3 years longer, when compared with 11.6 years for those with limitation in at least one activity of daily living [3]. A formidable challenge being faced by the cardiologists and the cardiac surgeons is the appropriate treatment of the 40% of the growing elderly population suffering from symptomatic cardiovascular disease [4]. The morbidity and mortality associated with cardiac surgical procedures in the elderly has substantially decreased since the late 1980s [5], although it is still higher than that of younger counterparts less than 70 years of age [6]. Reports of acceptable mortality rates and improved long-term quality of life justify cardiac operations in most symptomatic elderly patients. Only recently, large studies have been focused on risk analyses and outcomes in an effort to provide the clinician with as much evidence-based literature as possible to make the most appropriate decisions for many of these complex elderly patients.

Characteristics of the Elderly Cardiac Surgery Population

Despite the lack of consensus regarding the definition of "elderly," it has been found that perioperative cardiac surgery mortality rates rise significantly with patients older than 75 years of age [7]. For instance, an individual older than age 80 has more than three times the risk of death after coronary artery bypass than does a similar 50-year-old patient [8]. The increased risks of death and major complications are not only due to the natural processes of aging that result in associated comorbidities, but also due to the fact that cardiovascular disease, the major cause of death and disability among elderly patients, is diagnosed at a more advanced state in this older population.

The aging process is influenced by a variety of genetic and environmental factors and occurs at somewhat different rates in every individual. The older the patient, the more likely the presence of multiple chronic noncardiac diseases, increased tissue fragility, and limited organ reserves for stressful events [8]. Also, postoperative complications such as pneumonia, renal failure, stroke, and dementia are especially prevalent and contribute significantly to perioperative morbidity and

---

[1]Sections of this chapter are reprinted with permission from Camacho and Raval [1].

M.T. Camacho (✉)
Department of Cardiothoracic Surgery,
Newark Beth Israel Medical Center, 201 Lyons Avenue,
Suite G-5, Newark, NJ 07112, USA
e-mail: mcamacho@sbhcs.com

M.R. Katlic (ed.), *Cardiothoracic Surgery in the Elderly*, DOI 10.1007/978-1-4419-0892-6_30,
© Springer Science+Business Media, LLC 2011

mortality. More than 50% of elderly individuals have at least one or more chronic medical conditions [9]. In addition to the routine preoperative assessment, other issues that must be evaluated include the degree of cognitive, neurologic, renal, respiratory, and immune impairment and the presence of other noncoronary atherosclerosis. Approximately one in three patients older than age 80 has some degree of cognitive dysfunction [10], and it is important to establish a baseline level of performance prior to surgical intervention [11]. Tests with age-specific normative standards include the Wechsler Adult Intelligence Scale, the Controlled Oral Word Association, and the Multilingual Aphasia Examination [12]. Patients with previously compromised cognitive function are at highest risk for such postoperative complications such as delirium and progressive cognitive dysfunction. Depression is a common problem in patients of all ages, especially in those who have undergone cardiac surgery. It is significantly more pronounced in the elderly patient who may live alone and have few social support systems.

By age 80, there is a 25% decrease in kidney mass and 40% reduction in glomerular filtration rate (GFR) [11]. Because of the decrease in lean muscle mass, a decrease in GFR may not be reflected by an increase in serum creatinine concentration, and therefore a "normal" creatinine level in an octogenarian may be misleading. A more useful assessment of renal function in the elderly patient is the age-related creatinine clearance (Ccr)

$$\text{Ccr(mL/min)} = \frac{(140 - \text{age}) \times (\text{ideal body weight in kilograms})}{72 \times \text{serum creatinine}},$$

where normal values range from 75 to 125 mL/min. Renal function should be evaluated both before and after cardiac catheterization, and the amount of renally excreted dye used during angiography should be kept to an absolute minimum, employing nonionic contrast materials. The transient episodes of hypotension that inevitably occur during cardiopulmonary bypass may worsen any preexisting renal dysfunction; in this age group, perioperative renal insufficiency is a strong positive predictor of postoperative mortality [7, 13–15].

Older patients have declining cellular immunity and are therefore more predisposed to developing invasive bacterial and viral infections [11]. In addition to the bacterial colonization of the respiratory, urinary, and gastrointestinal tracts, there is a risk of infection from other monitoring lines and catheters used during cardiac surgery, such as central lines, Swan-Ganz catheters, and mediastinal drainage tubes. Leukocytosis is frequently absent or depressed in an elderly patient, who otherwise commonly exhibits atypical signs of infection such as hypothermia or confusion. Although most cardiac surgery patients are not cachexic or nutritionally depleted due to their cardiac disease, it is important to assess the preoperative nutritional status of an elderly individual whose other organ reserves are already limited. Adequate nutrition is vital for wound healing and for avoiding infection and ventilatory dependence. Ideally, the serum albumin concentration should be >3.5 mg/dL, and there should be no history of recent significant (>5%) weight loss.

Numerous physiologic changes affect the cardiovascular system with advancing age. There is a decrease in vascular elasticity: the aorta and large arteries become much less compliant, resulting in an increase in peripheral vascular resistance. Left ventricular stiffness increases [16], as does the ventricular septal thickness [17], and may require higher filling pressures to maintain adequate forward flow. During exercise, there is a decrease in peak heart rate and ejection fraction, likely because of reduced responsiveness to circulating catecholamines [18–20]. Autopsy studies of octogenarians revealed that atherosclerotic heart disease with more than 75% narrowing in at least one major coronary vessel was the most common abnormality (present in 60% of patients). In fact, coronary disease was the most common single cause of death, with the most frequent manifestation being acute myocardial infarction (MI) [17]. Finally, compared with younger age groups, the heart of the elderly individual has smaller ventricular cavities and tortuous coronary arteries [21–23]. In light of these morphologic findings, it is not surprising that by age 80, at least 20% of this population has an established clinical diagnosis of coronary artery disease and that eventually, 67% of elderly patients die from this disease.

Elderly patients tend to have more advanced coronary artery disease than their younger counterparts by the time they are referred for cardiac surgery. Compared with the Coronary Artery Surgery Study (CASS) with a patient population of mean age 68 years [24], octogenarians were found to have a higher incidence of three-vessel coronary disease (87 vs. 61%; $p<0.05$), left main or left main-equivalent disease (50 vs. 3%, $p<0.0001$), and significant left ventricular dysfunction (19 vs. 4% had an ejection fraction <35%, $p<0.01$) [25]. Older patients are more symptomatic on presentation; many series report that more than 90% of octogenarians are New York Heart Association (NYHA) functional class III–IV preoperatively [14, 26–32]. When compared with younger patients, a significantly higher percentage of elderly patients are referred for more urgent or emergent procedures, which carry substantially increased risks of major morbidity and mortality [8, 14, 25, 30, 32–35]. This underscores the need to prevent emergent and urgent surgical interventions.

A common finding in elderly patients is calcification and intimal disease of the aorta, which can crack and embolize when the ascending aorta is clamped or manipulated during coronary bypass operations. Such plaque embolization to cerebral vessels is the principal cause of perioperative stroke in this age group [36]. Another cause of surgery-related neurologic deficits is transient systemic hypotension during cardiopulmonary bypass and air embolism from procedures that necessitate opening great vessels, such as aortic valve operations. Aortic valve calcification is present in more than 55% of patients aged above 90, but only 5% eventually develop significant hemodynamic valvular stenosis [37]. Davis et al. [38] noted that 29% of elderly patients with significant aortic valve disease had concomitant disease of two or more coronary vessels. Concomitant aortic valve replacement (AVR) and coronary bypass surgery would increase stroke risk due to possible air embolization.

Predictors of Perioperative Morbidity and Mortality

As experience with the surgical treatment of cardiac disease in septuagenarians has grown, the resulting literature has focused on the surgical outcome in octogenarians (Table 30.1). Many of these studies have reported predictors of perioperative morbidity and mortality based on extensive univariate and multivariate analyses. This information has proved vital in identifying specific factors that may be optimized preoperatively and has provided physicians and patients with the ability to make timely treatment decisions based on expected short-term and long-term outcomes.

Several studies have shown that a decreased ejection fraction is a significant predictor of hospital mortality following coronary artery bypass surgery. This is even more predictive of an adverse outcome in octogenarians. A number of series have reported hospital mortality rates of 3–6, 5–13, and 24–43% in patients with normal, moderately impaired, and severely impaired (ejection fraction <0.30) left ventricular function, respectively [49–51]. In a multivariate analysis of factors involving 159 octogenarians who underwent isolated coronary artery bypass, Mullany et al. [45] found that an ejection fraction less than 0.50% was the most important predictor of adverse survival ($p < 0.01$). Ko et al., who analyzed 100 consecutive octogenarians undergoing isolated coronary artery bypass, also found a decreased ejection fraction to be the most significant predictor of perioperative mortality ($p < 0.002$). In fact, an ejection fraction less than 30% was associated with a mortality rate of 43% [29].

High NYHA functional cardiac class was highly predictive of hospital mortality in numerous studies [14, 17, 20, 23,

Table 30.1 Cardiac surgical procedures in the octogenarian: results and average length of hospital stay

Study	Year	No.	Procedure	Mortality (%)	Complication rate (%)	Mean postop. LOS	% Survival (years)
Deiwick et al. [35]	1997	101	Mixed	8	73		88 (1) 73 (5)
Gehlot et al. [39]	1996	322	AVR mixed	14	53	11.0	83 (1) 60 (5)
Sahar et al. [40]	1996	42	Mixed	7	24		
Logeais et al. [41]	1995	200	Mixed	12	35	12.7	82 (1) 75 (2) 57 (5)
Cane et al. [13]	1995	121	Mixed	9	49		
Klima et al. [42]	1994	75	Mixed	8	21		
Yashar et al. [43]	1993	43	Mixed	9	38		
Glower et al. [27]	1992	86	CABG	14	29	10.0	64 (3)
Freeman et al. [32]	1991	191	Mixed	20	30	16.4	92 (1) 87 (2) 82 (3) 78 (4)
Tsai et al. [44]	1991	157	CABG	7	20		85 (1) 62 (5)
Ko et al. [29]	1991	100	CABG	12	24		
Mullany et al. [45]	1990	159	CABG	11	73		84 (1) 71 (5)
Naunheim et al. [34]	1990	103	Mixed	17	71		90 (1)
Kowalchuk et al. [46]	1990	53	Mixed	11	38		81 (2)
Fiore et al. [47]	1989	25	Mixed valve	20	72	18.0	79 (1) 69 (2)
Naunheim et al. [25]	1987	23	Mixed	22	67	14.3	94 (1) 82 (2)
Rich et al. [48]	1985	25	Mixed	4	92	19.5	84 (2)

Mixed, series includes valve and coronary bypass procedures and/or valve + coronary bypass procedures
AVR aortic valve replacement; *CABG* coronary artery bypass grafting; *LOS* length of stay in hospital
Source: Reprinted with permission from Camacho and Raval [1]

26, 27, 32, 46]. In their series of 76 octogenarians undergoing a variety of cardiac surgery procedures, Tsai et al. [49] found that 94% of the hospital deaths were in patients who presented in NYHA functional class IV. In a study of 24,461 patients 80 years and older who underwent isolated coronary artery bypass, measures of more acute coronary disease, such as acute MI before bypass surgery, predicted higher procedural and long-term mortality rates [50]. This relation with acute coronary artery disease has been confirmed by numerous other authors [25, 27, 29].

Combined coronary surgical procedures and mitral valve replacement have been shown to carry significantly higher hospital mortality rates in the elderly population [20, 28, 33, 37, 38, 40, 43, 46]. In the early 1990s, Davis et al. reported operative mortality rates of 5.3% for AVR, 20.4% for mitral valve replacement, and 5.8% for isolated coronary artery bypass [38]. Several years earlier, Naunheim et al. reported even higher hospital mortality rates of 50% for mitral valve replacement, 9% for AVR, and 67% for double valve replacement combined with coronary revascularization [34]. More recent outcomes for those ages 75 and above at Newark Beth Israel Medical Center, a participant in The Society of Thoracic Surgeons 2004–2008 database, reveal mortality rates of only 4.8% for isolated AVR, 0% for isolated MVR, and 3.0% for isolated CABG (personal communication).

In addition to presenting with more advanced disease than their younger counterparts, a higher percentage of octogenarians are referred for urgent or emergent surgical intervention. As noted in Table 30.2, urgent and emergent operations are associated with extremely high mortality rates. These increased mortality rates reflect the progression and severity of the cardiac disease and the lack of functional reserve for stressful events in this older population. Another related factor, preoperative hemodynamic instability, was described by several authors as the need for an intraaortic balloon pump (IABP) [16, 20, 25, 26, 34, 40], preoperative admission to the coronary care unit [35, 39, 45], and preoperative use of inotropes and vasoactive medications [34, 51]. Each was found to be a significant predictor of hospital mortality. Multivariate analyses by Williams et al., who studied a group of 300 octogenarians who underwent isolated coronary artery bypass, revealed that preoperative renal dysfunction (creatinine >2.0 mg/dL), pulmonary insufficiency, and postoperative sternal wound infection were strong predictors of hospital mortality [14]. Tsai et al. found that 67% of the elderly patients with postoperative mediastinal bleeding necessitating reoperation ultimately died [49].

In a prospective study of 2,000 patients undergoing coronary artery bypass, Tuman et al. [52] studied the effect of age on neurologic outcome. The rate of neurologic complications rose significantly with age; patients <65-years old had a 0.9% stroke rate, whereas those of ages 65–74 and >75 had rates of 3.6 and 8.9%, respectively ($p = 0.0005$). Suspected causes of serious neurologic events (in patients unresponsive for more than 10 days) include atheromatous emboli from the ascending aorta, hypotension or low-flow state during cardiopulmonary bypass, and preexisting critical extracranial or intracranial cerebrovascular disease. The mortality rate in this group of patients who sustained significant strokes was 74% (Fig. 30.1) [52]. Perioperative

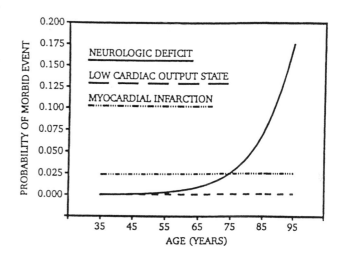

Fig. 30.1 Effect of advanced age on the predicted probability of neurologic and cardiac morbidity (reprinted with permission from Tuman et al. [52], Copyright Mosby 1992)

Table 30.2 Comparison of mortality rates by procedure status (elective vs. urgent vs. emergent)

Study	Year	No.	Procedure	Mortality (%)			
				Overall	Elective	Urgent	Emergency
Deiwick et al. [35]	1997	101	Mixed	7.9	4.7		23.5
Williams et al. [14]	1995	300	CABG	11.0	9.6	11.0	33.3
Diegeler et al. [30]	1995	54	Mixed	9.2	6.1		40.0
Freeman et al. [32]	1991	191	Mixed	18.8			35.9
Ko et al. [29]	1991	100	CABG	12.0	2.8	13.5	33.3
Naunheim et al. [34]	1990	103	Mixed	16.5		10.0	29.0
Naunheim et al. [25]	1987	23	Mixed	22.0	11.0		75.0

See Table 49.1 for explanation of abbreviations
Source: Reprinted with permission from Camacho and Raval [1]

mortality associated with perioperative stroke in younger patients, although still formidable, was less than half of this frequency (24–26%).

Quality of Life

Although the short-term and intermediate-term survival for elderly patients undergoing cardiac surgery is somewhat less than their younger cohorts, the long-term survival for octogenarians after open heart surgery compares favorably with survival for the general United States population of similar age. In a series of 600 consecutive patients 80 years or older undergoing various open heart procedures, the 5-year actuarial survival, including hospital mortality, was 63±2%. Survival in this group was identical to that for the simultaneous general U.S. octogenarian population [15]. Excellent long-term results have been achieved by several groups in octogenarians after mitral valve surgery, aortic valve surgery, and coronary artery bypass surgery [41, 53, 54].

Of as great importance to the elderly as survival is the associated quality of life. Several authors have shown that most (81–93%) of the octogenarians who survive open heart surgery "feel" as good and frequently better than as they did before their operations [15, 30, 41, 54]. An equally high percentage (75–84%) of octogenarians believed in retrospect that deciding to have a cardiac surgical procedure after age 80 had been a good choice [15, 55]. The precise and objective measurements of quality of life may be difficult to quantify.

Based on the well-studied populations, it is possible to construct instruments that reliably assess the various domains of daily living, thereby producing a meaningful reproducible measurement of quality of life [56–58].

The NYHA angina functional class and cardiac failure functional class reflect symptom-free living with regard to chest pain and dyspnea. Octogenarians have consistently demonstrated substantial improvement in their NYHA angina functional class and cardiac failure functional class after open heart surgery. In several reports, most (68–92%) of the octogenarians who survived open heart surgery were in NYHA functional class I or II during the long-term follow-up. This improvement was seen after isolated coronary artery bypass operations, valve operations, and combined operations (Table 30.3). When a well-validated health care index, the SF-36, was employed to prospectively study a cohort of elderly and nonelderly patients, those above 75 years of age enjoyed an identical long-term improvement in each of the seven domains of the SF-36. Indeed, as many of the elderly patients had low quality of life SF-36 scores preoperatively as their younger cohorts, the improvements in the older patients were even greater, as both populations produced with statistically identical SF-36 scores 6 months following surgery. Any neurologic injury associated with the diagnostic and surgical process dramatically affected their quality of life adversely when compared with those old patients who did not suffer any neurologic injury.

Many octogenarian patients live alone and consequently have impaired ability to carry out activities of daily living, which places them at a significant disadvantage. Karnofsky

Table 30.3 Change in functional class after cardiac surgical procedures

Study	Year	No.	Procedure	Functional class change (%) Preoperative FC III–IV	Postoperative FC I–II
Deiwick et al. [35]	1997	101	Mixed	88	83
Morris et al. [26]	1996	474	CABG	93	92
Gehlot et al. [39]	1996	322	Mixed	86	82
Sahar et al. [40]	1996	42	Mixed	87	90
Williams et al. [14]	1995	300	CABG	98	98
Logeais et al. [41]	1995	200	Mixed	74	99
Cane et al. [13]	1995	121	Mixed	69	84
Diegeler et al. [30]	1995	54	Mixed	100	92
Adkins et al. [59]	1995	42	Mixed	64	97
Tsai et al. [28]	1994	528	Mixed	99	70
Yashar et al. [43]	1993	43	Mixed	98	79
Tsai et al. [44]	1991	157	CABG	96	73
Ko et al. [29]	1991	100	CABG	100	94
McGrath et al. [31]	1991	54	Mixed	96	94
Mullaney et al. [45]	1990	159	CABG	97	89
Merrill et al. [60]	1990	40	Mixed	100	100
Edmunds et al. [61]	1988	100	Mixed	90	98
Naunheim et al. [25]	1987	23	Mixed	94	83

FC functional class
Source: Reprinted with permission from Camacho and Raval [1]

dependency category (KDC) and social support index (SSI) reflect the degree of help needed by the patients. Using the KDC, Glower et al. showed that the median performance status in a group of octogenarians undergoing isolated coronary artery bypass grafting improved from 20% preoperatively to 70% at hospital discharge, with 89% of survivors being discharged home [27]. Kumar et al. showed that when there was a significant decrease in the level of social support needed by octogenarians after open heart surgery, the mean KDC and mean SSI decreased significantly at the short-term follow-up (less than 2 years) [55]. These improvements were also present but significantly less evident at the long-term follow-up (more than 5 years). It is likely that significant comorbid conditions limit the ability of octogenarians to live independently long term, although they remain symptom-free from a cardiac point of view and thrive in the short term.

As mentioned earlier, the subjective indicators of quality of life for octogenarians after open heart surgery are complex and involve a number of modalities relating to various domains of life. In the study by Kumar et al., indices for satisfaction with marriage, children, and overall life, feelings about the present life, and general affect were assessed. In the short term, the indices for satisfaction with overall life and eight bipolar items assessing general affect showed significant improvements, although all these improvements became less evident at long-term follow-up [55]. Perhaps the symptomatic benefits and the value of cardiac surgery as seen subjectively by the patients lie in the question, "would you choose to undergo cardiac surgery again?" Virtually, all the current studies have shown that most octogenarians would have made the same decision to undergo open heart surgery retrospectively.

Possible Strategies to Decrease Operative Risk

Improvements in surgical techniques and anesthesia have increased the confidence of cardiac surgeons performing operations on an elderly population with increased perioperative risk. Awareness of the problems unique to this growing population of elderly patients, along with recent statistical data highlighting the impact of these problems on morbidity and mortality, can help the medical team recommend the most appropriate treatment choice and timing of intervention in each individual case.

The two principal causes of perioperative cerebrovascular accidents (CVAs) in elderly patients undergoing cardiac surgery are embolization (air, atheroma, calcific debris) and hypotension resulting in inadequate perfusion of the central nervous system. Preoperative evaluation of the ascending aorta and carotid arteries and intraoperative assessment of the proximal aorta using transesophageal or epiaortic echocardiography may alter the conduct of the procedure, minimize intraoperative manipulation, and thereby significantly reduce the incidence of stroke [35, 36, 40, 52, 62]. Such information enables the surgeon to avoid cannulation or direct manipulation of heavily diseased portions of the aorta where atheromas may dislodge or where plaque disruption may cause aortic dissection. The presence of extensive atheromatous or calcific disease, which precludes safe manipulation of the ascending aorta in patients with advanced coronary disease, leaves the surgeon with several choices.

1. Abandon the surgical procedure and consider nonoperative or nonbypass revascularization, such as angioplasty, transmyocardial revascularization, or angiogenesis.
2. Perform surgical revascularization on a beating heart, using one or both internal thoracic arteries or non-aortic-based grafts.
3. Establish cardiopulmonary bypass via the femoral, axillary, or other systemic nondiseased artery and perform graft replacement or endarterectomy of the ascending aorta [35, 36]. The latter alternative is an aggressive, complex procedure, and in the elderly population should be reserved for the very good risk patients with no significant comorbidities.

Diffuse systemic atherosclerosis is more prevalent in the elderly than in younger patients; as such, special precautions should be taken to ensure adequate cerebral and renal perfusion perioperatively. Maintaining high perfusion pressures while on cardiopulmonary bypass can help decrease the incidence of ischemic stroke [63, 64]. Control of atrial arrhythmias and avoidance of episodes of sustained arterial hypotension due to hypovolemia or medications are important during the immediate postoperative period. Although there is still controversy regarding the management of asymptomatic carotid disease, it is believed that known carotid disease in the elderly population is a risk factor for postoperative CVA [15, 35, 45, 52]. Morris et al. [26] recommended routine preoperative assessment of carotid artery disease in octogenarians and advocated carotid endarterectomy if significant disease is found. If symptomatic carotid artery disease is diagnosed prior to cardiac surgical intervention, consideration should be given to performing a staged or a combined procedure. If asymptomatic significant carotid disease is discovered by Doppler preoperatively (>75% stenosis bilaterally or lesser degrees of unilateral stenosis in the presence of an occluded contralateral artery), concomitant carotid endarterectomy may decrease the risk of perioperative stroke [62].

Because of the significant increase in mortality associated with urgent or emergent operative procedures (Table 30.2), all possible measures must be taken to optimize the elderly patient preoperatively and possibly convert an urgent or emergent situation to a more elective predicament. Careful selection of elderly patients in this setting is critical, and one must evaluate the patient's mental status and existing comorbidities when determining the potential for meaningful survival before recommending operation. Aggressive preoperative medical management includes the use, when needed, of intravenous nitroglycerin or heparin (or both), inotropic and ventilatory support, and if absolutely necessary, the IABP. Although numerous studies have reported that preoperative use of the IABP is a significant predictor of perioperative mortality [13, 15, 34, 51], it likely reflects the severity of the elderly patient's underlying cardiac disease, rather than any inherent risk in using the device. Sisto et al. [65] reported that in 25 consecutive octogenarians requiring IABP insertion, there were no significant complications related to device insertion; and of 20 patients who eventually underwent surgery after IABP, only 2 patients (10%) died in hospital. This operative mortality rate is significantly better than that reported by others for urgent/emergent cases (Table 30.2).

Prolonged ventilatory dependence can develop quickly in the elderly patient. As soon as the patient awakens from general anesthesia, respiratory muscles must be exercised. Pulmonary hygiene and physiotherapy must be aggressive with early and progressive ambulation. Unlike their younger counterparts, elderly patients have much less functional reserve, and therefore a successful first attempt at extubation and mobilization ensures the best outcome. Intraoperatively, exquisite care must be taken to avoid injury to the phrenic nerve during harvesting of the internal thoracic artery, and use of bilateral internal thoracic arteries should generally be avoided [66].

Nephrotoxic drugs should be also avoided or, if necessary, doses should be adjusted in light of the decreased renal function in elderly patients. Intravenous renal dosage dopamine hydrochloride (1–2 µg/kg/min) may prove to be beneficial when used for any patient with preexisting renal insufficiency. Because of the high mortality associated with perioperative renal failure in this population [14, 39, 44, 67, 68], an aggressive approach to optimize preoperative renal function is essential. Although rigorous studies demonstrating the benefit of "renal dopamine" are inconclusive, many centers use this drug to enhance urine flow during and immediately after cardiac surgery.

Cognitive function is one of the most important factors affecting overall outcome and is one of the most difficult neurologic outcome parameters to measure and assess. Delirium and confusion are common in the postoperative elderly individual and can hinder important initial attempts to extubate and mobilize a patient. Encephalopathy changes are seen in as many as 30% of all bypass patients and 50% of the elderly patients. Sensory deficits such as those due to hearing or vision impairments can be addressed as soon as the patient awakens by providing hearing aids and eyeglasses. Invasive lines and monitoring equipment should be removed as soon as medically possible to facilitate mobilization. Transfer out of an intensive care unit (ICU) setting, when possible, helps restore the sleep–wake cycle. Family members should stay with confused patients to offer reassurance and encouragement. Long-acting benzodiazepines should be avoided or other sedative/hypnotic medications should be altered to prevent excessive sedation, confusion, and respiratory depression. Haloperidol is a more appropriate drug for management of delirium in this patient population because of its short-acting effect and safety margin in the postoperative cardiothoracic patient. Small doses are usually effective, and the patient can be rapidly weaned in conjunction with professional and family encouragement.

Octogenarians are more likely to develop sternal dehiscence because of osteoporosis of the sternum. The use of bilateral internal thoracic arteries should be avoided. Sternal wound infection has been shown to be a positive predictor of mortality in this group of patients [14].

Aggressive management is essential and includes early institution of intravenous antibiotics, timely débridement, and either primary reconstruction or secondary closure with a wound vacuum device. Adequate nutrition and pulmonary physiotherapy are critical to success. Staged closures are to be avoided in this population, other than for the most advanced infections, which should then undergo coverage and secondary closure as rapidly as possible.

Utley and Leyland described a highly selective group of 25 patients above the age of 80 who underwent coronary artery bypass with no hospital deaths [69]. Patients were chosen on the basis of their ability to achieve acceptable functional recovery after operation. All patients were living at home alone or with relatives preoperatively, and they were ambulatory and capable of caring for their own personal needs. They were counseled preoperatively regarding the importance of early ambulation and self-care postoperatively. Four patients were rejected for surgery based on their mental or physical senility, previous debilitating strokes, or a history of long-term institutional care. Anesthetic management included the use of short-acting agents and minimal use of postoperative sedation. Patients were extubated within 9–48 h postoperatively, and many were ambulatory and eating on the first postoperative day. Although this restrictive degree of patient selection is not appropriate in most cases, it illustrates how outcome can be strongly influenced by preexisting functional status and meticulous perioperative care.

Nonsurgical Alternatives

During the current era of health care reform, there is considerable interest in providing the most appropriate care for patients aged above 80 at an "acceptable" cost [70]. As coronary bypass surgery is the most common major operation performed in the United States (more than 300,000 performed annually), the use of coronary bypass in the very elderly is an important issue in the present cost-conscious environment. Medicare data from 1987 to 1990 indicated that the use of this operation in patients more than 80 years of age increased by 67% during that time period [50]. The projected rise in the number of coronary bypass procedures to be done in these patients and associated costs is impressive [50]. Numerous studies have shown a considerable increase in length of stay (3–4 days longer) and hospital costs ($3,000–$6,000 more) in patients above 80-years old vs. their younger counterparts. However, failure to provide this service often results in repeated and prolonged hospitalization, the need for multidrug therapy, and poorer quality of life, not to mention the emotional impact on patients and their families [8, 50].

In one series of octogenarians, when coronary surgery was compared with medical therapy, the overall cost, annual reinterventions, coronary disease-associated readmissions, and mortality were favored in the surgical group. Several studies have attempted to compare the treatment results of less expensive alternatives to coronary bypass surgery. In elderly patients, percutaneous transluminal coronary angioplasty (PTCA) has the advantages of shorter hospital stay, less immobilization, and lower cost compared with coronary artery bypass; however, coronary bypass confers greater and more durable freedom from angina, less need for future repeat interventional measures, and overall improved quality of life [37, 71, 72]. Whereas Mick et al. [73] reported that the procedural complication rates in matched groups of patients undergoing coronary bypass vs. PTCA were similar, Braunstein et al. [71] observed that PTCA in the setting of unstable angina was associated with high initial morbidity but long-term survival roughly equivalent to that after coronary bypass surgery. As mentioned earlier, compared with medical noninterventional therapy, coronary artery bypass provides a significant survival advantage and improved quality of life. Ko et al. [72] compared 36 octogenarians who underwent coronary artery bypass with 29 octogenarians who continued medical noninterventional therapy and found that the functional class did not change in the latter group but improved significantly in the former group (NYHA functional class decreased from 3.4 to 1.2, $p < 0.01$). The 3-year survival rate of 77% for the surgical group was similar to the survival of octogenarians in the general US population and was significantly better than that of 55% for the medical group. Coronary bypass surgery provided improved long-term survival and functional benefit compared with medical therapy and improved the quality of life compared with PTCA.

More recent analyses by Likosky et al. at Dartmouth Medical School [74] and Mamoun et al. at the Cleveland Clinic [75] reveal even better outcomes after coronary bypass grafting in the very elderly (85 years and older),

likely because of improved perioperative technology and practice. Likosky et al. [74] conducted a large cohort study of 54,397 consecutive patients who underwent primary isolated coronary artery bypass between July 1, 1987 and June 30, 2006. Patients were identified by the voluntary New England Cardiovascular Disease Study Group registries and mortalities were linked to the Social Security Administration Death Master File. Fifteen years after coronary artery surgery, 10.4% of patients aged 80–84 were still alive, and 9.3% of patients aged 85 and above remained alive. Mamoun et al. [75] compared the outcomes after isolated coronary artery bypass in 132 patients aged 85 and older with 5,423 propensity score matched patients aged 55–65. The main outcome difference was a higher incidence of atrial arrhythmias in the older age group and longer ICU and hospital length of stay. However, major cardiac, neurologic, pulmonary, renal, gastrointestinal, hepatic and infectious morbidities, as well as hospital mortality, did not differ between the two age groups. We have entered a new era where the "elderly" population undergoing coronary artery surgery is 10–15 years older than the population from previous reports. In conclusion, coronary surgical revascularization is associated with acceptable outcomes in the very elderly aged 85 and older, and should be considered in the properly selected patient.

The New Era of Mechanical Circulatory Assist

In the mid-1980s, implantable mechanical circulatory assist devices were introduced in FDA clinical trials for patients with severe left ventricular dysfunction who were awaiting transplant and would otherwise not survive without such support. The most popular device in this early era, the HeartMate pneumatic left ventricular assist device (LVAD), enabled patients to ambulate and exercise on treadmills while in-hospital. The advantages of LVAD therapy for the often debilitated, deconditioned patients were significant and resulted in improved outcomes for heart transplant recipients who were able to optimize their physical and physiologic conditions prior to transplant. Since then, the LVADs have become smaller, more durable, and associated with increased survival rates than those of the earlier models [76]. The smaller size and decreased postoperative complications have enabled this technology to be offered to the elderly population with acceptable perioperative risk. The oldest patients with these smaller LVADs are octogenarians who, like their younger counterparts, are leading productive lives outside the hospital.

For a selective group of elderly but active patients who suffer hemodynamic compromise due to severe cardiac dysfunction, such as after a large MI, a temporary mechanical assist device can be implanted if there is hope of cardiac recovery. Newer devices in this category, such as the Thoratec CentriMag, have been associated with fewer complications and improved survival (personal communication). Percutaneously inserted assist devices such as the Tandem Heart and Impella can be implanted in the cardiac catheterization laboratory and may provide partial support with flow rates of 2.5–3.5 L/min (personal communication).

Guidelines for Therapy in the Elderly Cardiac Surgery Patient

During the process of deciding whether to offer cardiac surgical intervention to elderly patients, the relief of symptoms and improvement in quality of life should assume more importance than the issue of increased life expectancy. When surgical revascularization is considered in this patient population, numerous social, ethical, and clinical issues arise. Comorbidities, quality of life, and concerns raised by the patient's family should be acknowledged and factored into the decision-making process. It is important to integrate the patient's and family's wishes, but one must focus the therapeutic decisions on the patient's advance directives. Emergency cases in these patients may be associated with more than 70% mortality risk, and therefore nonoperative treatment must be strongly considered. Asymptomatic patients should continue medical treatment unless there is critical (>70%) left main coronary artery stenosis, which is associated with significantly reduced life expectancy. Numerous groups (Table 30.2) have observed significant increased mortality when combined procedures were performed. One study, comparing the operative mortalities for isolated AVR and isolated coronary artery bypass to combined AVR+coronary bypass, demonstrated five to sixfold increased operative mortality in the combined-procedure group [49]. In situations where two or three disease processes exist, the surgical plan should be modified to avoid such increased risks. For example, in an elderly patient with angina, severe coronary artery disease, and noncritical aortic stenosis, coronary revascularization alone may be the best option. Such patients are usually not at risk for a serious morbid event due to their aortic stenosis [37]. Conversely, in a patient with critical aortic stenosis, congestive heart failure, preserved or mildly impaired left ventricular function, and noncritical coronary lesions (<70–80% stenosis), valve replacement alone may be the best alternative. Fiore et al. [47] noted that of the early deaths of patients undergoing combined AVR+coronary bypass, 60% were due to low cardiac output; the patients who had died had little or no angina preoperatively, but each had considerable congestive heart failure and may have been better served by valve replacement alone.

In patients with advanced coronary artery disease who may be at high risk for complications arising from cardiopulmonary bypass, such as those with severe calcific disease of the ascending aorta (precluding safe insertion of cannulas), a history of stroke, or end-stage pulmonary or renal failure, an alternate option is surgical revascularization on a beating heart. Technological advances in pericardial retraction systems and stabilization devices have enabled the surgeon to perform anastomoses on a beating heart with the use of newer surgical techniques. However, there is a significant learning curve, as the surgical field is not nearly as optimal as that produced by cardiopulmonary bypass and ischemic arrest. Recent reports have observed a failure rate of 10%, even in experienced hands. Although it is a reasonable alternative for patients who would otherwise have no interventional options, the increased risk of technical failure must be kept in mind and discussed with the patient and family.

Finally, for elderly patients in previously good physical and mental condition, who suffer from acute or chronic severe ventricular dysfunction, both short-term and long-term mechanical circulatory assist devices are available at an acceptable operative risk, compared with their earlier counterparts.

Conclusions

As the elderly population has grown, so have the number of elderly patients being referred for cardiac surgery and their disease complexity. For the most part, these patients can be offered conventional surgical procedures with acceptable mortality, morbidity, and long-term quality of life expectations. Indeed, the perioperative complications are somewhat more numerous than for younger patients even when they are compared for procedure and matched for other risk factors.

This incremental morbidity and mortality is seen across the entire population but is most pronounced in emergently operated patients. With the availability of new and different techniques to accomplish myocardial revascularization, valvular repair and replacement, and the recent availability of mechanical assist devices, the range of procedures available for elderly patients with hemodynamically important heart disease is increasing at a rate almost faster than the population itself has grown. It is therefore critical that the health care professionals caring for these older patients are aware of ongoing developments in these areas and carefully stratify the preoperative risk factors to best select the least morbid and most effective procedure that is currently available.

Acknowledgments The authors wish to acknowledge the invaluable assistance of Gladys Madrid RN, in the creation of this manuscript.

References

1. Camacho MT, Raval PR. Cardiac surgery in the elderly. In: Rosenthal RE, Katlic MR, Zenilman ME, editors. Principles and practice of geriatric surgery. 2nd ed. New York: Springer; 2010.
2. US Census Bureau. Table 1: Annual estimates of the resident population by sex and five-year age groups for the United States: April 1, 2000 to July 1, 2008 (NC-EST2008-01). Source: Population Division, Release Date May 14, 2009 and Table 4: Annual Estimates of the Resident Population for the United States April 1, 2000 to July 1, 2008 (NST-EST 2008-01). Source: Population Division, US Census BUREAU. Release date 22 Dec 2008.
3. Lubitz J, Kiming C, Kramarow E, et al. Health, life expectancy and health cared spending among the elderly. N Engl J Med. 2003;349:1048–55.
4. Horvath KA, DiSesa VJ, Peigh PS, et al. Favorable results of coronary artery bypass grafting in patients older than 75 years. J Thorac Cardiovasc Surg. 1990;99:92–6.
5. Maganti M, Rao V, Brister S, et al. Decreasing mortality for coronary artery bypass surgery in octogenarians. Can J Cardiol. 2009; 25(2):e32–5.
6. Canver C, Nichols R, Cooler S, et al. Influence of increasing age on long-term survival after coronary artery bypass grafting. Ann Thorac Surg. 1996;62:1123–7.
7. Srinivasan A, Oo A, Grayson A, et al. Mid-term survival after cardiac surgery in elderly patients: analysis of predictors for increased mortality. Interact Cardiovasc Thorac Surg. 2004;3:289–93.
8. Alexander KP, Peterson ED. Coronary artery bypass grafting in the elderly. Am Heart J. 1997;134:856–64.
9. Kern LS. The elderly heart surgery patient. Crit Care Nurs Clin North Am. 1991;3:749–56.
10. Mezey MD, Rauckhorst LH, Stokes SA. Health assessment of the older individual. 2nd ed. New York: Springer; 1993.
11. Smith Rossi M. The octogenarian cardiac surgery patient. J Cardiovasc Nurs. 1995;9(4):75–95.
12. Sweet J, Finnin E, Wolfe P, et al. Absence of cognitive decline one year after coronary bypass surgery: comparison to non-surgical and healthy controls. Ann Thorac Surg. 2008;85:1571–8.
13. Cane ME, Chen C, Bailey BM, et al. CABG in octogenarians: early and late events and actuarial survival in comparison with a matched population. Ann Thorac Surg. 1995;60:1033–7.
14. Williams DB, Carrillo RG, Traad EA, et al. Determinants of operative mortality in octogenarians undergoing coronary bypass. Ann Thorac Surg. 1995;60:1038–43.
15. Akins CW, Daggett WM, Vlahakes GJ, et al. Cardiac operations in patients 80 years old and older. Ann Thorac Surg. 1997;64:606–15.
16. Iskandrian AS, Segal BL. Should cardiac surgery be performed in octogenarians? J Am Coll Cardiol. 1991;18:36–7.
17. Shirani J, Yousefi J, Roberts WC. Major cardiac findings at necropsy in 366 American octogenarians. Am J Cardiol. 1995;75:151–6.
18. Iskandrian AS, Hakki AH. The effects of aging after coronary artery bypass grafting on the regulation of cardiac output during upright exercise. Int J Cardiol. 1985;7:347–60.
19. Hakki AH, DePace NL, Iskandrian AS. Effect of age on left ventricular function during exercise in patients with coronary artery disease. J Am Coll Cardiol. 1983;2:645–51.
20. Iskandrian AS, Hakki AH. Age-related changes in left ventricular diastolic performance. Am Heart J. 1986;112:75–8.
21. Roberts WC. Ninety three hearts ≥90 years of age. Am J Cardiol. 1993;71:599–602.
22. Waller BF, Roberts WC. Cardiovascular disease in the very elderly: analysis of 40 necropsy patients aged 90 years or older. Am J Cardiol. 1983;51:403–21.
23. Roberts WC. The aging heart. Mayo Clin Proc. 1988;63:205–6.
24. Gersh BJ, Kronmal RA, Schaff HV, et al. Long-term (5 year) results of coronary bypass surgery in patients 65 years or older: a report from the coronary artery surgery study. Circulation. 1983;66(Suppl II):190–9.
25. Naunheim KS, Kern MJ, McBride LR, et al. Coronary artery bypass surgery in patients aged 80 years or older. Am J Cardiol. 1987;59:804–7.
26. Morris RJ, Strong MD, Grunewald KE, et al. Internal thoracic artery for coronary artery grafting in octogenarians. Ann Thorac Surg. 1996;62:16–22.
27. Glower DD, Christopher TD, Milano CA, et al. Performance status and outcome after coronary artery bypass grafting in persons aged 80 to 93 years. Am J Cardiol. 1992;70:567–71.
28. Tsai T, Chaux A, Matloff JM, et al. Ten-year experience of cardiac surgery in patients aged 80 years and over. Ann Thorac Surg. 1994;58:445–51.
29. Ko W, Krieger KH, Lazenby WD, et al. Isolated coronary artery bypass grafting in one hundred consecutive octogenarian patients. J Thorac Cardiovasc Surg. 1991;102:532–8.
30. Diegeler A, Autschbach R, Falk V, et al. Open heart surgery in the octogenarians: a study on long-term survival and quality of life. Thorac Cardiovasc Surg. 1995;43:265–70.
31. McGrath LB, Adkins MS, Chen C, et al. Actuarial survival and other events following valve surgery in octogenarians: comparison with age-, sex-, and race-matched population. Eur J Cardiothorac Surg. 1991;5:319–25.
32. Freeman WK, Schaff HV, O'Brien PC, et al. Cardiac surgery in the octogenarian: perioperative outcome and clinical follow-up. J Am Coll Cardiol. 1991;18:29–35.
33. Bashour TT, Hanna ES, Myler RK, et al. Cardiac surgery in patients over the age of 80 years. Clin Cardiol. 1990;13:267–70.
34. Naunheim KS, Dean PA, Fiore AC, et al. Cardiac surgery in the octogenarian. Eur J Cardiothorac Surg. 1990;4:130–5.
35. Deiwick M, Tandler R, Mollhoff TH, et al. Heart surgery in patients aged eight years and above: determinants of morbidity and mortality. Thorac Cardiovasc Surg. 1997;45:119–26.
36. Wareing TH, Davila-Roman VG, Barzilai B, et al. Management of the severely atherosclerotic ascending aorta during cardiac operations: a strategy for detection and treatment. J Thorac Cardiovasc Surg. 1992;103:453–62.
37. Cannon LA, Marshall JM. Cardiac disease in the elderly population. Clin Geriatr Med. 1993;9:499–525.
38. Davis EA, Gardner TJ, Gillinov AM, et al. Valvular disease in the elderly: influence on surgical results. Ann Thorac Surg. 1993;55:333–8.
39. Gehlot A, Mullany CJ, Ilstrup D, et al. Aortic valve replacement in patients aged eighty years and older: early and long-term results. J Thorac Cardiovasc Surg. 1996;111:1026–36.
40. Sahar G, Raanani E, Sagie A, et al. Surgical results in cardiac patients over the age of 80 years. Isr J Med Sci. 1996;32: 1322–5.
41. Logeais Y, Roussin R, Langanay T, et al. Aortic valve replacement for aortic stenosis in 200 consecutive octogenarians. J Heart Valve Dis. 1995;4 Suppl 1:S64–71.
42. Klima U, Wimmer-Greinecker G, Mair R, et al. The octogenarians: a new challenge in cardiac surgery? Thorac Cardiovasc Surg. 1994;42:212–7.
43. Yashar JJ, Yashar AG, Torres D, Hittner K. Favorable results of coronary artery bypass and/or valve replacement in octogenarians. Cardiovasc Surg. 1993;1:68–71.
44. Tsai T, Nessim S, Kass RM, et al. Morbidity and mortality after coronary artery bypass in octogenarians. Ann Thorac Surg. 1991; 51:983–6.

45. Mullany CJ, Darling GE, Pluth JR, et al. Early and late results after isolated coronary artery bypass surgery in 159 patients aged 80 years and older. Circulation. 1990;82(Suppl IV):229–36.

46. Kowalchuk GJ, Siu SC, McAuliffe LS, et al. Coronary artery bypass in octogenarians: early and late results. J Am Coll Cardiol. 1990;15:35A.

47. Fiore AC, Naunheim KS, Barner HB, et al. Valve replacement in the octogenarian. Ann Thorac Surg. 1989;48:104–8.

48. Rich MW, Sandza JG, Kleiger RE, et al. Cardiac operations in patients over 80 years of age. J Thorac Cardiovasc Surg. 1985;90: 56–60.

49. Tsai TP, Matloff JM, Gray RJ, et al. Cardiac surgery in the octogenarian. J Thorac Cardiovasc Surg. 1986;91:924–8.

50. Peterson ED, Cowper PA, Jollis JG, et al. Outcomes of coronary artery bypass graft surgery in 24,461 patients aged 80 years or older. Circulation. 1995;92(Suppl II):85–91.

51. Curtis JJ, Walls JT, Boley TM, et al. Coronary revascularization in the elderly: determinants of operative mortality. Ann Thorac Surg. 1994;58:1069–72.

52. Tuman KJ, McCarthy RJ, Najafi H, et al. Differential effects of advanced age on neurologic and cardiac risks of coronary artery operations. J Thorac Cardiovasc Surg. 1992;104:1510–7.

53. Lee EM, Porter JN, Shapiro LM, et al. Mitral valve surgery in the elderly. Heart Valve Dis. 1997;6:22–31.

54. Culliford AT, Galloway AC, Colvin SB, et al. Aortic valve replacement for aortic stenosis in persons aged 80 years and over. Am J Cardiol. 1991;67:1256–60.

55. Kumar P, Zehr KJ, Cameron DE, et al. Quality of life in octogenarians after open heart surgery. Chest. 1995;108:919–26.

56. Remington M, Tyrer PJ, Newson-Smith J, et al. Comparative reliability of categorical and analogue rating scales in the assessment of psychiatric symptomatology. Psychol Med. 1979;9:765–70.

57. Campbell A, Converse PE, Ridgers WL. The quality of American life. Russell Sage: New York; 1976. p. 1–583.

58. Bradburn NM. The structure of psychological well-being. Chicago: Aldine; 1969. p. 214–5.

59. Adkins M, Amalfitano D, Harnum NA, et al. Efficacy of combined coronary revascularization and valve procedures in octogenarians. Chest. 1995;108:927–31.

60. Merrill WH, Steward JR, Frist WH, et al. Cardiac surgery in patients age 80 years or older. Ann Surg. 1990;211:772–6.

61. Edmunds LH, Stephenson LW, Edie RN, et al. Open-heart surgery in octogenarians. N Engl J Med. 1988;319:131–6.

62. Berens ES, Kouchoukos NT, Murphy SF, et al. Preoperative carotid artery screening in elderly patients undergoing cardiac surgery. J Vasc Surg. 1992;15:313–23.

63. Grawlee GP, Cordell AR, Graham JE, et al. Coronary revascularization in patients with bilateral internal carotid occlusion. J Thorac Cardiovasc Surg. 1985;90:921–5.

64. Brener BJ, Bried DK, Alpert J, et al. The risk of stroke in patients with asymptomatic carotid stenosis undergoing cardiac surgery: a follow-up study. J Vasc Surg. 1987;5:269–79.

65. Sisto DA, Hoffman DM, Fernandes S, Frater RWM. Is use of the intraaortic balloon pump in octogenarians justified? Ann Thorac Surg. 1992;54:507–11.

66. He GW, Acuff TE, Ryan WH, et al. Determinants of operative mortality in elderly patients undergoing coronary artery bypass grafting. J Thorac Cardiovasc Surg. 1994;108:73–81.

67. Ennabli K, Pelletier LC. Morbidity and mortality of coronary artery surgery after the age of 70 years. Ann Thorac Surg. 1986;42:197–200.

68. Higgins TL, Estafanous FG, Loop FD, et al. Stratification of morbidity and mortality outcome by pre-operative risk factors in coronary artery bypass patients: a clinical severity score. JAMA. 1992;267:2344–8.

69. Utley JR, Leyland SA. Coronary artery bypass grafting in the octogenarian. J Thorac Cardiovasc Surg. 1991;101:866–70.

70. Weintraub WS. Coronary operations in octogenarians: can we select the patients? Ann Thorac Surg. 1995;60:875–6.

71. Braunstein EM, Bajwa TK, Andrei L, et al. Early and late outcome of revascularization for unstable angina in octogenarians. J Am Coll Cardiol. 1991;17:151A.

72. Ko W, Gold JP, Lazzaro R, et al. Survival analysis of octogenarian patients with coronary artery disease managed by elective coronary artery bypass surgery versus conventional medical treatment. Circulation. 1992;86(Suppl II):191–7.

73. Mick MJ, Simpfendorfer C, Arnold AZ, et al. Early and late results of coronary angioplasty and bypass in octogenarians. Am J Cardiol. 1991;68:1316–20.

74. Likosky DS, Dacey LJ, Baribeau YR, et al. Long-term survival of the very elderly undergoing coronary artery bypass grafting. Ann Thorac Surg. 2008;85:1233–7.

75. Mamoun NF, Meng XU, Sessler DI, et al. Comparison of outcomes in older and younger patients after coronary artery bypass graft surgery. Ann Thorac Surg. 2008;85:1974–9.

76. Camacho M, Baran D, Martin A, et al. Improved survival in high-risk patients with smaller implantable LVAD's: single-center experience over 3 years. J Heart Lung Transplant. 2009;28(2):S274.

these patients. We will also include non-CPB techniques for the relief of aortic stenosis including the left ventricle apex-to-descending aortic conduit and transcatheter aortic valve implantation [TAVI, via the transfemoral (TF) or transapical (TA) routes].

Nonsurgical Management

The natural history of untreated severe AS strongly suggests the need for surgical intervention. In 1968, Ross and Braunwald [23] reported that the average survival in AS patients is 3 years after the onset of angina or syncope and only 1.5 years after the onset of heart failure. More recently, the ACC/AHA guidelines estimate a patient's survival from initial AS symptoms to be less than 2–3 years [11]. However, the perception by the cardiac surgeon or referring cardiologist of associated co-morbidities, especially age greater than 80 years and low ejection fraction, on poor outcomes after AVR has led clinicians to pursue other nonsurgical options for this patient cohort [3, 24]. It is estimated that approximately 30–48% of high risk, elderly patients are denied AVR despite echocardiographic evidence of severe aortic stenosis [3, 24, 25]. In the Euro Heart Survey, it was noted that 33% of older patients with severe symptomatic AS were denied AVR. Although older age and left ventricular dysfunction were the most important factors associated with a decision not to operate, neurologic dysfunction also influenced the decision for nonoperative therapies [3]. Medical management alone is associated with poor outcomes with the large majority of symptomatic patients dying within 1–3 years if the structural valve disease is not treated surgically.

This has been more recently shown by Varadarajan et al. [10], who have noted a dismal survival for 453 nonsurgically managed patients with severe aortic stenosis with a 1-, 5-, and 10-year survival of 62, 32, and 18%, respectively. However, this report does not provide STS PROM scores and does not elucidate why such a large population of patients were nonsurgically managed. Furthermore, Varadarajan et al. [26] examined survival among 277 patients >80 years of age presenting with severe AS; 80 underwent AVR. Survival was significantly improved in the surgical patients. After AVR, 1-, 2-, and 5-year survival was 87, 78, and 68%, compared with 52, 40, and 22%, respectively, in the patients who were managed medically. They concluded that, when possible, surgery is the best alternative for survival in octogenarians with severe symptoms. Furthermore, Kojodjojo et al. [27] have noted a greater than 12-fold increase in mortality in patients greater than 80 years of age who were offered, but refused, AVR for personal reasons when compared to those patients undergoing surgical AVR. Kapadia et al. [28] studied 92 patients screened at one institution for percutaneous AVR. Of these patients, 30 underwent BAV; 8 patients were

bridged to TAVI, and 3 bridged to surgical AVR. Of the remaining 19 patients undergoing BAV, bridging to TAVI could not be accomplished because of death (47%), exclusion from the TAVI protocol (32%), and some improved and declined TAVI. The most common reasons for no intervention included death while awaiting definitive treatment (28%), uninterested in TAVI (28%), and questionable severity of symptoms or AS (25%). Patients not undergoing AVR had higher mortality compared with those undergoing AVR (44% vs. 14%) over a mean of 220 days [28].

Past studies have shown that although BAV can result in temporary relief of symptoms, restenosis is certain within 6–12 months [29, 30]. This led to clinical guidelines recommending BAV as a reasonable bridge to surgical intervention in hemodynamically unstable patients at high risk for AVR or as a palliative procedure in patients with AS at high risk for surgical AVR (class IIb indication) [11]. With the advent of TAVI and the rapid developments in this field, there has been a resurgence of interest in BAV procedures that otherwise offer little long-term benefit.

While BAV, left ventricular apex-to-descending aorta valve conduits, and percutaneous AVR techniques are feasible treatment alternatives to the traditional AVR in high risk surgical patients, these nontraditional techniques have not been adequately compared with modern outcomes of traditional open surgery.

Surgical Technique of Conventional AVR

New and improved pharmacological agents, operative techniques, and improved technology have advanced cardiac surgery since the late 1970s. Specifically, advances in cardiac anesthesia and myocardial protection during cardiac surgery and in surgical techniques have improved morbidity and mortality statistics for all patients, especially the elderly. The selection of candidates for cardiac operations is at the discretion of individual referring physicians, cardiologists, and cardiac surgeons. Meticulous preoperative and postoperative care, including aggressive early mobilization, is commonly utilized to minimize complications, shorten postoperative stay, and optimize survival.

Preoperative Assessment

Bearing in mind that age is an un-modifiable factor, the following have to be brought together to achieve this aim: (a) establishing a correct indication for surgery as a better alternative to other nonsurgical options; (b) identifying co-morbidities and the possibility of intervention; (c) assessing the suitability of the surgical techniques chosen in relation to the individual characteristics of the patient and the experience of the team itself; and (d) having a multi-disciplinary team available after the intervention that includes, together with healthcare professionals, the family, and a care-taker to ensure good short- and long-term follow-up [31]. The preoperative assessment in elderly patients with aortic stenosis commonly requires a thorough evaluation.

Standard preoperative testing for patients undergoing AVR includes a standard laboratory examination, transthoracic (TTE) or transesophageal (TEE) echocardiogram, cardiac catheterization, panorex, and chest X-rays. In addition, carotid duplex testing and pulmonary function testing should be performed in these patients. A noncontrast chest computed tomography may be performed to preoperatively assess ascending or arch aortic calcifications. Surgery should not be performed the day after cardiac catheterization to allow renal clearance of contrast dye and minimize postoperative renal dysfunction. A thorough discussion with the patient and family should include the risks of AVR including bleeding, infection, myocardial infarction, stroke, need for postoperative pacemaker, and renal/lung/liver failure.

Intraoperative Technique

Specific details of surgical technique and valve selection and implantation are to be determined by the individual cardiac surgeon. Generally, all patients should be performed with standard CPB techniques utilizing roller head pumps, membrane oxygenator, cardiotomy suction, arterial filters, cold antegrade and retrograde blood cardioplegia, and moderate systemic hypothermia ($\sim$32–34°C). Direct aortic clamping is utilized in all patients. Anti-fibrinolytics should be administered to all patients. It is without a doubt that cardiac tissue in elderly patients is more often friable; mandating careful handling of the heart and aorta by the surgeon during all aspects of the surgical procedure. Adjuncts such as routine intraoperative epi-aortic echocardiography, use of axillary artery cannulation in complex or redo surgery, soft-flow aortic cannulae, and CPB strategies favoring high-perfusion pressures in elderly patients may improve postoperative stroke rates.

Postoperative Care

The most common morbidities following AVR in elderly patients are similar to those undergoing all valve surgeries across the age groups. As expected, morbidity and resource utilization among elderly patients remain higher than their younger counterparts (Tables 31.1–31.3). In patients undergoing coronary surgery, octogenarians have been shown to have significantly higher rates of major adverse events, such as stroke, re-operation for bleeding, sepsis, and renal and

Table 31.1 Preoperative demographics for each age group

Characteristic	Ages 60–69 ($n=206$)	Ages 70–79 ($n=221$)	Ages 80–89 ($n=88$)	p Value
Age (mean $\pm$ SD)	64.1 $\pm$ 2.9	74.1 $\pm$ 2.8	82.8 $\pm$ 2.4	<0.001
Status				
Elective	192 (93.2%)	209 (94.6%)	80 (90.9%)	0.51
Urgent	13 (6.3%)	11 (5.0%)	8 (9.1%)	
Emergent	1 (0.5%)	1 (0.5%)	0	
Female gender	84 (40.8%)	115 (52.0%)	47 (53.4%)	0.03
Ejection fraction (mean % $\pm$ SD)	55.4 $\pm$ 12.9	54.6 $\pm$ 13.0	52.5 $\pm$ 12.2	0.29
Caucasian	164 (81.2%)	179 (83.3%)	71 (84.5%)	0.75
CCS class 4	4 (2.0%)	9 (4.3%)	3 (3.6%)	0.42
NYHA class 4	17 (12.8%)	19 (13.3%)	12 (21.1%)	0.29
Congestive heart failure	89 (43.2%)	99 (44.8%)	46 (52.3%)	0.35
Previous myocardial infarction	12 (5.8%)	28 (12.7%)	7 (8.0%)	0.05
Angina	46 (22.3%)	50 (22.6%)	27 (30.7%)	0.26
Preoperative CVA	12 (5.8%)	19 (8.6%)	9 (10.2%)	0.36
Cerebrovascular disease	23 (11.2%)	31 (14.0%)	15 (17.1%)	0.37
Peripheral vascular disease	6 (2.9%)	8 (3.6%)	3 (3.4%)	0.92
Chronic lung disease	30 (14.6%)	36 (16.3%)	10 (11.4%)	0.54
Current smoker	26 (12.6)	21 (9.5)	0 (0)	0.003
Diabetes mellitus	52 (25.2%)	57 (25.8%)	15 (17.1%)	0.24
Hypertension	139 (67.5%)	172 (77.8%)	62 (70.5%)	0.05
Infectious endocarditis	7 (3.4%)	0 (0)	3 (3.4%)	0.02
Last creatinine level (mean $\pm$ SD)	1.37 $\pm$ 1.4	1.31 $\pm$ 1.3	1.31 $\pm$ 1.0	0.90
Renal failure	24 (11.7%)	13 (5.9%)	7 (8.0%)	0.10
Dialysis	11 (5.3%)	4 (1.8%)	2 (2.3%)	0.10

CCS Canadian Cardiovascular Society classification; *NYHA* New York Heart Association; *CVA* cerebrovascular accident
Source: Thourani et al. [5]

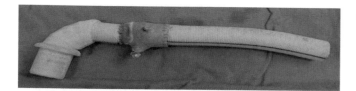

Fig. 31.2 Apical-aortic conduit (AAC) with interposed freestyle root

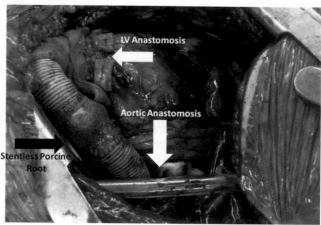

Fig. 31.3 Completed AAC with interposed freestyle root via a left thoracotomy

and the entire apex of the heart is exposed. Careful dissection is required to avoid injury to previous CABG when applicable. A left ventricular pacing wire is placed in the epicardium. The patient is heparinized to maintain an activated clotting time >250 s.

The AAC conduit is first assembled using a Hancock® apical connector interspersed with a 21 Freestyle® stentless porcine valve root (both from Medtronic Inc., Minneapolis, MN) (Fig. 31.2) using a 4-0 Prolene running suture. A partial occluding clamp is placed on the descending thoracic aorta above the diaphragm. An aortotomy is made and the distal end of the conduit is anastomosed end-to-side with the aorta using a 3-0 prolene suture. The conduit is de-aired by making the valve incompetent and through needle holes within the graft.

For the proximal end of the conduit, six pledgeted horizontal mattressed sutures (0 Ethibond, MH needle) are placed in a circular pattern around the apex of the heart allowing a central coring space equivalent to the 16 mm Hancock Trocar Blade Coring Device (Medtronic Inc., Minneapolis, MN) diameter. The 4 mattressed sutures are placed through the inferior portion of the sewing cuff of the apical connector so as to facilitate tying down of the knot after insertion of the connector into the LV. At this point, the two anterior suture sets are not placed through the sewing cuff to allow coring of the LV without entangling within the suture sets. Intravenous lidocaine (100 mg) is administered prior to placement of the left ventricular sutures. A stab incision is made into the LV with a size 11 blade through which a 12F Foley catheter is introduced. TEE echocardiography confirms that the Foley is within the left ventricle and not intertwined within the mitral apparatus [64]. Rapid left ventricular pacing is initiated at 180 beats/min and the LV coring device is placed over the Foley to remove an LV apex plug, which is sealed by inflating the catheter balloon with 9 cc of saline. After coring, the inflow cannula is placed into the LV apex and the rapid ventricular pacing is discontinued. The four sutures already placed within the sewing cuff are tied, followed by placing the anterior sutures within the sewing cuff. The heparin is reversed and the chest closed in routine fashion (Fig. 31.3). Although we had previously used a size 20 inflow cannula, in the past 11 cases more recently we have shifted to utilize a size 16 or 18 inflow device. On final evaluation, the transgastric 2-chamber TEE view tends to be

the most helpful since it allows clear visualization of the mitral sub-valvular apparatus and to ensure the cannula is in the center of the LV and unobstructed by papillary muscles or the septum [64].

Outcomes

In our series of 21 patients, the majority of patients were in their mid-70s and male. AACs were utilized for a porcelain aortas alone in 6 (28.6%) patients, previous CABG in 4 (19.0%), or both in 10 (47.6%). One patient (4.8%) had an AAC for severe cirrhosis and was thought not to be a candidate for CPB.

Postoperative complications were common among patients (61.9%). The most common morbidities were of pulmonary origin: pneumonia (23.8%) and prolonged ventilation (47.6%). Two patients had postoperative ventricular fibrillation and cardiac arrest and we have changed our practice such that lidocaine intravenous drip is administered till extubation and amiodarone 200 mg by mouth per day was administered for 1 month postoperatively. Since utilization of this regimen, no significant arrhythmias have occurred. In out 21 patients, the postoperative median length of stay was 9 days. Three patients died within hospitalization: one died of a pulmonary embolus prior to transfer to the wards, one died of a ventricular arrhythmia, and one died from multisystem organ failure secondary to sepsis.

In the adult population, a vast recent experience and excellent results with AAC have been reported from Indiana University and the University of Maryland [55, 57]. Collectively, they have performed 31 AAC patients in very high risk adult patients presenting with aortic stenosis. Similar to the Emory Series, the majority of patients were either prohibitive high risk for median sternotomy secondary to prior CABG or presented with a porcelain aorta. All three centers have a similar in-hospital mortality of 13–14%. In their most recent series, Gammie et al. [57] noted that 61% required CPB; however, they have used the CPB circuitry for a short period of time with a mean CPB time of 19 min. With similar mortality, it remains to be seen if off-pump AAC provides a significant benefit in mortality. It is plausible that in patients who have contra-indications to CPB (as in the patient with severe cirrhosis), off-pump AAC may provide expansion of the use of this technique.

Given the recent success several groups have experienced in implanting AACs in high-risk populations, we expect the indications for AAC to expand. With the avoidance of CPB documented by our technique, off-pump AAC insertion has evolved into an excellent option in patients who are unlikely to survive CPB or are not candidates for transcatheter valve implantation. For those patients who can tolerate CPB but have a porcelain aorta, AAC insertion offers the possibility of not only the avoidance of CPB but also deep hypothermic circulatory arrest and its associated complexities and added risks. Finally, AAC insertion may evolve into the procedure of choice in patients with aortic stenosis who have undergone prior CABG via a median sternotomy and have patent bypass grafts. Not only does AAC via left anterolateral thoracotomy avoid the use of CPB in this situation but, more importantly, the approach obviates any dissection whatsoever of pre-existing venous or arterial bypass grafts and thus prevents graft manipulation, plaque or atheroma embolization, or graft injury and thus avoids tissue ischemia or infarction.

Transcatheter Aortic Valve Implantation

In 1992, Andersen et al. [65] published their first results from experiments in which a balloon expandable stent valve was implanted into the descending aortas of pigs. This technology seemed promising for the treatment of degenerative aortic stenosis except for two major obstacles: removal of the native valve, which is often heavily calcified in the adult, and impedance of the coronary ostia by the stent valve [66]. The resurgence of interest in the balloon expandable stent valve for the treatment of aortic disease followed the first human implantation in an elderly patient with inoperable aortic stenosis by Cribier et al. [51]. The transcatheter heart valve, manufactured by Edwards LifeSciences (Fig. 31.4), was implanted safely in the sub-coronary position, using the calcified native valve as an anchor for the stent frame. Cribier had realized that removal of the native valve was not necessary to implant the percutaneous heart valve, and that the

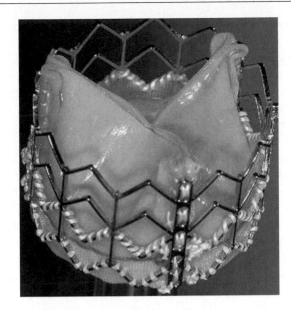

Fig. 31.4 Edwards SAPIEN® bioprosthetic valve

distance between the coronary ostia and the aortic annulus was larger and more forgiving in humans than in animals [66].

Since the first implant in 2002, TAVI has been limited to elderly patients with excessive co-morbidities who have been deemed ineligible for surgical valve replacement. The advent of TAVI (transfemoral and transapical) represents a tremendous advance in our ability to treat high-risk patients with severe AS. By avoiding the risks associated with aortic cross-clamping and CPB, it provides a treatment alternative for patients deemed too high risk for conventional AVR. Early implantation was accomplished by peripheral venous access, transseptal puncture and antegrade deployment [51]. However, technical difficulties associated with the complexity of this approach necessitated the development of alternative routes. Currently, there are two methods which represent the standard operative approaches. The transfemoral route utilizes arterial access through the femoral vessels and retrograde passage of the delivery system to the level of the aortic valve. Conversely, the transapical (TA) approach utilizes a small anterior left thoracotomy and direct access to the aortic valve through the left ventricle. Thus far the majority of clinical experience has been with two different valve prostheses: the Edwards SAPIEN® Valve and the Medtronic CoreValve®.

The SAPIEN® valve is a tri-leaflet pericardial valve mounted in a stainless steel stent, which is then balloon expanded and seated into place (Fig. 31.4). Currently available in 23 and 26 mm sizes which allows placement in any annulus ranging from 18 to 25 mm in size. The 26 mm requires a 24 fr introducer to be placed transfemorally while the 23 mm needs a 22 fr introducer. Clinical results using the SAPIEN® valve via both approaches have been promising.

In a study utilizing the transfemoral approach, Webb et al. [20] successfully implanted prosthetic aortic valves in 43 out of 50 high-risk patients who were not candidates for open surgery. As operator experience improved, rate of successful implantation increased to 96% among the second 25 patients. Treated patients demonstrated improved ventricular function as measured by left ventricular ejection fraction as well as improved functional status by NYHA class over the follow-up period. The overall 30-day mortality among treated patients was 12% which compared favorably to the expected mortality of 28% with open surgery. In successful implantations, the aortic valve area increases to 1.7 cm² and the mean transvalvular gradient is less than 10 mmHg [67, 68]. These results are already much better than those seen with BAV, where valve area increases to 1.0–1.1 cm² and mean transvalvular gradients are in the order of 50% of starting gradients (≤30 mmHg) [69–72]. Paravalvular leak is generally grade 2 insufficiency or less after valve implantation [68]. Long-term results have been tempered by the premorbid state of the patients, and no death has occurred as a result of device failure [67, 68].

In those patients with unsupported femoral or iliac arteries, the Edwards SAPIEN® valve is also available in a transapical implantation technique. Initial success with the transapical approach was reported in a series of 7 high-risk patients in 2006. Observed mortality in these patients was more than half the estimated mortality with open AVR (14% vs. 35%). Additionally, there were no procedural deaths and improvements in cardiac hemodynamic function paralleled that seen with the TF approach. A multi-center experience using the TA approach in 59 patients validated these findings and confirmed the potential benefit of this procedure. The authors reported a 93.2% successful implantation rate. Observed mortality was 13.6% compared to the expected rate of 26.8% for conventional AVR. The use of CPB in this series was 47.5% but was used disproportionately during the early, learning curve portion of the series.

A multi-center randomized trial involving over 20 North American centers recently completed enrolling high-risk AS patients. The Edwards LifeSciences US PARTNER trial (Placement of AoRTic traNscathetER) compares two groups of patients: inoperable patients who are randomized to either BAV or medical therapy, versus TAVI and high-risk patients who are randomized to open AVR or TAVI. The final comparison of over 1,000 high-risk patients with AS is expected within the next 6 months and will represent the definitive study in the literature to date regarding these complicated patients.

The second most commonly used valve, the Medtronic CoreValve® is also a tri-leaflet pericardial valve but is mounted in a Nitinol® stent (Fig. 31.5). The Medtronic CoreValve® is longer than the Edwards SAPIEN® valve, 55 mm for the 26 mm valve and 53 mm for the 29 mm valve. Initial results using the Medtronic CoreValve® demonstrated an early procedural learning curve as well [73]. Once initial design changes were implemented and the valve could be

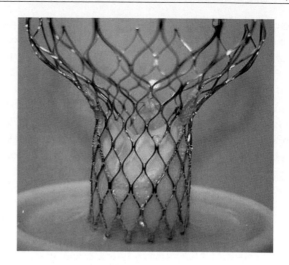

Fig. 31.5 Medtronic CoreValve® bioprosthetic valve

introduced via the TF approach using an 18 fr sheath the need for bypass was obviated and the procedure became truly percutaneous. Early results from the multi-center European registry demonstrated excellent procedural success (97%) and an impressive procedural mortality (1.5%). However, cardiac conduction abnormalities appear to be more common with the Medtronic CoreValve® (when compared with the Edwards SAPIEN® valve), with a subsequent series describing a 20% incidence of permanent pacemaker placement versus 7%, respectively.

Although both devices hold real promise in the treatment of valvular aortic disease, some of the limitations for their use are related to the size of the delivery systems that are used currently (18–24F introducers) in patients with peripheral arterial disease. Advances in nanotechnology might, however, provide another solution to this problem. With this new method of construction, a collapsible, mechanical aortic valve is compatible with an 8F system. Future devices might also have the advantage of retrievability before deployment, which is particularly important in cases of size mismatch or poor anchoring.

Pre-procedural planning is of paramount importance regardless of the planned placement route. High-quality computed tomography, echocardiography, and coronary angiography are all valuable tools to screen prospective TAVI patients. Accurate measurements of annular diameter by either CT or echocardiography are used for valve selection. Intraoperative echocardiography by an experienced operator is mandatory during valve positioning and deployment. When considering the TF route, special attention must be paid to the size and disease burden of the aorta over its entire length from the aortic valve down to both femoral arteries.

The major limitation affecting transfemoral deployments is related to vascular access. The minimal required diameter of the iliac and femoral arteries limits the use of the deployment sheaths required for the Edwards SAPIEN®

valve. Vascular complications account for the majority adverse events related to the TF approach. Even when the smaller sheath utilized by the Medtronic CoreValve® is employed, vascular complications still can be as high as 20% [17, 73].

Transcatheter aortic valves are steadily yet surely shifting the paradigm in the clinical management of aortic stenosis. Though currently limited to high-risk patient population, the technology is gaining popularity among the clinical community due to the ease of use and minimally invasive nature of the implantation. Both the Edwards SAPIEN® and Medtronic CoreValve® are CE mark in Europe and are under clinical investigation in the US. As access to this technology increases and is adopted in low-risk patients and patients with congenital bicuspid aortic valves, there is a need to characterize, understand, and address the long-term outcomes and engineering concerns with the current technologies.

Conclusions

Very important in selecting octogenarians for cardiac surgery is the surgeon's subjective impression after interviewing and examining the patient. Family history of longevity, intellectual function, and general level of fitness and activity are important predictors of outcome that cannot be easily quantified or reported. In summary, we believe that based on age alone, with minimal co-morbidities, conventional primary, isolated AVR remains the standard of care and can be performed with low morbidity and in-hospital mortality, and acceptable long-term survival. It is plausible that in patients with advanced age and additional co-morbidities, transcatheter (transfemoral or transapical) AVR or left ventricular apical to descending aorta conduits may provide potential benefits in postoperative morbidity and mortality.

Disclosures

Dr. Thourani is a consultant with Edwards LifeSciences, Medtronic Corporation, St. Jude Medical, Sorin, and Maquet. Dr. Guyton has no disclosures.

References

1. Census US. http://www.census.gov/population/www/projections/index.html. Accessed 20 Oct 2009.
2. Nkomo VT, Gardin JM, Skelton TN, Gottdiener JS, Scott CG, Enriquez-Sarano M, et al. Burden of valvular heart diseases: a population-based study. Lancet. 2006;368:1005–11.
3. Iung B, Cachier A, Baron G, et al. Decision-making in elderly patients with severe aortic stenosis: why are so many denied surgery? Eur Heart J. 2005;26:2714–20.
4. Filsoufi F, Rahmanian PB, Castillo JG, Chikwe J, Silvary G, Adams DH. Excellent early and late outcomes of aortic valve replacement in people aged 80 and older. J Am Geriatr Soc. 2008;56:255–61.
5. Thourani VH, Myung R, Kilgo P, et al. Long-term outcomes after isolated aortic valve replacement in octogenarians: a modern prospective. Ann Thorac Surg. 2008;86:1458–65.
6. Sundt TM, Bailey MS, Moon MR, et al. Quality of life after aortic valve replacement at the age of > 80 years. Circulation. 2000;102:III-70–4.
7. Chukwuemeka A, Borger MA, Ivanov J, Armstrong S, Feindel CM, David TE. Valve surgery in octogenarians: a safe option with good medium-term results. J Heart Valve Dis. 2006;15:191–6.
8. Stoica SC, Cafferty F, Kitcat J, et al. Octogenarians undergoing cardiac surgery outlive their peers: a case for early referral. Heart. 2006;92:503–6.
9. Kohl P, Kerzmann A, Lahaye L, Gerard P, Limet R. Cardiac surgery in octogenarians: peri-operative outcome and long-term results. Eur Heart J. 2001;22:1235–43.
10. Varadarajan P, Kapoor N, Bansal RC, Pai RG. Clinical profile and natural history of 453 nonsurgically managed patients with severe aortic stenosis. Ann Thorac Surg. 2006;82:2111–5.
11. Bonow RO, Carabello BA, Chatterjee K, et al. 2008 Focused update incorporated into the ACC/AHA 2006 guidelines for the management of patients with valvular heart disease: a report of the American College of Cardiology/American Heart Association Task Force on Practice Guidelines (Writing Committee to revise the 1998 guidelines for the management of patients with valvular heart disease). Endorsed by the Society of Cardiovascular Anesthesiologists, Society for Cardiovascular Angiography and Interventions, and Society of Thoracic Surgeons. J Am Coll Cardiol. 2008;52:e1–142.
12. Bramstedt KA. Aortic valve replacement in the elderly: frequently indicated yet frequently denied. Gerontology. 2003;49:46–9.
13. Asimakopoulos F, Edwards MB, Taylor KM. Aortic valve replacement in patients 80 years of age and older: survival and cause of death based on 1100 cases: collective results from the UK Heart Valve Registry. Circulation. 1997;96:3403–8.
14. Fruitman DS, MacDougall CE, Ross DB. Cardiac surgery in octogenarians: can elderly patients benefit? Quality of life after cardiac surgery. Ann Thorac Surg. 1999;68:2129–35.
15. Craver JM, Puskas JD, Weintraub WS, et al. 601 Octogenarians undergoing cardiac surgery: outcome and comparison with younger age groups. Ann Thorac Surg. 1999;67:1104–10.
16. Grossi EA, Schwartz CF, Yu P-J, et al. High-risk aortic valve replacement: are the outcomes as bad as predicted? Ann Thorac Surg. 2008;85:102–7.
17. Grube E, Schuler G, Buellesfeld L, et al. Percutaneous aortic valve replacement for severe aortic stenosis in high-risk patients using the second- and current third-generation self-expanding CoreValve prosthesis. J Am Coll Cardiol. 2007;50:69–76.
18. Walther T, Simon P, Dewey T, et al. Transapical minimally invasive aortic valve implantation: multicenter experience. Circulation. 2007;116 Suppl 1:I-240–5.
19. Webb JG, Chandavimol M, Thompson CR, et al. Percutaneous aortic valve implantation retrograde from the femoral artery. Circulation. 2006;113:842–50.
20. Webb JG, Pasupati S, Humphries K, et al. Percutaneous transarterial aortic valve replacement in selected high-risk patients with aortic stenosis. Circulation. 2007;116:755–63.
21. Shahian DM, O'Brien SM, Filardo G, et al. The Society of Thoracic Surgeons 2008 cardiac surgery risk models: part 3 – valve plus coronary artery bypass grafting surgery. Ann Thorac Surg. 2009;88(1 Suppl):S43–62.

technology for intra-operative TEE due to the lack of real time imaging. This problem has been solved and the pre-repair and post-repair intra-operative 3D TEE has proven a significant advancement for mitral valve repair surgery.

Management

Medical Therapy

Medical treatment of MR has limited efficacy although vasodilators and angiotensin-converting enzyme inhibitors have been used in the presence of hypertension and/or heart failure. In patients with severe LV dysfunction (ejection fraction [EF] <30% and/or end-systolic dimension >55 mm) and inability to repair the valve or preserve the subvalvular apparatus, patients may be managed medically as surgical intervention could lead to worsening or even fatal LV dysfunction.

Surgical Treatment

An attempt to preserve the native MV apparatus to maintain the normal shape, volume, and function of the LV by reparative surgery is always preferred to valve replacement. If successful, the risk of long-term anticoagulation and prosthetic valve complications are also avoided. Mitral valve repair leads to improved survival as compared to MV replacement. Mitral valve replacement with preservation of the subvalvular apparatus gives significantly better results as compared to MV replacement without preservation. Resection of the entire subvalvular apparatus should almost never be contemplated except in severely calcified valves. The Society of Thoracic Surgeons (STS) in 2005 reported an increase in MV repair in elderly and for the first time the number of MV repaired (3,966) exceeded the number replaced (3,854) [27]. For concomitant coronary artery bypass grafting (CABG), the same threshold was reached earlier in 2001 (3,171 mitral repair+CABG, 2,812 mitral replacement+CABG) [27]. Since 2003, for interventions involving the aortic and MV, MV repair exceeds MV replacement (8,386 MV repaired overall, 8,039 MV replaced) [28].

At the other end of the spectrum, with recent advances in surgical techniques and reduction in postoperative morbidity and mortality, asymptomatic elderly patients with severe MR and preserved LV function may benefit from surgical intervention. The recent American College of Cardiology/American Heart Association guidelines recommend surgical intervention for asymptomatic patients with any degree of

LV dysfunction (defined as EF <60% and/or ESD (end systolic dimension) >40 mm), and those with normal LV function (EF >60% and ESD <40 mm) with new-onset atrial fibrillation or pulmonary hypertension [16]. They also recommend that if MV repair is likely, that is, greater than 90% probability, asymptomatic patients with normal LV function and no atrial fibrillation or pulmonary hypertension should be referred for surgical intervention.

Surgical Techniques

Mitral Valve Replacement

Initially, mitral valve replacement with a mechanical or tissue prosthesis involved complete excision of the subvalvular apparatus, but subsequent studies revealed a detrimental effect on LV function with this technique [29]. Preservation of the entire subvalvular apparatus can usually be performed in MR patients because the MV leaflets and chordae are thin and pliable (Fig. 32.4). Subvalvular preservation results in maintenance of annulo-ventricular continuity and improved

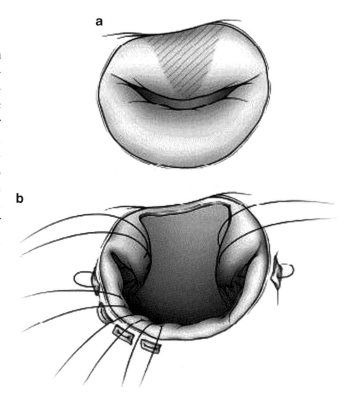

Fig. 32.4 Retention of the subvalvular apparatus during mitral valve replacement as described by Calafiore et al. [73]. Only a small portion of the anterior leaflet (*shaded area*) is resected. Calafiore et al. [73] recommend MV replacement when the distance between the coaptation point of the leaflets and the plane of the mitral annulus exceeds 10 mm (reprinted from Calafiore et al. [73], with permission from The Society of Thoracic Surgeons)

preservation of LV function [30]. An exception is in patients with rheumatic valvular disease. The secondary and tertiary chordae are often shortened and fused to the latter wall of the posterior ventricle. Therefore, resection of primary chordae and most of the valve leaflets can be done without hindering annular–ventricular continuity. Indeed it is often necessary to obtain space for an adequately sized valve.

Mitral Valve Repair

MV repair is preferred over replacement to treat mitral insufficiency with improved short-term and long-term survival [31–35]. The STS database indicates that MV repair is performed in only 36.1% of MV operations in patients older than 70 years nationally, significantly less than that in younger age populations [36]. There is discrepancy in the literature regarding the benefit of repair in elderly patients. Some authors cite improved in-hospital and long-term survival in elderly patients aged 70 years or older undergoing isolated MV repair [37], whereas others suggest MV repair provides no benefit in patients older than the age of 60 years [38].

The techniques for MV reconstruction were first introduced by Carpentier in the 1970s and these have proven to be durable and reproducible [31]. Newer techniques have been introduced in recent years such as the use of artificial neochordae (PTFE) and the edge-to-edge repair, leading to increased numbers of successful valve repairs worldwide. An annuloplasty ring or posterior band is generally used in combination with the repair to stabilize and correct annular dilatation to a normal size. The size of the annuloplasty ring or band is determined by measuring the anterior leaflet, inter-commissural distance, and/or inter-trigonal distance. If necessary, excision of prolapsing segments can be performed using either a triangular or quadrangular resection with or without leaflet sliding plasty. Abnormalities of the chordae can be treated by lengthening, shortening, transferring from a normal opposite leaflet segment, or more commonly, nowadays, by replacement (Fig. 32.5). This method has good long-term durability and is increasingly used.

Alfieri et al. [39] and Maisano et al. [40] have described an edge-to-edge MV leaflet repair technique by approximating the prolapsing segments of A2 and P2 for many different causes of MR. The technique is quick and relatively simple to perform. A suture is used to join the center of the anterior and posterior leaflets, creating a double orifice MV (Fig. 32.6). A mitral annuloplasty ring is inserted because long-term results without an annuloplasty ring are suboptimal [40].

In patients with ischemic mitral regurgitation, Messas et al. [41] proposed to reduce leaflet tethering by cutting a limited number of critically positioned second-order chordae tendinae to the anterior leaflet. This resulted in improved

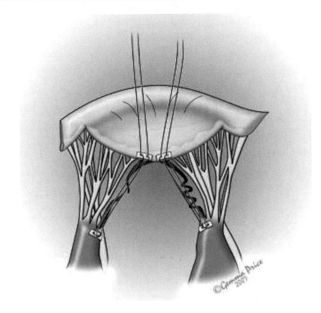

Fig. 32.5 Artificial neochordae can be implanted to repair ruptured or elongated chordae (adopted from Amirak et al. [74])

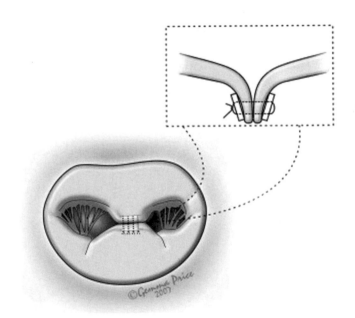

Fig. 32.6 The edge-to-edge (Alfieri) repair [39] (adopted from Amirak et al. [74])

leaflet coaptation and reduced MR, without leaflet prolapse or decline in LV ejection fraction [41]. Liel-Cohen et al. [42] devised an infarct placation procedure to reverse LV remodeling in sheep. The infarcted region of the LV is plicated with mattressed sutures to reduce myocardial bulging and to bring the displaced PM tips back toward the anterior mitral annulus. The plication process also reduces the proportion of LV circumference occupied by infracted myocardium. Kron et al. [43] have described another technique for the treatment of MR, particularly in patients with severe restriction of the

P3 segment of the MV. A suture is used to connect the posterior PM to the mitral annulus, adjacent to the right fibrous trigone, and a mitral annuloplasty ring is inserted (Fig. 32.7).

The suture between the PM and the mitral annulus is shortened to alleviate tethering of the P3 segment and to increase leaflet coaptation. Kron et al. [43] have performed this procedure in 18 patients, with all patients having no or trace MR 8 weeks postoperatively.

Fundaro et al. [44] devised a relatively simple technique to ameliorate posterior leaflet tethering and restore normal distance between the annulus and PM. An incision is made at the base of the posterior leaflet and the basal chordae are transected to increase posterior leaflet mobility (Fig. 32.8).

The detached portion of the mitral annulus is then plicated and the resulting defect in the posterior leaflet is closed with a running suture. The plicated annulus is reinforced with a short Gore-Tex strip or posterior annuloplasty band. The data on this procedure are sparse. We have done a similar technique but have additionally augmented the posterior leaflet by placing and elliptical patch of autologous pericardium, bovine pericardium, or decellularized pig submucosa to close the incision (unpublished). This additional leaflet substance creates a much larger zone of coaptation.

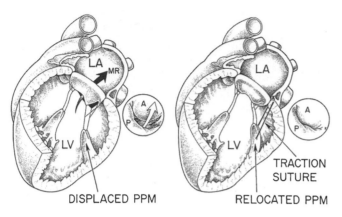

Fig. 32.7 Relocation of the posterior papillary muscle (PPM), as described by Kron et al. [43] (*A* anterior mitral leaflet; *LA* left atrium; *LV* left ventricle; *MR* mitral regurgitation [*arrow*]; *P* posterior mitral leaflet) (reprinted from Kron et al. [43], with permission from The Society of Thoracic Surgeons)

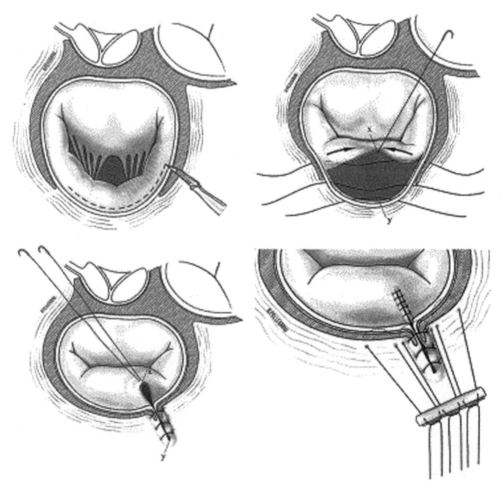

Fig. 32.8 Posterior mitral valve restoration, as described by Fundaro et al. [44] (reprinted from Fundaro et al. [44], with permission from The Society of Thoracic Surgeons)

Percutaneous MV repair techniques have recently been developed in large animal models and are now undergoing trials in patients. The Alfieri MV repair technique has been applied percutaneously [45] with a double-armed clip device, deployed through the femoral vessels. Percutaneous mitral annuloplasty has been described in large animal models where devices are inserted percutaneously into the coronary sinus in sheep [46] and dogs [47]. Both studies revealed acute reductions in MR, but long-term animal studies are pending. Percutaneous annuloplasty offers the advantage of avoiding an operation, but has the potential disadvantage of coronary sinus perforation or thrombosis, or injury to the adjacent circumflex artery [48]. In addition, the durability of this approach may be compromised by the coronary sinus having no fibrous connections to the mitral annulus.

MAC may present a formidable technical challenge to cardiac surgeons. Extensive calcification can prevent proper insertion of the prosthesis and give rise to periprosthetic leakage. Moreover, radical debridement of such calcification may cause cardiac rupture by atrio-ventricular groove separation or injury to the left circumflex coronary artery [18]. In these cases, several techniques have been proposed to undertake mitral valve replacement, such as enlarging the circumference of the prosthetic valve with a Dacron collar (polyethylene tereph-thalate fiber; Medi-Tech, Boston Scientific Corp, Natick, MA), ring reconstruction with a pericardial patch, and the plication of the left atrial wall, where the prosthesis is directly sutured for an intra-atrial insertion. In some cases, the calcium bar has been excised and a new annulus with pericardium has been created [49–52]. Using these techniques, the implantation of the prosthesis is supra-annular in most cases, which obliges the atrial wall to resist all the hemodynamic stress that can produce a tear of the suture with a consequent perivalvular leak. In such situations, Di Stefano et al. [53] suggested 2-0 polyester pledgeted mattress sutures between the free edges of the leaflets and the atrial wall, while avoiding passing through the calcified annulus (Fig. 32.9a) and creating a new ring inside the native annulus (Fig. 32.9b). The direction of the suture is not important and depends on the anatomic difficulty in accordance with the exposure of the valve, so that the placing of the pledget could be intraventricular or intraatrial. Depending on the extension of the calcification, the technique the authors [53] has described in the valve in its

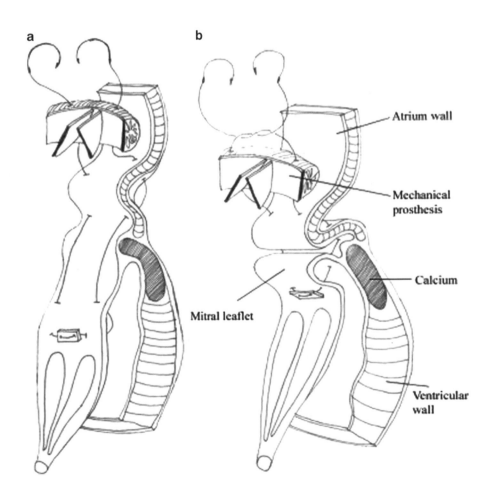

Fig. 32.9 Standard polyester pledgeted 2-0 U-shaped sutures crossing between (**a**) the free edges of the leaflet and the atrial wall (**b**) and the new created ring (reprinted from Di Stefano et al. [53], Copyright Elsevier 2009)

totality with both leaflets, or only in the calcified part, when normally posterior. Despite this, the anterior atrial wall is closely related to the right and left trigones and the inter-trigonal area, and above the annulus it maintains certain motility. Given the proximity of the aorta and the aortic valve to this area, special caution must be taken to avoid deep sutures in the inter-trigonal area, which could provoke injury to these structures. Both trigones can be used to anchor and give stability to the sutures.

Results of Surgery

Results of MV surgery continue to improve and in-hospital mortality especially in elderly patients with NYHA class I and II continue to decline. The STS reports overall mortality for isolated MV repair as less than 2% and for isolated MV replacement as 5% with a significant increase in mortality if either procedure is combined with CABG (7 and 11%, respectively, for repair and replacement) [27].

Mitral Repair vs. Replacement in Elderly

Major centers have documented an increase in the ability to repair valves in more recent times [54]. Though earlier, older patients are often not considered to be candidates for mitral repair because of (1) concerns of poor tolerance with return to cardiopulmonary bypass in the case of a failed repair, (2) unclear benefit of repair in elderly patients, and (3) the fact that valve repair can be difficult [55]. In our series, elderly patients fared better with MV repair compared with replacement with better 30-day and late survival [56]. Surgery performed in an early stage preceding the development of left ventricular dysfunction was associated with an improved freedom from late cardiac complications [56]. The improved late survival in elderly repair patients was admittedly in large part attributable to better operative mortality compared with replacement. Stroke, complication rate, and length of stay were improved in elderly patients undergoing repair compared to those undergoing replacement [56]. Enriquez-Sarano et al. [33] reported significantly less hospital mortality with MV repair over replacement for degenerative MV disease (2.6% vs. 10.3%). Ten-year survival rate was better for repair than replacement (68±6% vs. 52±4%; $p=0.0001$). A report from Gillinov et al. [32] supported long-term durability of MV repair for degenerative disease with 10-year freedom from reoperation of 93%. Patients with ischemic MR have also seen benefit to valve repair although this has been less well studied in part because of intrinsic disease that is inseparable from the process causing MR [57].

In a study evaluating patients with degenerative MR, Akins et al. [6] found a shorter length of stay (10 vs. 12 days) and less hospital mortality (3% vs. 12%) in patients who underwent MV repair versus replacement. Yet few studies have evaluated MV repair and replacement in elderly patients.

Earlier reports contrast more recent reports indicating the lower operative mortality in elderly patients undergoing MV repair compared with replacement. Gogbashian et al. [37] compared MV repair with replacement in 292 patients aged 70 years or older and showed that in-hospital mortality for isolated MV repair (0.7%) was significantly better than that for replacement (13.9%). Five-year survival also favored MV repair over replacement (MV repair, 81±3%; MV replacement, 63±3%). In the subset of patients aged 70 years or older in the report by Enriquez-Sarano et al. [33], operative mortality for repair patients was 6.8% compared with 30.8% in replacement patients. Thourani et al. [38] demonstrated that MV replacement and age were both independent predictors of in-hospital and long-term mortality. Despite documented superior outcomes with MV repair in elderly patients in these recent series, they concluded that MV repair does not provide long-term benefit in patients older than the age of 60 [38].

Improved Outcomes

Lower mortality documented in our study in elderly patients undergoing repair can be attributable to several reasons [29]. Preservation of the subvalvular apparatus improves long-term left ventricular function and survival [29, 58, 59]. Although techniques to preserve the subvalvular apparatus were used in the majority of patients undergoing replacement (71%) in our series, valve repair is still considered superior to replacement [37, 60]. Our experience describes shorter cardiopulmonary bypass times with valve repair, which may also be linked with lower mortality. Importantly, our experience of shorter cross-clamp and bypass times during mitral repair was seen in both elderly and young patients [56]. Unrepairable valves that require replacement may be a harbinger of more advanced heart disease and thus may bode worse outcomes [56]. Ailawadi et al. [61] indicate improved survival after MV repair over replacement in elderly patients (Fig. 32.10).

Operative mortality has been reported as low as 3.7% [62] and excellent long-term survival has been reported (generally comparable with an age- and gender-matched population) [62, 63]. Freedom from reoperation rates have been reported to be greater than 90% at 5 years [63, 64]. Others have reported postoperative symptomatic improvement to NYHA class I or II at follow-up and are experiencing favorable if not more than favorable results reoperatively [62, 63]. Quality of life scores are also reported as equal to or greater

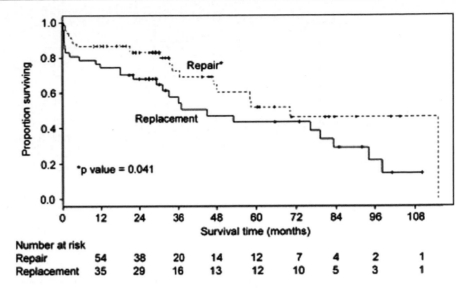

Fig. 32.10 Long-term survival with mitral valve repair (*dashed lines*) versus replacement (*solid line*) in elderly patients (reprinted with permission from Ailawadi et al. [61], Copyright Elsevier 2008)

than those of the age- and gender-matched population [65, 66]. However, these studies warrant a more aggressive approach.

Survival

Overall 1–5 year survival is reported to be 89.4% (95% CI: 81.4–97.4) and 61% (95% CI: 46.4–75.8) [44]. Bioprostheses have traditionally been considered a suitable choice for the elderly, given the higher freedom from structural deterioration evident in older patients compared to young patients and the lack of requirement for long-term anticoagulation [62, 64, 67]. Chordal sparing techniques for MVR might confer additional advantages by preserving left ventricular performance [68]. Recent data from the STS National Cardiac Database demonstrate that the proportion of patients with mitral disease who have their valve repaired rather than replaced decreases with age [36]. In contrast to the established practice, valve repair in older patients has been associated with favorable operative survival [41, 62] and shorter hospital stay [41] than valve replacement and indicates comparable long-term outcomes [41]. Our institutional policy was to repair the mitral valve whenever possible and to replace the valve only when adequate repair was not considered feasible.

Others

In elderly patients, it has been demonstrated that 1- and 5-year freedom from cardiac death, including mitral valve-related

deaths, is 94.6% (95% CI: 88.8–100) and 75.8% (95% CI: 61.6–90.9) (Fig. 32.11a) [56]. One- and five-year freedom from mitral valve-related death is 98 and 95%. One- and five-year freedom from thromboembolic complications in hospital survivors remains 96.6% (95% CI: 91.6–100) and 84.1% (95% CI: 70.9–96; Fig. 32.11b) [56]. One- and five-year freedom from bleeding events in hospital survivors is 96.1% (95% CI: 91–100) and 85.5% (95% CI: 72.3–97.7). One- and five-year freedom from heart-related hospitalization in hospital survivors remains 89.3% (95% CI: 81.3–97.8) and 78.3% (95% CI: 64.7–92.1). Preoperative LVEF greater than 40% is shown to be significantly associated with freedom from heart-related hospitalization (95% CI: 68–95) (p=0.01) [56].

Conclusion

Recent advances with regard to the comprehension of the natural history of mitral valve disease have changed the approach from a relatively passive response to the development of severe symptoms to an early surgery concept preceding the signs of left ventricular dysfunction [12, 69]. The discussion in this chapter suggests that the elderly should not be excluded from this concept because of age alone. Favorable preoperative NYHA class and favorable preoperative left ventricular function has been associated with favorable long-term survival in the elderly population [12, 59, 70]. When the surgical approach precedes the onset of left ventricular dysfunction, an improved freedom from late cardiac death and from the need for subsequent heart-related hospitalization is indicated. An observed survival rate comparable with the expected survival rate of the general population, the

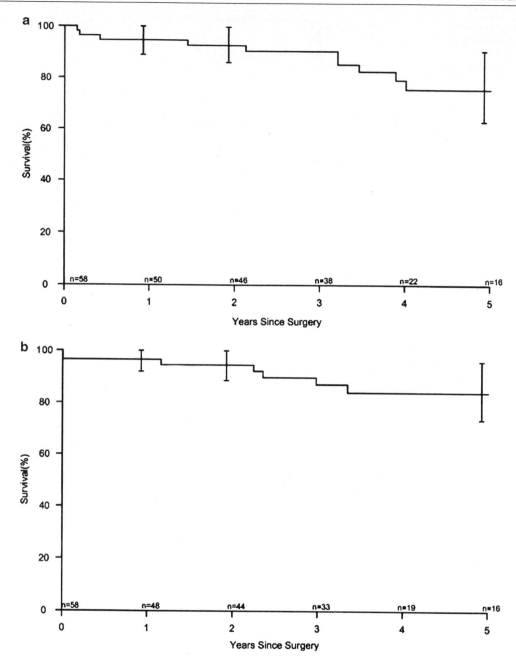

Fig. 32.11 (**a**) Freedom from cardiac death; (**b**) Freedom from thrombolic events (*n* = patients at risk) (reprinted with permission from DiGregorio et al. [56], Copyright Elsevier 2004)

improvement in the functional status of the patient, the low incidence of complications, and the absence of the need for reoperation provide evidence that octogenarians with MR can achieve beneficial results from mitral valve surgery. This chapter emphasizes on reparative techniques that do not argue in a survival advantage compared with replacement but do prove to be a reliable approach regarding elderly patients. We suggest that in elderly patients surgery performed at an early stage, preceding the development of left ventricular dysfunction is associated with an improved freedom from late cardiac complications.

References

1. Carpentier A. Cardiac valve surgery – the "French correction". J Thorac Cardiovasc Surg. 1983;86:323–37.
2. Singh JP, Evans JC, Levy D, Larson MG, Freed LA, Fuller DL, et al. Prevalence and clinical determinants of mitral, tricuspid, and aortic regurgitation (the Framingham Heart Study). Am J Cardiol. 1999;83:897–902.
3. Choong CY, Abascal VM, Weyman J, Levine RA, Gentile F, Thomas JD, et al. Prevalence of valvular regurgitation by Doppler echocardiography in patients with structurally normal hearts by two dimensional echocardiography. Am Heart J. 1989;117:636–42.

4. Wilcken DE, Hickey AJ. Lifetime risk for patients with mitral valve prolapse of developing severe valve regurgitation requiring surgery. Circulation. 1988;78:10–4.

5. Northrup III WF, Kshettry VR, DuBois KA. Trends in mitral valve surgery in a large multi-surgeon, multi-hospital practice, 1979–1999. J Heart Valve Dis. 2003;12:14–24.

6. Akins CW, Daggett WM, Vlahakes GJ, Hilgenberg AD, Torchiana DF, Madsen JC, et al. Cardiac operations in patients 80 years old and older. Ann Thorac Surg. 1997;64:606–15.

7. Edwards MB, Kenneth MT. Outcomes in nonagenarians after heart valve replacement operation. Ann Thorac Surg. 2003;75:830–4.

8. Bacchetta MD, Ko W, Girardi LN, Mack CA, Krieger KH, Isom OW, et al. Outcomes of cardiac surgery in nonagenarians: a 10-year experience. Ann Thorac Surg. 2003;75:1215–20.

9. Tsai TP, Chaux A, Matloff JM, Kass RM, Gray RJ, DeRobertis MA, et al. Ten-year experience of cardiac surgery in patients aged 80 years, and over. Ann Thorac Surg. 1994;58:445–51.

10. Mehta RH, Eagle KA, Coombs LP, Peterson ED, Edwards FH, Pagani FD, et al. Society of Thoracic Surgeons National Cardiac Registry. Influence of age on outcomes in patients undergoing mitral valve replacement. Ann Thorac Surg. 2002;74:1459–67.

11. Scott ML, Stowe CL, Nunnally LC. Mitral valve reconstruction in the elderly population. Ann Thorac Surg. 1989;48:213–7.

12. Enriquez-Sarano M. Timing of mitral valve surgery. Heart. 2002;87:79–85.

13. Tribouilloy CM, Enriquez-Sarano M, Schaff HV, Orszulak TA, Bailey KR, Tajik AJ, et al. Impact of preoperative symptoms on survival after surgical correction of organic mitral regurgitation. Circulation. 1999;99:400–5.

14. Boon A, Cheriex E, Lodder J, Kessels F. Cardiac valve calcification: characteristics of patients with calcification of the mitral annulus or aortic valve. Heart. 1997;78:472–4.

15. Al-Absi AI, Wall BM, Aslam N, Mangold TA, Lamar KD, Wan JY, et al. Predictors of mortality in end-stage renal disease patients with mitral annulus calcification. Am J Med Sci. 2006;331:124–30.

16. Carpentier AF, Pellerin M, Fuzellier J, Relland JYM. Extensive calcification of the mitral anulus: pathology and surgical management. J Thorac Cardiovasc Surg. 1998;111:718–30.

17. de Vrey EA, Scholte AJ, Krauss XH, Dion RA, Poldermans D, van der Wall EE, et al. Intracardiac pseudotumor caused by mitral annular calcification. Eur J Echocadiogr. 2006;7:62–6.

18. Feindel CM, Tufail Z, David TE, Ivanov J, Armstrong S. Mitral valve surgery in patients with extensive calcification of the mitral annulus. J Thorac Cardiovasc Surg. 2003;126:777–82.

19. Chirillo F, Salvador L, Cavallini C. Medical and surgical treatment of chronic mitral regurgitation. J Cardiovasc Med (Hagerstown). 2006;7:96–107.

20. Ling LH, Enriquez-Sarano M, Seward JB, Tajik AJ, Schaff HV, Bailey KR, et al. Clinical outcome of mitral regurgitation due to flail leaflet. N Engl J Med. 1996;335:1417–23.

21. Bonow RO, Carabello BA, Kanu C, de Leon AC Jr, Faxon DP, Freed MD, et al. ACC/AHA 2006 guidelines for the management of patients with valvular heart disease: a report of the American College of Cardiology/American Heart Association Task Force on Practice Guidelines (writing committee to revise the 1998 Guidelines for the Management of Patients With Valvular Heart Disease): developed in collaboration with the Society of Cardiovascular Anesthesiologists: endorsed by the Society for Cardiovascular Angiography and Interventions and the Society of Thoracic Surgeons. Circulation. 2006;114:e84–231.

22. Monin JL, Dehant P, Roiron C, Monchi M, Tabet JY, Clerc P, et al. Functional assessment of mitral regurgitation by transthoracic echocardiography using standardized imaging planes diagnostic accuracy and outcome implications. J Am Coll Cardiol. 2005;46:302–9.

23. Agricola E, Oppizzi M, Pisani M, Maisano F, Margonato A. Accuracy of realtime 3D echocardiography in the evaluation of functional anatomy of mitral regurgitation. Int J Cardiol. 2008;127:342–9.

24. Sharma R, Mann J, Drummond L, Livesey SA, Simpson IA. The evaluation of real-time 3-dimensional transthoracic echocardiography for the preoperative functional assessment of patients with mitral valve prolapse: a comparison with 2-dimensional transesophageal echocardiography. J Am Soc Echocardiogr. 2007;20:934–40.

25. Müller S, Müller L, Laufer G, Alber H, Dichtl W, Frick M, et al. Comparison of three-dimensional imaging to transesophageal echocardiography for preoperative evaluation in mitral valve prolapse. Am J Cardiol. 2006;98:243–8.

26. Stork A, Franzen O, Ruschewski H, Detter C, Müllerleile K, Bansmann PM, et al. Assessment of functional anatomy of the mitral valve in patients with mitral regurgitation with cine magnetic resonance imaging: comparison with transesophageal echocardiography and surgical results. Eur Radiol. 2007;17:3189–98.

27. Society of Thoracic Surgeons. Society of Thoracic Surgeons Adult Cardiovascular Surgery National Database – Fall 2005 Report Executive Summary. http://www.sts.org/documents/pdf/STSExecutiveSummaryFall2005.

28. Society of Thoracic Surgeons. Society of Thoracic Surgeons Adult Cardiovascular Surgery National Database – Fall 2006 Report Executive Summary. http://www.sts.org/documents/pdf/STSExecutiveSummaryFall2006.

29. David TE, Uden DE, Strauss H. The importance of the mitral apparatus in left ventricular function after correction of mitral regurgitation. Circulation. 1983;68:76–82.

30. David TE, Armstrong S, Sun Z. Left ventricular function after mitral valve surgery. J Heart Valve Dis. 1995;4:175–80.

31. Braunberger E, Deloche A, Berrebi A, Abdallah F, Celestin JA, Meimoun P, et al. Very long-term results (more than 20 years) of valve repair with Carpentier's techniques in nonrheumatic mitral valve insufficiency. Circulation. 2001;104:I-8–11.

32. Gillinov AM, Cosgrove DM, Blackstone EH, Diaz R, Arnold JH, Lytle BW, et al. Durability of mitral valve repair for degenerative disease. J Thorac Cardiovasc Surg. 1998;116:734–43.

33. Enriquez-Sarano M, Schaff HV, Orszulak TA, Tajik AJ, Bailey KR, Frye RL. Valve repair improves the outcome of surgery for mitral regurgitation. A multivariate analysis. Circulation. 1995;91:1022–8.

34. Suri RM, Schaff HV, Dearani JA, Sundt TM 3rd, Daly RC, Mullany CJ, et al. Survival advantage and improved durability of mitral repair for leaflet prolapsed subsets in the current era. Ann Thorac Surg. 2006;82:819–26.

35. Gillinov AM, Wierup PN, Blackstone EH, Bishay ES, Cosgrove DM, White J, et al. Is repair preferable to replacement for ischemic mitral regurgitation? J Thorac Cardiovasc Surg. 2001;122:1125–41.

36. Savage EB, Ferguson TB Jr, DiSesa VJ. Use of mitral valve repair: analysis of contemporary United States experience reported to the Society of Thoracic Surgeons National Cardiac Database. Ann Thorac Surg. 2003;75:820–5.

37. Gogbashian A, Sepic J, Soltesz EG, Nascimben L, Cohn LH. Operative and long-term survival of elderly is significantly improved by mitral valve repair. Am Heart J. 2006;151:1325–33.

38. Thourani VH, Weintraub WS, Guyton RA, Jones EL, Williams WH, Elkabbani S, et al. Outcomes and long-term survival for patients undergoing mitral valve repair versus replacement: effect of age and concomitant coronary artery bypass grafting. Circulation. 2003;108:298–304.

39. Alfieri O, Maisano F, De Bonis M, Stefano PL, Torracca L, Oppizzi M, et al. The double orifice technique in mitral valve repair: a simple solution for complex problems. J Thorac Cardiovasc Surg. 2001;122:674–81.

40. Maisano F, Caldarola A, Blasio A, De Bonis M, La Canna G, Alfieri O. Midterm results of edge-to-edge mitral valve repair without annuloplasty. J Thorac Cardiovasc Surg. 2003;126:1987–97.

41. Messas E, Pouzet B, Touchot B, et al. Efficacy of chordal cutting to relieve chronic persistant ischemic mitral regurgitation. Circulation. 2003;108:111–5.

42. Liel-Cohen N, Guerrero JL, Otsuji Y, Handschumacher MD, Rudski LG, Hunziker PR, et al. Design of a new surgical approach for ventricular remodeling to relieve ischemic mitral regurgiation: insights from three-dimensional echocardiography. Circulation. 2000;101:2756–63.

43. Kron IL, Green GR, Cope JT. Surgical relocation of the posterior papillary muscle in chronic ischemic mitral regurgitation. Ann Thorac Surg. 2002;74:600–1.

44. Fundarò P, Pocar M, Moneta A, Donatelli F, Grossi A. Posterior mitral valve restoration for ischemic regurgitation. Ann Thorac Surg. 2004;77:729–30.

45. Fann JI, St Goar FG, Komtebedde J, Oz MC, Block PC, Foster E, et al. Beating heart catheter-based edge-to-edge mitral valve procedure in a porcine model: efficacy and healing response. Circulation. 2004;110:988–9.

46. Daimon M, Shiota T, Gillinov AM, Hayase M, Ruel M, Cohn WE, et al. Percutaneous mitral valve repair for chronic ischemic mitral regurgitation: a real-time three-dimensional echocardiographic study in an ovine model. Circulation. 2005;111:2183–9.

47. Maniu CV, Patel JB, Reuter DG, Meyer DM, Edwards WD, Rihal CS, et al. Acute and chronic reduction of functional mitral regurgitation in experimental heart failure by percutaneous mitral annuloplasty. J Am Coll Cardiol. 2004;44: 1652–61.

48. Singh SK, Borger MA. Percutaneous valve replacement: fact or fiction? Can J Cardiol. 2005;21:829–32.

49. Konstantinov IE, Carter M, Saxena P, Koniuszko MD, Singh T, Alvarez J, et al. Prosthesis replacement in a calcified mitral annulus with reconstruction of the intervalvular fibrous body: the value of an alternative repair. Tex Heart Inst J. 2006;33:232–4.

50. Fukada Y, Matsui Y, Sasaki S, Yasuda K. A case of mitral valve replacement with a collar-reinforced prosthetic valve for heavily calcified mitral annulus. Ann Thorac Cardiovasc Surg. 2005;11: 260–3.

51. Nataf P, Pavie A, Jault F, Bors V, Cabrol C, Gandjbakhch I. Intraatrial insertion of a mitral prosthesis in a destroyed or calcified mitral annulus. Ann Thorac Surg. 1994;58:163–7.

52. Iida H, Mochizuki Y, Matsushita Y, Mori H, Yamada Y, Miyoshi S. A valve replacement technique for heavily calcified mitral valve and annulus. J Heart Valve Dis. 2005;14:209–11.

53. Di Stefano S, López J, Flórez S, Rey J, Arevalo A, San Román A. Building a new annulus: a technique for mitral valve replacement in heavily calcified annulus. Ann Thorac Surg. 2009;87:1625–7.

54. Detaint D, Sundt TM, Nkomo VT, Scott CG, Tajik AJ, Schaff HV, et al. Surgical correction of mitral regurgitation in the elderly: outcomes and recent improvements. Circulation. 2006;114:265–72.

55. Cohn LH, Kowalker W, Bhatia S, DiSesa VJ, St John-Sutton M, Shemin RJ, et al. Comparative morbidity of mitral valve repair versus replacement for mitral regurgitation with and without coronary artery disease. 1988. Updated in 1995. Ann Thorac Surg. 1995;60:1452–3.

56. DiGregorio V, Zehr KJ, Orszulak TA, Mullany CJ, Daly RC, Dearani JA, et al. Results of mitral surgery in octogenarians with isolated nonrheumatic mitral regurgitation. Ann Thorac Surg. 2004;78:807–13.

57. Gazoni LM, Kern JA, Swenson BR, Dent JM, Smith PW, Mulloy DP, et al. A change in perspective: results for ischemic mitral valve repair are similar to mitral valve repair for degenerative disease. Ann Thorac Surg. 2007;84:750–7.

58. Komeda M, David TE, Rao V, Sun Z, Weisel RD, Burns RJ. Late hemodynamic effects of the preserved papillary muscles during mitral valve replacement. Circulation. 1994;90:190–4.

59. Lee EM, Shapiro LM, Wells FC. Importance of subvalvular preservation and early operation in mitral valve surgery. Circulation. 1996;94:2117–23.

60. Jebara VA, Dervanian P, Acar C, Grare P, Mihaileanu S, Chauvaud S, et al. Mitral valve repair using Carpentier techniques in patients more than 70 years old. Early and late results. Circulation. 1992;86:53–9.

61. Ailawadi G, Swenson BR, Girotti ME, Gazoni LM, Peeler BB, Kern JA, et al. Is mitral valve repair superior to replacement in elderly patients? Ann Thorac Surg. 2008;86:77–85.

62. Lee EM, Porter JN, Shapiro LM, Wells FC. Mitral valve surgery in the elderly. J Heart Valve Dis. 1997;6:22–31.

63. Grossi EA, Zakow PK, Sussman M, Galloway AC, Delianides J, Baumann G, et al. Late results of mitral valve reconstruction in the elderly. Ann Thorac Surg. 2000;70:1224–6.

64. Pupello DF, Bessone LN, Hiro SP, Lopez-Cuenca E, Glatterer MS Jr, Angell WW, et al. Bioprosthetic valve longevity in the elderly: an 18-year longitudinal study. Ann Thorac Surg. 1995;60:S270–5.

65. Khan JH, Magnetti S, Davis E, Zhand J. Late outcomes of open heart surgery in patients 70 years or older. Ann Thorac Surg. 2000;69:165–70.

66. Fruitman DS, MacDougall CE, Ross DB. Cardiac surgery in octogenarians: can elderly patients benefit? Quality of life after cardiac surgery. Ann Thorac Surg. 1999;68:2129–35.

67. Rizzoli G, Bottio T, Thiene G, Toscano G, Casarotto D. Long-term durability of the Hancock II porcine bioprosthesis. J Thorac Cardiovasc Surg. 2003;126:66–74.

68. Yun KL, Sintek CF, Miller DC, Pfeffer TA, Kochamba GS, Khonsari S, et al. Randomized trial comparing partial versus complete chordal-sparing mitral valve replacement: effects on left ventricular volume and function. J Thorac Cardiovasc Surg. 2002;123:707–14.

69. Smolens IA, Pagani FD, Deeb GM, Prager RL, Sonnad SS, Bolling SF. Prophylactic mitral reconstruction for mitral regurgitation. Ann Thorac Surg. 2001;72:1210–6.

70. David TE, Ivanov J, Armstrong S, Rakowski H. Late outcomes of mitral valve repair for floppy valves: implications for asymptomatic patients. J Thorac Cardiovasc Surg. 2003;125:1143–52.

71. Butany J, Vaideeswar P, Dixit V, Feindel C. Massive mitral annular calcification: a stone in the heart. Can J Cardiol. 2009;25:e18.

72. Bito Y, Shibata T, Yasuoka T, Inoue K, Ikuta T. Mitral valve replacement for extensive calcification: half and half technique. Gen Thorac Cardiovasc Surg. 2008;56:526–8.

73. Calafiore AM, Di Mauro M, Gallina S, Di Giammarco G, Iacò AL, Teodori G, et al. Mitral valve surgery for chronic ischemic mitral regurgitation. Ann Thorac Surg. 2004;77:1989–97.

74. Amirak E, Chan KM, Zakkar M, Punjabi PP. Current status of surgery for degenerative mitral valve disease. Prog Cardiovasc Dis. 2009;51:454–9.

Chapter 33
Surgical Treatment of Thoracic Aortic Disease in the Elderly

Arnar Geirsson

Abstract Management of thoracic aortic diseases remains complex but has made tremendous progress over the last decades. Although thoracic aortic diseases affect patients of all ages, the older age group predominates. Clinical decision making can be particularly challenging in the elderly patients whether being an elective circumstances for asymptomatic aneurysm evaluation or under emergent situation in patient presenting with aortic emergencies such as aortic dissection or degenerative aortic aneurysm rupture. Even under the best circumstances, the operations are associated with well-know set of complications and risk of mortality that is generally higher than other operations performed by cardiothoracic surgeons. Advances both in surgical techniques, intraoperative management, and postoperative care have reduced both mortality and morbidity in recent years in all age groups. Concomitant with that increasing number of elderly patients are being evaluated and undergo complex aortic operations. This chapter will focus on the surgical treatment of thoracic aortic disease as it pertains to the elderly patients. It will not attempt to address the general management of multiple thoracic aortic syndromes that the cardiothoracic surgeon faces in detail but instead highlight studies that specifically refer to the elderly patients and the specific and unique issues that relate to that group of patients. This includes decision making in the elderly patient presenting with symptomatic and asymptomatic thoracic aortic aneurysm, acute aortic dissection, as well as addressing the issue of use of endovascular treatment of thoracic aortic aneurysm in the elderly.

Keywords Aortic disease • Thoracic aortic aneurysm • Aortic dissection • Penetrating atherosclerotic ulcer • Intramural hematoma • Ascending aorta • Descending aorta • Hypothermic circulatory arrest • Aortic surgery • Emergency surgery

Cardiovascular Surgery in the Aging Population

The absolute and relative number of the older population continues to rise in the US and the developed countries. The group that has experienced the most rapid change in numbers are individuals aged 85 years and older. Over the last century, their number increased 34-fold from 122,000 in the year 1900 to 4.2 millions in the year 2000. It is projected that by 2050 this group will have reached 20.9 million individuals. The life expectancy of elderly individual also continues to increase. In 1900, an 85-year old individual had a life expectancy of 4.0 years. According to the most recent census data, the life expectancy of a 75-year old male or female is 10.8 and 12.8 years, respectively. For an 85-year old, the life expectancy is 6.1 years for males and 7.2 years for females [1, 2]. Comprehensive knowledge of patient life expectancy is extremely important part of clinical decision making when taking care of the elderly patient. The main goals for surgical interventions for aneurysm disease should be to prolong life, alleviate symptoms, and/or improve quality of life. There are numerous studies that have demonstrated acceptable perioperative risk in elderly patients undergoing other cardiovascular operation than on the thoracic aorta. These studies have demonstrated that although the elderly patient undergoing coronary artery bypass grafting, valve surgery and abdominal aortic aneurysm repair are at slightly higher risk of complication and require longer hospital stay compared with younger patients, the long-term survival normalized and becomes similar to the general population [3–6].

Aneurysmal Disease of the Thoracic Aorta

The prevalence and incidence of thoracic aortic disease is increasing both as a result of aging of the population and more frequent use of CT scans and echocardiography for diagnosis of various conditions. There are limited number of population studies to accurately determine the incidence of

A. Geirsson (✉)
Yale University School of Medicine, 333 Cedar Street, FMB 121, New Haven, CT 06520, USA
e-mail: arnar.geirsson@yale.edu

M.R. Katlic (ed.), *Cardiothoracic Surgery in the Elderly*, DOI 10.1007/978-1-4419-0892-6_33,
© Springer Science+Business Media, LLC 2011

both thoracic aortic aneurysm and aortic dissection. The most contemporary data originates from nationwide population-based study from Sweden. The incidence of thoracic aortic disease diagnosis (aneurysm and dissection) in men rose by 52% from 10.7 per 100,000 per year in 1987 to 16.3 per 100,000 per year in 2002. In women the incidence was lower but also increased 28% from 7.1 per 100,000 per year in 1987 to 9.1 per 100,000 per year in 2002. Relative risk of diagnosis of thoracic aortic disease was strongly correlated with age. The mean age was 70 years for the whole registry but the median age decreased from 73 years in the 1987–1990 period to 71 years in the 1999–2002 period ($p < 0.0001$). The annual incidence of operative intervention also increased over the study period by sevenfold in male and 15-fold in women [7]. The overall incidence of thoracic aortic aneurysm in Olmsted County in the period of 1990–1994 was 10.99 per 100,000 per year compared with the 1951–1955 period when the incidence was 2.41 per 100,000 per year [8]. Increased awareness of aneurysmal disease and improved diagnostic tools account for large portion of the earlier increase in incidence but there is indication that the true incidence of thoracic aortic aneurysm is increasing because of the increasing age of the population.

Size of the thoracic aortic aneurysm is the strongest predictor for complication such as dissection, rupture, or death. This has been well defined by the Yale Center for Thoracic Aortic Disease. In their database, the average growth rate is 0.12 cm per year (0.10 for ascending aorta and 0.30 for descending aorta) [9]. The median size at the time of rupture or dissection was 6.0 cm for ascending aneurysm and 7.2 cm for descending aortic aneurysm. Once the size of an ascending aneurysm reached 6.0 cm, the risk of rupture or dissection increased by 32.1% points. For descending aneurysm, there was 43.0% increase in risk once aneurysm reached 7.0 cm in size [10]. Once the size of thoracic aortic aneurysm (both ascending and descending) reaches 6.0 cm in size the average yearly rate of rupture or dissection is 6.9%, and the average yearly risk of death becomes 11.8% with 5-year survival of only 56%. Patient who underwent elective operative repair restored life expectancy to normal [11]. Based on these findings, the current size recommendations for operative intervention is 5.0–5.5 cm for ascending and 6.0–6.5 cm for descending aneurysm in asymptomatic patients. Patients with connective tissue disorder such as Marfan disease are at increased risk of complication and should be offered operation when ascending aorta or root aneurysm reaches 4.5 cm. Patients with strong family history or aneurysm associated with bicuspid aortic valve are also at increased risk and should be considered for operation once aorta reaches 5.0 cm. Aneurysm growth of more than 1 cm/year, pain consistent with rupture or unexplained by other causes are also considered indications for surgery. The data for saccular aneurysm generally located in the descending aorta are not as clear but sac with over 2 cm and total diameter more than 5 cm are considered indications for surgery. These recommendations should certainly be extended to elderly patients but individual approach is paramount. Risk of aneurysm rupture, dissection, or death have to be weighed against the risk of perioperative death and complications as well as the overall expected long-term survival. This is particularly important in patients who have asymptomatic thoracic aneurysm where prolonging patient survival should be the primary goal.

Surgery of the Ascending Aorta and Aortic Arch

Aneurysmal surgery of the ascending aorta and aortic arch generally requires the use of profound hypothermic circulatory arrest to perform a direct open repair. These complex operations are associated with significant morbidity such as stroke and neurological dysfunction and significantly higher mortality rates compared with other cardiac operations. Debates have arisen whether these operations should be offered to the elderly patient. Age has been identified to be an independent risk factor for stroke and transient neurological dysfunction defined as postoperative confusion, agitation, and transient delirium in patient undergoing hypothermic circulatory arrest [12, 13]. Age above 60 has also been defined as a risk factor for death or permanent neurological injury in same series [12]. The Swedish heart surgery registry of patients undergoing operations on the ascending aorta found that age (HR = 1.05), aortic dissection (HR = 1.54), emergency operation (HR = 2.80), coronary artery bypass grafting (HR = 2.03), postoperative stroke (HR = 1.84) and postoperative renal failure (HR = 2.45) were all independently associated with surgical mortality. Only age was an independent but a weak risk factor associated with long-term mortality with HR = 1.06 per 1 year increment [14]. A large Japanese series demonstrated that early mortality, postoperative stroke, transient neurological dysfunction, and respiratory complication were all higher in patient over the age of 70. That series included all types of thoracic aortic operations and demonstrated that emergency operations were associated with very high mortality rates [15]. However, majority of studies that have specifically addressed the use of hypothermic circulatory arrest in the elderly demonstrate favorable outcomes. However, these studies are all retrospective, contain few cases, and probably are affected by significant selection bias where preferably "good risk" elderly patients were offered operation but others excluded and therefore not studied further. Incidence of stroke was between 8 and 20% and early mortality was between 5 and 16% [16–18]. Only one of the studies demonstrated increased risk of stroke compared with younger patients or elderly patients undergoing other cardiovascular operations [17], while other demonstrated the protective role of retrograde cerebral perfusion

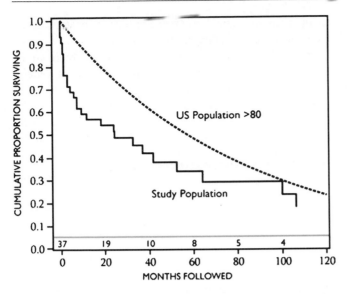

Fig. 33.1 Survival analysis of octogenarians undergoing ascending and transverse aortic arch repair compared to the US population. Survival in the study population was 56% vs. 86% ($p=0.02$) at year 1, 48% vs. 76% ($p=0.03$) at year 2, 36% vs. 48% at year 5, and 20% vs. 20% at year 10 ($p=0.10$) (reprinted with permission from Shah et al. [18], Copyright Elsevier 2008)

as an adjunct during hypothermic circulatory arrest [18]. Predictors of stroke in octogenarians were prior history of stroke and increased cardiopulmonary bypass time, while predictors of early mortality included low glomerular filtration rate, long cardiopulmonary bypass time, and emergency operations. Long-term survival in these elderly patients did not differ from age-matched US population (Fig. 33.1) [18]. It is therefore safe to conclude that elective operations on the ascending aorta and aortic arch can be safely performed with the use of hypothermic circulatory arrest in octogenarians with acceptable morbidity and mortality.

Surgery of the Descending and Thoracoabdominal Aorta

Operative repair of the descending aortic and thoracoabdominal aortic aneurysm remain highly complex and associated with numerous significant complications and high mortality. Operative mortality for open repair of descending aortic aneurysm is between 2.8 and 8.8% in contemporary series where incidence of spinal cord ischemia was 2.6–2.7% [19, 20]. For thoracoabdominal repairs, the incidence of spinal cord ischemia is higher between 3.8 and 9.5%, and perioperative mortality has remained mostly unchanged between 5.0 and 8.2% for years in experienced centers despite improvements in operative techniques and perioperative care [21, 22]. In addition to spinal cord ischemia with resulting paraplegia both pulmonary and renal complication are common and when they occur they are associated with significant

increase in postoperative mortality. Various operative strategies and adjuncts are used in attempt to decrease complication aimed most specifically to decrease complication of spinal, renal, and visceral ischemia. Cerebrospinal fluid drainage, reimplantation of critical spinal arteries, neuromonitoring (evoked-potential), epidural cooling, moderate hypothermia, visceral and renal perfusion, and atriofemoral bypass have all been demonstrated to be beneficial adjuncts in these complex operations. Most recently introduction of endovascular approaches have demonstrated improved short-term outcome in high-risk patient, although long-term outcome is not clear (see Endovascular treatment of thoracic aneurysmal disease).

There are only few numbers of studies specifically addressing open surgery of descending thoracic and thoracoabdominal aneurysm in the elderly. Huynh et al. described their experience of 56 patients between the ages of 79 and 88 years at the time of surgery who underwent replacement of the descending aorta or thoracoabdominal aorta. The cohort had significant number of comorbidities including hypertension (61%), chronic obstructive pulmonary disease (23%), coronary artery disease (23%), congestive heart failure (5%), history of cerebrovascular disease (20%), diabetes (9%), or chronic renal insufficiency or dialysis (5%). Patient with at least one of the three factor, emergent presentation, diabetes, or congestive heart failure, were categorized as high risk and had 50% 30-day mortality compared with 17% in group of patients considered low risk. Age was not a risk factor by univariate analysis. However, there was only comparison within the group of elderly patients (79–88 years). Importantly, the 5-year actuarial survival was 48% [23]. The Baylor group presented their data comprising of 39 octogenarians undergoing thoracoabdominal aortic aneurysm repair ranging from 80 to 89 years of age. They also had significant preoperative risk factors including hypertension (61%), chronic obstructive pulmonary disease (36%), coronary artery disease (33%), renal occlusive disease (31%), aneurysm rupture (18%), renal insufficiency (15%), diabetes (9%), history of cerebrovascular accident (5%). They had excellent results with in-hospital mortality of only 10.3% and all patients with ruptured aneurysm survived to discharge. There was fairly high rate of postoperative complication including paraplegia (5.1%) all occurring in Crawford extent III aneurysm, cerebrovascular accidents (5.1%), renal failure (18%), pulmonary complications (36%), and cardiac events (18%). Univariate risk factors predictive for death were tracheostomy, myocardial infarction, and hemodialysis. The median length of stay was 15 days with a range of 10–86 days. The 5-year actuarial survival was 50% demonstrating that despite long and complicated hospital stay the long-term outcome is quite acceptable [24]. Although these studies demonstrate that thoracic and thoracoabdominal operations can be performed with moderate operative risks of mortality when performed in the elective setting they are all results from high volume aortic surgery centers and may not properly represent the true operative outcome. Information from the National Inpatient Sample database report a staggering 22.3% overall mortality for thoracoabdominal aneurysm repair, with higher-volume centers and surgeons having much improved results [25]. Also state-wide registry demonstrates that the early mortality underestimates that long-term risk of thoracoabdominal repair where the 1-year mortality rates following elective operation was 34.7% in 70–79 years old and 40% in 80–89 years old. If emergency operation was performed, the long-term outcome was markedly worse with 62.4% one-year mortality in 70–79 years old and 68.8% in the oldest group (Fig. 33.2) [26]. Emergency surgery in this population of patients is associated with very high risk of stroke and mortality especially when hypothermic circulator arrest is required (Fig. 33.3) [16, 23]. It brings up the issue whether open operative treatment should be offered in the emergency setting for ruptured descending or thoracoabdominal aortic

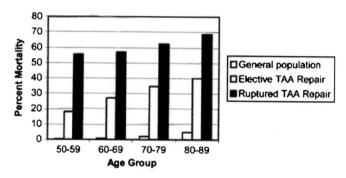

Fig. 33.2 One-year mortality following operative treatment of elective or ruptured thoracoabdominal aortic aneurysms (TAA) compared to the general population. The results are stratified into groups by increasing decade of life. Data are from the National Vital Statistic report (reprinted with permission from Rigberg et al. [26] Copyright Elsevier 2006)

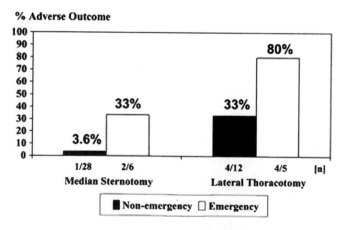

Fig. 33.3 The risk of adverse outcome (death or permanent stroke) in octogenarians following aortic surgery requiring hypothermic circulatory arrest was highest in patients undergoing lateral thoracotomy and emergency surgery (reprinted with permission from Hagl et al. [16], Copyright Elsevier 2001)

aneurysm in this patient group and argues for earlier elective operative repair. Quality of life following these complex operations is important to address but currently there are no good data available regarding quality of life of elderly patients surviving complex descending thoracic or thoracoabdominal aneurysm repair.

Penetrating Atherosclerotic Ulcers

Penetrating atherosclerotic ulcers are caused by rupture of an atherosclerotic aortic plaque that results in initial hematoma formation and then ulcer formation between the media and the adventitia. It is most commonly located in the descending aorta and can be associated with both intramural hematoma and localized type B dissection. It is generally an indicator of severe atherosclerotic disease of the aorta and frequently more than single ulcers are noted. The proper treatment of penetrating atherosclerotic ulcer has been debated and pendulum has swung between operative and nonoperative management. Two large centers have presented opposite school of thoughts. Investigators at Yale presented their series of 26 patients where more than one-third presented with rupture and two thirds underwent surgery. Early rupture was especially high when associated with intramural hematoma but also later complications such as aneurysm formation and rupture where also high [27]. On the contrary, the Mayo Clinic group presented a series where majority of patients were managed medically with success [28]. It is not clear what explains these differences expect a possible difference in patient characteristics where the Yale group were all symptomatic and had much higher incidence of ascending aortic ulcers. Also no incidental atherosclerotic ulcers were included in that study. So management needs to be individualized both in respect to patient comorbidities and characteristics of the ulcers. Symptomatic penetrating ulcers, atherosclerotic ulcers with surrounding hematoma or with evidence of enlargement or impending rupture should be managed operatively. Patients at high-risk for surgery can probably be managed medically with anti-impulse therapy and close radiographic follow-up. Surgical treatment consists of either open operative repair with replacement of aortic segment containing the ulcer or endovascular stent grafting that has shown promise especially when the aortic ulcer is localized [29].

Aortic Dissection Syndromes

Aortic dissection is characterized by separation of the aortic intima and adventitia to various extents. Generally the initiating event is a hypertensive episode resulting in primary intimal tear. The inflow of blood then propagates the dissection both proximally and distally creating a false lumen that communicates with the true aortic lumen at one or more secondary intimal tear sites. Stanford type A involves the entire aorta (DeBakey type I) or only the ascending aorta up to the level of the aortic arch (DeBakey type II). The tear is most commonly in the ascending aorta or proximal arch. Stanford type B involves dissection in the descending thoracic aorta extending into abdominal aorta where the primary tear is in the proximal descending aorta. Risk factors for aortic dissection include hypertension, thoracic aortic aneurysm, atherosclerotic disease, bicuspid aortic valve, aortic coarctation, and connective tissue disorders such as Marfan syndromes [30].

Acute Type A Aortic Dissection

Acute type A aortic dissection remains one of the most challenging diseases the cardiothoracic surgeon faces. In the early days of cardiac surgery, early mortality without surgical treatment was considered to be 1–2% per hour with less than 10% surviving 3 days [31]. Current operative mortality ranges from 12.7 to 32.5% while in-hospital mortality for nonoperative treatment is 58% [32–36]. Therefore, all patients presenting with acute type A aortic dissection should be considered for operative intervention. Probably the most contentious issue that has been extensively investigated in the elderly undergoing cardiac surgery is the appropriateness of surgical intervention for acute aortic dissection. Most of the literature focuses on acute type A aortic dissection, and several groups have reported dismal surgical outcomes in octogenarians, while others have reported acceptable results. Arguing against offering operation for type A dissection in octogenarians, Neri et al. reported on 24 patient aged 80 years and older with intraoperative mortality of 33% and overall hospital mortality of 83%. All patients who survived the operation had one or more postoperative complication, and the mean hospital stay was 37 days and no patient survived beyond 6 months [37]. Piccardo et al. reported on 57 consecutive octogenarians that underwent operation for type A aortic dissection with 45.6% in-hospital mortality and 5-year survival of 44% [38]. Japan contains one of the largest proportions of the elderly population in the world and have demonstrated remarkably good surgical results. Shiono et al. reported on 24 octogenarians where hospital mortality was only 13% but significantly higher than the 6% mortality seen in patients younger than 80 years of age. The same goes with 5- and 10-year survival that was significantly lower in octogenarians, 55 and 42%, respectively, than in the younger age group of 83 and 73%, respectively. However, age over 80 was not an independent risk factor on univariate or multivariate analysis [39]. In an attempt to address the issue

of quality of life following repair of type A dissection, another Japanese report described the results of 58 octogenarians. Thirty patients (Group I) underwent emergency operation, while 28 patients (Group II) did not undergo and operation and were treated conservatively according to patient or family wishes. Hospital mortality was very acceptable of 13.3% in group I while 60.7% of group II died in the hospital. Ten of the patients in group I remained either bedridden or highly dependent on assistance or care following discharge from the hospital. There was no difference in actuarial 5-year survival between operated and conservatively treated cases [40]. The study concluded that emergency surgery can be performed with acceptable hospital mortality; however, surviving patients are at high risk of complications, dementia, depression, and immobility, and operative intervention does not improve long-term survival, which needs to be addressed in discussing treatment options with patient and family. The International Registry of Acute Aortic Dissection (IRAD) database has reported on the difference in outcome of patients 70 years or older and patients younger than 70 years. Elderly patient had higher incidence of diabetes, prior cardiac surgery, hypertension, atherosclerosis, iatrogenic dissection, and preexisting ascending aortic aneurysm. They were less likely to present with typical symptoms of acute onset of chest or back pain. In the database only 64.4% of elderly patients underwent surgical intervention. Reasons for nonoperative management included comorbid conditions, age, patient refusal, and intramural hemotoma. In-hospital mortality was significantly higher in the elderly cohort, 42.8% vs. 28%. Interestingly, medically managed patients had mortality of only 52.5% similar to the operated group. Age >70 was identified to be an independent predictor of mortality by multivariate analysis. The study concluded that age alone should not be used as a sole criterion to exclude patients from undergoing repair of type A aortic dissection [41]. Other studies describe in-hospital mortality of 17.6–37.3% in patients aged 70 and older following operation for acute type A dissection [42–44].

So should the elderly patient be offered an operation when he/she presents with acute type A dissection? The general answer should be yes if preexisting comorbidity and clinical presentation are not considered to present a prohibitive operative risk. The rational for offering operation for acute type A dissection in octogenarians is primarily that age is not a strong risk factor for mortality. Therefore, age per se should not be the primary factor determining whether operation should be offered or not. The condition of the patient at the time of presentation is the primary determinant of mortality regardless of age. Patients with evidence of circulatory collapse indicating rupture, pericardial tamponade, and coronary malperfusion are at high risk for mortality. Patients with evidence of malperfusion syndromes especially cerebral malperfusion (stroke and coma) but also mesenteric, renal,

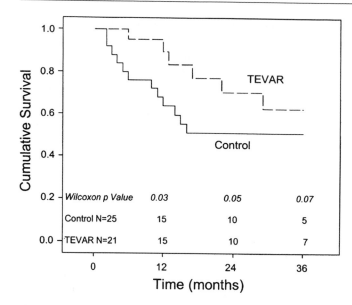

Fig. 33.5 Survival analysis in high-risk groups demonstrates that endovascular thoracic aortic repair (TEVAR) results in an early-term to intermediate-term survival advantage compared with nonoperated group (control). The long-term survival is not significantly different (reprinted with permission from Patel et al. [58], Copyright Elsevier 2007)

44 patients with mean age of 84 years demonstrated that there was no difference in complication rates in octogenarians and younger patients. Survival was similar in early and mid-term follow-up and it was not until after 5 years following the treatment that the group diverged and survival of the older group decreased [60]. There is only one publication specifically comparing open vs. endovascular repair of the descending aorta in patient older than 75 years of age. The study included 41 patients undergoing open repair and 52 patients undergoing endovascular repair. The endovascular group was older, 80.6 years vs. 76.9 years, had more significant comorbidities, where 80.8% of them were prospectively identified as too high risk for open repair. The 30-day mortality appeared higher in the open group 17.1% vs. 5.7% but was not significant ($p = 0.1$). Composite end-point of 30-day mortality, stoke, paralysis, or dialysis was similar between the two groups as well as the 4-year survival [61]. The conclusion to be drawn from studies of endovascular repair in high-risk patients and the elderly is that endovascular repair can be safely performed in those patient groups with acceptable rates of complications. There is improved short and mid-term survival but no difference in long-term survival.

Palliative Care in Elderly Patients with Terminal Thoracic Aortic Condition

The decision when not to offer an elderly patient an operation for a thoracic aortic condition generally falls on the shoulder of the cardiovascular surgeon in situations of emergency conditions such as acute type A aortic dissection, frank rupture, or contained rupture of descending aortic aneurysm. It is often an easier decision for the surgeon and also the patient and the family to consent for an operation rather than elect for nonoperative management. Negative operative outcome is then attributed to patient preoperative condition but affected individuals "feel better" that they gave their elderly family member a chance. Denying patient treatment may bring up ethical concerns from both the patient and surgeon. Obviously, the surgeon has to give their own consent to accept and endure the responsibility of their recommendations and decisions in and out of the operating room. It is important to inform the family that side effects of surgery can be associated with degrading and disabling effect as well as pain. It is also important to be fluent in the current literature and operative outcomes to properly explain to patient and relative the expected outcome of surgery as has been attempted in this chapter. Acute type A dissection without symptoms of malperfusion or hypotension/shock has similar outcome in the young and the elderly, and unless there are prohibitive comorbidities, patient should be offered surgery. However, emergent operations of the thoracoabdominal aorta have extremely poor outcome and generally should not be offered unless the elderly patient is highly functional and with minimal comorbidities. Certainly respect of patient wishes or written advance directives is paramount in emergency situations. Sudden change in patient condition especially when patient is incapacitated tends to push family toward operative intervention that sometimes goes against patients own wishes. The ethical values and principles that need to be applied in those circumstances are respect, beneficence, discernment, and justice [62]. Once a decision has been made not to offer patient operative treatment, patient comfort and dignity at end of life is paramount. Anti-impulse therapy should be given in addition to opioids for pain relief if needed. Some individual patients will survive toward improved clinical condition or even to hospital discharge. In those circumstances, caution should be applied when reconsideration of management strategy is suggested. Although it has not been studied specifically, it is unlikely that operative risk changes significantly in the course of few days or even weeks.

Conclusion

Surgical treatment of thoracic aortic disease has changed dramatically over the last two decades both with respect to outcome and operative strategies. This has occurred concurrently with increased number of elderly patients undergoing those complex operations. Although few studies have indicated that older age as a categorical variable is a predictor of survival, old age should not be the main factor determining appropriateness of operative treatment for thoracic aortic conditions. When age is analyzed as a continuous variable, it is actually a very weak independent predictor of operative outcome when compared with other comorbidities and clinical presentation. Most elective operations can be safely performed in the elderly with acceptable short-term complication and return to normal life expectancy. Emergency operations such as repair of acute type A dissection should generally be performed but emergency treatment of descending aortic conditions remains associated with high morbidity and needs to be individualized. Endovascular treatment of thoracic aortic condition is promising but will need further evaluation prior to be considered as the standard of care in the elderly patient.

References

1. Health, United States, 2008, in US Department of Health and Human Services, Centers for Disease Control and Prevention.
2. Older Americans 2008: Key indicators of well-being, in http://www.aoa.gov/agingstatsdotnet/Main_Site/Data/2008_Documents/tables/Tables.aspx.
3. Adkins MS et al. Efficacy of combined coronary revascularization and vavle procedures in octogenarians. Chest. 1995;108:927–31.
4. Dean RH et al. Operative treatment of abdominal aortic aneurysm in octogenarians. When is it too much too late? Ann Surg. 1993;217:721–8.
5. Melby SJ et al. Aortic valve replacement in octogenarians: risk factors for early and late mortality. Ann Thorac Surg. 2007;83:1651–7.
6. Peterson E et al. Outcomes of coronary artery bypass graft surgery in 24, 461 patients aged 80 years or older. Circulation. 1995;92 (9 Suppl):II85–95.
7. Olsson C et al. Thoracic aortic aneurysm and dissection. Increasing prevalence and improved outcomes reported in a nationwide population-based study of more than 14000 cases from 1987–2002. Circulation. 2006;114:2611–8.
8. Clouse WD et al. Improved prognosis of thoracic aortic aneurysms. JAMA. 1998;280:1926–9.
9. Coady MA et al. Surgical intervention criteria for thoracic aortic aneurysm: a study of growth rates and complications. Ann Thorac Surg. 1999;67:1922–6.
10. Coady MA et al. What is the appropriate size criterion for resection of thoracic aortic aneurysm. J Thorac Cardiovasc Surg. 1997;113:476–91.
11. Davies RR et al. Yearly rupture or dissection rates for thoracic aortic aneurysms: simple prediction based on size. Ann Thorac Surg. 2002;73:17–28.
12. Ehrlich MP et al. Predictors of adverse outcome and transient neurological dysfunction after ascending aorta/hemiarch replacement. Ann Thorac Surg. 2000;69:1755–63.
13. Hagl C et al. Neurological outcome after ascending aorta-aortic arch operations: effect of brain protection technique in high-risk patients. J Thorac Cardiovasc Surg. 2001;121:1107–21.
14. Olsson C et al. Surgical and long-term outcome in 2634 consecutive patients operated on the proximal thoracic aorta. Eur J Cardiothorac Surg. 2007;31:963–9.
15. Okita Y et al. Early and long-term results of surgery for aneurysms of the thoracic aorta in septuagenerians and octogenerians. Eur J Cardiothorac Surg. 1999;16:317–23.
16. Hagl C et al. Is aortic surgery using hypothermic circulatory arrest in octogenerians justifiable? Eur J Cardiothorac Surg. 2001;19:417–23.
17. Liddicoat JR et al. Hypothermic circulatory arrest in octogenarians: risk of stroke and mortality. Ann Thorac Surg. 2000;69:1048–52.
18. Shah PJ et al. Analysis of ascending and transverse aortic arch repair in octagenarians. Ann Thorac Surg. 2008;86:774–9.
19. Coselli JS et al. Left heart bypass during descending thoracic aortic aneurysm repair does not reduce the incidence of paraplegia. Ann Thorac Surg. 2004;77:1298–303.
20. Estrera AL et al. Descending thoracic aortic aneurysm: Surgical approach and treatment using the adjuncts cerebrospinal fluid drainage and distal aortic perfusion. Ann Thorac Surg. 2001;72:481–6.
21. Conrad MF et al. Thoracoabdominal aneurysm repair: a 20 year perspective. Ann Thorac Surg. 2007;83:S856–61.
22. Coselli JS, Bozinovski J, LeMarie S. Open surgical repair of 2286 thoracoabdominal aortic aneurysms. Ann Thorac Surg. 2007;83:S862–4.
23. Huynh TTT et al. Thoracoabdominal and descending thoracic aortic aneurysm surgery in patients aged 79 years or older. J Vasc Surg. 2002;36:469–75.
24. Girardi LN, Coselli JS. Repair of thoracoabdominal aortic aneurysm in octogenarians. Ann Thorac Surg. 1998;65:491–5.
25. Cowan JJ et al. Surgical treatment of intact thoracoabdominal aortic aneurysms in the United States: hospital and surgeon volume-related outcomes. J Vasc Surg. 2003;37:1169–74.
26. Rigberg DA et al. Thirty-day mortality statistics underestimate the risk of repair of thoracoabdominal aortic aneurysm: a statewide experience. J Vasc Surg. 2006;43:217–23.
27. Tittle SL et al. Midterm follow-up of penetrating ulcer and intramural hematoma of the aorta. J Thorac Cardiovasc Surg. 2002;123(6):1051–9.
28. Cho KR et al. Penetrating atherosclerotic ulcer of the descending thoracic aorta and arch. J Thorac Cardiovasc Surg. 2004;127(5):1393–401.
29. Demers P et al. Stent-graft repair of penetrating atherosclerotic ulcers in the descending thoracic aorta: mid-term results. Ann Thorac Surg. 2004;77:81–6.
30. Golledge J, Eagle KA. Acute aortic dissection. Lancet. 2008;372:55–66.
31. Anagnopoulos C, Prabhakar M, Kittle C. Aortic dissections and dissecting aneurysm. Am J Cardiol. 1972;30:263–73.
32. Erasmi A et al. Up to 7 years' experience with valve-sparing aortic root remodeling/reimplantation for acute type A aortic dissection. Ann Thorac Surg. 2003;76:99–104.
33. Geirsson A et al. Fate of the residual distal and proximal aorta after acute type A dissection repair using a contemporary surgical reconstruction algorithm. Ann Thorac Surg. 2007;84:1955–64.
34. Hagan PG et al. The international registry of acute aortic dissection (IRAD): new insights into an old disease. JAMA. 2000;283(7):897–903.
35. Kirsch M et al. Risk factor analysis for proximal and distal reoperations after surgery for acute type A aortic dissection. J Thorac Cardiovasc Surg. 2002;123:318–25.
36. Sabik J et al. Long-term effectiveness of operations for ascending aortic dissections. J Thorac Cardiovasc Surg. 2000;119:946–62.
37. Neri E et al. Operation for acute type A aortic dissectio nin octogenarians: is it justified. J Thorac Cardiovasc Surg. 2001;121:259–67.
38. Piccardo A et al. Outcomes after surgical treatment for type A acute aortic dissection in octagenarians: a multicenter study. Ann Thorac Surg. 2009;88:491–7.
39. Shiono M et al. Emergency surgery for acute type A aortic dissection in octogenarians. Ann Thorac Surg. 2006;82:554–9.
40. Hata M et al. Should emergency surgical intervention be performed for an octogenerian with type A aortic dissection? J Thorac Cardiovasc Surg. 2008;135:1042–6.
41. Mehta RH et al. Acute type A aortic dissection in the elderly: clinical characteristics, management, and outcomes in the current era. J Am Coll Cardiol. 2002;40:685–92.

42. Caus T et al. Clinical outcome after repair of acute type A dissection in patients over 70 years-old. Eur J Cardiothorac Surg. 2002;22:211–7.

43. Chiappini B et al. Surgery for acute type A aortic dissection: is advanced age a contraindication? Ann Thorac Surg. 2004;78: 585–90.

44. Shrestha M et al. Is treatment of acute type A aortic dissection in septuagenarians justifiable. Asian Cardiovasc Thorac ann. 2008;16: 33–6.

45. Augoustides JG et al. Observational study of mortality risk stratification by ischemic presentation in patients with acute type A aortic dissection: the Penn classification. Nat Clin Pract Cardiovasc Med. 2009;6:1–7.

46. Geirsson A et al. Significance of malperfusion syndromes prior to contemporary surgical repair for acute type A dissection: outcomes and need for additional revascularizations. Eur J Cardiothorac Surg. 2007;32:255–62.

47. McKneally MF. "We don't do that here": Reflections of the Siena experience wtih dissection aneurysms of the thoracic aorta in octogenarians. J Thorac Cardiovasc Surg. 2001;121:202–3.

48. Mehta RH et al. Acute type B aortic dissection in elderly patients: clinical features, outcome, and simple risk stratification rule. Ann Thorac Surg. 2004;77:1622–9.

49. Trimarchi S et al. Role and results of surgery in acute type B aortic dissection: insights from the international registry of acute aortic dissection (IRAD). Circulation. 2006;114(1 suppl): I357–64.

50. Parker JD, Golledge J. Outcome of endovascular treatmetn of acute type B aortic dissection. Ann Thorac Surg. 2008;86:1707–12.

51. Maraj R et al. Meta-analysis of 143 reported cases of aortic intramural hemotoma. Am J Cardiol. 2000;86:661–8.

52. Porcellini M et al. Intramural hematoma of the thoracic aorta in octogenarians: is non operation justified? Eur J Cardiothorac Surg. 1999;16:414–7.

53. Dake MD et al. Transluminal placement of endovascular stent-grafts for the treatment of descending thoracic aortic aneurysms. N Engl J Med. 1994;331(26):1729–34.

54. Conrad MF, Cambria RP. Contemporary management of descending throacic and thoracoabdominal aortic aneurysm: endovascular versus open. Circulation. 2008;117:841–52.

55. Orandi BJ et al. A population-based analysis of endovascular versus open thoracic aortic aneurysm repair. J Vasc Surg. 2009;49:1112–6.

56. Walsh SR et al. Endovascular stenting versus open surgery for thoracic aortic disease: systematic review and meta-analysis of perioperative results. J Vasc Surg. 2008;47:1094–8.

57. Demers P et al. Midterm results of endovascular repair of descending thoracic aortic aneurysms with first-generation stent grafts. J Thorac Cardiovasc Surg. 2004;127(3):664–73.

58. Patel HJ et al. Survival benefit of endovascular descending thoracic aortic repair for the high-risk patient. Ann Thorac Surg. 2007;83: 1628–34.

59. Kern JA et al. Thoracic aortic endografting is the treatment of choice for elderly patients with thoraic aortic disease. Annals of Surgery. 2006;243:815–23.

60. Kpodonu J et al. Endovascular repair of the thoracic aorta in octogenerians. Eur J Cardiothorac Surg. 2008;34:630–4.

61. Patel HJ et al. A comparison of open and endovascular descending thoracic aortic repair in patients older than 75 years of age. Ann Thorac Surg. 2008;85:1597–604.

62. McKneally MF. "We didn't expect dementia and diapers": reflection on the Nihon experience with type A dissection in octogenarians. J Thorac Cardiovasc Surg. 2008;135:984–5.

Chapter 34
Surgical Treatment of Pericardial Disease in the Elderly

Joshua Kindelan and Alberto de Hoyos

Abstract Published data on pericardial disease in the elderly population are scarce. There are microanatomic changes that occur with aging that reduce the elasticity of the pericardial sac, which are presumed to make the elderly more hemodynamically sensitive to the ill effects of pericardial effusion. Certain diseases, such as postpericardiotomy syndrome, Dressler's syndrome, and neoplasms, are more frequently seen in the elderly patients. Although not historically a disease of the elderly, constrictive pericarditis is becoming just that due to a shift in etiology away from tuberculosis in much of the industrialized world. Optimal management of any pericardial disease in the elderly must take into account frequent and occasionally severe comorbidities, as well as occasionally complex social situations requiring careful hospital discharge planning.

Keywords Cardiac tamponade • Constrictive pericarditis • Echocardiography in acute tamponade • Echocardiography in constrictive pericarditis • Pericardial effusion • Pericardial neoplasm • Pericardiectomy(f) • Pericardiocentesis (f) • Pericarditis • Pericardium • Postpericardiectomy syndromes

Anatomy

The visceral pericardium is made up of a thin monocellular serosal layer, while the thicker parietal pericardium is composed of a fibrous outer layer covered with a lining of the same monocellular serosal layer that comprises the visceral pericardium. The serosal layer is composed of mesothelial cells, while the fibrosa is composed of fibrocollagenous tissue that demonstrates age-related decreases in the "waviness" of collagen bundles and elastin content [1]. Therefore, it is expected that the pericardium will become less forgiving of volume increases as a person ages [2].

J. Kindelan (✉)
Northwestern University, Feinberg School of Medicine, Chicago, Illinois Fellow, Division of Cardiothoracic Surgery, USA
e-mail: joshua.kindelan@yahoo.com

The pericardial reflection is at the base of the heart in association with the great vessels. This serosal reflection forms sinuses to allow passage of vessels. The transverse sinus is between the aorta and the pulmonary artery trunk and the atria, while the oblique sinus allows entry of the vena cavae and pulmonary veins [2].

The inferior and anterior parietal pericardium is fixed at the diaphragm and sternum by the pericardiophrenic and sternopericardial ligaments, while the posterior pericardium is anchored by loose connective tissue to the posterior mediastinum [3].

The arterial blood supply to the pericardium derives from the pericardiophrenic branches of the internal thoracic arteries and small aortic branches. The venous drainage is via pericardiophrenic veins that drain into the brachiocephalic veins [3].

Innervation of the pericardium is mainly through the phrenic nerve, while the vagus nerves contribute some posterior branches [2].

The pericardium normally contains between 20 and 60 mL of serous fluid [1]. Radiographic enlargement of the cardiac silhouette usually does not occur until more than 250 mL of fluid is present [4]. Smaller amount can be detected by echocardiogram, computed tomography (CT), or magnetic resonance (MR).

Physiology

Pericardial physiology is relatively complex, but can be simplified by defining its three general functions: mechanical, membranous, and ligamentous. The mechanical functions of the pericardium include limiting acute chamber dilation and maintaining normal ventricular compliance. The membranous function includes reducing external friction and creating a barrier to inflammation. The ligamentous function serves to limit cardiac displacement [2].

The pericardium does have a small capacitance reserve of approximately 150–250 mL in which only small increases in intrapericardial pressure will accompany increases in fluid accumulation [3]. Beyond this capacitance reserve, the intrapericardial pressure increases exponentially with even small increases in volume, interfering with mechanical myocardial function. Compensatory mechanisms are set in motion that delay or prevent the development of clinical tamponade [5], explaining the occurrence of acute tamponade with saline instillation into experimental animals' pericardia of 200–300 mL of fluid [6], while chronic effusions may contain two liters without demonstrating signs of tamponade [5].

Pericardial Diseases

Acute Pericarditis

The causes of acute pericarditis comprise an extensive list, some of which are more common in the elderly. Among the causes of acute pericarditis in the general population are infections such as tuberculosis, streptococcus, staphylococcus, coxsackie virus, vasculitides and other connective-tissue diseases, neoplasms, trauma, metabolic problems such as uremia or gout, postpericardiotomy syndrome, and pulmonary embolism [4, 7]. In the past, the cause was rarely identified; however, the diagnostic yield has improved to the point that only about 30% of cases remain idiopathic [4]. Some causes of acute pericarditis that are more specific to an elderly population are primary and secondary malignancy, postinfraction pericarditis (Dressler's syndrome), and postpericardiotomy syndrome following median sternotomy and cardiac operations [7].

Diagnosis of acute pericarditis in the elderly population is complicated by the overlap of symptoms of pericarditis and acute myocardial infarction (AMI). The pleuritic nature of the chest pain in pericarditis is unusual in AMI. Ischemic myocardial pain is not exacerbated by movement as is the pain of acute pericarditis. Chest pain from pericarditis is exacerbated by laying supine and relieved by leaning forward. Unlike in ischemia, nitrates do not alleviate the pain of pericarditis. Pericardial friction rub is pathognomonic for pericarditis but is not heard in all, or even most cases [8]. Myocardial enzymes can be elevated in both pericarditis and AMI making their specificity unreliable. The 12-lead electrocardiogram is probably the most useful diagnostic modality. In the earliest stage of acute pericarditis, the ECG will demonstrate elevated j-point, upward concave ST elevations, and the corresponding PR depression [9].

Pericardiocentesis with fluid evaluation in the setting of pericarditis is indicated for cardiac tamponade, purulent pericarditis, suspicion of malignancy, or for diagnostic clarification. The fluid evaluation should include glucose, lactate dehydrogenase, protein, cell count, gram stain, bacterial and viral cultures, staining for acid-fast bacilli and cytology. Immunohistochemistry techniques may help clarify autoimmune causes. Adenosine deaminase activity is diagnostic for tuberculosis [10], while carcinoembryonic antigen elevations are quite specific for malignant pericarditis [11].

The basic first-line treatment of noninfectious acute pericarditis is nonsteroidal antiinflammatory drugs (NSAIDS). Ibuprofen is a good first choice, while colchicine is a useful adjunct for recurrent disease. Colchicine is also an acceptable alternative for those who cannot tolerate NSAIDS [10]. Indomethacine is effective but is associated with an increased risk of cardiovascular events [12]. Corticosteroids have been shown to decrease the amount of effusion and effusion recurrence in the treatment of tuberculous pericarditis [13]. Otherwise, corticosteroids should be reserved for pericarditides caused by diseases specifically treated with steroids and severe pericarditis resistant to NSAIDS [9]. Pericardial drainage is not routinely indicated for pericarditis complicated by effusion except for purulent pericarditis, large effusions refractory to medical therapy, persistent unexplained effusions (>3 months), tuberculous effusions, or tamponade [14].

Complications of acute pericarditis are effusion recurrence, tamponade, and constrictive pericarditis. Recurrent pericarditis occurs in 30% of patients, and can be seen after Dressler's and postpericardiotomy syndromes [10]. Colchicine is recommended in recurrent disease [15]. Pericardiectomy may ultimately be required for recurrent disease refractory to nonsurgical therapy.

Constrictive Pericarditis

Constrictive pericarditis is defined as thickened, scarred, often calcified pericardium that limits diastolic ventricular filling [16]. Processes that can result in acute pericarditis can eventually cause constrictive pericarditis. Common causes include infection (especially tuberculosis), radiation therapy, postcardiac surgical procedures, traumatic hemopericardium, neoplasm, and renal failure [14]. In the last few decades, there has been a shift to more iatrogenic causes than infectious etiologies [17]. Because of this shift in etiology from tuberculosis to postcardiac surgery and mediastinal irradiation [3], the median age of patients with constrictive pericarditis has increased from 45 to 61 years [17]. This shift in demographics to an older population with more comorbidities increases the risk of pericardiectomy. Advanced age has been shown to be an independent predictor of decreased late survival following pericardiectomy. In addition, certain etiologies independently may increase the risk of pericardiectomy as is the case with mantle irradiation [17].

The crucial diagnostic task is to distinguish between constrictive pericarditis and restrictive cardiomyopathy. This requires a multimodality diagnostic evaluation, including clinical presentation, echocardiography, some form of axial imaging, endomyocardial biopsy, and cardiac catheterization as indicated.

The signs and symptoms of constrictive pericarditis are essentially those of right heart failure and include peripheral edema (76%), abdominal swelling, gastrointestinal symptoms related to hepatic and bowel congestion, elevated jugular venous pulsations (93%), hepatomegaly (53%), ascites (37%), S3 heart sound (47%), concomitant left heart failure (69%), and exertional dyspnea [3, 17].

Classic echocardiographic findings that differentiate constrictive pericarditis from restrictive cardiomyopathy are dramatic respiratory variations in mitral inflow and pulmonary vein flow. These findings are present only in constrictive pericarditis. Combining newer modalities of color M-mode echo and doppler echo with transesophageal echo has resulted in improved percentage of correct diagnoses from 74 to 95%. On transesophageal echocardiography, a respiratory variation ≥18% for peak pulmonary vein diastolic flow velocity is 79% sensitive, and 91% specific for constrictive pericarditis, while a respiratory variation ≥ 10% for peak early mitral filling is 84% sensitive, and 94% specific for constrictive pericrditis. On M-mode echocardiography, a first aliasing slope ≥100 cm/s has a sensitivity of 74%, and specificity of 94% for constrictive pericarditis. Finally, on doppler echocardiography, a peak early velocity of longitudinal axis mitral annulus expansion ≥8 cm/s is 89% sensitive, and 100% specific for constrictive pericarditis [18].

Axial imaging with CT or MR is not diagnostic of constrictive pericarditis but provides supporting evidence for the diagnosis and can be used to ensure that no concomitant thoracic pathology is present. CT typically demonstrates calcification associated with constrictive pericarditis, as will MRI but without the use of iodinated contrast or ionizing radiation [19].

Hemodynamic testing in the cardiac catheterization laboratory can provide several characteristic findings of constrictive pericarditis, the most reliable of which is ventricular discordance. This is demonstrated by a reciprocal increase in RV and decrease in LV pressure on inspiration due to fixed cardiac volume caused by the constrictive disease process [3].

Endomyocardial biopsy is utilized to evaluate for restrictive cardiomyopathy [20].

Treatment for constrictive pericarditis is ultimately surgical; however, medical therapy plays a limited but important role. Pericardial constriction may improve or resolve within a few months of development; although early operation is considered, a period of observation should be recommended to allow spontaneous resolution. Medical therapy consists of NSAIDS, corticosteroids, and antibiotics [21]. Surgical treatment consists of radical pericardiectomy (Figs. 34.1 and 34.2). Heart

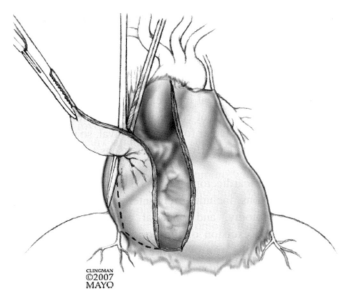

Fig. 34.1 Pericardiectomy for constrictive pericarditis. Anterior dissection (from Villavicencio et al. [24], reprinted by permission of Mayo Foundation for Medical Education and Research. All rights reserved)

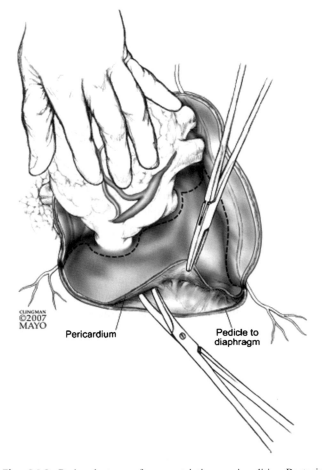

Pericardium   Pedicle to diaphragm

Fig. 34.2 Pericardectomy for constrictive pericarditis. Posterior dissection (from Villavicencio et al. [24], reprinted by permission of Mayo Foundation for Medical Education and Research. All rights reserved)

13. Dooley DP, Carpenter JL, Rademacher S. Adjunctive corticosteroid therapy for tuberculosis: a critical reappraisal of the literature. Clin Infect Dis. 1997;25(4):872–87.

14. Hoit BD. Management of effusive and constrictive pericardial heart disease. Circulation. 2002;105(25):2939–42.

15. Adler Y, Finkelstein Y, Guindo J, Rodriguez de la Serna A, Shoenfeld Y, Bayes-Genis A, et al. Colchicine treatment for recurrent pericarditis. A decade of experience. Circulation. 1998; 97(21):2183–5.

16. Fowler NO. Constrictive pericarditis: new aspects. Am J Cardiol. 1982;50(5):1014–7.

17. Ling LH, Oh JK, Schaff HV, Danielson GK, Mahoney DW, Seward JB, et al. Constrictive pericarditis in the modern era: evolving clinical spectrum and impact on outcome after pericardiectomy. Circulation. 1999;100(13):1380–6.

18. Rajagopalan N, Garcia MJ, Rodriguez L, Murray RD, Apperson-Hansen C, Stugaard M, et al. Comparison of new Doppler echocardiographic methods to differentiate constrictive pericardial heart disease and restrictive cardiomyopathy. Am J Cardiol. 2001;87(1): 86–94.

19. Wang ZJ, Reddy GP, Gotway MB, Yeh BM, Hetts SW, Higgins CB. CT and MR imaging of pericardial disease. Radiographics. 2003;23 Spec No:S167–80.

20. Schoenfeld MH, Supple EW, Dec Jr GW, Fallon JT, Palacios IF. Restrictive cardiomyopathy versus constrictive pericarditis: role of endomyocardial biopsy in avoiding unnecessary thoracotomy. Circulation. 1987;75(5):1012–7.

21. Oh JK, Hatle LK, Mulvagh SL, Tajik AJ. Transient constrictive pericarditis: diagnosis by two-dimensional Doppler echocardiography. Mayo Clin Proc. 1993;68(12):1158–64.

22. McCaughan BC, Schaff HV, Piehler JM, Danielson GK, Orszulak TA, Puga FJ, et al. Early and late results of pericardiectomy for constrictive pericarditis. J Thorac Cardiovasc Surg. 1985;89(3): 340–50.

23. Chowdhury UK, Subramaniam GK, Kumar AS, Airan B, Singh R, Talwar S, et al. Pericardiectomy for constrictive pericarditis: a clinical, echocardiographic, and hemodynamic evaluation of two surgical techniques. Ann Thorac Surg. 2006;81(2):522–9.

24. Villavicencio MA, Dearani JA, Sundt TM. Op Techs T CV Surg. 2008 Spring 13(1):2–13.

25. Spodick DH. Images in cardiology. Truly total electric alternation of the heart. Clin Cardiol. 1998;21(6):427–8.

26. Spodick DH. Electric alternation of the heart. Its relation to the kinetics and physiology of the heart during cardiac tamponade. Am J Cardiol. 1962;10:155–65.

27. Becit N, Unlü Y, Ceviz M, Koçogullari CU, Koçak H, Gürlertop Y. Subxiphoid pericardiostomy in the management of pericardial effusions: case series analysis of 368 patients. Heart. 2005;91(6):785–90.

28. Allen KB, Faber LP, Warren WH, Shaar CJ. Pericardial effusion: subxiphoid pericardiostomy versus percutaneous catheter drainage. Ann Thorac Surg. 1999;67(2):437–40.

29. Georghiou GP, Stamler A, Sharoni E, Fichman-Horn S, Berman M, Vidne BA, et al. Video-assisted thoracoscopic pericardial window for diagnosis and management of pericardial effusions. Ann Thorac Surg. 2005;80(2):607–10.

30. O'Brien PK, Kucharczuk JC, Marshall MB, Friedberg JS, Chen Z, Kaiser LR, et al. Comparative study of subxiphoid versus video-thoracoscopic pericardial "window". Ann Thorac Surg. 2005; 80(6):2013–9.

31. Asensio JA, Berne JD, Demetriades D, Chan L, Murray J, Falabella A, et al. One hundred five penetrating cardiac injuries: a 2-year prospective evaluation. J Trauma. 1998;44(6):1073–82.

32. Warren WH. Malignancies involving the pericardium. Semin Thorac Cardiovasc Surg. 2000;12(2):119–29.

33. Shepherd FA. Malignant pericardial effusion. Curr Opin Oncol. 1997;9(2):170–4.

34. Maruyama R, Yokoyama H, Seto T, Nagashima S, Kashiwabara K, Araki J, et al. Catheter drainage followed by the instillation of bleomycin to manage malignant pericardial effusion in non-small cell lung cancer: a multi-institutional phase II trial. J Thorac Oncol. 2007;2(1):65–8.

35. Prince SE, Cunha BA. Postpericardiotomy syndrome. Heart Lung. 1997;26(2):165–8.

36. Imazio M, Cecchi E, Trinchero R, COPPS Investigators. Colchicine for the prevention of the postpericardiotomy syndrome: the COPPS trial. Int J Cardiol. 2007;121(2):198–9.

Chapter 35
Pacemakers and Implantable Cardioverter Defibrillators in the Elderly

Luciana Armaganijan and Jeff S. Healey

Abstract Permanent pacemakers, implantable cardioverter defibrillators (ICDs) and cardiac resynchronization (CRT) devices are commonly used in the management of cardiovascular disease. Sick sinus syndrome and atrio-ventricular block are the two most common indications for permanent pacemaker implantation, representing more than 90% of the cases, and are both strongly associated with increasing age. Understanding the cardiovascular physiology among elderly patients is critical to the selection of the optimal surgical technique and reduction of complications. In this chapter, the role of pacemakers, ICDs, CRTs as well as technical issues for cardiac rhythm device implantation, including risk of device-related complications and appropriate programming in elderly patients, is discussed.

Keywords Pacemaker • Implantable cardioverter-defibrillator • Cardiac resynchronization • Elderly • Epidemiology • Complications randomized trials

Introduction

Permanent pacemakers, implantable cardioverter defibrillators (ICDs) and cardiac resynchronization devices are commonly used in the management of cardiovascular disease. There is abundant clinical evidence that these devices either improve patients' symptoms, improve their survival, or both [1–4]. As with other surgical interventions, clinicians carefully consider the use of these technologies in elderly patients, paying particular attention to the likelihood that elderly patients will derive a similar benefit to patients evaluated in clinical trials, the potential for an increased risk of adverse outcomes in the elderly, technical issues of surgery specific to the elderly and the possible unique roles for these

devices in elderly patients. However, age is not unique and is just one of many important patient characteristics. For example, patient gender and a history of renal insufficiency requiring dialysis are also strong predictors of adverse outcomes in patients receiving ICDs [5, 6]. Thus, clinicians must always consider the totality of each patient's medical history, demographic information and prior interventions when contemplating any medical surgical interventions.

Epidemiology of Pacemaker and Implantable Cardioverter Defibrillator Use

The use of both pacemakers and ICDs is more common with advancing age, although this is particularly true for pacemakers. Surveys have shown that up to 80% of pacemakers are implanted in the elderly [7, 8] and the average age of pacemaker recipients in the randomized trials of pacing mode was 75 ± 10 years [1]. This is not surprising as sick sinus syndrome and atrio-ventricular block are the two most common indications for permanent pacemaker implantation, representing more than 90% of the cases [7] and are both strongly associated with increasing age. Also, there are additional indications for pacing such as carotid sinus hypersensitivity and non-accidental falls which although much less prevalent, are strongly associated with increasing age [9, 10]. As a result of this epidemiology, it would be fair to consider any discussion about the role of pacemakers in general to be highly representative of their role in the elderly. As opposed to the evaluation of many new medical and surgical interventions, the majority of patients in pacemaker trials are elderly, thus, there is little or no concern about the application of the results of pacemaker trials to elderly patients. In fact, some pacing trials such as PASE [11] and UK-PACE [12] restricted enrolment to elderly patients. Thus, in interpreting the results of pacemaker trials, one should generally reverse the usual way of thinking about "how do the results of this trial apply to elderly patients?" and consider "how do the results of this pacemaker trial apply to the young?"

L. Armaganijan (✉)
Department of Medicine, McMaster University,
237 Barton Street East, Hamilton, ON L8L2X2, Canada
e-mail: luciana_va@hotmail.com

M.R. Katlic (ed.), *Cardiothoracic Surgery in the Elderly*, DOI 10.1007/978-1-4419-0892-6_35,
© Springer Science+Business Media, LLC 2011

Table 35.2 Implant complication rates by age group. Previously unpublished data from the meta-analysis of clinical trials of pacing mode [1]

Complication	Age <75 years (n = 1,790) (%)	Age ≥75 years (n = 3,024) (%)	p value
Pneumothorax	0.8	1.6	0.07
Hematoma	0.2	0.2	0.97
Lead dislodgment	0.9	1.7	0.11
Loss of capture	0.2	0.5	0.08
Pacemaker infection	0.7	0.9	0.52
Peri-operative death	0.7	0.5	0.55
Any implant complication[a]	3.4	5.1	0.006

[a]May be more than one per patient

Table 35.3 Late issues following pacemaker implantation based on age: previously unpublished data from the meta-analysis of clinical trials of pacing mode [1]

Complication	Age <75 years (n = 1,790) (%)	Age ≥75 years (n = 3,024) (%)	p value
Lead fracture	3.6	2.7	0.08
Need for generator replacement	3.7	2.2	0.008

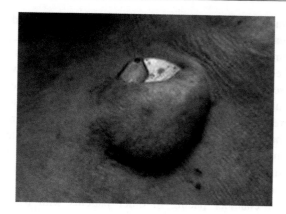

Fig. 35.1 Example of skin erosion in a patient with pacemaker

illnesses that may limit their life-expectancy, so their pacemaker or ICD system does not have time to experience chronic system issues such as battery depletion or lead insulation failure. In the case of lead fracture, the elderly may also be at lower risk of this complication anyway, as their limited mobility and lower body mass exert less stress on their leads, causing less breakdown of insulation.

In elderly patients, several issues must be considered in selecting the appropriate location for a pulse generator, particularly for an ICD, as the size of the generator is much larger. Many elderly patients have arthritis, other orthopedic issues or prior stroke and it is not uncommon that elderly patients have limited use of one of their upper extremities. In such cases, it is usually wise to implant the new pacemaker or ICD on the side with the limitation, as implantation on the contra-lateral side could significantly disable the patient (at times with loss of independence) during the early post-operative period. At this time, their mobility on the side of the pacemaker or ICD will be limited by both pain as well as the restriction in range of motion prescribed to reduce the risk of lead dislodgement. Perhaps the only exception to this rule would be a patient who is actively undergoing rehabilitation of an upper extremity with the hope of significant recovery of function. In such a case, the implantation of a pulse generator could impede their progress.

The next issue with cardiac rhythm device implantation is the selection of the optimal tissue plane for the pulse-generator, either sub-cutaneous or sub-pectoral. In general, sub-cutaneous implantation is preferred as it is simpler, causes less pain during the implant procedure and is associated with

a lower risk of late complications such as generator migration and generator compromise/header separation [49]. However, many elderly patients may be quite thin, without sufficient sub-cutaneous tissue to avoid generator erosion and associated infection (Fig. 35.1). In the PASE trial, which compared single versus dual-chamber pacing among elderly patients, skin erosion and pocket infection occurred in 1% of patients. If there is any concern about potential of skin erosion, it is generally preferable to implant the pulse generator in the sub-pectoral position. The risk of generator/header damage in the sub-pectoral position is probably lower in elderly patients as they have substantial less force exerted on the generator by their pectoral muscles than in younger, more robust patients. Also, accessing the sub-pectoral plane in elderly patients is often easier than in younger patients as there is much less muscle mass to traverse. Finally, if the generator is placed in the sub-pectoral position, care should be taken to suture the header to the fascia as generator migration is otherwise common in this plane.

Another option to facilitate successful placement of a pulse generator in a thin elderly patient is to implant a smaller device. Most pacemaker manufacturers do make smaller sized pacemakers by limiting the size (and hence longevity) of the battery. However, in elderly patients, limitation in battery life may not be a major concern, particularly if the patient is very old, has a limited life-expectancy or is predicted to require very little pacing during follow-up. Even with the devices of the 1980s and 1990s, up to 50% of implanted pacemakers would "out-live" the patients in whom they were implanted [50]. Thus, the rationale use of small-volume, "short-life" pacemakers in properly selected, thin elderly patients is a reasonable strategy.

The next consideration for cardiac rhythm device implant is venous access. There is a higher rate of pneumothorax in elderly patients (Table 35.2), particularly those who are small, have chronic lung disease or are agitated/confused at the time of implantation. Pneumothorax (Fig. 35.2) was the second most common complication among the elderly patients in the

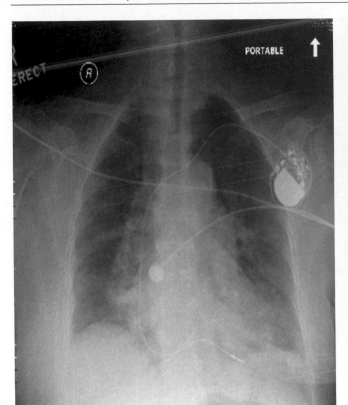

Fig. 35.2 Chest X-ray showing large left pneumothorax post pacemaker insertion

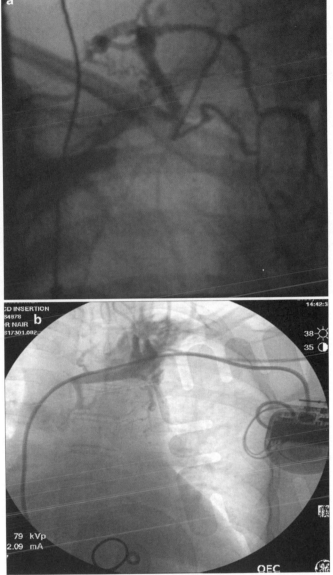

Fig. 35.3 (**a**, **b**) Right sub-clavian vein and left sub-clavian vein-SVC junction occlusion in same patient

PASE trial, occurring in 2% of patients [11]. Risk factors included age over 75 ($p=0.01$) and lower body mass indices ($p=0.04$). Females also exhibited a trend toward an increased risk of pneumothorax ($p=0.07$). Although it was seen only in cases of sub-clavian venous access, there was no significant difference between sub-clavian and cephalic approaches (chi-square, $p=0.21$); however, this was likely an issue of low statistical power, as relatively few implants were done via the cephalic vein [11]. Multivariate analysis showed older age to be the main risk factor ($p=0.04$) [7]. Notwithstanding the results of PASE [11], many implanters attempt to minimize the risk of pneumothorax by implanting leads via the cephalic vein or via the axillary vein, with or without the use of ultrasound or micro-puncture techniques to facilitate safe placement. However, in elderly patients it is not infrequent that the cephalic vein may be too small to accept a lead or is thrombosed.

Once the venous system is accessed, the state of the sub-clavian, inominate vein and superior vena cava must be assessed. In elderly patients, these vessels (particularly the former two) often have a serpiginous course, which is felt to be the result of folding of these vessels in response to loss of vertebral height with advancing age. This may result in challenges advancing a lead to the heart and maintaining torque control once there. Also, appreciation of this tortuosity is

important as it may be quite dynamic and as the vessel "straightens" when the patient stands up, the amount of "redundant" lead in the vessel may decrease significantly, even to the point of causing lead dislodgement.

Another challenge with venous access is the issue of venous obstruction in patients with existing cardiac rhythm devices who require lead replacement or system up-grade (Fig. 35.3a, b). These patients are often elderly as they would have survived long-enough after their initial implant to have depleted their battery or suffered lead fracture. In such cases, lead extraction or venoplasty (Fig. 35.4) can be used to overcome the obstruction; however, in the frail elderly, one must appreciate that there may be an increased risk of complications with these more aggressive interventions [51]. Thus, in

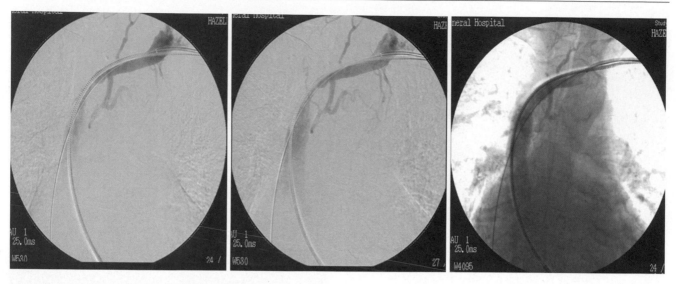

Fig. 35.4 Successful relief of obstruction with venoplasty

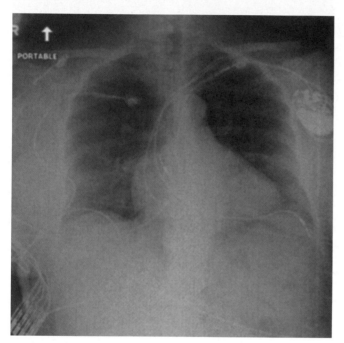

Fig. 35.5 Lead perforation

certain cases, it may be preferable to insert a new device on the contra-lateral side if this is feasible.

Lead perforation is another complication which may be more common in elderly patients. Although uncommon, lead perforation is an important and potential fatal complication (Fig. 35.5) and may be more frequent in the elderly due to a thin-walled right ventricle. In the PASE trial, 1% of elderly patients experienced lead perforation [11]. In a large cohort series, the risk factors for perforation included older age, presence of a temporary trans-venous pacemaker, body mass index <20 kg/m², recent right ventricular infarction, use of an active-fixation lead, steroid therapy and longer fluoroscopy

time (probably indicative of the need to repeatedly deploy the helix in an attempt to find a good pacing site) [52]. Right ventricular systolic pressure >35 mmHg was protective. In elderly patients with additional risk factors for perforation, the use of passive fixation leads or the placement of active-fixation leads in a septal position may help mitigate this risk.

Implantable Cardioverter Defibrillators in Elderly Patients

There is now robust clinical trial evidence that implantable cardioverter defibrillators prolong life in patients with a history of sustained ventricular arrhythmias or with severe left ventricular dysfunction [3, 13, 53]. However, these devices are expensive [54] and are associated with important peri-operative and long-term complications and inconvenience [55, 56]. Furthermore, with the exception of cardiac resynchronization devices [4], they do not improve quality of life. For these reasons, many have questioned the value of these devices, particularly for primary prevention, among elderly individuals.

This debate centers on several key issues: (1) Do elderly patients derive the same benefit from an ICD as younger patients? (2) Are elderly patients at increased risk of dying from non-arrhythmic causes? (3) Is quality of life the same among elderly recipients as younger patients and are the complications and inconveniences of ICD therapy more significant among elderly patients? (4) Do elderly view the potential risk of sudden death differently than younger patients?

In interpreting studies of the ICD in "elderly" patients, it is important to note the differences in age used to define "elderly" as there is no standard, and various reports have used anything from 65 to 80 years [14, 57]. The lower the cut-off used, the more likely the "elderly" patient group will be similar to the younger group and to the overall results of the study. Conversely, a very high cut-off will certainly define a unique group of patients; however, the number of patients studied in such a group is likely to be small, limiting any inferences.

In patients with a history of ventricular tachycardia or cardiac arrest, the three main clinical trials, AVID, CIDS and CASH, demonstrate a 30% reduction in all-cause mortality, which is driven by a 50% reduction is arrhythmic death [53]. Among these three trials, there were 252 patients ≥75 years old [57]. This represents only 13% of patients enrolled in these three trials. Compared to younger patients, those ≥75 years old were twice as likely to die of both non-arrhythmic death (8.74% per year vs. 3.96% per year, $p = 0.001$) and arrhythmic death (6.73% per year vs. 3.84% per year, $p = 0.03$) [57]. Their excess in non-arrhythmic death was due to both an increase in heart failure death and non-cardiac death [57]. When one looks at the benefit of ICD therapy by age group, although there is no significant statistical interaction between age <75 and ≥75 years (suggesting a similar treatment benefit in both groups), it is provocative that, among patients ≥75 years, there is no observed reduction in all-cause mortality (HR = 1.06, 95% CI: 0.69–1.64, $p = 0.79$) or even arrhythmic mortality (HR = 0.90, 95% CI: 0.42–1.95, $p = 0.79$) with ICD therapy.

The data from these three trials do not suggest that ICD therapy should be withheld from patients based on age alone; however, they do suggest that physicians should carefully consider a patient's overall prognosis and specifically the risk of non-arrhythmic death before recommending an ICD. It is well known that the ratio of arrhythmic to all-cause mortality decreases with age from 0.51 at age 50 to 0.26 after age 80 [58]; thus, as the ICD is only effective against arrhythmic mortality, the likelihood of an ICD reducing all-cause mortality is lower among elderly patients. The implication is that, in some elderly patients who have survived a cardiac arrest, co-morbidities may make the risk of non-arrhythmic death so high that withholding ICD therapy could be justified on the basis that it is unlikely to offer the patient a meaningful likelihood of improved survival.

Data on the use of the ICD for primary prevention among elderly patients paint a slightly different picture [14]. In the MADIT-II trial, there were 204 patients ≥75 years old, and those randomized to receive an ICD experienced a 46% reduction in the relative risk of all-cause mortality [14]. Conversely, data from the SCD-HeFT [13] and COMPANION [2] trials do not show a clear reduction in all-cause mortality among the small numbers of patients ≥65 years old. How does one reconcile the seemingly disparate results of all these analyses? First, it should be appreciated that the total number of elderly patients included in these secondary analyses is small,

and thus statistical play of chance could explain many of the differences. However, it is quite plausible that it is differences in the patient populations studied that account for this heterogeneity of outcome differences and that understanding the differences in populations can lead the clinician to an understanding of how to use the data.

The COMPANION and SCD-HeFT trials were trials of patients with advanced heart failure symptoms, thus patients at high risk of both arrhythmic but, more importantly, heart failure mortality. Thus, it is not surprising that elderly patients in heart failure trials may not have derived as much benefit from the ICD as they were likely to die of heart failure, relatively soon after enrolment. In contrast, 71% of patients in MADIT-II had NYHA class I or II [3] and were, therefore, at lower risk of non-arrhythmic, heart failure death. Also, as MADIT-II was a primary prevention trial, it is highly likely that elderly patients recruited for this study were selected from the healthier, more active patients in the practices of participating physicians and are not representative of the general population of elderly patients with severe left-ventricular dysfunction. This is in contrast to the secondary prevention trials [57] where patients were in-hospital survivors of cardiac arrest or sustained ventricular arrhythmias, thus less likely to have undergone the same degree of selection as for primary prevention, where recruitment is generally in the outpatient setting.

Taken together, these data suggest that properly selected elderly patients may derive similar relative benefits from the ICD as younger patients. Results from observational registries suggest that this is this case [59–61]. However, care should be taken not to overstate the benefits of the ICD among elderly patients with severe co-morbidities and limited prognosis. Although there is a tendency among the elderly not to recommend the ICD for primary prevention but to always consider for secondary prevention, the data would suggest a different approach: that in carefully selected elderly patients, the ICD may be useful in primary prevention but, in poorly selected secondary prevention patients, the ICD may be of no benefit. Thus, the medical history and functional status of patients should dictate the appropriate place for ICD therapy, not simply the age of the patient.

Finally, although ICD therapy may prolong life in appropriately selected elderly patients, one must also consider the quality of that patient's life and their preferences with respect to therapy. Elderly patients are often afflicted by conditions that may be painful, limit their mobility and social interaction and overall quality of life. Thus, even if ICD therapy can prolong life, the reduction in quality of life results in ICD therapy not being cost-effective [54]. As such, society would deem this to be inappropriate use of scarce health-care resources. Still, more importantly, the patient in question may also feel that ICD therapy is undesired. Depending on their quality of life, elderly patients may be more likely to decline appropriately indicated ICD therapy as they may perceive a sudden, arrhythmic death to be preferable to a non-sudden death, or even continued life with significant pain or disability. Their views on death will also be heavily influenced by issues such as lack of dependents, loss of spouse, diminished social network and the need for institutional care.

Appropriate Programming of Pacemakers and Defibrillators in Elderly Patients

Differences in the physiology and habits of elderly individuals require a tailored approach to the appropriate selection and programming of pacemakers and implantable defibrillators. The key issues are reduced activity levels, lower peak sinus heart rate, higher prevalence of sinus node and atrioventricular node dysfunction and higher incidence of atrial arrhythmias such as atrial fibrillation [62].

A patient's anticipated peak heart rate is inversely correlated with advancing age, approximated by the formula: 220 beats/minute minus their age in years. Accordingly, elderly patients will require programming of lower upper-tracking rates (for dual-chamber devices) and upper sensor rates (for those with the rate response function activated). Although there is clearly variability between individual elderly patients, an upper tracking rate of 110–120 beats/minute is reasonable for most. The issue of rate-response sensor activation is also age specific. As the majority of current devices use accelerometer-based sensors for their rate-response function, patients must be active to cause the pacemaker to accelerate. However, activity levels among elderly patients are often quite reduced, particularly in those requiring institutional care. Such patients would not generally have any modulation of pacing rate due to lack of activity. Even if these sensors did produce a modulation of heart rate, the benefits associated with this rate-response are not all that clear. In an observational, secondary analysis of the CTOPP trial, although the use of rate-response sensor did result in a significant, albeit very small 2–3 beat/minute increase in heart rate while performing a 6-min hall walk test, this did not translate into an increased in the distance walked [63].

Even more striking are the results from the UK-PACE trial, which enrolled patients with a mean age of 80 years (and restricted enrolment to those over 70 years) [12]. These trial randomized patients between dual-chamber pacing, single-chamber/rate-adaptive pacing and fixed-rate single chamber pacing and found no differences between the three groups with respect to mortality and the majority of clinical outcomes studied. However, UK-PACE did suggest a trend toward an early increase in atrial fibrillation with dual-chamber pacing and a trend towards an increased risk

stroke/thrombo-embolism/TIA among patients assigned to fixed-rate ventricular pacing [12]. The discordance of these secondary outcomes may simply reflect the statistical play of chance, and the totality of the results from UK-PACE suggest no clear benefit in important clinical events with the use of more complex pacing systems in elderly patients. Thus, the selection of the appropriate mode should be based on patient-specific factors such as the presence of normal sinus rhythm, activity levels and other factors.

For the programming of both ICDs and pacemakers, it is important to understand that the risk of atrial fibrillation increases with age and may exceed 10% in patients over the age of 80 years [62]. For this reason, particular care must be taken to program on mode-switching, to avoid inappropriate tracking of atrial tachy-arrhythmias and, in the case of ICDs, the use of SVT-discrimination algorithms to avoid inappropriate shocks.

Conclusions

The use of pacemakers, implantable-cardioverter defibrillators and cardiac resynchronization devices can now offer patients improvement in their survival and/or quality of life. Elderly patients make up a growing proportion of patients receiving these devices, including the majority of patients receiving pacemakers. Proper selection of patients, devices, surgical technique and device programming can result in excellent patient outcomes with these devices, even among the very old.

References

1. Healey JS, Toff WD, Lamas GA, et al. Cardiovascular outcomes with atrial-based pacing compared with ventricular pacing: meta-analysis of randomized trials, using individual patient data. Circulation. 2006;114(1):11–7.
2. Bristow MR, Saxon LA, Boehmer J, et al. Cardiac-resynchronization therapy with or without an implantable defibrillator in advanced chronic heart failure. N Engl J Med. 2004;350:2140–50.
3. Moss AJ, Zareba W, Hall WJ, et al. Prophylactic implantation of a defibrillator in patients with myocardial infarction and reduced ejection fraction. N Engl J Med. 2002;346(12):877–83.
4. Cleland JG, Daubert J-C, Erdmann E, et al. The effect of cardiac resynchronization on morbidity and mortalilty in heart failure. N Engl J Med. 2005;352:1539–49.
5. Curtis JP, Rathore SS, Wang Y, et al. The association of 6-minute walk performance and outcomes in stable outpatients with heart failure. J Card Fail. 2004;10:9–14.
6. Aggarwal A, Wang Y, Rumsfeld JS, Curtis JP, Heidenreich PA. Clinical characteristics and in-hospital outcome of patients with end-stage renal disease on dialysis referred for implantable cardioverter defibrillator implantation. Heart Rhythm. 2009;6(11): 1565–71.

7. Bernstein AD, Parsonnet V. Survey of cardiac pacing and defibrillation in the United States in 1993. Am J Cardiol. 1996;78:187–96.

8. Kozak LJ, Owings MF, Hall MJ. National Hospital Discharge Survey: 2002 annual summary with detailed diagnosis and procedure data. Vital Health Stat. 2005;13(158):1–199.

9. Healey J, Connolly SJ, Morillo CA. The management of patients with carotid sinus hypersensitivity: is pacing the answer? Clin Auton Res. 2004;14 Suppl 1:80–6.

10. McIntosh S, da Costa D, Kenny RA. Benefits of an integrated approach to the investigation of dizziness, falls and syncope in the elderly. Age Ageing. 1993;22:53–8.

11. Lamas GA, Orav J, Stambler BS, et al. Quality of life and clinical outcomes in elderly patients treated with ventricular pacing as compared with dual-chamber pacing. N Engl J Med. 1998;338: 1097–104.

12. Toff WD, Camm AJ, Skehan JD. Single-chamber versus dual-chamber pacing for high-grade atrioventricular block. N Engl J Med. 2005;353(2):145–55.

13. Bardy GH, Lee KL, Mark DB, et al. Amiodarone or an implantable cardioverter-defibrillator for congestive heart failure. N Engl J Med. 2005;352:225–37.

14. Huang DT, Sesselberg HW, McNItt S, et al. Improved survival associated with prophylactic implantable defibrillators in elderly patients with prior myocardial infarction and depressed ventricular function: a MADIT-II substudy. J Cardiovasc Electrophysiol. 2007;18(8):833–8.

15. Peterson PN, Daugherty SL, Wang Y, et al. Gender differences in procedure-related adverse events in patients receiving implantable cardioverter-defibrillator therapy. Circulation. 2009;119(8):1078–84.

16. Bradley DJ, Bradley EA, Baughman KL, et al. Cardiac resynchronization and death from progressive heart failure: a meta-analysis of randomized controlled trials. JAMA. 2003;289:730–40.

17. Birnie D, Wiliams K, Guo A, et al. Reasons for escalating pacemaker implants. Am J Cardiol. 2006;98(1):93–7.

18. Shen WK, Hammill SC, Hayes DL, et al. Long-term survival after pacemaker implantation for heart block in patients >65 years. Am J Cardiol. 1994;74(6):560–4.

19. Sutton R, Chatterjee K, Leatham A. Heart-block following acute myocardial infarction. Treatment with demand and fixed-rate pacemakers. Lancet. 1968;2(7569):645–8.

20. Alpert MA, Curtis JJ, Sanfilippo JF, et al. Comparative survival after permanent ventricular and dual chamber pacing for patients with chronic high degree atrioventricular block with and without pre-existing congestive heart failure. J Am Coll Cardiol. 1986;7:925–32.

21. Shen WK, Hayes DL, Hammill SC, Bailey KR, Ballard DJ, Gersh BJ. Survival and functional independence after implantation of a permanent pacemaker in octogenarians and nonagenarians. A population-based study. Ann Intern Med. 1996;125(6):476–80.

22. Lipsitz LA, Wei JY, Rowe JW. Syncope in elderly, institutionalized population: prevalence, incidence and associated risk. Q J Med. 1985;55:45–55.

23. Hale WA, Delaney MJ, McGaghie WC. Characteristics and predictors of falls in elderly patients. J Fam Pract. 1992;34:577–81.

24. O'Laughlin JL, Robitaille Y, Boivin JF, Suissa S. Incidence and risk factors for falls and injurious falls among the community-dwelling elderly. Am J Epidemiol. 1993;137:342–5.

25. Parry SW, Baptist M, Kenny R-A. Drop attacks in older adults: systematic assesment has high diagnostic yield. J Am Geriatr Soc. 2005;53:74–8.

26. McIntosh SJ, Lawson J, Kenny RA. Clinical characteristics of vasodepressor, cardioinhibitory and mixed carotid sinus syndrome in the elderly. Am J Med. 1993;95:203–8.

27. Crilley JG, Herd B, Khurana CS, et al. Permanent cardiac pacing in elderly patients with recurrent falls, dizziness and syncope and a hypersensitive cardioinhibitory reflex. Postgrad Med J. 1997;73: 415–8.

28. Davies AJ, Kenny RA. Falls presenting to the accident and emergency department: types of presentation and risk factor profile. Ageing. 1996;25:362–5.

29. Parry SW, Richardson D, O'Shea D, et al. Diagnosis of carotid hypersensitivity in older adults: carotid sinus massage in the upright position is essential. Heart. 2000;83:22–3.

30. Parry SW, Steen IN, Baptist M, et al. Amnesia for loss of consciousness in patients with carotid sinus syndrome. J Am Coll Cardiol. 2005;45:1840–3.

31. Kenny RA, Richardson DA, Steen N, et al. Carotid sinus syndrome: a modifiable risk factor for non-accidental falls in older adults (SAFE PACE). J Am Coll Cardiol. 2001;38:1491–6.

32. Richardson DA, Bexton RS, Shaw FE, Kenny R-A. Prevalence of cardio-inhibitory carotid sinus hypersensitivity in patients 50 years or over presenting to the accident and emergency department with "unexplained" or "recurrent" falls. Pacing Clin Electrophysiol. 1997;3(2):820–3.

33. Morley CA, Perrins EJ, Grant P, et al. Carotid sinus syncope treated by pacing. Analysis of persistent symptoms and role of atrioventricular sequential pacing. Br Heart J. 1982;47:411–8.

34. Fitzpatrick A, Theodorakis G, Ahmed R, Williams T, Sutton R. Dual chamber pacing aborts vasovagal syncope induced by head-up tilt. Pacing Clin Electrophysiol. 1991;4:13–9.

35. Brignole M, Menozzi C, Lolli G, Oddone D, Gianfranchi L, Bertulla A. Validation of a method of pacing mode in carotid sinus syndrome with or without sinus bradycardia. Pacing Clin Electrophysiol. 1991;14:196–203.

36. Brignole M, Menozzi C, Lolli G, Bottoni N, Gagglioli G. Long-term outcome of paced and nonpaced patients with severe carotid sinus syndrome. Am J Cardiol. 1992;69:1039–43.

37. McAnulty J. Carotid sinus massage in patients who fall: will it define the role of pacing? J Am Coll Cardiol. 2001;38:1497.

38. Parry SW, Steen N, Bexton RS, Tynan M, Kenny R-A. Pacing in elderly recurrent fallers with carotid sinus hypersenstivity: a randomised, double-blind, placebo controlled crossover trial. Heart. 2009;95(5):405–9.

39. Sheldon R. Components of clinical trials for vasovagal syncope. Europace. 2001;3:233–40.

40. Connolly SJ, Sheldon R, Roberts RS, Gent M. The North American vasovagal pacemaker study (VPS): a randomized trial of permanent cardiac pacing for the prevention of vasovagal syncope. J Am Coll Cardiol. 1999;33(1):16–20.

41. Connolly SJ, Sheldon R, Thorpe KE, et al. Pacemaker therapy for prevention of syncope in patients with recurrent severe vasovagal syncope: second vasovagal pacemaker study (VPS II): a randomized trial. JAMA. 2003;289(17):2224–9.

42. Ammirati F, Colivicchi F, Santini M. Permanent cardiac pacing versus medical treatment for the prevention of recurrent vasovagal syncope: a multi-centre, randomized-controlled trial. Circulation. 2001;104:52–7.

43. Sutton R, Brignole M, Menozzi C, et al. The vasovagal syncope international study (VASIS) investigators. Dual-chamber pacing in the treatment of neurally mediated tilt-positive cardioinhibitory syncope: pacemaker versus no therapy: a multi-centre randomized study. Circulation. 2000;102:294–9.

44. Raviele A, Giada F, Menozzi C, et al. A randomized, double-blind, placebo-controlled study of permanent cardiac pacing for the treatment of recurrent tilt-induce vasovagal syncope. The vasovagal syncope and pacing trial (SYNPACE). Eur Heart J. 2004;25:1741–8.

45. Aggarwal RK, Connelly DT, Ray SG, Ball J, Charles RB. Early complications of permanent pacemaker implantation: no difference between dual and single chamber systems. Br Heart J. 1995;73: 571–5.

46. Chauhan A, Grace AA, Newell SA, et al. Early complications after dual-chamber versus single chamber pacemaker implantation. Pacing Clin Electrophysiol. 1994;17:2012–5.

47. Lee DS, Birinie D, Cameron D, et al. Design and implementation of a population-based registry of implantable cardioverter defibrillators (ICDs) in Ontario. Heart Rhythm. 2008;5(9):1250–6.

48. Curtis JP, Leubbert JJ, Wang Y, et al. Association of physician certification and outcomes among patients receiving an implantable cardioverter-defibrillator. JAMA. 2009;301(16):1661–70.

49. Pickett 3rd RA, Saavedra P, Ali MF, Darbar D, Rottman JN. Implantable cardioverter-defibrillator malfunction due to mechanical failure of the header connection. J Cardiovasc Electrophysiol. 2004;15(9):1095–9.

50. Gillis AM, MacQuarrie DS, Wilson SL. The impact of pulse generator longevity on the long-term costs of cardiac pacing. Pacing Clin Electrophysiol. 1996;19:1459–68.

51. Rusanov A, Spotnitz HM. A 15-year experience with permanent pacemaker and defibrillator lead and patch extractions. Ann Thorac Surg. 2010;89(1):44–50.

52. Mahapatra S, Bybee KA, Bunch TJ, et al. Incidence and predictors of cardiac perforation after permanent pacemaker placement. Heart Rhythm. 2005;2(9):907–11.

53. Connolly SJ, Hallstrom AP, Cappato R, et al. Meta-analysis of the implantable cardioverter defibrillator secondary prevention trials. Eur Heart J. 2000;21:2071–8.

54. Sanders GD, Hlatky MA, Owens DK. Cost-effectiveness of implantable cardioverter-defibrillators. N Engl J Med. 2005;353:1471–80.

55. Mark DB, Anstrom KJ, Sun JL, et al. Quality of life with defibrillator therapy or amiodarone in heart failure. N Engl J Med. 2008;359(10):1058–9.

56. Poole JE, Johnson GW, Hellkamp AS, et al. Prognostic importance of defibrillator shocks in the sudden cardiac death in heart failure trial. N Engl J Med. 2008;359:1009–17.

57. Healey JS, Hallstrom AP, Kuck KH, et al. Role of the implantable defibrillator in elderly patients with a history of life-threatening ventricular arrhythmias. Eur Heart J. 2008;28(14):174–1749.

58. Krahn A, Connolly SJ, Roberts RS, Gent M, ATMA Investigators. Diminishing proportional risk of sudden death with advancing age: implications for prevention of sudden death. Am Heart J. 2004;147(5):837–40.

59. Duray G, Richter S, Manegold J, Israel CW, Gronefeld G, Hohnloser SH. Efficacy and safety of ICD therapy in a population of elderly patients treated with optimal background medication. J Interv Card Electrophysiol. 2005;14:169–73.

60. Kleman JM, Pinski SL, Morant VA. ICDs in the very elderly: short and long-term outcome. Pacing Clin Electrophysiol. 1994;17:835.

61. Noseworthy PA, Lashevsky I, Dorian P, Greene M, Cvitkovic S, Newman D. Feasibility of implantable cardioverter-defibrillator use in elderly patients. Pacing Clin Electrophysiol. 2004;27:373–8.

62. Feinberg WM, Blackshear JL, Laupacis A, Kronmal R, Hart RG. Prevalence, age distribution and gender of patients with atrial fibrillation: analysis and implications. Arch Intern Med. 1995;155:469–73.

63. Baranchuk A, Healey JS, Thorpe KE, et al. The effect of atrial-based pacing on exercise capacity as measured by the 6-minute walk test: a sub-study of the Canadian trial of physiologic pacing (CTOPP). Heart Rhythm. 2007;4(8):1024–8.

Chapter 36
Heart Transplantation and Mechanical Assistance in the Elderly

Edwin C. McGee Jr.

Abstract Heart failure is a major source of morbidity and mortality in the population 65 and older. While medications offer benefit, many patients progress to end-stage heart failure. Heart transplantation and mechanical assistance offer the hope of improved quality and length of life in patients with end-stage heart failure.

Keywords Heart failure • Heart transplantation • Ventricular assist device

Introduction

Heart failure is a syndrome caused by an impairment of ventricular filling or ejection and is characterized by breathlessness, loss of energy, and fluid retention [1]. It affects five million Americans and poses a tremendous public health crisis which is becoming more apparent as the baby boomer generation ages. Heart failure is the most frequently utilized Medicare diagnosis- related group (DRG), and yearly costs for caring for patients afflicted with heart failure are conservatively estimated to amount up to 39 billion dollars [2]. Coronary artery disease, hypertension, obesity, and diabetes are common predisposing factors [2]. The life time risk of developing heart failure is one in five for individuals over the age of 40 [2]. Without a history of myocardial infarction, the lifetime risk is one in nine for males and one and six for females [2]. Seventy-five percent of patients with heart failure have a history of hypertension. The incidence of heart failure in the population aged 65 and older approaches 10 per 1,000 [2]. Despite improvements in medical therapy, heart failure remains a highly lethal condition with an overall 1 year mortality of 20% [2]. The 30 day, 1 year, and 5 year mortality rates after a hospital admission for heart failure are 10.4, 22, and 42.3%, respectively [2]. In 2006, heart failure was listed as the cause of death in 282, 754 individuals and was mentioned on one in eight death certificates [2].

Heart Failure is commonly classified by the New York Heart Association (NYHA) classification or American Heart Association (AHA) classification. Like many diseases heart failure exists as a spectrum of severity. The worst stages of heart failure (NYHA IIIb or IV or Stage D) account for nearly 10% of patients that carry the diagnosis. Individuals with Stage D heart failure have extremely limited survival and extremely poor quality of life.

Appropriate medial therapy is the cornerstone of treatment for heart failure. Medications like Angiotensin converting enzyme inhibitors (ACEI) and Beta Blockers have been shown to decrease morbidity and mortality in patients with heart failure [3–5]. Cardiac resynchronization has also been shown to enhance survival in individuals with heart failure [6]. However, heart failure is a progressive disease in many patients. Often individuals with heart failure progress to intolerance of ACE inhibitors or Beta Blockers or become "nonresponders" to therapies like biventricular pacing. Mortality is particularly high in this group of patients [7]. It was once thought that either intermittent or continuous infusion of inotropic drugs like milrinone or dobutamine would benefit the population with stage D heart failure. While patients may feel better on inotropes, survival is worsened. In a series of 36 patients who were referred for transplantation but subsequently turned down, Hershberger demonstrated a median survival of 3.4 months and 1-year survival of 6% in patients supported with inotropes [8]. Gorodeski reported the outcomes of 112 patients who were supported on milrinone or dobutamine. At 130 days of follow-up 85 (76%) patients had died; of those surviving, 7 (6%) received VADS and 12 (11%) underwent heart transplant [9].

While conventional cardiac surgery like coronary bypass or aortic valve replacement can benefit certain patient with heart failure, many with advanced heart failure do not have lesions which are repairable and have hearts which have progressed to the point of no return. In such individuals, heart transplantation and/or mechanical assistance are the only therapies that can improve both the length and quality of life.

E.C. McGee Jr. (✉)
Department of Cardiac Surgery, Northwestern Memorial Hospital, Bluhm Cardiovascular Institue, Chicago, IL 60611, USA
e-mail: emcgee@nmh.org

M.R. Katlic (ed.), *Cardiothoracic Surgery in the Elderly*, DOI 10.1007/978-1-4419-0892-6_36,

In this chapter, we will examine the indications, results, and overall status of heart transplantation and mechanical assistance both as a bridge to transplant and stand alone therapy for the elderly patient with advanced heart failure.

Heart Transplantation

Heart transplantation is the gold standard surgical therapy for patients with Stage D heart failure. In the modern era, 1-year survival approaches 90%, and of those patients living a year, half are alive at 13 years [10]. However, transplantation remains a donor limited therapy. Approximately 2,300 transplants are performed each year in North America, with around 4,000 being performed worldwide [10]. These totals fall far short in terms of making a meaningful epidemiologic impact in the overall treatment of stage D heart failure.

To fully understand the option of transplantation for any particular patient with advanced heart failure, it is first necessary to have some understanding of the process of listing, and the matching algorithm used to place donor hearts with potential recipients on the waiting list.

Screening for absolute and relative contraindications is done in all potential heart transplant recipients, but is of particular importance in the older patient referred for transplant as comorbidities are common. A list of commonly referenced contraindications can be found in Table 36.1. Judgment must be exercised in assessing the impact of a particular comorbidity in terms of the impact it will have on posttransplant morbidity and mortality. Listing decisions are typically made by a multidisciplinary team of physicians, surgeons, nurses, social workers, and psychologists and must be made on an individual patient basis.

Currently four wait list status levels exist for heart transplantation (www.unos.org). Requirements for listing at a particular status can be found in Table 36.2. In general, listing status is determined by the severity of heart failure at presentation. Status 2 patients have advanced heart failure but typically have preserved cardiac output and hemodynamics and can be maintained as outpatients. Measurement of peak oxygen consumption (V02) is commonly utilized to identify these patients. A VO2 max of ≤14 mL/kg/min was shown by Mancini and colleagues to have a 1-year survival of 70% at 1 year in potential transplant candidates, and is typically the value viewed as the cutoff value for listing the ambulatory heart failure patient for transplant. Right heart catheterization typically demonstrates preserved cardiac output in the ambulatory population.

Traditionally patients with a depressed cardiac index (<2.2 L/min/m²) qualify for intravenous inotropes and fulfill the requirements for status 1b if only one agent is utilized in a moderate dose. The presence of a ventricular assist device (VAD) also qualifies the patient as being at least a status 1b. Status 1a is the most critical patient designation of the heart transplant waiting list. Historically, 1a patients have required

Table 36.1 Contraindications to cardiac transplantation

General contraindications

Presence of any noncardiac condition that would itself shorten life expectancy or increase the risk of death from rejection or complications of immunosuppression

Specific contraindication[a]

Old age (> about 65 years) (program variability)

Active infection

Active peptic ulcer disease

Severe diabetes mellitus with end organ damage

Severe peripheral vascular or cerebrovascular disease

Coexisting active neoplasm

Morbid obesity (>140% predicted ideal body weight)

Creatinine clearance <40–45 mL/min, ERPF < 200 mL/min[b]

Bilirubin >2.5 mg/dL(when not due to reversible hepatic congestion), transaminases >2× normal[c]

Severe pulmonary dysfunctionwith FVC and FEV₁ < about 40% of predicted , especially with predicted lung disease

Pulmonary artery systolic pressure >60 mm Hg, and/or pulmonary vascular resistance >5 Wood units[d]

Acute pulmonary thromboembolism

Active diverticulitis

History of smoking within last 6 months

High risk of life-threatening noncompliance

  Inability to make strong commitment to transplantation

  Cognitive impairment severe enough to limit comprehension of medical regimen

  Psychiatric instability severe enough to jeopardize incentive for adherence to medical regimen

  History of recurring alcohol or drug abuse

  Failure of established stable addressor telephone number

  Previous demonstration of repeated noncompliance with medication or follow-up

  Lack of independent family or social support system

  History of marked depression or emotional instability

Source: Reprinted with permission from Kirklin et al. [35]. Copyright Elsevier (2002)

ERPF effective renal plasma flow

[a] May be relative or absolute, depending on severity or program philosophy

[b] May be suitable for cardiac transplantation if inotropic support and hemodynamic management produce a creatinine <2 mg/dL and creatinine clearance >50 mL/min. Transplantation may also be advisable as combined heart-kidney transplant

[c] Requires lives biopsy to exclude cirrhosis or other intrinsic liver disease

[d] These apply only if the increased resistance is largely nonreactive (fixed). See text for details

one high dose or two moderate level inotropes to maintain hemodynamics. The presence of an intraaortic balloon pump (IABP) also qualifies a patient as 1a. Individuals that have in place a VAD also qualify for 30 days of 1a time, which can be arbitrarily assigned. When these 30 days elapse the patient reverts back to 1b unless a VAD related complication occurs.

Some patients may initially be listed as status two and progress to 1b and subsequently 1a if they are not transplanted at an earlier status. Other patients may present in cardiogenic shock initially and be listed up front as a 1a. Status 7 patients are not entered into match runs and as such are considered an inactive status.

Table 36.2 Heart transplant recipient status

UNOS Medical Urgency Status Categories

Status Level	Category
Status 1A	Patient is admitted to the listing transplant center hospital and has at least one of the following devices or therapies in place: 1. Mechanical circulatory support for acute hemodynamic decompensation that includes at least one of the following: left or right ventricular device, total artificial heart, IABP, ECMO 2. Mechanical circulatory support with evidence of significant device-related complications 3. Mechanical ventilation 4. Continuous infusion of a single high-dose intravenous inotrope 5. Life expectancy < 7 days
Status 1B	At least one of the following devices or therapies in place: 1. Left or right ventricular device 2. Continuous infusion of intravenous inotropes
Status 2	All other actively listed patients
Status 7	Patient is temporarily removed from active waiting list

Source: Sellke et al. [36]. Reprinted with permission from Elsevier

Several factors must be taken into consideration when contemplating transplantation in an individual over 65 years of age. Some regions or programs have age restrictions and do not consider individuals older than 65 as being appropriate transplant candidates. Several series have looked at the outcomes of heart transplant patients over the age of 65. In general results are good but long-term outcomes typically fall short of the younger patients.

Marelli and colleagues recently reported the outcome of 182 patients, aged 62–75 who underwent transplantation at the University of California- Los Angeles from 1995 to 2001 [11]. Follow-up at 100 months demonstrated 55% survival for the elderly cohort and 63% for controls (*P*=0.051) [11]. Freedom from malignancy was 68% for the elderly and 95% for the younger cohort. Freedom from dialysis was 81% for the elderly and 87% for control [11]. The authors argued that while overall mortality was acceptable for elderly patients, complications of immunosuppression are more of a problem for older patients. As such they argue that long-term mechanical circulatory support should be considered as an adjunct to heart transplantation in this population.

Another recent large series from the Netherlands by Tjang et al. looked at a group of 1,262 recipients who underwent transplantation from 1989 to 2004 [12]. Outcomes of recipients age 55 and older were compared to those of patients younger than 55. One and fifteen year survival was 84 and 50% for patients less than 55, and 73 and 35% for patients 55 and older. Cardiac allograft vasculopathy, rejection and infection were the leading cause of late mortality in the younger cohort while for malignancies, rejection and infection were the leading cause of late mortality in patients 55 and older.

The authors conclude that heart transplantation should be undertaken with caution in patients older than 55 [12].

Other groups come to different conclusions when studying transplant in older patients. Blanche and colleagues demonstrated 1 and 4-year survival rates of 93 and 74% in a group of 15 patients 70 years and older transplanted from 1994 to 1999 [13]. Short and intermediate term survival was comparable with a younger cohort of patients and the authors concluded that age alone should not be considered as an exclusion for heart transplant. Demers and colleagues from Stanford compared the outcome of 81 patients between age 60–70 with 403 adults less than 60 [14]. Overall survival out to 10 years was not statistically different. Potentially due to a less active immune system, the older cohort suffered fewer rejection episodes (*P*=0.003) but had a higher incidence of malignancy (*P*=0.002) [14].

The "alternate list" strategy has been evoked to deal with potential ethical considerations that arise when transplantation is offered to nonstandard recipients such as the elderly. It is an approach taken by some centers where extended criteria donor hearts are matched with recipients with less than ideal characteristics. The goal of the alternate list strategy is to expand the donor pool and offer life saving hearts to more patients with end-stage heart failure. Several groups have reported excellent results using this strategy. Laks and colleagues from UCLA compared the outcomes of 22 patients (age 47–71; mean 67 years) transplanted off the alternate list from 1991 to 1996 with 266 patients transplanted from the standard list [15]. Early mortality and actuarial survival was not statistically different for the two groups.

Felker and colleagues reported the outcomes of 50 patients transplanted from the alternate list and compared them to 195 patients from the standard list [16]. Age >65 (*N*=28) was the most common reason for alternate listing in this study. Two year survival was 70% for the alternate list patients as compared to 88% for the standard list recipients (*P*=0.02). The authors concluded that alternate listing achieved outcomes much better than standard medical therapy.

Chen and colleagues form Columbia looked at 90 day mortality in a group of patients transplanted off the alternate list from 2001 to 2004 [17]. 37 pts (14%) of transplants during this time were from the alternate list which included patients older than 65 as well as patients with HIV, peripheral vascular disease, amyloidosis as well as severe diabetes. Overall survival for both groups was the same, but the alternate list patients had longer ventilator times and suffered more sternal wound infections.

There has been an understandable push to prioritize hearts for the sickest patients. The United Network of Organ Sharing (UNOS) implemented an allocation policy change (APC) in 2006 which has had a significant effect on the chance of lower status patients receiving an organ. The essence of the APC is that hearts are offered to all status 1 patients within a 500 mile radius of the donor in question prior to being offered to status 2 patients. As such, in most regions, status 2 patients are infrequently transplanted unless they are very small or have blood type AB. This trend was recently studied in a series that looked at recipient listing status at the time of transplant 2 years prior to and 2 years after the APC [18]. After the 2006 APC the proportion of status 1A patients transplanted increased from 24 to 43% (*P*=0.015) and the proportion of status 2 transplanted decreased from 56 to 24% (*P*=0.001). Procurement costs, ischemic time (196–223 *P*=0.02), and percentage of patients with VADs (17–31% *P*=0.036) all increased [18]. Waitlist mortality stayed the same (6–5% *P*=0.75) [18].

The trend towards a higher percentage of VAD usage as a bridge to transplant has primarily been driven by the improved outcomes demonstrated by newer generation devices. Continuous-flow pumps have proven to be less morbid to implant and more durable than the previous generation of pulsatile VADs. The Heartmate II (Thoratec Corp. Pleasanton, CA) is a small implantable axial flow pump (Fig. 36.1). 133 transplant eligible patients were implanted with the Heartmate II device in the United States Food and Drug Administration (FDA) pivotal bridge to transplant trial from March 2005 to May 2006 [19]. Principal outcome was determined at 180 days by the number of patients who had been transplanted, were currently listed awaiting transplant, or had been explanted for recovery. 100 (75%) patients achieved the principal outcome. 25 (19%) had died at 180 days. Complications included: bleeding requiring surgery (31%), right ventricular failure (17%), sepsis (20%), drive line infection (14%) renal failure (14%), ischemic stroke (6%), hemorrhagic stroke, (2%) and pump thrombosis (1.5%). The results of this trial lead to FDA approval of the Heartmate II for the indication of bridge to transplantation.

Pagani and colleagues reported the 18 month follow-up of 281 patients enrolled in the pivotal and continuing access arm of the bridge to transplant Heartmate II trial (Fig. 36.2). At 18 month follow-up, 222(79%) patients had undergone

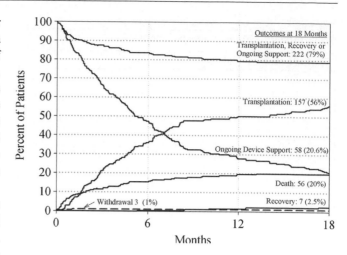

Fig. 36.2 Heartmate II bridge to transplant survival. Outcomes for 281 patients after implantation of the continuous-flow left ventricular assist device (VAD). Competing outcomes analysis of patients undergoing implantation of the continuous-flow left VAD for the first 18 months after device implantation (reprinted with permission from Pagani et al. [20], Copyright Elsevier 2009)

transplant, device explant for recovery, or were currently being supported with the device [20]. Actuarial survival with VAD support was 72% at 18 months. Quality of life scores and NYHA functional class were significantly improved. Pump thrombosis occurred in four patients (1.4%).

There is clear evidence that earlier implantation of VADS leads to improved early outcomes. A number of groups are now advocating for VAD implantation not only for inotrope dependant patients, but also for patients who have become intolerant to ACEI or Beta blockers, and for those who require hospital admissions despite maximal medical therapy.

Because heart failure typically progresses and because fewer patients are being transplanted as a status 2, in most regions many patients first undergo VAD placement prior to transplantation. In the second report from the Interagency Registry for Mechanical Circulatory Support (INTERMACS), older age was shown to be a risk factor for mortality with a relative risk of 1.41 (*P*<0.001) [21]. It should be noted that all of the devices implanted in adults in this report were first generation pulsatile pumps. In the most recent report from INTERMACS, the outcomes of 1,092 patients undergoing primary LVAD were reported (Fig. 36.3). 564 (51.6%) of the pumps implanted were the continuous-flow Heartmate II [22]. A hazard ratio (HR) was generated to describe the risk of VAD implantation for patients age 60–70. In the entire cohort, the HR for older age was 2.42 (*P*<0.0001) in the postoperative period and was 1.55 (*P*<0.0005) in the constant phase. It is noteworthy that in the early phase, older age was a greater risk than cardiogenic shock, elevated right atrial pressure, and higher bilirubin [22]. In the 100 patients undergoing implantation of destination VADs, which at the time of the report were all Heartmate XVE devices, older age

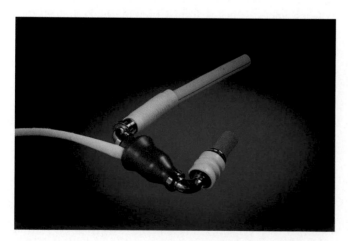

Fig. 36.1 Heartmate II (reprinted with permission of Thoratec Corporation)

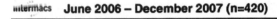

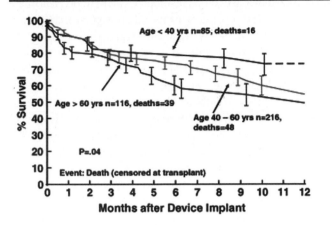

Fig. 36.3 Intermacs survival after VAD implantation by age (reprinted with permission from Holman et al. [21], Copyright Elsevier 2009)

was the only risk factor with a HR of 2.76 [22]. The INTERMACS reports provide clear evidence that VAD implantation becomes more morbid as patients age. In addition, a VAD explant/transplant is also a bigger operation for the older patient to endure than just a transplant alone. Certainly treatment has to be individualized to the patient, but it could be argued that such older patients would be better served by keeping their VAD and foregoing the risk of the explant/transplant.

To summarize, transplantation remains a donor limited therapy. Even if the number of available hearts were tripled by such measures as increased donation and the use of extended criteria organs, the numbers would fall far short of the number of potential salvageable patients with stage D heart failure. While research in xenotransplantation offers hope, the clinical reality of large scale implantation of non-human hearts to address the all too real epidemic of heart failure remains years away. Transplantation will continue to be a therapy for select individuals with advanced heart failure. Super selective criteria should be applied to potential recipients 65 and older. With the improvements in VADS, mechanical assistance will play an increasingly important role in this population not only as a bridge to transplant but also as permanent long-term therapy. As VADS continue to improve it is likely that the indication of long-term destination therapy will supplant that of bridge to transplantation in individuals 65 and older in the not too distant future.

Destination Therapy

Long-term mechanical assistance for patients who are not transplant candidates has been termed destination therapy. The vision of long-term mechanical assistance grew out of

the initial dismal results encountered during the early experience of heart transplantation. The first VAD was placed in 1963 by Dr Michael DeBakey in a patient with postcardiotomy failure [23]. Dr. DeBakey was instrumental in establishing the NIH sponsored Artificial Heart Program. Modern VADs arose out of this initial work on complete heart replacement.

The determination of which patient is or is not a potential transplant candidate is potentially complex and is best made by a multidisciplinary team that factors in not only medical and surgical factors, but also psychological and social issues. The truly dismal results of medical therapy in Stage D patients together with limited applicability of heart transplantation led to the study of VADs as sole therapy in this population.

Rematch

The Randomized Evaluation of Mechanical Assistance for the Treatment of Congestive Heart Failure (REMATCH) was a prospective randomized multicenter trial that examined the outcomes of Stage D heart failure patients, ineligible for transplant, who received either optimal medical management or mechanical assistance with the first generation pulsatile Heartmate XVE [24]. In this study, 68 patients received a VAD while 61 were randomized to the optimal medical management arm. The average age of patients receiving a VAD was 66 ± 9 years. A 48% reduction in the rate of death for the group that received a VAD as well as improved quality of life was demonstrated (Fig. 36.4). The majority of patients not

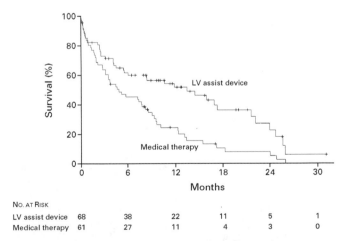

Fig. 36.4 REMATCH trial patient survival Kaplan–Meier analysis of survival in the group that received left ventricular (LV) assist devices and the group that received optimal medical therapy. Crosses depict censored patients. Enrollment in the trial was terminated after 92 patients had died; 95 deaths had occurred by the time of the final analysis (reprinted with permission from Rose et al. [24]. Copyright © 2001 Massachusetts Medical Society. All rights reserved)

receiving the device died of heart failure, while sepsis (40%) and complications of device failure (17%) most commonly led to the demise of patients undergoing VAD implantation (Fig. 36.2). Higher rates of adverse events (relative risk 2.35) such as sepsis, bleeding, and device malfunction were seen in the VAD patients. The authors concluded that mechanical assistance was an acceptable therapy in patients not candidates for heart transplant [24]. Based on the outcomes of REMATCH, the Heartmate XVE received FDA approval in 2003 for long-term implantation and became the first VAD to receive approval for destination therapy.

Despite the results of REMATCH and FDA approval, adoption of destination therapy with the Heartmate XVE was slow and limited to only a few centers. The failure of destination therapy with the Heartmate XVE to catch on was largely due to the morbidity of the implant and the durability of the device, which begins to fail predictably after 18 months [25]. Widespread adoption of implantation of the mechanical assist devices in nontransplant patients would have to wait until of development of a less morbid more durable VAD.

Heartmate II Destination Trial

Shortly after it entered into trial in the bridge to transplant arena, the Heartmate II destination therapy trial was initiated (Fig. 36.5). In this prospective multicenter trial, 200 patients

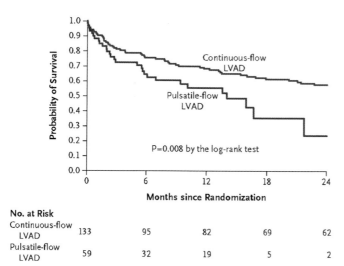

Fig. 36.5 Outcomes of the heartmate II destination therapy trial. Kaplan–Meier estimates of survival from the as-treated analysis, according to treatment group. The data shown are for the 192 patients who received a left ventricular assist device (LVAD). Of the 59 patients who had a pulsatile-flow LVAD, 20 had the device replaced during the study period, with 18 (31%) receiving a continuous-flow LVAD instead of another pulsatile-flow LVAD. By 2 years, only two patients had a pulsatile-flow LVAD, both of whom had replacement devices (reprinted with permission from Slaughter et al. [26]. Copyright © 2009 Massachusetts Medical Society. All rights reserved)

(median age 64) who were not transplant eligible were randomized in a two to one fashion (134 HMII: 66 Heartmate XVE) [26]. The leading reasons for transplant ineligibility were age >65, diabetes with end organ dysfunction, and chronic renal failure with a creatinine >2.5. The primary composite endpoint of the trial was 2-year survival with freedom from disabling stroke or device replacement [26]. 46% (62/134) of patients with the Heartmate II achieved this endpoint as opposed to 11% (7/66) of those with the Heartmate XVE (P<0.001) [26]. 20 of 59 patients receiving the Heartmate XVE underwent 21 pump replacements. Twelve patients required replacement of the Heartmate II secondary to percutaneous lead fracture (10/13), pump thrombosis (2/13), and outlet elbow disconnection (1/13). As a result of this trial, the Heartmate II was approved for implantation as destination therapy in January, 2010.

An interesting caveat of the Heartmate II destination therapy trial is the fact that in a trial of patients not eligible for transplantation, 26 patients (17 Heartmate II: 9 Heartmate XVE) were actually transplanted [26]. The authors state that this occurred as the contraindication to transplant resolved while on device support. While this is certainly true, it is likely that outcomes may have been positively impacted by the fact that over 10% of the patients in the study were ultimately transplanted. When these patients were transplanted, they completed the trial and were not subject to developing pump related adverse events.

In many aspects, the notion of transplant eligibility and how it relates to mechanical assistance is somewhat artificial and is primarily a vehicle for insurance coverage and FDA approval. While the distinction of transplant ineligibility is obvious in some patients, it may be very murky in others. By definition, relative contraindications are open to interpretation and the aggressiveness and overriding philosophies of the physicians in terms of transplantation and VAD support is a tremendously important factor. Whatever the case, one cannot dispute that VADs have proven themselves to be effective in treating the vast majority of patients with Stage D heart failure.

Patient Selection for Destination Therapy

Not all patients with advanced heart failure are candidates for VAD therapy. Patient selection remains one of the most important aspects of a successful mechanical assistance program. It must be remembered that currently approved pumps for destination therapy are available only in an LVAD configuration. As such, the right ventricle functions to pump blood through the lungs to in effect fill the LVAD. VADs can only pump what they get and if the right ventricle fails, the LVAD will be unable to supply the body with adequate perfusion.

The chronically elevated central venous pressure (CVP) that is the hallmark of right ventricular failure leads to renal and splanchnic congestion which in turn contributes to renal and hepatic dysfunction and fosters bacterial translocation from the gut. Multisystem organ failure (MSOF) often is the end result. Right ventricular failure complicates fifteen to twenty percent of all LVAD implantations and remains a significant source of morbidity and mortality.

Identifying patients preoperatively that are predisposed to RV failure is important if RV failure is to be avoided. Elevated right sided filling pressures with relatively low left side filling pressures are often found on right heart catheterization in the patient suffering predominantly of right sided heart failure. Typically, the left ventricle is small or only mildly dilated. With the current state of the art, these patients are at high risk for isolated LVAD implantation. Many patients with heart failure have end organ dysfunction that can be reversed once the cardiac output is restored with a VAD [27, 28]. However, once patients develop irreversible end organ failure and severe cachexia, VAD implantation is associated with near prohibitive morbidity and mortality [29, 30]. In addition, certain anatomic issues such as aortic insufficiency and intracardiac shunts must be surgically managed in order to achieve a successful implant.

Certification

To receive reimbursement for implantation of destination therapy, CMS now requires that a hospital achieves VAD certification of distinction as outlined by the Joint Commission. (http://www.jointcommission.org/CertificationPrograms/LeftVentricularAssistDevice/).

In addition to providing evidence of having a track record of providing care for cardiac surgery patients, the center must have a cardiologist with some training in heart transplantation and a surgeon who has performed 10 VAD implants in the last 36 months with a current implant in the last year. The program must also be part of a database that tracks outcomes of VAD patients, and must demonstrate the usual regulatory quality approval benchmarks required by all Joint Commission programs.

Conclusion

Heart Failure is a highly lethal condition that affects millions of Americans. The incidence of heart failure increases with age. Currently, the best therapy for end-stage heart failure is heart transplantation. Heart transplantation is limited by the availability of donor hearts. The survival after heart transplantation is diminished in patients older than 65, primarily by preexisting comorbidities and the risk of malignancy. Many programs have age limitations and do not offer transplantation to individuals >65. While heart transplantation remains an option for select individuals >65, it is certainly not a widely applicable solution.

Results with mechanical assistance have improved using the new generation continuous-flow pumps. Such pumps are less morbid to implant and have increased durability when compared to earlier generation pulsatile devices. The currently FDA approved Heartmate II provides acceptable long-term outcomes both in terms of quality and length of life. However, there is much room for improvement. The field is in no way static and several devices are currently in trial that offer the promise of improved outcomes. The Jarvik 2000 flowmaker has been in trial for the bridge to transplant and destination therapy indications for some time and has supported a patient over 7 years [31]. The Heartware HVAD is a miniaturized centrifugal pump that is designed for intrapericardial implantation which leads to less bleeding as it does not require construction of an abdominal wall pocket. It has recently completed a bridge to transplant trial and is projected to start a destination therapy trial in late 2010 [32]. The Terumo Duraheart is a fully magnetically levitated centrifugal pump that is currently the subject of a bridge to transplant trial and will ultimately enter trial as long-term therapy [33]. The Worldheart Levacor is another fully magnetically levitated pump that is scheduled to enter trial in the not too distant future [34].

Trials are exceedingly expensive, and the therapy is expensive to implement and maintain. Mechanical assistance is a costly therapy and requires a large specific infrastructure at the hospital level to care for the patients in question. The profit margin for the hospitals involved is very tight, largely due to the cost of the pumps and accessory equipment. It remains to be seen what the overall volume of destination therapy implants will be. Given the state of healthcare finances, it is not yet clear whether mechanical assistance as destination therapy will gain traction and be accepted into the mainstream. Certainly mechanical assistance has been proven to be a therapy that improves length and quality of life for patients with advanced heart failure.

We are grateful to Ms. Angela Green for her assistance in the preparation of this manuscript.

References

1. Hunt SA, Abraham WT, Chin MH, Feldman AM, Francis GS, Ganiats TG, et al. Focused update incorporated into the ACC/AHA 2005 Guidelines for the diagnosis and management of heart failure in adults a report of the American College of Cardiology Foundation/American Heart Association Task Force on Practice

Chapter 37
Invited Commentary

Joseph LoCicero III

Abstract For cardiac and thoracic surgeons, elderly patients with their unique physiology and social problems are becoming an increasing proportion of their practice. Also, they are faced with a dwindling workforce and rapid changes in surgical approaches and competing technologies. These chapters make insightful observations and practical suggestions to guide the surgeon through delicate procedures on these fragile patients.

Keywords Cardiac surgery • Thoracic surgery • Minimally invasive surgery • Elderly

Cardiothoracic surgery in the elderly is a pain. It is a pain for our country to observe the meteoric rise in the elderly population with all of its attendant implications. It is a pain to note that many of these individuals have accelerating rates of cardiac and thoracic diseases. It is a pain trying to predict the appropriate size of the cardiothoracic surgical workforce which is diminishing due to attrition, early retirement, and sluggish applications of young physicians to undertake the long and arduous training required to become a competent practitioner of the art.

It is a pain to discuss deadly diseases with older patients who, despite their age, are stunned to realize they are facing their own mortality. It is a pain to prepare a patient and family for a major surgical procedure, especially in relation to the significant chance of debilitating complications. It is a pain to break the news to the patient that there are more than just the two options of cure and death – that living a life of diminished capacity is a distinct possibility. It is a pain to realize that the better, or at least the more attractive, option may be performed percutaneously rather than with a knife.

Central to all cardiothoracic surgery is pain. Regardless of the size of our incisions, thoracic surgical pain is significant. Everyday, we work to minimize the body invasion and to minimize the effects on physiology and on the production of pain. For many reasons, the elderly do not deal well with pain. They have altered sensation and they tend to underreport their level of pain. Healthcare workers tend to underdose pain-relieving medicines or underutilize pain-relieving techniques. Pain relief is essential in preventing complications, yet very few meaningful trials exist to direct us. We constantly must adapt our methods to balance optimal pain relief and rehabilitation.

Each of the chapters in this section discusses these painful facts and other significant problems and potential solutions to a greater or lesser degree. Each brings insightful observations and practical suggestions to make our practice optimal based upon our current knowledge. Cardiothoracic surgery began in earnest after Sauerbruch's negative pressure chamber just over a century ago and evolved into a major discipline with the invention of a safe cardiac bypass machine. Now, cardiothoracic surgery is evolving rapidly again as we work to make it safe and effective for the elderly. It is at once exciting, daunting, exhilarating, frustrating, and rewarding. Cardiothoracic surgery is a pain, but pain and reward are opposite sides of the same coin. With diligence, hard work, thoughtful clinical trials, and luck, it will flip soon.

J. LoCicero III (✉)
Department of Surgery, SUNY Downstate, 1158 Church Street,
Mobile, AL 36604, USA
e-mail: lociceroj@comcast.net

M.R. Katlic (ed.), *Cardiothoracic Surgery in the Elderly*, DOI 10.1007/978-1-4419-0892-6_37,
© Springer Science+Business Media, LLC 2011

Chapter 38
Preoperative Evaluation and Preparation in the Elderly Thoracic Surgery Patient

Ticiana Leal, Noelle K. LoConte, Anai Kothari, and Tracey L. Weigel

Abstract The United States population is aging and median life expectancy is increasing as well. Older age is one of the strongest predictors for heart disease and cancer that require cardiothoracic surgery. The traditional preoperative evaluation has been unsuccessful in risk stratifying the older patient fit for elective surgery. This chapter is innovative, focusing on the preoperative assessment of the geriatric patient prior to cardiothoracic surgery, with a particular emphasis on novel assessment methods, incorporating elements of the comprehensive geriatric assessment, meant to identify geriatric syndromes and ways to potentially modulate the higher risks of surgery present for some patients.

Keywords Preoperative • Geriatric • Thoracic • Surgery

Introduction

The United States population is rapidly aging with Baby Boomers now reaching retirement age (see Fig. 38.1). Median life expectancy has increased dramatically in all industrialized countries and is still increasing. In the United States, the number of patients older than 65 years of age is predicted to increase by 13.3% by 2010 and by 53.2% by 2020 [1].

Older age is one of the strongest predictors for heart disease and cancer that require cardiothoracic surgery [2]. In addition, aging is associated with loss of pulmonary and/or cardiac functional capacity coupled with increased likelihood of competing comorbidities and functional impairment that may lead to increased risk of cardiothoracic surgical complications [3]. Interestingly, to illustrate the variability in treatment recommendations for the older patient, a reluctance to recommend a surgical intervention for the older cancer patient is often unrelated to impaired functional status and comorbidities and more likely associated with age [4]. However, evidence suggests that many older patients may benefit from standard treatment and should not be denied optimal treatment based on chronological age alone [3, 5].

The traditional preoperative evaluation has been unsuccessful in risk stratifying the older patient fit for elective surgery, and also in strategically planning for preoperative risk reduction, rehabilitation or informing the patient of anticipated outcomes of surgery. In this regard, a more robust tool that incorporates modified elements of the comprehensive geriatric assessment (CGA) to better assess preoperative risk and predict clinical outcomes would be useful to individualize management.

This chapter will outline the preoperative assessment of the geriatric patient prior to cardiothoracic surgery, with a particular emphasis on novel assessment methods meant to identify geriatric syndromes and ways to potentially modulate the higher risks of surgery present for some patients.

Indications for Surgery in the Older Patient

Indications for common cardiothoracic surgeries in older adults include thoracic malignancies, coronary artery disease (CAD), and valvular disease.

Lung cancer is the leading cause of cancer death [6]. The average age at diagnosis is increasing as the population ages and the peak incidence in the United Kingdom is now between 75 and 79 years of age [7]. This is also the trend in the United States according to analysis of the Surveillance Epidemiology and End Results (SEER)-Medicare database from 2002 to 2006, the median age at diagnosis for lung cancer was 71 years of age [8]. Using the SEER-Medicare database, Farjah et al. [9] hypothesized that the proportion of patients with stages I, II and IIIA nonsmall cell lung cancer (NSCLC) operated on over time would increase coinciding

T. Leal (✉)
Department of Medicine, University of Wisconsin Hospitals and Clinics, 600 Highland Avenue, Mail Code 5669, Madison, WI 53792-5669, USA
e-mail: tbleal@medicine.wisc.edu

M.R. Katlic (ed.), *Cardiothoracic Surgery in the Elderly*, DOI 10.1007/978-1-4419-0892-6_38,
© Springer Science+Business Media, LLC 2011

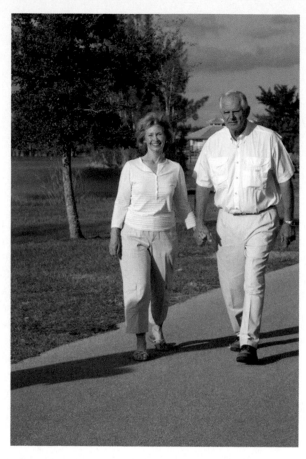

Fig. 38.1 The fit older adult (reprinted with permission from Shutterstock Images, LLC)

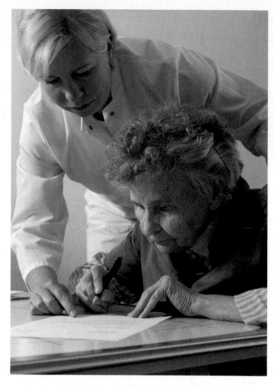

Fig. 38.2 Discharge planning is an important component of the preoperative informed consent process (reprinted with permission from Shutterstock Images, LLC)

with improved adherence to guidelines and better patient/provider education. Unexpectedly, between 1992 and 2002, the use of resection for lung cancer decreased dramatically over time, and this decline was not fully accounted for by an older cohort with more comorbid conditions [9].

More than 800,000 patients undergo cardiac operations annually, with a growing number of procedures in octogenarians [10, 11], with a 67% increase in cardiac surgical procedures for this age group observed nationwide between 1987 and 1990 [12]. This trend is observed in part due to the recent advances in myocardial preservation and perioperative management, which have permitted acceptable outcomes in the older patient, despite notably higher risk compared with younger counterparts [13, 14].

A national retrospective study of octogenarians undergoing cardiac surgery (predominantly coronary artery bypass grafting [CABG] with or without aortic valve replacement, and a smaller number of mitral valve procedures) reported that although the risk of complications is notably higher in octogenarians compared with younger patients, the overall morbidity and mortality and resource utilization is acceptable to continue to offer thoracic surgeries to appropriate patients [15]. In this descriptive study, older patients appear to have longer lengths of hospital stays, need placement in a skilled nursing facility after hospitalization, and have longer intensive care unit stays relative to younger patients.

Another study utilizing the 2004 National Surgical Inpatient Sample (NIS) database identified octogenarians who underwent CABG and reported outcomes and discharge status after the inpatient hospitalization. Only 21% of patients had a routine discharge to home; the remainder of the patients were transferred to another health care facility or received some form of professional home health care after discharge [16]. This study reinforces the need to inform the patient and family in the preoperative informed consent process of the real and likely possibility of additional care prior to discharge to home in order to facilitate the transition after acute hospitalization for older patients. It also suggests that the surgical team will need to focus closely on discharge planning for the older patient (see Fig. 38.2).

Traditional Preoperative Assessment Prior to Cardiothoracic Surgery

The traditional preoperative physiologic assessment for elective procedures should include a cardiovascular and pulmonary evaluation, as well as an evaluation of the patient's functional reserve.

Amongst older patients, the risk of perioperative morbidity and mortality is highest amongst those who need emergent surgery, a major surgical procedure, and have poor preoperative functional or nutritional status [17].

Pulmonary Risk and Evaluation

Thoracic surgery holds the highest risk of pulmonary complications [18], which may include postoperative pneumonia, respiratory failure, reactive airway disease, and exacerbation of an underlying lung condition, such as chronic obstructive pulmonary disease (COPD). Underlying cancer, subjective complaints of dyspnea, obesity, COPD, and asthma all increase the risk of postoperative pulmonary complications [18, 19]. The more severe these conditions are, the higher the risk to the patient from surgery. Smoking also increases the surgical risk [19]. Several surgical factors also appear to increase the risk of pulmonary complications, including prolonged operative time, the need for general anesthesia, and the use of pancuronium [18].

The initial preoperative pulmonary evaluation includes a careful history and physical exam to identify medical comorbidities, the patient's functional capacity, and the degree of limitation of activity. In the case of a lung cancer patient, a history of smoking and symptoms of COPD should be documented and explored. This may lead to an opportunity for preoperative intervention with the use of bronchodilators and/or steroids and smoking cessation counseling, which may lead to some degree of reversal of airway obstruction, decreased risk of postoperative pneumonia, and facilitate weaning from the ventilator postoperatively [20] (Fig. 38.3). In addition, this same population (due to the history of smoking) is also at risk for atherosclerotic cardiovascular disease, which will further increase the perioperative risk.

Age has been considered a factor that might increase perioperative risks. For patients >70 years of age, the reported mortality rate is 4–7% for lobectomy and approximately 14% for pneumonectomy [21, 22]. These mortality rates are higher than those for patients <70 years of age (lobectomy, 1–4%; pneumonectomy, 5–9%) [23]. The difference has been largely attributed to increasing comorbidities in older patients. However, a systematic review [24] estimated the impact of age on postoperative pulmonary complications

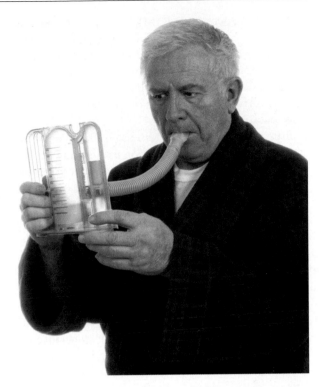

Fig. 38.3 Incentive spirometry involves deep breathing facilitated by a simple mechanical device and has been shown to reduce postoperative pulmonary complications (reprinted with permission from Shutterstock Images, LLC)

among studies that used multivariable analysis to adjust for age-related comorbidities. This review concluded that age >50 years was an important independent predictor of risk. When compared with patients <50-years old, patients aged 50–59 years, 60–69 years, 70–70 years, and ≥80 years had odds ratios (OR) of 1.50 (CI 1.31–1.71), 2.28 (CI 1.86–2.80), 3.90 (CI 2.70–5.65), and 5.63 (CI 4.63–6.85), respectively. Based on this review, even healthy older patients carry a substantial risk of pulmonary complications after surgery. One should be cautious when interpreting these results because there was significant variability among the studies with respect to the cutoff ages used to define age strata. For example, some studies reported only one age category stratification, i.e., >65 years or older, and the authors arbitrarily grouped this within the category 60–69 years of age stratification to facilitate analysis, and using sensitivity analysis it was demonstrated that this had little effects in the results.

Regarding the preoperative pulmonary-specific evaluation, the first test to be performed should be a spirometry [23]. Spirometry is a simple, inexpensive, standardized, and readily available test. Spirometric indexes that have been extensively studied include forced expiratory volume in 1 s (FEV1), forced vital capacity (FVC), forced expiratory flow, midexpiratory phase (FEF$_{25–75\%}$), and maximum voluntary ventilation (MVV). FVC reflects lung volume, while FEV1 and $FEF_{25-75\%}$ reflect airflow. MVV represents respiratory muscle strength and correlates with postoperative morbidity. However, the FEV1, $FEF_{25-75\%}$, and MVV are very dependent on patient effort. Of all these indexes, FEV1 is regarded as being the best for predicting complications of lung resection in the initial assessment, and it is one of the most commonly used for decision making [25].

If diffuse parenchymal lung disease is identified on imaging or if there is dyspnea on exertion that is clinically out of proportion to the FEV1, the diffusing capacity of the lung for carbon monoxide (DLCO) should also be measured. According to American College of Chest Physicians (ACCP) evidence-based clinical practice guidelines [23], in patients with either an FEV1 or DLCO <80% predicted, the predicted postoperative pulmonary reserve should be estimated by either the perfusion scan method for pneumonectomy or the anatomic method, based on counting the number of segments to be removed (for lobectomy). Datta et al. reported that an FEV1 and DLCO over 60% indicate a low surgical risk from lung cancer surgery [20]. An estimated postoperative FEV1 or DLCO <40% predicted indicates an increased risk for perioperative complications, including death, from a standard lung cancer resection (such as lobectomy). In these cases, cardiopulmonary exercise testing (CPET) to measure maximal oxygen consumption (VO_2max) should be performed to further define the perioperative risk of surgery. A VO_2max <15 mL/kg/min indicates an increased risk of perioperative complications, and these patients are probably best managed by nonsurgical modalities [20].

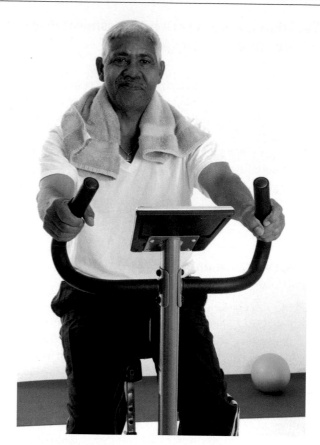

Fig. 38.4 Assessment of cardiac functional status can provide valuable prognostic information (reprinted with permission from Shutterstock Images, LLC)

Cardiac Risk and Evaluation

Cardiovascular complications pose significant risks to older patients undergoing cardiothoracic surgeries [17]. The most common postoperative cardiac complications associated with surgery in the elderly patients include myocardial infarction and myocardial ischemia. The risk of these events is highest in patients with unstable cardiac conditions (such as recent myocardial infarction, decompensated heart failure, poorly controlled arrhythmias, and severe valvular disease) [17].

There are many tools that can be used for preoperative cardiac evaluation, and the importance of a detailed history of the patient's symptoms, comorbidities, and exercise capacity is essential for a more accurate preoperative risk assessment. In particular, a history of previous CAD, angina, heart failure, aortic stenosis, severe hypertension, and peripheral arterial disease should be investigated.

Next an assessment of cardiac functional status can provide valuable prognostic information, since patients with good functional status are known to have a lower risk of complications [26] (see Fig. 38.4). A patient's functional status is usually expressed in metabolic equivalents (METs). For the purpose of definition, 1 MET is defined as 3.5 mL O_2 uptake/kg per min, which is the resting oxygen uptake in a sitting position. Perioperative cardiac and long-term risk is increased in patients who are unable to meet a 4-MET demand during the most normal daily activities [27–29]. One important indicator of poor functional status and an increased risk of postoperative cardiopulmonary complications after major noncardiac surgery is the inability to climb two flights of stairs or walk four blocks. In a prospective evaluation of 83 patients undergoing several types of surgeries (included 31 lobectomies, 6 wedge resections, 3 pneumonectomies, 3 substernal thymectomies, 1 substernal thyroidectomy, and other surgeries), postoperative complications occurred in 25% of patients overall. No patient able to climb the maximum of seven flights of stairs had a postoperative complication. The inability to climb two flights of stairs was associated with a positive predictive value of 82% for the development of a postoperative complication [30].

Many anesthesiologists also assess patients utilizing the American Society of Anesthesiology (ASA) classification, and the risk of perioperative adverse events is highest among patients with ASA classification III or IV [17]. Lower levels of serum albumin and higher levels of total bilirubin have been associated with higher rates of morbidity and mortality following cardiac surgery [31].

There are also several different risk indices developed by Goldman [32], Detsky [33, 34], and Eagle [35], which can be used to estimate the risk of cardiac complications in patients undergoing noncardiac surgery. Based on an algorithmic approach, decision for further noninvasive testing (such as stress testing) and cardiac catheterization may affect the timing of surgery in selected patients.

Informed Consent and Capacity to Consent

Informed consent is an essential part of clinical care, especially in the older patient population. Meaningful informed consent requires that the patient understands the risks and benefits of a proposed intervention and then voluntarily gives authorization to proceed. This can be challenging to accomplish in the older patient population because of the interaction between the complex medical problems, cognitive issues, and social barriers that may accompany the aging process (see Figs. 38.5 and 38.6).

It has been proposed by ACOVE-3 (Assessing Care of Vulnerable Elders) that documentation of the patient's capacity to understand the risks and benefits of the proposed procedure before the operative consent form is presented for signature should be a measure of quality of care [36].

There are few studies in the literature addressing informed consent in older patients. In a systematic review of the literature, older age and fewer years of education were associated

with poorer understanding of informed consent information [37]. In a chart review involving hospitalized patients who had developed delirium, 19% of the charts did not have any documentation of consent, and 20% used surrogate consent [38].

It is evident that effective strategies to improve the understanding of the informed consent process should be further developed.

Geriatric Assessment

Evaluation of Geriatric Assessment Prior to Cardiothoracic Surgery

In primary care, geriatric assessments, such as the CGA, are widely used to evaluate the older patient, but there is no widely accepted tool for surgeons or medical oncologists [39]. Although these assessments are generally very thorough and include assessments of mobility, nutrition, cognition, functional status, mood, polypharmacy, and comorbid illness, they can be time consuming, making it challenging to apply these comprehensive assessments in a busy practice.

A briefer instrument applicable to a busy thoracic surgery practice would be valuable to assist with treatment

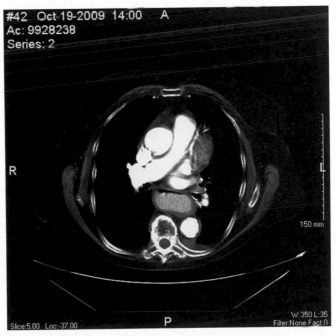

Fig. 38.6 Seventy-five-year old woman with history of comorbid Amyotrophic lateral sclerosis and esophageal cancer was deemed not to be a surgical candidate, but underwent definitive chemotherapy/radiation and has been disease-free for 2 years. The image illustrates a large hiatal hernia that mimics appearance of esophagectomy (reprinted with permission from Shutterstock Images, LLC)

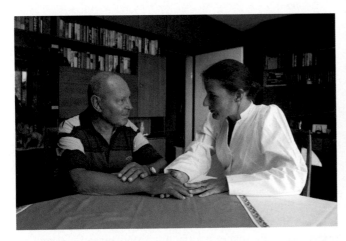

Fig. 38.5 Meaningful informed consent requires that the patient understands the risks and benefits of a proposed intervention and then voluntarily gives authorization to proceed (reprinted with permission from Shutterstock Images, LLC)

recommendations for or against surgery for the older patient and to assist in counseling patients about the likely outcomes after surgery (including risk of complications, or likelihood of being discharged to a nursing home, for example).

Most of the studies to date regarding geriatric assessment prior to elective surgery have included mainly older cancer patients undergoing thoracic surgery for a variety of thoracic malignancies. As cardiac surgery in the older population is an increasing trend, studies in this setting are also warranted.

One prospective study performed in Japan evaluated 120 patients ≥60 years undergoing thoracic surgery for a variety of diseases (lung cancer: 85 patients; mediastinal tumor: 14; bullas: 12; and other diseases: 9) demonstrated that preoperative CGA is helpful to inform the patient and provider about the risks of surgery. Dependence in activities of daily living (ADL) and the Mini-Mental State Examination (MMSE) were strongly predictive of postoperative complications, particularly when the operative time was longest [40].

The necessary preoperative physiologic evaluation need not be cumbersome. One elegant study by Brunelli and colleagues [41] demonstrated that the relatively simple test of symptom-limited stair climbing applied to older patients predicted postoperative cardiopulmonary complications after lobectomy for lung cancer, after controlling for spirometry and comorbid illnesses.

Pope et al. [42] created a preoperative assessment of cancer in the elderly (PACE). This encompasses the validated CGA [43] and measures of surgical risk assessment such as the ASA grade [44] and fatigue using the Brief Fatigue Inventory (BFI) [45] providing a thorough evaluation of onco-geriatric fitness for surgery [46]. Their group subsequently conducted an international prospective study with 460 elderly cancer patients (216 breast, 146 GI, 71 GU, 27 other) receiving PACE prior to elective surgery. A multivariate analysis identified instrumental activities of daily living (IADLs), BFI, and ASA to be the most important predictors of comorbidities. In a follow-up publication [47], they reported further results of this study in respect to whether PACE would be predictive of short-term postoperative outcomes (hospital stay, 30-day morbidity and 30-day mortality). Poor health in relation to disability (assessed using IADL), fatigue, and performance status (PS) were associated with a 50% increase in the relative risk of postoperative complications. Multivariate analysis identified moderate/severe fatigue, a dependent IADL and an abnormal PS as the most important independent predictors of postsurgical complications. Disability assessed by ADLs, IADL s, and PS were associated with an extended hospital stay.

Our group has been developing a reliable, physician and patient-friendly, pre-operative Thoracic Oncology Geriatric Assessment (TOGA) (Table 38.1) to predict surgical risk and outcomes in geriatric oncology patients with thoracic

Table 38.1 Pre-operative thoracic oncology geriatric assessment (TOGA)

Screening test	Measure	Normal range
Activities of daily living (ADL)/ instrumental	Functional status	0
Activities of daily living (IADL)		
Geriatric depression score (GDS)	Mood	Less than 5
Brief fatigue inventory (BFI)	Fatigue, function	0–3
Eastern cooperative oncology Group/Zubrod performance status (PS)	Performance	0–1
Mini mental state exam (MMSE)	Cognition	25 or greater
Mini nutritional assessment (MNA)	Nutrition	5 or less

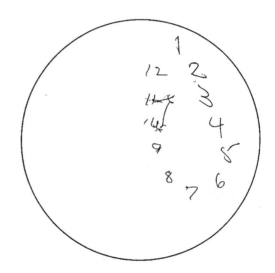

Fig. 38.7 Abnormal clock drawing test indicative of cognitive changes after treatment in a 78-year-old male with esophageal cancer (reprinted with permission from Shutterstock Images, LLC)

neoplasms, including cancer of the lung, esophagus, pleura, and thymus, modeled upon existing CGA tools including (PACE) [48–50] (see Fig. 38.7).

We are currently conducting a prospective study to investigate how these different tools, independently and in combination, predict postoperative morbidity/complications, length of hospital stay, and change in residential status after discharge. Eligible patients are age 70 years and older with lung, esophageal, pleural, or thymic neoplasms with a target accrual of 62 patients. The TOGA includes parts of the PACE [49], involving assessment of ADLs [51] (including toileting, feeding, dressing, grooming, ambulation, and bathing), IADLs [52] (including use of a telephone, shopping, food preparation, housekeeping, laundry, transportation, medication management, and finances), geriatric depression screen (GDS [53]), BFI [54], PS, MMSE [55], the ASA and Mini Nutritional Assessment (MNA [56]). PS and ASA were

Table 38.2 Total length of stay

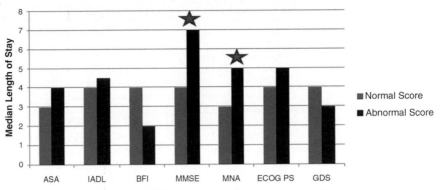

Length of stay (median values)	ASA	IADL	BFI	MMSE	MNA	ECOG PS	GDS
Normal score	3	4	4	4	3	4	4
Abnormal score	4	4.5	2	7	5	5	3
p Value	0.54	0.92	0.41	0.08	0.04	0.39	0.51

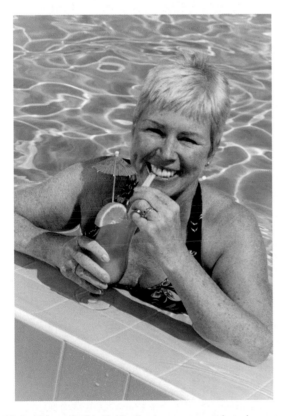

Fig. 38.8 The goal of individualized management is to improve outcomes and maintain quality of life (reprinted with permission from Shutterstock Images, LLC)

predictors of major surgical complications. IADL, PS, and MNA were predictors of place of discharge. MMSE and MNA were predictors of length of stay (see Table 38.2). A clinical applicable TOGA can be composed of PS, ASA, IADL, MNA, MMSE to predict surgical outcomes of thoracic cancer surgery in older patients.

Conclusion

The lack of evidence-based approach to the preoperative assessment of the older patient negatively impacts clinical practice with a substantial number of older patients being excluded from optimal treatment.

A valid and reliable multidimensional assessment of geriatric patients undergoing thoracic surgery to provide detailed information about the functional reserve is increasingly important to aid individualized management (see Fig. 38.8).

References

1. Etzioni D, Liu J, Maggard M, Ko C. The aging population and its impact on the surgery workforce. Annals of Surgery. 2003;238:170–7.
2. Yancik R. Cancer burden in the aged: an epidemiologic and demographic overview. Cancer. 1997;80(7):1273–83.
3. Ramesh HS, Boase T, et al. Risk assessment for cancer surgery in elderly patients. Clin Interv Aging. 2006;1(3):221–7.
4. Samet J, Hunt WC, Key C, Goodwin JS. Choice of cancer therapy varies with age of patient. J Am Med Assoc. 1986;255:3385–90.
5. Repetto L, Fratino L, Audisio RA, Venturino A, et al. Comprehensive geriatric assessment adds information to Eastern Cooperative Oncology Group performance status in elderly cancer patients: an Italian Group for Geriatric Oncology Study. JCO. 2002;20:494–502.
6. Jemal A, Siegel R, Ward E, Murray T, Xu J, Thun MJ. Cancer statistics. CA Cancer J Clin. 2007;57:43–66.
7. Statistics. OfN. Cancer statistics registrations: registrations of cancer diagnosed in 2006, England. 2009.
8. http://seer.cancer.gov/
9. Farjah F, Wood DG, Yanez III D, Symons RG, Krishnadasan B, Flum DR. Temporal trends in the management of potentially resectable lung cancer. Ann Thorac Surg. 2008;85:1850–6.

10. Specer G. US bureau of the Census: Projections of the Population of the United States, by Age, Sex, and Race: 1988 to 2080 Washington, DC: US Government Printing Office. Current Population Reports 1989 Series P-25:No. 1018; 1989.

11. Statistics NCfH. United States life tables: US decennial life tables for 1979–1981. Washington DC: US Government Printing Office 1985 (DHHS publication (PHS) vol 1, no. 1:85-1150-1.

12. Peterson ED, Cowper PA, Jollis JG, et al. Outcomes of coronary artery bypass graft surgery in 24, 461 patients aged 80 years and older. Circulation. 1995;92 Suppl 2:85–91.

13. Alexander KP, Anstrom KJ, Muhlbaier LH, et al. Outcomes of cardiac surgery in patients age 80 years: results from the National Cardiovascular Network. J Am Coll Cardiol. 2000;35:731–8.

14. Craver JM, Puskas JD, Weintraub WW, et al. 601 Octogenarians undergoing cardiac surgery: outcomes and comparison with younger age groups. Ann Thorac Surg. 1999;67:1104–10.

15. Avery GJ, Ley SJ, Hill JD, Hershon JJ, Dick SE. Cardiac surgery in the octogenarian: evaluation of risk, cost and outcome. Ann Thor Surg. 2001;71:591–96.

16. Gopaldas RR, Chu D, Dao TK, et al. Predictors of surgical mortality and discharge status after coronary artery bypass grafting in patients 80 years and older. Am J Surg. 2009;198(5):633–8.

17. Jin F, Chung F. Minimizing perioperative adverse events in the elderly. Br J Anaesth. 2001;87(4):608–24.

18. Smetana GW. Preoperative Pulmonary Evaluation. N Engl J Med. 1999;340(12):937–44.

19. Dales RE, Dionne G, Leech JA, Lunau M, Schweitzer I. Preoperative prediction of pulmonary complications following thoracic surgery. Chest. 1993;104(1):155–9.

20. Datta D, Lahiri B. Preoperative evaluation of patients undergoing lung resection surgery. Chest. 2003;123(6):2096–103.

21. Damhuis RA, Schutte PR. Resection rates and postoperative mortality in 7, 899 patients with lung cancer. Eur Respir J. 1996;9:7–10.

22. Yellin A, Hill LR, Lieberman Y. Pulmonary resections in patients over 70 years of age. Isr J Med Sci. 1985;21:833–40.

23. Colice GL, Shafazand S, Griffin JP, Keenan R, Bolliger CT. Physiologic evaluation of the patient with lung cancer being considered for resectional surgery: ACCP evidenced-based clinical practice guidelines (2nd edition). Chest. 2007;132(3 Suppl): 161S–77S.

24. Smetana GW, Lawrence VA, Cornell JE. Preoperative pulmonary risk stratification for noncardiothoracic surgery: systematic review for the American College of Physicians. Ann Intern Med. 2006;144(8):581–95.

25. Datta D, Lahir B. Preoperative evaluation of patients undergoing lung resection surgery. Chest. 2003;123(6):2096–103.

26. Mangano DT, Goldman L. Preoperative assessment of patients with known or suspected coronary disease. N Engl J Med. 1995;333:1750.

27. Reilly DF, McNeely MJ, Dea D. Self-reported exercise tolerance and the risk of serious perioperative complications. Arch Intern Med. 1999;159:2185–92.

28. Older P, Hall A, Hader R. Cardiopulmonary exercise testing as a screening test for perioperative management of major surgery in the elderly. Chest. 1999;116:355–62.

29. Bartels C, Bechtel JF, Hossmann V, Horsch S. Cardiac risk stratification for high-risk vascular surgery. Circulation. 1997;95: 2473–5.

30. Girish M, Trayner EJ, Damman O, Pinto-Plata V, Celli B. Symptom-limited stair climbing as a predictor of postoperative cardiopulmonary complications after high-risk surgery. Chest. 2001;120(4):1147–51.

31. Rady MY, Ryan T, Starr N. Perioperative determinants of morbidity and mortality in elderly patients undergoing cardiac surgery. Crit Care Med. 2001;29(9):S163–72.

32. Goldman L, Caldera DL, Nussbaum SR, et al. Multifactorial index of cardiac risk in noncardiac surgical procedures. N Engl J Med. 1977;297(16):845–50.

33. Detsky AS, Abrams HB, McLaughlin JR, et al. Predicting cardiac complications in patients undergoing non-cardiac surgery. J Gen Intern Med. 1986;1(4):211–9.

34. Detsky AS, Abrams HB, Forbath N, Scott JG, Hilliard JR. Cardiac assessment for patients undergoing noncardiac surgery. A multifactorial clinical risk index Arch Intern Med. 1986;146(11):2131–4.

35. Eagle KA, Coley CM, Newell JB, et al. Combining clinical and thallium data optimizes preoperative assessment of cardiac risk before major vascular surgery. Ann Intern Med. 1989;110(11):859–66.

36. Arora VM, McGory ML, Fung CH. Quality Indicators for Hospitalization and Surgery in Vulnerable Elders. JAGS. 2007;55:S347–S58.

37. Sugarman J, McCrory DC, Hubal RC. Getting meaningful informed consent from older adults: a structured literature review of empirical research. J Am Geriatr Soc. 1998;46:517–24.

38. Auerswald KB, Charpentier PA, Inouye SK. The informed consent process in older patients who developed delirium: a clinical epidemiologic study. Am J Med. 1997;103:410–8.

39. Repetto L, Fratino L, Audisio RA, et al. Comprehensive geriatric assessment adds information to Eastern Cooperative Oncology Group performance status in elderly cancer patients: an Italian Group for Geriatric Oncology Study. J Clin Oncol. 2002;20:494–502.

40. Fukuse T, Satoda N, Hijiya K, Fujinaga T. Importance of a comprehensive geriatric assessment in prediction of complications following thoracic surgery in elderly patients. Chest. 2005;127(3):886–91.

41. Brunelli A, Monteverde M, Al Refal M, Flanchini A. Stair climbing test as a predictor of cardiopulmonary complications after pulmonary lobectomy in the elderly. Ann Thor Surg. 2004;77(1): 266–70.

42. Pope D, Ramesh H, Gennar R, et al. Pre-operative assessment of cancer in the elderly (PACE): a comprehensive assessment of underlying characteristics of elderly cancer patients prior to elective surgery. Surg Oncol. 2007;15:189–97.

43. Mofardini S, Ferucci L, Fratino L, et al. Validation of a multidimensional scale for use in elderly cancer patients. Cancer. 1996;77: 395–401.

44. Anesthesiologists AS. New classification of physical status. Anesthesiology. 1963;24:111.

45. Mendoza TR, Wang XS, Cleeland CS, et al. The rapid assessment of fatigue severity in cancer patients: use of the Brief Fatigue Inventory. Cancer. 1999;85:1186–96.

46. Audisio R, Gennari R, Sunouchi K, Pope DP. Preoperative assessment of cancer in elderly patients: a pilot study. Support Cancer Ther. 2003;1:55–60.

47. Audisio RA, Pope D, Ramesh HS, et al. Shall we operate? Preoperative assessment in elderly cancer patients (PACE) can help. A SIOG surgical task force prospective study. Crit Rev Oncol Hematol. 2008;65(2):156–63.

48. Pope D, Ramesh H, Gennari R, et al. Pre-operative assessment of cancer in the elderly (PACE): a comprehensive assessment of underlying characteristics of elderly cancer patients prior to elective surgery. Surg Oncol. 2006;15:189–97.

49. Audisio RA, Pope D, Ramesh HS, et al. Shall we operate? Preoperative assessment in elderly cancer patients (PACE) can help. A SIOG surgical task force prospective study. Crit Rev Oncol Hematol. 2008;65:156–63.

50. Audisio RA, Gennari R, Sunouchi K, et al. Preoperative assessment of cancer in elderly patients: a pilot study. Support Cancer Ther. 2003;1:55–60.

51. Katz S, Akpom CA. 12. Index of ADL. Med Care. 1976;14:116–8.

52. Lawton MP, Brody EM. Assessment of older people: self-maintaining and instrumental activities of daily living. Gerontologist. 1969;9:179–86.

53. Yesavage JA. Geriatric depression scale. Psychopharmacol Bull. 1988;24:709–11.

54. Mendoza TR, Wang XS, Cleeland CS, et al. The rapid assessment of fatigue severity in cancer patients: use of the Brief Fatigue Inventory. Cancer. 1999;85:1186–96.

55. Folstein MF, Folstein SE, McHugh PR. "Mini-mental state". A practical method for grading the cognitive state of patients for the clinician. J Psychiatr Res. 1975;12:189–98.

56. DiMaria-Ghalili RA, Guenter PA. The mini nutritional assessment. Am J Nurs. 2008;108:50–9; quiz 60.

Chapter 39
Thoracic Anesthesia in the Elderly

Anne C. Kolker

Abstract Projections are that the elderly population is increasing by as much as 50% by 2025. Increasing age and noncardiac thoracic surgery are both risk factors for increased morbidity and mortality. Thoracic anesthesia for the elderly patient requires optimization of medical status when possible. Coexisting diseases and subtle changes in physiology can affect the stability of an anesthetic. Drug metabolism may be decreased or brain sensitivity may be increased leading to more profound effects of various anesthetic drugs. Cardiovascular and respiratory complications as well as delirium increase morbidity. Short acting drugs and minimally invasive techniques may allow for a rapid return to preoperative function. No single anesthetic technique has been found to improve outcome. Further studies will help elucidate what factors are important in the anesthetic care of the elderly.

Keywords Thoracic anesthesia • Elderly • Geriatric • Co-morbidity • Physiology • Risk factors • Cardiovascular • Pulmonary • Renal • Hepatic • Nervous system • Temperature regulation • Positioning • Anesthetic • Inhaled anesthesia • Propofol • Fentanyl • Alfentanil • Remifentanil • Midazolam • Muscle relaxants • VATS • Pain control • Epidural • Postoperative • Pneumonia • Myocardial infarction • Delirium • Morbidity • Mortality

Introduction

Recognizing that elderly Americans are an enlarging population that is projected to increase by as much as 50% by 2025, a group of anesthesiologists started the Society for the Advancement of Geriatric Anesthesia (SAGA) in 2000. Its stated purpose was to better understand the implication of aging for our future and how it relates to the continuum of the perioperative period. Increasing age and noncardiac thoracic surgery are both risk factors for increased morbidity and mortality. Many factors that affect the outcome from anesthesia and surgery in the aging population are being identified and may then be studied.

A task force met to define what changes must take place within organized medicine to provide good care for the elderly outside of internal medicine [1]. Aging is associated with progressive loss of functional reserve and reduced ability to compensate for physiologic stress [1]. However, there is individual variation as to onset and extent of these changes. In addition to physiologic changes, the elderly patients often have multiple comorbid conditions, which affect their care. Preoperative evaluation and optimization of preexisting medical conditions reduce postoperative morbidity and mortality. Maintenance of cognitive function and independence are important goals for recovery from surgery and anesthesia in the geriatric patient.

In 1995, adults aged ≥65 years composed 13% of the population but accounted for 35% of total personal health care dollars spent ($310 billion), and real per capita personal health-care expenditure for this age group increased at an average annual rate of 5.8% during 1985–1995. Projections for 2000 and beyond are substantially higher [2]. Mortality associated with anesthesia and surgery increases with age. Mortality in the general population is 1.2%, compared with 2.2% in patients aged 60–69, 2.9% in patients 70–79, 5.8–6.2% in patients over 80, and 8.4% in those over 90 [3]. Risk factors for postoperative mortality in the elderly are shown in Table 39.1 [3]. Age, American Society of Anesthesiologists (ASA) classification, surgical risk, and emergency surgery have been found to be independent predictors of adverse postoperative outcomes [4–7]. Since ASA classification is based on existing preoperative medical status and classification greater than ASA II is associated with increased risk of adverse outcome, optimization of preoperative medical status is imperative to the extent possible.

A.C. Kolker (✉)
Department of Anesthesia, Memorial Sloan Kettering Cancer Center, 1275 York Avenue, New York, NY 10065, USA
e-mail: kolkera@mskcc.org

M.R. Katlic (ed.), *Cardiothoracic Surgery in the Elderly*, DOI 10.1007/978-1-4419-0892-6_39,
© Springer Science+Business Media, LLC 2011

Table 39.2 Clinical pharmacology of anesthetic agents in elderly patients

Drug	Brain sensitivity	Pharmacokinetics	Dose
Inhaled agents	↑	–	↓
Thiopental	–	↓ Initial distribution volume	↓
Etomidate	–	↓ Initial distribution volume ↓ Clearance	↓
Propofol	↑	↓ Clearance	↓
Midazolam	↑	↓ Clearance	↓
Morphine	↑	↓ Clearance	↓
Sufentanil	↑		↓
Alfentanil	↑		↓
Fentanyl	↑		↓
Remifentanil	↑	↓ Clearance ↓ Central compartment volume	–
Pancuronium	NA	↓	↓[a]
Atracurium	NA	–	–
Cisatracurium	NA	–	–
Vecuronium	NA	↓ Clearance	↓

NA not applicable

[a] See text

Source: Reprinted with permission from Miller [4], Copyright Elsevier 2009

Hypnotics

Several drugs commonly used either for induction of anesthesia or amnesia have age-related changes in potency. Thiopental requirements for induction of anesthesia for an 80-year old are approximately 85% of the dose required for a 20-year old. The increased sensitivity of elderly patients to thiopental is the result of a reduction in the volume of distribution and, therefore, higher concentrations exist for any given dose [24].

Elderly patients may show a 30–50% increased sensitivity to Propofol, which is widely used in anesthesia practice [25]. The intrinsic potency of propofol increases with age because of the increased brain sensitivity to the drug. Recovery from a 1 h propofol infusion in the elderly patient is nearly identical for a 20 and 80-year old patient. However, in the elderly patient, recovery after a 4 h infusion may double due to decreased clearance as well as increased brain sensitivity [24].

The pharmacokinetics and pharmacodynamics of midazolam are profoundly influenced by age. Plasma concentrations fall slowly in elderly patients due to reduced clearance [24]. Sedation studies show a 75% decrease in dose from age 20 to 90 when used for intravenous sedation in endoscopic procedures. Small doses, usually 1–2 mg, used as anxiolytics prior to anesthesia induction, are likely less to have long lived effects such as prolonged sedation unless the surgical procedure is a brief diagnostic one.

Muscle Relaxants

Age does not generally affect the pharmacodynamics of muscle relaxants. Both atracurium and cis-atracurium are unaffected by age mainly because of the elimination by hydrolysis and Hofmann degradation, which are intrinsic properties of the drugs. Vecuronium clearance during infusion is reduced by about 30% but the difference in recovery time is small (~10 min). Pancuronium clearance is variable relying primarily on renal function. Therefore, pancuronium might best be avoided in elderly patients, in whom renal function is often impaired.

Narcotics

Existing data suggest that for the elderly population, increased brain sensitivity to narcotics and decreased clearance account for lower dose requirements. Morphine-6-glucuronide is an active morphine metabolite that depends on renal excretion. Elderly patients with renal insufficiency may have impaired elimination of morphine glucuronides and resultant enhanced analgesia from a given morphine dose. Sufentanil, alfentanil, and fentanyl are approximately twice as potent in elderly patients primarily due to an increase in brain sensitivity to opioids with aging [26]. In contrast, slower onset and offset of remifentanil effects are seen in elderly patients compared with 20-year olds. About half the dose used in younger patients is required to achieve the same drug level effect. This is entirely due to increased brain sensitivity, as with fentanyl and alfentanil [24].

Positioning

No specific complications of positioning occur uniquely in the geriatric patient. However, elderly patients are, in general, less flexible than younger patients, so that surgical positioning can be problematic. In addition, loss of subcutaneous tissue and diminished skin elasticity may predispose to skin damage. Bony abnormalities can also require attention and careful padding to reduce risk of postoperative neuropathies [27].

Comorbidity

In addition to physiologic changes associated with advanced age, elderly patients presenting for thoracotomy often have a variety of comorbidities, which complicate their

Table 39.3 Cohort patients: comorbidities, according to the outcomes [28]

Comorbidities	SG n(%)	DG n(%)	p-Value
Hypertension	213 (58)	24 (73)	0.09
Anemia	100 (27)	17 (52)	0.004
Diabetes mellitus	76 (21)	7 (21)	0.93
Dyslipidemia	39 (11)	8 (24)	0.04
Coronary disease	21 (06)	8 (24)	≤0.001
Cardiac failure	25 (07)	3 (09)	0.47
Hypothyroidism	27 (07)	0	0.15
COPD[a]	24 (06)	1 (03)	0.70
Stroke	19 (05)	3 (09)	0.40
Atrial fibrillation	17 (05)	4 (12)	0.08
Chronic kidney disease stage ≥3	11 (03)	7 (21)	≤0.001
Depression	13 (04)	2 (06)	0.35
Body mass index <16	6 (02)	5 (16)	≤0.001
Dementia	6 (02)	2 (06)	0.13
Heart valve disease	1 (0.3)	3 (09)	≤0.001

SG survivor group; DG death group

[a]Chronic obstructive pulmonary disease

Source: Reprinted with permission from Machado et al. [28]

anesthetic care. As shown in Table 39.3, some comorbid states affect outcome. Preoperative comorbid disease is a stronger determinant of postoperative morbidity than is anesthetic management. As already stated, preoperative optimization of medical status reduces postoperative mortality. Comorbidities do not correlate with mortality [6, 28]. Various authors have found that tachycardia [6], hypothermia [3], and fluid overload [3] can increase morbidity. ASA status, emergency surgery, and increasing age are all risk factors for morbidity and mortality [5].

Surgical Population

The hazards of anesthesia cannot be separated from the risk of surgery [8, 29]. Multiple studies confirm that increasing age is associated with increased risk for postoperative morbidity and mortality in the general surgical population. In a large scale prospective study that examined anesthesia and surgical mortality, of 7,306 general surgical patients [8], it was found that 0.05% (1:1,800) died during anesthesia, 0.1% (1:730) died during the recovery period, and the overall mortality rate in hospital was 1.2% (1:81). Perioperatively, the period of greatest risk appears to be the postoperative period [8]. Most deaths occurred in the elderly (greater than or equal to 70 years of age) and were unavoidable due to progression of the presenting condition, such as advanced cancer, or to coexisting diseases such as cardiopulmonary or renal failure. Of the patients who developed MI following anesthesia, 67% (8/12) died in the postoperative period. It was determined that within the same group, a left ventricular ejection fraction

less than 50% or greater than 70% was associated with a 58% risk of complications when compared with 12% risk in the 50–70% ejection fraction group. A prospective study of 5-year survival among 900 patients aged 65 years and above who were undergoing a general surgical procedure revealed that high early mortality was associated with nonelective admissions, age 75 years and above, ASA grade 4–5 and major surgery.

Patients aged 65 and above comprise at least one quarter of the surgical population. Studies of elderly surgical patients have focused largely on the lung cancer population, as there is an increasing worldwide incidence of the disease [30]. Although surgery for lung cancer is only one aspect of thoracic surgical practice, generalizations from the published literature can be made for other conditions requiring thoracotomy. Although surgery for benign thoracic disease states, including treatment of esophageal disorders as well as diagnostic procedures, is a component of thoracic surgical practice, the geriatric population comprises only a small part of the affected population. Minimally invasive techniques have been increasingly used for both benign and malignant conditions in the general population. In terms of benign disease, laparoscopy has been successfully used in repair of paraesophageal hernias, although the focus is not specifically the elderly population [31]. Reports of thoracoscopic Belsey fundoplication include elderly patients [32]. There are isolated reports of surgical repair of esophageal perforation on elderly subjects [33].

Both surgical and anesthetic choices have been examined to determine the best approach for minimizing morbidity and mortality in the elderly population. A retrospective study of 68 octogenarians with non small cell lung cancer (NSCLC) who underwent lung resection found that health status and tumor stage were more important than chronologic age in determining outcome and survival [34]. ASA class greater than 2, FEV_1 of less than 1.5 L and advanced stage of disease were found to be strong independent negative predictors of long-term survival [34]. Another large retrospective study found that among elderly patients with good performance status and no comorbidity, perioperative mortality and prognosis were similar to those in younger patients [35]. A retrospective study of patients 70 and older concluded that age was a risk factor for overall but not major morbidity [36]. Analysis of data collected for the Society of Thoracic Surgeons on patients undergoing esophagectomy concluded that age above 75 is a significant predictor for major morbidity [37].

Respiratory complications are the major cause of morbidity and mortality after pulmonary resection in the elderly. A study designed to develop and validate risk factors for postoperative pneumonia after major noncardiac surgery found that thoracic surgery has a greater relative risk value for development of pneumonia than emergency procedures or those requiring more than 4 units transfusion [38]. Each decade after the seventh decade increases the risk for postoperative pneumonia. Numerous studies have evaluated the benefit of video-assisted thoracic surgery (VATS) in the elderly population, with emphasis on octogenarians [39]. With appropriately selected patients, the risk of surgery and anesthesia is acceptable. By comparison with standard thoracotomy, VATS treatment of lung malignancy in the elderly appears to have parallel oncologic efficacy and may confer improved pulmonary function [30, 40]. A study of 138 patients comparing postoperative pain-related morbidity in video-assisted thoracoscopic surgery (VATS) or limited lateral thoracotomy found that VATS patients experienced less postop pain, reduced requirements for narcotics, and improved early pulmonary function. Shoulder girdle strength was equally impaired following VATS or thoracotomy at day 3 but recovered more rapidly (by 3 weeks) in VATS patients [41]. Minimally invasive surgical techniques seem to allow for improved recovery from a variety of procedures.

Anesthetic Management

Anesthesia goals for the elderly patient should be to maintain homeostasis during surgery, to preserve myocardial and hemodynamic function, and to provide adequate pain control postoperatively. Careful monitoring during surgery as well as attention to issues related to preexisting medical conditions are part of standard anesthetic care. Additionally, maintaining intact neuro-cognitive function as well as the ability to function independently are two important desired postoperative outcomes. Preexisting level of function appears to predict long-term outcome in geriatric patients [42].

As previously stated, no one anesthetic technique has been found to have improved outcome over another. Studies attempting to demonstrate benefits of regional over general anesthesia have been conflicting. One study found no significant difference [18], while another concluded that regional anesthesia reduces postoperative mortality and other serious complications [43]. Thoracic epidural anesthesia has been shown in vascular surgery, coronary artery bypass grafting, and abdominal surgical procedures to attenuate the perioperative stress response, improve myocardial oxygenation, reduce the release of troponin T, and effectively control refractory unstable angina as a result of sympatholysis [44–46]. Epidural analgesia has also been shown to provide superior pain management over systemic narcotics in the postoperative period [47]. Use of short acting drugs and modalities such as epidural analgesia for postoperative pain relief appears to have some theoretical and practical merit. Further studies will help to delineate the relative importance of the combined epidural-general technique.

Interestingly, patients who received 100% oxygen were found to have better proinflammatory and antimicrobial responses of alveolar macrophages than those given minimal oxygen [48]. Although this study was performed on patients undergoing orthopedic surgery and was not limited to the elderly population, it is interesting to consider that patients for thoracic procedures often receive 100% oxygen during surgery and might therefore similarly benefit from the improved alveolar macrophage responses.

Pain Control and Delirium

Delirium in surgical patients has been reported to increase the length of stay as well as the cost of care [49]. A large scale international study found that only age correlated with late postoperative cognitive dysfunction [19]. Unfortunately, recognition of delirium and definition of postoperative cognitive decline (POCD) are often ambiguous and unrecognized so that studies are difficult to assess. Noncardiac thoracic surgery is a defined risk factor for postoperative delirium [50]. Additionally, adequate pain control with appropriate routes of administration of pain medicine is important to minimize adverse events and limit morbidity due to postoperative delirium. Although combining general anesthesia with epidural placement for postoperative analgesia has an intrinsic appeal to limit systemic exposure to narcotics, no evidence exits as yet that there is any decrease in postoperative delirium or POCD [51]. Recent studies have evaluated pain and pain management modalities as they relate to postoperative delirium or POCD. In one study [52], age, moderate and severe preoperative resting pain, and increased pain from baseline were independently associated with a greater risk for development of postoperative delirium. Meperidine was associated with increased risk of delirium in elderly surgical patients but morphine, fentanyl, and hydromorphone were not found to have significant difference in risk of delirium [51]. According to the analysis of a literature search [51], available studies do not differentiate between IV or epidural techniques in terms of cognitive function in elderly patients.

Summary

The geriatric patient population comprises a highly varied group in terms of functional status. The onset and extent of loss of functional reserve is individual. As the elderly population is increasing, the anesthetic care of this group is being studied to better understand what factors can be identified that impact outcome from surgery and anesthesia.

Known risk factors for perioperative complications have been and will continue to be elucidated. Optimization of the patient's preoperative medical status, when possible, reduces morbidity and mortality. Elective surgery, as opposed to emergency surgery, also reduces relative risk of morbidity and mortality. Organ function declines with increasing age and concomitant ability to metabolize drugs or equilibrate fluid balance after surgery is reduced. Risk of cardiac and pulmonary complications increases with aging. Noncardiac thoracic surgery includes a high relative risk for complications in the elderly.

Although no single anesthetic technique has been shown to be superior to another in terms of outcome, combined epidural and general anesthesia has been found to provide superior pain relief and to reduce narcotic requirement postoperatively. As yet, no evidence exists that an anesthetic technique is associated with reduced incidence of postoperative delirium. Certainly minimizing delirium in the elderly is important for reducing morbidity and allowing a return to preoperative functional state. VATS and minimally invasive techniques also improve rapid return to function when compared with standard thoracotomy. Studies targeting a reduction in morbidity and mortality from anesthesia and surgery in the geriatric population will continue to guide the development of safer and better techniques in the care of this large diverse group.

References

1. Cook DJ, Rooke GA. Priorities in perioperative geriatrics. Anesth Analg. 2003;96(6):1823–36.
2. Desai MM, Zhang P, Hennessy CH. Surveillance for morbidity and mortality among older adults – United States, 1995–1996. MMWR CDC Surveill Summ. 1999;48(8):7–25.
3. Jin F, Chung F. Minimizing perioperative adverse events in the elderly. Br J Anaesth. 2001;87(4):608–24.
4. Miller RD. Anesthesia. 7th ed. New York: Churchill Livingstone; 2009.
5. John AD, Sieber FE. Age associated issues: geriatrics. Anesthesiol Clin North America. 2004;22(1):45–58.
6. Leung JM, Dzankic S. Relative importance of preoperative health status versus intraoperative factors in predicting postoperative adverse outcomes in geriatric surgical patients. J Am Geriatr Soc. 2001;49(8):1080–5.
7. Dzankic S, Pastor D, Gonzalez C, Leung JM. The prevalence and predictive value of abnormal preoperative laboratory tests in elderly surgical patients. Anesth Analg. 2001;93(2):301–8.
8. Pedersen T, Eliasen K, Henriksen E. A prospective study of mortality associated with anaesthesia and surgery: risk indicators of mortality in hospital. Acta Anaesthesiol Scand. 1990;34(3):176–82.
9. Rooke GA. Autonomic and cardiovascular function in the geriatric patient. Anesthesiol Clin North America. 2000;18(1):31–46, v–vi.
10. Redfield MM, Jacobsen SJ, Burnett Jr JC, Mahoney DW, Bailey KR, Rodeheffer RJ. Burden of systolic and diastolic ventricular dysfunction in the community: appreciating the scope of the heart failure epidemic. JAMA. 2003;289(2):194–202.
11. Ashton CM, Petersen NJ, Wray NP, et al. The incidence of perioperative myocardial infarction in men undergoing noncardiac surgery. Ann Intern Med. 1993;118(7):504–10.
12. Fleisher LA, Beckman JA, Brown KA, et al. 2009 ACCF/AHA focused update on perioperative beta blockade incorporated into the ACC/AHA 2007 guidelines on perioperative cardiovascular evaluation and care for noncardiac surgery. J Am Coll Cardiol. 2009;54(22):e13–118.
13. Erskine RJ, Murphy PJ, Langton JA, Smith G. Effect of age on the sensitivity of upper airway reflexes. Br J Anaesth. 1993;70(5):574–5.
14. Pedersen T, Eliasen K, Henriksen E. A prospective study of risk factors and cardiopulmonary complications associated with anaesthesia and surgery: risk indicators of cardiopulmonary morbidity. Acta Anaesthesiol Scand. 1990;34(2):144–55.
15. Nicholson G, Pereira AC, Hall GM. Parkinson's disease and anaesthesia. Br J Anaesth. 2002;89(6):904–16.
16. Schmucker DL. Age-related changes in liver structure and function: Implications for disease? Exp Gerontol. 2005;40(8–9):650–9.
17. Martin JE, Sheaff MT. Renal ageing. J Pathol. 2007;211(2): 198–205.
18. Rasmussen LS, Johnson T, Kuipers HM, et al. Does anaesthesia cause postoperative cognitive dysfunction? A randomised study of regional versus general anaesthesia in 438 elderly patients. Acta Anaesthesiol Scand. 2003;47(3):260–6.
19. Levine WC, Mehta V, Landesberg G. Anesthesia for the elderly: selected topics. Curr Opin Anaesthesiol. 2006;19(3):320–4.
20. Frank SM, Fleisher LA, Breslow MJ, et al. Perioperative maintenance of normothermia reduces the incidence of morbid cardiac events. A randomized clinical trial. JAMA. 1997;277(14):1127–34.
21. Liu LL, Leung JM. Predicting adverse postoperative outcomes in patients aged 80 years or older. J Am Geriatr Soc. 2000;48(4): 405–12.
22. Roy RC. Choosing general versus regional anesthesia for the elderly. Anesthesiol Clin North America. 2000;18(1):91–104, vii.
23. Bates DW, Cullen DJ, Laird N, et al. Incidence of adverse drug events and potential adverse drug events. Implications for prevention. ADE Prevention Study Group. JAMA. 1995;274(1):29–34.
24. Shafer SL. The pharmacology of anesthetic drugs in elderly patients. Anesthesiol Clin North America. 2000;18(1):1–29, v.
25. Schnider TW, Minto CF, Shafer SL, et al. The influence of age on propofol pharmacodynamics. Anesthesiology. 1999;90(6):1502–16.
26. Minto CF, Schnider TW, Shafer SL. Pharmacokinetics and pharmacodynamics of remifentanil. II. Model application. Anesthesiology. 1997;86(1):24–33.
27. Martin JT. Positioning aged patients. Anesthesiol Clin North America. 2000;18(1):105–21.
28. Machado AN, Sitta Mdo C, Jacob Filho W, Garcez-Leme LE. Prognostic factors for mortality among patients above the 6th decade undergoing non-cardiac surgery: cares – clinical assessment and research in elderly surgical patients. Clinics (Sao Paulo). 2008;63(2):151–6.
29. Finlayson EV, Birkmeyer JD. Operative mortality with elective surgery in older adults. Eff Clin Pract. 2001;4(4):172–7.
30. Heerdt PM, Park BJ. The emerging role of minimally invasive surgical techniques for the treatment of lung malignancy in the elderly. Anesthesiol Clin. 2008;26(2):315–24, vi–vii.
31. Luketich JD, Raja S, Fernando HC, et al. Laparoscopic repair of giant paraesophageal hernia: 100 consecutive cases. Ann Surg. 2000;232(4):608–18.
32. Champion JK. Thoracoscopic Belsey fundoplication with 5-year outcomes. Surg Endosc. 2003;17(8):1212–5.
33. Sobrino MA, Kozarek R, Low DE. Primary endoscopic management of esophageal perforation following transesophageal echocardiogram. J Clin Gastroenterol. 2004;38(7):581–5.
34. Brock MV, Kim MP, Hooker CM, et al. Pulmonary resection in octogenarians with stage I nonsmall cell lung cancer: a 22-year experience. Ann Thorac Surg. 2004;77(1):271–7.
35. Sawada S, Komori E, Nogami N, et al. Advanced age is not correlated with either short-term or long-term postoperative results in

lung cancer patients in good clinical condition. Chest. 2005; 128(3):1557–63.

36. Pagni S, McKelvey A, Riordan C, Federico JA, Ponn RB. Pulmonary resection for malignancy in the elderly: is age still a risk factor? *Eur J Cardiothorac Surg.* 1998;14(1):40–4; discussion 44–5.

37. Wright CD, Kucharczuk JC, O'Brien SM, Grab JD, Allen MS. Predictors of major morbidity and mortality after esophagectomy for esophageal cancer: a Society of Thoracic Surgeons General Thoracic Surgery Database risk adjustment model. *J Thorac Cardiovasc Surg.* 2009;137(3):587–95; discussion 596.

38. Arozullah AM, Khuri SF, Henderson WG, Daley J. Development and validation of a multifactorial risk index for predicting postoperative pneumonia after major noncardiac surgery. Ann Intern Med. 2001;135(10):847–57.

39. Koizumi K, Haraguchi S, Hirata T, et al. Lobectomy by video-assisted thoracic surgery for lung cancer patients aged 80 years or more. Ann Thorac Cardiovasc Surg. 2003;9(1):14–21.

40. Kaseda S, Aoki T, Hangai N, Shimizu K. Better pulmonary function and prognosis with video-assisted thoracic surgery than with thoracotomy. Ann Thorac Surg. 2000;70(5):1644–6.

41. Landreneau RJ, Hazelrigg SR, Mack MJ, et al. Postoperative pain-related morbidity: video-assisted thoracic surgery versus thoracotomy. Ann Thorac Surg. 1993;56(6):1285–9.

42. Inouye SK, Peduzzi PN, Robison JT, Hughes JS, Horwitz RI, Concato J. Importance of functional measures in predicting mortality among older hospitalized patients. JAMA. 1998;279(15): 1187–93.

43. Rodgers A, Walker N, Schug S, et al. Reduction of postoperative mortality and morbidity with epidural or spinal anaesthesia: results from overview of randomised trials. BMJ. 2000;321(7275):1493.

44. Kapral S, Gollmann G, Bachmann D, et al. The effects of thoracic epidural anesthesia on intraoperative visceral perfusion and metabolism. Anesth Analg. 1999;88(2):402–6.

45. Loick HM, Schmidt C, Van Aken H, et al. High thoracic epidural anesthesia, but not clonidine, attenuates the perioperative stress response via sympatholysis and reduces the release of troponin T in patients undergoing coronary artery bypass grafting. Anesth Analg. 1999;88(4):701–9.

46. Olausson K, Magnusdottir H, Lurje L, Wennerblom B, Emanuelsson H, Ricksten SE. Anti-ischemic and anti-anginal effects of thoracic epidural anesthesia versus those of conventional medical therapy in the treatment of severe refractory unstable angina pectoris. Circulation. 1997;96(7):2178–82.

47. Block BM, Liu SS, Rowlingson AJ, Cowan AR, Cowan Jr JA, Wu CL. Efficacy of postoperative epidural analgesia: a meta-analysis. JAMA. 2003;290(18):2455–63.

48. Kotani N, Hashimoto H, Sessler DI, et al. Supplemental intraoperative oxygen augments antimicrobial and proinflammatory responses of alveolar macrophages. Anesthesiology. 2000;93(1):15–25.

49. Franco K, Litaker D, Locala J, Bronson D. The cost of delirium in the surgical patient. Psychosomatics. 2001;42(1):68–73.

50. Marcantonio ER, Goldman L, Orav EJ, Cook EF, Lee TH. The association of intraoperative factors with the development of postoperative delirium. Am J Med. 1998;105(5):380–4.

51. Fong HK, Sands LP, Leung JM. The role of postoperative analgesia in delirium and cognitive decline in elderly patients: a systematic review. Anesth Analg. 2006;102(4):1255–66.

52. Vaurio LE, Sands LP, Wang Y, Mullen EA, Leung JM. Postoperative delirium: the importance of pain and pain management. Anesth Analg. 2006;102(4):1267–73.

Chapter 40
Postoperative and Critical Care in the Elderly Thoracic Surgery Patient

Brannon R. Hyde and Joseph B. Zwischenberger

Abstract Citizens over the age of 65 constitute the fastest growing segment of the population of the United States. Consequently, patients older than 65 years of age will constitute a growing segment of an average thoracic surgeon's practice. Treating physicians must understand the normal physiologic changes associated with aging to accurately construct a risk versus benefit analysis specifically tailored to the elderly patient, taking into account the patient's life expectancy and quality of life both before and after a procedure. A surgeon must be cognizant of the special postoperative needs and concerns in the elderly population, including pain control, end-of-life issues, and the potential need for rehabilitation or nursing home placement in the postoperative period. The challenge for the future will be to continue to improve perioperative and postoperative care, patient selection, and operative techniques to lower the morbidity and mortality rates among the elderly, and will require coordination between the family, patient, physician, surgeon, and critical care teams.

Keywords Risk assessment • Benefit analysis • Risk-benefit ratio • End-of-life issues • Palliative care • Pain management • Mechanical ventilation • Oxygenation • Pneumonia • Atelectasis • Comorbidities • Atrophy • Chronic obstructive pulmonary disease (COPD) • Cardiovascular disease • Acute respiratory distress syndrome (ARDS) • Acute renal failure (ARF) • Glomerular filtration rate (GFR) • Arrhythmia • Cardiac assessment • Atrial fibrillation (AF) • Myocardial infarction (MI) • Beta blockers • Blood transfusion • Exercise capacity • Lung volume reduction surgery (LVRS) • Anesthesia • Thoracotomy • Video-assisted thoracoscopic surgery (VATS) • Muscle sparing thoracotomy (MST) • Lung cancer • Esophagectomy • Cognitive impairment • Analgesia • Pain relief • Depression • Cognitive dysfunction • Delirium • Postoperative delirium • Postoperative cognitive disorder (POCD) • Life expectancy

B.R. Hyde (✉)
Department of Surgery, University of Kentucky, A301 KY Clinic, Lexington, KY 40536-0284, USA
e-mail: brhy222@uky.edu

Introduction

Citizens over the age of 65 constitute the fastest growing segment of the population of the United States. Although projections continue to rise, the U.S. Census Bureau currently estimates the elderly population (age >65) will rise from 40 million in 2010 to 81 million by 2040 and 89 million by 2050, doubling the elderly population in the US in just 30 years. Elderly persons over 85 years are also estimated to double in number, from five million in 2010 to over 11 million by 2035. Worldwide, the 65 and older population is estimated at 506 million as of 2008 with projections of 1.3 billion by the year 2040. Consequently, the number of elderly over 65 years of age could double from 7 to 14% of the world's population in just 30 years, paralleling the percentage growth in the United States. By 2030, estimates are that 19% of the population will be older than 65 years of age [1]. After 80 years of age, men, on average, live another 7.62 years and women live another 9.16 years [2].

Consequently, patients older than 65 years of age will constitute a growing segment of an average thoracic surgeon's practice. Fifty percent of newly diagnosed non-small-cell lung cancers are in patients over 65 years old with 30–40% in patients over 70 years old. The median age at diagnosis is now 69 years [3]. With average life expectancy between 87 and 89 years for individuals alive at 80, cancer management in the octogenarian should focus on quality of life [4] and take into consideration the individual's comorbidities and underlying physiologic reserve. The challenge for the future will be to continue to improve perioperative and postoperative care, patient selection, and operative techniques to lower the morbidity and mortality rates among the elderly. This will require coordination between the family, patient, physician, surgeon, and critical care teams. Advanced age alone is not a contraindication to operative treatment, even for higher risk procedures in thoracic and vascular surgery [5–7]. The elderly should not be considered simply as older adults any more than a surgeon would consider a baby a little adult. Treating physicians must understand the normal physiologic changes associated with aging to accurately construct a risk

M.R. Katlic (ed.), *Cardiothoracic Surgery in the Elderly*, DOI 10.1007/978-1-4419-0892-6_40,
© Springer Science+Business Media, LLC 2011

versus benefit analysis specifically tailored to each patient. Risk assessment should focus on identifying the physiologic state and reserve of specific organ systems to treat, or anticipate compromised function. Benefit analysis should take into account a patient's life expectancy and quality of life both before and after a procedure. Finally, a surgeon must be cognizant of the special postoperative needs and concerns in the elderly population, especially pain control issues. The surgeon should anticipate end-of-life issues, and the potential need for rehabilitation or nursing home placement in the early postoperative period. Standards of critical care that do not change with respect to the adult patient's age, such as nutritional support, fluid and electrolyte management, endocrine dysfunction, glucose control, antimicrobial therapy, and sepsis, are not discussed in this chapter.

Cardiovascular Physiology

Eighty percent of patients older than 80 years have identifiable cardiovascular disease. Men and women over 75 years old account for 36% of myocardial infarctions (MI) and 60% of MI-related deaths [8]. Age-related changes of the cardiovascular system, from small arterioles to large vessels and even the heart itself, play an important role in the loss of physiologic reserve. Most patients show no obvious sign of impaired hemodynamic performance. Stresses of anesthesia and the inflammatory response of an operation (increased myocardial oxygen demand from tachycardia or loss of vascular tone from the vasodilatory effects of anesthetic agents, for example) will often uncover the limited cardiac reserve of a patient.

As blood vessels age, the intimal layer gradually becomes less smooth and causes turbulent flow patterns, endothelial damage, and has an increased number of potential sites for lipid deposition. A complex cascade is initiated with endothelial damage which leads ultimately to intimal deposition of increased connective tissue, calcium, and lipid. The media also collects increased calcium, with thickening elastic fibers and hypertrophy of smooth muscle cells. These changes lead to stiffening of the vascular wall and increased peripheral vascular resistance [9].

Increased peripheral vascular resistance causes elevated blood pressure. With prolonged exposure to higher afterload pressures, myocyte turnover through apoptosis is accelerated with subsequent hypertrophy of the remaining cells and development of interstitial fibrosis. Resultant ventricular hypertrophy causes impaired diastolic function of the heart. The thickened ventricle wall, together with increased impedance through the aortic outflow tract, results in prolonged myocardial contraction and delayed relaxation. The ventricle

remains stiff during the early passive phases of diastolic filling when the mitral valve opens, reducing end diastolic volume and cardiac output [10]. The early diastolic filling of an 80-year-old patient is one-third to one-half that of a 20-year-old [10, 11]. The left atrium enlarges to augment late diastolic filling [12]. The nonstressed heart in normal sinus rhythm can compensate for some diastolic dysfunction, but tachycardia or hypertension may additionally reduce diastolic filling beyond the ability of the heart to compensate. A patient who develops atrial fibrillation loses the atrial contraction (or kick) leading to more reduced end diastolic volume and cardiac output [13]. These pathophysiologic changes underscore the importance of maintaining the heart and vascular systems in a nonstressed, normotensive, sinus rhythm during surgical procedures.

Cardiac output is a primary determinant of oxygen delivery and of aerobic metabolism in the body [14]. Even without severe cardiovascular disease, aging causes a decrease in cardiac output, beginning at age 30 years, of 1% per year [15]. Similarly, the maximum rate of oxygen use (VO_2 max) by the body declines steadily at 10% per decade, or about 50% between the ages of 20 and 80 years [13]. Congestive heart failure (CHF) is present in 10% of individuals over 65 years of age [16], and is the leading cause of postoperative morbidity and mortality after surgical procedures. Patients with CHF have an increased rate of cerebral stroke, myocardial infarction, and postoperative renal failure. To minimize adverse outcomes, preoperative recognition of impaired cardiac function and reserve is essential to maintain proper fluid balance and limit myocardial work intra- and postoperatively. Estimate of cardiac reserve also greatly impacts risk assessment.

Pulmonary Physiology

Pulmonary complications account for a majority of the morbidity encountered after thoracic operation. Atelectasis, pneumonia, air leaks, and prolonged mechanical ventilation account for a 7–33% morbidity rate after thoracic procedures in the elderly [17–19].

Pulmonary changes associated with aging are evident by a loss of elastic recoil of the lung and impaired chest wall movement from muscle atrophy, resulting in decreased intrathoracic volume displacement [20]. Impaired elasticity also causes air trapping and ventilation-perfusion mismatching, leading to decreased oxygen transfer reflected by an increased alveolar-arterial oxygen gradient [21]. Oxygenation is additionally impaired by an increased closure volume of small airways, and decreased surface area for gas exchange, as lung parenchyma is destroyed or thickened by aging [22]. The amount of lung volume not ventilated during normal respiration can double between the ages of 20 and 65 years. Vital capacity decreases with age, reflecting an increase in dead space ventilation [23]. Loss of parenchymal elasticity, joint stiffening, weakening of inspiratory muscles, and early small airway collapse also change gas flow characteristics. The forced expiratory volume in 1 s (FEV_1) progressively declines with aging resulting in an FEV_1: VC ratio <70% by age 70. The sum of the respiratory changes associated with aging ultimately limits the maximal breathing capacity by age 70–50% of that at age 30 [24].

Chronic obstructive pulmonary disease (COPD) is the primary diagnosis in 18% of all hospital admissions in patients older than 65 years [25] and accounts for two to three admissions per year averaging 12 hospital days per admission [26]. COPD affects approximately 16 million Americans [27] and is the fourth leading cause of death in the US [28]. Though the age-adjusted death rate for stroke and coronary artery disease has declined in the last 30 years, the death rate for COPD has increased by 70% [29]. With early diagnosis and aggressive preoperative pulmonary treatment, complication rates in the elderly with COPD can be minimized [30].

Prevalence of acute respiratory distress syndrome (ARDS) among hospitalized patients has been estimated to be as high as 40% in high-risk patients [31]. Mortality rates in patients younger than age 60 are 12–45%, although rates in patients older than age 60 are 64–72% [32–34]. One study examined the relationship between age and outcomes in ARDS and found a progressive decline in survival for each increasing age group at 28 days of hospitalization (Fig. 40.1). Mortality at 28 days was 25.4% in patients less than age 70, and 50.3% in those older than age 70 [35]. Age as an independent risk factor for mortality in ARDS has been challenged recently. When 343 patients (*n*=210 >65 years old) developed ARDS at a single institution, there was no significant difference in mortality between the group over age 65 years (51.9%) and the group under age 65 years (41.7%). Only Acute Physiology

and Chronic Health Evaluation III and nonpulmonary multiple organ dysfunction scores were statistically significant predictors of mortality [36]. Consequently, treatment strategies do not differ among age groups, and should focus on identification of the underlying causes for ARDS combined with ventilator management based on low tidal volume protective strategies to minimize ongoing ventilator-induced lung injury [37].

Pain associated with thoracic and abdominal operations can have profound effects on pulmonary mechanics and tip a marginal patient to failure or prolonged mechanical ventilation. Splinting from inadequate pain control restricts lung expansion and prevents adequate cough to clear secretions, leading to increased risk for atelectasis, pneumonia, and hypoxia. Functional residual capacity can be suppressed up to 70% from baseline and remain severely suppressed for as long as a week postoperatively [38]. To lower the incidence of pulmonary complications, an aggressive pulmonary toilet regimen of coughing, deep breathing, and early ambulation should be implemented immediately after the operation [39].

Renal Physiology

Acute renal failure (ARF) occurs in approximately 5–6% of ICU admissions and has an associated 60% in-hospital mortality. In an analysis of over 29,000 patients in 23 countries, 34% of patients had ARF after major surgery. In 47.5% of the study patients, ARF was associated with septic shock, and each year of advancing age was shown to be statistically significant for an increased risk of hospital mortality on multivariate analysis [40]. Consequently, avoiding kidney injury increases survival in surgical patients and has an even greater effect among the elderly.

Avoiding acute kidney injury is predicated on understanding the numerous age-related changes in renal morphology and physiology (Table 40.1) [41]. A progressive reduction in renal mass results in kidney weight decreasing to 75–80% of young adult weight by 80–90 years of age. By 70 years of age, 30–50% of cortical glomeruli have been lost secondary to ischemic changes or glomerulosclerosis [24, 41, 42]. Glomerulosclerosis results in a decline in renal plasma flow and in glomerular filtration rate (GFR) [43]. Moreover, the number and size of tubules decreases, leading to increased tubulointerstitial fibrosis, glomerular filtering surface area decreases because of increased mesangial cells, increased thickness of glomerular and tubular basement membranes, arteriosclerosis, and decreased cross-sectional area of afferent arterioles. From age 20–80 years, renal blood flow decreases 50%, resulting in a decreased GFR [41]. Additionally, the age-related decline in cardiac output also

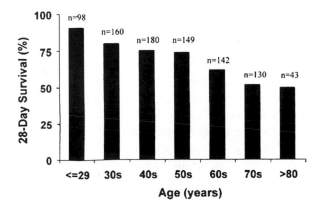

Fig. 40.1 Decreased 28-days survival in patients with acute lung injury by decade of age (Reprinted from Cheng and Matthay [37])

Table 40.1 Anatomic and physiologic changes in the aging kidney

Anatomic

Loss of renal mass

Glomerular drop out and glomerulosclerosis

Diminished glomerular filtering surface area

Decreased tubular size and number

Increased tubulointerstitial fibrosis

Thickened glomerular and tubular basement membranes

Decreased afferent arteriolar luminal area

Increased arteriosclerosis

Physiologic

Decreased renal blood flow

Decreased glomerular filtration rate

Diminished urinary concentrating and diluting capacity

Diminished capacity for sodium conservation

Decreased plasma renin and aldosterone levels

Decreased prostaglandin production

Increased vasoconstrictive response to stimuli (e.g., volume depletion)

Source: Reprinted with permission from Abdel-Kader and Palevsky [41]

negatively impacts renal plasma flow and GFR. All elderly patients have decreased GFR, and are susceptible to volume overload and accumulation of metabolic substances and drugs that rely on renal clearance for excretion [44]. Slowed drug elimination can lead to prolonged sedative effects of anesthetic and narcotic medication, and a propensity to drug-induced ARF after administration of nonsteroidal antiinflammatory medications, diuretics, and antibiotics [24]. Impaired renal sodium conservation can lead to electrolyte imbalances that could potentially affect cardiac conduction and lead to arrhythmia [13]. The plasma level of creatinine is an unreliable marker of GFR in the elderly. In the critically ill elderly patient, GFR should be calculated using serum-creatinine based equations, such as the modification of diet in renal disease formula. GFR may also be estimated using cystatin C, a serum marker more reliable than creatinine in the elderly. However, the cystatin C assay is not widely available [45].

Adjuncts necessary to avoid acute kidney injury include providing hydration and volume loading (normal saline or isotonic sodium bicarbonate), maintaining renal perfusion pressure, avoiding nephrotoxin exposure (aminoglycosides, amphotericin B, and radiocontrast), and judicious use of *N*-acetylcysteine. Fenoldopam may help avoid septic acute kidney injury, but evidence is lacking. Theophylline, likewise, will need further trials before its role in avoidance of contrast nephropathy is elucidated [46].

Preoperative Assessment

Coexisting disease has more impact on morbidity and mortality than age alone in the geriatric population [47]. Likewise, age alone is not an independent risk factor for

morbidity and mortality after a thoracic operation [5]. A barrage of laboratory tests is generally not indicated, and has been shown to be of no benefit in the elderly [48]. A workup should begin with basic laboratory screening based on an individual's known comorbidities. Symptoms of ongoing infection should prompt an inquiry to identify the source and clear the infection before any elective procedure. Recent weight loss is important and the nutritional state of the patient should be evaluated and corrected if possible. The National Veteran's Affairs Surgical Risk Study has identified albumin level as the most important independent risk factor predicting postoperative morbidity and mortality [49]. Mortality was <1% for albumin levels >46 g/L and rose exponentially to 29% for levels <21 g/L. Age ranked fifth for predicting mortality and tenth for morbidity [49, 50].

Cardiac Evaluation

Cardiac assessment usually begins with an ECG, and 75% of patients over 70 years of age have some abnormality on ECG. No correlation exists between ECG abnormalities alone and life expectancy [51]. Arrhythmias have been shown to adversely impact postoperative cardiac morbidity in elderly patients [18], possibly leading to hemodynamic instability or stoke. Atrial fibrillation (AF) is the most common arrhythmia, estimated to be present in 10% of patients over 80 years of age and accounting for 75,000 thromboembolic events per year. AF is common after thoracic surgery, occurring in approximately 12–15% of all types of thoracic surgery [13, 52], but is reported as high as 22% in patients over 70 years [52], 12–30% for lobectomy, and 24–67% for pneumonectomy [53]. Older age is the strongest predictor of AF after thoracic surgery. Patients with AF have a higher incidence of pneumonia, respiratory failure, and mortality [13, 54]. Furthermore, AF incidence rises with increasing age, comorbidities, or increased thoracic dissection. On a multivariate analysis of 2,588 patients, the relative risk of AF was significant for male sex (1.72), age 50–59 (1.7, vs. age <50), age 60–69 (4.49, vs. age <50), age >70 (5.30, vs. age <50), history of CHF (2.51), history of arrhythmias (1.92), lobectomy (3.89, vs. single wedge), bilobectomy (7.16, vs. single wedge), and pneumonectomy (8.91, vs. single wedge) [52]. Obviously, the incidence of AF rises with increasing age and increased intrathoracic dissection. New onset AF requires rate control and attempted restoration of normal rhythm, but there is no survival benefit to converting chronic AF to sinus rhythm preoperatively in asymptomatic patients. Rate control and anticoagulation are still the mainstays of treatment in chronic atrial fibrillation. One recent randomized trial reports a decreased incidence of AF after lobectomy, bilobectomy, or pneumonectomy when patients were given prophylactic amiodarone (32.3% in control group versus 13.8% in amiodarone group, $p=0.02$). The amiodarone group also had a significantly shorter length of ICU stay [53]. Prophylactic amiodarone therapy, however, still requires further investigation before becoming standard care. In one retrospective analysis, VATS versus thoracotomy for lung resection did not significantly impact on the incidence of AF [55].

Cardiac complications in the elderly occur in 10.3–12.5% of patients with preexisting heart disease [17, 56]. Preexisting CHF can lead to a two- to fourfold increase in postoperative cardiovascular complications, including MI, supraventricular tachycardia, hypo- or hypertension, and cardiac arrest [56, 57]. Estimation of cardiac reserve can be difficult because most elderly patients with cardiac dysfunction are compensated, and will only show signs of disease when stressed. Physical reserve of elderly patients is difficult to estimate under circumstances of a sedentary lifestyle or general debility. Provocative testing with either thallium scans or dobutamine stress test is helpful to identify patients with reversible ischemic heart disease. Of course, reversible ischemia should be treated before elective or even urgent (cancer-related) thoracic surgery.

Patients with coronary artery disease are at particular risk for perioperative myocardial ischemia. Tachycardia and hypertension during the operation can increase cardiac work and decrease coronary blood flow leading to ischemia [57]. Implementation of β-adrenergic blocking agents should begin before a planned procedure and continue throughout the perioperative period. Intraoperative IV nitroglycerine dilates the coronary circulation and reduces cardiac stress to prevent myocardial ischemia. Patients with known CHF should have their fluid balance and hypertension well controlled before any elective procedure.

Blood transfusions are associated with increased 30-day mortality, surgical-site infection, pneumonia, and sepsis [58] in general surgery patients, and an increased mortality, morbidity, and cost in cardiac surgery patients [59]. However, in elderly populations with acute MI, blood transfusion is associated with a lower short-term mortality rate when given to patients with a hematocrit less than 30% on admission [60]. Consequently, although current trends are justifiably toward a restrictive transfusion practice, a higher hematocrit may be needed in the elderly postoperative thoracic surgery patient with a MI.

Pulmonary Evaluation

Pulmonary complications account for the highest morbidity after thoracic procedures in all age groups. Especially at risk are patients with a history of smoking, reactive airway disease, and recent pneumonia. Smoking cessation can reduce surgical

risk in as little as 2 weeks [61, 62]. Predicting pulmonary recovery relies on formal pulmonary function testing with both volume and flow studies and assessment of exercise capability and reserve. Among the various pulmonary function tests, FEV_1 has shown good correlation with predicting morbidity in thoracic surgery patients. An FEV_1 >1.5 L predicted good outcomes in patients older than 70 years [63]. A predicted postoperative FEV_1 <55% has been shown to be the strongest independent predictor of pulmonary complications after pulmonary resection [19]. Subsequently, using this predictor as exclusion criteria, pulmonary morbidity decreased from 33 to 9.8%, and mortality from 10 to 0% in elderly patients undergoing resection for lung cancer [19].

Exercise tolerance has also proved excellent in predicting morbidity in elderly patients. Simply having the patient walk flights of stairs can give a valuable functional assessment in the clinic. Brunelli and colleagues [4] studied 109 patients over 70 years of age undergoing lobectomy for cancer. Patients who could climb more than four flights of stairs had a <20% cardiopulmonary complication rate, although those who could not climb at least three flights of stairs had a 57% complication rate [4]. Achieving an exercise capacity of only 2 min with a heart rate of 99 beats per minute can lower an elderly patient's complication rate from 42 to 9%, and mortality rate from 7 to 1% [63]. A quantified measurement of exercise capacity is a patient's maximal oxygen consumption per kilogram body weight (VO_2 max). A VO_2 max <60% is an independent risk factor associated with higher cardiopulmonary morbidity and mortality after pulmonary resection [64, 65].

Many groups have studied the effects of preoperative pulmonary rehabilitation on patients undergoing lung volume reduction surgery (LVRS). A structured pulmonary rehabilitation program includes detailed one-on-one patient education about the chronicity of their disease, instruction in respiratory and chest physiotherapy techniques, psychosocial support, and exercise training to promote muscle strengthening and aerobic endurance [66]. Most studies show only minimal improvement in quantitative lung function testing. Six-minute walk distances, dyspnea, and patient-perceived pulmonary function all show improvement with pulmonary rehabilitation. Patients who show improvement with pulmonary rehabilitation report a quicker return to activity, and some have sustained improvement in exercise capacity for up to 5 years postoperatively [67]. The NIH-sponsored National Emphysema Treatment Trial, which compared medical treatment to LVRS in patients with severe emphysema, showed select patient groups experienced improved quality of life and increased exercise capacity after surgery [68]. A 2009 follow-up study showed that twelve months after LVRS, patients during exercise show improved carbon dioxide elimination and dead space, improved respiratory rate and depth of breathing, and reported less dyspnea (Borg dyspnea scale) [69].

Intraoperative Approaches to Minimize Morbidity

Anesthesia

Physiologic changes seen in the elderly and their effects on drug bioavailability and side effect profiles can define the type and dose of agent used for anesthesia in the elderly patient. For instance, a decrease in total body water seen with aging leads to higher peak drug concentrations after bolus or rapid infusion [70]. The progressive decrease in cardiac output observed in the elderly has many anesthetic considerations. Lower tissue perfusion can lengthen the time required to transport drugs to tissues and delay the time-to-peak effect. A relative reduction in perfusion to organs such as the liver and kidneys can prolong a drug's duration of action by slowing metabolism and excretion [71]. Most anesthetic drugs have some degree of cardiac depressant activity, so the dose delivered must be reduced in the elderly. In a patient with CHF, using drugs such as midazolam or opioids that have minimal effects on cardiac contractility and heart rate can reduce the likelihood of hypotension or arrhythmia at induction [72, 73]. For patients with minimal cardiac functional reserve, tachycardia has deleterious effects. Avoiding drugs like pancuronium, which induce tachycardia, can help avoid cardiac ischemia [57]. Epidural anesthesia decreases perioperative cardiac stress and decreases tachycardia-induced cardiac ischemia [74, 75].

Minimally Invasive Operation

The traditional posterolateral thoracotomy used for exposure in thoracic procedures involves a large incision from the anterior midclavicular line to the transverse process of the vertebrae and divides the serratus anterior, latissimus dorsi, and part of the trapezius muscles. This incision results in severe pain and splinting postoperatively, especially in elderly patients with limited pulmonary reserve. Two alternative approaches, the muscle-sparing open incision and video-assisted thoracoscopic surgery (VATS), can minimize postoperative pain and speed recovery after thoracic procedures.

A muscle-sparing thoracotomy (MST) incision is usually between 8 and 10-cm long and located in the anterior axilla or anterior chest. The serratus anterior muscle fibers are split, not divided, and the latissimus dorsi muscle is retracted posteriorly to gain exposure to the thoracic cavity. The ribs are spread to the minimum amount to allow only instruments (i.e., chopstick operation), or for the surgeon to insert fingers or one hand into the chest. Although seroma formation appears higher in these patients as opposed to a standard thoracotomy [76],

postoperative pain and muscle function are improved with MST [77, 78]. The number of lymph nodes sampled through MST and long-term outcomes for lung cancer are equivalent stage-for-stage to those obtained with a standard posterolateral thoracotomy. When VATS, MST, and standard posterolateral thoracotomy were compared, posterolateral thoracotomy patients showed marked impairment in vital capacity up to 24 weeks postoperatively, and in 6-min walk distance compared with VATS and MST groups [79].

Reported benefits from VATS include decreased postoperative pain [73], improved pulmonary function tests [80, 81], and decreased cytokine release [80, 82]. VATS is ideally suited to treat nonneoplastic conditions such as bullous disease, decortication, chronic pleural effusion, and wedge biopsy of unknown pulmonary nodules. Operative times for these procedures average less than 1 h and length of stay is between 2 and 4 days [83] in patients over 80 years, significantly less than open procedures. Major morbidity, such as postoperative bleeding, air leak requiring hospitalization, and prolonged ventilatory support, can be reduced from between 11 to 30 to 5% and perioperative mortality is 2–5% [83, 84].

Equivalent results between VATS and conventional thoracotomy have been reported for local tumor control rates and 1 and 3-year survival for stage I and II disease [85–89]. Reluctance to use VATS for early lung cancer treatment results from a lack of long-term data on local recurrence rates and overall survival. In addition, there has been no prospective randomized trial comparing VATS or robot-assisted surgery to conventional thoracotomy [90]. A cohort study of over 12,000 patients from the SEER Medicare database showed that the use of VATS segmentectomy or lobectomy for early stage lung cancer increased from 1 to 9% from 1994 to 2002. When compared with thoracotomy, VATS was not associated with a difference in long-term survival [91]. In one prospectively kept database, VATS was used for clinical stage IA lung cancer with a conversion rate of 18% (others report 14% [92]), shorter hospital stays by 2 days ($p < 0.001$), fewer complications ($p = 0.06$), and similar 5-year survivals ($p = 0.08$ on intent-to-treat analysis) [93]. For elderly patients, VATS offers improved morbidity over open thoracotomy for treatment of early lung cancer or benign thoracic disease.

Outcomes

Previously published morbidity and mortality rates for pulmonary resections in the elderly led many to believe age itself was a prohibitive factor [94, 95]. In the 1960s and 1970s, morbidity rates of 40–50% and mortality rates of 20–30% for pulmonary resections in the elderly were discouraging [96]. Over the last three decades, morbidity and mortality rates have steadily declined, although complication and death rates

Table 40.2 Thirty-days morbidity and mortality in patients >70-years-old after lung resection for non-small cell lung cancer

Author	n	Year	Morbidity (%)	Mortality (%)
Ishida et al. [111]	167	1990	21	3
Roxburgh et al. [112]	43	1991	NA	7
Thomas et al. [113]	47	1993	38	13
Gebitekin et al. [114]	145	1993	19	9
Massard et al. [103]	210	1996	NA	7
Morandi et al. [102]	85	1997	55	1
Ciriaco et al. [115]	76	1998	19	1
Thomas et al. [116]	500	1998	57	7
Pagni et al. [117]	385	1998	34	4
Hanagiri et al. [118]	18	1999	50	0
Oliaro et al. [119]	258	1999	39	3
Sioris et al. [120]	75	1999	29	9
Dyszkiewicz et al. [105]	90	2000	58 (non-pneumonectomy) 79 (pneumonectomy)	0 (non-pneumonectomy) 16 (pneumonectomy)
Aoki et al. [121]	35	2000	60	0
Conti et al. [122]	151	2002	10	3
Birim et al. [7]	126	2003	57 minor, 13 major	3
Brock et al. [123]	68	2004	44	9
Port et al. [124]	61	2004	38	2
Sawada et al. [125]	73	2005	NA	4
Matsuoka et al. [126]	40	2005	20	0
Sullivan et al. [127]	25	2005	48	1
Sirbu et al. [128]	273	2005	48	5
Cerfolio [129]	726	2006	20	2
Berry et al. [130]	338	2009	47	4

NA not available electronically or not recorded; some citations from Table 1 in Pallis [3], all data independently verified

still do not equal those for younger patients. Improvements in imaging and preoperative staging help to better select patients with potentially curable disease. The quality of ICU care and improved perioperative monitoring has also influenced outcomes for the elderly. Overall, perioperative mortality rates in the ICU have declined from >20% in the 1960s to around 10% in the 1970s, and 5% in the past 20 years [97–100]. Mortality after lung resection in patients older than 70 years of age has declined steadily from upwards of 11% in the 1970s [101] to anywhere from 0–5% in most series over the last two decades (Table 40.2). Recent series that report higher mortality rates (7–16%) attribute death to a high incidence of cardiovascular disease, pulmonary disease, or advanced stage lung cancer (requiring extended resection or pneumonectomy) [3]. Age alone is not an independent risk factor for mortality in the absence of comorbidities [102–104]. Survival in the elderly for thoracic procedures based on stage of disease and extent of resection have shown mixed results. Mortality rates for pneumonectomy continue to be highest among the elderly, varying between 12 and 20% [105–107]. The British Thoracic Society and other authors have cited these results in recommendations against pneumonectomy in the elderly [101, 108, 109]. Continuous monitoring capabilities, improved cardiovascular pharmacotherapies, and gentle

mechanical ventilation strategies have played a role in improving perioperative care. Introduction of the pulmonary artery catheter was heralded as a great breakthrough in the early 1970s, but critical analysis has failed to show improved outcomes. In fact, many speculate it has contributed to poorer results from overtreatment of the numbers [110]. Routine use of the pulmonary artery catheter is not warranted in the elderly, but pulmonary artery monitoring is beneficial in select patients with cardiopulmonary comorbidities.

Morbidity after thoracic procedures is a direct function of the patient's preoperative comorbidities, length of operation, and extent of operation. In younger patients, the most common complications are usually pulmonary in nature and include atelectasis, prolonged air leak, and prolonged ventilatory support occurring in 7–18% of patients. Morbidity in the elderly population is usually divided into minor (non–life-threatening) and major (life-threatening) complications (Table 40.3). Minor complications, including atelectasis, bronchospasm, hemodynamically stable arrhythmia, and prolonged air leak, are reported to occur between 10 and 57% in patients over 65 years of age [7, 101, 116, 122, 131]. Major complications, including myocardial infarction, pulmonary embolus, stroke, acute limb ischemia, and arrhythmia

Table 40.3 Common complications arising in patients aged 70 years or older after thoracic procedures

Complication	%
Minor	
Supraventricular arrhythmia	13–30
Prolonged air leak	7–21
Atelectasis	2–7
Pneumonia	2–6
Urinary infection	5–6
Chylothorax	1–11
Recurrent nerve injury	1–6
Major	
Prolonged mechanical ventilation	1–12
Myocardial infarction	2–3
Bronchopleural fistula	1–8
Empyema	1–5
Cardiac failure	1–2
Ventricular arrhythmia	1–2
Pulmonary embolism	1–3
ARDS	<1
Stroke	<1
Renal failure	<1

requiring cardioversion, occur between 11 and 38% in patients over 65 years of age [7, 101, 116, 131]. Risk factors for postoperative cardiopulmonary morbidity include myocardial infarction within 6 months, preoperative use of supplemental oxygen, low FEV_1, and smoking history.

Stage of lung cancer is still the most important factor in determining long-term survival in the elderly [102, 116]. Stage-for-stage results in the elderly are comparable with those for the general population of thoracic-operation patients with early disease. Elderly patients with Stages I and II disease should be considered for operation as first-line therapy. For patients over 70 years of age, 5-year survival for Stage I disease ranges from 57 to 79% [101, 116, 132], compared with 70% for younger patients. Elderly patients with more advanced lung cancer do not show comparable long-term survival after surgical resection. Five-year survival for Stage III disease ranges from 0 to 15% and is an independent risk factor for poor long-term outcomes [7, 101]. However, given the absence of prospective data that verify decreased survival due to lung cancer-attributable death in the elderly, age alone should not exclude individuals from extended resection. Competing therapies, especially stereotactic radiotherapy, show promise. In one series of 38 octogenarians with Stage I NSCLC, stereotactic radiotherapy achieved survival of 65% at 1 year and 44% at 2 years; local tumor control was 100% at 2 years [133]. While prospective trials are ongoing, stereotactic radiotherapy is an alternative treatment for high-risk surgical candidates [134].

For patients with esophageal cancer, age alone has been shown to be an independent risk factor for poor outcomes. Patients over 70 years tend to have a higher mortality rate after esophagectomy when compared with younger patients [135]. The Veterans' Administration analyzed the largest patient cohort to date and found that in over 1,700 esophagectomies, advanced age was among the independent risks factors predicting a higher rate of pulmonary morbidity and mortality [136, 137]. A patient's poor preoperative performance status has also been shown to correlate with increased cardiopulmonary morbidity after esophagectomy in the elderly, thereby prompting many to advocate a period of cardiopulmonary rehabilitation before esophagectomy in select patients [136, 137].

Pain Management

A physician's bias toward the elderly patient's perception of pain is associated with many misconceptions. The elderly are often incapable of complaining of pain, because of intubation or cognitive impairment ,or they simply do not report pain for fear of being a "bad patient," or becoming addicted to pain medication [138, 139]. Physicians may perceive this as evidence that elderly patients are not feeling pain, or that they feel less pain than younger patients after similar procedures [140]. Many physicians believe either a higher incidence of respiratory compromise follows administration of pain medicine in older patients, or they require less pain medication to treat the same amount of pain seen in younger patients. In fact, these misconceptions have caused untreated pain to be the most frequent complaint in hospitalized elderly patients. The hospitalized elderly longitudinal project reported 45% of hospitalized patients felt their pain was undertreated, and 53% of patients continued to experience considerable pain 1 year after discharge from the hospital [141].

A surgeon should be aware of the psychological aspects of pain and age-related physiologic changes that affect drug distribution and metabolism to adequately treat pain. With aging, the body loses muscle mass and increases body fat, resulting in overall loss of total body water and a smaller volume of distribution for drugs [142]. The loss of adequate compensatory mechanisms of the cardiovascular system leads to slower delivery of drugs to the liver and kidneys for metabolism. Renal mass and blood flow are reduced with aging, which can alter metabolism and excretion of drugs and drug metabolites [143]. These age-related changes lead to higher circulating plasma drug levels with longer duration of action and potential side effects [142, 144]. Pain has a strong psychological component. Inadequately treated pain can lead to depression and anxiety and ultimately prolong hospital stay. Many physicians are reluctant to give elderly patients pain medicine for fear of causing cognitive impairment; postoperative delirium is less frequent in elderly who have lower pain scores [145].

Adequate postthoracotomy pain control not only increases patient satisfaction but can decrease morbidity and mortality.

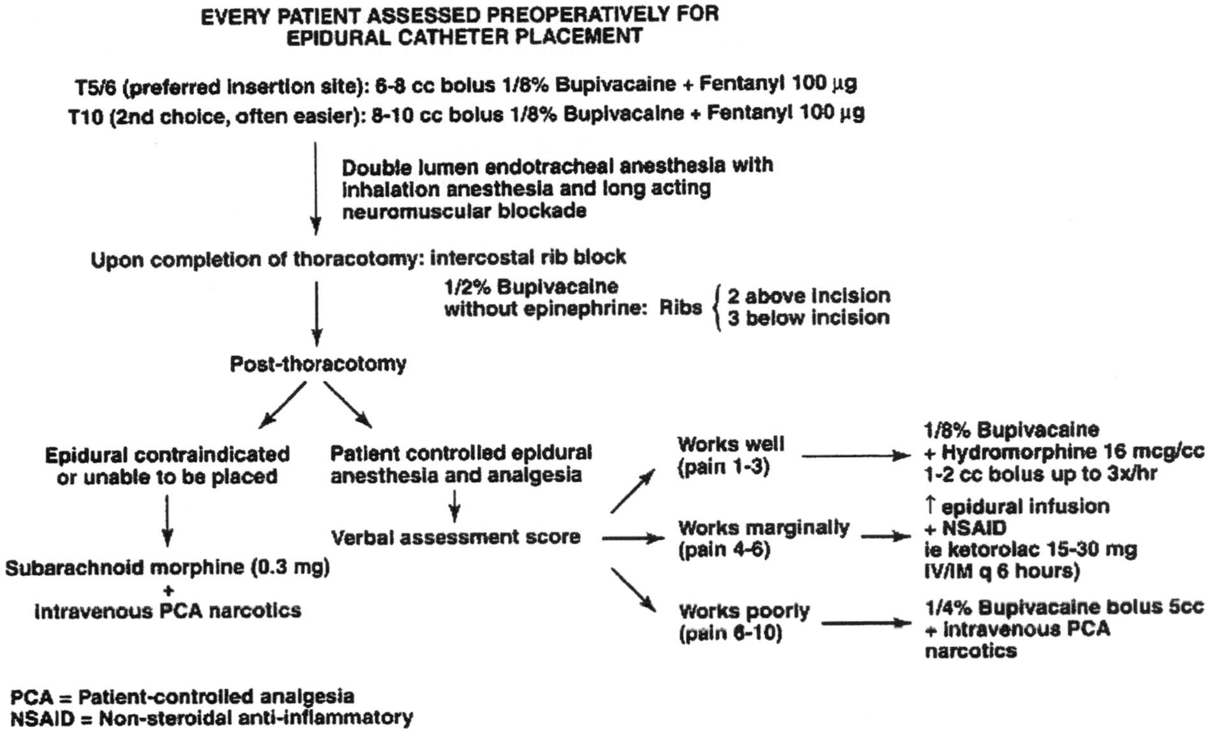

**EVERY PATIENT ASSESSED PREOPERATIVELY FOR
EPIDURAL CATHETER PLACEMENT**

T5/6 (preferred insertion site): 6-8 cc bolus 1/8% Bupivacaine + Fentanyl 100 μg
T10 (2nd choice, often easier): 8-10 cc bolus 1/8% Bupivacaine + Fentanyl 100 μg

Double lumen endotracheal anesthesia with
inhalation anesthesia and long acting
neuromuscular blockade

Upon completion of thoracotomy: intercostal rib block

1/2% Bupivacaine
without epinephrine: Ribs { 2 above incision
                             3 below incision

Post-thoracotomy

Epidural contraindicated
or unable to be placed

Patient controlled epidural
anesthesia and analgesia

Verbal assessment score

Subarachnoid morphine (0.3 mg)
+
Intravenous PCA narcotics

Works well
(pain 1-3) → 1/8% Bupivacaine
+ Hydromorphine 16 mcg/cc
1-2 cc bolus up to 3x/hr

Works marginally
(pain 4-6) → ↑ epidural infusion
+ NSAID
ie ketorolac 15-30 mg
IV/IM q 6 hours)

Works poorly
(pain 6-10) → 1/4% Bupivacaine bolus 5cc
+ intravenous PCA
narcotics

PCA = Patient-controlled analgesia
NSAID = Non-steroidal anti-inflammatory

Fig. 40.2 Algorithm for post-thoracotomy pain control emphasizing epidural and regional anesthesia (Reprinted from Savage et al. [146], with permission from Elsevier)

Numerous intermittent or on-demand approaches to pain management have proved to be ineffective. These include intermittent IM narcotic injection, interpleural analgesia, and postoperative intercostal nerve block [146]. Continuous epidural anesthesia has been associated with a lower incidence of pulmonary embolism, deep vein thrombosis, respiratory depression, and pulmonary complications [147, 148]. In addition, adequate pain relief allows patients to become mobile earlier in the recovery period. A recommended method for controlling postoperative pain is continuous epidural anesthesia followed by IV narcotic administration through a patient-controlled analgesia device [146, 149]. Figure 40.2 illustrates an algorithm for postthoracotomy pain management based on the use of epidural and regional anesthesia to provide adequate postoperative pain relief and encourage early ambulation while minimizing respiratory depression and sedation.

Neurocognitive Dysfunction

Cognitive dysfunction has been increasingly recognized as a postoperative complication after thoracic and other noncardiac operations [150]. Postoperative cognitive impairment can be classified into postoperative delirium (PD) or postoperative neurocognitive disorder. PD is characterized by fluctuating levels of consciousness and abnormalities in memory and perception that are temporary, lasting 30 days or less [151]. With PD, emotional disturbances can be prominent with labile symptoms of anxiety, fear, anger, and depression [152]. Postoperative neurocognitive disorder is a condition characterized by impaired concentration, language comprehension, and social integration, which can become evident days to weeks after the operation and may become permanent [153]. Many of these patients lose their ability to live independently and are ultimately discharged to long-term care facilities.

Incidence of PD in the elderly varies widely from 3 to 50% and its cause is believed to be multifactorial [151]. Several theories about the pathophysiologic mechanisms of PD are being studied. Some suggest a reduced cerebral oxidative metabolism may lead to abnormalities in the levels of neurotransmitters, such as cerebral acetylcholine, which has been implicated in the regulation of memory and alertness [154, 155]. Also, perioperative alterations in stress hormones, such as reduced thyroid hormone, increased cortisol, and cytokine release, may alter amino acid and neurotransmitter concentrations, thereby provoking PD [156]. Risk factors for PD include preoperative factors such as severe illness, impaired cognitive functioning, physical debilitation, and a history of dementia [157, 158]. Advanced age has consistently been found to be an independent risk factor for PD [158]. Perioperative factors associated with PD include

60. Wu WC, Rathore SS, Wang Y, Radford MJ, Krumholz HM. Blood transfusion in elderly patients with acute myocardial infarction. N Engl J Med. 2001;345:1230–6.

61. Mason DP, Subramanian S, Nowicki ER, et al. Impact of smoking cessation before resection of lung cancer: a society of thoracic surgeons general thoracic surgery database study. Ann Thorac Surg. 2009;88:362–70; discussion 370–1.

62. Warner MA, Offord KP, Warner ME, Conover LRL, MA Jansson-Schumacher U. Role of preoperative cessation of smoking and other factors in postoperative pulmonary complications: a blinded prospective study of coronary artery bypass patients. Mayo Clin Proc. 1989;64:609–16.

63. Gerson MC, Hurst JM, Hertzberg VS, Baughman R, Rouan GW, Ellis K. Prediction of cardiac and pulmonary complications related to elective abdominal and noncardiac thoracic surgery in geriatric patients. Am J Med. 1990;88:101–7.

64. Brutsche MH, Spiliopoulos A, Bolliger CT, Licker M, Frey JG, Tschopp JM. Exercise capacity and extent of resection as predictors of surgical risk in lung cancer. Eur Respir J. 2000;15:828–32.

65. Villani F, De Maria P, Busia A. Exercise testing as a predictor of surgical risk after pneumonectomy for bronchogenic carcinoma. Respir Med. 2003;97:1296–8.

66. Connors G, Hilling L. American Association of Cadiovascular and Pulmonary Rehabilitation Guidelines for pulmonary rehabilitation programs. Champeign, IL: Human Kinetics; 1993.

67. Yusen RD, Lefrak SS, Gierada DS, et al. A prospective evaluation of lung volume reduction surgery in 200 consecutive patients. Chest. 2003;123:1026–37.

68. Fishman A, Martinez F, Naunheim K, et al. A randomized trial comparing lung-volume-reduction surgery with medical therapy for severe emphysema. N Engl J Med. 2003;348:2059–73.

69. Criner GJ, Belt P, Sternberg AL, et al. Effects of lung volume reduction surgery on gas exchange and breathing pattern during maximum exercise. Chest. 2009;135:1268–79.

70. Norris AH, Lundy T, Shock NW. Trends in selected indicis of body composition in men between the ages of 30 and 80 years. Ann NY Acad Sci. 1963;110:608–22.

71. Sadean MR, Glass PS. Pharmacokinetics in the elderly. Best Pract Res Clin Anaesthesiol. 2003;17:191–205.

72. Bailey JM, Mora CT, Shafe SL. Pharmacokinetics of propofol in adult patients undergoing coronary revascularization. The Multicenter Study of Perioperative Ischemia Research Group. Anesthesiology. 1996;84:1288–97.

73. Thomson IR, Harding G, Hudson RJ. A comparison of fentanyl and sufentanil in patients undergoing coronary artery bypass graft surgery. J Cardiothorac Vasc Anesth. 2000;14:652–6.

74. Kessler P, Neidhart G, Lischke V, et al. Coronary bypass operation with complete median sternotomy in awake patients with high thoracic peridural anesthesia. Anaesthesist. 2002;51:533–8.

75. Loick HM, Schmidt C, Van Aken H, et al. High thoracic epidural anesthesia, but not clonidine, attenuates the perioperative stress response via sympatholysis and reduces the release of troponin T in patients undergoing coronary artery bypass grafting. Anesth Analg. 1999;88:701–9.

76. Akcali Y, Demir H, Tezcan B. The effect of standard posterolateral versus muscle-sparing thoracotomy on multiple parameters. Ann Thorac Surg. 2003;76:1050–4.

77. Kutlu CA, Akin H, Olcmen A, Biliciler U, Kayserilioglu A, Olcmen M. Shoulder-girdle strength after standard and lateral muscle-sparing thoracotomy. Thorac Cardiovasc Surg. 2001;49:112–4.

78. Hazelrigg SR, Landreneau RJ, Boley TM, et al. The effect of muscle-sparing versus standard posterolateral thoracotomy on pulmonary function, muscle strength, and postoperative pain. J Thorac Cardiovasc Surg. 1991;101:394–401.

79. Nomori H, Ohtsuka T, Horio H, Naruke T, Suemasu K. Difference in the impairment of vital capacity and 6-minute walking after a lobectomy performed by thoracoscopic surgery, an anterior limited thoracotomy, an anteroaxillary thoracotomy, and a posterolateral thoracotomy. Surg Today. 2003;33:7–12.

80. Nagahiro I, Andou A, Aoe M, Sano Y, Date H, Shimzu N. Pulmonary function, postoperative pain, and serum cytokine level after lobectomy: a comparison of VATS and conventional procedure. Ann Thorac Surg. 2001;72:362–5.

81. Nakata M, Saeki H, Yokoyama N, Kurita A, Takiyama W, Takashima S. Pulmonary function after lobectomy: video-assisted thoracic surgery versus thoracotomy. Ann Thorac Surg. 2000;70:938–41.

82. Yim AP, Wan S, Lee TW, Arifi AA. VATS lobectomy reduces cytokine responses compared with conventional surgery. Ann Thorac Surg. 2000;70:243–7.

83. Koren JP, Bocage JP, Geis WP, Caccavale RJ. Major thoracic surgery in octogenarians: the video-assisted thoracic surgery (VATS) approach. Surg Endosc. 2003;17:632–5.

84. Koizumi K, Haraguchi S, Hirata T, et al. Lobectomy by video-assisted thoracic surgery for lung cancer patients aged 80 years or more. Ann Thorac Cardiovasc Surg. 2003;9:14–21.

85. McKenna RJ, Jr., Houck W, Fuller CB. Video-assisted thoracic surgery lobectomy: experience with 1,100 cases. Ann Thorac Surg. 2006;81:421–5; discussion 425–26.

86. Tomaszek SC, Cassavi SD, Sheri KR, et al. Clinical outcomes of video-assisted thoracoscopic lobectomy. Mayo Clin Proc. 2009;84:509–13.

87. Walker WS, Codispoti M, Soon SY, Stamenkovic S, Carnochan F, Pugh G. Long-term outcomes following VATS lobectomy for non-small cell bronchogenic carcinoma. Eur J Cardiothorac Surg. 2003;23:397–402.

88. Gharagozloo FTempesta B, Margolis M, Alexander EP. Video-assisted thoracic surgery lobectomy for stage I lung cancer. Ann Thorac Surg. 2003;76:1009–15.

89. Koizumi K, Haraguchi S, Hirata T, et al. Video-assisted lobectomy in elderly lung cancer patients. Jpn J Thorac Cardiovasc Surg. 2002;50:15–22.

90. Flores RM, Alam N. Video-assisted thoracic surgery lobectomy (VATS), open thoracotomy, and the robot for lung cancer. Ann Thorac Surg. 2008;85:S710–5.

91. Farjah F, Wood DE, Mulligan MS, et al. Safety and efficacy of video-assisted versus conventional lung resection for lung cancer. J Thorac Cardiovasc Surg. 2009;137:1415–21.

92. Swanson SJ, Herndon JE, D'Amico TA, et al. Video-assisted thoracic surgery lobectomy: report of CALGB 39802 – a prospective, multi-institution feasibility study. J Clin Oncol. 2007;25:4993–7.

93. Flores RM, Park BJ, Dyoco J, et al. Lobectomy by video-assisted thoracic surgery (VATS) versus thoracotomy for lung cancer. J Thorac Cardiovasc Surg. 2009;138:11–8.

94. Weiss W. Operative mortality and five year survival rates in patients with bronchogenic carcinoma. Am J Surg. 1974;128:799–804.

95. Breyer RH, Zippe C, Pharr WF, Jenski RJ, Kittle CF, Faber LP. Thoracotomy in patients over age seventy years: ten-year experience. J Thorac Cardiovasc Surg. 1981;81:187–93.

96. Yellin A, Benfield JR. Surgery for bronchogenic carcinoma in the elderly. Am Rev Respir Dis. 1985;131:197.

97. Herron PW, Jesseph JE, Harkins HN. Analysis of 600 major operations in patients over 70 years of age. Ann Surg. 1960;152:686–98.

98. Burnett W, McCaffrey J. Surgical procedures in the elderly. Surg Gynecol Obstet. 1972;134:221–6.

99. Djokovic JL, Hedley-Whyte J. Prediction of outcome of surgery and anesthesia in patients over 80. JAMA. 1979;242:2310–6.

100. Hosking MP, Warner MA, Lobdell CM, Offord KP, Melton 3rd LJ. Outcomes of surgery in patients 90 years of age and older. JAMA. 1989;261:1909–15.

101. Pagni S, Federico JA, Ponn RB. Pulmonary resection for lung cancer in octogenarians. Ann Thorac Surg. 1997;63:785–9.

102. Morandi U, Stefani A. Golinelli, et al. Results of surgical resection in patients over the age of 70 years with non small-cell lung cancer. Eur J Cardiothorac Surg. 1997;11:432–9.

103. Massard G, Moog R, Wihlm JM, et al. Bronchogenic cancer in the elderly: operative risk and long-term prognosis. Thorac Cardiovasc Surg. 1996;44:40–5.

104. Kamiyoshihara M, Kawashima O, Ishikawa S, Morishita Y. Long-term results after pulmonary resection in elderly patients with non-small cell lung cancer. J Cardiovasc Surg (Torino). 2000;41:483–6.

105. Dyszkiewicz W, Pawlak K, Gasiorowski L. Early post-pneumonectomy complications in the elderly. Eur J Cardiothorac Surg. 2000;17:246–50.

106. de Perrot M, Licker M, Reymond MA, Robert J, Spiliopoulos A. Influence of age on operative mortality and long-term survival after lung resection for bronchogenic carcinoma. Eur Respir J. 1999;14:419–22.

107. Mizushima Y, Noto H, Sugiyama S, Kusajima Y, et al. Survival and prognosis after pneumonectomy for lung cancer in the elderly. Ann Thorac Surg. 1997;64:193–8.

108. British Thoracic Society; Society of Cardiothoracic Surgeons of Great Britain and Ireland Working Party. BTS guidelines: guidelines on the selection of patients with lung cancer for surgery. Thorax. 2001;56:89–108.

109. Au J, el-Oakley R, Cameron EW. Pneumonectomy bronchogenic carcinoma elderly. Eur J Cardiothorac Surg. 1994;8:247–50.

110. Peters SG, Afessa B, Decker PA, Schroeder DR, Offord KP, Scott JP. Increased risk associated with pulmonary artery catheterization in the medical intensive care unit. J Crit Care. 2003;18:166–71.

111. Ishida T, Yokoyama H, Kaneko S, Sugio K, Sugimachi K. Long-term results of operation for non-small cell lung cancer in the elderly. Ann Thorac Surg. 1990;50:919–22.

112. Roxburgh JC, Thompson J, Goldstraw P. Hospital mortality and long-term survival after pulmonary resection in the elderly. Ann Thorac Surg. 1991;51:800–3.

113. Thomas P, Sielezneff I, Ragni J, Guidicelli R, Fuentes P. Is lung cancer resection justified in patients aged over 70 years? Eur J Cardiothorac Surg. 1993;7:246–50; discussion 250–1.

114. Gebitekin C, Gupta NK, Martin PG, Saunders NR, Walker DR. Long-term results in the elderly following pulmonary resection for non-small cell lung carcinoma. Eur J Cardiothorac Surg. 1993;7:653–6.

115. Ciriaco P, Zannini P, Carretta A, et al. Surgical treatment of non-small cell lung cancer in patients 70 years of age or older. Int Surg. 1998;83:4–7.

116. Thomas P, Piraux M, Jacques LF, Gregoire J, Bedard P, Deslauriers J. Clinical patterns and trends of outcome of elderly patients with bronchogenic carcinoma. Eur J Cardiothorac Surg. 1998;13:266–74.

117. Pagni S, McKelvey A, Riordan C, Federico JA, Ponn RB. Pulmonary resection for malignancy in the elderly: is age still a risk factor? Eur J Cardiothorac Surg. 1998;14:40–4; discussion 44–5.

118. Hanagiri T, Muranaka H, Hashimoto M, Nagashima A, Yasumoto K. Results of surgical treatment of lung cancer in octogenarians. Lung Cancer. 1999;23:129–33.

119. Oliaro A, Leo F, Filosso PL, Rena O, Parola A, Maggi G. Resection for bronchogenic carcinoma in the elderly. J Cardiovasc Surg (Torino). 1999;40:715–9.

120. Sioris T, Salo J, Perhoniemi V, Mattila S. Surgery for lung cancer in the elderly. Scand Cardiovasc J. 1999;33:222–7.

121. Aoki T, Yamato Y, Tsuchida M, Watanabe T, Hayashi J, Hirono T. Pulmonary complications after surgical treatment of lung cancer in octogenarians. Eur J Cardiothorac Surg. 2000;18:662–5.

122. Conti B, Brega Massone PP, Lequaglie C, Magnani G, Cataldo I. Brega Massone PP, Lequaglie C, Magnani G, Cataldo I. Major surgery in lung cancer in elderly patients? Risk factors analysis and long-term results. Minerva Chir. 2002;57:317–21.

123. Brock MV, Kim MP, Hooker CM, et al. Pulmonary resection in octogenarians with stage I nonsmall cell lung cancer: a 22-year experience. Ann Thorac Surg. 2004;77:271–7.

124. Port JL, Kent M, Korst RJ, et al. Surgical resection for lung cancer in the octogenarian. Chest. 2004;126:733–8.

125. Sawada S, Komori E, Nogami N, et al. Advanced age is not correlated with either short-term or long-term postoperative results in lung cancer patients in good clinical condition. Chest. 2005;128:1557–63.

126. Matsuoka H, Okada M, Sakamoto T, Tsubota N. Complications and outcomes after pulmonary resection for cancer in patients 80 to 89 years of age. Eur J Cardiothorac Surg. 2005;28:380–3.

127. Sullivan V, Tran T, Hlmstrom A, et al. Advanced age does not exclude lobectomy for non-small cell lung carcinoma. Chest. 2005;128:2671–6.

128. Sirbu H, Schreiner W, Dalichau H, Busch T. Surgery for non-small cell carcinoma in geriatric patients: 15-year experience. Asian Cardiovasc Thorac Ann. 2005;13:330–6.

129. Cerfolio RJ, Bryant AS. Survival and outcomes of pulmonary resection for non-small cell lung cancer in the elderly: a nested case-control study. Ann Thorac Surg. 2006;82:424–9; discussion 429–30.

130. Berry MF, Hanna J, Tong BC, et al. Risk factors for morbidity after lobectomy for lung cancer in elderly patients. Ann Thorac Surg. 2009;88:1093–9.

131. Limmer S, Hauenschild L. Eckmann, et al. Thoracic surgery in the elderly – co-morbidity is the limit. Interact Cardiovasc Thorac Surg. 2009;8:412–6.

132. Shirakusa T, Tsutsui M, Iriki N, et al. Results of resection for bronchogenic carcinoma in patients over the age of 80. Thorax. 1989;44:189–91.

133. van der Voort van Zyp NC,van der Holt B, can Klaveren RJ, Pattynama P, Maat A, Nuyttens JJ. Stereotactic body radiotherapy using real-time tumor tracking in octogenarians with non-small cell lung cancer. Lung Cancer. 2010;69(3):296–301.

134. Banki F, Luketich JD, Chen H, Christie N, Pennathur A. Stereotactic radiosurgery for lung cancer. Minerva Chir. 2009;64:589–98.

135. Naunheim KS, Hanosh J, Zwischenberger J, et al. Esophagectomy in the septuagenarian. Ann Thorac Surg. 1999;56:880–4.

136. Bailey SH, Bull DA, Harpole DH, et al. Outcomes after esophagectomy: a ten-year prospective cohort. Ann Thorac Surg. 2003;75:217–22.

137. Ferguson MK, Durkin AE. Preoperative prediction of the risk of pulmonary complications after esophagectomy for cancer. J Thorac Cardiovasc Surg. 2002;123:661–9.

138. Crook J, Rideout E, Browne G. The prevalence of pain complaints in a general population. Pain. 1984;18:299–314.

139. Ferrell BA, Ferrell BR, Osterweil D. Pain in the nursing home. J Am Geriatr Soc. 1990;38:409–14.

140. The management of chronic pain in older persons: AGS Panel on Chronic Pain in Older Persons. American Geriatrics Society. J Am Geriatr Soc. 1998;46:635–51.

141. Desbiens NA, Mueller-Rizner N, Connors Jr AF. Hamel MB, Wenger NS. Pain in the oldest-old during hospitalization and up to one year later. HELP Investigators. Hospitalized Elderly Longitudinal Project. J Am Geriatr Soc. 1997;45:1167–72.

142. Vuyk J. Pharmacodynamics in the elderly. Best Pract Res Clin Anaesthesiol. 2003;17:207–18.

143. Hall LG, Oyen LJ, Murray MJ. Analgesic agents. Pharmacology and application in critical care. Crit Care Clin. 2001;17:899–923, viii.

Table 41.1 Select relevant adjuvant trials in NSCLC

Trial	Regimen	Stage	N	Survival adjuvant group	Survival control group
ANITA	CDDP + Vinorelbine	I 36% II 22% IIIa 41% IIIb-IV <1%	840	65.7 months	43.7 months
JBR.10	CDDP + Vinorelbine	IB 45% II 55%	242	94 months*	73 months
IALT	CDDP + Choice of Etoposide, Vinorelbine, Vinblastine, Vindesine	I 36.5% II 24.2% III 39.3%	1,867	2 year OS of 70.3%* 5 year OS of 44.5%*	2 year OS of 66.7% 5 year OS of 40.4%
ALPI	Mitomycin C + Vindesine + Cisplatin	(reported for adjuvant group) I 39% II 31% IIIa 29%	1,209	55.2 months*	48 months
Big lung	CDDP + Videsine or Mitomycin + Ifosfamide + Cisplatin or Mitomycin + Vinblastine + Cisplatin or CDDP + Vinorelbine	Stage I 27% Stage II 38% Stage III 34%	381	33.9 months	32.6 months
CALGB 9633	Carboplatin + Paclitaxel	All had stage IB	344	95 months[a]	78 months

* Statistically significant
[a] Significant only in subgroup >4 cm

restricted to node positive disease, with a strong trend toward benefit in node-negative disease >4 cm (5-year overall survival of 79% vs. 59%, p 0.13).

The divergent results of these trials have resulted in sustained therapeutic controversy. Thus, the Lung Adjuvant Cisplatin Evaluation (LACE) metaanalysis pooled individual patient results from these five trials, combining a total of 4,584 patients. In aggregate, a 5-year absolute benefit of 5.4% from chemotherapy was observed. Benefit was significantly different by stage (HR for stage IA 1.4, HR for stage IB 0.93, HR for stage II 0.83, HR for stage III 0.83). Those with stage IA disease actually had a survival decrement, while those with node (+) disease experienced a statistically significant improvement in survival. There was a trend for greater benefit from vinorelbine-based therapies (HR for vinorelbine adjuvant therapy 0.8, HR for etoposide or vinca alkaloid therapy 0.92, and HR for other 0.97); the confidence intervals for those receiving vinorelbine did not cross unity, denoting a statistical advantage. There was no interaction between chemotherapy effect and age.

Cancer and leukemia group B (CALGB) 9633 was contemporaneous with LACE and is important for two reasons: it was the only major adjuvant trial to utilize carboplatin instead of cisplatin, and it exclusively enrolled early stage disease; only patients with stage IB were eligible. Although the trial initially reported a 12% four-year survival advantage (p = 0.028) [10], it "turned negative" with subsequent follow-up with the p value rising to 0.10, although the HR of 0.83 reported in later follow-up was consistent with the HRs of better powered trials such as ANITA and IALT [11]. In an unplanned subgroup analysis of patients with tumors greater than 4 cm the survival benefit remained significant (p=0.04) with a HR of 0.66. A similar analysis of JBR.10 in patients with T2N0M0 also suggested that 4 cm was the crucial cut-off with an identical HR of 0.66 for those receiving chemotherapy with vinorelbine and cisplatin compared with observation. Those with T2N0 tumors under this size derived no benefit whatsoever from adjuvant chemotherapy. Although the relative merits of cisplatin vs. carboplatin remain controversial, there has been general acceptance of 4 cm, as a cutoff for adjuvant therapy, The ongoing Eastern Cooperative Oncology Group (ECOG) 1505 trial requires either this T size or node positivity for eligibility [12].

Ultimately, a consensus has emerged to recommend adjuvant therapy for stage IB tumors 4 cm and larger, and for any node positive disease after R0 resection. Although the degree of absolute benefit is uncertain, it is probably close to 10% with the use of optimal modern chemotherapy regimens and appropriate patient selection. These trials are reviewed in Table 41.1.

Elderly-Specific Data

Although lung cancer is largely a disease of the elderly, clinical trials of adjuvant therapy have frequently included age cutoffs or failed to accrue the elderly [13]. Both the ANITA and IALT trials explicitly excluded patients over the age of 75. Further, there is a paucity of elderly-specific trials. Thus, the oncologist must question the applicability of the general trial results to elderly patients. Subgroup analyses to date suggest that the findings are indeed applicable.

JBR.10 provides the best data to address the merits of adjuvant therapy in the elderly. Of the 482 patients randomized in JBR.10, 155 were above 65 years of age and 327 were below 65 [14]. The hazard ratio for survival in the elderly was 0.61, comparable with that of younger patients, 0.77. This translates into an 8% overall survival advantage at 5 years [15]. Results for overall survival (OS) and disease free survival (DFS) are shown in Fig. 41.1. Dose-delivery was inferior in the elderly with fewer delivered doses of cisplatin and vinorelbine as well as a lower rate of treatment completion and a higher rate of treatment refusal. Nonetheless, there were no significant differences in toxicities, hospitalizations, or treatment-related death by age group. As would also be expected in the general population, the younger patients on average lived longer than the older patients, with the effect particularly pronounced in those above 75 years of age. The results for the above 75 group must be interpreted with caution. The poor survival was not echoed by the disease-specific survival, suggesting that the results may not have been due to failure of adjuvant therapy; further, the numbers

analyzed are small with only 23 patients over the age of 75. Thus, the safety and efficacy of adjuvant chemotherapy in those over 75 years of age must be considered relatively unaddressed by existing data.

Subgroup analyses from the two major metaanalyses support the conclusions of the elderly subgroup analysis of JBR.10. The 2000 update to the Non-small Cell Lung Cancer Collaborative Group metaanalysis [16] showed similar hazard ratios for improved survival with adjuvant chemotherapy regardless of age: 0.87 for less than 54 years, 0.89 for 55–59 years, 0.83 for 60–64 years, and 0.86 for more than 64 years. In this analysis, poor performance status (PS) did not predict less benefit from adjuvant chemotherapy. In fact, patients with poor PS paradoxically derived greater benefit (OR 0.54) when compared with those with good PS (OR 0.89), suggesting that even poor PS should not represent an absolute contraindication to appropriate therapy.

Subgroup analysis from LACE [17] reached similar conclusions. In LACE, 901 patients (20%) were aged 60–65 years and 414 (9%) at least 70 years. Elderly patients did not

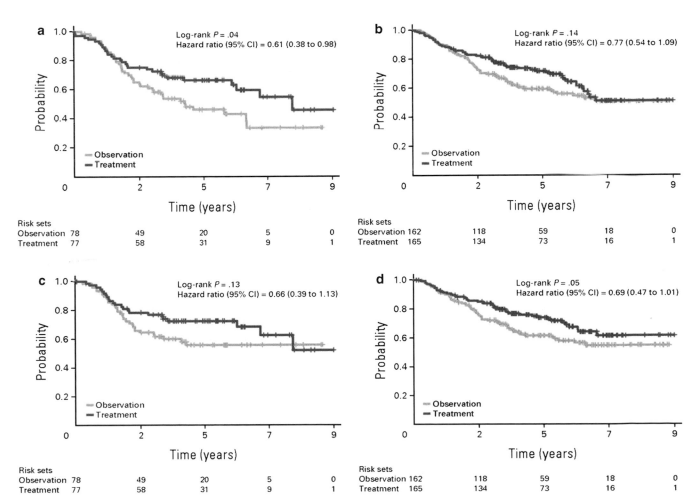

Fig. 41.1 Overall and disease-specific survival by treatment arm from JBR.10. (Reprinted with permission from Pepe, C. et al. J Clin Oncol; 25:1553–1561 2007. © 2007 American Society of Clinical Oncology. Overall survival by treatment arm (A) age > 65 and (B) ≤ 65 years; disease-specific survival by treatment arm (C) age > 65 and (D) ≤ 65 years

for expression of the MAGE-A3 antigen, and only patients expressing it are eligible. Prior to randomization to the study vaccine or to placebo, patients may receive standard-of-care adjuvant chemotherapy, or they may choose to forgo it. The RADIANT trial also allows, but does not require, adjuvant chemotherapy prior to study therapy. To be eligible, the patient's tumor must be positive for the epidermal growth factor receptor by either immunohistochemistry or fluorescence in-situ hybridization. Patients are randomized to receive erlotinib, a small-molecule inhibitor of the epidermal growth factor tyrosine kinase, or placebo. Both the MAGE and RADIANT trials are nearing their enrollment goals as of the time of authorship of this chapter (November 2009).

References

1. Ries LAG, Melbert D., Krapcho M, Stinchcomb DG, Howlader N, Horner MJ, Mariotto A, Miller BA, Feuer EJ, Altekruse SF, Lewis DR, Clegg L, Eisner MP, Reichman M, Edwards BK, editors. SEER Cancer Statistics Review, 1975-2005, National Cancer Institute. Bethesda, MD, http://seer.cancer.gov/csr/1975_2005/, based on November 2007 SEER data submission, posted to the SEER web site, 2008.
2. Owonikoko TK, Ragin CC, Belani CP, et al. Lung cancer in elderly patients: an analysis of the surveillance, epidemiology, and end results database. J Clin Oncol. 2007;25(35):5570–7.
3. Anon. Chemotherapy in non-small cell lung cancer: a meta-analysis using updated data on individual patients from 52 randomised clinical trials. Non-small Cell Lung Cancer Collaborative Group. BMJ 1995;311(7010):899–909.
4. Arriagada R, Bergman B, Dunant A, Le Chevalier T, Pignon JP, Vansteenkiste J. Cisplatin-based adjuvant chemotherapy in patients with completely resected non-small-cell lung cancer. N Engl J Med. 2004;350(4):351–60.
5. Scagliotti GV, Fossati R, Torri V, et al. Randomized study of adjuvant chemotherapy for completely resected stage I, II, or IIIA non-small-cell Lung cancer. J Natl Cancer Inst. 2003;95(19):1453–61.
6. Waller D, Peake MD, Stephens RJ, et al. Chemotherapy for patients with non-small cell lung cancer: the surgical setting of the Big Lung Trial. Eur J Cardiothorac Surg. 2004;26(1):173–82.
7. Douillard JY, Rosell R, De Lena M, et al. Adjuvant vinorelbine plus cisplatin versus observation in patients with completely resected stage IB-IIIA non-small-cell lung cancer (Adjuvant Navelbine International Trialist Association [ANITA]): a randomised controlled trial. Lancet Oncol. 2006;7(9):719–27.
8. Winton T, Livingston R, Johnson D, et al. Vinorelbine plus cisplatin vs. observation in resected non-small-cell lung cancer. N Engl J Med. 2005;352(25):2589–97.
9. Vincent MD, Butts C, Seymour L, Ding K, Graham B, Twumasi-Ankrah P, Gandara D, Schiller J, Green M, Shepherd F. Updated survival analysis of JBR.10: A randomized phase III trial of vinorelbine/cisplatin versus observation in completely resected stage IB and II non-small cell lung cancer (NSCLC). J Clin Oncol. 2009;27:15s, (suppl; abstr 7501).
10. Strauss GM, Herndon J, Maddaus MA, et al. Randomized Clinical Trial of adjuvant chemotherapy with paclitaxel and carboplatin following resection in Stage IB non–small-cell lung cancer (NSCLC): report of cancer and leukemia Group B (CALGB) Protocol 9633. J Clin Oncol 22:621s, 2004 (suppl; abstr 7019), 2004.
11. Strauss GM, Herndon II JE, Maddaus MA, et al. Adjuvant paclitaxel plus carboplatin compared with observation in stage IB non-small-cell lung cancer: CALGB 9633 with the Cancer and Leukemia Group B, Radiation Therapy Oncology Group, and North Central Cancer Treatment Group Study Groups. J Clin Oncol. 2008;26(31):5043–51.
12. Chemotherapy with or without bevacizumab in treating patients with stage IB, stage II, or stage IIIA non-small lung cancer that was removed by surgery. [cited 2009 September 30]; Available from: http://clinicaltrials.gov/ct2/show/NCT00324805`?term=ecog+1505&rank=1.
13. Talarico L, Chen G, Pazdur R. Enrollment of elderly patients in clinical trials for cancer drug registration: a 7-year experience by the US Food and Drug Administration. J Clin Oncol. 2004;22(22):4626–31.
14. Pepe C, Hasan B, Winton TL, et al. Adjuvant vinorelbine and cisplatin in elderly patients: National Cancer Institute of Canada and Intergroup Study JBR.10. J Clin Oncol. 2007;25(12):1553–61.
15. Pepe C, Hasan B, Winton T, Seymour L, Pater J, Livingston R, Johnson D, Rigas J, Ding K, Shepherd F. National Cancer Institute Of Canda Clinical Trials, Adjuvant chemotherapy in elderly patients: An analysis of National Cancer Institute of Canada Clinical Trials Group and Intergroup BR.10. J Clin Oncol. 2006, ASCO Annual Meeting Proceedings Part I. 2006;24(18S) (June 20 Suppl): 7009.
16. Non-small Cell Lung Cancer Collaborative Group. Chemotherapy for non-small cell lung cancer. Cochrane Database of Syst Rev. 2000, Issue 2. Art. No.: CD002139. DOI: 10.1002/14651858.CD002139.
17. Fruh M, Rolland E, Pignon JP, et al. Pooled analysis of the effect of age on adjuvant cisplatin-based chemotherapy for completely resected non-small-cell lung cancer. J Clin Oncol. 2008;26(21):3573–81.
18. Felip E, Massuti B, Alonso G, González-Larriba JL, Camps C, Isla D, Costas E, Sánchez JJ, Griesinger F, Rosell R. Surgery (S) alone, preoperative (preop) paclitaxel/carboplatin (PC) chemotherapy followed by S, or S followed by adjuvant (adj) PC chemotherapy in early-stage non-small cell lung cancer (NSCLC): results of the NATCH multicenter, randomized phase III trial. J Clin Oncol. 2009;27:15s (suppl; abstr 7500).
19. K. Pisters EV, Bunn PA, Crowley J, Chansky K, Ginsberg, R, Gandara DR. Southwest Oncology Group *S9900: Surgery alone or surgery plus induction (ind) paclitaxel/carboplatin (PC) chemotherapy in early stage non-small cell lung cancer (NSCLC): Follow-up on a phase III trial.* Journal of Clinical Oncology, 2007 ASCO Annual Meeting Proceedings Part I. Vol 25, No. 18S (June 20 Supplement), 2007:7520.
20. Scagliotti GV, on behalf of Ch.E.S.T. investigators. A phase III study of surgery alone or surgery plus preoperative gemcitabine-cisplatin in clinical early stages non-small cell lung cancer (NSCLC). J Clin Oncol. 2005, ASCO Annual Meeting Proceedings Part I of II. 23(16S) (June 1 Suppl):7023.
21. Lim E, Harris G, Patel A, Adachi I, Edmonds L, Song F. Preoperative versus postoperative chemotherapy in patients with resectable non-small cell lung cancer: systematic review and indirect comparison meta-analysis of randomized trials. J Clin Oncol. 2008;26:(abstr 7546).
22. Fossella F, Pereira JR, von Pawel J, et al. Randomized, multinational, phase III study of docetaxel plus platinum combinations versus vinorelbine plus cisplatin for advanced non-small-cell lung cancer: the TAX 326 study group. J Clin Oncol. 2003;21(16):3016–24.
23. Fossella FV, Belani CP, for the TAX 326 Study Group. Phase III study (TAX 326) of docetaxel-cisplatin (DC) and docetaxel-carboplatin (DCb) versus vinorelbine-cisplatin (VC) for the first-line treatment of advanced/metastatic non-small-cell lung cancer (NSCLC): analyses in elderly patients. Proc Am Soc Clin Oncol. 22: 2003 (abstr 2528).

24. Weiss J, Evans T, Eaby B, Stevenson J, Kucharczuk J, Cooper J, Kaiser L, Shrager J, Rengan R, Langer C. Adjuvant cisplatin and docetaxel (CDDP-Doc) for non small cell lung cancer (NSCLC): the hospital of the university of Pennsylvania (HUP) experience. 13th World Conference on Lung Cancer: San Francisco, CA; 2009.

25. Scagliotti GV, Parikh P, von Pawel J, et al. Phase III study comparing cisplatin plus gemcitabine with cisplatin plus pemetrexed in chemotherapy-naive patients with advanced-stage non-small-cell lung cancer. J Clin Oncol. 2008;26(21):3543–51.

26. Schmid-Bindert G, Chemaissani A, Fischer JR, Schütte W, Mazières J, Viñolas N, Wolf M, Thareau Vaury A, Leschinger M, Reck M. Pemetrexed in combination with cisplatin or carboplatin as adjuvant chemotherapy in early-stage NSCLC. J Clin Oncol. 2009;27:15s (suppl; abstr 7565).

27. Lynch TJ, Patel T, Dreisbach L, McCleod M, Heim W, Hermann RC, Paschold E, Pautret V, Weber MR, L.L.H. Overall survival (os) Results from the Phase III Trial BMS 099: cetuximab+taxane/carboplatin as 1st-line treatment for advanced NSCLC. Multidisciplinary Symposium in Thoracic Oncology. Chicago, IL; 2008.

28. Rajeswaran A, Trojan A, Burnand B, Giannelli M. Efficacy and side effects of cisplatin- and carboplatin-based doublet chemotherapeutic regimens versus non-platinum-based doublet chemotherapeutic regimens as first line treatment of metastatic non-small cell lung carcinoma: a systematic review of randomized controlled trials. Lung Cancer. 2008;59(1):1–11.

29. Langer CJ, Manola J, Bernardo P, et al. Cisplatin-based therapy for elderly patients with advanced non-small-cell lung cancer: implications of Eastern Cooperative Oncology Group 5592, a randomized trial. J Natl Cancer Inst. 2002;94(3):173–81.

30. Olaussen KA, Dunant A, Fouret P, et al. DNA repair by ERCC1 in non-small-cell lung cancer and cisplatin-based adjuvant chemotherapy. N Engl J Med. 2006;355(10):983–91.

31. Randomized study of customized adjuvant chemotherapy based on BRCA1 mRNA levels in completely resected stages II-IIIA in non-small cell lung cancer (GECP-SCAT). [cited; Available from: http://clinicaltrials.gov/ct2/show/NCT00478699?term=scat&rank=1].

32. Filipits M, Pirker R, Dunant A, et al. Cell cycle regulators and outcome of adjuvant cisplatin-based chemotherapy in completely resected non-small-cell lung cancer: the International Adjuvant Lung Cancer Trial Biologic Program. J Clin Oncol. 2007;25(19):2735–40.

33. Cobo M, Massuti B, Morán T, Chaib I, Pérez-Roca L, Jiménez U, Aguiar Bujanda D, González-Larriba J, Gómez J, Rosell R. Spanish customized adjuvant trial (SCAT) based on BRCA1 mRNA levels. J Clin Oncol. 2008;26:(May 20 Suppl; abstr 7533).

34. Tsao MS, Aviel-Ronen S, Ding K, et al. Prognostic and predictive importance of p53 and RAS for adjuvant chemotherapy in non small-cell lung cancer. J Clin Oncol. 2007;25(33):5240–7.

35. Vansteenkiste J, Zielinski M, Linder A, Dahabre J, Esteban E, Malinowski W, Jassem J, Passlick B, Lehmann F, Brichard VG. Final results of a multi-center, double-blind, randomized, placebo-controlled phase II study to assess the efficacy of MAGE-A3 immunotherapeutic as adjuvant therapy in stage IB/II non-small cell lung cancer (NSCLC). J Clin Oncol. 2007 ASCO Annual Meeting Proceedings Part I. 2007,25(18S) (June 20 Supplement): 7554.

36. GSK1572932A Antigen-specific cancer immunotherapeutic as adjuvant therapy in patients with non-small cell lung cancer. [cited; Available from: http://clinicaltrials.gov/ct2/show/NCT00480025?term=mage+lung&rank=4.

37. RADIANT: A study of tarceva after surgery with or without adjuvant chemotherapy in NSCLC patients who have EGFR-positive tumors (adjuvent).

Lung Cancer Treatment in the Elderly

There are multiple studies that draw attention to the tendency to limit the treatment of elderly cancer patients [7]. In the surgical treatment of lung cancer, an analysis of the SEER database showed that the frequency of limited resections increases with age, with a decline of pneumonectomies and lobectomies with age. Approximately 30% of the most elderly patients in the database were denied surgery or were offered only palliative surgery, in contrast with only 8% of the youngest patients [8]. Although this may in part represent an appropriate treatment strategy for a patient population with declining functional reserves and increased comorbidities, it may also signify a general reluctance for surgeons to operate on those with a relatively limited lifespan. However, by 2004 data, the life expectancy of an 80-year old in the United States is 9.1 years (8.2 years for males, 9.8 years for females), whereas the median survival for elderly patients with untreated early stage lung cancer is only 14 months [9]. This suggests that life limitation for an 80-year old with lung cancer is likely to be cancer related, and argues for treatment of well-selected elderly cancer patients [10].

Case Study

Mr. Joseph is an 82-year-old male with a past medical history of coronary artery disease status post a coronary artery bypass graft 15 years ago and a right thigh Merkel cell carcinoma that was excised and irradiated 4 years ago without recurrence. He developed a cough that did not improve with antibiotics, and a chest X-ray suggested a left upper lobe mass. A chest CT revealed two left upper lobe nodules, which were subsequently found to be FDG avid by PET. A head MRI was negative for metastases and a trans-bronchial biopsy was consistent with adenocarcinoma. He now presents for consideration of surgical resection.

On evaluation in your office, you find him to be a sharp, energetic octogenarian. He is functionally independent and is the primary caregiver for his wife. He does the shopping and cooking at home. He volunteers at the local library and enjoys going to classical music concerts. His son, who is available to offer support in the perioperative period, accompanies him to the visit. Mr. Joseph states that he tries to walk every day; however, recently he noticed that he gets short of breath after several blocks. He does not require mobility aids to ambulate. He smoked one pack per day for 55 years; however, he quit tobacco use 15 years prior. He denies recent weight loss. He understands the risk of surgery but "wants to fight" his newly diagnosed cancer.

Pulmonary function tests show preserved lung function with a forced expiratory volume in 1 second (FEV1) of 2.00 L

(83% predicted) and an FVC of 2.57 L (82% predicted). He is able to walk 1,425 ft in 6 min; however, he becomes moderately short of breath during the examination. You thus refer him to his cardiologist, who performs a cardiac stress test. His stress test is negative for ischemia, and you and the patient decide to go forward with a thoracoscopic resection.

Two weeks later he undergoes a video-assisted lingular sparing left upper lobectomy with mediastinal lymph node sampling. Postoperatively he was noted to have persistent high chest tube output of 100–250 cc/h, and was thus taken back to the operating room for reexploration. About 600 cc of clot was removed from his left hemi-thorax; however, no source for the hemorrhage was identified. Postoperatively, he was placed in the intensive care unit overnight; however, he continued to progress in his recovery and was discharged home with a visiting nurse on postoperative day 6.

His pathology returned with two foci of moderately differentiated adenocarcinoma, the largest measuring 2.9 cm. His margins and lymph nodes were negative (T2 N0 Mx). At the time of this writing, Mr. Joseph is now 91-years old and 9 years after surgery. He has no evidence of disease.

Preoperative Evaluation

Mr. Joseph's presentation and management illustrate the importance of a thorough preoperative assessment. Elderly patients are at increased risk for perioperative morbidity and mortality because of both decreased ability to recover physiologic homeostasis after surgical stress and increased prevalence of comorbid conditions. Older patients represent a heterogeneous population. A preoperative assessment should establish whether a patient is an appropriate surgical candidate and forewarn clinicians about potential for certain postoperative complications.

All patients in consideration for lung cancer resection surgery, regardless of age, require a complete history and physical exam with particular attention to characterization of symptoms, functional status, smoking history, and weight loss. At a minimum, patients should undergo an electrocardiogram, pulmonary function tests for patients undergoing lung resection, basic laboratory work, and a complete staging evaluation. Elderly patients should be assessed for functional status, independence, social support, and any cognitive impairment that may impact their treatment or recovery.

Accurate diagnosis and staging is of utmost importance to ensure appropriate selection of patients for operative resection. Similar to younger patients, elderly patients with lung cancer should have chest CT scans to image suspected lung nodules, PET scans to assess for metastatic disease, brain CT or MRI to look for occult metastases and, if indicated, cervical mediastinoscopy to stage mediastinal nodes. Elderly patients with suspected lung nodules should undergo

Table 42.1 Components of the preoperative assessment in elderly lung cancer patients

Preoperative evaluation of the elderly lung cancer patient
History and physical exam with attention to symptoms, smoking history, and comorbidities
Basic preoperative studies: EKG, basic lab work, chest X-ray
Complete staging workup: chest CT, PET scan, CT or MRI of the brain, and cervical mediastinoscopy if indicated
Geriatric: functional status, performance status, independence, social supports
Cardiac: symptoms, ability to climb stairs or walk one block, cardiac risk factors and previous history
Pulmonary: PFTs, workup as described in Fig. 42.1
Additional workup to be guided by symptoms or past medical history
Adaptations of the preoperative exam for the elderly

this standard workup unless their functional status is so impaired that treatment is not possible. Further workup can be determined based on symptoms or the existence of comorbid conditions. A summary of necessary requirements of a preoperative examination for an elderly lung cancer patient is shown in Table 42.1.

The preoperative visit with an elderly patient should first begin with a discussion with the patient about their personal values and goals for cancer care. It is often helpful to engage family members in the discussion of treatment options and give all involved parties the opportunity to ask questions. If the patient is clearly in favor of pursing surgical resection, the workup proceeds rapidly. In the event that a patient is unable to decide whether or not to pursue surgical management, our practice is to have the patient return in 2–4 weeks in order to provide the patient and their family time to digest the diagnosis of cancer and to clarify their goals before proceeding forward.

The patient and their family may not realize the degree of compensation for functional impairments that can slowly evolve over time. Our practice is to assess the patient's extent of impairment with a series of questions aimed at determining the patient's physical and cognitive reserves. For example, we will ask questions such as: Do you do your own shopping and cooking? Are you active in any civic or church groups? How do you spend your time on a typical day? Answers to these questions can illuminate impairments that the patient and their family may not even recognize.

One of the most important outcomes for an elderly patient is maintenance of baseline physical and mental function after surgery. Although patients and their families understand that there will be a postoperative recovery time in the hospital or rehabilitation setting, it is difficult council patients about longer-term effects of surgery such as the potential to cause permanent functional declines. There is limited data assessing changes in quality of life after thoracic surgery in the elderly, and few studies that assess whether surgery triggers loss of independence such as the need for increased assistance or more supportive living arrangements.

More immediately, patients with preoperative cognitive declines are at risk for postoperative morbidity. Karneko et al. determined that preoperative dementia was a risk factor for postoperative delirium [11]. Furthermore, Fukuse et al. found that thoracic surgery patients with preoperative dementia, as estimated by the mini-mental status exam (MMS), were fourfold more likely to have postoperative complications [12].

Functional and Performance Status

Preoperative functional and performance status are two of the most predictive indices of postoperative outcomes in elderly patients. Functional status describes the ability to perform self-care, self-maintenance, and physical activities. Traditional measures used to assess functional status are activities of daily living (ADLs) and instrumental activities of daily living (IADLs). ADLs are six basic self-care skills, such as the ability to dress or bathe, while IADLs include higher functioning skills that are used to maintain independence in the community. Need for assistance in these tasks has been predictive of prolonged hospital stay, nursing home placement, and home care requirements [13, 14]. Poor nutritional status, defined as a BMI of less than 22 kg/m squared, has been associated with increased need for assistance with ADLs and a decreased 1-year survival [15]. A lower ADL score is associated with postoperative complications [16].

Performance status is a standardized scale designed to measure the ability of a cancer patient to perform ordinary tasks. There are two scales, the Karnofsky performance scale, which ranges from 0 (dead) to 100 (normal) and the ECOG scale that ranges from 0 (normal) to 5 (dead). Comparisons of the two scales have been validated with a large sample of patients [17]. Performance status has been used to select patients for entry into chemotherapy trials; however, it is also well accepted to be associated with postoperative morbidity [18–20].

Cardiac Assessment and Perioperative Cardiac Management

A preoperative cardiac history should focus on the assessment of coronary risk factors and exercise tolerance including the ability to climb two flights of stairs or walk one block. In general, patients with poor exercise tolerance, or patients with a history of angina or claudication, should undergo noninvasive testing. Elderly patient may have mobility impairments such as arthritis that prevent assessment of functional reserve. Additionally, it may be difficult to determine whether symptoms such as shortness of breath or chest pain are due to cardiac or pulmonary etiology, and thus it is appropriate to have a low threshold for additional cardiac workup and assessment by a cardiologist to assist with perioperative risk stratification. Additionally, older patients are at increased risk for postoperative supraventricular tachycardias and should be considered for beta-blockade to reduce perioperative cardiac risk and to decrease postoperative atrial fibrillation [21, 22].

Pulmonary Assessment

Pulmonary function tests form the backbone of the preoperative pulmonary assessment and should be performed on all patients under consideration for lung resection surgery. Patients with marginal PFT results should undergo further evaluation with exercise testing, ventilation/perfusion scans to calculate predicted postoperative (PPO) lung function or VO_2 max testing as outlined in Fig. 42.1. [23]

The FEV1 by spirometry is most commonly used to determine a patient's suitability for surgery. The diffusion capacity for carbon monoxide (DLCO) and spirometry may be used as complimentary tests, particularly in patients with diffuse parenchymal disease or dyspnea that is out of proportion to the FEV1, with a low DLCO prompting further evaluation [24].

Exercise testing evaluates the cardiopulmonary system under induced physiological stress, and also has been found to be predictive of postoperative complications. Although simple exercise testing such as stair climbing or the six-minute walk test (6MWT) are easy to perform, their use in elderly patients may be limited by orthopedic or neurological impairments, or peripheral vascular insufficiency. The 6MWT measures the distanced walked over a period of 6 min. A normal patient is able to cover at least 1,400 ft in 6 min.

A recommended preoperative evaluation for an elderly patient considering pulmonary resection should consist of spirometry, pulmonary diffusion capacity of the lung for carbon monoxide (DLCO), room air ABG, and exercise tolerance tests including stair climbing and 6-min walk. Patients with an FEV1 > 1L and no major abnormality of other tests (FEV1/FVC > 50%, DLCO > 50% predicted, ABG paO_2 > 45 mmHg, tolerance of exercise tests) may safely proceed with surgery, including pneumonectomy [25].

Patients who do not meet these criteria should undergo further testing, including ventilation/perfusion scans to calculate PPO lung function or VO_2 max testing. Multiple studies have suggested that morbidity increases at a threshold % PPO FEV1 of <40%, or a % PPO DLCO of <40% [26–30]. A maximal oxygen consumption (VO_2 max) of <10 mL/kg/min has been shown to be associated with very high operative morbidity (26% total in combined data) in several small case series. VO_2 max values of 10–15 mL/kg/min has an intermediate perioperative morbidity (8.3% total) whereas patients with >15 mg/kg/min can undergo resection with an acceptable morbidity and mortality rate (25% morbidity and 0% mortality in a small series) [23, 31].

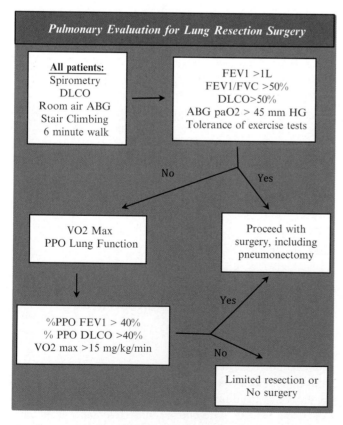

Fig. 42.1 Recommended pulmonary evaluation for patients undergoing lung resection surgery. *DLCO* diffusion capacity for carbon monoxide; *ABG* arterial blood gas; *FEV1* forced expiratory volume in 1 second; *FVC* forced vital capacity; *VO_2 Max* maximal oxygen consumption; *PPO* predicted postoperative (adapted from Jaklitsch and Billmeier [23], with permission)

Nonsmall Cell Lung Cancer in the Elderly

Histology

About 80–85% of all primary lung cancers are nonsmall cell histology [4]. Of the nonsmall cell subtypes, elderly patients are more likely to be diagnosed with squamous cell carcinoma (SCC) than younger lung cancer patients [6, 32, 33]. Relative to nonsquamous cell cancers, SCCs are associated with a higher incidence of localized disease, tend to have lower recurrence rates, and may have longer survival times than nonsquamous cell cancers [34–36]. However, squamous cell tumors are more likely to be centrally located, and thus are more likely to require pneumonectomy for curative resection. Mery et al. analysis of the SEER database showed that the frequency of SCC increased from 27% in patients less than 65-years old, to 38% in patients 75 and older, with parallel decreases in frequency of adenocarcinoma from 61 to 50% in corresponding age groups [35].

Stage at Presentation

Elderly patients are more commonly diagnosed with early stage disease, and are thus more likely to have surgically resectable tumors. An analysis of 22,874 patients revealed that the percent of lung cancer patients with local stage NSCLC increased from 15.3% in those aged 54 years or younger, to 25.4% of those aged 75 years or older [37]. Data published from the Surveillance, epidemiology, and end results (SEER) database in 2005 examining a cohort of 14,555 patients with early stage NSCLC showed that the frequency of stage I disease increased from 79% in patients <65 to 87% in patients age 75 or more [8]. Thus, although the elderly are at higher risk of developing lung cancer, a higher proportion present at a potentially curable stage of disease relative to a younger aged cohort.

Surgical Planning

Surgical resection for early stage nonsmall cell lung cancer offers the best chance for cure. In the elderly population, surgeons must balance the potential for long-term oncologic remission vs. the risk of short-term morbidity and mortality associated with surgery. The operative risk of death after pulmonary resection is largely attributable to two anatomical insults. First, there is the loss of functional lung tissue. Second, there is the morbidity and mortality introduced by the access thoracotomy. Operative strategies particular to the elderly population address both disruptions, with use of video-assisted thoracoscopic surgery (VATS) to minimize the chest wall disruption of a thoracotomy and by consideration of limited resections for the most elderly.

Surgical Approach

There are multiple studies that indicate that advanced age is a risk factor for death after thoracotomy. Several small single institution studies in the 1960s and 1970s indicated operative mortality rates of 14–27% for the elderly depending on age and type of surgery [38–41]. These findings were confirmed by a multi-institution study by the Lung Cancer Study Group in 1983. Ginsberg et al. reviewed 2,200 cases of lung

resection for cancer and found that operative mortality increased proportionally with age. Patients with age less than 60 had a 1.3% 30-day mortality rate, with increasing rates of 4.1, 7.0, and 8.1% mortality rates for the 60–69, 70–79, and 80 or greater age groups, respectively [42].

In a more modern analysis of 14,555 patients who had undergone curative resections for treating stage I or II NSCLC between 1992 and 1997, Mery et al. determined the effect of age on 30-day postoperative mortality. Including all types of resections, there was a 0.45% mortality rate for those below the age of 65 years, 0.6% for ages 65–74, and 1.2% for patients aged 75 or older. Mortality differences were found to be primarily due to differences in survival of patient undergoing lobectomy, with 0.3, 0.5, and 1.5% mortality for corresponding age groups ($p = 0.0001$), respectively. The difference in perioperative mortality was statistically similar for patients undergoing limited resection [43]. Studies have not shown an improvement in expected operative mortality if lung-sparing operations are performed via an access thoracotomy [44–46].

In 2006, the American College of Surgeons Oncology Group (ACOSOG) Z0030 Study published morbidity and mortality data for 1,023 clinically resectable T1 or T2, N0 or non-hilar N1 NSCLC patients randomized over a period from 1999 to 2004 to undergo pulmonary resection with lymph node sampling vs. mediastinal lymph node dissection. Overall mortality was 1.4%, improved from Ginsberg's reported 3.8%, and was not statistically associated with age [47]. However, the complication rate did rise as the age increased, with 49% of patients in the age group 80 and above experiencing one or more complication. Ninety percent of patients in the ACOSOG Z0030 study underwent resection via a thoracotomy, with the remaining procedures performed as VATS or VATS-assisted resections. Operative mortality reported by Ginsberg for pneumonectomy and lobectomy was 6.2 and 2.9%, respectively, compared with 0 and 1.3%, in the ACOSOG study. Notably, the pneumonectomy rate of the earlier study was 25.6, vs. 4% in ACOSOG, likely in part explaining the higher mortality rate of the earlier study.

VATS is defined as surgery performed through two or three incisions that are 2 cm in length. A utility incision less than 10 cm long may be used, without spreading of the ribs. VATS procedures in the elderly have been shown to have lower morbidity, lower rates of postoperative delirium, and result in earlier ambulation, a lower narcotic requirement, and a quicker recovery time [48–52].

Extent of Resection

The extent of NSCLC resection in elderly patients has been extensively debated, with advocates for limited resections for the aged to reduce associated morbidity and mortality risk.

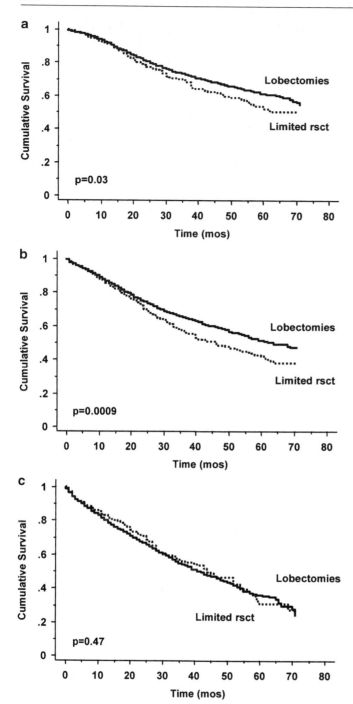

Fig. 42.2 Overall survival for patients <65 years (*top*, **a**), 65–74 years (*middle*, **b**), and ≥75 years (*bottom*, **c**) undergoing lobectomies (*solid line*) and limited resections (*dashed line*) (reprinted from Mery et al. [8], with permission. Copyright Elsevier 2009)

Lobectomy has generally been considered as standard of care for surgical resection of early stage NSCLC for the past 50 years [24, 53]. Lobectomy has traditionally been performed via thoracotomy; however, it is now often approached via VATS. Limited resections, consisting of either a sementectomy or wedge resection, remove less lung tissue and can usually be performed without a thoracotomy. These operations are associated with less perioperative morbidity and mortality; however, they do not completely remove draining lymphatics and may be associated with higher rates of local recurrence. A randomized trial by the Lung Cancer Study Group of limited resection vs. lobectomy for T1 N0 disease revealed a tripling of locoregional recurrence with limited resection, and a trend toward improved survival in the lobectomy group [54]. However, divergence of the survival curves between lobectomy and limited resection did not occur until 3 years after surgery, indicating a potential role for limited resection in patients with a shorter expected life span. Additional studies have concluded that limited resection remains an option for those unable to tolerate a lobectomy due to age or limited cardiopulmonary reserve [55, 56]. An age stratified analysis of 14,555 patients in the SEER database showed no benefit for lobectomy over limited resection in patients above age 71, as shown in Fig. 42.2 [35]. The decision to perform a limited resection vs. a lobectomy must take into account the patient's ability to tolerate a larger surgery and potential associated complications vs. a smaller resection with less durable oncologic outcomes.

Advances in Technology and the Elderly

Advances in technology will continue to alter the approach to management of nonsmall cell cancer in the elderly. Lobectomy is now commonly performed via VATS, allowing for a complete oncologic resection without requiring a full access thoracotomy. The elderly patient population is a clear benefactor of this technical progress. An illustration of VATS lobectomy is shown in Fig. 42.3.

Emerging technology involving radioactive seed placement at the resection margin has the potential to decrease the local recurrence associated with limited resections. Radioactive ^{125}I strands are sewn into a custom mesh that is then sutured in place along the resection margin [57]. Multiple small studies combining sublobar resection and planar ^{125}I seed implants have shown a decrease in local recurrence [58, 59]. A multicenter retrospective study of 291 patients with T1 N0 disease compared sublobar resections with lobar resections. Brachytherapy was used in 48% of the sublobar resections and was found to significantly decrease the local recurrence rate from 17.2 to 3.3%. For tumors less than 2 cm, there was no difference in survival between sublobar and lobar resection groups; however, median survival was better in the lobar resection group for larger tumors [60]. In elderly patients with small tumors and insufficient reserve to undergo a lobectomy, limited resection with staple line brachytherapy may prove to limit local recurrence and produce similar long-term outcomes.

In patients who are not surgical candidates, there are multiple options for achieving some measure of local control, including stereotactic radiosurgery (such as Cyberknife (Accuray, Inc, Sunnyvale, CA)), brachytherapy, and radiofrequency ablation (RFA). Initially found effective for brain metastases, stereotactic radiosurgery has been adapted to primary lung metastases with some success in small series [61, 62]. This technique aims to deliver a high radiation dose to the tumor while minimizing radiation exposure to the surrounding normal lung and adjacent tissues [63]. Although not a first-line therapy for lung tumors, image-guided percutaneous RFA can also offer some element of local control [64]. Since first described in 2000, several small case series have been published, with improvement of local control and

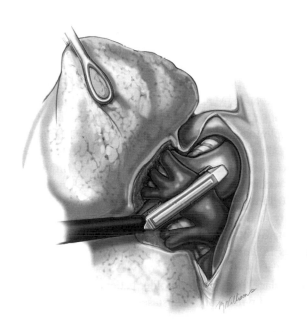

Fig. 42.3 Right upper VATS lobectomy, illustrating division of the superior pulmonary vein and exposure of the pulmonary artery. Artwork by Marcia Williams

survival relative to historical controls [65–67]. However, RFA is not without complications, including pneumothoraces, hemoptysis, and postprocedure pleuritic pain. Prospective randomized trials are needed to compare these therapies to conventional treatments.

Recommended Treatment Algorithm

Based on the accumulation of data and personal experience, we recommend the treatment approach outlined in Table 42.2 for elderly patients with nonsmall cell lung cancer. The approach is modified based on functional status, lung function, and lesion size. Clinical stage I or II patients with normal lung function and preserved functional status with lesions less than 1 cm in size are treated with a VATS wedge resection and thoracoscopic hilar lymph node sampling whenever possible. If the lesion is too centrally located to perform a wedge, then our preferred approach is a VATS lobectomy. If the lesion is larger than 1 cm then we routinely perform VATS lobectomy. In the elderly patient population, we do not perform pneumonectomies unless the patient is unusually well selected as, according to our opinion, chemoradiation without surgery is similar in long-term outcome compared to pneumonectomy. Clinical stage I or II patients with impaired functional status are managed with VATS wedge, RFA, or Cyberknife depending on the ability of the surrounding tissue to tolerate radiation effect. Patients with severely impaired lung function or hypoxic respiratory disorders are managed with VATS wedge or RFA to limit risk of pulmonary failure due to radiation pneumonitis.

In stage IIIa patients with normal lung function and preserved functional status, we prefer neoadjuvant chemotherapy followed by lobectomy with adjuvant radiation, with or without additional chemotherapy. We do not perform pneumonectomies in elderly stage IIIa patients. If a patient with stage IIIa disease has impaired functional status or poor

Table 42.2 Recommended treatment algorithm for elderly nonsmall cell cancer patients

Stage	Condition		Treatment
Clinical stage I or II	Preserved functional status and normal lung function	Lesion size <1 cm	VATS wedge resection if possible, with thoracoscopic hilar lymph node sampling
			If deep in lobe then perform VATS lobectomy
		Lesion size >1 cm	VATS lobectomy. Avoid pneumonectomy unless highly selected patient
	Impaired functional status		VATS wedge, RFA or Cyberknife
	Impaired lung function		VATS wedge or RFA
Clinical stage IIIa	Preserved functional status and normal lung function		Prefer neoadjuvant chemotherapy followed by lobectomy followed by adjuvant radiation ± chemotherapy
			Avoid pneumonectomy
	Impaired functional status or poor lung function		Chemotherapy/radiation only, prefer staggered administration
Stage IIIb or IV			Nonsurgical management

mortality and morbidity after lung resection. Am Rev Respir Dis. 1989;139:902–10.

28. Bolliger CT, Wyser C, Roser H, Soler M, Perruchoud AP. Lung scanning and exercise testing for the prediction of postoperative peformance in lung resection candidates at increased risk of complications. Chest. 1995;108:341–8.

29. Holden DA, Rice TW, Stefmach K, Meeker DP. Exercise testing, 6-min walk, and stair climb in the evaluation of patients at high risk for pulmonary resection. Chest. 1992;102:1774–9.

30. Wahi R, McMurtrey MJ, DeCaro LF, Mountain CF, Ali MK, Smith TL, et al. Determinants of perioperative morbidity and mortality after pneumonectomy. Ann Thorac Surg. 1989;48:33–7.

31. Morice RC, Peters EJ, Ryan MB, Putnam JB, Ali MK, Roth JA. Exercise testing in the evaluation of patients at high risk for complications from lung resection. Chest. 1992;101(2):356–61.

32. Weinmann M, Jeremic B, Toomes H, Friedel G, Bamberg M. Treatment of lung cancer in the elderly. Part I. Non-small cell lung cancer. Lung Cancer. 2003;39:233–53.

33. Morandi U, Stefani A, Golinelli M, Ruggiero C, Brandi L, Chiapponi A, et al. Results of surgical resection in patients over the age of 70 years with non small-cell lung cancer. Eur J Cardiothorac Surg. 1997;11:432–9.

34. Gail MH, Eagan RT, Feld R, Ginsberg R, Goodell B, Hill L, et al. Prognostic factors in patients with resected state I non-small cell lung cancer: a report from the Lung Cancer Study Group. Cancer. 1984;54:1802–13.

35. Mountain CF, Lukeman JM, Hammar SP, Chamberlain DW, Coulson WF, Page DL, et al. Lung cancer classification: the relationship of disease extent and cell type to survival in a clinical trials population. J Surg Oncol. 1987;35:147–56.

36. Deslauriers J, Gregoire J. Surgical therapy of early non-small cell lung cancer. Chest. 2000;117(Suppl):104S–9S.

37. O'Rourke MA, Feussner JR, Feigl P, Laszlo J. Age trends of lung cancer stage at diagnosis: implications for lung cancer screening in the elderly. JAMA. 1987;258:921–6.

38. Bates M. Results of Surgery for bronchial carcinoma in patients aged 70 and over. Thorax. 1970;25:77–8.

39. Evans EW. Resection of bronchial carcinoma in the elderly. Thorax. 1973;28:86–8.

40. Kirsh MM, Rotman H, Bove E, Argenta L, Cimmino V, Tashian J, et al. Major pulmonary resection for bronchial carcinoma in the elderly. Ann Thorac Surg. 1976;22:369–73.

41. Harviel JD, McNamara JJ, Straehley CJ. Surgical treatment of lung cancer in patients over the age of 70 years. J Thorac Cardiovasc Surg. 1978;75:802–5.

42. Ginsberg RJ, Hill LD, Eagan RT, Thomas P, Mountain CF, Deslauriers J, et al. Modern thirty-day operative mortality for surgical resections in lung cancer. J Thorac Cardiovasc Surg. 1983;86:654–8.

43. Mery CM, Jaklitch MT. Lung resection in the elderly, correspondence. Chest. 2006;129:496–7.

44. Albano WA. Should elderly patients undergo surgery for cancer. Geriatrics. 1977;32:105–8.

45. Breyer RH, Zippe C, Pharr WF, Jensik RJ, Kittle CF, Faber LP. Thoracotomy in patients over age seventy years: ten-year experience. J Thorac Cardiovasc Surg. 1981;81:187–93.

46. Zapatero J, Madrigal L, Lago J, Baschwitz B, Penalver R, Candelas J. Thoracic surgery in the elderly: review of 100 cases. Acta Chir Jung. 1990;31:227–34.

47. Allen MS, Darling GE, Pechet TT, Mitchell JD, Herndon II JE, Landreneau RJ, et al. ACOSOG Z0030 Study Group. Morbidity and mortality of major pulmonary resections in patients with early-stage lung cancer: initial results of the randomized, prospective ACOSOG Z0030 trial. Ann Thorac Surg. 2006;81(3):1013–9.

48. Decamp Jr MM, Jaklitsch MT, Mentzer SJ, Harpole DH Jr, Sugarbaker DJ. The safety and versatility of video-thoracoscopy: a prospective analysis of 895 cases. J Am Coll Surg. 1995;181:113–20.

49. McKenna R. Thoracoscopic lobectomy with mediastinal sampling in 80 year-old patients. Chest. 1994;106:1902–4.

50. Landreneau RL, Hazelrigg SR, Mack MJ, Dowling RD, Burke D, Gavlick J, et al. Postoperative pain-related morbidity: video-assisted thoracic surgery versus thoracotomy. Ann Thorac Surg. 1993;56:1285–9.

51. Jaklitsch MT, DeCamp MM Jr, Liptay MJ, Harpole DH Jr, Swanson SJ, Mentzer SJ, et al. Video-assisted thoracic surgery in the elderly: a review of 307 cases. Chest. 1996;110:751–8.

52. Cattaneo SM, Park BJ, Wilton AS, Seshan VE, Bains MS, Downey RJ, et al. Use of video-assisted thoracic surgery for lobectomy in the elderly results in fewer complications. Ann Thorac Surg. 2008;85:231–6.

53. Faulkner SL. Is lobectomy the gold standard for stage I lung cancer in year 2000? [abstract]. Chest. 2000;118(4 Suppl):119S.

54. Ginsberg RJ, Rubinstein LV. Randomized trial of lobectomy versus limited resection for T1 N0 non-small cell lung cancer. Lung Cancer Study Group. Ann Thorac Surg. 1995;60(3):615–22; discussion 622–3.

55. Landreneau RJ, Sugarbaker DJ, Mack MJ, Hazelrigg SR, Luketich JD, Fetterman L, et al. Wedge resection versus lobectomy for stage I (T1 N0 M0) non-small-cell lung cancer. J Thorac Cardiovasc Surg. 1997;113(4):691–700.

56. Sugarbaker DJ. Lung cancer • 6: the case for limited surgical resection in non-small cell lung cancer. Thorax. 2003;58(7):639–41.

57. Mutyala S, Devlin PM. Innovative radiation techniques: role of brachytherapy and intraoperative radiotherapy in treatment of lung cancer. In: David Sugarbaker J, editor. Adult chest surgery. New York: Mcgraw Hill; 2009. p. 639–40.

58. Lee W, Daly BD, DiPetrillo TA, Morelli DM, Neuschatz AC, Morr J, et al. Limited resection for non-small cell lung cancer: observed local control with implantation of I-125 brachytherapy seeds. Ann Thorac Surg. 2003;75(1):237–42.

59. Santos R. Comparison between sublobar resection and 125Iodine brachytherapy after sublobar resection in high-risk patients with stage I nonsmall-cell lung cancer. Surgery. 2003;134(4):691–7.

60. Fernando HC, Santos RS, Benfield JR, Grannis FW, Keenan RJ, Luketich JD, et al. Lobar and sublobar resection with and without brachytherapy for small stage IA non-small cell lung cancer. J Thorac Cardiovasc Surg. 2005;129(2):261–7.

61. Uematsu M, Shioda A, Suda A, Fukui T, Ozeki Y, Hama Y, et al. Computed tomography-guided frameless stereotactic radiotherapy for stage I non-small cell lung cancer: a 5-year experience. Int J Radiat Oncol Biol Phys. 2001;51(3):666–70.

62. Wulf J, Haedinger U, Oppitz U, Thiele W, Mueller G, Flentje M. Stereotactic radiotherapy for primary lung cancer and pulmonary metastases: a noninvasive treatment approach in medically inoperable patients. Int J Radiat Oncol Biol Phys. 2004;60(1):186–96.

63. Whyte RI, Crownover R, Murphy MJ, Martin DP, Rice TW, DeCamp MM, et al. Stereotactic radiosurgery for lung tumors: preliminary report of a phase I trial. Ann Thorac Surg. 2003;75(4):1097–101.

64. van Sonnenberg E, Morrison PR, Silverman SG, Shankar S, Tuncali K, Nair RT, et al. Percutaneous thoracic tumor ablation. In: David Sugarbaker J, editor. Adult chest surgery. New York: Mcgraw Hill; 2009. p. 652–9.

65. Dupuy DE, Zagoria RJ, Akerley W, Mayo-Smith WW, Kavanagh PV, Safran H. Percutaneous radiofrequency ablation of malignancies in the lung. Am J Roentgenol. 2000;174(1):57–9.

66. Hiraki T, Gobara H, Iishi T, Sano Y, Iguchi T, Fujiwara H, et al. Percutaneous radiofrequency ablation for clinical stage I non-small cell lung cancer: results in 20 nonsurgical candidates. J Thorac Cardiovasc Surg. 2007;134(5):1306–12.

67. Lee JM, Jin GY, Goldberg SN, Lee YC, Chung GH, Han YM, et al. Percutaneous radiofrequency ablation for inoperable non–small cell

lung cancer and metastases: preliminary report. Radiology. 2004;230(1):125–34.

68. Kulke MH, Mayer RJ. Carcinoid tumors. N Engl J Med. 1999;340(11):858–68.

69. Marty-Ane C, Costes V, Pujol J, Alauzen M, Baldet P, Mary H. Carcinoid tumors of the lung: do atypical features require aggressive management? Ann Thorac Surg. 1995;59(1):78–83.

70. Mezzetti M, Raveglia F, Panigalli T, Giuliani L, Lo Giudice F, Meda S, et al. Assessment of outcomes in typical and atypical carcinoids according to latest WHO classification. Ann Thorac Surg. 2003;76(6):1838–42.

71. Jaklitsch MT, Mery CM, Lukanich JM, Richards WG, Bueno R, Swanson SJ, et al. Sequential thoracic metastasectomy prolongs survival by re-establishing local control within the chest. J Thorac Cardiovasc Surg. 2001;121(4):657–67.

72. Inoue M, Ohta M, Iuchi K, Matsumura A, Ideguchi K, Yasumitsu T, et al. Benefits of surgery for patients with pulmonary metastases from colorectal carcinoma. Ann Thorac Surg. 2004;78(1):238–44.

73. Weiser MR, Downey RJ, Leung DH, Brennan MF. Repeat resection of pulmonary metastases in patients with soft-tissue sarcoma. J Am Coll Surg. 2000;191(2):184–90; discussion 190–1.

74. Saito Y, Omiya H, Kohno K, Kobayashi T, Itoi K, Teramachi M, et al. Pulmonary metastasectomy for 165 patients with colorectal carcinoma: a prognostic assessment. J Thorac Cardiovasc Surg. 2002;124(5):1007–13.

75. Pfannschmidt J. Prognostic factors and survival after complete resection of pulmonary metastases from colorectal carcinoma: experiences in 167 patients. J Thorac Cardiovasc Surg. 2003; 126(3):732–9.

76. Carballo M, Maish M, Jaroszewski D, Holmes C. Video-assisted thoracic surgery (VATS) as a safe alternative for the resection of pulmonary metastases: a retrospective cohort study. J Cardiothorac Surg. 2009;4(1):13.

77. Pastorino U, Buyse M, Friedel G, Ginsberg RJ, Girard P, Goldstraw P, et al. Long-term results of lung metastasectomy: Prognostic Analyses based on 5206 cases. J Thorac Cardiovasc Surg. 1997;113(1):37–49.

78. Collie DA, Wright AR, Williams JR, Hashemi-Malayeri B, Stevenson AJM, Turnbull CM. Comparison of spiral-acquisition computed tomography and conventional computed tomography in the assessment of pulmonary metastatic disease. Br J Radiol. 1994;67(797):436–44.

79. McCormack PM, Bains MS, Begg CB, Burt ME, Downey RJ, Panicek DM, et al. Role of video-assisted thoracic surgery in the treatment of pulmonary metastases: results of a prospective trial. Ann Thorac Surg. 1996;62(1):213–6.

80. Nakajima J, Takamoto S, Tanaka M, Takeuchi E, Murakawa T, Fukami T. Thoracoscopic surgery and conventional open thoracotomy in metastatic lung cancer. Surg Endosc. 2001;15(8):849–53.

81. Reinhardt M, Wiethoelter N, Matthies A, Joe A, Strunk H, Jaeger U, et al. PET recognition of pulmonary metastases on PET/CT imaging: impact of attenuation-corrected and non-attenuation-corrected PET images. Eur J Nucl Med Mol Imaging. 2006;33(2):134–9.

82. Mutsaerts E, Zoetmulder F, Meijer S, Baas P, Hart A, Rutgers E. Long term survival of thoracoscopic metastasectomy vs metastasectomy by thoracotomy in patients with a solitary pulmonary lesion. Eur J Surg Oncol. 2002;28(8):864–8.

Chapter 43
Benign Thoracic Disease in the Elderly[1]

Rita A. Mukhtar and Pierre R. Theodore

Abstract The spectrum of noncancerous diseases of the chest in elderly patients includes both diseases that affect younger patients, as well as processes exacerbated by the underlying physiological changes of aging. Structural alterations, immunological changes, decreases in physiologic reserve, and comorbid disease processes all affect the presentation and response to disease in the elderly. Benign disorders of the thorax in the elderly include diseases of the chest wall and pleura, thoracic spine deformities which affect pulmonary function, benign masses, rheumatological disorders, infectious processes such as pneumonia and emypema, and chronic obstructive pulmonary disease. When caring for elderly patients, clinicians must be aware of signs and symptoms of these disorders, options for management, and potential complications in this population.

Keywords Benign • Thoracic disease • Elderly • COPD • Pleural effusion • Pneumonia • Kyphosis

Introduction

Elderly patients present challenges in diagnosis and treatment of various disease processes. While they may develop thoracic diseases seen in other age groups, older patients often have atypical presentations of these diseases, and may be vulnerable to thoracic pathology as a result of comorbid diseases. Pulmonary function testing of the elderly population shows increased ventilation-perfusion mismatch, decreased forced expiratory volumes, and decreased diffusion capacities. Combined with increased chest wall rigidity, decreasing muscle mass, impaired mucocilary clearance, blunted perception of dyspnea, and possible increased aspiration risk due to underlying neurological dysfunction, these physiological changes associated with aging make this population particularly vulnerable to thoracic disease [2].

Disease of the Chest Wall and Pleura

Mondor's Disease

Mondor's disease is a benign thrombophlebitis usually involving the thoracoepigastric and lateral thoracic veins. Three fourths of patients are women. Although the anterior and lateral chest wall are most commonly affected, Mondor's disease has been reported in the antecubital fossa, inguinal region, axilla, penis, abdomen, and lower limbs [3].

The pathogenesis involves formation of venous thrombi, with resultant venous occlusion and fibrosis. The overlying skin retracts, creating characteristic cord-like structures, often starting from the areola or axilla. While the etiology is unknown, there is an association with hypercoagulable states, thoracic surgical procedures, breast infections, hyperextension of the upper extremity, and intravenous drug abuse. Patients typically present with localized chest pain, and palpable cords on the chest wall. Although Mondor's disease itself is a benign, self-limited disease, it has been associated with the presence of carcinoma of the breast.

Treatment involves local application of heat, systemic or topical nonsteroidal antiinflammatories, and rest of the affected limb. Pain usually resolves in about 10 days, while skin changes may take longer to resolve. For chronic or subacute cases, resection of the thrombotic vessels can be considered. There is no clear benefit of anticoagulation.

[1]Sections of this text are reproduced from Mukhtar and Theodore [1]. Review. Copyright © 2009, with permission from Elsevier.

R.A. Mukhtar (✉)
Department of General Surgery, University of California, San Francisco, 513 Parnassus Avenue, S321, San Francisco, CA 94143, USA
e-mail: Rita.Mukhtar@ucsfmedctr.org

Lung Herniation

Lung herniation occurs when the lung parenchyma and pleural membranes protrude through a defect in the thoracic wall. This can result from congenital abnormalities, trauma, underlying disease, or thoracic surgical procedures. Spontaneous lung herniation secondary to vigorous coughing or playing a wind instrument has been reported [4]. Patients may be asymptomatic, or present with a bulge on the chest wall, hemoptysis due to strangulation of herniated lung, or recurrent pulmonary infections. In patients undergoing minimally invasive thoracic surgery, the anterior approach appears to have a higher incidence of postoperative lung hernia development, likely due to inherent weakness in the thoracic cage where there is only a single layer of intercostals muscles [5].

Predisposing factors for lung herniation include chronic obstructive pulmonary disease (COPD), inflammatory or neoplastic processes, and chronic steroid use. Lung herniation is unlikely to recover spontaneously, but surgical treatment is not mandatory for all lung hernias. Indications for operative intervention include strangulated lung, hemoptysis, and pain. Some authors advocate repair for all anterior hernias, even if asymptomatic, to avoid extension into the abdominal wall. Surgical treatment involves identification of the hernia sac, freeing the lung from adhesions, and patch repair. Minimally invasive repairs with videoscopic techniques have been described.

Pneumomediastinum

The primary development of free air in the mediastinum, or spontaneous pneumomediastinum, must be distinguished from secondary pneumomediastinum, as the two processes have very different clinical implications. Spontaneous pneumomediastinum results from a sudden increase in intrathoracic pressure, leading to increased intraalveolar pressure. Alveolar rupture then allows air to track along the bronchovascular tissue sheath toward the mediastinum [6].

The most common cause of spontaneous pneumomediastinum is forceful emesis, although intense coughing, screaming, childbirth, and bronchospasm have been reported as causative events. Predisposing factors include asthma and idiopathic pulmonary fibrosis. Patients can present with chest pain, shortness of breath, subcutaneous emphysema, or Hammon's sign, crepitus heard with the heart beat on auscultation of the chest.

Spontaneous pneumomediastinum is a benign condition for which treatment is usually expectant. The diagnosis of spontaneous pneumomediastinum is one of exclusion however, and the presence of free air on chest radiographs mandates differentiation from secondary pneumomediastinum. By contrast, secondary pneumomediastinum, which results most commonly from blunt or penetrating trauma, interventions in the esophagus or tracheobronchial tree, or infectious processes, is associated with life threatening injury to the aerodigestive tract, and carries a high mortality rate.

Kyphosis

Kyphosis is a common problem, and may contribute to pulmonary dysfunction in the elderly. It is an exaggerated posterior convexity of the thoracic spine, which increases with aging. This spinal deformity results from the combined effects of osteoporotic vertebral fractures, arthritis, intervertebral disk thinning, and reduced muscular tone. Vertebral compression fractures are estimated to occur in one-third of women over 65 years of age, and half of women over 80 years. One study found that over 80% of patients greater than 80 years of age had kyphosis [7].

As with younger patients with spinal deformities, older patients with kyphosis suffer increased mortality from pulmonary disease, and measurable differences in spirometric evaluation. Women with radiographically evident vertebral fractures have double the mortality from pulmonary causes compared to women without vertebral fractures. Additionally, severe kyphosis is strongly predictive of pulmonary death.

Kyphosis resulting from osteoporotic vertebral fractures is thought to result in pulmonary impairment, resulting in a restrictive pattern evident in pulmonary function testing. In one study, kyphotic participants reported more dyspnea, and had restrictive and obstructive ventilatory patterns on spirometric testing [8]. With worsening kyphosis, or a Cobb's angle greater than 55°, impairment is considerable. Cobb's angle is calculated by drawing lines parallel to the vertebral body at the superior aspect of the spinal curvature and the vertebral body at the inferior aspect of the spinal curvature, and then measuring the angle formed by the intersection of two lines perpendicular to these.

While results are mixed, some randomized trials of physical rehabilitation programs for patients over the age of 60 have shown improvements in Cobb's angle [9, 10]. Minimally invasive vertebroplasty and kyphoplasty are surgical procedures which are typically offered for intractable pain, progressive kyphosis, or neurological compromise. After kyphoplasty, forced vital capacity (FVC) and maximum voluntary ventilation have been shown to improve. It is unclear whether this is related to improved pain, or improved pulmonary mechanics. Difficulties in interpretation of existing studies include inconsistencies in methods used to measure height and kyphosis, as well as variability in tested pulmonary function parameters. However, given its high prevalence and association with poor pulmonary outcomes, kyphosis may be an under-recognized contributor to dyspnea in the elderly population [11].

Neoplastic Disease

Benign Lung Tumors

Benign neoplasms of the lung are uncommon tumors. Either epithelial or mesenchymal in origin, they can present with cough, pneumonia, hemoptysis, or be completely asymptomatic. In asymptomatic patients, the use of diagnostic imaging techniques identifies these lesions, often resulting in their resection for diagnostic purposes. Lack of progression of a pulmonary lesion over a minimum of 2 years is required to radiographically rule out a malignant process.

When surgical excision is needed, minimally invasive techniques such as video-assisted thoracic surgery have been shown to result in significantly shorter hospital stays and decreased complications compared to thoracotomy in patients aged 70 or older [12]. Older age is a risk factor for postoperative atrial fibrillation following pneumonectomy [13].

Reviews of surgical series of patients with benign lung tumors show hamartomas to be the most prevalent. The age range is wide, with most benign tumors of adulthood presenting at a median age of 52 years. Below, various epithelial and mesenchymal benign neoplasms are described (Table 43.1) [14, 15].

Epithelial Tumors

Papillomas

Papillomas occasionally occur in the lower airway. These are generally exophytic tumors, affecting men more often than women, and children most commonly. Papillomas have been classified as squamous, glandular, and mixed. Squamous papillomas are associated with human papilloma virus (HPV), while the more rare glandular papillomas are not. Squamous papillomas are thought to result from ororespiratory HPV exposure during vaginal delivery. As with other lesions caused by HPV infection, those papillomas caused by high risk strains of the virus are at risk for malignant transformation to squamous carcinoma [16].

Papillomas often present as thin-walled cysts and nodules with postobstructive atelectasis on chest radiograph. Histologically, exophytic papillomas have an epithelial layer covering a central fibrovascular core which protrudes into the airway lumen. Stratified squamous epithelium lines the squamous papillomas, while a single layer of columnar nonciliated epithelial cells line the glandular papillomas.

Recurrent respiratory papillomatosis is managed by endoscopic cryotherapy, laser, or microdebrider treatment. Attempts at management with TGF-beta cytokine blockade have met with some success in younger patients, but most are managed with local ablative techniques rather than systemic therapy.

Sclerosing Hemangioma (Pneumocytoma)

Benign lung neoplasms with a female predominance, these lesions are thought to arise from type II pneumocytes. They are well-circumscribed, containing two morphologic populations, cuboidal epithelium resembling type II pneumocytes, and round to oval stromal cells.

Alveolar Adenoma

Alveolar adenomas are unusual neoplasms typically found in the lung periphery with no gender predilection. They are usually identified as solitary asymptomatic pulmonary nodules in adults, and classified as epithelial neoplasms, although mesenchymal origin has also been suggested.

Table 43.1 Benign tumors of the lower respiratory tract, World Health Organization Classification 2004

Epithelial	Mesenchymal	Miscellaneous	Tumorlike conditions
Papilloma	Hamartoma	Thymoma	Minute meningothelial nodules
Squamous	Localized fibrous tumor	Mature teratoma	Nodular lymphoid hyperplasia
Glandular	Chondroma		Inflammatory pseudotumor
Mixed	Leiomyoma		Localized organizing pneumonia
Sclerosing hemangioma	Lipoma		Nodular amyloid
Alveolar adenoma	Clear cell tumor		Hyalinizing granuloma
Papillary adenoma	Other soft tissue tumors		Bronchial inflammatory polyp
Mucous gland adenoma			Micronodular penumocyte hyperplasia
Pleomorphic adenoma			Endometriosis
Mucinous cystadenoma			Others – rounded atelectasis and congenital lesions

Source: data from reference [15]. Reprinted from Mukhtar and Theodore [1]. Review. Copyright © 2009, with permission from Elsevier

Type II Pneumocyte Papilloma

These are rare, benign neoplasms composed of type II pneumocyte-lined papillae. They are typically solitary, well-circumscribed lesions in the periphery.

Mucous Gland Adenomas

Mucous gland adenomas are benign epithelial neoplasms of the lung. Previous nomenclature includes adenomatous polyps of the bronchus, bronchial cystadenomas, bronchial adenomas of the mucous gland type, mucous cell adenomas, and papillary cystadenomas. They occur sporadically, affecting men more than women.

Amongst reported cases, most patients presented with coughing, shortness of breath, and wheezing. Most mucous gland adenomas occur in the mainstem airways and trachea. Although chest radiographs can show a nodular density, or distal atelectasis, imaging studies are often unrevealing. Computed tomography can identify obstructing bronchial lesions, although it may underestimate the amount of submucosal invasion. Pathologic examination shows mucus-filled glandular and tubular spaces with an epithelial cell lining. These benign tumors are treated with lung parenchyma sparing resection (i.e., bronchial sleeve resection), generally without the need for lobectomy. Those smaller than 3 cm with low mitotic activity are more likely to have a benign course [17].

Mucinous Cystadenoma

These are epithelial neoplasms typically found as asymptomatic, peripheral, cystic nodules. While some are benign, many are malignant or have atypical features. They are often positive for thyroid transcription factor and cytokeratin 7. Because of the high incidence of atypia, complete excision is recommended.

Mesenchymal Tumors

Hamartoma

The term hamartoma was first applied to benign tumors in the lung composed of fat and cartilage by Goldsworthy in 1934 [18]. Lung hamartomas are the most common benign lung tumors, most commonly discovered as asymptomatic radiographic findings.

Hamartomas are generally nonneoplastic, disordered collections of benign tissue normally present in a given organ.

In the lung, however, pulmonary hamartomas are benign neoplasms composed of at least two types of mesenchymal tissue. They are typically found in the periphery, although endobronchial hamartomas are occasional seen (<10%) [19]. Chest radiographs classically show a "popcorn" pattern of calcification in 30% of cases. On histopathology, they are often lobulated, and contain a mixture of cartilage, fat, myxoid connective tissue, smooth muscle, or epithelium. The presence of only one type of mesenchymal tissue suggests lipoma, leiomyoma, or chondroma. Cytogenetic abnormalities have been identified in pulmonary hamartomas. Pulmonary hamartomas can be managed either nonoperatively with serial imaging, or with wedge resection.

Solitary Fibrous Tumor of the Lung

These are typically pleural-based tumors containing bland spindled cells with ingrowths of epithelial cells. Vimentin and CD34 histopathology markers confirm the diagnosis of solitary fibrous tumor. Importantly, solitary fibrous tumors can be mistaken for mesothelioma if thorough immunohistochemistry panels are not employed. While 80% are benign, there is some malignant potential, and resection is generally recommended [20].

Clear Cell (Sugar Tumor)

Clear cell tumors of the lung are rare asymptomatic nodules. Histologically, they are uniform proliferations of clear and granular cells. They must be distinguished from metastatic renal cell carcinoma. Unlike renal cell carcinoma, clear cell tumors of the lung are cytokeratin negative, vimentin negative, and HMB-45 positive. They are not mitotically active, and generally benign.

Other Mesenchymal Tumors

Nerve Sheath Tumors – rare intrapulmonary tumors histologically similar to schwannomas of other sites. Nerve sheath tumors are often associated with the dorsal root ganglia of spinal nerves, and may present with posterior pleural or mediastinal mass.

Leiomyomas – smooth muscle tumors which can be endobronchial or parenchymal

Chrondromas – cartilaginous tumors without epithelial elements

Lipomas – composed of adipose tissue, they are more commonly endobronchial in location, but can be parenchymal

Infectious and Rheumatologic Disease

Pneumonia

Pneumonia is the fifth leading cause of death in the United States among adults 65 years of age and older. Physiologic changes that occur with aging predispose to the development of pneumonia, including impaired mucociliary clearance, increased risk of aspiration due to diminished swallowing reflexes, increased rigidity of the chest wall, and atrophy of respiratory muscles and chronic obstructive airway disease. Elderly patients with pneumonia often present with nonspecific or atypical symptoms such as failure to thrive, confusion, frequent falling, and decreased ability to perform usual daily activities, particularly if they have some level of underlying dementia. The most commonly reported symptom in one study of patients over the age of 65 with community-acquired pneumonia was dyspnea, followed by cough and fever [2].

Community acquired pneumonia remains a substantial cause of morbidity, with about 915,000 cases in the elderly population each year. *Streptococcus pneumoniae* is thought to be the leading cause. Among adults aged 50 or older, there are 24,000 cases of invasive pneumococcal disease, (defined by isolation of *Streptococcus pneumoniae* from a normally sterile site, e.g., blood or cerebrosprinal fluid), resulting in 4,500 deaths [21].

Nursing home acquired pneumonia typically occurs in an even older, more debilitated population, with resulting higher morality rates. A study of microbial causes of pneumonia in patients aged 85 or older found *Chlamydophila pneumoniae* to be the most common cause of nursing home acquired pneumonia, followed by *Streptococcus pneumoniae* and viral pathogens such as *Cytomegalovirus*. Mortality was associated with performance status, albumin, and blood urea nitrogen [22].

Increasing age confers greater risk of invasive pneumococcal disease, that is, pneumococcal bacteremia. Compared to adults aged 65–74, adults 85 or older have 3 times the risk of invasive disease. While the pneumococcal polysaccharide vaccine (PPV) has been shown to be effective in reducing the risk of invasive pneumococcal disease in immunocompetent older adults, its efficacy at preventing nonbacteremic pneumococcal pneumonia has not been firmly established, nor has its efficacy in preventing invasive pneumococcal disease in immunocompromised older adults. Currently, the Advisory Committee on Immunization Practices recommends that all adults receive a dose of PPV at or after age 65. While patients over 85 have increased risk of invasive pneumococcal disease, a study of 221 elderly patients with community acquired pneumonia found that those over 85 had a significantly lower rate of acute respiratory distress syndrome than patients aged 65–85 [23]. This was thought to be due to impaired host reaction to infection with aging, with a resulting decrease in circulating inflammatory cytokines, dampening the expected systemic inflammatory response.

The introduction of a conjugate vaccine for young children targeting seven pneumococcal serotypes has resulted in a decreased incidence of pneumococcal disease in older adults. Among adults aged 50 and older, the incidence of disease caused by the seven conjugate vaccine serotypes decreased by 55% in the period after introduction of the vaccine for children, presumably due to decreased pneumococcal carriage and transmission by young children [24].

As the epidemiology of community acquired pneumonia changes, particularly since the advent of the pneumococcal conjugate vaccine in children, so does the potential benefit of the PPV in older adults. From 1998 to 1999, there were 51.7 of invasive pneumococcal disease due to the 23 serotypes in the PPV per 100,000 older adults; in 2004, there were 26.9 cases per 100,000 older adults.

When pneumonia is complicated by para-pneumonic effusion, chest tube drainage may be necessary. Of note, pleural effusion can be seen as opacification on chest radiograph, in which case a mass effect leads to mediastinal shift away from the affected side. Atelectasis however, while also causing an opacification, results in volume loss and a mediastinal shift towards the affected side. Distinguishing the two clinical scenarios is important in preventing complications of inappropriate chest tube placement for atelectasis, which can result in the rare but reported circumstance of chest tube placement into the ventricle [25].

Empyema

Thoracic infections can be complicated by the development of pleural empyemas: loculated fibrinopurulent collections in the pleural space. Empyemas carry considerable morbidity, and are associated with mortality of up to 20%. Most empyemas result from parapneumonic effusions in patients with pneumonia, with nearly half resulting from infection with gram-positive bacteria (Table 43.2). If untreated, these effusions progress from freely flowing exudates to multiloculated collections. Empyema can result in sepsis, respiratory compromise, and trapped lung [26].

Thoracic empyema affects roughly 65,000 people annually. A retrospective study of 132 patients in Taiwan compared community acquired empyema in patients under 65 years of age to those over 65. Risk factors for the development of empyema in older patients included chronic lung

Table 43.2 Bacterial isolates in empyema in patients aged 65 or older, excluding mycobacterium, both community and nursing home acquired

Organism	Percent of positive pleural cultures	
	Tsai et al. (%)	El Solh et al. (%)
Aerobic gram-positive	46	49
Streptococcus milleri		
Viridans streptococci		
Staphylococcus aureus		
Streptococcus pneumoniae		
Aerobic gram-negative	24	27
Escherichia coli		
Klebsiella pneumoniae		
Proteus mirabilis		
Pseudomonas aeruginosa		
Anaerobic	21	26
Peptostreptococcus species		
Bacteroides species		
Prevotella species		
Fusobacterium species		
Fungal	9	
Candida albicans		
Nonalbicans *Candida*		

disease, central nervous system disease, malignancy, and diabetes mellitus. Most thoracic empyemas develop as a complication of bronchopulmonary infection, but they can also result from intra-abdominal infection, esophageal fistula, chest trauma, retropharyngeal or periodontal abscesses, and mycotic aortic aneurysms. Older patients were less likely to present with high fevers and chest pain, but more likely to have dyspnea. Microbiology data did not differ significantly from the younger group of patients. Although the older group had increased incidence of respiratory failure, renal failure, shock, and longer hospital stays, the overall mortality was the same. While earlier surgical intervention led to faster recovery in the younger group of patients, early intervention did not alter the recovery course for older patients [27].

Given the high incidence of pneumonia in the elderly population, older patients are at an attendant increased risk of developing empyemas. Those elderly patients who reside in nursing homes are at particular risk of developing empyemas following aspiration pneumonia, and presenting with more indolent, subtle symptoms.

A comparison of community-acquired vs. nursing-home acquired empyemas found that community-dwelling patients typically presented with dyspnea, fever, and cough, while nursing home residents were more likely to present with dyspnea and weight loss. More nursing home residents had multiloculated effusions on computed tomography. Not surprisingly, the success rate of nonsurgical intervention was significantly lower for the nursing-home patients.

Anaerobic bacteria were more frequently isolated from the pleural cultures of nursing home residents compared to community dwellers, suggesting that swallowing abnormalities, as one might develop from dementia or cerebrovascular accident, put the patient at high risk of aspiration pneumonia and subsequent empyema development. Oral and dental hygiene thus remains a potentially modifiable risk factor in the elderly nursing home patient population. Speech and language specialists can be indispensible in detecting patients at high risk for aspiration.

Elderly patients undergoing thoracoscopic or open evacuation of empyema and pneumolysis have higher mortality rates than younger patients. One study found surgery-related mortality rates of 3.46% in patients under 70, vs. 18.3% in patients over 70 years undergoing surgical treatment of thoracic empyema. Risk factors for surgery related mortality in the elderly population included the presence of lung abscess, necrotizing pneumonitis, and preoperative ventilatory dependency. This is perhaps related to decreased physiologic reserve, with respiratory muscle atrophy, and resultant reduced force-generating capacity of the respiratory muscles [28].

Rheumatoid Pleural Effusions

Although rare, pleural effusions can develop as a complication of rheumatoid arthritis (RA). While clinically significant effusions are uncommon, pleural involvement is the most frequent manifestation of RA in the chest, and pleural effusions can be the initial presentation of previously undiagnosed RA. Men with high rheumatoid factor titers are most likely to be affected.

Rheumatoid pleural effusions result from rheumatoid nodules on the parietal pleural surface, increasing the permeability of pleural capillaries and decreasing egress of fluid from the pleural cavity. These nodules are occasionally seen during thoracoscopic biopsies as numerous small vesicles or granules, giving the parietal pleura a "gritty" appearance. Mesothelial cells are replaced by a pseudo-stratified epithelioid cell layer which is easily detached, leaving an inflamed pleural surface with impaired pleural fluid absorption. Rheumatoid pleural effusions are exudative, with lymphocytic predominance. Tadpole cells (likely of macrophage origin), palisades of epithelioid cells, and a lack of mesothelial cells in the pleural fluid are suggestive of rheumatoid effusion.

Most rheumatoid pleural effusions resolve in an average of 14 months, and they are typically treated with repeated aspiration if clinically indicated. However, some patients will require pleurectomy for nonexpanding lung. Pleural biopsy is only indicated in atypical cases of rheumatoid pleural effusion – those patients without arthritis, with a chylous effusion, or when tuberculosis or malignancy is suspected.

Ruling out infection and malignancy are critical, particularly since therapy for RA involves immunosuppressive agents as well as new biologic therapies [29, 30].

Chronic Obstructive Pulmonary Disease in the Elderly

COPD is characterized as symptomatic impairment of airflow due to progressive degradation of the alveoli or chronic inflammation of the more proximal bronchi. As a result of an aging population and the often delayed onset of severe symptoms that result from smoking, an increasing prevalence of COPD has been observed [31]. Historically, COPD has been divided into the categories chronic bronchitis and emphysema, with the former characterized by a productive cough for at least 3 months per year for two or more consecutive years. COPD is the fourth leading cause of overall mortality nationwide [32].

Tobacco use remains the most significant risk factor for COPD in the elderly despite recent promising trends of decreasing smoking rates. The cumulative effects of smoking and age related diminution in lung function conspire to cause progressive symptomatic pulmonary disease, particularly in the elderly population. Both functional and structural changes are observed in the elderly lung including alveolar dilation, reduction in elastic recoil of the lung, changes in the compliance of the chest wall, and reduced respiratory muscle capacity [33]. The net results are impaired expiratory volumes (FEV1) with increased residual volumes of the lung and decreased FVC. Classic emphysema involves destruction of the distal airways with enzymatic degradation of the alveolar walls. In a population already experiencing the normal effects of aging on the lung, this loss of alveolar wall integrity results in progressive airflow obstruction and air trapping that is not reversible with medical treatments [34]. Those with genetic risk factors, such as alpha-1-antitrypsin (AAT) deficiency are more susceptible to the effects of smoking. AAT deficiency is a risk factor identified in fewer than 5% of patients with COPD. AAT acts a protease inhibitor of alveolar elastase released from inflammatory cells [35]. The clinical effects of the variant forms of AAT are variable and no clear natural history has been determined. However, the link between smoking and AAT associated COPD is well established.

Pulmonary function testing is used to assess and follow disease severity in COPD. Significant airflow obstruction is considered present when the ratio FEV1/FVC falls to less than 0.7. An FEV1 less than 50% of what is predicted is considered severe, and measures of decline in FEV1 are often used to evaluate decline in lung function or response to intervention [36]. As airflow limitations become more pronounced and

FEV1/FVC ratios decrease, the response to bronchodilators is lessened and therapeutic options become limited. The chronically hyperinflated lungs ultimately lead to flattening of the diaphragms which become atrophic and weakened. Clinically, COPD is characterized by acute periods of decompensation often brought on by pulmonary infection, fluid overload, allergies, or pulmonary thromboembolism which may be present in up to 25% of patients with COPD [37].

Initial medical therapy for COPD involves elimination of the noxious effects of cigarette smoking. Cessation of smoking can slow the rate of decline of lung function in COPD patients. Thus, even in elderly patients it is important for physicians to screen patients for tobacco use when obtaining a medical history. Common medical approaches include daily bronchodilators, and inhaled corticosteroids in addition to supplemental oxygen. In limited clinical trials trans-tracheal oxygenation through pinpoint tracheostomies has been used with success [38].

Emphysema patients are often under-nourished. Age related decline in appetite coupled with the work of breathing associated with the decline in normal lung function may result in inadequate caloric intake. Screening for nutritional insufficiencies by following weights or daily calorie counts should be considered [39].

Pulmonary rehabilitation is effective for patients with progressive respiratory impairment. Efforts such as resistance training and disciplined aerobic training are associated with measurable improvements in spirometry [40]. Such measures are an important intermediate step before proceeding to more aggressive surgical interventions.

Three principle interventional techniques exist for COPD: lung volume reduction surgery (LVRS), lung transplantation, and endobronchial approaches.

First introduced in the 1950s by Brantigan, lung volume reduction therapy has been associated with inconsistent success in improving lung function and symptoms in emphysema patients [41]. The National Emphysema Treatment Trial (NETT) was a randomized, prospective trial comparing lung volume reduction to medical therapy in patients with severe emphysema. Reported in 2003, this trial showed no difference in overall survival between the two treatment groups [42]. However, subgroups with high surgical risk and those who had benefit from surgery were identified. Patients with FEV1 less than 20% of expected had high surgical mortality, while those with upper lobe predominant disease and impaired 6 min walk tests had improved pulmonary function following lung volume reduction surgery. While the trial was "negative" with respect to overall survival, the subgroup analysis has served to frame surgical opinion regarding the proper patient selection for the procedure [43]. Since the inception of the NETT trial, several advances in surgical therapy have been introduced including near routine use of minimally invasive techniques and better

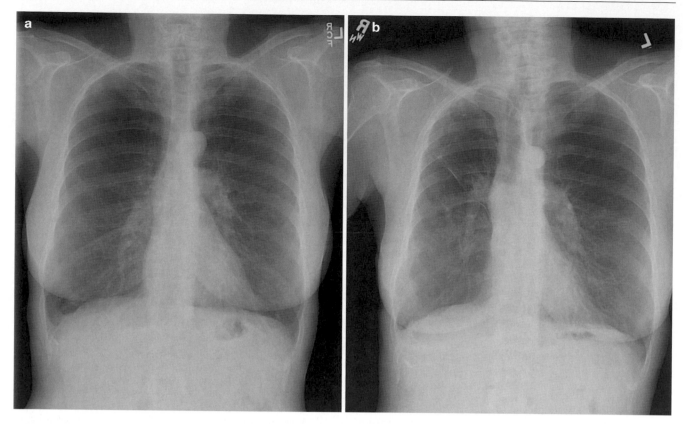

Fig. 43.1 Chest X-rays of a patient before and after lung volume reduction surgery. (**a**) This preoperative chest radiograph shows right sided, heterogeneous, apical dominant emphysema in a 65-year-old-woman.

(**b**) Six months after the patient underwent lung volume reduction surgery, the chest radiograph shows a reduction in right sided lung volume with improved distribution of pulmonary parenchyma

options for sealants of air leaks. As a result of better patient selection and techniques, mortality rates from the procedure have fallen [44] (Fig. 43.1a, b).

Lung transplantation in the elderly has been employed on a limited basis. While many centers have limited the age of the recipients to 60 years and younger, several centers have published good results in selected patients 70 years and over. Perioperative mortality does not appear to differ significantly in these older patients presumably because they are more carefully selected among potential recipients [45]. Elderly emphysema patients with well compensated emphysema have relatively low allocation scores used to determine the priority of transplant recipients [46].

Endobronchial techniques in COPD have met with varying levels of success [47]. These approaches include bronchial blockers, airway bypass, endobronchial valves, biologic sealants, and thermal ablative technologies. The principle advantage of bronchoscopic approaches to COPD is a lower procedure associated mortality and morbidity in comparison to surgery. While demonstration of objective improvement in lung function through spirometry has been inconsistent, subjective measures such as dyspnea scores appear to improve after intervention. One potential advantage of bronchoscopic

technology is the ability to select target segments of the tracheo-bronchial tree in non upper lobe predominant COPD [48]. LVRS with heterogeneous disease is associated with high treatment related morbidity and mortality, and a less invasive approach for this subset of patients is desirable. In frail elderly patients in whom surgical risk may be prohibitive, endobronchial technologies represent viable treatment options.

Summary

The spectrum of benign thoracic disease in the elderly includes structural abnormalities, infectious disease and their complications, benign neoplastic growths, auto-immune disease and, progressive decline in pulmonary function. Differences in physiologic reserve in this population make diagnosis difficult, as elderly patients may not present in the classic fashion, and complicate treatment. Thus, benign thoracic disease in the elderly can pose a challenging clinical problem. Older patients with comorbid diseases may have poor tolerance of unnecessary surgical interventions.

However, in well selected patients with partially reversible conditions, surgery can provide improved quality of life and relief of dyspnea. Benign disorders of the chest associated with symptoms due to effusion or obstruction of airways can limit quality of life, and COPD may progress to severe impairment. Minimally invasive techniques (such as video-assisted thoracoscopic surgery) can limit the morbidity associated with intervention. Additionally, prompt intervention may spare the patient more invasive treatments. For example, early effusions can be managed with simple drainage rather than thoracotomy and decortication.

With respect to suspected benign thoracic lesions in the elderly, guiding principles for management include avoiding unnecessary interventions while not overlooking potential malignancies. Close surveillance of progressive symptoms, assuring no radiographic change in the size of the lesion over 2 years, and use of positron-emission tomography remain the diagnostic keys to accurate management.

References

1. Mukhtar RA, Theodore PR. Benign thoracic disease in the elderly. Thorac Surg Clin. 2009;19(3):313–9.
2. Torres M, Moayedi S. Evaluation of the acutely dyspneic elderly patient. Clin Geriatr Med. 2007;23(2):307–25; vi.
3. de Godoy JM, Godoy MF, Batigalia F, Braile DM. The association of Mondor's disease with protein S deficiency: case report and review of literature. J Thromb Thrombolysis. 2002;13(3):187–9.
4. Sulaiman A, Cottin V, De Souza Neto EP, Orsini A, Cordier J-F, Gamondes J-P, et al. Cough-induced intercostal lung herniation requiring surgery: report of a case. Surg Today. 2006;36(11):978–80.
5. Athanassiadi K, Bagaev E, Simon A, Haverich A. Lung herniation: a rare complication in minimally invasive cardiothoracic surgery. Eur J Cardiothorac Surg. 2008;33(5):774–6.
6. Caceres M, Ali SZ, Braud R, Weiman D, Garrett Jr HE. Spontaneous pneumomediastinum: a comparative study and review of the literature. Ann Thorac Surg. 2008;86(3):962–6.
7. Di Bari M, Chiarlone M, Matteuzzi D, Zacchei S, Pozzi C, Bellia V, et al. Thoracic kyphosis and ventilatory dysfunction in unselected older persons: an epidemiological study in Dicomano, Italy. J Am Geriatr Soc. 2004;52(6):909–15.
8. Harrison RA, Siminoski K, Vethanayagam D, Majumdar SR. Osteoporosis-related kyphosis and impairments in pulmonary function: a systematic review. J Bone Miner Res. 2007;22(3):447–57.
9. Kado DM. The rehabilitation of hyperkyphotic posture in the elderly. Eur J Phys Rehabil Med. 2009;45(4):583–93.
10. Bautmans I, Van Arken J, Van Mackelenberg M, Mets T. Rehabilitation using manual mobilization for thoracic kyphosis in elderly postmenopausal patients with osteoporosis. J Rehabil Med. 2010;42(2):129–35.
11. Yang HL, Zhao L, Liu J, et al. Changes of pulmonary function for patients with osteoporotic vertebral compression fractures after kyphoplasty. J Spinal Disord Tech. 2007;20(3):221–5.
12. Cattaneo SM, Park BJ, Wilton AS, Seshan VE, Bains MS, Downey RJ, et al. Use of video-assisted thoracic surgery for lobectomy in the elderly results in fewer complications. Ann Thorac Surg. 2008;85(1):231–5; discussion 235–6.
13. Mansour Z, Kochetkova EA, Santelmo N, Meyer P, Wihlm J-M, Quoix E, et al. Risk factors for early mortality and morbidity after pneumonectomy: a reappraisal. Ann Thorac Surg. 2009;88(6):1737–43.
14. Beasley MB, Brambilla E, Travis WD. The 2004 World Health Organization classification of lung tumors. Semin Roentgenol. 2005;40(2):90–7.
15. Borczuk AC. Benign tumors and tumorlike conditions of the lung. Arch Pathol Lab Med. 2008;132(7):1133–48.
16. Ruan SY, Chen KY, Yang PC. Recurrent respiratory papillomatosis with pulmonary involvement: a case report and review of the literature. Respirology. 2009;14(1):137–40.
17. Milenkovic B, Stojsic J, Mandaric D, Stevic R. Mucous gland adenoma simulating bronchial asthma: case report and literature review. J Asthma. 2007;44(9):789–93.
18. Goldsworthy N. Chondroma of the lung (Hamartoma chondromatosum pulmonis). J Pathol Bacteriol. 1934;39(2):291–8.
19. Cosio BG, Villena V, Echave-Sustaeta J, de Miguel E, Alfaro J, Hernandez. L, et al. Endobronchial hamartoma. Chest. 2002;122(1):202–5.
20. Jenkins LA, OY AH. Solitary fibrous pleural tumor. J Am Osteopath Assoc. 2008;108(6):307–9.
21. Jackson LA, Janoff EN. Pneumococcal vaccination of elderly adults: new paradigms for protection. Clin Infect Dis. 2008;47(10):1328–38.
22. Maruyama T, Gabazza EC, Morser J, Takagi T, D'Alessandro-Gabazza C, Hirohata S, et al. Community-acquired pneumonia and nursing home-acquired pneumonia in the very elderly patients. Respir Med. 2010;104(4):584–92.
23. Toba A, Yamazaki M, Mochizuki H, Noguchi T, Tsuda Y, Kawate E, et al. Lower incidence of acute respiratory distress syndrome in community-acquired pneumonia patients aged 85 years or older. Respirology. 2010;15(2):319–25.
24. Lexau CA, Lynfield R, Danila R, Pilishvili T, Facklam R, Farley MM, et al. Changing epidemiology of invasive pneumococcal disease among older adults in the era of pediatric pneumococcal conjugate vaccine. JAMA. 2005;294(16):2043–51.
25. Drury NE, Moro C, Cartwright N, Ali A, Nashef SA. A unilateral whiteout: when not to insert a chest drain. J R Soc Med. 2010;103(1):31–3.
26. El Solh AA, Alhajjhasan A, Ramadan FH, Pineda LA. A comparative study of community- and nursing home-acquired empyema thoracis. J Am Geriatr Soc. 2007;55(11):1847–52.
27. Tsai TH, Jerng JS, Chen KY, Yu CJ, Yang PC. Community-acquired thoracic empyema in older people. J Am Geriatr Soc. 2005;53(7):1203–9.
28. Hsieh MJ, Liu YH, Chao YK, Lu MS, Liu HP, Wu YC, et al. Risk factors in surgical management of thoracic empyema in elderly patients. ANZ J Surg. 2008;78(6):445–8.
29. Balbir-Gurman A, Yigla M, Nahir AM, Braun-Moscovici Y. Rheumatoid pleural effusion. Semin Arthritis Rheum. 2006;35(6):368–78.
30. Avnon LS, Abu-Shakra M, Flusser D, Heimer D, Sion-Vardy N. Pleural effusion associated with rheumatoid arthritis: what cell predominance to anticipate? Rheumatol Int. 2007;27(10):919–25.
31. Mannino DM, Homa DM, Akinbami LJ, Ford ES, Redd SC. Chronic obstructive pulmonary disease surveillance – United States, 1971–2000. MMWR Surveill Summ. 2002;51(6):1–16.
32. Heron M, Hoyert DL, Murphy SL, Xu J, Kochanek KD, Tejada-Vera B. Deaths: final data for 2006. Natl Vital Stat Rep. 2009;57(14):1–134.
33. O'Donnell DE, Laveneziana P. The clinical importance of dynamic lung hyperinflation in COPD. COPD. 2006;3(4):219–32.
34. Calverley PM, Burge PS, Spencer S, Anderson JA, Jones PW. Bronchodilator reversibility testing in chronic obstructive pulmonary disease. Thorax. 2003;58(8):659–64.

35. Kelly E, Greene CM, Carroll TP, McElvaney NG, O'Neill SJ. Alpha-1 antitrypsin deficiency. Respir Med. 2010;104(6):763–72.

36. Haruna A, Oga T, Muro S, Ohara T, Sato S, Marumo S, et al. Relationship between peripheral airway function and patient-reported outcomes in COPD: a cross-sectional study. BMC Pulm Med. 2010;10:10.

37. Tillie-Leblond I, Marquette CH, Perez T, Scherpereel A, Zanetti C, Tonnel AB, et al. Pulmonary embolism in patients with unexplained exacerbation of chronic obstructive pulmonary disease: prevalence and risk factors. Ann Intern Med. 2006;144(6):390–6.

38. Folch E, Mehta AC. Airway interventions in the tracheobronchial tree. Semin Respir Crit Care Med. 2008;29(4):441–52.

39. Man WD, Kemp P, Moxham J, Polkey MI. Skeletal muscle dysfunction in COPD: clinical and laboratory observations. Clin Sci (Lond). 2009;117(7):251–64.

40. Rubi M, Renom F, Ramis F, Medinas M, Centeno MJ, Górriz M, et al. Effectiveness of pulmonary rehabilitation in reducing health resources use in chronic obstructive pulmonary disease. Arch Phys Med Rehabil. 2010;91(3):364–8.

41. Young J, Fry-Smith A, Hyde C. Lung volume reduction surgery (LVRS) for chronic obstructive pulmonary disease (COPD) with underlying severe emphysema. Thorax. 1999;54(9):779–89.

42. Fishman A, Martinez F, Naunheim K, Piantadosi S, Wise R, Ries A. A randomized trial comparing lung-volume-reduction surgery with medical therapy for severe emphysema. N Engl J Med. 2003;348(21):2059–73.

43. Carino T, Sheingold S, Tunis S. Using clinical trials as a condition of coverage: lessons from the National Emphysema Treatment Trial. Clin Trials. 2004;1(1):108–14; discussion 115–21.

44. Lim E, Ali A, Cartwright N, Sousa I, Chetwynd A, Polkey M. Effect and duration of lung volume reduction surgery: mid-term results of the Brompton trial. Thorac Cardiovasc Surg. 2006;54(3):188–92.

45. Pizanis N, Heckmann J, Tsagakis K, Tossios P, Massoudy P, Wendt D. Lung transplantation using donors 55 years and older: is it safe or just a way out of organ shortage? Eur J Cardiothorac Surg. 2010;38(2):192–7.

46. Takahashi SM, Garrity ER. The impact of the lung allocation score. Semin Respir Crit Care Med. 2010;31(2):108–14.

47. Ernst A, Anantham D. Endoscopic management of emphysema. Clin Chest Med. 2010;31(1):117–26; Table of Contents.

48. Hopkinson NS. Bronchoscopic lung volume reduction: indications, effects and prospects. Curr Opin Pulm Med. 2007;13(2):125–30.

Chapter 44
Lung Transplantation in the Elderly

Juan J. Fibla, Sandra C. Tomaszek, and Stephen D. Cassivi

Abstract Although lung transplantation became clinically widespread only during the 1990s, it is currently considered a standard treatment for a growing list of end-stage chronic lung diseases. With increasing experience, the range of ages of potential candidates for lung transplantation has been extended to now include more elderly patients. Although long term survival data shows an overall increased relative risk associated with elderly patients as compared with younger counterparts, lung transplantation remains a viable option for certain highly selected elderly patients. As is the case with most diseases, potential lung transplant patients at the upper extremes of age appropriately receive increased scrutiny in the preoperative evaluation process. Furthermore, in an effort to expand the donor organ pool, the age of potential cadaveric multiorgan donors considered for lung transplantation has extended into the elderly population. Considerations in lung transplantation particular to elderly recipients and elderly donors, including issues of patient selection as well as technical aspects relevant to lung transplantation in the elderly are the subject of this chapter.

Keywords Acute rejection • Alpha-1 antitrypsin deficiency emphysema • Anastomosis • Bronchiolitis obliterans syndrome • Cardiopulmonary bypass • Chronic obstructive pulmonary disease • Chronic rejection • Emphysema • Idiopathic pulmonary arterial hypertension • Idiopathic pulmonary fibrosis • Immunosuppression • Lung allocation score • Lung transplant donor • Lung transplant recipient • Lung transplantation

Introduction

In 1963, Hardy and associates reported on the first human lung transplantation, which resulted in only an 18-day survival, but illustrated the technical feasibility of the procedure [1].

J.J. Fibla (✉)
Lung Transplant Program, William J. von Liebig Transplant Center, Mayo Clinic, 200 First Street SW, Rochester, MN 55905, USA
e-mail: fibla.juan@mayo.edu

Over the next 20 years, multiple further attempts remained unsuccessful until 1983, when the University of Toronto group, under the leadership of Joel Cooper and Alec Patterson, achieved the first long term survival following single lung transplantation [2]. This was followed in 1986 with the first successful double lung transplantation, again at the University of Toronto [3]. Since these first successes, the field of lung transplantation has grown in both the number of procedures performed, and the scope of chronic lung disease that is treated. In 2007, over 2,700 lung transplants were reported worldwide to the registry of the International Society of Heart and Lung Transplantation (ISHLT) [4].

Lung transplantation currently is a viable treatment option for a wide spectrum of chronic end-stage lung diseases as presented in Table 44.1. By far, the two most frequent of these indications are chronic obstructive pulmonary disease (COPD) and idiopathic pulmonary fibrosis (IPF), typically affecting patients in their sixth to eighth decades [4]. In fact, the age range of lung transplant recipients has been increasing to include both pediatric and elderly patients. Similarly, the age range of multiorgan donors, including those being considered to be potential lung donors for transplantation has been increasing in an effort to expand the lung donor organ pool.

Elderly Lung Transplant Recipients

In the early days of lung transplantation, the age range of recipients was initially very restrictive. In fact, the University of Toronto group, which had initially the largest successful experience in clinical lung transplantation, for a number of years in the late 1980s and early 1990s, restricted the upper age limit for lung transplant recipients to 50 years of age [5]. Nevertheless, it was recognized early on that this restrictive upper limit would exclude a major portion of the very patients suffering from end-stage chronic lung diseases such as COPD and IPF. Efforts began soon thereafter to experiment with extending the upper age limit for potential recipients in order to meet the obvious need of that particular age group.

M.R. Katlic (ed.), *Cardiothoracic Surgery in the Elderly*, DOI 10.1007/978-1-4419-0892-6_44,
© Springer Science+Business Media, LLC 2011

Table 44.1 Indications for lung transplantation and percentage of cases by diagnosis

Diagnosis	% of lung transplants
COPD/emphysema	36
Idiopathic pulmonary fibrosis	21
Cystic fibrosis	16
Alpha-1 antitrypsin deficiency emphysema	7
Idiopathic pulmonary arterial hypertension	3
Sarcoidosis	3
Bronchiectasis	1
Lymphangioleiomyomatosis	1
Congenital heart disease	1
Retransplantation – obliterative broncholitis	1
Nonretransplantation – obliterative bronchiolitis	1
Retransplantation – not obliterative bronchiolitis	1
Connective tissue diseases	1
Other	7

COPD chronic obstructive pulmonary disease
Source: data from Ref [4]

At first, concerns regarding older lung transplant recipients related to deaths due to cardiac morbidity and the initial requirement for cardiopulmonary bypass (CPB) in double lung transplants and patients with pulmonary hypertension [5]. This lead to initially stretching the age range upwards into ages 50–55 years by offering exclusively single lung transplantation [6]. Eventually it was shown that CPB was not always necessary for double lung transplantation with the technique of bilateral sequential lung transplantation [7].

With further improvements in surgical technique and more in depth experience in the critical care and immunosuppression of lung transplant recipients, the upper age limit has continued to be gradually extended. The mean age of lung transplant recipients has continued to increase since 1989, when the average recipient was approximately 40 years old. In 2008, the average lung transplant recipient was 50.8 years old. Most markedly, the proportion of recipients 60 years of age or older has increased from 15% in 1998 to 35% in 2008. The proportion in the age group of 65 years of age and older was as high as 9% of the overall lung transplant recipient cohort. This upward trend in the upper age limit for lung transplantation is seen globally, but is more prevalent in North American lung transplant centers [4]. Nevertheless, it should be noted that the most recent publication of the international guidelines for the selection of lung transplant recipients continues to include age older than 65 as a relative but not absolute contraindication [8].

The two most common indications for lung transplantation in the general population as well as the elderly are COPD and IPF. In the cohort of lung transplant recipients over the age of 60, COPD and IPF account for more than 80% of all registry reports and case series [4, 9–13]. In our own institutional series (1990–2009), recipients 60 years of age and over accounted for 25% of our lung transplant cases. COPD accounted for

47% of these cases while IPF, Alpha-1 antitrypsin deficiency emphysema, and pulmonary fibrosis due to connective tissue disease accounted for 35, 9 and 9% respectively. Conversely, in our cohort of recipients less than 60 years of age, COPD and IPF accounted for only 29 and 16% of the diagnoses leading to transplantation.

The choice of single vs. bilateral lung transplantation remains a controversial issue [14]. The prevailing consensus during the early experience in lung transplantation was that bilateral lung transplantation was perhaps too rigorous a procedure for older patients, and this was manifested in the observation that significantly more bilateral lung transplants were being done in the younger patient cohorts, while older patients were receiving predominantly single lung transplants. Indeed, the 1998 ISHLT guidelines specified the upper age limit of 65 years for single lung transplantation and 60 years for bilateral lung transplantation [15]. Nevertheless, increasing experience with bilateral lung transplantation has been observed and accounted for 69% of all transplants in 2007 as reported by the ISHLT registry [4]. In particular, distinct increases in the proportion of bilateral lung transplantations have been seen in both COPD and IPF cohorts in recent years. This has occurred in parallel with the aforementioned increase in the proportion of elderly lung transplant recipients.

It is clear from the ISHLT registry data as well as multiple large single institution reports that bilateral lung transplantation confers a statistically significant long term survival advantage [4, 16–19]. Median survival for bilateral lung transplantation was 6.6 years as compared with 4.6 years for single lung transplantation. Even more striking is the median survival conditional on 1-year survival which was 9.0 years and 6.4 years for bilateral and single lung transplants respectively [4]. This long term survival advantage for bilateral lung transplant recipients is likely the most important factor in the continuing increase in the proportion of this approach as compared with single lung transplantation. In the case of elderly lung transplant candidates with COPD or IPF, who could receive either a single or bilateral lung transplant, the controversy regarding the appropriate role of these two approaches remains. Nevertheless, there appears, in recent years, to be an increasing experience with bilateral procedures. In our own institutional series, we have employed bilateral lung transplantation in 37.5% of our recipients 60 years of age or older.

When considering survival outcomes of lung transplantation in the elderly, analysis of the data from the ISHLT registry demonstrates that age of recipient is a significant factor in both short and long term survival [4]. One-year survival for recipients younger than 50 was 80% as compared to 72% for those older than 65. Five-year survival was 56% for recipients aged 35–49, while it was only 37% for those above 65. Whereas median survival for patients aged 35–49 is 6.3 years and for patients aged 50–59 was 5.1 years, for patients in the elderly age cohorts of 60–65 years and those 66 years and above the median survival was 4.2 years and 3.2 years respectively. One caveat that was noted in interpreting these results is that these comparisons between age cohorts, although statistically significant, were not adjusted for other possible confounding factors. The authors of the ISHLT registry report noted that since the majority of lung transplantation in the elderly has taken place in the more modern era of lung transplantation and that overall survival has generally improved in the more recent cohorts of patients, the negative age-related effects may be in reality more profound if adjusted for era of transplantation. However, it could also be argued in a similar fashion that since bilateral lung transplants are more often reserved for younger patients and that this approach is known to have improved long term survival, adjustment for type of lung transplant (single vs. bilateral) may in fact reduce the gradient of survival difference seemingly related to age.

Apart from the overall ISHLT registry data, a small number of single institution series of lung transplantation in the elderly have been reported [10, 11, 13, 20–22]. Admittedly, these studies report on much smaller cohorts of patients than the overall international registry kept by the ISHLT and therefore none of them come close to having the same statistical power as the data from the ISHLT registry. Both a combination of this lack of statistical power (increased likelihood of a type II error) as well as a reporting bias that favors reports from institutions that have had a favorable experience likely explains the contradictory findings of equal success with lung transplant in the elderly in these recent single institution series. In our institutional case series, comprising 32 patients aged 60–73 years of age, 30-day, 90-day, and 5-year survival was 93.7, 91.3 and 47.3% respectively. No difference was found in these outcomes as compared with our lung transplant recipients younger than 60 years of age.

Although most of these case series report favorable experience in lung transplantation in the elderly, one of these reports notes worsening survival outcomes for lung transplant recipients over the age of 60 [11]. In this series, 11 of 42 patients (26.2%) died within 6 months of transplantation, with ten of these early deaths (90.9%) attributed to infectious causes. A similar finding of a large proportion of infection related deaths (6 of 8) in this population within 1 year of transplant was reported [10]. More information regarding the causes of death for elderly lung transplant recipients was ascertained by the Duke University group who investigated the United Network for Organ Sharing (UNOS) database. They found that in recipients over the age of 65, as compared with their younger lung transplant recipient counterparts, there were trends toward increased cerebrovascular, cardiovascular and malignancy related deaths with rates of 4.4, 7.6, and 9.6% respectively [23].

Notwithstanding their small number of cases, these single institution case series do have the value of emphasizing the potential success of lung transplantation in the elderly. They also, in some cases, shed some light on the very critical aspect of recipient selection, and equally important notion of tailoring postoperative care including immunosuppression strategies. Furthermore, these case series currently provide the most informative data regarding complications and morbidity specific to elderly lung transplant recipients.

As noted previously, infectious complications appear to be notably prevalent for elderly lung transplant patients in the first year following transplantation, and carry significant consequences on survival [10, 11]. This may be a further emphasis of the increased risk of infection, particularly pulmonary infections ,known to be preferentially manifested to some extent in older patients in general [24].

It is also recognized that lung transplant recipients, in general, are at a higher risk of developing renal dysfunction with rates of 25% within the first year [4]. This is associated with a 4-times higher relative risk of death [25]. Elderly recipients are potentially at a further increased risk due to a concomitant increased rate of hypertension, hyperlipidemia, and diabetes mellitus in this age group.

In terms of rejection episodes within the first year after lung transplantation, elderly recipients, in general, do not demonstrate an overall increased risk when compared to younger lung transplant recipients [4]. Within this age group, however, there are differences in the incidence of rejection episodes within the first year according to induction therapy strategy. Whereas the proportion of elderly transplant recipients (66 years of age and older) experiencing a rejection episode in the first year after transplantation is approximately 30% for those receiving interleukin 2 receptor antagonists as induction agents, it is 59% for those receiving polyclonal induction therapy [4]. Maintenance immunotherapy options also are associated with significantly different percentages of patients having a rejection episode within 1 year of lung transplantation. Whereas only about 25% experience a within 1-year rejection episode with tacrolimus and mycophenolate treatment, 70% of those receiving cyclosporine and azathioprine will develop acute rejection within 1 year of lung transplant [4].

Selection of Elderly Candidates for Lung Transplantation

Lung transplantation causes significant physiologic stress to the recipient, requiring considerable ability to recover physiologic homeostasis.Also,, there is a recognized relative scarcity of appropriate donor lungs for transplantation, along with a tremendous amount of resources required for successful lung transplantation. A deliberate selection of appropriate candidates for lung transplantation is therefore of critical importance for patients of all ages. It becomes increasingly important in patients of advanced age due to the increased potential prevalence of major comorbidities.

The initial investigations and consultations recommended during the pretransplant evaluation of elderly lung transplant candidates are presented in Table 44.2. Specific attention in elderly patients is emphasized in certain areas of well-defined increased risk. Further targeted investigations may be warranted according to the findings of the initial tests.

In the pulmonary system, beyond confirming the underlying pulmonary process leading to end-stage lung disease and the need for transplantation, there should be an assessment

of the potential atrophy of respiratory musculature, and the degree of age-related stiffening of the chest wall due calcified costal cartilages, narrowing of intervertebral disc spaces and kyphosis. These are not usually reversible after transplantation, and will all negatively affect chest wall mechanics potentially causing sufficient impairment to compromise or even negate the benefit of lung transplantation.

Special attention must be given to the cardiovascular system. Identification of pulmonary hypertension is essential, as this will significantly influence the need for CPB during the transplant procedure. Although advanced age is not a contraindication for the use of CPB, the requirement for its assistance during lung transplantation has been associated with increased morbidity and mortality [16]. Furthermore, it has been shown that neither the presence of mild to moderate coronary artery disease, nor the need to undergo concomitant coronary artery bypass grafting at the time of lung transplantation, have adversely affected survival outcomes. These findings however emanate from small single institution studies where age of the recipient was not considered [26, 27].

In the elderly population, particular attention to issues related to osteoporosis, renal dysfunction, and diabetes are essential as these patients are at increased risk for these comorbidities. A specific consultation with an endocrinologist specializing in transplantation is advised. As the prevalence of cancer increases substantially with advancing age, we find it prudent to specifically investigate for this. Apart from the requisite history and physical exam, we recommend the addition of a fused positron emission tomography and computed tomography scan as a noninvasive screening test.

Specific geriatric assessment is essential in order to completely assess potential elderly lung transplant candidates. In particular, this includes an assessment of the candidate's ability to perform activities of daily living (ADLs) such as bathing, dressing and feeding one's self, going to the toilet and maintaining continence, and transferring from a bed to a chair. The inability to perform these basic functions has been associated with increased perioperative morbidity, albeit in nontransplant situations [28]. Higher functioning skills are tested by so-called instrumental activities of daily living (IADLs) which include the ability to use a telephone, shop for one's self, prepare food, perform housekeeping and laundry, use various forms of transportation, assume responsibility for medications, and manage personal finances. When an elderly patient requires assistance with these tasks, this has been predictive of prolonged hospital stay, and increased dependance on postdischarge resources and services, such as home care or nursing home placement [29]. These would be considered surrogates for decreased benefit following lung transplantation. The transplant candidacy of a patient who has difficulty with these tasks should be seriously questioned.

Table 44.2 Recommended investigations for evaluation of potential elderly lung transplant candidates

General	History and physical examination
	Screening bloodwork (CBC, electrolytes, AST, ALT, alkaline phosphatase, INR
Pulmonary system	Pulmonary function tests (spirometry and diffusing capacity)
	Arterial blood gas analysis
	High definition computed tomography scan of chest and upper abdomen
	Fused computed tomography-positron emission tomography scan
	Quantitative ventilation-perfusion scan (V/Q scan)
	Cotinine blood level
Cardiovascular system	Electrocardiogram
	Echocardiogram
	Right heart catheterization
	Coronary angiogram
	Carotid artery doppler ultrasound
	Six minute walk test
Infectious disease evaluation	Serology – cytomegalovirus, Ebstein–Barr virus, toxoplasma
Renal system	Serum creatinine
	Urinalysis
	Corrected iothalamate clearance
Endocrine system	Bone densitometry
	Fasting glucose, hemoglobin A-1C
Immunology system	ABO Blood typing
	Single bead antigen HLA typing
Cognitive and psychosocial evaluation	Transplant psychiatry evaluation
	Social work evaluation of social support network
Geriatric assessment	ADLs assessment
	IADLs assessment

CBC complete blood count; *AST* aspartate transaminase; *ALT* alanine transaminase; *INR* international normalized ratio; *HLA* human leukocyte antigen; *ADLs* activities of daily living (ability to bathe, dress, go to the toilet, maintain continence, feed one's self, transfer from bed to chair); *IADLs* instrumental activities of daily living (ability to use telephone, ability to shop for oneself, prepare food, perform housekeeping and laundry, use various forms of transportation, assume responsibility for medications, manage personal finances)

Technical Considerations for Elderly Lung Transplant Recipients

The technique for lung transplantation has evolved since its first successful clinical cases. Early concerns regarding airway anastomotic complications were managed with the use of omental flap coverage, requiring entry into the abdomen. With more tailored immunosuppression strategies available in recent times, a more judicious use of perioperative steroids has been possible. Furthermore, technical refinements such as circumferentially covering the bronchial anastomosis with native peribronchial tissue, and limiting the length of the donor bronchus to 1–2 cartilaginous rings proximal to the lobar bifurcation, thus minimizing the length of ischemic donor airway, have resulted in a decrease in postoperative airway complications.

The technical aspects of the lung transplantation procedure in the elderly recipients are similar to those in younger recipients. Consideration of certain aspects particular to elderly recipients are nevertheless advisable. As an example, because of the higher incidence of osteopenia and osteoporosis in the elderly population, the ability, when possible, to limit the incision and exposure, in the case of a bilateral lung transplant, to bilateral anterior thoracotomies is preferred. This avoids the significant potential morbidity associated with the transverse sternotomy inherent in the full "clamshell" approach. When the transverse sternotomy is needed, as in the case where CPB is planned or required, some centers have used metal struts embedded longitudinally across the transverse sternal closure to support this postoperatively and avoid complications of sternal instability.

The trend in the use of single or bilateral lung transplant in the elderly has evolved over time, with an increasing use of bilateral lung transplantation being seen in recent years. In our Mayo Clinic series we elected to use bilateral lung transplantation in 37.5% of patients who were 60 years of age or older. We observed no increase in associated morbidity or mortality in this highly selected group of patients. Ultimately, the decision to proceed with single or bilateral lung transplantation must be individualized in keeping with the realities of organ availability, individual patient characteristics and urgency, as well as transplant center-specific expertise.

When contemplating bilateral lung transplantation, in patients of any age, the increased potential need for CPB should be taken into consideration. As mentioned above, although it is associated with increased morbidity and mortality, the requirement for CPB is not an absolute contraindication to lung transplantation in the elderly. Nevertheless, it is advisable to avoid CPB if feasible. Therefore, at the time of evaluation of an elderly candidate for lung transplantation, it is important to specifically review the possible need for CPB, and consider this in the decision to proceed to wait listing that particular patient. This is especially the case if there is known preoperative pulmonary hypertension, which would increase the likelihood of requiring CPB at the time of lung transplantation.

As with all patients, but potentially more critically important in the elderly patients awaiting lung transplantation, it is imperative that they be encouraged to maintain or improve their overall level of fitness in preparation for their procedure. Admittedly, this may be difficult due to their underlying lung disease. It has been observed that notwithstanding the severity of lung disease, the intensity of the exercise program is determined for the most part by the individual's symptom limitation, and the acknowledgment that adequate rest between exercises is necessary to provide for recovery [30]. It is our policy to enlist our patients awaiting lung transplantation in a structured pulmonary rehabilitation program. This has the dual effect of enhancing fitness leading up to lung transplantation and providing the basis for further beneficial exercise rehabilitation postoperatively [31].

A further consideration in the postoperative management of elderly lung transplant recipients revolves around immunosuppression issues. As mentioned earlier, elderly patients have a more marked response to different immunosuppression strategies. The ISHLT registry records almost double the proportion of patients over the age of 65 experiencing a rejection episode within the first year of lung transplantation when they have received polyclonal induction therapy (59%) vs. an interleukin 2 receptor antagonist (30%) [4]. Furthermore, in terms of maintenance immunosuppression, for the same group of elderly patients, 70% experience a rejection episode within the first year after lung transplantation when treated with cyclosporine and azathioprine vs. 25% in the group treated with tacrolimus and mycophenolate ($p < 0.0001$) [4]. These observations appear as a more striking contrast in the elderly recipient population as compared with younger recipient groups. The reasons for this difference are not completely elucidated, but they underline the challenges and opportunities in targeting postoperative strategies for the elderly cohort.

Elderly Lung Transplant Donors

It should first be noted that although living lobar lung transplantation has been successfully implemented in certain specialized centers, its widespread adoption has been limited [32, 33]. Therefore, the vast majority of lung transplants depend on the availability of brain-dead donors and more recently nonheart beating donors.

As the age of lung transplant recipients has increased over time, so too has an increase in the age of lung donors been observed. In 2008, the average age of lung donors was 35.5 years [4]. In 2007,

References

Chapter 45
Esophageal Surgery for Malignant Disease in the Elderly

Philip A. Rascoe and John C. Kucharczuk

Abstract Neoplasms of the esophagus and gastroesophageal junction are aggressive tumors that often present at an advanced stage, and that historically have been associated with poor survival despite therapy. 16,470 Americans are diagnosed with and 14,280 die of esophageal cancer annually, and the incidence is increasing. In fact, the incidence of esophageal adenocarcinoma (EAC) has increased in the last 25 years, greater than the incidence of any other major malignancy in the United States. Esophageal cancer is primarily a disease of the elderly. The median age at diagnosis is 69 years, with 61.5% of those diagnosed being age 65 or older. While surgery remains the best single modality of therapy in terms of survival and durable control of dysphagia, careful patient selection and medical optimization of existing comorbidities is of paramount importance in maintaining acceptable surgical outcomes, especially in the elderly. Whether postsurgical outcome in the elderly is worse than for younger patients remains controversial. It seems likely that the best possible surgical outcomes are obtained in elderly patients who are meticulously screened, medically optimized with regards to existing comorbidities, and undergo surgery in a high-volume tertiary referral center. Recent data suggest that elderly patients with early EAC have improved survival following surgery rather than chemoradiation. Palliative esophagectomy for advanced stage malignancy is associated with mortality rates in excess of 20% and morbidity rates as high as 50% and should therefore be avoided. Very effective palliation can be obtained with chemotherapy, radiation therapy, and endoscopic interventions such as stenting.

Keywords Esophageal adenocarcinoma • Esophageal squamous cell carcinoma • Esophagogastric junction adenocarcinoma • Siewert classification • Tylosis • Barrett's metaplasia • Columnar-lined esophagus • Gastroesophageal reflux disease • Endoscopic ultrasonography • Positron emission tomography • Photodynamic therapy • Radiofrequency ablation • Transhiatal esophagectomy • Ivor Lewis esophagectomy • Thoracoabdominal esophagectomy • Three-hole esophagectomy • Minimally invasive esophagectomy • Neoadjuvant therapy • Palliative chemoradiation • Endoscopic palliation • Esophageal stent

Neoplasms of the esophagus and gastroesophageal junction are aggressive tumors that often present at an advanced stage, and that historically have been associated with poor survival despite therapy. Surveillance, Epidemiology and End Results (SEER) data from the National Cancer Institute estimate that 16,470 Americans are diagnosed with and 14,280 die of esophageal cancer annually. Moreover, the incidence of esophageal cancer is increasing, with an annual percentage change of +0.5% between 1975 and 2005. SEER data also demonstrate that esophageal cancer is primarily a disease of the elderly. From 2001 to 2005, the median age at diagnosis for cancer of the esophagus was 69 years, with 61.5% of those diagnosed being age 65 or older (Fig. 45.1) [1]. According to U.S. Census Bureau projections, we can expect our population to be older by midcentury. In 2000, 12% of the population was 65 or older. In 2030, when all of the baby boomers will be 65 or older, this age group will represent 20% of the U.S. population. Furthermore, this age group is projected to increase to 88.5 million in 2050, more than doubling the number in 2008 (38.7 million) [2]. It is apparent that surgeons should expect to see an ever-increasing number of patients with esophageal cancer. With earlier identification due to surveillance of premalignant disease and improved treatment strategies, some improvement in 5-year survival has been made over the past two decades (Fig. 45.2). However, most patients still present at an advanced stage. Surgeons will continue to play a significant role in the management of these patients, performing potentially curative extirpation in those with early-stage disease, and palliative procedures in those with advanced malignancy.

P.A. Rascoe (✉)
Division of Cardiothoracic Surgery, Texas A&M University Health Science Center College of Medicine, Scott & White Memorial Hospital and Clinic, Olin E. Teague Central Texas VA Medical Center, Temple, TX 76508, USA
e-mail: rascoe@uphs.upenn.edu

M.R. Katlic (ed.), *Cardiothoracic Surgery in the Elderly*, DOI 10.1007/978-1-4419-0892-6_45,
© Springer Science+Business Media, LLC 2011

Table 45.2 Risk factors for the development of esophageal cancer with their relevant contribution to both squamous cell and adenocarcinoma of the esophagus

Risk factor	Squamous cell carcinoma	Adenocarcinoma
Tobacco use	+++	++
Alcohol use	+++	–
Barrett's esophagus	–	++++
Weekly reflux symptoms	–	+++
Obesity	–	++
Poverty	++	–
Achalasia	+++	–
Caustic injury to the esophagus	++++	–
Nonepidermolytic palmoplantar keratoderma (tylosis)	++++	–
Plummer-Vinson syndrome	++++	–
History of head and neck cancer	++++	–
History of breast cancer treated with radiotherapy	+++	+++
Frequent consumption of extremely hot beverages	+	–
Prior use of beta-blockers, anticholinergic agents, or aminophyllines	–	±

+ Increase in the risk by a factor of less than two; ++ increase by a factor of two to four; +++ increase by a factor of more than four to eight; ++++ increase by a factor of more than eight; ± conflicting results have been reported; – no proven risk
Source: from Enzinger and Mayer [9] Copyright © 2003 Massachusetts Medical Society. All rights reserved

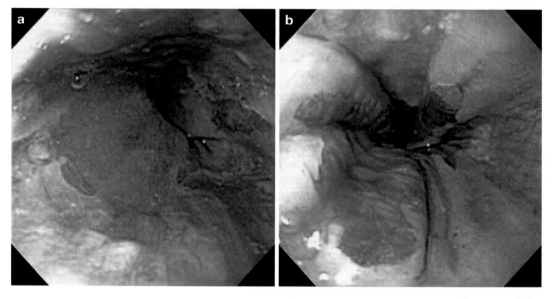

Fig. 45.5 (**a**) The typical endoscopic appearance of Barrett's metaplasia at the GE junction. Note the "salmon-colored" areas of erosion extending proximally from the GE junction. Also note the intervening areas of normal appearing mucosa. (**b**) Vital staining with methylene blue. Vital stains are used to highlight the mucosal changes at the time of endoscopy (images courtesy of Micheal L. Kochman, M.D., Professor of Medicine, University of Pennsylvania)

genetic predisposition to esophageal cancer, tylosis is the only recognized familial syndrome that predisposes to the development of esophageal cancer. This is an autosomal dominant disorder, which has been mapped to chromosome 17q25 [18]. Patients have hyperkeratosis of the palms of their hands and the soles of their feet. The risk of developing squamous cell carcinoma of the esophagus by age 70 is 95% in this cohort of patients [19].

Barrett's metaplasia (columnar-lined esophagus) and obesity are associated with an increased risk of developing adenocarcinoma of the esophagus. Chronic gastroesophageal reflux disease (GERD) is considered the predominant contributor to the development of Barrett's metaplasia. The frequency, severity, and duration of reflux symptoms are correlated with an increased risk of developing EAC [20]. Patients with recurring symptoms of reflux have an eightfold increase in the risk of EAC. Barrett's esophagus develops in about 5% of patients with GERD. Endoscopically, it is recognized by inflamed salmon-colored mucosa extending proximally from the GE junction. Often there are intervening areas of normal appearing mucosa, or so-called skip areas. Figure 45.5a shows the typical endoscopic appearance; Fig. 45.5b shows the same patient with methylene blue vital stain, which can be used to highlight the mucosal changes. Microscopic evaluation reveals replacement of the normal stratified squamous epithelium of the esophagus with columnar epithelium more typical of other parts of the gastrointestinal tract. Thus, these changes are often referred to as "intestinalization" of the mucosa. With progression to dysplasia, the nuclei become "crowded," and the normal glandular architecture is lost (Fig. 45.6). Histologically,

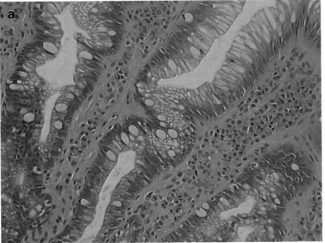
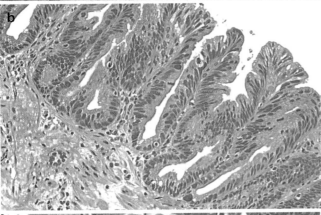
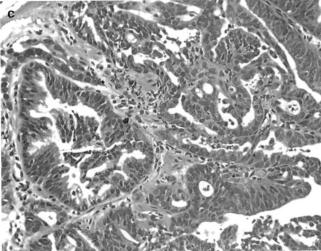

Fig. 45.6 Distal esophageal biopsy specimens (stained with hematoxylin and eosin). Histologic progression of Barrett's metaplasia (**a**) to Barrett's esophagus with dysplasia (**b**) to esophageal adenocarcinoma (**c**)

patients with high-grade dysplasia carry a significant risk for esophageal carcinoma and should be considered candidates for resection. 10–30% of patients with high-grade dysplasia will develop invasive adenocarinoma within 5 years of the initial diagnosis; moreover, in patients undergoing esophagectomy for presumed high-grade dysplasia, invasive carcinoma is identified in 30–40% of the pathologic specimens [21]. Barrett's esophagus increases the risk of EAC thirty to fortyfold when compared with the general population [22]. The annual rate of neoplastic transformation to adenocarcinoma in patients with Barrett's is 0.5% [23]. A great deal of progress has been made in understanding columnar-lined esophagus since the entity was first described by Barrett in 1950 [24]. However, many questions remain including why Barrett's esophagus and adenocarcinoma affect primarily Caucasian men, why only some patients progress to dysplasia and adenocarcinoma, and how long this process takes?

Diagnosis

Unfortunately, early esophageal carcinoma is largely asymptomatic. As a distensible muscular tube, a significant portion of the esophageal lumen must be obstructed to impede passage of a food bolus and produce symptoms. Dysphagia is the primary manifestation of esophageal cancer in 80% of patients and up to 20% have odynophagia. Vague symptoms of retrosternal discomfort and transient dysphagia are often overlooked by the patient and the physician. On retrospective evaluation, many patients have significantly altered their eating habits by avoiding foods such as meats and breads, while increasing their intake of semisolid foods and liquids. About one half of patients have significant weight loss. Weight loss of more than 10% of body mass is an independent predictor of poor prognosis [25].

Pulmonary symptoms may be caused by aspiration of regurgitated food or by direct invasion of the airway by esophageal tumor, often resulting in esophagorespiratory fistula. Direct invasion through the membranous airway can occur with locally advanced lesions, usually involving the trachea or left mainstem bronchus as it passes anterior to the esophagus. Patients with cancers involving the upper thoracic esophagus must undergo preoperative bronchoscopy to rule out airway involvement as this precludes resection. Although flexible bronchoscopy may demonstrate gross airway invasion, rigid bronchoscopy is much more sensitive in determining adherence to the membranous trachea. Loss of the normal "ripple" effect as the rigid scope slides over the membranous trachea and left main bronchus suggests the tumor is fixed to the airway and is not resectable.

New hoarseness due to vocal cord paralysis is indicative of left recurrent nerve involvement and suggests unresectability. Virchow's node, a palpable left supraclavicular lymph

patients older than 70 who were deemed surgical candidates was statistically lower than younger patients. Overall morbidity, mortality, and survival were equivalent in the two surgical groups, with only atrial fibrillation and myocardial infarction being increased in the elderly [54].

Retrospective analysis of a large cohort of esophagectomy patients at M.D. Anderson Cancer Center demonstrated that increasing age was an independent prognosticator of poor overall survival. Approximately 90% of these 600 patients had adenocarcinoma, and greater than 2/3 received neoadjuvant therapy. In addition to poorer survival, patients older than 70 years had statistically significantly higher rates of aspiration pneumonia, ARDS, cardiovascular complications, and neurologic complications [55].

Experience at Memorial Sloan-Kettering Cancer Center revealed that older patients had longer length of hospital stay and worse postoperative mortality. In particular, their octogenarian cohort had a perioperative mortality of almost 20%, as well as an overall shorter disease-free survival [56].

In analyzing surgical outcome in 1,777 esophagectomy patients from the Veterans Affairs (VA) Medical Centers, the largest cohort to date, Bailey et al. documented a 10% mortality and 50% morbidity rate. Multivariate analysis revealed increasing age to be one of eight preoperative and intraoperative variables predictive of 30-day mortality [57].

In a retrospective cohort study analyzing outcomes from two large national databases, Finlayson and colleagues demonstrated higher mortality, lower 5-year survival, and greater probability of transfer to extended-care facilities among octogenarians undergoing esophagectomy for cancer when compared to patients aged 65–69 [58]. They identified similar results for patients undergoing pancreatectomy and lung resection for malignancy.

Ra and colleagues similarly analyzed the SEER-Medicare national database and found that age greater than 80, increasing Charlson comorbidity index, and operation at a low esophagectomy volume hospital were statistically significant predictors of postoperative mortality after esophagectomy for cancer [59].

Finally, a recent query of the Society of Thoracic Surgeons (STS) General Thoracic Surgery Database revealed that in 2,315 esophagectomies for cancer performed by STS surgeons at 73 centers, age (75 vs. 55) was one of ten important predictors of major morbidity (including death) [33].

The above-mentioned studies demonstrate well the ongoing controversy regarding surgical outcome in elderly esophageal cancer patients. Series of highly selected elderly patients at tertiary referral centers appear to demonstrate equivalent outcome when compared to younger patients. However, when national series are obtained from retrospective analyses of the VA, SEER-Medicare, and STS databases, increasing age appears to be an independent predictor of morbidity and mortality. It seems likely that the best possible surgical outcomes are obtained in elderly patients who are meticulously screened, medically optimized with regards to existing comorbidities, and undergo surgery in a high-volume tertiary referral center.

Neoadjuvant Therapy

The role of preoperative therapy followed by operation for Stage II and III disease remains ill-defined and hotly debated. The current information on neoadjuvant treatment can be divided into studies evaluating preoperative radiation, preoperative chemotherapy, and combined preoperative chemoradiation therapy. In operable patients with resectable tumors, the results of any preoperative therapy, followed by resection must be compared with the results of primary resection alone. Importantly, this analysis must take into account the toxicities associated with multimodality therapy and the impact on the intended resection and quality of life.

A number of randomized trials have failed to show any benefit from preoperative radiation therapy alone. Proponents of preoperative radiotherapy argue that the trials are too small to demonstrate the advantages of this approach. A meta-analysis of available randomized trials comprising 1,147 patients, however, found no improvement in survival with preoperative radiotherapy alone in patients with resectable esophageal cancer [60]. At this time, there is no indication for preoperative radiation therapy alone followed by resection.

The utility of preoperative chemotherapy alone is much more poorly defined. A large multicenter randomized trial in the United States (Intergroup Trial) of 440 patients failed to show any improvement in survival after three cycles of combined cisplatin and fluorouracil followed by surgery and two postoperative cycles when compared to surgery alone [61]. This is in contrast to a large randomized European study (Medical Research Council, or MRC), which suggested that neoadjuvant chemotherapy resulted in nearly a 10% improvement in survival at 2 years [62]. Unfortunately, the preoperative staging techniques and duration of treatments were quite different, making the two studies difficult to compare. More recently, another European neoadjuvant chemotherapy trial (MAGIC trial) demonstrated improved survival with perioperative chemotherapy vs. surgery alone (36 vs. 23% at 5 years) [63]. Of note, 75% of the MAGIC trial participants had gastric cancer, while only 25% had either distal esophageal or GE junction adenocarcinoma. Also, only 41.6% of patients randomized to perioperative chemotherapy were able to complete all six prescribed cycles of therapy. In the most recent Cochrane Review of the topic, 11 randomized controlled trials with 2,051 patients suggested that preoperative chemotherapy plus surgery may offer a survival advantage compared to surgery alone for resectable esophageal cancer [64]. There was no demonstrable difference in the rate of resection, tumor recurrence, or postoperative morbidity. There was some chemotherapy-related morbidity. Presumably based on the relative success of the MRC and MAGIC trials, chemotherapy alone is utilized quite commonly as neoadjuvant therapy in Europe, while combined chemotherapy and radiation is utilized more commonly in the United States.

Several small randomized trials have evaluated combined preoperative chemoradiation followed by surgical resection. The most widely cited trial to justify the use of combined treatment followed by surgery was published by Walsh et al. in 1996 [65]. This study demonstrated a 3-year survival of 32% in the neoadjuvant treatment group as compared to 6% in the surgery alone group for patients with EAC. Critics were quick to point out the lack of appropriate staging, the poor survival in the surgical group as compared with other surgical series, and the small study size. A more recent study found equivalent median and 3-year survival in patients with squamous cell carcinoma of the esophagus randomized to either preoperative chemoradiation followed by surgery or surgery alone [66]. An increased complication rate was noted in the patients undergoing preoperative chemoradiation therapy. The Cancer and Leukemia Group B (CALGB) 9,781 trial randomized patients to either surgery alone, or trimodality therapy with neoadjuvant chemoradiation followed by surgery. Unfortunately, this trial closed early after accruing only 56 patients. Median survival (21.5 vs. 53.8 months) and 5-year survival (16 vs. 39%) favored the patients receiving trimodality therapy [67]. A recent meta-analysis of ten randomized controlled trials of neoadjuvant chemoradiotherapy vs. surgery alone demonstrated an absolute survival advantage of 13% at 2 years favoring neoadjuvant therapy [68]. Preoperative chemoradiation, postoperative chemoradiation, and perioperative chemotherapy have never been compared with each other in a clinical trial. Despite a paucity of conclusive data, there seems to be an evolving consensus at most centers that patients with T3 and/or N1 disease should receive neoadjuvant chemoradiation. This issue remains unresolved, and operation remains the standard treatment for localized esophageal cancer outside of a clinical trial.

Very little data exists regarding neoadjuvant chemoradiation in the elderly. Elderly patients are often not offered neoadjuvant therapy due to concerns of susceptibility to treatment-related toxicities. Moreover, octogenarians are often excluded from neoadjuvant trials. The M.D. Anderson Cancer Center group has reported their experience with combined modality therapy in elderly patients. They compared three groups of patients: (1) patients 70 years or older who received neoadjuvant chemoradiation; (2) patients younger than 70 who received neoadjuvant chemoradiation; and (3) patients 70 years or older who received surgery alone. Elderly patients receiving preoperative chemoradiation were more likely to require perioperative blood transfusions and had a higher incidence of postoperative atrial arrhythmias. Otherwise, postoperative outcome as well as median, 1-year, and 3-year survival were similar in the 3 groups [69].

Surgery vs. Chemoradiation in the Elderly

A recent retrospective review of the SEER-Medicare database was performed to compare outcomes of elderly patients with early esophageal cancer who received chemoradiation or underwent esophagectomy. Seven hundred and thirty patients with stage I or II esophageal cancer treated between 1991 and 2002 were identified. In multivariate analysis, chemoradiation was associated with worse disease-specific and overall survival than esophagectomy. When histology-specific comparisons were made, receipt of chemoradiation was associated with worse survival in patients with adenocarcinoma (5-year disease-specific survival 7.5 vs. 50.2%), while there was no difference in survival between treatment groups in patients with squamous cell carcinoma (Fig. 45.10) [70]. This review contains inherent selection bias, as increasing age was associated with increased odds of receiving chemoradiation. Despite its limitations, this study certainly suggests that elderly patients with early stage EAC should be considered for surgery.

Palliation

The goal of esophageal resection, whether as primary treatment or as part of a multimodality plan, is cure, though this goal remains elusive. Palliative esophagectomy is associated with mortality rates in excess of 20% and morbidity rates as high as 50% and should therefore be avoided [71]. Very effective palliation can be obtained with chemotherapy, radiation therapy, and endoscopic interventions such as stenting. The intent of palliation is to maintain comfort, restore swallowing function, and support nutrition. Establishment of alternative enteral access is helpful in maintaining nutritional status and hydration. When possible, this is provided by a percutaneous gastrostomy (PEG) tube placed under endoscopic guidance. For patients with bulky obstructing lesions who cannot undergo PEG, an open or laparoscopic gastrostomy or jejunostomy tube is required.

Radiation

Palliative radiotherapy relieves dysphagia in up to 75% of patients. The dose is 4,000–5,000 cGy delivered over 4 weeks. This allows patients with advanced disease and severe dysphagia to handle secretions, and to swallow liquids as well as dietary supplements. Unfortunately, relief is not

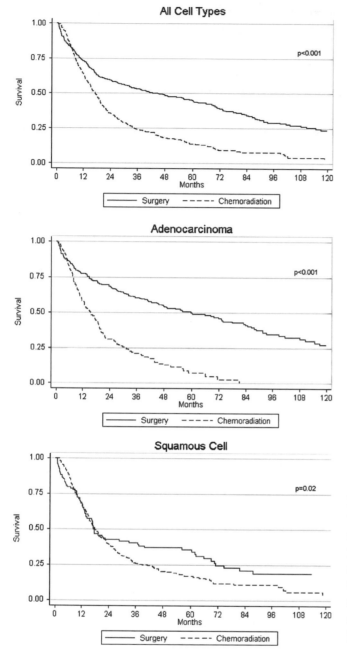

Fig. 45.10 These Kaplan-Meier curves for overall survival compare esophagectomy with chemoradiation in elderly patients with stage I and II esophageal cancer for (*top*) all cell types, (*middle*) adenocarcinoma only, and (*bottom*) squamous cell carcinoma only (from Abrams et al. [70], with permission from John Wiley & Sons)

Chemotherapy

Esophageal cancers are usually responsive to chemotherapeutic drugs, providing some palliation. Agents currently in use include fluorouracil and taxanes either alone or in combination with platinum-based agents. Palliative chemotherapy requires time to effectively reduce symptoms of dysphagia and must be balanced with the associated risks of systemic treatment in usually debilitated, malnourished patients. Chemotherapy has been used in combination with radiation therapy with the goal of increasing response rates, lengthening the disease-free interval, and improving survival. The Radiation Therapy Oncology Group (RTOG) compared four cycles of cisplatinum +5-fluorouracil (5-FU) + 50 Gy of radiation to radiotherapy alone with 64 Gy [72]. The trial was stopped early because the interim results demonstrated a significant survival advantage in the chemotherapy group, with median survival of 12.5 and 8.9 months and 2-year survival of 50 and 38% for the chemoradiation and radiotherapy groups, respectively. Therefore patients with locally advanced disease who are not considered surgical candidates as a result of unresectable tumors or medical risks should be considered for chemoradiation therapy rather than irradiation alone.

Endoscopic Palliation

Endoscopic techniques to restore luminal patency are palliative procedures that may be used in patients who are not candidates for primary surgical therapy, in an adjuvant setting for patients receiving combination therapy, or in the setting of locally recurrent cancer following surgery. Endoscopic techniques include dilatation, thermal ablation with laser or coagulation probes, intubation with self-expanding stents, and PDT. The variables that must be considered when selecting the specific method are cost, tumor location and length, whether the tumor is circumferential, and the presence or absence of an esophagorespiratory fistula.

Stenting

Palliative endoscopic intubation of inoperable malignant esophageal strictures was first described in the 1970s [73]. Currently, self-expanding coated and uncoated nitinol stents are utilized for palliation. These stents can be inserted either radiologically or endoscopically on an outpatient basis. Following insertion, the lumen can be balloon-dilated to an acceptable diameter to provide palliation. Cook and Dehn [74] cited four major benefits of covered expandable stent

immediate and maximal improvement occurs at about 4 weeks following completion of treatment. In patients with a life expectancy greater than 3 months, combined chemotherapy with radiation is utilized. Short-term side effects from radiation therapy include skin irritation and erythema. Esophagitis with painful swallowing also occurs with some frequency. Additional complications include stricture formation, radiation pneumonitis, and fistulization to the airway.

use: (1) shorter hospital stay compared with rigid tube insertion; (2) single hospital stay; (3) lack of readmission for recurrent obstruction from tumor ingrowth or food impaction; and (4) no procedure-related morbidity or mortality.

Neodymium: Yttrium-Aluminum-Garnet Laser Fulguration

Endoscopic neodymium:yttrium-aluminum-garnet (Nd: YAG) laser fulguration can be used to provide temporary relief of esophageal obstruction in patients with unresectable obstructing tumors. A flexible quartz fiber is passed through the working channel of the esophagoscope to deliver the laser energy at the fiber tip. Multiple sessions are usually required to achieve debulking and functional success. Laser fulguration is often combined with endoluminal stenting and radiation therapy. It can also be useful in patients who have undergone uncovered stenting procedures with ingrowth of tumor through the stent. To be a candidate for this therapy, the endoscope must be able to traverse the tumor. Contraindications for laser therapy include completely obstructing cancers and esophagorespiratory fistulae.

Photodynamic Therapy

Intraluminal PDT is a nonthermal ablative technique that can be used to palliate patients. This technique requires the systemic administration of a hematoporphyrin, which is concentrated within the malignant cells. Approximately 48 h after administration of the photosensitizer, patients undergo endoscopy, and an argon-pump dye-laser is used to deliver endoluminal light at a wavelength of 630 nm. This results in the generation of oxygen radicals, which quickly lead to tumor necrosis. The depth of penetration is relatively limited, and this decreases the risk of full-thickness necrosis with perforation. Unfortunately, the photosensitizing agents are retained by the reticuloendothelial system in skin; thus, patients are sensitive to infrared wavelength light, including sunlight, radiant heat, fluorescent light, and strong incandescent light. Depending on the photosensitizing agent used, this sensitivity can persist up to 3 months, a challenging problem in patients with short life expectancies.

A recent series of 215 patients treated with palliative endoluminal PDT revealed a procedure-related mortality rate of 1.8%, effective palliation for patients with obstructing cancers in 85% of the treatment courses, and median survival of 4.8 months [75]. A number of patients in this series also required stenting, suggesting that PDT has a role in multimodality palliation of obstructing esophageal cancers.

References

1. Surveillance, Epidemiology and End Results. 2008. http://seer.cancer.gov/statfacts/html/esoph.html. Accessed 2 Nov 2008.
2. U.S. Census Bureau. 2008. http://www.census.gov/Press-Release/www/releases/archives/population/012496.html. Accessed 2 Nov 2008.
3. Pohl H, Welch G. The role of overdiagnosis and reclassification in the marked increase of esophageal adenocarcinoma incidence. J Natl Cancer Inst. 2005;97:142–6.
4. Postlethwaite RW. Squamous cell carcinoma of the esophagus. In: Surgery of the esophagus. 2nd ed. Norwalk: Appleton & Lange; 1986. p. 369–42.
5. Ming S. Adenocarcinoma and other epithelial tumors of the esophagus. In: Ming S, Goldman H, editors. Pathology of the gastrointestinal tract. Philadelphia: Saunders; 1992. p. 459–77.
6. Ibrahim NB, Briggs JC, Corbishley CM. Extrapulmonary oat cell carcinoma. Cancer. 1984;54:1645–61.
7. Siewert JR, Stein HJ. Classification of adenocarcinoma or the oesophagogastric junction. Br J Surg. 1998;85:1457–9.
8. Von Rahden BHA, Stein HJ, Siewert JR. Sugical management of esophagogastric junction tumors. World J Gastroenterol. 2006;12(41):6608–13.
9. Enzinger C, Mayer J. Esophageal cancer. N Engl J Med. 2003; 349:2241–52.
10. Newcomb PA, Carbone PP. The health consequences of smoking. Med Clin North Am. 1992;76:305–31.
11. Choi SY, Kahyo H. Effect of cigarette smoking and alcohol consumption in the etiology of cancers of the digestive tract. Int J Cancer. 1991;49:381–6.
12. Franceschi S, Talamini R, Barra S, et al. Smoking and drinking in relation to cancers of the oral cavity, pharynx, and esophagus in northern Italy. Cancer Res. 1990;50:6502–7.
13. DeStefani E, Munoz N, Esteve J, et al. Mate drinking, alcohol, tobacco, diet, and esophageal cancer in Uruguay. Cancer Res. 1990;50:426–31.
14. Gray JR, Coldman AJ, MacDonald WC. Cigarette and alcohol use in patients with adenocarcinoma of the gastric cardia or lower esophagus. Cancer. 1992;69:2227–31.
15. Christen AG, McDonald Jr JL, Olsen BL, Christen JA. Smokeless tobacco addiction: a threat to the oral and systemic health of the child and adolescent. Pediatrician. 1989;16:170–7.
16. Adami HO, McLaughlin JK, Hsing AW, et al. Alcoholism and cancer risk: a population-based cohort study. Cancer Causes Control. 1992;3:419–25.
17. Kato I, Nomura AM, Stemmermenn GN, Chyon PH. Prospective study of the association of alcohol with cancer of the upper aerodigestive tract and other sites. Cancer Causes Control. 1992; 3:145–51.
18. Risk JM, Mills HS, Garde J, et al. The tylosis esophageal cancer (TOC) locus: more than just a familial cancer gene. Dis Esophagus. 1999;12:173–6.
19. Ellis A, Field JK, Field EA, et al. Tylosis associated with carcinoma of the oesophagus and oral leukoplakia in a large Liverpool family – a review of six generations. Eur J Cancer B Oral Oncol. 1994;30:102–12.
20. Lagergren J, Bergström R, Lindgren A, et al. Symptomatic gastroesophageal reflux as a risk factor for esophageal adenocarcinoma. N Engl J Med. 1999;340:825–31.
21. Spechler SJ. Dysplasia in Barrett's esophagus: limitations of current management strategies. Am J Gastroenterol. 2005;100(4): 927–35.
22. Solaymani-Dodaran M, Logan RF, West J, et al. Risk of oesophageal cancer in Barrett's oesophagus and gastro-oesophageal reflux. Gut. 2004;53:1070–4.

23. Shaheen N, Ransohoff DF. Gastroesophageal reflux, Barrett esophagus, and esophageal cancer: scientific review. JAMA. 2002; 287:1972–81.

24. Barrett NR. Chronic peptic ulcer of the oesophagus and "oesophagitis". Br J Surg. 1950;38:175–82.

25. Fein R, Kelsen DP, Geller N, et al. Adenocarcinoma of the esophagus and gastroesophageal junction: prognostic factors and results of therapy. Cancer. 1985;56:2512–8.

26. Puli SR, Reddy JB, Bechtold ML, et al. Staging accuracy of esophageal cancer by endoscopic ultrasound: a meta-analysis and systematic review. World J Gastroenterol. 2008;14(10):1479–90.

27. Flamen P, Lerut A, Van Cutsem E, et al. Utility of positron emission tomography for the staging of patients with potentially operable esophageal carcinoma. J Clin Oncol. 2000;18:3202–10.

28. Swisher SG, Maish M, Erasmus JJ, et al. Utility of PET, CT, and EUS to Identify Pathologic Responders in Esophageal Cancer. Ann Thorac Surg. 2004;78:1152–60.

29. Cerfolio RJ, Bryant AS, Buddhiwardhan O, et al. The accuracy of endoscopic ultrasonography with fine-needle aspiration, integrated positron emission tomography with computed tomography, and computed tomography in restaging patients with esophageal cancer after neoadjuvant chemoradiotherapy. J Thorac Cardiovasc Surg. 2005;129:1232–41.

30. Krasna MJ, Flowers JL, Attar S, et al. Combined thoracoscopic/laparoscopic staging of esophageal cancer. J Thorac Cardiovasc Surg. 1996;111:800–6; discussion 806–7.

31. Esophagus. In: American joint committee on cancer. AJCC cancer staging manual. 7th ed. New York: Springer; 2010. p. 103–15.

32. Loran DB, Zwischenberger JB. Thoracic surgery in the elderly. J Am Coll Surg. 2004;199(5):773–84.

33. Wright CD, Kucharczuk JC, O'Brien SM, et al. Predictors of major morbidity and mortality after esophagectomy for esophageal cancer: a society of thoracic surgeons general thoracic surgery database risk adjustment model. J Thorac Cardiovasc Surg. 2009;137:587–96.

34. Overholt B, Lightdale C, Wang K, et al. Photodynamic therapy (PDT) with porfimer sodium for the ablation of high-grade dysplasia in Barrett's esophagus (BE): international, partially blinded randomized phase III trial. Gastrointest Endosc. 2005;62:488–98.

35. Shaheen NJ, Sharma P, Overholt BF, et al. Radiofrequency ablation in Barrett's esophagus with dysplasia. N Engl J Med. 2009; 360:2277–88.

36. Prasad GA, Wang KK, Buttar NS, et al. Long term survival following endoscopic and surgical treatment of high grade dysplasia following endoscopic and surgical treatment of high grade dysplasia in Barrett's esophagus. Gastroenterology. 2007;132:1226–33.

37. Orringer MB, Sloan H. Esophagectomy without thoracotomy. J Thorac Cardiovasc Surg. 1978;76:643–54.

38. Lewis I. The surgical treatment of carcinoma of the esophagus with special reference to a new operation for growths of the middle third. Br J Surg. 1946;34:18.

39. McKeown KC. Total three-stage esophagectomy for cancer of the esophagus. Br J Surg. 1976;51:259–62.

40. Bolten JS, Teng S. Transthoracic or transhiatal esophagectomy for cancer of the esophagus – does it matter. Surg Oncol Clin North Am. 2002;11:365–75.

41. Dimick JB, Pronovost PJ, Cowan JA, et al. Surgical volume and quality of care for esophageal resection: do high-volume hospitals have fewer complications? Ann Thor Surg. 2003;75:337–41.

42. Rizk NP, Bach PB, Schrag D, et al. The impact of complications on outcomes after resection for esophageal and gastroesophageal junction carcinoma. J Am Coll Surg. 2004;198:42–50.

43. Davis PA, Law S, Wong J. Colonic Interposition after esophagectomy for cancer. Arch Surg. 2003;138:303–8.

44. Orringer MB, Marshall B, Iannettoni MD. Eliminating the cervical esophagogastric anastomotic leak with a side-to-side stapled anastomosis. J Thorac Cardiovasc Surg. 2000;119:277–88.

45. Orringer MB, Marshall B, Iannettoni MD. Transhiatal esophagectomy: clinical experience and refinements. Ann Surg. 1999;230: 392–400; discussion 400–3.

46. Orringer MB, Marshall B, Chang AC, et al. Two thousand transhiatal esophagectomies: changing trends, lessons learned. Ann Surg. 2007;246:363–74.

47. Altorki N, Kent M, Ferrara C, Port J. Three-field lymph node dissection for squamous cell and adenocarcinoma of the esophagus. Ann Surg. 2002;236:177–83.

48. Hulscher JB, van Sandick JW, de Boer AG, et al. Extended transthoracic resection compared with limited transhiatal resection for adenocarcinoma of the esophagus. N Engl J Med. 2002;374:1662–9.

49. Hulscher JB, Tijssen JG, Obertop H, van Lanschot JJ. Transthoracic versus transhiatal resection for carcinoma of the esophagus: a meta-analysis. Ann Thorac Surg. 2001;72:306–13.

50. Peyre CG, Hagen JA, DeMeester SR, et al. The number of lymph nodes removed predicts survival in esophageal cancer: an international study on the impact of extent of surgical resection. Ann Surg. 2008;248:549–56.

51. Heitmiller RF. Results of standard left thoracoabdominal esophagogastrectomy. Semin Thorac Cardiovasc Surg. 1992;4:314–9.

52. Luketich JD, Alvelo-Rivera M, Buenaventura PO, et al. Minimally invasive esophagectomy: outcomes in 222 patients. Ann Surg. 2003;238:486–94.

53. Ruol A, Portale G, Zaninotto G, et al. Results of esophagectomy for esophageal cancer in elderly patients: age has little influence on outcome and survival. J Thorac Cardiovasc Surg. 2007;133:1186–92.

54. Sabel MS, Smith JL, Nava HR, et al. Esophageal resection for carcinoma in patients older than 70 years. Ann Surg Oncol. 2002;9(2):210–4.

55. Braiteh F, Correa AM, Hofstetter WL, et al. Association of age and survival in patients with gastroesophageal cancer undergoing surgery with or without preoperative therapy. Cancer. 2009;115(19):4450–8.

56. Moskovitz AH, Rizk NP, Venkatraman E, et al. Mortality increases for octogenarians undergoing esophagogastrectomy for esophageal cancer. Ann Thorac Surg. 2006;82:2031–6.

57. Bailey SH, Bull DA, Harpole DH, et al. Outcomes after esophagectomy: a ten-year prospective cohort. Ann Thorac Surg. 2003;75: 217–22.

58. Finlayson E, Fan Z, Birkmeyer JD. Outcomes in octogenarians undergoing high-risk cancer operation: a national study. J Am Coll Surg. 2007;205:729–34.

59. Ra J, Paulson EC, Kucharczuk J, et al. Postoperative mortality after esophagectomy for cancer: development of a preoperative risk prediction model. Ann Surg Oncol. 2008;15(6):1577–84.

60. Arnott SJ, Duncan W, Gignoux M, Girling DJ, Hansen HS, Launois B, Nygaard K, Parmar MKB, Rousell A, Spiliopoulos G, Stewart LA, Tierney JF, Wang M, Rhugang Z (Oesophageal Cancer Collaborative Group). Preoperative radiotherapy for esophageal carcinoma. Cochrane Database of Systematic Reviews 2005, Issue 4. Art. No.: CD001799. DOI: 10.1002/14651858.CD001799.pub2.

61. Kelsen DP, Ginsberg R, Pajak TF, et al. Chemotherapy followed by surgery compared with surgery alone for localized esophageal cancer. N Engl J Med. 1998;339:1979–84.

62. Medical Research Council Oesophageal Cancer Working Group. Surgical resection with or without postoperative chemotherapy in oesophageal cancer: a randomised controlled trial. Lancet. 2002;359:1727–33.

63. Cunningham D, Allum WH, Stenning SP, et al. Perioperative chemotherapy versus surgery alone for resectable gastroesophageal cancer. N Engl J Med. 2006;355(1):11–20.

64. Malthaner RA, Collin S, FenlonD. Preoperative chemotherapy for resectable thoracic esophageal cancer. CochraneDatabase of Systematic Reviews 2006, Issue 3. Art. No.: CD001556. DOI: 10.1002/14651858.CD001556.pub2.

65. Walsh T, Noonan N, Hollywood D, et al. A comparison of multimodal therapy and surgery for esophageal adenocarcinoma. N Engl J Med. 1996;335:462–7.

66. Bosset J-F, Gignoux M, Triboulet J-P, et al. Chemoradiotherapy followed by surgery compared with surgery alone in squamous-cell cancer of the esophagus. N Engl J Med. 1997;337:161–7.

67. Tepper J, Krasna MJ, Niedzwiecki D, et al. Phase III trial of trimodality therapy with cisplatin, flourouracil, radiotherapy, and surgery compared with surgery alone for esophageal cancer: CALGB 9781. J Clin Oncol. 2008;26:1086–92.

68. Gebski V, Burmeister B, Smithers BM, et al. Survival benefits from neoadjuvant chemoradiotherapy or chemotherapy in oesophageal carcinoma: a meta-analysis. Lancet Oncol. 2007;8:33–4.

69. Rice DC, Correa AM, Vaporciyan AA, et al. Preoperative chemoradiotherapy prior to esophagectomy in elderly patients is not associated with increased morbidity. Ann Thorac Surg. 2005;79:391–7.

70. Abrams JA, Buono DL, Strauss J, et al. Esophagectomy compared with chemoradiation for early stage esophageal cancer in the elderly. Cancer. 2009;115(21):4924–33.

71. Orringer MB. Substernal gastric bypass of the excluded esophagus–results of an ill-advised operation. Surgery. 1984;96:467–70.

72. Herskovic A, Martz K, Al-Sarraf M, et al. Combined chemotherapy and radiotherapy compared with radiotherapy alone in patients with cancer of the esophagus. N Engl J Med. 1992;326:1593–8.

73. Atkinson M, Ferguson R. Fibreoptic endoscopic palliative intubation of inoperable oesophagogastric neoplasms. Br Med J. 1997;1:266–7.

74. Cook TA, Dehn CB. Use of covered expandable metal stents in the treatment of oesophageal carcinoma and tracheo-oesophageal fistula. Br J Surg. 1996;83:1417–8.

75. Litle VR, Luketich JD, Christie NA, et al. Photodynamic therapy as palliation for esophageal cancer: experience in 215 patients. Ann Thorac Surg. 2003;76:1687.

76. Orringer MB. Transhiatal esophagectomy without thoracotomy. Oper Tech Thorac Cardiovasc Surg. 2005;10:63.

Chapter 46
Esophageal Surgery for Benign Disease in the Elderly

Rose E. Hardin, Katie S. Nason, and James D. Luketich

Abstract Benign esophageal disease in elderly patients can present unique diagnostic and therapeutic challenges to physicians and surgeons. While benign esophageal diseases may be associated with classic presentations of dysphagia, heartburn, and regurgitation, recognition that atypical symptoms are also quite common in the elderly population is crucial. Atypical symptoms, such as chest pain and pulmonary complaints, often co-exist with known cardiac and pulmonary dysfunction, and can lead to misinterpretation of symptoms if the physician and surgeon do not consider esophageal disorders in the differential diagnosis. This chapter will briefly summarize the pathophysiology of the aging esophagus, including discussions of dysphagia and changes in esophageal motility. Manometric findings will be highlighted. Finally, surgical management of specific benign esophageal disorders, including paraesophageal hernia, gastroesophageal reflux disease, and esophageal diverticulum, will be discussed. Careful consideration of benign esophageal disease will improve patient quality of life through earlier intervention for relief of symptoms and prevent subsequent complications, including aspiration pneumonia and severe malnutrition.

Keywords Esophageal achalasia • Esophageal spasm • Diffuse • Gastroesophageal reflux • Hernia • Hiatal

Introduction

Benign esophageal disease in elderly patients can present unique diagnostic and therapeutic challenges to physicians and surgeons. Symptoms associated with benign esophageal diseases, such as difficulty swallowing (dysphagia), cough, and chest pain, are common. More importantly, these symptoms are not unique to esophageal diseases and are often attributed to other causes, such as stroke, myocardial ischemia, and primary pulmonary dysfunction. Failure to recognize these signs and symptoms results in delayed evaluation and treatment of the underlying esophageal disorder, and contributes to poor quality of life and further decline in the patient's physiologic reserve.

The average age for the population of the United States has been steadily increasing over the past several decades. In 2000, people 65 and older comprised 12% of the United States population, totaling ~35 million people. Looking forward to 2030, population projections released in 2008 predict that this same age group will increase to >71 million people and account for >20% of the total population [1]. Considering that approximately 10% of people over the age of 50, and up to 30–40% of patients confined to care facilities have swallowing difficulties [2], it is anticipated that there will be a growing number of geriatric patients who will be referred for surgical evaluation. Knowledge of benign esophageal diseases within this population is crucial to the appropriate evaluation and proper delivery of optimal surgical care to these patients. Proper care of geriatric patients with esophageal disorders is of particular importance, because esophageal symptoms often go undetected in hospitalized or institutionalized geriatric patients [3].

This chapter will briefly summarize the pathophysiology of the aging esophagus, including discussions of dysphagia, and changes in esophageal motility. Manometric findings will be highlighted. Finally, surgical management of specific benign esophageal disorders, including paraesophageal hernia (PEH), gastroesophageal reflux disease (GERD), achalasia, and esophageal diverticulum, will be discussed.

Pathophysiology of the Aging Esophagus

Over the past 50 years, improvements in diagnostic testing have improved our understanding of the changes in esophageal physiology attributable to increasing age. Once considered an inevitable result of aging, esophageal dysfunction was first described in 1964 as *presbyesophagus* [4].

R.E. Hardin (✉)
Department of Heart, Lung and Esophageal Surgery Institute,
University of Pittsburgh Medical Center, Pittsburgh, PA 15213, USA
e-mail: hardinre@upmc.edu

M.R. Katlic (ed.), *Cardiothoracic Surgery in the Elderly*, DOI 10.1007/978-1-4419-0892-6_46,
© Springer Science+Business Media, LLC 2011

Presbyesophagus was a constellation of age-related changes including decreased esophageal body peristaltic pressures, incomplete lower esophageal sphincter (LES) relaxation, nonpropulsive or tertiary contractions, and dilation of the esophagus in patients over the age of 90 years. Since that time, diagnostic testing, including esophageal manometry, esophageal impedance monitoring, barium esophagography, and upper gastrointestinal endoscopy, has shown that the majority of patients with symptomatic complaints have a specific esophageal disorder [5]. In particular, manometric evaluation of elderly patients with esophageal symptoms has helped to diagnose the majority of these patients with achalasia, diffuse esophageal spasm (DES), or nonspecific dysmotility syndromes. Interestingly, up to 36% of elderly patients without esophageal symptoms will have radiographic evidence of esophageal dysfunction [5]. Normal changes that occur with aging include a diminished number of ganglion cells of Auerbach's plexus, which can result in decreased strength and tonicity of the esophageal musculature. This loss of strength and tone leads to diminished amplitude of peristaltic contractions [6]. Furthermore, laxity of the phrenoesophageal membrane causes upward traction on the LES, and can lead to progressively enlarging hiatal hernias and gastroesophageal reflux (Table 46.1).

These age-related changes impact both the physiologic function of the esophagus, and the clinical presentation of esophageal disorders in elderly patients. Motility disorders in the elderly may also be related to existing medical problems, such as diabetes mellitus, neurological disorders, and to adverse effects of the multiple medications that elderly patients are often prescribed. A careful evaluation is vital to making accurate diagnoses, and planning for appropriate surgical intervention. A comprehensive evaluation should include a thorough history of the onset, timing, and changes in esophageal symptoms; appropriate objective radiographic studies; upper endoscopy; and manometry.

Table 46.1 Changes in esophageal physiology with aging

Upper esophageal sphincter (UES) and pharynx
  Impaired coordination
  Lower UES pressure
  Incomplete UES relaxation with swallowing
Esophageal body
  Impaired secondary peristalsis
  Increased frequency of failed primary peristalsis (possibly reflux related)
  More patients with ineffective esophageal motility (IEM)
Lower esophageal sphincter (LES)
  More hiatal hernias (subsequently low LES pressure)
Sensory function
  Impaired sensation with balloon distention
  Impaired sensation with acid perfusion (Bernstein test)
  Impaired pharyngeal sensation (decreases swallow initiation)

Source: Reprinted from Achem et al. [2] with permission from Lippincott Williams & Wilkins

Dysphagia in the Elderly

The act of swallowing is a carefully coordinated neuromuscular process that sequentially transfers a food or liquid bolus from the pharynx to the stomach. When this motility process becomes disordered, patients complain of dysphagia, odynophagia, regurgitation of undigested food or liquid, and atypical chest pain. Indeed, a high index of suspicion for benign esophageal motility disorders is necessary when elderly patients complain of atypical chest pain, especially when evaluations for cardiac etiologies of atypical chest pain are negative or inconclusive. A firm understanding of these disorders will guide the clinician toward the correct diagnosis and facilitate provision of effective treatment.

Dysphagia, defined as a difficulty or partial inability to swallow, is one of the most common presenting symptoms of esophageal motility disorders in the elderly population. It can also result from injury to the brain, such as cerebral vascular accidents (stroke), or from mechanically obstructing lesions. Benign mechanical causes of esophageal dysphagia in the elderly may include peptic strictures, rings or webs, vascular lesions, or medication-induced esophageal mucosal injury [2]. The impact of dysphagia on the quality of life and well-being of the elderly patient can be quite significant, resulting in severely decreased caloric intake and malnutrition, as well as interfering with the social aspects of eating. Indeed, elderly patients living in nursing homes who have swallowing difficulties are 3 times more likely to suffer from malnutrition than elderly patients without swallowing difficulties [7], and are significantly more likely to die within the next 6 months, compared with elderly patients who are independent in their ability to feed themselves [8]. It is difficult to know whether this excess in mortality is directly related to these feeding difficulties; however, the findings do suggest that interventions designed to improve swallowing may result in improved outcomes for elderly patients. Although oropharyngeal dysphagia (i.e., disordered swallowing mechanism) contributes significantly to these swallowing difficulties, this chapter focuses specifically on the contribution of esophageal motility disorders to dysphagia complaints.

Esophageal Motility in the Elderly Patient

Upper Esophageal Sphincter (UES)

The upper esophageal sphincter (UES), or pharygoesophageal sphincter, is the superior most portion of the esophagus. It consists of striated muscle and, in normal circumstances, is under conscious control. During swallowing, the cricopharyngeus portion of the inferior pharyngeal constrictor relaxes, the UES opens, and bolus solid or liquid passes into the esophagus. It then closes, thereby preventing backflow into the hypopharynx. With age, this coordinated swallowing mechanism can become disordered and lead to dysphagia. Studied extensively, the data, though not conclusive, suggest that changes to the UES are not inevitable, but that elderly patients with dysphagia do have changes in the function of the UES that contribute to the swallowing difficulties [9, 10]. For example, the function of the pharynx, resting UES pressure, and the ability of UES to relax were assessed in a comparison of asymptomatic patients greater than 75 years of age, with a younger cohort of patients (20–35 years). Resting UES pressure and UES relaxation decreased in the older patients compared with the younger patients [5]. Meier-Ewert et al. confirmed these findings in another study of elderly patients with dysphagia compared with elderly patients without dysphagia and with a younger cohort. These investigators found that elderly patients with dysphagia had decreased peak pharyngeal pressure and impaired relaxation of the UES [11]. Other investigators found that UES function in asymptomatic elderly patients was not significantly different from younger patients without dysphagia [12].

The exact etiology of these changes is unclear, but may be the result of a loss of connective tissue compliance that occurs with aging. Another possible etiology is laryngopharyngeal reflux, causing spasm of the UES due to reflux of gastrointestinal secretions to the level of the pharynx [13]. Regardless of etiology, failure of the UES to relax predisposes elderly patients to dysphagia, due to a functional obstruction to food and liquid boluses. Over time, even though the overall pressures in the esophagus just proximal to the UES are diminished, the failure of the UES to relax leads to increased pressure just proximal to the cricopharyngeus muscle, and contributes to the formation of Zenker's diverticulum.

Body of the Esophagus

The primary function of the esophagus is to transport boluses of food and liquid from the oropharynx to the stomach. The body of the esophagus is the muscular tube, located between the UES and the LES, responsible for this bolus transfer. The esophageal body propagates the bolus through primary and secondary peristalsis. Triggered by swallowing, primary peristalsis is a voluntary contraction of the esophageal body that begins at the UES and progresses to the LES in a coordinated wave. This peristaltic wave moves the bolus rapidly through the esophagus with intra-luminal pressures that range from 20 to 100 mmHg. Secondary peristalsis is initiated if the primary peristalsis fails to completely clear the esophagus. Caused by distention or irritation, these secondary peristaltic waves are involuntary, but also progressive and sequential.

When primary and secondary peristalsis become disordered, such as occurs with simultaneous "tertiary" contractions or low-amplitude contractions, esophageal complaints, such as dysphagia, odynophagia and chest pain, become common. Tertiary contractions have no known physiologic function and occur more often in elderly people [3].

Common esophageal body motility disorders in elderly patients include achalasia, DES and scleroderma. Several potential theories exist regarding the underlying physiologic mechanism of esophageal motility dysfunction in elderly patients. Dysmotility disorders in elderly patients may be secondary to the decreased number of myenteric neurons with aging, which results in denervation of the esophagus. This loss of innervation may then lead to loss of secondary peristalsis triggered by the distension of the esophagus [5]. It has also been noted that the pathologic changes seen in the aging esophagus are similar to changes that occur with spastic esophageal motility disorders. A significant decrease in esophageal amplitude pressures have been reported in elderly patients in the 8th and 9th decade of life [5].

Lower Esophageal Sphincter (LES)

The LES consists of a ring of smooth muscle fibers in the distal few centimeters of the esophageal body and proximal stomach. This ring of muscle fibers normally remains constricted, creating a 3–5 cm zone of increased pressure at the junction of the esophagus and the gastric cardia. When the LES pressure is decreased, reflux of gastrointestinal contents into the distal esophagus occurs. GERD is quite common in the general population, and the majority of studies suggest that there are minimal-to-no changes in LES pressure with aging [2, 3]. Indeed, at least one investigator has found that diagnoses related to failure of the LES are more frequent in patients younger than 80 years of age [14].

Manometry in the Elderly Patient

After exclusion of intrinsic structural esophageal pathology with upper endoscopy and barium swallow, elderly patients with esophageal dysphagia should undergo manometry for evaluation for underlying motility disorder. Despite the early identification of "presbyesophagus" in nonagenarians, more recent studies have found that manometric findings are helpful in diagnosing specific motility abnormalities in older patients [14, 15] (Tables 46.2 and 46.3).

Motility disorders, such as achalasia, nutcracker esophagus or nonspecific disorders, have been diagnosed in up to 50% of patients without intrinsic esophageal pathology who undergo manometry testing, making manometry an

Table 46.2 Esophageal motility disorders in older and younger patients

Diagnosis	Older patients (%)	Younger patients (%)
Normal	30.3	44.3
Achalasia	15.2[a]	4.1
Diffuse spasm	16.6[a]	4.1
Incomplete LES relaxation	1.5[b]	9.8
NEMD	22.7	13.9
Nutcracker esophagus	9	5.7
Scleroderma esophagus	3	10.7
Low LES pressure	0	5.7
Abnormal UES/pharynx	1.5	1.6

LES lower esophageal sphincter; *NEMD* nonspecific esophageal motility disorder

[a]$p < 0.005$ (older compared with younger patients)

[b]$p < 0.05$

Source: Reprinted with permission from Ribeiro et al. [3], Copyright Elsevier 1998

Table 46.3 Manometric characteristics of esophageal motility disorders

Achalasia	Aperastaltic esophageal body with incomplete lower esophageal sphincter (LES) relaxation; ±elevated LES resting pressure (>40 mmHg)
Diffuse esophageal spasm (DES)	Simultaneous contractions with prolonged duration of contractions (>8 s)
Hypertensive esophagus ("nutcracker esophagus")	Mean amplitude in the distal esophagus >180 mmHg with increased duration of distal contractions (>8 s)
Hypotensive esophagus	Resting LES pressure <15 mmHg
	Ineffective motility: abnormal peristalsis occurring >30% with low distal amplitude (<30 mmHg) or failed non transmitted contractions

Source: Modified from Robson and Glick [15], with permission from Springer Science+Business media

invaluable tool in evaluation of dysphagia in elderly patients. In a recent study, comparing esophageal motility studies of patients >65 years of age presenting with dysphagia, to motility studies of matched dysphagic younger patients, no differences were identified in LES pressure, residual pressure after deglutition, LES relaxation or peristalsis, or amplitude of esophageal body contractions [15]. Interestingly, the main difference between these age groups was the prevalence of presenting symptoms; elderly patients are more likely to present with dysphagia, unlike younger patients, who are more likely to present with heartburn. This may simply reflect the finding that older patients are more likely to have spastic disorders underlying their dysphagia, and younger patients more likely to have motor dysfunction related to reflux disease as the underlying etiology for their dysphagia [14].

Esophageal Surgery for Benign Esophageal Disorders

Paraesophageal Hernia/Hiatal Hernia

PEH accounts for approximately 5–10% of all hiatal hernias. They are more prevalent in elderly patients and are especially common among elderly women. PEHs are classified into four main types: type 1 PEH is a sliding-type hiatal hernia; type 2 PEH involves true "paraesophageal" herniation of the stomach, posterolateral to the esophagus, with the gastroesophageal junction remaining in the normal intra-abdominal position; type 3 PEH involves proximal migration of the gastroesophageal junction into the posterior mediastinum along with the cardia (or more) of the stomach; and type 4 PEH (Fig. 46.1) involves the stomach, and at least one other visceral organ migrating into the chest [16]. Type 4 PEH is associated with the highest morbidity and mortality. It is likely that PEHs progress from type 1 sliding hiatal hernias to type 3 and 4 PEH over time. Not surprisingly, type 4 PEHs are more likely to occur in patients over the age of 70 years [16]. Sliding type 1 hiatal hernias are associated with incompetence of the gastroesophageal sphincter and subsequent development of symptomatic GERD [17–21]. The development of PEH involves the progressive weakening of the phrenoesophagal membrane, attenuation of the muscles of the diaphragmatic hiatus, and subsequent hiatal enlargement. PEH development progresses with age [19, 20].

PEH is associated with a variety of symptoms and patients can present electively or emergently. While symptoms often

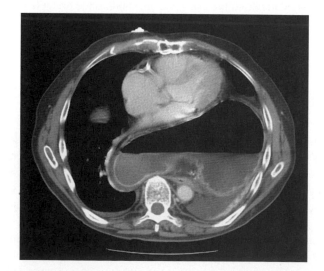

Fig. 46.1 Contrast CT scan of the chest demonstrating a type 4 paraesophageal hernia with migration of the entire stomach into the chest. This is a giant paraesophageal hernia because greater than one third of the stomach is intrathoracic

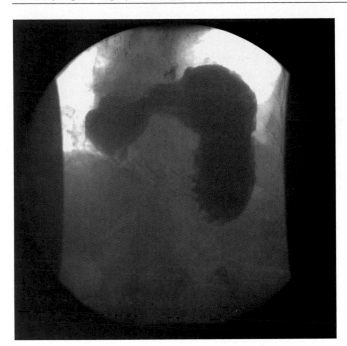

Fig. 46.2 Barium swallow examination in a patient presenting with dysphagia and anemia secondary to a giant paraesophageal hernia; anemia resulted from chronic low grade bleeding from herniated intrathoracic stomach

include classic gastroesophageal reflux complaints of heartburn and regurgitation, patients also frequently complain of postprandial fullness, bloating, retrosternal chest pain (which may be misdiagnosed as cardiac angina), and dysphagia. Anemia can result from chronic bleeding from the herniated stomach, and gastrointestinal bleeding can be a source of major morbidity and even mortality (Fig. 46.2). Patients can be minimally symptomatic for years despite a significant herniation of stomach into the mediastinum. The symptoms are often misdiagnosed as cardiac or pulmonary in origin, or are treated with antireflux medications. As such, PEH progressively enlarge. Over time, herniation of the entire stomach into the chest can occur, and is often associated with organo- or meso-axial volvulus. Referral for surgical repair is often delayed until the patient suffers a major complication. When the predominant symptoms are dysphagia, chest pain, aspiration (often leading to pneumonia), or bleeding, the underlying cause is mechanical obstruction. As such, these symptoms are not responsive to medical management. Surgical delay in this situation is of no benefit [22].

Because large PEH can occupy a significant amount of space in the thorax, chronic lung compression may compromise pulmonary function in patients with large PEH. Mechanical obstruction with regurgitation and aspiration can further compromise respiratory status. Indeed, patients with long-standing, large PEHs may present with significant

progressive dyspnea and pulmonary dysfunction, which may dissuade surgical intervention because of the high risk for complications associated with general anesthesia and surgery. Despite the fact that patients are frequently aware that they have a PEH with a large herniation of stomach into the chest, their progressive pulmonary dysfunction is still often mistakenly attributed to comorbid conditions, such as COPD or heart failure. It is important, however, that clinicians be aware of the contribution of PEH to dyspnea, as well as the risk for aspiration, and to consider referral of the patient for operative evaluation and possible repair. Low and Simchuk studied the relationship between pulmonary function and PEH repair, and found that repair was associated with improved basic spirometry values, up to 16% above baseline. Repair was also associated with increases in FEV1 (forced expiratory volume in 1 s) and forced vital capacity [23]. In fact, the degree of improvement after PEH correction correlated with the increasing size of the hernia and was attributed to relief of the mechanical compression. Many patients have reported improved dyspnea, reduced aspiration, and better quality of life postoperatively [23, 24]. This is due to relief of mechanical compression, improved diaphragmatic function, and reduced atelectasis. Furthermore, mechanical compression may also transiently affect cardiac function, which contributes to the sensation of dyspnea and to decreased exercise capacity. Significant respiratory dysfunction may in fact be an indication for surgery in patients with large PEH and should be carefully assessed.

The repair of PEH in elderly patients, as with younger patients, requires strict attention to complete dissection of the hernia sac from the mediastinum, reduction of the herniated contents back into the abdomen, recognizing and managing a shortened esophagus, and closing a large hiatal defect without tension [25]. Because the surgical dissection disrupts the phrenoesophageal ligament, many surgeons routinely include an antireflux procedure as a part of the repair. PEH is often associated with esophageal shortening, necessitating extensive esophageal mobilization and, when necessary, collis-gastroplasty to achieve an adequate length of intra-abdominal esophagus. Repair can be achieved with a laparoscopic approach in centers of excellence with outcomes that compare favorably to open repair [24, 26].

The management of asymptomatic or minimally symptomatic PEHs remains a highly debated topic, in part because the true natural history of this disease entity is yet to be determined. Morbidity is substantial among elderly patients, in part because of advanced disease and associated comorbid conditions [16, 22, 27], and raises the question of the best therapeutic strategy for patients with asymptomatic or minimally symptomatic PEHs. However, many surgeons advocate elective laparoscopic repair. The laparoscopic approach for PEH repair is now the standard of care, enabling these hernias to be fixed with less pain, faster recovery and reduced morbidity and mortality. The benefits of laparoscopy may be most pronounced in elderly patients who are less able to tolerate operative intervention due to the effects of age and greater comorbid burden. The morbidity associated with PEH repair in elderly patients may dissuade surgical referral. However, the morbidity and mortality associated with emergent presentations secondary to acute strangulation, volvulus or perforation are considerable higher [22, 27]. In our center, patients requiring hospitalization and nonelective repair for significant symptoms related to PEH were significantly older than those treated with elective repair. Octogenarians were nearly 5 times more likely to receive nonelective repair, with a postoperative mortality of 16% compared to 0.7% for elective repair. The combined effect of age >80, nonelective operation and a Charlson comorbidity index score of 3 or greater increased the risk of postoperative mortality to 40 times that of the patient undergoing elective operation at an age less than 80 years with lower comorbidity scores. Based on these findings, and supported by recent reports by others, we strongly recommend that patients with large hiatal hernia be carefully assessed for symptoms by a qualified surgeon once the large hiatal hernia has been identified. The surgeon must weigh the patient's functional status, comorbid conditions, symptoms, and the potential for life-threatening complications due to the herniated stomach to determine whether operative intervention is needed, rather than waiting for an acute presentation as the morbidity and mortality associated with nonelective presentation is substantial [28].

Gastroesophageal Reflux Disease (GERD)

GERD is a constellation of symptoms that occur as the result of gastric contents regurgitating from the stomach back into the esophagus. GERD results from three distinct aberrations in normal physiology: (1) impaired esophageal motility; (2) impaired function of the LES; and (3) delayed gastric emptying. Patients with GERD typically have at least one of these three mechanisms underlying their disease process. In the elderly, all three factors are often present and, when combined with the age-related changes described below, contribute to increased disease severity. Indeed, while the prevalence of GERD within the elderly population is similar to the entire population, elderly patients are more likely to suffer from complications of GERD, more likely to be under- or misdiagnosed, and more likely to be under-treated. Delays in diagnosis and appropriate therapy contribute to more severe esophagitis and 20% of elderly patients have grade 3 or 4 esophagitis at endoscopy [29]. Historically, the increased morbidity and mortality of open surgery in elderly patients limited the number of referrals for surgical intervention.

However, with the advent of advanced laparoscopic techniques and experience, antireflux surgery is now considered a safe option for elderly patients, and should be considered in patients with complications of GERD, or whose GERD symptoms are not adequately resolved by medication.

There are several factors associated with the aging process that have been implicated in the etiology of GERD in elderly patients. In particular, with aging, there is increased gastric acid secretion, decreased esophageal mucosal regeneration, and decreased esophageal protective mechanisms (namely impaired esophageal clearance and reduced bicarbonate secretions) [30]. With advancing age, salivary bicarbonate production decreases, while physiologic levels of gastric acid secretion remain constant. The reduction in the bicarbonate buffer within the stomach results in an overall increase in gastric acidity. When gastric contents reflux into the esophagus, the result is increased esophageal acid exposure [29]. In a recent study, the percentage of time with pH <4 was as high as 32.5% in elderly patients, significantly higher than the 12.9% in younger counterparts with GERD [31].

The impact of GERD on esophageal mucosal injury can be further exacerbated by certain medications that are taken with greater frequency by the elderly. Several common medications can cause direct esophageal mucosal injury (such as nonsteroidal anti-inflammatory drugs (NSAIDs), potassium tablets and bisphosphonates), while others cause decreased LES pressure (including nitrates, calcium-channel blockers, benzodiazepines, anticholinergics, and antidepressants). As with younger patients, decreased LES pressure increases acid exposure in the distal esophagus. In the elderly, this acid exposure is accentuated by delayed esophageal acid clearance that occurs due to disturbances of esophageal motility. Compared with younger patients, the elderly are more likely to have a significant decrease in the amplitude of peristaltic contraction, and an increase in the frequency of nonpropulsive contractions [4, 32–34]. Furthermore, many comorbid conditions can adversely affect esophageal motility, such as Parkinson's disease, cerebrovascular disease, and diabetes mellitus, all of which occur with greater prevalence in the elderly. Combined with the diminished regenerative capability of esophageal mucosal cells, the decrease in esophageal protective mechanisms significantly increases the vulnerability of elderly patients to mucosal injury and esophagitis [6].

Despite increased vulnerability to esophageal mucosal injury, elderly patients are less likely to experience the classic reflux symptoms of heartburn and regurgitation than are younger patients. Atypical presentations of GERD, such as dysphagia, chest pain and pulmonary complications, including asthma-like symptoms and aspiration pneumonia, may be more common. These atypical GERD symptoms can mimic symptoms of underlying coronary artery disease and chronic lung disorders, and are another important reason why GERD is easily misdiagnosed in the elderly. Anemia may also be an atypical presentation of GERD within the elderly population.

The phenomenon of reduced heartburn symptom severity with advancing age may be explained by age-related decreases in esophageal pain perception. Fass et al. prospectively analyzed GERD symptoms, and response to acid infusion in patients over 60 years of age compared to patients less than 60 years. All patients complained of GERD symptoms and GERD was confirmed with 24-h pH monitoring and endoscopy. The elderly patients were significantly less likely to complain of severe heartburn (17.6 vs. 52%) despite the fact that 74% of the elderly cohort had erosive esophagitis compared with only 64% of the younger group. Importantly, the elderly patients had a significantly longer lag time to initial symptom perception in response to acid infusion, and a significantly lower acid perfusion sensitivity score [35]. This decrease in esophageal pain perception may, in fact, be a factor in the increased rate of GERD complications in the elderly, because it can lead to more advanced acid injury without the usual warning symptoms.

Several diagnostic tests are available for the evaluation of GERD and, as with younger patients, are extremely useful in the evaluation of elderly patients with GERD. Because of the increased prevalence of atypical symptoms in the elderly, including dysphagia, noncardiac chest pain and pulmonary manifestations, the indications for GERD evaluation should be expanded to include these symptoms in older patients. The complications associated with untreated GERD in the elderly can be severe and life threatening, making an aggressive approach to diagnosis important. Barium swallow and upper GI endoscopy are used to evaluate dysphagia and mucosal injury. Barium swallow examination utilizing a double contrast technique is useful to characterize anatomy and provide qualitative information on esophageal function. The barium swallow is particularly important in elderly patients whose symptoms may be related to an underlying motility disorder, Zenker's diverticulum, esophageal neoplasm, or peptic stricture [36]. In contrast to younger patients, endoscopy should be considered earlier, as an initial diagnostic test, in elderly patients with heartburn, regardless of the severity or duration of complaints, to evaluate for erosive esophagitis and esophageal malignancy. However, the definitive diagnosis of GERD in the elderly remains ambulatory esophageal 24-h pH monitoring, as in younger patients. Ambulatory esophageal 24-h pH monitoring quantifies the degree of reflux but, more importantly, can be used to correlate symptoms with documented reflux episodes, which is critical for determining the etiology of atypical symptoms [36]. Esophageal manometry is often used in patients with markedly atypical symptoms, for locating the LES for pH testing, and in those for whom surgery is contemplated.

Treatment of GERD in the elderly is essentially the same as in all adults. The treatment goals for GERD include elimination of symptoms, healing of esophagitis, managing or preventing complications, and maintaining remission. The vast majority of people with GERD can be treated successfully with the noninvasive methods of lifestyle modification and medication. Approximately a decade ago, proton pump inhibitors (PPIs) were introduced for management of GERD and have provided considerable relief of heartburn in both older and younger patients. However, despite considerable enthusiasm for their use, PPIs have not proven to be the perfect panacea for management of GERD, particularly in the elderly. First, PPIs have little effect on regurgitation and respiratory symptoms and, therefore, may be less effective for symptom control in elderly patients. They are extremely effective at neutralizing the acid, but several studies utilizing esophageal impedance have demonstrated that acid-reducing medications allow reflux and regurgitation of gastric contents with a neutral PH through the incompetent sphincter [37, 38]. Symptoms that are secondary to volume regurgitation, such as pulmonary aspiration, pneumonia, and chronic sinusitis, persist in this setting, despite the resolution of heartburn. Second, the Food and Drug Administration (FDA) issued a warning in 2009 regarding the interaction between drugs that inhibit the CYP2C19 enzyme, the target for PPIs and the anti-platelet medication, clopidogrel [39]. According to the FDA, CYP2C19 enzyme inhibiting drugs significantly reduce the active metabolite levels of patients taking clopidogrel. Taken with omeprazole, the active metabolite levels were reduced by 45%, and the anti-platelet effect reduced by 47%. They recommend that patients requiring clopidogrel and acid-reducing agents use antacids or H2 antagonists, such as ranitidine or similar medications. The warning from the FDA will likely have a significant impact on the ability to effectively manage symptoms of heartburn in the elderly.

Laparoscopic fundoplication is safe and effective for management of GERD in elderly patients and is not associated with a higher incidence of intraoperative or postoperative complications [40]. The procedure is very effective at eliminating heartburn, similar to the effectiveness of PPI, but also eliminates volume regurgitation. This is an important distinction and warrants serious consideration in the management of elderly patients with atypical GERD symptoms, particularly nocturnal regurgitation and pulmonary aspiration, as these can lead to irreversible lung damage [40]. When performed laparoscopically, fundoplication carries a morbidity rate of 8–20% and a mortality rate of less than 1%. These rates do not differ significantly in elderly patients [29, 36, 41, 42]. It is now well-accepted that age alone should not be a contraindication to antireflux surgery, especially in properly selected patients. Furthermore, minimally invasive Nissen fundoplication is safe and efficacious in the elderly population with added benefit of decreased postoperative pain, shortened length of hospital stay, and faster return to normal activity [43, 44].

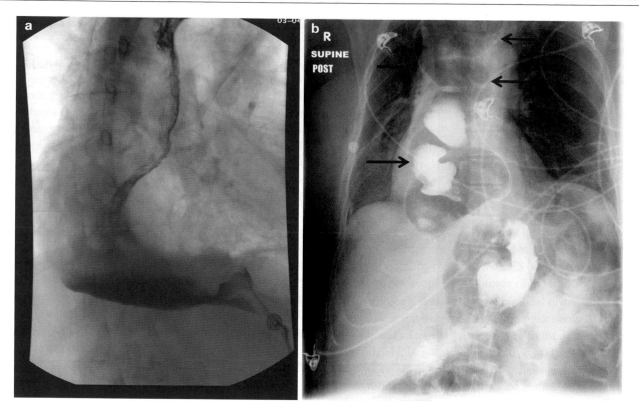

Fig. 46.5 (a) Barium swallow representing the classic changes in an older patient with long standing achalasia resulting in extreme dilation and tortuosity of the esophagus, referred to as sigmoid esophagus. (b) Chest X-ray following contrast examination demonstrating an extremely dilated and tortuous sigmoid esophagus. The *red arrows* indicate the contour of the esophagus, which is similar in appearance to sigmoid colon

perforation, also identified and treated intra-operatively, 3 pleural effusions, 1 case of pneumonia, and 3 other minor complications (ileus, *Clostridium difficile* infection and respiratory insufficiency). All complications were appropriately managed without significant morbidity. The average length of stay was 3 days. At a mean follow up of 23.5 months, 96% of patients experienced significant symptomatic relief; mean dysphagia score improved from 3.28 to 1.36 following minimally invasive myotomy ($p < 0.001$). These results have been replicated by other centers of excellence in minimally invasive surgery, and suggest that minimally invasive myotomy, performed by experienced surgeons, is an excellent option for long-term and durable management of achalasia, even in elderly patients [65–70].

Diffuse Esophageal Spasm and Hypercontracting "Nutcracker" Esophagus

DES accounts for approximately 3–5% of all esophageal motility disorders, and predominant symptoms are dysphagia and severe chest pain. DES is characterized by normal peristalsis interrupted by simultaneous contractions of unclear etiology [71]. Possible etiologic factors for DES are neural dysfunction, hypersensitive esophagus, gastroesophageal reflux, and stress-induced contractions. Concomitant GERD is present in approximately 30–50% of patients suffering with DES and 24-h ambulatory pH studies may provide useful information in these patients. Patients with DES can generally be categorized by the amplitude of distal esophageal contractions. As the amplitude of distal contractions increases, higher pressures are generated within the esophagus, causing significant chest discomfort [71–73] (Fig. 46.6). Chest pain can be particularly confusing in an elderly patient with concomitant coronary artery disease and angina. Of particular interest, not only does the chest pain of DES mimic cardiac angina, it can also be alleviated by administration of nitroglycerin. However, the chest pain characteristic of DES is rarely exertional and is often precipitated by meals. Therefore, careful history and physical examination and an appropriate subsequent diagnostic workup are crucial to providing effective treatment to elderly patients with DES. It is also important to remember that manometric evaluation of these patients can vary from day to day depending on the amount of spastic activity, which does not necessarily correlate well with occurrence of symptoms.

Although DES can occur at any age, it is far more common in patients older than 50 years of age. Treatment of DES is predominately nonsurgical, and patients can be reassured

Fig. 46.6 Esophageal amplitude pressures in diffuse esophageal spasm (reprinted with permission from Bremner [82], p. 83)

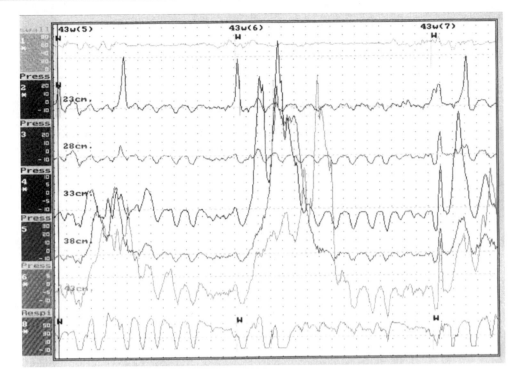

that their chest pain is not of cardiac origin. GERD should be identified and aggressively treated and may result in resolution or alleviations of symptoms of DES. Other medical therapies with varied success include long-acting nitrates, calcium channel blockers, and anticholinergics. More aggressive interventions are limited to a specific subset of patients. For patients with DES whose predominant complaint is dysphagia, pneumatic dilation or Botox injection may be helpful, especially for those patients whose manometry shows abnormal relaxation of the LES. Extensive surgical myotomy may help some patients with symptomatic relief of chest pain, however, this should be undertaken with caution since symptomatic relief is highly variable [71]. Nonoperative measures should be optimized, and the decision to proceed with surgery made after careful counseling of the patient regarding the risks of major surgery, often involving a transthoracic approach. Options for surgical intervention include long myotomy, roux-en-y near-esophagojejunostomy, and esophagectomy and should be performed by surgeons who have extensive experience in esophageal surgery, as the risks for adverse outcomes and poor quality of life postoperatively are not inconsequential.

Nutcracker esophagus is defined by mean distal esophageal peristaltic amplitudes exceeding 180 mmHg, mean distal duration greater than 6 s, and a hypertensive LES with resting pressures greater than 45 mmHg (Fig. 46.7). The main presenting complaint in patients with nutcracker esophagus is chest pain; dysphagia is uncommon. In fact, approximately 27–48% of patients who undergo manometry secondary to complaint of atypical chest pain are later determined to have nutcracker esophagus. Treatment of nutcracker esophagus is similar to treatment of DES. Relief of chest pain, as with DES, does not always coincide with pharmacological or surgical therapy.

Esophageal Diverticula

An esophageal diverticulum is a sac or outpouching from the tubular esophagus. Esophageal diverticula are found most commonly in the elderly population, as they are typically acquired rather than congenital. Esophageal diverticula in the elderly are most commonly classified by anatomic location (e.g., hypopharyngeal or distal esophageal), and by pathogenesis (e.g., pulsion or traction). Knowledge of the symptom complex associated with esophageal diverticula and the underlying pathophysiology of esophageal diverticula are critical for early diagnosis and appropriate treatment. As with other benign esophageal disorders in the elderly, progressively worsening dysphagia is a common presentation of esophageal diverticula and can lead to adverse consequences, such as aspiration, pneumonia, and malnutrition. Patients complain of regurgitation of undigested food, halitosis, hoarseness and weight loss and, as a result, impaired quality of life.

Fig. 46.7 Esophageal amplitude pressures in Nutcracker Esophagus (reprinted with permission from Bremner [82], p. 85)

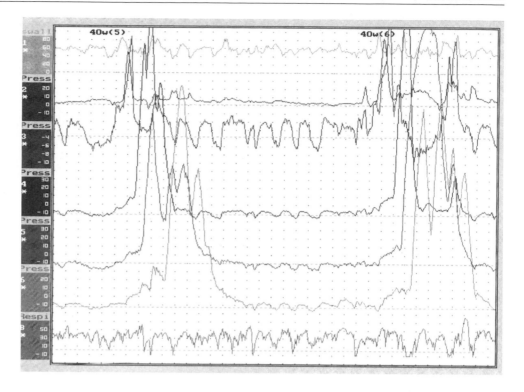

Zenker's Diverticulum

Pharyngoesophageal diverticula, commonly known as Zenker's diverticula, are acquired, false, pulsion diverticula that frequently affect elderly patients. A Zenker's diverticulum is an outpouching in the posterior pharyngeal wall immediately above the UES (Killian's triangle), and is found almost exclusively in patients older than 50 years of age. Zenker's diverticula progressively enlarge leading to worsening of symptoms with time. The etiology of Zenker's diverticulum remains unclear,. However, it is proposed to involve dysfunction or dyscoordination of the UES with increased association in patients with hiatal hernia and GERD [74]. Zenker's diverticula likely results from decreased compliance and inadequate opening of the cricopharyngeus muscle. Histopathologic changes in the cricopharyngeus muscle, with features of fibrosis and inflammation, have been identified in some patients with Zenker's diverticula. This inadequate upper esophageal response leads to a high intrabolus swallowing pressure in the pharynx and subsequently to a diverticulum [75, 76].

The diagnosis of Zenker's diverticulum is based on clinical presentation and confirmed with barium swallow (Fig. 46.8). Rarely is any other evaluation necessary [74]. The traditional open procedures include diverticulectomy and myotomy, myotomy alone for small diverticula<4 cm or diverticuloplexy. They are all well tolerated in elderly patients. Over the last decade, minimally invasive, transoral

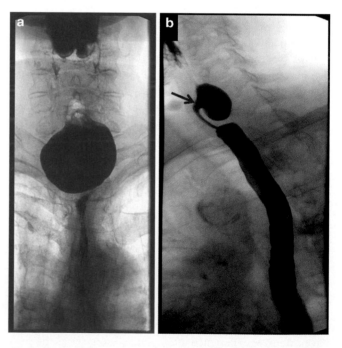

Fig. 46.8 (**a**) Barium swallow demonstrating an acquired Zenker's diverticulum in a 72-year old female who presented with worsening dysphagia and regurgitation of undigested food. (**b**) Lateral view, from another patient, that clearly demonstrates the neck of a diverticulum that is amendable to minimally invasive stapled diverticular exclusion

stapled diverticulostomy has been developed as a suitable option for treatment of Zenker's diverticula in well selected patients. Originally described by Collard in 1993, transoral stapling of a Zenker's diverticulum is accomplished with the patient under general anesthesia [77]. Using a Weerda diverticuloscope, the diverticulum can be visualized and divided using endoscopic staplers passed transorally [77]. The Weerda diverticuloscope is a specially designed, bivalved fiberoptic instrument, which can be passed through the patient's mouth into the esophagus. By positioning one blade of the instrument in the esophageal lumen and the other in the diverticulum, the diverticular septum can be clearly identified. A suture placed in the septum of the diverticulum is very useful for providing counter-traction, and preventing the septum from being pushed away from the stapler as it is deployed. Because the endostapler places a double line of staples on either side of the transected mucosa and underlying cricopharyngeus muscle, postoperative leaks are extremely rare, and short-term relief of symptoms is excellent.

Multiple studies now show that transoral stapling of Zenker's diverticula is effective in relieving dysphagia and regurgitation with short operative times (ranging from 30 min to 1.5 h), minimal morbidity, and reduced length of hospital stay [77–80]. Several studies, however, report recurrent symptoms requiring re-intervention due to incomplete diverticulostomy. For optimal results, the diverticulum should be at least 2 cm in size to enable complete transaction of the muscle fibers of the cricopharyngeus muscle [77, 78, 80]. In addition, the patient cannot have a small oral cavity or degenerative neck disease that limits range of motion, as these factors inhibit passage of the stapling device. Despite the need for reintervention in approximately 10% of patients, the reduced morbidity and excellent, durable symptom relief obtained in the majority of patients makes transoral stapled diverticulostomy an excellent option for management of Zenker's diverticulum in elderly high-risk patients. The short length of stay and the early resumption of oral intake with stapled diverticulotomy are also clearly advantageous in the geriatric population.

Epiphrenic Diverticulum

In contrast to Zenker's diverticula, epiphrenic diverticula are diverticula that occur in the distal 10 cm of the esophagus (Fig. 46.9). Epiphrenic diverticula are also pulsion diverticula that occur in the setting of increased intraluminal pressure due to underlying neuromuscular motility disorders. Ideal management of epiphrenic diverticula remains controversial but transthoracic resection, either with a traditional open technique or laparoscopic technique, along with a long esophagomyotomy and an antireflux procedure provides reliable functional results with relatively low morbidity and mortality. Various guidelines have been developed for indications for surgical intervention, such as diverticulum size greater than 5 cm; however, because symptoms and clinical progression correlate poorly with diverticular size, a more

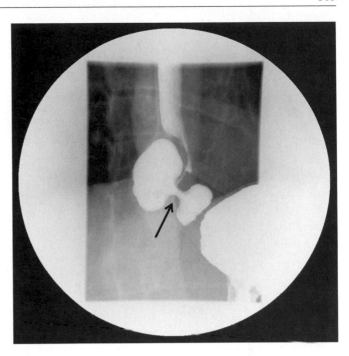

Fig. 46.9 Barium swallow demonstrating an epiphrenic diverticula involving the distal esophagus. The neck of the diverticulum is indicated by the *red arrow*

aggressive approach may limit complications, in particular pulmonary morbidity which has been associated with epiphrenic diverticulum. Of particular note, despite the typical occurrence of epiphrenic diverticula on the right side, a left transthoracic approach remains the best approach for surgical correction. The left transthoracic approach allows access to the diverticulum, distal esophagus, and esophagogastric junction, enables adequate mobilization and resection of the diverticulum, and provides adequate exposure to perform esophagomyotomy and an antireflux procedure [81]. Resection is favored to simple diverticuloplexy, particularly for large diverticula, as resection is associated with better functional outcomes and eliminates the risk of malignant transformation, which can occur in large, chronic diverticula, of the squamous epithelium into invasive squamous cell cancer. It is critical to recognize that epiphrenic diverticula result from motility disorders of the esophagus. In the majority of cases, morbidity results when the underlying esophageal motility disorder is not recognized and appropriately addressed. Diverticulectomy without a concomitant esophagomyotomy has been associated with a high rate of recurrence and suture line leakage, reportedly as high as 20% [81].

Summary

A thorough understanding of the evaluation and management of benign esophageal disease is increasingly important for primary physicians, gastroenterologists, and surgeons.

While benign esophageal diseases may be associated with classic presentations of dysphagia, heartburn and regurgitation, recognition that atypical symptoms are also quite common in the elderly population is crucial. These atypical symptoms, such as chest pain and pulmonary complaints, often co-exist with known cardiac and pulmonary dysfunction, and can lead to misinterpretation of symptoms if the physician and surgeon do not consider esophageal disorders in the differential diagnosis. Careful consideration of benign esophageal disorders in the diagnosis and management of these symptoms will improve patient quality of life through earlier intervention for relief of symptoms and prevent subsequent complications, including aspiration pneumonia and severe malnutrition.

References

1. P.D. U.S. Census Bureau. 2008 National population projections. 2008.
2. Achem SR, Devault KR. Dysphagia in aging. J Clin Gastroenterol. 2005;39(5):357–71.
3. Ribeiro AC et al. Esophageal manometry: a comparison of findings in younger and older patients. Am J Gastroenterol. 1998;93(5):706–10.
4. Soergel KH, Zboralske FF, Amberg JR. Presbyesophagus: esophageal motility in nonagenarians. J Clin Invest. 1964;43:1472–9.
5. DeVault KR. Presbyesophagus: a reappraisal. Curr Gastroenterol Rep. 2002;4(3):193–9.
6. Sheth N, Diner WC. Swallowing problems in the elderly. Dysphagia. 1988;2(4):209–15.
7. Suominen M et al. Malnutrition and associated factors among aged residents in all nursing homes in Helsinki. Eur J Clin Nutr. 2005;59(4):578–83.
8. Siebens H et al. Correlates and consequences of eating dependency in institutionalized elderly. J Am Geriatr Soc. 1986;34(3):192–8.
9. Dejaeger E et al. Manofluorographic analysis of swallowing in the elderly. Dysphagia. 1994;9(3):156–61.
10. Hurwitz AL, Nelson JA, Haddad JK. Oropharyngeal dysphagia manometric and cine esophagraphic findings. Am J Dig Dis. 1975;20(4):313–24.
11. Meier-Ewert HK et al. Effect of age on differences in upper esophageal sphincter and pharynx pressures between patients with dysphagia and control subjects. Am J Gastroenterol. 2001;96(1): 35–40.
12. Kendall KA, Leonard RJ. Pharyngeal constriction in elderly dysphagic patients compared with young and elderly nondysphagic controls. Dysphagia. 2001;16(4):272–8.
13. Celik M et al. Cricopharyngeal muscle electromyography in laryngopharyngeal reflux. Laryngoscope. 2005;115(1):138–42.
14. Andrews JM et al. Is esophageal dysphagia in the extreme elderly (>or=80 years) different to dysphagia younger adults? A clinical motility service audit. Dis Esophagus. 2008;21(7):656–9.
15. Robson KM, Glick ME. Dysphagia and advancing age: are manometric abnormalities more common in older patients? Dig Dis Sci. 2003;48(9):1709–12.
16. Larusson HJ et al. Predictive factors for morbidity and mortality in patients undergoing laparoscopic paraesophageal hernia repair: age, ASA score and operation type influence morbidity. World J Surg. 2009;33(5):980–5.
17. Hazebroek EJ et al. Laparoscopic paraesophageal hernia repair: quality of life outcomes in the elderly. Dis Esophagus. 2008;21(8):737–41.
18. Kahrilas PJ et al. Increased frequency of transient lower esophageal sphincter relaxation induced by gastric distention in reflux patients with hiatal hernia. Gastroenterology. 2000;118(4):688–95.
19. Kahrilas PJ et al. The effect of hiatus hernia on gastro-oesophageal junction pressure. Gut. 1999;44(4):476–82.
20. Kahrilas PJ et al. Attenuation of esophageal shortening during peristalsis with hiatus hernia. Gastroenterology. 1995;109(6):1818–25.
21. Lin S et al. The phrenic ampulla: distal esophagus or potential hiatal hernia? Am J Physiol. 1995;268(2 Pt 1):G320–7.
22. Polomsky M et al. Should elective repair of intrathoracic stomach be encouraged? J Gastrointest Surg. 2010;14(2):203–10.
23. Low DE, Simchuk EJ. Effect of paraesophageal hernia repair on pulmonary function. Ann Thorac Surg. 2002;74(2):333–7. discussion 337.
24. Luketich JD. Outcomes after a decade of laparoscopic giant paraesophageal hernia repair. J Thorac Cardiovasc Surg. 2010; 139(2):395–404.
25. Gangopadhyay N. Outcomes of laparoscopic paraesophageal hernia repair in elderly and high-risk patients. Surgery. 2006;140(4): 491–8. discussion 498–9.
26. Nason KS. Laparoscopic repair of giant paraesophageal hernia results in long term patient satisfaction and a durable repair. J Gastrointest Surg. 2008;12(12):2066–75. discussion 2075–7.
27. Polomsky M et al. A population-based analysis of emergent vs. elective hospital admissions for an intrathoracic stomach. Surg Endosc. 2010;24:1250–5.
28. Nason KS, et al. Adverse outcomes after non-elective giant paraesophageal hernia repair are significantly higher than after elective repair. American College of Surgeons Papers Forum, 2009. Paper presentation, 11 Oct 2009.
29. Pizza F et al. Influence of age on outcome of total laparoscopic fundoplication for gastroesophageal reflux disease. World J Gastroenterol. 2007;13(5):740–7.
30. Brunt LM et al. Is laparoscopic antireflux surgery for gastroesophageal reflux disease in the elderly safe and effective? Surg Endosc. 1999;13(9):838–42.
31. Zhu H et al. Features of symptomatic gastroesophageal reflux in elderly patients. Scand J Gastroenterol. 1993;28(3):235–8.
32. Schoeman MN, Holloway RH. Integrity and characteristics of secondary oesophageal peristalsis in patients with gastro-oesophageal reflux disease. Gut. 1995;36(4):499–504.
33. Iwakiri K et al. Defective triggering of secondary peristalsis in patients with non-erosive reflux disease. J Gastroenterol Hepatol. 2007;22(12):2208–11.
34. Wallner G. Esophageal motility impairment – the cause or consequence of gastroesophageal reflux disease? Przegl Lek. 2000;57 Suppl 5:89–91.
35. Fass R et al. Symptom severity and oesophageal chemosensitivity to acid in older and young patients with gastro-oesophageal reflux. Age Ageing. 2000;29(2):125–30.
36. Linder JD, Wilcox CM. Acid peptic disease in the elderly. Gastroenterol Clin North Am. 2001;30(2):363–76.
37. Vela MF et al. Simultaneous intraesophageal impedance and pH measurement of acid and nonacid gastroesophageal reflux: effect of omeprazole. Gastroenterology. 2001;120(7):1599–606.
38. Gerson LB et al. Oesophageal and gastric pH profiles in patients with gastro-oesophageal reflux disease and Barrett's oesophagus treated with proton pump inhibitors. Aliment Pharmacol Ther. 2004;20(6):637–43.
39. United States Food and Drug Administration. Public health advisory: updated safety information about a drug interaction between Clopidogrel Bisulfate (marketed as Plavix) and Omeprazole (marketed as Prilosec and Prilosec OTC). 2009.

40. Tedesco P. Laparoscopic fundoplication in elderly patients with gastroesophageal reflux disease. Arch Surg. 2006;141(3):289–92. discussion 292.

41. Trus TL et al. Laparoscopic antireflux surgery in the elderly. Am J Gastroenterol. 1998;93(3):351–3.

42. Khajanchee YS et al. Laparoscopic antireflux surgery in the elderly. Surg Endosc. 2002;16(1):25–30.

43. Peters MJ. Meta-analysis of randomized clinical trials comparing open and laparoscopic anti-reflux surgery. Am J Gastroenterol. 2009;104(6):1548–61. quiz 1547, 1562.

44. Ackroyd R et al. Randomized clinical trial of laparoscopic versus open fundoplication for gastro-oesophageal reflux disease. Br J Surg. 2004;91(8):975–82.

45. Pregun I et al. Peptic esophageal stricture: medical treatment. Dig Dis. 2009;27(1):31–7.

46. Heitmiller RF, Redmond M, Hamilton SR. Barrett's esophagus with high-grade dysplasia. An indication for prophylactic esophagectomy. Ann Surg. 1996;224(1):66–71.

47. Wang VS et al. Low prevalence of submucosal invasive carcinoma at esophagectomy for high-grade dysplasia or intramucosal adenocarcinoma in Barrett's esophagus: a 20-year experience. Gastrointest Endosc. 2009;69(4):777–83.

48. Konda VJ et al. Is the risk of concomitant invasive esophageal cancer in high-grade dysplasia in Barrett's esophagus overestimated? Clin Gastroenterol Hepatol. 2008;6(2):159–64.

49. Morganstern B, Anandasabapathy S. GERD and Barrett's esophagus: diagnostic and management strategies in the geriatric population. Geriatrics. 2009;64(7):9–12.

50. Meshkinpour H, Haghighat P, Dutton C. Clinical spectrum of esophageal aperistalsis in the elderly. Am J Gastroenterol. 1994;89(9):1480–3.

51. Ho KY, Tay HH, Kang JY. A prospective study of the clinical features, manometric findings, incidence and prevalence of achalasia in Singapore. J Gastroenterol Hepatol. 1999;14(8):791–5.

52. Sonnenberg A et al. Epidemiology of hospitalization for achalasia in the United States. Dig Dis Sci. 1993;38(2):233–44.

53. Clouse RE, Abramson BK, Todorczuk JR. Achalasia in the elderly. Effects of aging on clinical presentation and outcome. Dig Dis Sci. 1991;36(2):225–8.

54. Eckardt VF, Stauf B, Bernhard G. Chest pain in achalasia: patient characteristics and clinical course. Gastroenterology. 1999;116(6):1300–4.

55. Kilic A et al. Minimally invasive myotomy for achalasia in the elderly. Surg Endosc. 2008;22(4):862–5.

56. Hulselmans M et al. Long-term outcome of pneumatic dilation in the treatment of achalasia. Clin Gastroenterol Hepatol. 2010;8(1):30–5.

57. Tuset JA et al. Endoscopic pneumatic balloon dilation in primary achalasia: predictive factors, complications, and long-term follow-up. Dis Esophagus. 2009;22(1):74–9.

58. Chuah SK et al. Clinical remission in endoscope-guided pneumatic dilation for the treatment of esophageal achalasia: 7-year follow-up results of a prospective investigation. J Gastrointest Surg. 2009;13(5):862–7.

59. Katsinelos P et al. Long-term results of pneumatic dilation for achalasia: a 15 years' experience. World J Gastroenterol. 2005;11(36):5701–5.

60. Eckardt VF, Gockel I, Bernhard G. Pneumatic dilation for achalasia: late results of a prospective follow up investigation. Gut. 2004;53(5):629–33.

61. Neubrand M et al. Long-term results and prognostic factors in the treatment of achalasia with botulinum toxin. Endoscopy. 2002;34(7):519–23.

62. Schuchert MJ et al. Minimally-invasive esophagomyotomy in 200 consecutive patients: factors influencing postoperative outcomes. Ann Thorac Surg. 2008;85(5):1729–34.

63. Gaissert HA et al. Transthoracic Heller myotomy for esophageal achalasia: analysis of long-term results. Ann Thorac Surg. 2006;81(6):2044–9.

64. Frantzides CT et al. Minimally invasive surgery for achalasia: a 10-year experience. J Gastrointest Surg. 2004;8(1):18–23.

65. Sharp KW. 100 consecutive minimally invasive Heller myotomies: lessons learned. Ann Surg. 2002;235(5):631–8. discussion 638–9.

66. Pellegrini C. Thoracoscopic esophagomyotomy. Initial experience with a new approach for the treatment of achalasia. Ann Surg. 1992;216(3):291–6. discussion 296–9.

67. Zaninotto G et al. Four hundred laparoscopic myotomies for esophageal achalasia: a single centre experience. Ann Surg. 2008;248(6):986–93.

68. Patti MG. Minimally invasive surgery for achalasia: an 8-year experience with 168 patients. Ann Surg. 1999;230(4):587–93. discussion 593–4.

69. Wright AS et al. Long-term outcomes confirm the superior efficacy of extended Heller myotomy with Toupet fundoplication for achalasia. Surg Endosc. 2007;21(5):713–8.

70. Roll GR et al. Excellent outcomes of laparoscopic esophagomyotomy for achalasia in patients older than 60 years of age. Surg Endosc. 2010;24:2562–6.

71. Richter JE. Oesophageal motility disorders. Lancet. 2001;358(9284):823–8.

72. Allen ML, DiMarino Jr AJ. Manometric diagnosis of diffuse esophageal spasm. Dig Dis Sci. 1996;41(7):1346–9.

73. Stein HJ. Ambulatory 24-hour esophageal manometry in the evaluation of esophageal motor disorders and noncardiac chest pain. Surgery. 1991;110(4):753–61. discussion 761–3.

74. Crescenzo DG et al. Zenker's diverticulum in the elderly: is operation justified? Ann Thorac Surg. 1998;66(2):347–50.

75. Cook IJ et al. Pharyngeal (Zenker's) diverticulum is a disorder of upper esophageal sphincter opening. Gastroenterology. 1992;103(5):1229–35.

76. Lerut T et al. Zenker's diverticulum: is a myotomy of the cricopharyngeus useful? How long should it be? Hepatogastroenterology. 1992;39(2):127–31.

77. Morse CR et al. Preliminary experience by a thoracic service with endoscopic transoral stapling of cervical (Zenker's) diverticulum. J Gastrointest Surg. 2007;11(9):1091–4.

78. Chiari C et al. Significant symptomatic relief after transoral endoscopic staple-assisted treatment of Zenker's diverticulum. Surg Endosc. 2003;17(4):596–600.

79. Peracchia A et al. Minimally invasive surgery for Zenker diverticulum: analysis of results in 95 consecutive patients. Arch Surg. 1998;133(7):695–700.

80. Rizzetto C. Zenker's diverticula: feasibility of a tailored approach based on diverticulum size. J Gastrointest Surg. 2008;12(12):2057–64. discussion 2064–5.

81. Varghese Jr TK. Surgical treatment of epiphrenic diverticula: a 30-year experience. Ann Thorac Surg. 2007;84(6):1801–9. discussion 1801–9.

82. Bremner CG. Esophageal motility testing made easy. St. Louis: Quality Medical Publishing; 2001. p. 61.

Chapter 47
Surgery for Mediastinal Disease in the Elderly

Cameron D. Wright

Abstract Mediastinal masses present throughout the decades of life but certainly occur with relative frequency in the older population. Furthermore, with the increasing frequency of obtaining pulmonary embolism chest CT scans, there are more incidentally discovered mediastinal abnormalities that require investigation. Relatively common conditions encountered include substernal and intrathoracic goiters, anterior mediastinal masses suspicious for lymphoma, mediastinal lymphadenopathy, thymomas, and posterior mediastinal neurogenic tumors. Mediastinal cysts-pericardial, bronchogenic, and esophageal duplication are all uncommon in the elderly, rarely require any treatment in the elderly population and so will not be discussed.

Keywords Substernal goiter • Anterior mediastinal mass • Lymphoma • Thymoma • Posterior mediastinal neurogenic tumor

Mediastinal masses present throughout the decades of life but certainly occur with relative frequency in the older population. Furthermore, with the increasing frequency of obtaining pulmonary embolism chest CT scans, there are more incidentally discovered mediastinal abnormalities that require investigation. Relatively common conditions encountered include substernal and intrathoracic goiters, anterior mediastinal masses suspicious for lymphoma, mediastinal lymphadenopathy, thymomas, and posterior mediastinal neurogenic tumors. Mediastinal cysts-pericardial, bronchogenic and esophageal duplication are all uncommon in the elderly, rarely require any treatment in the elderly population and so will not be discussed.

C.D. Wright (✉)
Department of Thoracic Surgery, Massachusetts General Hospital,
32 Fruit Street, Blake 1570, Boston, MA 02114-2698, USA
e-mail: wright.cameron@mgh.harvard.edu

Thymoma and Thymic Carcinoma

Thymomas represent the most common mediastinal neoplasm as well as the most common anterior mediastinal compartment neoplasm, constituting about 20 and 50% of all mediastinal and anterior compartment tumors occurring in the adult population, respectively. The overall incidence of thymoma is rare, however; with 0.15 cases/100,000, based upon data from the National Cancer Institute Surveillance, Epidemiology and End Results Program [1]. Thymoma is an epithelial tumor generally considered to have an indolent growth pattern but malignant nonetheless because of potential for local invasion, pleural dissemination, and even systemic metastases. Most patients are between the ages of 40 and 60 years at the time of diagnosis with an equal gender distribution. There is a sizable proportion of thymoma patients over the age of 70, however, 22% in our series. Approximately one-third of patients with localized disease at presentation are symptomatic, most commonly reporting cough or vague chest discomfort. With increasing use of routine CT screening, one would anticipate that a higher percentage of patients will present with asymptomatic disease. Patients demonstrating either locally advanced or disseminated thymoma at the time of presentation are usually symptomatic with significant chest pain, shortness of breath from lung involvement, phrenic nerve paralysis, pleural effusions, and/or SVC syndrome.

Of unique interest, several immune disorders have been associated with thymoma. Myasthenia gravis is the most common autoimmune disease associated with thymoma. Approximately 30–65% of patients with thymoma have been diagnosed with myasthenia gravis in reported series [2, 3]. Conversely only 10–15% of patients with myasthenia gravis will have a thymoma. Patients with thymoma-associated myasthenia gravis can produce autoantibodies to a variety of neuromuscular antigens, particularly the acetylcholine receptor and titin, a striated muscle antigen [4, 5]. Up to 28% of thymoma patients will present with an immune disorder other than myasthenia gravis, the most common include pure red cell aplasia, lupus erythematosus, and hypogammaglobulinemia [2, 3].

M.R. Katlic (ed.), *Cardiothoracic Surgery in the Elderly*, DOI 10.1007/978-1-4419-0892-6_47,
© Springer Science+Business Media, LLC 2011

Diagnosis

Patients presenting with the commonly associated diseases such as myasthenia gravis, red blood cell aplasia, or hypogammaglobulinemia should prompt investigation with a screening chest CT scan to rule out the presence of an asymptomatic thymoma. Conversely, symptoms which may be consistent with myasthenia gravis such as easy fatigability, muscular weakness, diploplia, ptosis, and dysarthria, should be elicited from any patient presenting with a mass in the anterior mediastinal compartment. Neurologic consultation should be considered if there is suspicion of myasthenia particularly for any patient being evaluated for diagnostic and/or therapeutic surgical intervention as severe respiratory morbidity can be minimized with appropriate perioperative management [6–8].

Chest CT scanning with intravenous contrast is the radiographic examination of choice for evaluation of all mediastinal masses in the anterior compartment (Figs. 47.1 and 47.2). CT not only precisely defines size, density characteristics, and relationship to surrounding intrathoracic organs such as the great vessels, lungs, pericardium, and heart but also defines the presence of pleural parietal pleural deposits or so-called "droplet metastases" most frequently found in the posterior basilar pleural space and diaphragm. As this tendency to metastasize in the posterior basilar pleural space is rather unique to thymomas, the radiographic presence of both an anterior compartment mass and "droplet" metastases is highly suggestive of the diagnosis. The edge characteristics of the mass should be carefully studied to look for evidence of invasion. Abutment to important structures should be noted and can help plan surgery to enhance the likelihood

of a complete resection. The internal architecture of the mass should be noted as calcification, hemorrhage, and necrosis are often associated with a more aggressive tumor. CT/PET scans are often used for locally advanced cases and it appears that B3 and thymic carcinomas are quite PET avid [9]. The position of the diaphragm should be noted and if there is any question as to whether the diaphragm is paralyzed a sniff test should be performed.

In general, the differential diagnoses of patients presenting with a mass in the anterior mediastinal compartment are typically initially guided by patient's age, gender, associated symptoms, and CT appearance. Malignant germ cell tumors occur primarily in young adult males and can essentially be ruled out by measuring the serum tumor marker levels of alpha fetoprotein and the beta subunit of human chorionic gonadotropin [10]. Thyroid lesions involving the anterior mediastinal compartment are readily identified on CT scan as contiguous with the thyroid gland. The two main differential diagnoses of most anterior compartment masses are therefore lymphoma and thymoma. In general, thymoma patients are older as compared to patients presenting with lymphoma originating in the anterior mediastinal compartment. Constitutional symptoms such as night sweats, fever, weight loss, and malaise are more consistent with lymphomas. Physical examination including careful palpation of lymph bearing areas such as the neck, axillae, and groins for adenopathy amenable to excisional biopsy, which might establish a diagnosis of lymphoma, is indicated. Anterior mediastinal masses that are associated with surrounding lymphadenopathy are usually lymphomas and should be biopsied rather than excised for diagnosis. A small anterior mediastinal compartment mass in a patient with a history of an associated immune disorder has a high probability of representing a thymoma. In general, we believe that wide surgical

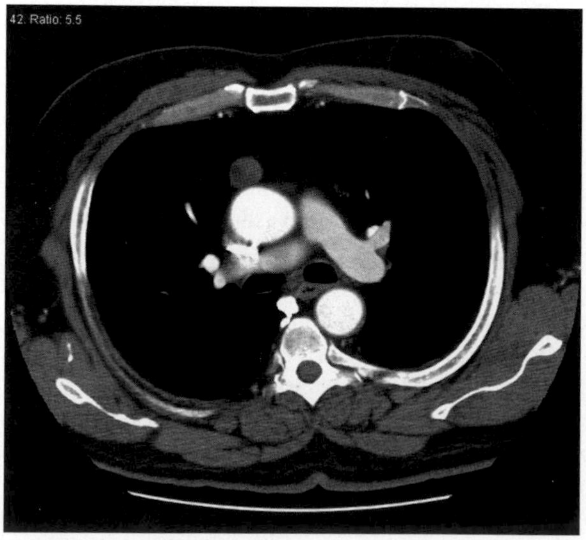

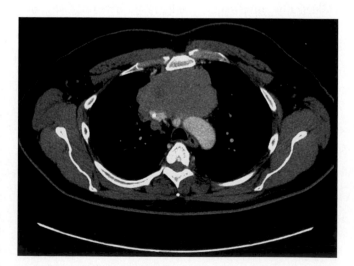

Fig. 47.1 CT scan of a patient with an encapsulated Masaoka stage I thymoma

Fig. 47.2 CT scan of a patient with an invasive Masaoka stage III thymoma

excision including en-bloc thymectomy without biopsy is justified for both diagnostic and likely therapeutic purposes in patients with small anterior mediastinal masses that are clinically thought to be thymomas.

Following initial clinical and CT scan evaluation, biopsy of the anterior compartment mass may be indicated when lymphoma is suspected or a locally advanced thymoma is suspected. The least invasive technique is CT-guided FNA. Cytokeratin staining is a useful diagnostic marker for epithelial type cells in this regard [11]. It must be emphasized, however, that cytology not only lacks sensitivity but also can be misleading with respect to differentiating thymomas and lymphomas [12]. Moreover, a substantial tissue sample for genetic marker studies including flow cytometry is considered optimal prior to treatment for lymphoma. Accordingly, we have become less reliant on CT-guided FNA cytology for diagnosis. In our experience, CT-guided core needle biopsy can usually be safely performed for most larger masses in the anterior compartment particularly if a large bore needle can be passed into the mass without traversing lung parenchyma. Core needle biopsies allow histologic examination of the tumor and immunohistochemical stains can be performed to allow accurate diagnosis. If core needle biopsy is not possible or is non-diagnostic, then two surgical options exist for further diagnostic evaluation. For larger and/or invasive masses, we consider anterior mediastinotomy (Chamberlain procedure) the next diagnostic procedure of choice. The Chamberlain procedure may be performed on either side and at any level which best provides the access to any given anterior mediastinal tumor. Video-assisted thoracic surgery (VATS) does provide excellent exposure to the anterior compartment for biopsy purposes using minimally invasive technology; however, the pleural space is traversed and if thymoma is a diagnostic possibility, pleural space seeding could theoretically occur during VATS biopsy efforts. VATS is very helpful to document pleural disease and obtain a biopsy when patients present with apparent pleural metastases. For small solid masses identified in the anterior mediastinal compartment not amenable to core needle biopsy, several diagnostic options exist. Although open Chamberlain or VATS biopsy could be performed, in otherwise healthy patients, we would advocate complete surgical excision including total thymectomy as a reasonable approach for both diagnostic and therapeutic purposes.

Pathology

Many histological classifications have been described for thymoma and thymic neoplasms in general. Rosai and Levine in 1976 suggested "the definition of thymoma should be restricted to neoplasms of the thymic epithelial cells, regardless of the presence or absence of a lymphoid component or the abundance of the latter." Bernatz proposed the first widely used histologic thymoma classification scheme with the following types: predominantly lymphocytic, predominantly epithelial, predominantly mixed, and predominantly spindle cell type lymphoma. This classification system did not separate the various histologic types into prognostically relevant groups. Levine and Rosai in 1978 proposed a more clinically useful classification system. Benign (noninvasive) thymomas were distinguished from malignant (invasive) thymomas. Malignant thymomas were subdivided into Type I (no or minimal atypia) and Type II (moderate to marked atypia). Type II thymomas were considered thymic carcinomas. This classification system was clinicopathologic since both invasion and the degree of cellular atypia were taken into consideration. Muller-Hermelink and colleagues described a histogenetic classification in 1985. They classified thymomas into medullary and cortical types that reflected the architecture of the normal thymus. This system was of prognostic value but its use was not widespread. More recently, the World Health Organization (WHO) reached a consensus on histologic classification based on both morphology and lymphocyte to epithelial cell ratio using letters and numbers in 1999 and was updated in 2003 [13]. In the WHO system, there are two types of thymomas based on the shape of the neoplastic cell – Type A (spindle or oval) and Type B (dendritic or epithelioid) (Table 47.1). Type B thymomas are subdivided on the basis of the proportional increase (in relation to the number of lymphocytes) in thymocytes and cellular atypia. B1 thymomas are richest in lymphocytes and B3 thymomas have atypia and sparse lymphocytes. Thymomas that have a combination of Type A and B1 features are termed Type AB. Thymic carcinomas (Type C) are named according to their differentiation (squamous cell, neuroendocrine, mucoepidermoid, basaloid, lymphoepithelioma like, sarcomatoid, clear cell, papillary). Type A thymomas have the best prognosis and are usually low stage (Table 47.2). Type B thymomas may recur and are typically higher stage. The WHO classification system is an independent prognostic factor after resection.

Table 47.1 WHO classification of thymomas

WHO type	Traditional nomenclature
Type A	Medullary, spindle cell
Type AB	Mixed
Type B1	Organoid, predominately cortical, lymphocyte predominant
Type B2	Cortical
Type B3	Well-differentiated thymic carcinoma, epithelial predominant, squamoid
Type C	Thymic carcinoma

also be a role for lung sealants, although this has not been well studied. We reserve the instillation of sclerosing agents through thoracostomy tubes for patients who are exceedingly poor operative candidates.

Figures 48.1a and b show preoperative CT images of a 76-year-old male COPD patient with a recurrent and persistent pneumothorax transferred with a thoracostomy tube in-situ. He underwent VATS bullectomy, pleurectomy, and talc pleu-

rodesis with good results. Figure 48.1c shows his CXR on postoperative day four after removal of his drain tubes.

Management of pneumothoraces secondary to malignancy is also more common in elderly patients than in the younger population. An individual approach taking into consideration the patient's prognosis from the underlying disease and their operative risks is advocated.

Table 48.1 Classification of pneumothorax

Spontaneous
Primary
Secondary
  Chronic obstructive pulmonary disease (COPD)
  Malignant – including NSCLC, sarcomas
  Infectious – including abscesses, TB
  Miscellaneous – including sarcoidosis, CF

Acquired
Iatrogenic
Traumatic
  Blunt
  Penetrating

Fluid: Pleural Effusions

Classification and causes of pleural effusions are listed in Table 48.2. The pleural space continuously produces and absorbs fluid with daily transit estimated between 1 and 2 L despite there being only 5 mL in each hemithorax at any one time [7]. Any disruption in the absorption channels of the pleura, or any excess production secondary to changes in osmotic or hydrostatic pressure gradients can result in an effusion. Effusions of varying magnitude and the resulting complications often present in elderly patients, particularly in those with multiple comorbidities. The first principles of

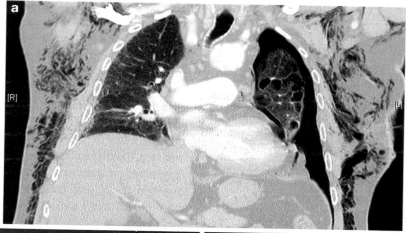

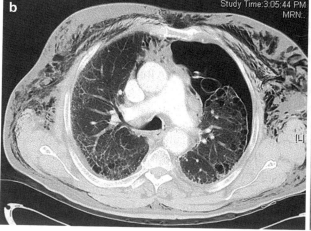

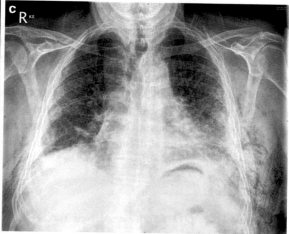

Fig. 48.1 (**a**) Secondary spontaneous pneumothorax – CT Coronal; (**b**) secondary spontaneous pneumothorax – CT axial; (**c**) secondary spontaneous pneumothorax – CXR POD 3 following VATS bullectomy, pleurectomy, and pleurodesis

Table 48.2 Classification of pleural effusions

Transudate
Congestive heart failure
Renal or hepatic failure

Exudate
Benign
  Infectious
  Transudate
  Congestive heart failure
  Miscellaneous – including collagen vascular diseases, drug induced
Malignant

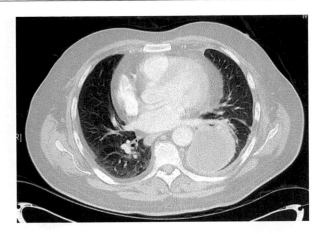

Fig. 48.2 Posterior empyema – CT

management include biochemical analysis via aspiration to ascertain if the fluid is transudative or exudative. Surgery is generally not warranted in the management of transudative effusions. In the elderly, surgeons will most commonly be involved in the management of infectious collections (parapneumonic effusions or empyemas) and malignant effusions.

Pleural Space Infections

Pleural effusions may accompany over 50% of pneumonias, the majority of which are sterile and are referred to as simple parapneumonic effusions that resolve with antibiotics alone [8]. Occasionally these simple effusions progress secondary to bacterial contamination of the pleural space and subsequent fibrin deposition. These complex parapneumonic effusions are more common in the elderly and often require surgical intervention [9]. Risk factors for development of complex parapneumonic effusions include diabetes, rheumatoid arthritis, and gastroesophageal reflux [10, 11].

Surgeons are generally involved after the diagnosis is made. In addition to adequate antibiotic therapy and maintenance of nutritional status, the goals of surgery in the elderly remain the same, evacuation of infected material and the obliteration of any remaining pleural space. Imaging plays an important role in the choice of intervention. Nonloculated lateral or anterior collections can often be treated with tube thoracostomy alone with good results. The size of the drainage tube may be influenced by the nature of the fluid with smaller diameter tubes appropriate for thin effusions, and larger bore tubes placed for frankly purulent collections. Collections that are posterior, particularly in the costo-diaphragmatic recess (Fig. 48.2), are difficult to drain percutaneously due to the narrow intercostal spaces and consideration of more invasive surgical procedures should be entertained.

Patients with frank empyema or complex multiloculated collections should have some form of open drainage particularly if they remain septic after tube thoracostomy. In patients with acceptable anesthetic risk, some form of decortication (VATS or thoracotomy) is the preferred therapy [12–19].

Figure 48.3a–c show a complex loculated effusion in an 83-year-old female with sputum and blood cultures positive for *Pseudomonas aeruginosa*. She underwent VATS decortication with rapid improvement. A CXR on postoperative day 3 is shown in Fig. 48.3d with resolution of the infection and re-expansion of the lung. We have found VATS procedures particularly helpful in managing elderly patients. In a 4-year period (09/2005 – 09/2009), at one of our institutions (NA) we have performed 75 decortications (72 VATS and 3 Open) in patients over the age of seventy for various indications including empyema, retained hemothorax following cardiac surgery or blunt trauma, and mesothelioma (palliative). There was one death for an operative mortality of 1.3% (unpublished data).

Some older patients do have prohibitive anesthetic risks which require other strategies. Trials of fibrinolytic therapy through drain tubes can be considered in this cohort of patients [8]. A number of studies using urokinase and streptokinase have been published suggesting they are safe, but the randomized trials have been underpowered to detect effects on mortality or any decrease in the need for further surgery [20–22]. Another strategy is to employ the old technique of rib resection and drainage under local anesthesia, with placement and gradual withdrawal over a number of weeks of an empyema tube [12, 23]. This method has some merit in those patients deemed too unwell for general anesthesia keeping in mind the time honored thoracic surgical dictum, "No space, no problem."

Malignant Pleural Effusions

Malignant pleural effusions cause considerable distress to elderly oncology patients and are occasionally the first presentation of malignancy. More than 75% of malignant effusions are caused by carcinomas of the lung, breast or ovary, and lymphomas with adenocarcinoma the most common histological subtype overall [24–29]. The median survival for all-comers is only 4 months after presentation. Palliation of

with surgery reserved for patients who do not have progression of disease after chemotherapy. Surgery is either extrapleural pneumonectomy (EPP) or pleurectomy/decortication (P/D) depending on the burden of disease. Hemithoracic irradiation is administered following surgery.

We have previously published results on a cohort of 663 patients that underwent either EPP or P/D [53]. A greater proportion of elderly patients underwent P/D. Patient selection prior to surgery based on cardiopulmonary function and performance status is essential. However, on multivariate analysis age demonstrated a hazard ratio of 1, suggesting that age plays a minimal role in outcome as long as patients are selected properly.

The treatment of MPM in the elderly is subject to the same caveats as that for younger patients. Curative treatment approaches should be undertaken with multidisciplinary teams in high volume centers with specialist expertise, preferably under the auspices of a clinical trial. The role and even the extent of surgery in this disease remains undefined for patients of all ages. However, age alone should not prevent patients from undergoing treatment.

References

1. Melton LJ, Hepper NCG, Offord KP. Incidence of spontaneous pneumothorax in Olmstead County, Minnesota: 1950 to 1974. Am Rev Respir Dis. 1979;120:1379–82.
2. Light RW, O'Hara VS, Moritz TE, et al. Intrapleural tetracycline for the prevention of recurrent spontaneous pneumothorax. JAMA. 1990;264:2224–30.
3. Miller AC, Harvey JE. Guidelines for the management of spontaneous pneumothorax. BMJ. 1993;307:114–6.
4. Baumann MH, Strange C, Heffner JE, et al. Management of spontaneous pneumothorax. Chest. 2001;119:590–2.
5. Videau V, Pillgram-Larsen J, Oyvind E, et al. Spontaneous pneumothorax in COPD: complications, treatment and recurrences. Eur J Respir Dis. 1987;71:365–71.
6. Shen KR, Cerfolio RJ. Decision making in the management of secondary spontaneous pneumothorax in patients with severe emphysema. Thorac Surg Clin. 2009;19:233–8.
7. Little AG. The management of pleural space problems. In: Franco KL and Putnam JB, editors. Advanced Therapy in Thoracic Surgery. 2nd ed. Hamilton: BC Decker; 2005. p 205–14.
8. Chapman SJ, Davies RJO. The management of pleural space infections. Respirology. 2004;9:4–11.
9. Davies CW, Kearney SE, Gleeson FV, Davies RJ. Predictors of outcome and long-term survival in patients with pleural infection. Am J Respir Crit Care Med. 1999;160:1682–7.
10. Chen KY, Hsueh PR, Liaw YS, Yang PC, Luh KT. A 10-year experience with bacteriology of acute thoracic empyema: emphasis on *Klebsiella pneumoniae* in patients with diabetes mellitus. Chest. 2000;117:1685–9.
11. Maskell NA, Davies CW, Jones E, Davies RJO. Characteristics of the first 150 patients participating in the MRC/BTS MIST empyema trial. Thorax. 2001;56(Suppl III):40–1.
12. Katariya K, Thurer RJ. Surgical management of empyema. Clin Chest Med. 1998;19:395–406.
13. Angelillo Mackinlay TA, Lyons GA, Chimondeguy DJ, Piedras MA, Angaramo G, Emery J. VATS debridement versus thoracotomy in the treatment of loculated postpneumonia empyema. Ann Thorac Surg. 1996;61:1626–30.
14. Waller DA, Rengarajan A. Thoracoscopic decortication: a role for video-assisted surgery in chronic postpneumonic pleural empyema. Ann Thorac Surg. 2001;71(6):1813–6.
15. Landreneau RJ, Keenan RJ, Hazelrigg SR, Mack MJ, Naunheim KS. Thoracoscopy for empyema and hemothorax. Chest. 1996;109:18–24.
16. Podbielski FJ, Maniar HS, Rodriguez HE, Hernan MJ, Vigneswaran WT. Surgical strategy of complex empyema thoracis. JSLS. 2000;4:287–90.
17. Cunniffe MG, Maguire D, McAnena OJ, Johnston S, Gilmartin JJ. Video-assisted thoracoscopic surgery in the management of loculated empyema. Surg Endosc. 2000;14:175–8.
18. Powell LL, Allen R, Brenner M, Aryan HE, Chen JC. Improved patient outcome after surgical treatment for loculated empyema. Am J Surg. 2000;179:1–6.
19. Lackner RP, Hughes R, Anderson LA, Sammut PH, Thompson AB. Video-assisted evacuation of empyema is the preferred procedure for management of pleural space infections. Am J Surg. 2000;179:27–30.
20. Davies RJO, Traill ZC, Gleeson FV. Randomised controlled trial of intra-pleural streptokinase in community acquired pleural infection. Thorax. 1997;52:416–21.
21. Bouros D, Schiza S, Tzanakis N, Chalkiadakis G, Drositis J, Siafakas N. Intrapleural urokinase versus normal saline in the treatment of complicated parapneumonic effusions and empyema. Am J Respir Crit Care Med. 1999;159:37–42.
22. Thomson AH, Hull J, Kumar MR, Wallis C, Balfour Lynn IM. Randomised trial of intrapleural urokinase in the treatment of childhood empyema. Thorax. 2002;57:343–7.
23. Ali I, Unruh H. Management of empyema thoracis. Ann Thorac Surg. 1990;50(3):355–9.
24. Henschke CI, Yankelevitz DF, Davis SD. Pleural diseases: multimodality imaging and clinical management. Curr Probl Diagn Radiol. 1991;20:155–81.
25. Anderson CB, Philpott GW, Ferguson TB. The treatment of malignant pleural effusions. Cancer. 1974;33:916–22.
26. Storey DD, Dines DE, Coles DT. Pleural effusion. A diagnostic dilemma. JAMA. 1976;236:2183–6.
27. Martinez-Moragon E, Aparicio J, Sanchis J, Menendez R. Cruz Rogado M et al. Malignant pleural effusion:prognostic factors for survival and response to chemical pleurodesis in a series of 120 cases. Respiration. 1998;65:108–13.
28. Hausheer FH, Yarbro JW. Diagnosis and treatment of malignant pleural effusion. Cancer Metastasis Rev. 1987;6:23–40.
29. Awasthi A, Gupta N, Srinivasan R, Nijhawan R, Rajwanshi A. Cytopathological spectrum of unusual malignant pleural effusions at a tertiary care centre in north India. Cytopathology. 2007;18:28–32.
30. Heffner JE. Diagnosis and management of malignant pleural effusions. Respirology. 2008;13:5–20.
31. Lee YC, Baumann MH, Maskell NA, Waterer GW, Eaton TE, et al. Pleurodesis practice for malignant pleural effusions in five English-speaking countries: survey of pulmonologists. Chest. 2003;124:2229–38.
32. Tan C, Sedrakyan A, Browne J, Swift S, Treasure T. The evidence on the effectiveness of management for malignant pleural effusion: a systematic review. Eur J Cardiothorac Surg. 2006;29:829–38.
33. Katlic MR. Video-assisted thoracic surgery utilizing local anesthesia and sedation. Eur J Cardiothorac Surg. 2006;30:529–32.
34. Shaw P, Agarwal R. Pleurodesis for malignant pleural effusions. Cochrane Database Syst Rev. 2004;1:CD002916.

35. Dresler CM, Olak J, Herndon II JE, Richards WG, Scalzetti E, et al. Phase III intergroup study of talc poudrage vs talc slurry sclerosis for malignant pleural effusion. Chest. 2005;127:909–15.

36. Arapis K, Caliandro R, Stern JB, Girard P, Debrosse D, et al. Thoracoscopic palliative treatment of malignant pleural effusions: results in 273 patients. Surg Endosc. 2006;20:919–23.

37. Brega-Massone PP, Lequaglie C, Magnani B, Ferro F, Cataldo I. Chemical pleurodesis to improve patients' quality of life in the management of malignant pleural effusions. The 15 year experience of the National Cancer Institute of Milan. Surg Laparosc Endosc Percutan Tech. 2004;14:73–9.

38. Cardillo G, Facciolo F, Carbone L, Regal M, Corzani F, et al. Long-term follow-up of video-assisted talc pleurodesis in malignant recurrent pleural effusions. Eur J Cardiothorac Surg. 2002;21:302–5; discussion 5–6.

39. Crnjac A. The significance of thoracoscopic mechanical pleurodesis for the treatment of malignant pleural effusions. Wien Klin Wochenschr. 2004;116 Suppl 2:28–32.

40. Gasparri R, Leo F, Veronesi G, Depas T, Colleoni M, et al. Video-assisted management of malignant pleural effusion in breast carcinoma. Cancer. 2006;106:271–6.

41. Marrazzo A, Noto A, Casa L, Taormina P, Lo Gerfo D, et al. Video-thoracoscopic surgical pleurodesis in the management of malignant pleural effusion: the importance of an early intervention. J Pain Symptom Manage. 2005;30:75–9.

42. Trotter D, Aly A, Siu L, Knight S. Video-assisted thoracoscopic (VATS) pleurodesis for malignant effusion: an Australian teaching hospital's experience. Heart Lung Circ. 2005;14:93–7.

43. van den Toorn LM, Schaap E, Surmont VF, Pouw EM, van der Rijt KC, et al. Management of recurrent malignant pleural effusions with a chronic indwelling pleural catheter. Lung Cancer. 2005;50:123–7.

44. Putnam Jr JB, Light RW, Rodriguez RM, Ponn R, Olak J, et al. A randomized comparison of indwelling pleural catheter and doxycycline pleurodesis in the management of malignant pleural effusions. Cancer. 1999;86:1992–9.

45. Putnam Jr JB, Walsh GL, Swisher SG, Roth JA, Suell DM, et al. Outpatient management of malignant pleural effusion by a chronic indwelling pleural catheter. Ann Thorac Surg. 2000;69:369–75.

46. Pollak JS, Burdge CM, Rosenblatt M, Houston JP, Hwu WJ, et al. Treatment of malignant pleural effusions with tunneled long-term drainage catheters. J Vasc Interv Radiol. 2001;12:201–8.

47. Tremblay A, Michaud G. Single-centre experience with 250 tunnelled pleural catheter insertions for malignant pleural effusion. Chest. 2006;129:362–8.

48. Pien GW, Gant MJ, Washam CL, Sterman DH. Use of an implantable pleural catheter for trapped lung syndrome in patients with malignant pleural effusion. Chest. 2001;119:1641–6.

49. Musani AI, Haas AR, Seijo L, Wilby M, Sterman DH. Outpatient management of malignant pleural effusions with small-bore, tunneled pleural catheters. Respiration. 2004;71:559–66.

50. Ohm C, Park D, Vogen M, Bendick P, Welsh R, et al. Use of an indwelling pleural catheter compared with thorascopic talc pleurodesis in the management of malignant pleural effusions. Am Surg. 2003;69:198–202; discussion.

51. Flores RM, Rusch VW. Diffuse malignant mesothelioma. In: Shields TW, Ponn LJ, RB RVW, editors. General thoracic surgery. 6th ed. Philadelphia: Lippincott Williams & Wilkins; 2005. p. 901–21.

52. Vogelzang NJ, Rusthoven JJ, Symanowski J, et al. Phase III study of pemetrexed in combination with cisplatin versus cisplatin alone in patients with malignant pleural mesothelioma. J Clin Oncol. 2003;21:2636–44.

53. Flores RM, Pass HI, Seshan VE, Dycoco J, Zakowski M, Carbone M, et al. Extrapleural pneumonectomy versus pleurectomy/decortications in the surgical management of malignant pleural mesothelioma: results in 663 patients. J Thorac Cardiovasc Surg. 2008;135(3):620–6.

Chapter 49
Surgery for Chest Wall Disease in the Elderly

Daniel L. Miller

Abstract Surgery for chest wall disease in the elderly can be a challenge. A comprehensive preoperative evaluation to determine the risks and benefits prior to proceeding with chest wall resection and reconstruction is warranted. A team approach of thoracic surgeons, plastic surgeons, critical care specialists, and oncologist is necessary to maximize the successful outcome with minimal morbidity and mortality in elderly patients who undergo surgery for chest wall diseases.

Keywords Chest wall resection • Muscle flaps • Chest wall reconstruction • Soft tissue • Ribs • Sternum

Chest wall reconstruction has been a challenge that surgeons have been confronted with much apprehension for over 100 years. Improvements in surgical technique and anesthesia, critical care, antibiotics, and the development and refinement in reconstruction techniques have allowed extensive chest wall resections to be performed in all patients, even the elderly, with acceptable morbidity and mortality.

Chest wall reconstruction techniques were first introduced in the 1940s. Watson and James [1] described the use of fascia lata grafts for closure of chest wall defects. Maier treated large anterior defects with cutaneous flaps that included the remaining breast, while Pickrell et al. advanced surgical treatment of recurrent breast carcinoma by resecting a portion of chest wall [2, 3]. Bisgard and Swenson [4] were the first to use rib grafts as horizontal struts for reconstruction after sternal resection.

Use of a muscle flap was originally described by Tansini in 1906 when he used a latissimus dorsi muscle flap for coverage of the anterior chest wall after radical mastectomy, whereas Campbell in 1950 first introduced the latissimus dorsi muscle as a chest wall reconstruction flap of a full-thickness anterior thorax defect when the muscle was covered immediately with a split-thickness skin graft (STSG) [5, 6]. Kiricuta [7] from Rumania was the first to describe transposition of the great omentum for reconstruction of chest wall defects.

These methods of soft tissue reconstruction went unnoticed for nearly 20 years, until interest in muscle transposition was revived. Muscle and musculocutaneous flaps of the latissimus dorsi, pectoralis major, serratus anterior, rectus abdominis, and external oblique muscles are now used frequently. The clarification of the functional anatomy and blood supply of these muscles have resulted in more aggressive resections in the treatment of chest wall tumors and in the surgical amelioration of the ravages of radiation therapy; the latter being common in older patients. Reports by McCormack and Larson and their colleagues, as well as by Arnold and Pairolero, and by Pairolero and Arnold confirmed that aggressive resection of the chest wall with immediate, dependable reconstruction is reasonable for managing these problems in the elderly [8–17].

Indications

The most common indications for a chest wall resection include primary or metastatic chest wall neoplasms, tumors contiguous from breast and lung cancer, radiation necrosis, congenital defects, trauma, infectious processes from osteomyelitis or median sternotomy or lateral thorocotomy incisions (Table 49.1). The chest wall defect produced by resection of most neoplasms involve loss of the skeleton and frequently the overlying soft tissues as well, while infection, radiation necrosis, and trauma produce partial- or full-thickness defects, depending on their severity.

Preoperative Evaluation

Chest wall resection and reconstruction is a major undertaking and has the full potential for life-threatening complications. As discussed by Azarow et al. [18], accurate preoperative assessment is critical because it will allow the detection and

D.L. Miller (✉)
Section of General Thoracic Surgery, Emory University School of Medicine, 1365 Clifton Road, NE, Atlanta, GA 30322, USA
e-mail: dlmill2@emory.edu

M.R. Katlic (ed.), *Cardiothoracic Surgery in the Elderly*, DOI 10.1007/978-1-4419-0892-6_49,
© Springer Science+Business Media, LLC 2011

Table 49.1 Indications for chest wall reconstruction

Neoplasms
  Primary
  Metastatic
  Direct extension
    Breast
    Lung
  Recurrent
Infection
  Median sternotomy incision
  Thoracotomy incision
  Osteomyelitis
  Costochondritis
Radiation injury
Trauma

treatment of correctable problems. The patient at high risk for developing postoperative complications can often be identified by history and physical examination, radiographic assessment, routine laboratory examinations, and cardiopulmonary function analysis. The importance of a careful respiratory history cannot be overemphasized. The patient's smoking habits, occupational exposure, and other possible exposure to pulmonary irritants should also be established. The presence of dyspnea, cough, sputum, and wheeze should be thoroughly evaluated. The extent of any underlying lung disease should be documented. Routine pulmonary function testing should be performed in all patients to determine the pulmonary status of the patient to anticipate postoperative complications, predict the need for ventilatory support, and maximize the patient's recovery.

Although the majority of patients do not undergo concomitant lung and chest wall resections (34% present in our series), the loss in ventilatory capacity in those with a preexisting marginal respiratory function may lead to prolonged respiratory support and pulmonary complications in the postoperative period [19]. After careful preoperative screening and as indicated, we do not hesitate to perform concomitant pulmonary resections with chest wall resection. This is also the philosophy of the thoracic surgeons at the Mayo Clinic and Memorial Sloan Kettering Cancer Center that in patients who have lung cancer and concomitant chest wall involvement that a combined chest wall and lung resection is warranted to achieve long-term survival [20, 21]. Non-pulmonary risk factors, such as cardiovascular and renal disease, are equally important. Age itself, however, is relatively unimportant if the patient is otherwise in good health.

Principles of Reconstruction

In the treatment of patients requiring chest wall resection, three principles of surgical resection should be maintained [22]. First, a sufficient amount of tissue must be resected to dispose of all devitalized tissue. Second, in segments of large chest wall resections, replacement must be found to restore the rigid chest wall to prevent physiologic flail. Third, healthy soft tissue coverage is essential to seal the pleural space, to protect the viscera and great vessels, and to prevent infection. A combined multidisciplinary approach with plastic and reconstruction surgeons, thoracic surgeons, and critical care specialist provides an acceptable functional result after chest wall resections.

A basic rule prior to the institution of chest wall reconstruction is an appropriate and thorough chest wall resection that leaves healthy, viable margins to which materials and tissues used in a reconstruction may be anchored securely. Careful preoperative assessment for the extent of disease in patients with primary or metastatic malignancies is necessary prior to chest wall resection or reconstruction [19]. This is particularly important in patients with breast and lung cancer locally invading the chest wall and in patients with metastasis to the ribs or the sternum. More recently, PET scanning has been utilized to determine the presence of non-thoracic metastatic disease which is not infrequent in these patients and in the majority of cases negate an extensive chest wall resection.

Chest wall resection for local failure provides palliation for pain and removal of an ulcerated occasionally pungent mass, thus potentially improving quality of life even if age is a factor. Moreover, it may give the best opportunity for local control when combined with adjuvant chemotherapy and radiation. However, we caution that careful preoperative selection should be exercised in patients with recurrent local tumor owing to their high mortality rate [23]. In the era of superb technologic advances in radiation and chemotherapy and if no distant metastatic disease is present, we believe that chest wall resection and reconstruction after or before chemoradiation should be the standard of care in patients with chest wall tumors regardless of the cell type.

The ability to close large chest wall defects is the main consideration in the surgical treatment of most chest wall problems. Excision should not be undertaken if the surgeon does not have the confidence and ability to close the defect. The critical questions of whether or not the reconstructed thorax will support respiration and protect the underlying organs must be answered when considering both the extent of resection and the method of reconstruction. This is true whether the thorax is involved with a neoplasm, an infection, or radiation necrosis. Adequate resection and dependable reconstruction are the mandatory ingredients for successful treatment. These two important items are accomplished most safely, as Arnold and Pairolero [11] noted, by the joint efforts of a thoracic surgeon and a plastic surgeon.

Reconstruction of chest wall defects involves consideration of many factors (Table 49.2). The location and size are of utmost importance, but the past medical history and local conditions of the wound may drastically alter a reconstructive choice. Primary closure remains the best option available

Table 49.2 Reconstruction factors

Location
Size
Depth
  Partial thickness
  Full thickness
Duration
Condition of tissue
  Radiation
  Infection
  Recurrent cancer
  Residual cancer
  Redo (scarring)
Performance status
  Nutrition
  Pulmonary
  Cardiac
  Corticosteroid use
  Diabetes mellitus
  Immunocomprized
  Chronic infection
Quality of life/work profession
Prognosis

when possible. If the defect is partial thickness and will accept and support a skin graft, reconstruction in this manner is quite reasonable. If a partial-thickness defect will not reliably accept a skin graft, a situation that frequently occurs with radiation necrosis, omental transposition with skin grafting should be used. If full-thickness reconstruction is required, both the structural stability of the thorax and soft tissue coverage must be considered.

Radiation therapy has undoubtedly saved many lives and benefited countless other patients. However, the reconstructive surgeon is rarely, if ever, asked to see a recipient of such therapy who has had absolutely no problems. Rather, most patients have impending or actual chest wall ulceration, or complicated by the ever-present possibility of recurrent cancer, or the presence of active infection. Certainly, situations arise when resection and reconstruction are reasonable alternatives despite the possible presence of metastatic disease. In many of these patients, the quality of life can be vastly improved with such a procedure. It is also important to understand the extent of radiation injury in adjacent tissues. Computed tomography (CT) and magnetic resonance (MR) imaging are helpful because they more accurately delineate the condition of the underlying lung and mediastinum. Such information may, in fact, be more important than the presence or absence of distant metastases. Knowledge of the presence of a mediastinal abscess or destroyed lung is critical for successful chest wall resection and reconstruction. If a history of chest wall bleeding is present, consideration should be given to angiography if there is any suspicion of involvement of the heart or great vessels. Similarly, parasternal ulceration deserves careful evaluation because of potential erosion into the mammary vessels, with severe hemorrhage as its sequelae.

Reconstruction of acquired thoracic defects requires attention to management of: (1) pleural cavity, (2) skeletal support, and (3) soft tissue coverage. In elderly patients, the main focus is usually on the actual chest wall reconstruction (skeletal support and soft tissue coverage); however, the management of the pleural cavity is also essential and may be the single component that adversely affects the ultimate recovery of elderly patients.

Management of Pleural Cavity

Transposition of muscle flaps or vascularized tissue into the chest cavity is widely used to obliterate post-pneumonectomy empyema space, closure of bronchopleural, or tracheoesophageal fistulas. Excellent local flap options include extrathoracic muscles (latissimus dorsi, serratus, and pectoralis major) and omentum previously described at our institution. These muscles are easily passed through a 4–5 cm chest wall defect with a one- to two-rib resection, location of which depends on the muscle used and its dominant blood supply. These defects are then closed over chest tubes for drainage with appropriate antibiotic usage. The maintenance of chest wall mechanics relies on both an air-tight seal within the pleural cavity as well as skeletal support over the thorax. One exception to this end is that the severely debility is controlled by creating an Eloesser flap to drain the pleural cavity until appropriate for closure. Another important issue in the management of these pleural cavity infections is the timing of the reconstruction. The success rate is higher if treatment is instituted early, prior to maturation of the empyema cavity. Thoracoplasty or total collapse of the chest wall with obliteration of the remaining pleural cavities is reserved as a last resort for chronic empyema.

Management of Skeleton

The management of chest wall defects requires similar logic with a thorough analysis of the defect and understanding of respiratory mechanics. Restoration of skeletal stability is often required to protect intrathoracic contents as well as to preserve the mechanical forces that allow respiration. Integrity of the diaphragm and accessory muscles of inspiration should always be considered when accessing the skeletal defect, and when deciding on appropriate local flap coverage if needed.

In cases where structural integrity is necessary for preventing chest wall collapse, methyl methacrylate sandwich, silicone, Teflon, or acrylic materials have been utilized.

While it is still unclear of the importance of the rigidity of the chest wall reconstruction, observations of chest wall trauma give much significance to the presence of paradoxical motion of the chest wall. However, this uncoordinated motion during respiration is seen in almost every major resection of the chest wall, but it is not associated with pulmonary insufficiency, which is seen with its traumatic counterpart, flail chest. A methyl methacrylate sandwich (Fig. 49.1) is commonly used with Prolene or Marlex mesh with excellent physiologic and aesthetic success [19, 24]. Daigeler et al. [25] observed that pulmonary function was only moderately reduced and was not significantly affected by the resection size or location. They concluded that thoracic wall reconstruction provides excellent thoracic wall stability to maintain pulmonary function, but postoperative pain and sensation disorders were considerable. Although a variety of synthetic materials can be used to reconstruct the chest wall defect, there is no consensus on the most physiologic or efficacious material [24, 26].

Historically, bone, diced cartilage, metal sheets, autogenous rib graft, fascia lata, Teflon, and numerous other substances have been used with minimal success. With modern surgical technique a wide range of reconstructive options are at the surgeon's disposal and hence it is imperative that the appropriate procedure be selected in a given patient. In general, all full-thickness skeletal defects that have the potential for paradox should be reconstructed. The decision not to reconstruct the skeleton depends on the size and location of the defect. For small defects (less than 5 cm) or those located posteriorly under the scapula above the fourth rib (after resection of Pancoast tumors), the skeleton component can be ignored and the defect closed with only soft tissue. For patients undergoing large chest wall defects (greater than

5 cm), stabilization of the chest wall defect is indicated. Arnold and Pairolero [14] state that most patients can tolerate sternectomy or resection of four to six ribs at the cartilage level without experiencing flail chest or respiratory insufficiency postoperatively. Although the number of resected ribs is an important indicator for mesh usage, there does not appear to be a direct association between the number of ribs resected and the need for mesh reconstruction. This is likely to be due to the presence of additional factors that influence chest wall stability and subsequently the decision process regarding the necessity for mesh reconstruction. Such factors include defect location and history of radiation. Location of the chest wall defect did appear to influence the need for skeletal stabilization, with mesh reconstruction being required more often for the lateral defects. The lack of sternal or spinal stability in that location renders the patient more prone to flail chest deformities which can be detrimental in elderly patients.

Reconstruction can be with autogenous tissue such as fascia lata or ribs (Table 49.3) or synthetic prosthetic materials (Table 49.4). LeRoux and Shama have set fourth the ideal characteristics of a prosthetic material: *rigidity* to abolish paradoxical chest motion, *inertness* to allow in-growth of fibrous tissue and decrease the likelihood of infection, *malleability* so that it can be fashioned to the appropriate shape at the time of operation, and *radiolucency* to allow radiographic follow-up of the underlying problem [27].

Because no substance has been found to fulfill all the criteria, synthetic or alloplastic materials can used if chest

Table 49.3 Autogenous tissue

Fascia lata
Rib
Muscle
Latissimus dorsi
Pectoralis major
Rectus abdominis
Serratus anterior
External oblique
Trapezius
Deltoid
Omentum
STSG

STSG Split-thickness skin graft

Table 49.4 Synthetic material

Prolene mesh
Marlex mesh
Vicryl mesh
PTFE soft tissue patch
Methyl methacrylate sandwich
Bovine pericardium

PTFE Polytetrafluoroethylene

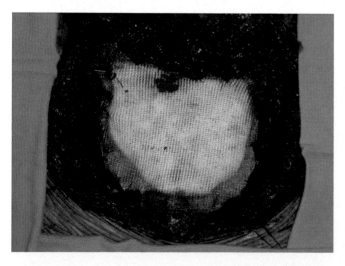

Fig. 49.1 Methyl methacrylate marlex mesh sandwich reconstruction after an anterior sternal and chest wall resection for an angiosarcoma related to radiation therapy for breast cancer

wall integrity is compromised. Synthetic mesh (e.g., Marlex [knitted polypropylene] by Davol and Bard, Cranston, RI; Prolene by Ethicon, Inc, Somerville, NJ; 2-mm PTFE [polytetrafluoroethylene] soft tissue patch by W.L. Gore and Associates, Inc, Flagstaff, AZ; Vicryl [polyglactin 910] by Ethicon, Inc., Somerville, NJ; methyl methacrylate sandwich [polymethyl methacrylate] by Stryker Howmedica Osteonics, Mahwah, NJ) can be utilized for attaining rib or sternal stability. Placing either of these materials under tension improves the rigidity of the prosthesis in all directions. Sutures are often placed in an interrupted fashion around the ribs for added strength and support. The PTFE soft tissue patch (Fig. 49.2) is superior because it prevents movement of fluid and air across the reconstructed chest wall. Marlex mesh is used less frequently because when placed under tension, it is rigid in one direction only. Although Pairolero and Arnold [15, 16] believe that reconstruction with rigid material such as methyl methacrylate impregnated meshes is not necessary. McCormack and Mansour and colleagues have been strong advocates of this reconstruction technique with excellent results [19, 22]. For the most part, the choice of prosthetic material is based on surgeon's preferences as Deschamps et al. [28] have shown that there was no significant difference in the rate of postoperative success or complications exist between the use of Prolene mesh and PTFE soft tissue patch for chest wall reconstruction.

Full-thickness skeletal defects resulting from excision of tumors of both the sternum and lateral chest wall should be reconstructed if the wound is not contaminated. If the wound is contaminated from previous radiation necrosis or necrotic neoplasm, reconstruction with prosthetic material is usually not advised, because the prosthesis may subsequently become infected, resulting in obligatory removal. Two materials may be used in this situation as a temporary device, Vicryl (Ethicon Inc., Summerville, NJ) mesh or bovine pericardium (Synovis,

Inc., St Paul, MN). A combination of materials can be used in these situations such as bioabsorbable PDS bars (Acute Innovations, Los Angeles, CA) (Fig. 49.3) or titanium struts (Stratos, Inc., Stratosburg, France) (Fig. 49.4) for skeletal rigidity and covered with remodeled bovine pericardium (Veritas-Synovis Surgical Innovations, St Paul MN) (Figs. 49.5 and 49.6) to close the pleural cavity. Also, reconstruction with a musculocutaneous flap alone can also be performed. Similarly, resection of the bony thorax in a patient who

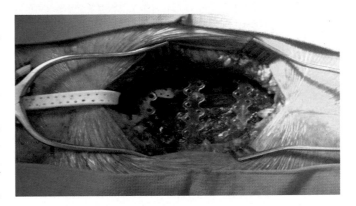

Fig. 49.3 PDS strut reconstruction after sternal resection

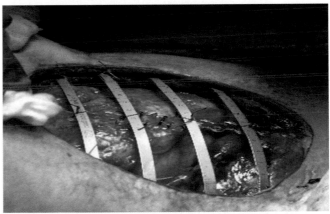

Fig. 49.4 Titanium strut reconstruction of lateral chest wall

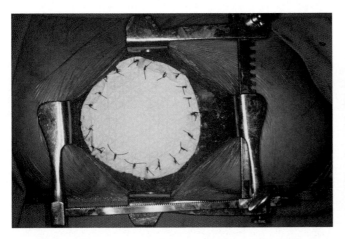

Fig. 49.2 PTFE soft tissue patch reconstruction of the lateral chest wall after resection for lung cancer

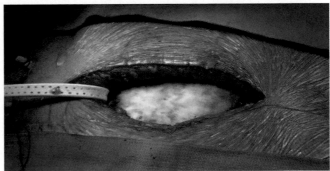

Fig. 49.5 Bovine (Veritas) pericardial patch coverage of sternal PDS struts

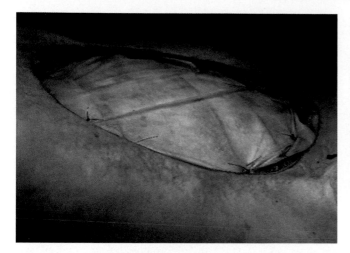

Fig. 49.6 Bovine (Veritas) pericardial patch coverage of lateral chest wall titanium struts

has been previously irradiated may not require skeletal reconstruction because the lung frequently adheres to the underlying parietal pleura and paradox does not occur. Covering radiation skin necrosis with soft tissue is frequently adequate.

Management of Soft Tissue

Whereas superficial defects of the chest wall are easily closed with local flaps or skin grafts, full thickness defects are more challenging and often require close interaction between the thoracic and plastic surgeons. The indications for soft tissue free or pedicle muscle reconstruction are to provide vascularized tissue to cover a thoracic wound, control infection, obliterate dead space, and to potentially provide coverage of synthetic mesh used to stabilize the chest wall. The availability of numerous reconstructive techniques with well-vascularized tissue enables the extirpative surgeon then to take the wide and appropriate resections to ensure quick healing, rehabilitation, cosmesis, and successful long-term management. A variety of techniques including pedicle muscle transposition, free muscle or omental flaps have been used to provide adequate wound coverage (Table 49.4).

Muscle is the tissue of choice for soft tissue coverage of full-thickness defects for which skeletal reconstruction is not required. Muscle can be transposed as muscle alone or as a musculocutaneous flap (Fig. 49.7). As noted by Matsuo et al. [29], combinations of different muscle flaps can be used to reconstruct larger chest wall defects that a single flap would not cover. The omentum should be reserved for partial-thickness reconstruction or as a backup procedure for muscle transposition that has failed in full-thickness defects. Such complex reconstructions should thoroughly be considered as last resort in elderly patients.

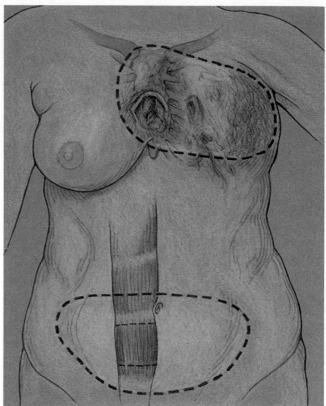

Fig. 49.7 Drawing for planned resection of recurrent breast cancer with chest wall involvement and reconstruction with transverse rectus abdominis musculocutaneous (TRAM) flap

Muscle Transposition

Latissimus Dorsi. The latissimus dorsi muscle is the largest flat muscle of the thorax. Its dominant thoracodorsal neurovascular leash has an arc of rotation that allows coverage of the lateral and central back as well as the anterolateral and central front of the thorax as Bostwick et al. [30] have described. Its dependable musculocutaneous vascular connections also make it a reliable musculocutaneous flap. This muscle flap can cover huge chest wall defects because virtually one half of the back can be elevated on the blood supply of a single latissimus dorsi muscle in the uninjured, non-irradiated patient. The donor site may need skin grafts when large musculocutaneous flaps are elevated, but this represents a small disadvantage when considering that large, robust flaps can be transposed to either the anterior or posterior chest for full-thickness reconstruction. If the dominant blood supply has been compromised from previous trauma or surgery, Fischer et al. [31] have shown that the muscle can still dependably be transposed on the branch of the adjacent serratus anterior muscle.

Pectoralis Major. The pectoralis major muscle is the second largest flat muscle on the chest wall and in many respects in the mirror image of the latissimus dorsi muscle. As Arnold and Pairolero [10] reported, its dominant thoracoacromial neurovascular bundle, which enters posteriorly about midclavicle, allows both elevation of the muscle, either as a muscle or as musculocutaneous flap, and rotation centrally for chest wall reconstruction. The pectoralis major muscle is equally as reliable as the latissimus dorsi flap. Pairolero and Arnold [17, 32] showed that it is beneficial in reconstructing anterior chest wall defects such as those resulting from sternal tumor excisions and infected medial sternotomy wounds. Generally, only the muscle is transposed, and the skin can be closed primarily, thereby avoiding the distortion created by centralizing the breast. Reconstruction in this manner is more symmetric and aesthetically acceptable. If central skin must be excised, symmetry of the breast can still be maintained, because the transposed muscle readily accepts and supports an overlying skin graft. If necessary, the muscle can also be transposed on its secondary blood supply through the perforators from the internal mammary vessels.

Rectus Abdominis. Use of the rectus abdominis muscle for chest wall reconstruction is based on the internal mammary neurovascular bundle. The inferior epigastric vessels must be divided to allow rotation to the chest wall. This muscle can be mobilized and moved either as a muscle or as a musculocutaneous flap with the skin component oriented either horizontally or vertically, or both, as described by Coleman and Bostwick [33]. The vertical skin flap, however, is more reliable because it is oriented along the long axis of the muscle and thus maintains more musculocutaneous perforators. The donor site is usually closed primarily.

Pairolero and Arnold [15] believe that the transverse rectus abdominis musculocutaneous (TRAM) flap is most useful in reconstruction of lower sternal wounds. Either muscle can be used, because their arcs of rotation are identical. The muscle that has patent and uninjured internal mammary vessels must be chosen. Angiographic demonstration of vessel patency may help determine which musculocutaneous unit would be most reliable, particularly in sternotomy wounds. Also, in many infected sternotomy wounds, the internal mammary artery may have previously been used for coronary artery bypass.

Serratus Anterior. The serratus anterior muscle is a small flat muscle located in the midaxillary line between the latissimus dorsi and pectoralis major muscles. Its blood supply comes from the serratus branch of the thoracodorsal vessels and form the long thoracic artery and vein. This muscle can be used alone or as an adjunctive muscle with the pectoralis major or the latissimus dorsi muscles. The muscle also augments the skin-carrying ability of either adjacent muscle. Greason et al. [34] have also found that this muscle is particularly useful as an intrathoracic muscle flap.

External Oblique. The external oblique muscle can also be transposed as a muscle or musculocutaneous flap, and it is most useful in closing defects of the upper abdomen and lower thorax. It reaches the inframammary fold without tension but, as Hodgkinson and Arnold [35] noted, does not readily extend higher. The primary blood supply is from the lower thoracic intercostal vessels. With this muscle, lower chest wall defects can be closed without distorting the breast.

Trapezius Muscle. The trapezius muscle has been useful to close defects at the base of the neck or the thoracic outlet but is not consistently useful for other chest wall reconstructions. Its primary blood supply is the dorsal scapular vessels.

Deltoid Muscle. The deltoid muscle is usually used for reconstruction when an interscapulothoracic amputation (removal of the entire upper extremity, the shoulder girdle, and its muscular attachments) also known as a four-quarter amputation is undertaken for malignant tumors of the upper arm, shoulder, and scapula [36]. Its primary blood supply is a dual system from the deltoid branch of the thoracoacromial artery and the posterior humeral circumflex artery. The deltoid muscle is mobilized with the skin and soft tissue from the upper arm after the amputation for coverage of the defect. This myocutaneous flap reconstruction technique has been well described by Mansour and Powell [37]. This reconstruction method can be a lifesaving procedure even in the elderly patient, but an extensive preoperative evaluation and comprehensive education of the patient about the procedure is warranted in this life-changing reconstruction.

Omental Transposition

Omental transposition, as Jurkiewicz and Arnold [38] noted, has been most useful in reconstructing partial-thickness chest wall defects, particularly in radiation necrosis that does not involve tumor. In this situation, the skin and soft tissue are debrided down to what remains of the thoracic skeleton, which may be either bone or cartilage but frequently is only irradiated ischemic scar. The transposed omentum with its excellent blood supply from the gastroepiploic vessels adheres to the irradiated wound and readily accepts and supports an overlying skin graft. Because the omentum has no structural stability of its own, it is not particularly useful in full-thickness defects because additional support, such as fascia lata, bone, or prosthetic material, is necessary.

Omental transposition is helpful when planned muscle flaps have failed with partial necrosis. Generally, this results in only a soft tissue defect, and pleural seal with respiratory stability is not required, as noted by Fix and Vasconez [39], thus allowing a most threatening situation to be salvaged. Although infections of the lower sternum are best treated with a rectus abdominis muscle flap, the blood supply, based on the distal aspect of the internal mammary artery, may have been interrupted previously either by use of this artery for coronary revascularization or by ligation with sternal resection. If the internal mammary artery is not intact or if the wound is large, omental transposition is performed, followed by STSG immediately or after 48 h.

The numerous advances in chest reconstruction over the years with the introduction of muscle and musculocutaneous flaps have made them the mainstay in chest wall reconstruction, even in the elderly where the blood supply is dependable. The thoracic trunk is well suited for vascularized coverage given the many local muscle flaps (e.g., latissimus dorsi, pectoralis major, rectus abdominis, trapezius, or deltoid muscles) or greater omentum (used alone or in combination as options for wound coverage). With the bountiful methods of pedicles muscle transfer and uncommon pedicle muscle flap loss, the necessity for free flap in the reconstruction of the thoracic wall defect is minimal. Free tissue transfer flap is seldom utilized in the elderly for chest wall reconstruction and is generally used only when pedicle flaps are unavailable. In the rare situation of pedicles muscle flap loss, the pedicle omental flap has been useful as a salvage procedure in those instances.

Clinical Experience

Mansour et al. and Losken et al. have reported on 200 patients who underwent chest wall reconstruction within the Emory University Healthcare system over a 25-year period [19, 40]. The most common indication for chest wall resection in our series was lung cancer in 75 patients (38%), chest wall tumors in 53 (27%), breast cancer in 43 (22%), infection in 31 (16%), and radiation necrosis in 29 (15%) (Table 49.5). Chest wall resections included the ribs in 118 patients (79%), sternum in 56 patients (28%), and a forequarter amputation in 14 (7%) (Table 49.6); 46 patients underwent reoperations (23%) and 68 patients (34%) had combined lung and chest wall resection. Immediate closure was performed in 195 patients (98%) and 5 patients underwent delayed closure at an average of 10 days after chest wall resection (Table 49.7).

Table 49.5 Indications for chest wall resection

Indication	Number of patients (%)
Lung cancer	75 (38)
Chest wall tumor	53 (27)
Breast cancer	43 (22)
Chest wall infections	31 (16)
Radiation necrosis	29 (15)
Miscellaneous tumors	23 (12)
Pectus repair	6 (3)

Delayed repairs were performed secondary to hemodynamic instability and ongoing infectious process.

Primary repair of the soft tissue and skin was performed in 43 patients (22%). Synthetic materials were used for chest wall integrity reconstruction in 93 patients (47%); Prolene mesh in 49, Marlex mesh in 21, methyl methacrylate sandwich in 11, Vicryl mesh in 11, and PTFE in 1 (Table 49.8). Muscle flap transposition was performed in 113 patients (57%); 96 patients (48%) underwent pedicle muscle flap and 17 patients (9%) underwent a free muscle flap. The most common muscle groups utilized were latissimus dorsi in 40 patients, TRAM flap in 33 patients, and pectoralis in 31 (Table 49.9). Fourteen patients (12%) required more than

Table 49.6 Chest wall resections

Type	Number of patients (%)
Recurrent surgery	46 (23)
Combined lung and chest wall	68 (34)
Rib defects	66 (33)
Sternal defects	56 (28)
Forequarter amputation	14 (7)

Table 49.7 Chest wall reconstruction

Type	Number of patients (%)
Immediate reconstruction	195 (98)
Delayed reconstruction	5 (3)
Primary chest wall closure	43 (22)
Prosthetic replacement	49 (25)
Autogenous replacement	96 (48)

Table 49.8 Prosthetic material

Type	Number of patients (%)
Prolene mesh	49 (25)
Marlex mesh	21 (11)
Methyl methacrylate	11 (6)
Vicryl mesh	11 (6)
PTFE	1 (0.5)

PTFE Polytetrafluoroethylene

Table 49.9 Autogenous material

Type	Number of patients (%)
Pedicle flap	96 (48)
Free flap	17 (9)
Latissimus muscle	40 (20)
TRAM flap	40 (20)
Pectoralis muscle	31 (16)
Serratus muscle	17 (9)
Deltoid muscle	4 (2)
Trapezius muscle	3 (2)
Omentum muscle	20 (10)
STSG	23 (12)

TRAM Transverse rectus abdominis musculocutaneous; *STSG* split-thickness skin graft

Table 49.10 Outcomes

Overall length of stay (median)	10 Days (3–99 days)
Postoperative length of stay (median)	6 Days (2–98 days)
Intensive care stay postoperatively	168 Patients (84%)
Intensive care length of stay (median)	3 Days (1–83 days)
Hospital mortality	13 Patients (7%)
Combine lung and chest wall resection	5 of 68 Patients (7%)
Forequarter amputation	1 of 14 Patients (7%)

Table 49.11 Complications

Complication	Number of patients (%)
Pneumonia	27 (14)
ARDS	11 (6)
Flap loss	10 (3)
Infection/sepsis	9 (5)
Atrial fibrillation	5 (3)
Flap hematoma	3 (2)
Mesenteric ischemia	1 (0.5)
Pancreatitis	1 (0.5)
Acute renal failure	1 (0.5)
Donor site hernia	1 (0.5)

ARDS Acute respiratory distress syndrome

one muscle flap for complete reconstruction. The omentum was used in 20 patients (10%) and STSG were utilized in 23 patients (12%).

Hospital outcomes are summarized in Table 49.10. The median overall hospital stay was 10 days (range, 3–99 days) and the median postoperative stay was 6 days (range, 2–98 days). A total of 168 patients (84%) required intensive care unit stay postoperatively for a median of 3 days (range, 1–83 days). Thirteen of the 200 patients (7%) died during their hospital stay; most commonly from multi-system organ failure (MSOF). Forty-seven patients (24%) had complications (Table 49.11); the most common complication was pneumonia in 27 (14%), acute respiratory distress syndrome (ARDS) in 11 (6%), and flap loss in 10 (6%). Only 14 patients (7%) had a complication related to their flap, the most common unfortunately was flap death in 10 patients. There was no difference with regard to morbidity, mortality, or overall success based on advanced age.

Conclusion

In conclusion, the key to a successful outcome in these complex cases is the coordinated effort by the surgical teams in individualizing the care of the elderly patient utilizing total resection of the disease process, reconstruction of the chest

wall integrity, and soft tissue coverage of the defect. The team of surgeons should be well versed in chest wall reconstruction utilizing prosthetic and biological materials as well as pedicle muscle flaps and must plan and work together to achieve optimal results.

Chest wall reconstruction is both safe and effective in the immediate setting with the majority of defects being closed using synthetic mesh, regional muscle, or myocutaneous flaps. Although this chapter is a helpful guide, the complexity of each individual patient needs to be taken into account, and numerous variables will influence the decision process regarding the most appropriate management. Close interaction with the plastic surgeon and critical care physician is important, so that all teams must completely understand the ablative goals and reconstructive options to avoid unnecessary morbidity and ensure a successful outcome in the elderly patient.

References

1. Watson WL, James AG. Fascia lata grafts for chest wall defects. J Thorac Surg. 1947;14:399–406.
2. Maier HC. Surgical management of large defects of the thoracic wall. Surgery. 1947;22:169–74.
3. Pickrell KL, Kelley JW, Marzoni FA. The surgical management of recurrent carcinoma of the breast and chest wall. Plast Reconstr Surg. 1948;3:156–60.
4. Bisgard JD, Swenson Jr SA. Tumors of the sternum: report of a case with special operative technic. Arch Surg. 1948;56:570–2.
5. Tansini I. Sopra il mio nuovo processo di amputazione della mammella. Gazz Med Ital. 1906;57:141–3.
6. Campbell DA. Reconstruction of the anterior thoracic wall. J Thorac Surg. 1950;19:456–61.
7. Kiricuta I. L'empoli du grand epiploon dans la chirugie du sein canereux. Presse Med (Paris). 1963;71:15–8.
8. McCormack P, Bains MS, Beattie Jr EJ, et al. New trends in skeletal reconstruction after resection of chest wall tumors. Ann Thorac Surg. 1981;31:45–52.
9. Larson DL, McMurtery MJ, Howe HJ, et al. Major chest wall reconstruction after chest wall irradiation. Cancer. 1982;49:1286–91.
10. Arnold PG, Pairolero PC. Use of pectoralis major muscle flaps to repair defects of the anterior chest wall. Plast Reconstr Surg. 1979;63:205–13.
11. Arnold PG, Pairolero PC. Chest wall reconstruction: experience with 100 consecutive patients. Ann Surg. 1984;199:725–32.
12. Arnold PG, Pairolero PC. Surgical management of the radiated chest wall. Plast Reconstr Surg. 1986;77:605–12.
13. Arnold PG, Pairolero PC. Reconstruction of the radiation-damaged chest wall. Surg Clin North Am. 1989;69:1081–9.
14. Arnold PG, Pairolero PC. Chest wall reconstruction: an account of 500 consecutive patients. Plast Reconstr Surg. 1996;98:804–10.
15. Pairolero PC, Arnold PG. Chest wall tumors: experience with 100 consecutive patients. J Thorac Cardiovasc Surg. 1985;90:367–72.
16. Pairolero PC, Arnold PG. Thoracic wall defects: surgical management of 205 consecutive patients. Mayo Clin Proc. 1986;61:557–63.
17. Pairolero PC, Arnold PG. Chondrosarcoma of the manubrium: resection and reconstruction with pectoralis major muscle. Mayo Clin Proc. 1978;53:54–7.

18. Azarow KS, Molloy M, Seyfer AE, et al. Preoperative evaluation and general preparation for chest wall operations. Surg Clin North Am. 1989;69:899–910.

19. Mansour KA, Thourani VH, Losken A, et al. Chest wall resections and reconstruction: a 25-year experience. Ann Thorac Surg. 2002;73:1720–6.

20. Burkhart HM, Allen MS, Nichols III FC, et al. Results of en bloc resection for bronchogenic carcinoma with chest wall invasion. J Thorac Cardiovasc Surg. 2002;123:670–5.

21. Weyant MJ, Bains MS, Venkatraman E, et al. Results of chest wall resection and reconstruction with and without rigid prosthesis. Ann Thorac Surg. 2006;81:279–85.

22. McCormack PM. Use of prosthetic material in chest-wall reconstruction. Surg Clin North Am. 1989;69:965–76.

23. Mansour KA, Anderson TM, Hester TR. Sternal resection and reconstruction. Ann Thorac Surg. 1993;55:838–43.

24. Kilic D, Gungor A, Kavukcu S, et al. Comparison of mersilene mesh-methyl methacrylate sandwich and polytetrafluoroethylene grafts for chest wall reconstruction. J Invest Surg. 2006;19:353–60.

25. Daigeler A, Druecke D, Hakimi M, et al. Reconstruction of the thoracic wall long-term follow-up including pulmonary function. Langenbecks Arch Surg. 2008;66:1–25.

26. Kroll SS, Walsh G, Ryan B, et al. Risks and benefits of using Marlex mesh in chest wall reconstruction. Ann Plast Surg. 1993;31:303–6.

27. Le Roux BT, Shama DM. Resection of tumors of the chest wall. Curr Probl Surg. 1983;20:345–86.

28. Deschamps C, Tirnaksiz BM, Darbandi R, et al. Early and long-term results of prosthetic chest wall reconstruction. J Thorac Cardiovasc Surg. 1999;117:588–92.

29. Matsuo K, Hirose T, Havashi R, et al. Reconstruction of large chest wall defects using a combination of a contralateral latissimus dorsi and rectus abdominis musculocutaneous flap. Br J Plast Surg. 1991;44:102–5.

30. Bostwick III J, Nahai F, Wallace JG, et al. Sixty latissimus dorsi flaps. Plast Reconstr Surg. 1979;63:31–41.

31. Fischer J, Bostwick III J, Powell RW. Latissimus dorsi blood supply after thoraodorsal vessel division: the serratus collateral. Plast Reconstr Surg. 1983;72:502–4.

32. Pairolero PC, Arnold PG. Management of recalcitrant median sternotomy wounds. J Thorac Cardiovasc Surg. 1984;88:357–64.

33. Coleman III JJ, Bostwick III J. Rectus abdominis muscle – musculocutaneous flap in chest wall reconstruction. Surg Clin North Am. 1989;69:1007–27.

34. Greason KG, Miller DL, Johnson CH, et al. Management of the irradiated bronchus after lobectomy for lung cancer. Ann Thorac Surg. 2003;76:180–5.

35. Hodgkinson DJ, Arnold PG. Chest wall reconstruction using the external oblique muscle. Br J Plast Surg. 1980;33:216–9.

36. Berger P. Bull Mém Soc Chir Paris. 1883;9:656.

37. Mansour KA, Powell RW. Modified technique for radical transmediastinal forequarter amputation and chest wall resection. J Thorac Cardiovasc Surg. 1978;76:358–63.

38. Jurkiewicz MJ, Arnold PG. The omentum: an account of its use in the reconstruction of the chest wall. Ann Surg. 1977;185:548–54.

39. Fix RJ, Vasconez LO. Use of the omentum in chest-wall reconstruction. Surg Clin North Am. 1989;69:1029–46.

40. Losken A, Thourani VH, Carlson GW, et al. A reconstructive algorithm for plastic surgery following extensive chest wall reconstruction. Br J Plast Surg. 2004;57:295–302.

Chapter 50
Surgery of the Trachea and Bronchi in the Elderly

Douglas J. Mathisen and Ashok Muniappan

Abstract This chapter describes the various pathologic conditions that might affect the trachea and bronchi in the elderly. Diseases considered include airway neoplasms, benign tracheoesophageal fistulae, and tracheal stenoses. Appropriate operative techniques to address these problems are described. The results obtained in the elderly are also presented. Airway surgery in the elderly may be safely and effectively performed.

Keywords Trachea • Bronchus • Tracheal stenosis • Tracheoesophageal fistula • Tracheal resection • Sleeve resection • Bronchoplasty

Introduction

The development of modern airway surgery owes a great deal to the efforts of Dr. Hermes Grillo, who studied, practiced, and perfected techniques that permit safe and effective correction of airway pathology. The culmination of his work is the text *Surgery of the Trachea and Bronchi* [1], which presents a survey of the pathology that can affect the airways, and the surgical approaches to manage it. We will summarize the standard techniques in this chapter, keeping in mind how the elderly patient can present specific challenges and what outcomes can be expected in this patient population.

Anatomy of the Trachea

A thorough understanding of normal tracheal anatomy is necessary before planning and performing tracheal surgery. The average length of the adult human trachea is 11.8 cm (range 10–13 cm), measuring from the bottom of the cricoid cartilage to the carina. There are approximately 18–22 C-shaped cartilaginous rings making up the length of the trachea, with about 2 rings every centimeter. The transverse and anteroposterior diameters are on average 2.3 and 1.8 cm, respectively [2]. There are no significant changes to normal tracheal dimensions in the elderly.

The position of the trachea is variable and greatly affected by the positioning of the neck. With the neck extended, as in the case of normal positioning for a thyroidectomy, the upper half of the trachea is cervical and the lower half is mediastinal. However, with the neck flexed, the entire trachea may become mediastinal, as the cricoid cartilage descends to the level of the thoracic inlet. In elderly patients, especially those with prominent cervical kyphosis, this may be the fixed position of the trachea (Fig. 50.1). Accurate measurements and a clear operative plan are necessary for selecting either a cervical approach (the majority of tracheal operations) or a transthoracic approach (pathology typically centered at the distal trachea or carina).

Anteriorly, at the level of the second tracheal ring, the thyroid isthmus crosses the trachea. The thyroid lobes are apposed to the trachea at this level, and the blood supply delivered by the inferior thyroid arteries are shared. Posteriorly, the esophagus is intimately associated with the membranous trachea, although the plane is typically easily developed between these two structures, in the normal situation. The blood supply of the trachea is segmental and shared with the esophagus. The arteries approach laterally and divide to give anterior branches to the trachea and posterior branches to the esophagus [3]. Extensive circumferential dissection of the trachea is avoided as disrupting the lateral blood supply risks devascularization. The distal tracheal and mainstem bronchi share the blood supply delivered by the bronchial arteries.

Airway Pathology

Airway pathology includes tumors, acquired stenoses, and tracheoesophageal fistulae. The most common tracheal disorders requiring operative management are acquired stenoses followed

D.J. Mathisen (✉)
Department of Surgery, Division of Thoracic Surgery,
Massachusetts General Hospital, Blake 1570, 55 Fruit Street,
Boston, MA 02114, USA
e-mail: dmathisen@partners.org

M.R. Katlic (ed.), *Cardiothoracic Surgery in the Elderly*, DOI 10.1007/978-1-4419-0892-6_50,
© Springer Science+Business Media, LLC 2011

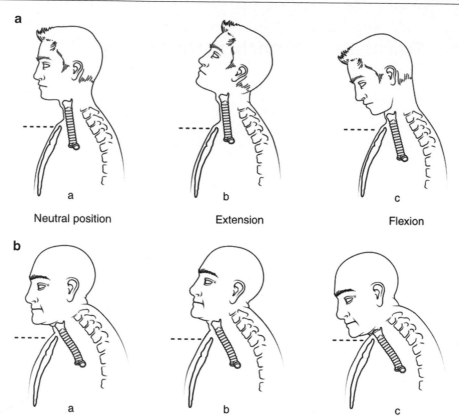

Fig. 50.1 Tracheal position is altered in the elderly and kyphotic. (**a**) The position of the trachea with the neck in neutral (a), extended (b), and flexed (c) positions in youth. In neutral position (a), one-third of the trachea is in the neck. With cervical extension (b), more than one half of the trachea is present in the neck. With cervical flexion (c), most of the trachea is intrathoracic. In the elderly (**b**), most of the trachea may be intrathoracic, and does not change its position whether the neck is neutral (a), extended (b), or flexed (c) (from Grillo [1], used with permission)

by tracheal neoplasms, of which, squamous cell carcinoma (SCC) and adenoid cystic carcinoma are the most common. Both palliative and curative approaches to these disorders have been developed. The approach that has been developed at Massachusetts General Hospital, and shared by a number of other centers expert at airway surgery, incorporates techniques that strive to completely deal with the pathology in the safest manner possible. With respect to stenoses, while palliative measures such as tracheostomies and T-tubes have their role, every effort is made to resect and reconstruct the airway to restore the airway and permit normal function. Likewise, with respect to neoplasms, a complete resection of the tumor is always considered, typically requiring a formal resection and reconstruction of the airway. The age of the patient is one of the many variables the airway surgeon must consider in planning an operation, but it certainly is not a contraindication to proceeding in of itself.

Tracheal and Bronchial Neoplasms

While there are a variety of neoplasms that can affect the airways (Table 50.1), only a few present commonly. The exact incidence of primary airway neoplasms is unknown,

Table 50.1 Primary tracheal tumors

Malignant neoplasms
Adenoid cystic carcinoma
Squamous cell carcinoma (SCC)
Intermediate grade neoplasms
Carcinoid
Mucoepidermoid
Benign tracheal neoplasms
Squamous papilloma
Pleomorphic adenoma
Granular cell tumor (myoblastoma)

given their relative rarity. Rather, data are available from a variety of centers regarding the frequency of different neoplasms presenting for operative management. At MGH, the majority of primary tracheal tumors are found to be malignant. Looking at a 26-year period at MGH, 40% of patients with primary tracheal tumors ($n=198$) presented with adenoid cystic carcinoma and 36% of patients presented with primary SCC. The remaining 24% of patients had other malignant tumors (4%), intermediate character tumors such as carcinoid and mucoepidermoid tumor (9%), and benign tumors (11%) [4].

SCC of the trachea presents either as an exophytic or as ulcerative lesion, with or without symptoms. The lesion may infiltrate locally or longitudinally along the tracheal wall, with possible involvement of structures adjacent to the trachea. Metastasis to adjacent peritracheal lymph nodes is possible, while hematogenous spread to distant organs is less common. Virtually all patients have a significant smoking history, and the age at presentation is similar to lung cancer, typically between 50 and 70 years. The mean age of presentation is 61 years [5].

Adenoid cystic carcinoma presents across a wider age group, from 20 to 70 years. The mean age of presentation is significantly younger than SCC, at 49 years, but it still may be encountered in the elderly [5]. The lesion may occur anywhere in the trachea, but is most likely to be centered at the distal trachea or carina. The gross appearance of the lesion is variable, and the borders may or may not be distinct. The tumor has a propensity to infiltrate the tracheal wall submucosally and perineurally, remote from the visible mass. This feature is what makes complete resection of this tumor more difficult. The tumor may have a large extra-tracheal component, but is less prone to invasion of adjacent structures. Peritracheal lymph nodes may be involved, and metastasis to the lungs is possible.

Intermediate grade tumors presenting with some frequency, but still relatively rarely, are mucoepidermoid and carcinoid tumors of the trachea and bronchi. Mucoepidermoid tumors can occur anywhere in the trachea as well as the bronchi. Mucoepidermoid tumors can behave in a very malignant fashion, while others respond very favorably to resection without recurrence. In a series of 18 patients with mucoepidermoid tumors of the airway, managed at MGH, the mean age of the patients was 37 years, with a range of 9–62 years [6]. Carcinoid tumors are more typically encountered in the bronchi, but can also present in the peripheral lung and rarely in the trachea. They present typically in the fifth to the sixth decades, but can be encountered in the very young and the elderly. Typical carcinoid responds very favorably to resection, and recurrence is rare. Atypical carcinoid may present with metastasis to lymph nodes, and exhibit a more aggressive behavior. Endobronchial treatment of carcinoid tumors with modalities such as the laser is occasionally used by some centers. At MGH, we have espoused resectional techniques to completely eradicate the disease and prevent recurrence. The carcinoid tumor has its origin deeper than the mucosa, and endobronchial treatment is incapable of removing the disease completely, and may complicate definitive resectional therapy. We will review bronchoplastic "sleeve" techniques later in this chapter. Again, we emphasize that age is not a contraindication to attempting cure of these tumors with resection and reconstruction of the airway.

Of the possible secondary tracheobronchial tumors that may be encountered, invasive thyroid carcinoma and bronchogenic carcinoma involving the carina or proximal mainstem bronchus are the ones that are most likely in the elderly population. Well-differentiated thyroid carcinoma is found to invade the trachea between 1 and 10% of patients [7]. Invasion is more likely with advancing age of the patient. In the MGH experience, the mean age of patients undergoing a tracheal resection for invasive thyroid cancer was 64 years, with patients as old as 79 years [8]. Poorly differentiated and anaplastic thyroid carcinoma, in particular, are prone to tracheal invasion. There is no widely implemented staging system that takes into account tracheal invasion, although an attempt at staging has been made [9]. As a result, outcomes of different approaches to thyroid carcinoma invading the trachea are difficult to compare. The two primary surgical approaches are shave resection of the trachea and formal tracheal resection and reconstruction at the time of thyroidectomy. Again, the approach at MGH has been to undertake, whenever possible, complete eradication of the disease by resection of the involved segment of the trachea. The goals of tracheal resection for patients with invasive thyroid carcinoma are to prevent tracheal obstruction by the slowly growing tumor, alleviate the potential for chronic and debilitating hemorrhage, and potentially to cure the patient. When tracheal resection is undertaken at the time of thyroidectomy or soon after, very good outcomes are obtained with minimal morbidity [8]. Even when tracheal resection is undertaken for local recurrence after thyroidectomy, palliation can be achieved; however, cure and prolonged survival are harder to achieve. Given the location of the thyroid gland and its isthmus, the tumor may involve the larynx as well as the trachea. As a result, laryngotracheal resection, rather than a more straightforward tracheal resection, may be necessary. Even more radical surgery such as cervical exenteration and mediastinal tracheostomy may be necessary in the rare patient.

Bronchogenic carcinoma may involve the proximal mainstem bronchi or carina. The initial experience with surgical management of proximal bronchogenic carcinoma was poor, with mortality exceeding long-term survival. However, more recent experiences, with careful patient selection and improved operative and postoperative management, significantly improved outcomes are expected, justifying operative management in selected patients. The operation that is typically performed is a right carinal pneumonectomy. The tumor typically originates in the right upper lobe; left-sided tumors are less likely to involve the proximal left mainstem bronchus given its longer length, and thus left carinal pneumonectomies are rarely necessary. In the MGH experience for carinal pneumonectomies for bronchogenic carcinoma, the mean age of patients was 56 years, with the oldest patient being 73 years old [10]. The operative mortality was 15%, and 5-year survival was 42%. Lymph node involvement had a very significant effect on long-term survival, and not unexpectedly, N2 or N3 disease was associated with extremely poor survival rates.

Airway Stenosis

The two most common etiologies for tracheal stenosis requiring resection and reconstruction are post-intubation stenosis and idiopathic tracheal stenosis. The latter disorder almost exclusively affects women, typically in their 40s, and is unlikely to be the cause of stenosis in the elderly. Post-intubation stenosis is likely secondary to stomal complications from a prior tracheostomy or cuff injury from an orotracheal or tracheostomy tube. Both stomal complications and cuff injuries occur less frequently with attention to proper tracheostomy placement and the introduction of low-pressure high-volume cuffs, respectively. The kyphotic neck of the elderly makes tracheostomy placement more complicated, as the trachea has a tendency to descend into the thorax. As a consequence, the rigid tube has a tendency to erode into the anterior aspect of the cricoid cartilage. The stenosis that results from this injury is high, and typically requires a laryngotracheal resection and reconstruction. Cuff injuries should be eliminated with proper cuff inflation pressures and monitoring, but are still encountered.

Patients present with dyspnea only when the degree of narrowing exceeds 50% of the normal cross-sectional area. The presence of granulation tissue, tracheal wall flaps proximal to the stoma, and malacia with dynamic collapse of the tracheal wall all can contribute to airway obstruction and symptoms. The most common stomal lesion, however, is anterolateral stenosis, which produces a characteristic "A"-shaped airway stenosis. The patients may become symptomatic immediately upon decannulation or present more remotely. Most patients can be stabilized in an intensive care setting with conservative measures such as humidification, supplemental oxygen, Heliox, and suctioning to keep the patient breathing spontaneously. Rarely, intubation above the stenosis may be necessary, and ventilation with Venturi-like flow through the stenosis can maintain the patient. The airway surgeon must be prepared to also re-establish an airway with rigid bronchoscopy and tracheal dilation. This is typically a temporizing maneuver, as these lesions will tend to contract spontaneously. Tracheal dilation can be expected to be effective for days to weeks, which permits time for planning. It is preferable not to establish a new tracheostomy, as this will only reduce the length of normal trachea available for reconstruction after resection of the stenosis.

In our experience, there are very few contraindications to definitive repair of these lesions. The most important contraindication to undertaking tracheal resection and reconstruction would be anticipated need for postoperative mechanical ventilation. These patients are usually better served by permanent tracheostomy or delayed tracheal resection at a time when they are likely to breathe spontaneously. Stable coronary artery disease has not been a barrier to safe airway reconstruction. Likewise, we have successfully operated on patients with significant COPD or limited pulmonary reserve; in these cases, the patient and the surgeon must be prepared to accept the need for permanent tracheostomy after reconstruction if the patient does not do well. The MGH has presented its series of tracheal and laryngotracheal resections for post-intubation stenosis in 503 patients from 1965 to 1992 [11]. While the mean age of patients was 44 years old, the oldest patient was 85 years old. Moreover, 97 patients were in their 60s, 45 patients were in their 70s, and 4 patients were in their 80s. Ninety-four percent of the patients were judged to have good or satisfactory outcomes, and mortality was 2.4% in this series. Age was not studied as a risk factor. The most important barrier to success, in this report, was failed prior attempt at tracheal resection, emphasizing that success at the first operation is paramount.

Acquired Airway Esophageal Fistulae

Fistulae between the airway and the esophagus may be classified as either malignant or benign. Malignant fistulae are predominantly due to esophageal cancer that has progressed to involve the airway. The prognosis is grim, and palliative measures such as esophageal stenting are recommended. Benign fistulae are secondary to a variety of causes, including granulomas of the membranous tracheal or bronchial wall, trauma, iatrogenic injury at procedures such as cervical spine fixation, and most commonly from post-intubation injury. The lesions typically arise from an over distended endotracheal or tracheostomy tube cuff pushing against an indwelling hard nasogastric tube. These lesions may present while the patient is mechanically ventilated as saliva contaminates the airway or tidal volume is lost via the enteric route. Bronchoscopy confirms the diagnosis. The fistulae from post-intubation injuries are typically "giant," as the entire membranous wall of the trachea may be deficient. Along with the fistula, a significant tracheal stenosis also accompanies this lesion, secondary to the cuff injury. The need for mechanical ventilatory support makes immediate repair inadvisable, and the situation is temporized by placing a new tracheostomy tube with a cuff that is distal to the fistula. The nasogastric tube is removed, a gastrostomy is placed for drainage, and a jejunostomy is performed for enteral nutrition. Once the patient weans from the ventilator and pulmonary sepsis has been controlled, a repair of the fistula may be undertaken. The technique is described later in this chapter. In a recent series of patients successfully managed with this problem, the mean age of patients was 52 years old, while the oldest patient was 84 years old [12]. In an earlier report from MGH, 38 patients with an acquired non-malignant tracheoesophageal fistula were managed. In this series, there was a 10% mortality. Results were judged to be excellent in the surviving patients, with all but one able to aliment themselves orally and all but two able to breathe without a tracheal appliance [13].

Tracheobronchial Malacia and Saber-Sheath Trachea

Tracheobronchial malacia and saber-sheath abnormality of the trachea are two other airway problems that rarely need operative intervention, but are not infrequently identified in the elderly. Tracheobronchial malacia is most typically associated with advanced COPD, although idiopathic cases may also be encountered. It is manifest by expiratory collapse of the trachea or mainstem bronchi, and represents an intrinsic defect in the rigidity of the cartilaginous rings. The expiratory collapse is typically documented bronchoscopically in the awake patient as well as by dynamic computed tomography scans in both inspiratory and expiratory phases of breathing. In a 10-year period at MGH, fourteen patients underwent a tracheoplasty procedure that splints the posterior membranous wall of the trachea and mainstem bronchi with a strip of Marlex mesh [14]. In this series, 8 of 10 patients with long-term follow-up had good results. Two of the patients were elderly at 79 and 84 years old; both patients had good results, although one required 2 days of ventilatory assistance. Although the results of this series were considered good, it was in a highly selected group of patients. Most patients with some degree of tracheomalacia likely do not need any operative intervention.

The saber-sheath trachea is often identified incidentally on plain chest radiography, which reveals marked coronal narrowing of the intrathoracic trachea. In one cohort of patients with saber-sheath trachea seen at MGH, the mean coronal diameter of the intrathoracic trachea was 10.5 mm as compared to a mean saggital diameter of 23 mm [15]. The majority of these patients had a significant smoking history and suffered from COPD. The age of the patients ranged from 52 to 75 years old, and they were predominantly male. Although the association with COPD is strong, most patients with COPD do not develop the saber-sheath abnormality. While the pathophysiology of this disorder is uncertain, there has been speculation that the abnormality develops as a consequence of excessive coughing and repetitive injury of the tracheal cartilage, which are not malaciac per se. The clinical significance of the abnormality is typically minimal, and as with tracheobronchial malacia, operative management is usually unnecessary. For the rare patient with severe saber-sheath abnormality, tracheal stenting or a tracheal T-tube may be required to maintain airway patency. Awake bronchoscopy, careful analysis of flow-volume loops, and dynamic inspiration–expiration CT scanning all help to select the patient that would benefit from airway stenting.

Extrinsic Airway Compression

Extrinsic compression of the airways can occur in a variety of circumstances. One particular disorder that may afflict the elderly is thyroid goiter that descends into the thorax and wraps posteriorly around the trachea [16]. Substernal goiter, as this is often referred to, is associated with dyspnea or dysphagia in as much as one-third of patients; these patients require thyroidectomy to prevent progression of symptoms, which may even lead to mortality. The surgical approach for substernal goiter is typically via a low-collar incision and rarely is sternotomy necessary. It is important to keep in mind that a recurrent laryngeal nerve on either side may be compromised preoperatively, and that intraoperative dissection may result in both nerves being compromised at the conclusion of the procedure. Careful extubation is necessary, and preparation for restoring an airway in the setting of a closed glottis is necessary. Another problem to anticipate is that the chronic goiter may have caused tracheomalacia, and with the removal of the thyroid, expiratory collapse of the airway may become evident. If the degree of tracheomalacia is significant and pulmonary compromise develops, it may be overcome by re-intubation and a repeat attempt at extubation in a few days. Rarely, a tracheostomy or T-tube may be necessary to maintain the airway.

Preoperative Diagnostic Procedures

After a thorough history and physical examination, radiographic and bronchoscopic examinations are performed to characterize the nature of the airway lesion. In benign disease, such as post-intubation stenosis, non-contrast soft tissue plain radiographs of the neck are sufficient. With potential for malignancy, CT scanning is essential to delineate the extent of disease and possible involvement of adjacent structures and regional lymphadenopathy. A combination of flexible and rigid bronchoscopy is used to define the type and extent of pathology. Rigid bronchoscopy can also alleviate tracheal obstruction by coring out tumor or dilating a benign stenosis. Rigid bronchoscopy may require a set of pediatric bronchoscopes starting with a size 3, and also Jackson dilators that may be passed through a stenosis under direct vision through a rigid scope. Biopsy and histopathological assessment of potentially neoplastic lesions also can aid in planning treatment.

As discussed in earlier chapters, the physiologic assessment of the elderly patient must also be thorough, as comorbidities must be well defined and the patient's status optimized. On the other hand, most stable comorbidities, such as coronary artery disease, do not preclude elective airway surgery. An interesting case performed recently at MGH was an elderly patient who presented with tracheal stenosis (due to prior laryngotracheal trauma) that had progressively become more symptomatic. Moreover, he had symptomatic three-vessel coronary disease. He underwent coronary artery bypass grafting, after rigid bronchoscopy and dilation. He failed extubation and underwent tracheostomy (performed through the diseased tracheal segment). He had an uneventful recovery from his bypass surgery, and returned for definitive laryngotracheal resection and reconstruction 8 weeks after CABG, from which he recovered without issues.

Anesthesia

We refer the reader to the excellent chapter on thoracic anesthesia in this text and also make some points specific to anesthesia for airway surgery. With a compromised airway, it is essential that it is under complete control at all times. Induction of anesthesia is slow and deliberate, and paralysis is avoided unless definitive control of the airway is obtained. A slow inhalational anesthetic or total intravenous anesthetic (TIVA) technique may be used. Prompt reversal of the anesthetic and return of spontaneous ventilation at the conclusion of the procedure is necessary, as even brief intubation and presence of a cuffed tube is to be avoided after tracheal resection and reconstruction. If the tracheal lumen is less than 5 mm in the stenotic segment, dilatation via rigid bronchoscopy may be necessary to permit endotracheal tube intubation. During tracheal resection, the endotracheal tube is drawn back into the proximal airway while the trachea is divided and "cross-field" ventilation is established by intubating the distal trachea in the surgical field. The tube used for cross-field ventilation is typically an "armored" tube that is made of wire reinforced plastic to prevent kinking. This tube may be removed intermittently to permit further dissection and placement of sutures. Close coordination with the anesthesiologist is necessary. Cardiopulmonary bypass, although utilized in various reports of airway surgery, has not been required in most airway reconstructive cases at MGH.

Tracheostomy in the Elderly

Although tracheostomy placement is perhaps the simplest of airway operations, even it has the potential for significant complications. The technique we have favored is an open surgical technique that carefully positions the tracheostomy tube at the appropriate level and avoids the potential for hemorrhage and injury to adjacent structures. An orotracheal airway is established, realizing that this may require the use flexible or rigid bronchoscopy. The patient is positioned with the neck slightly extended. The elderly patient may have a cervical spine that does not permit much if any extension, and appropriate padding of the occiput is necessary. The incision is made not with respect to the sternal notch, but rather should be about 1 cm below the level of the cricoid cartilage. After going through the platysma and making small flaps, the strap muscles are separated. The thyroid isthmus is isolated and divided between heavy silk ligatures. Division of the isthmus, which typically lies over the second tracheal ring, ensures that stomal placement is performed through the appropriate rings. Care is taken to preserve the tissue surrounding the innominate artery, which may be high in some patients. Just prior to making the tracheotomy, the cuff is deflated. Our preference is the use of a vertical tracheotomy through the second and third, and if necessary fourth tracheal rings. The incision is kept to the minimum necessary, in order to minimize the injury to the trachea and potential for scarring. A scissor may be necessary to extend the incision, as calcification of the tracheal cartilage is common in the elderly. It is important not to make the incision into the first tracheal ring, as that is the buffer between the tube and the cricoid cartilage. Erosion of the tube into the cricoid cartilage has the potential for causing laryngotracheal stenosis. A stoma that is too low increases the risk of tracheoinnominate fistula, and this is also to be avoided. Flaps and resection of tracheal wall are typically avoided. The endotracheal tube is withdrawn so that its tip lies just above the stoma. Retractors, such as the thyroid pole retractor, or tracheal dilators may be used as the appropriate tracheostomy tube is introduced. The cuff is inflated, and a swivel connector is attached and connected to the ventilator circuit. Traction sutures in the trachea are typically not necessary. The skin is closed around the tracheostomy tube with interrupted nylon sutures. The flange of the tracheostomy tube is sutured to the skin at four corners, to prevent accidental extubation.

Care of the tracheostomy tube can be just as important in avoiding complications. The cuff must never be overinflated, as the low-pressure high-volume cuff can easily become a high-pressure cuff with over distention. Diligent monitoring of the cuff pressure whenever air is added to the cuff can prevent this problem. The swivel, accordion style circuit tubing, and suspension of circuit tubing to avoid undue traction on the tracheostomy tube, also help avoid stomal complications. Adherence to these details should virtually eliminate these problems.

The elderly patient undergoing almost any major operation or recovering from a critical medical illness may need prolonged mechanical ventilation. Tracheostomy is typically considered once intubation extends beyond 7–14 days, and sometimes even earlier. The advantages of a tracheostomy are well established and include: improved pulmonary toilet, easier nursing, reduced dead space and airway resistance, easier weaning from ventilation, and possibility of eating while weaning from the vent. What is less certain in the elderly patient population is whether or not tracheostomy is justified in the face of a likely poor outcome. One of the few studies of tracheostomy in the elderly (mean age 77 years) found that over 50% of patients died after tracheostomy, with a mean time to death of 31 days [17]. Moreover, a large proportion of patients surviving after tracheostomy never realized the potential advantages of tracheostomy, such as ventilator independence and eating (many had undergone gastrostomy placement). The authors speculated that age was not necessarily the primary predictor of the poor results in this study, but rather the severity and nature of the illness the patients were suffering. Tracheostomy should not be avoided in the elderly; rather, it should be selectively and safely used in patients with reasonable chance for recovery.

Tracheal T-Tubes and Airway Stents

Airway surgeons should be experienced with the placement and management of tracheal T-tubes and airway stents. T-tubes possess a number of advantages compared to tracheostomy tubes and airway stents. In most cases, T-tubes permit speech more effectively than tracheostomy tubes. Moreover, they are not as rigid, and are less likely to injure the airway. Unlike silicone airway stents, T-tubes are significantly less likely to migrate. Specific indications for placement of tracheal T-tubes include need for temporary airway stenting, management of complications after airway reconstruction, and definitive palliation of airway stenosis. In one large series of patients managed with T-tubes, the oldest patient was 95 years old [18]. The series described very effective management of airway stenoses with T-tubes, with approximately one-third of patients tolerating T-tubes for longer than 1 year.

While the list of indications for airway stenting is long, some sophistication and judgment is necessary to decide whether or not a patient will benefit from the procedure. Stents are particularly useful in the palliative setting, where the patient's life expectancy is short. This makes stent complications such as migration, obstruction, and granulation production less likely.

Laryngotracheal and Tracheal Resection for Airway Stenosis and Tumors

There are a number of variables that need to be examined before determining how much trachea may be safely resected and reanastomosed. Arbitrary numbers such as 5 cm or one half of the trachea are not sufficient guidelines when planning an operation for the individual patient. Experience and judgment are necessary to take into consideration a number of variables such as age, body habitus, nature of the disease, and history of prior airway or mediastinal surgery. Having said that lengths of up to 4–5 cm are often resected safely, the approach for most benign stenoses and tumors of the upper half of the trachea is through a cervical or cervicomediastinal approach. The transthoracic approach, through a right thoracotomy usually, is reserved for tumors or pathology at the distal trachea, carina, or mainstem bronchi.

For a benign stenosis or tumor of the upper trachea, the patient has an orotracheal airway established using techniques reviewed above. The patient is positioned supine with a bag inflated under the shoulders to slightly extend the neck. The hips and knees are slightly flexed. A low-collar incision is made for most upper tracheal and laryngotracheal resections. If there is a tracheal stoma, the incision incorporates it, as long as the stoma is not too high in the neck. Skin and plastysmal flaps are raised cephalad and caudad to the cricoid cartilage and sternal notch, respectively. Two Gelpi retractors are used to hold the flaps open. The strap muscles are mobilized laterally, and the midline established. Normal tracheal anatomy may be lost, particularly in the presence of a stoma and significant peristomal scarring. Dissection over more normal trachea either proximal or distal to the stoma or scar can usually establish some anatomical landmarks. It is important to restrict this dissection to the anterior aspect of the trachea to avoid injury to the recurrent laryngeal nerves and disruption of the lateral blood supply of the trachea. The thyroid isthmus should be divided if it has not been previously, and the thyroid lobes mobilized off of the trachea. Again, meticulous dissection just on the tracheal wall is necessary. There is no attempt made to visualize the recurrent nerves, which are often obscured by the fibrosis. Lesions that are mid-tracheal or lower may require a partial sternotomy to increase exposure. A vertical skin incision to the Angle of Louis is made perpendicular to the low-collar incision. A partial sternotomy is made with the Liebsche knife, after carefully making sure the retrosternal space is free of adhesions. A complete sternotomy does not increase exposure, and is unnecessary. A pediatric chest retractor is used to hold apart the sternal edges. With a partial sternotomy, even the distal trachea may be approached.

The initial dissection may or may not expose the extent of pathology. At some point, bronchoscopy may be performed by the surgeon, and an assistant may introduce a 25-gauge needle from the field to mark the location of the stenosis. Circumferential dissection may be carefully attempted at the distal aspect of the stenosis, where division of the trachea is anticipated (Fig. 50.2). If the scar is too dense and makes this difficult, the posterior dissection is delayed until after the trachea is partially divided.

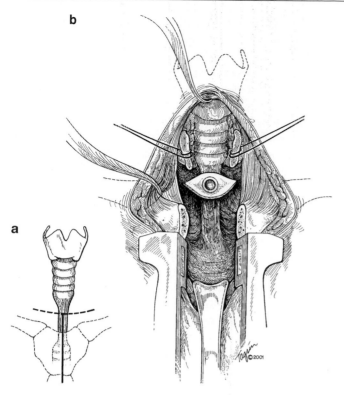

Fig. 50.2 Cervicomediastinal exposure. (**a**) A low-collar cervical incision (*dashed line*) is used for most tracheal and laryngotracheal resections. Additional exposure of the middle and distal trachea is gained by adding a vertical extension to the angle of Louis (*solid line*) and performing a partial sternotomy. (**b**) The completed incision and partial sternotomy, as well as division of the thyroid isthmus (shown with traction sutures) exposes the stoma, stenotic trachea, and normal distal trachea in this patient (from Grillo [1], used with permission)

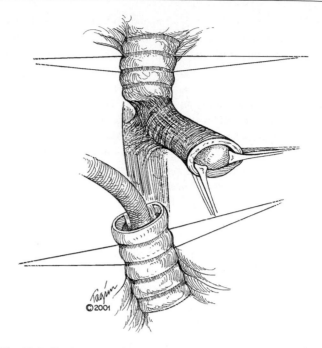

Fig. 50.3 Tracheal transection and dissection of stenosis. The trachea has been dissected circumferentially just distal to the stenosis, then divided and intubated distally for cross-field ventilation. Traction sutures (shown in figure) are placed in the mid-lateral wall that assists dissection. The traction sutures are tied together when the anastomosis is completed (from Grillo [1], used with permission)

In preparation for tracheal division, sterile tubing for ventilation and an appropriately sized armored endotracheal tube are prepared on the field. The trachea is opened anteriorly just distal to the stenosis or tumor. Especially with benign strictures, the point of distal division is kept very close to the lesion as more trachea can always be resected, but never restored. A 2-0 Vicryl traction suture is placed in both midlateral tracheal walls about 1 cm below the cut edge of distal trachea. These are used to assist further dissection posteriorly, as the membranous wall is separated from the esophagus. The distal divided trachea is intubated with the armored endotracheal tube, and cross-field ventilation is begun (Fig. 50.3). Circumferential dissection around the lesion is carefully performed, and no more than 1 cm of trachea beyond the cut ends should be mobilized. If the proximal point of tracheal division is at the cricoid, it should be noted that no attempt is made to dissect posterior to the cricoid cartilage. 2-0 traction sutures are placed in the proximal divided trachea as well. With tracheal tumors, pathologic assessment of margins is made by frozen section analysis. With adenoid cystic carcinoma, microscopically positive margins are acceptable so as to not exceed safe limits of

tracheal resection. This tumor has a tendency to have microscopic spread along distances that cannot be safely resected; moreover, it is very radiosensitive, and most patients will receive radiation postoperatively.

The tension with which the two ends will come together is tested by having the anesthesiologist flex the neck by picking up the head, and bringing the two sets of traction sutures together. With experience, it will be easy to judge whether or not there is excessive tension. There are maneuvers, such as a suprahyoid release, which give some mobility to the larynx and reduce some tension; however, these are not routinely required. The 4-0 Vicryl anastomotic sutures are placed next, starting with a suture in the middle of the membranous wall. These sutures are clamped to the drapes, as they will be tied in the reverse order of placement. Once all sutures are placed, the orotracheal tube is advanced across the anastomosis. The head is supported with blankets in order to flex the neck. The traction sutures are brought together and tied. The anterior sutures are tied first, with the assistant crossing the leading sutures to reduce tension while tying (Fig. 50.4). The posterior sutures are then tied. The anastomosis is tested by deflating the endotracheal cuff and applying 30 cm H_2O of pressure through it. The anastomosis should be submerged in saline to assess for any air leak. The anastomosis is covered by either re-approximating the thyroid isthmus or mobilizing a strap muscle and suturing it over its anterior aspect. The sternum is re-approximated with wires, if it was divided. The skin is

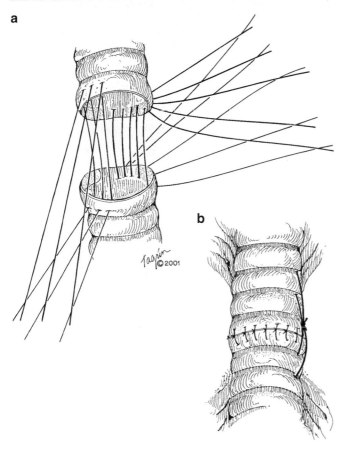

Fig. 50.4 Anastomotic suture placement. (**a**) The posterior sutures are placed first, with each additional suture being placed anterior to the previously placed suture. The sutures are tied in reverse order of placement. In this diagram, the right posterolateral sutures and stay sutures are omitted for clarity. A few anterior sutures are also shown. (**b**) The completed anastomosis (only the left traction sutures tied together are shown) (from Grillo [1], used with permission)

closed over a closed suction drain. A "guardian" stitch from the submental skin crease to the presternal skin is placed and tied, so that the neck is held in moderate flexion. This stitch is to prevent the patient from suddenly extending the neck and placing excessive tension on the anastomosis.

The patient is usually extubated at the conclusion of the procedure. The airway may be inadequate if there is significant laryngeal edema, which may require a brief period of intubation; a short course of steroids may be used, and extubation attempted again in 24–48 h. Rarely, a small tracheostomy distal to the anastomosis may be necessary to provide an adequate airway. Patients are typically monitored in the intensive care unit overnight. They are kept upright to minimize the risk of aspiration and reduce edema. Moreover, talking is discouraged. Racemic epinephrine nebulizer therapy and judicious use of diuretics also have a role.

Some of the expected outcomes are discussed above in the section on airway pathology. Specific complications that may occur include granulation at the anastomosis, anastomotic

dehiscence, tracheal restenosis, and wound infection. Recently, a retrospective analysis was performed of over 900 tracheal and laryngotracheal resections at MGH [19]. In this study, age under 17 years was identified as a risk factor for anastomotic complications, while being elderly was not. The mean age of patients in this series was 47 years, and the oldest patient was 86 years. Significant risk factors that were identified included diabetes, resections longer than 4 cm, reoperation, and need for tracheostomy preoperatively.

Laryngotracheal resection may be required for lesions that involve the distal larynx and the proximal trachea. Post-intubation stenosis often involves the cricoid cartilage, especially when the tracheostomy tube erodes through the first tracheal ring and into the anterior cricoid. Tumors such as invasive thyroid carcinoma also have a tendency to involve the inferior larynx, given the location of disease. The goal of laryngotracheal resection is to perform an adequate resection, while still preserving laryngeal competence and function. This requires sufficient space beneath the vocal cords to place anastomotic sutures. It is also dependent on adequate glottic function, and otolaryngologic assessment is typically advised. When the lesion only involves the anterior cricoid, this section of the larynx is resected, preserving the posterior cricoid cartilage. Anastomosis requires the distal trachea to be slightly beveled to match the proximal airway, as the anterior sutures will be placed in the thyroid cartilage, and the posterior sutures will be placed in the slightly caudal cricoid cartilage. When there is a cuff injury to the circumference of the subglottic space, and the posterior cricoid cartilage is not spared, more specialized techniques are necessary [20].

Resection and Reconstruction for Airway Esophageal Fistula

The operation for a tracheoesophageal fistula caused by an indwelling tracheostomy or endotracheal tube requires a single stage procedure in which both an airway stenosis and a large tracheoesophageal defect must be simultaneously addressed (Fig. 50.5). The patient should be weaned from mechanical ventilation, and airway sepsis must have been adequately treated. The patient usually has a tracheostomy tube whose cuff resides distal to the tracheoesophageal fistula. An orotracheal tube is placed, usually under bronchoscopic guidance, with care not to intubate the esophagus. A low-collar incision that incorporates the stoma is made as described above. The initial dissection is also similar. The division of the trachea is followed by on-field intubation of the divided trachea and cross-field ventilation. Division of the trachea gives excellent visualization of the defect, and dissection proceeds proximally. The proximal limit of the posterior dissection is the cricoid cartilage, as the aerodigestive tract cannot be

Fig. 50.5 Post-intubation
tracheoesophageal fistula.
(**a**) Anterior view of tracheoesophageal fistula with cricoid
cartilage (a), stoma (b), fistula
(c), and circumferential tracheal
stenosis (d) identified. (**b**)
Saggital view of tracheoesophageal fistula (from Grillo [1], used
with permission)

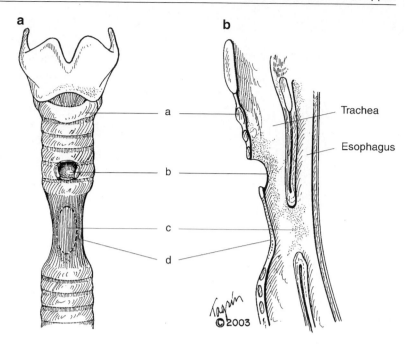

separated safely above that level. At times, the length of
trachea that is affected is too long for resection, and it may be
prudent to consider a repair of the posterior aspect of the
trachea rather than resecting a long segment of trachea. In this
case, relatively normal esophagus is left attached to the
tracheal walls laterally, and brought together by interrupted
4-0 Vicryl sutures in the posterior midline, fashioning a new
membranous trachea. The esophagus is typically redundant,
and the esophageal lumen will be adequate after the remaining
esophagus is closed. In other cases, a segment of trachea may
be safely resected. The esophagus is repaired with two layers
of interrupted 4-0 silk or Vicryl sutures, which is similar to the
Sweet technique for esophageal anastomosis. The esophageal
repair should be buttressed with a strap muscle that has been
mobilized for this purpose. A tracheal or laryngotracheal
anastomosis is performed as discussed previously.

An even rarer lesion is an acquired bronchoesophageal fistula
from inflammatory etiologies such as tuberculosis or iatrogenic
trauma. These lesions are approached via thoracotomy.
Resectional therapy is typically not necessary, as the esophagus
and bronchus may be repaired primarily [21]. Intercostal muscle
flap interposition between the bronchial and esophageal suture
lines is considered vital to the success of this repair. A thoracotomy is the typical approach for this procedure.

Carinal Reconstruction

The pathologic entities that may require carinal resection are
bronchogenic cancer, other neoplasms (such as adenoid cystic carcinoma and mucoepidermoid tumor), and benign or

inflammatory strictures, in descending order of frequency.
Specialized techniques have been developed to manage these
lesions, which are relatively rare.

Patient evaluation and preparation is important, as for any
other airway or pulmonary resection. Steroid therapy, especially high dose, should be tapered prior to resection, and is
a relative contraindication. Likewise, any prior radiation to
the mediastinum should be concerning, and provisions for
omental mobilization to wrap the anastomosis must be made.
The patient must be able to tolerate a thoracotomy, and
mechanical ventilation ought to be avoided postoperatively.
CT scanning to assess the extent and nature of airway
involvement, local invasion, and possible metastatic lymphadenopathy is essential. A careful metastatic survey should
also be performed. Cervical mediastinoscopy as a separate
prior operation should be avoided, as fibrosis of the tissues
surrounding the trachea will impair its mobility, which is
important for reducing tension on the anastomosis. While
some lesions may be amenable to simple carinal resection
and anastomosis of a neo-carina (fashioned from the orifices
of the mainstem bronchi) to the distal trachea (Fig. 50.6),
other lesions will require resection of distal trachea, proximal bronchi, or both. There are strict limits to how much
airway can be resected and safely reconstructed; certain
extensive tumors in this region may be better served by
definitive radiotherapy.

Mediastinoscopy is performed to assess for resectability,
and to develop the pretracheal plan, which enhances tracheal
mobility and reduces tension on the anastomosis. The
approach to the carina is typically via a right thoracotomy,
although a left thoracotomy or a clamshell incision will be
necessary to operate in the circumstance of the rare left

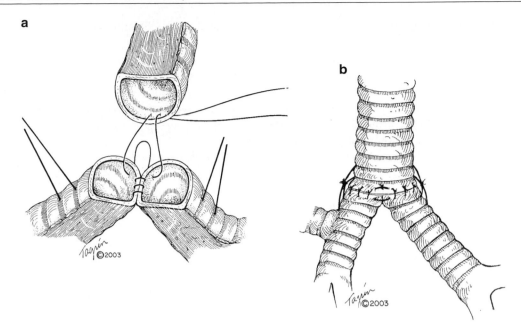

Fig. 50.6 Carinal reconstruction after resection of the carina alone. (**a**) Interrupted sutures joining the two mainstem orifices are placed to construct a neo-carina. A mattress suture then is placed to join the anterior trachea wall with the neo-carina. Simple interrupted sutures are placed proportionally between the anterior tracheal wall and the bronchi. Further sutures are placed between the membranous wall of the trachea and bronchi. Finally, another mattress suture will be required at the confluence of the membranous wall of the trachea and the two bronchi. (**b**) Completed anastomosis (tied sutures, including traction sutures, are shown) (from Grillo [1], used with permission)

carinal pneumonectomy. Although some surgeons have advocated using median sternotomy for approaching the carina, at MGH we have found access through this incision lacking and only useful for the simplest of carinal reconstructions. Assessment for resectability of a tumor should be made at this time. There are cases in which concomitant superior vena cava or esophageal resection may be necessary. If resection appears feasible, the inferior pulmonary ligament is divided, and a U-shaped incision is made in the infrahilar pericardium. This maneuver, an infrahilar release, provides some mobility to the proximal bronchus, reducing tension on the anastomosis. Suprahyoid release, in our experience, does not increase mobility of the distal trachea, and is not useful.

Jet ventilation should be available and may be necessary, especially when completing the anastomosis. Initially, an extra-long single-lumen tube is advanced bronchoscopically, allowing for single-lung ventilation. After the airway is divided, the away or "down" bronchus may be intubated on the field and cross-field ventilation is used. Intermittent ventilation and other strategies, such as jet ventilation, may be necessary during certain parts of the dissection and creation of the anastomosis.

The distal trachea and proximal mainstem bronchi are dissected and isolated, usually with umbilical tape. Care is taken not to injure the left recurrent nerve or the aortic arch, when dissection of the left mainstem bronchus is performed. Extensive lymphadenectomy is avoided, out of concern for devascularization of the airway, and the risk to the anastomosis. A pulmonary resection (either lobectomy or pneumonectomy) may be combined with the carinal resection, depending on the extent of tumor. Once the carinal resection is complete, the surgeon must determine the best way to reconstruct the airway. If any amount of trachea is resected along with the carina, the reconstruction will typically require an end-to-end anastomosis of the distal trachea to a mainstem bronchus, and an end-to-side anastomosis between the remaining bronchus and the trachea or contralateral bronchus. The most common reconstruction in cases of carinal resection without pneumonectomy is an end-to-end anastomosis of trachea to the left mainstem bronchus, and end-to-side anastomosis of the right mainstem bronchus to the trachea. The anastomotic technique is similar to that of the tracheal anastomosis, with 3-0 Vicryl traction sutures and interrupted 4-0 Vicryl sutures to complete the anastomosis. The anastomosis should be wrapped with a flap. While a pedicled pericardial fat pad is usually sufficient, in patients who have received preoperative radiation, a pedicled omental flap is recommended.

Although the mortality from carinal resections performed at MGH is acceptable at 12.7%, it is significantly higher than that of isolated tracheal resections or bronchoplastic resections. The primary risk factors were need for postoperative mechanical ventilation, extent of resected airway, and the occurrence of an anastomotic complication. Age, in this series, was examined, and was not an independent risk factor for complications [22].

Main and Lobar Bronchoplasty

The ideal lesion suitable for main or lobar bronchoplasty is the benign or low-grade lesion that affects a lobe or bronchus that is anatomically suitable for "sleeve" resection. Bronchoplasty may also be utilized in resecting malignant lesions, as long as basic oncologic principles are not violated. The goal is to preserve physiologically functioning lung that would have otherwise been sacrificed by resection of the airway.

Sleeve resection may be "obligatory" in patients with minimal pulmonary reserve, and advanced age should not be a contraindication. As with carinal resection, high-dose corticosteroid use, active bronchial inflammation, and significant radiation history are all relative contraindications to bronchoplasty. Steroids can typically be weaned to very low doses or eliminated prior to bronchoplasty. Bronchial inflammation, especially with tuberculosis, must be limited and controlled with medical therapy. With respect to radiation, the more remote the radiation history, especially with doses greater than 5,000 Gy, the more likely that postoperative dehiscence or stenosis may complicate bronchoplasty. Neoadjuvant therapy that is administered several weeks before bronchoplasty has not been associated with increased complications in most series. Anastomotic complications should be ameliorated by the liberal use of flaps. Pericardial fat pad flaps are appropriate and sufficient for most bronchoplasties. Omentum, however, is more robust and should be considered for resections considered to be at higher risk. Post-obstructive pneumonia or atelectasis also should not be considered contraindications. Coring out of tumor and aspiration bronchoscopy can be used to improve the state of lung that will be saved by bronchoplasty.

The techniques for bronchoplasty are similar to that used for any airway resection. Meticulous and gentle dissection is necessary to avoid injury to the bronchial ends that are to be anastomosed. Although there might be a size discrepancy between the two bronchial ends being anastomosed, no attempt is made to specially tailor the ends. Rather, proportional spacing of sutures, and possible intussuception of the airway are used to complete the anastomosis. We have relied on an interrupted suture technique with absorbable sutures (Vicryl) that have virtually eliminated granulation, and are ideal for placement and tying. Traction sutures, 3-0 Vicryl rather than 2-0 Vicryl that is used for tracheal resections, are placed in the midlateral walls of the bronchial ends. Interrupted sutures are placed, so that the knots will be tied on the outside. Sutures are placed in an ordered fashion so that tying will be systematic and not be impeded by previously placed sutures. The traction sutures are tied first, and then typically the anterior sutures, followed by the posterior sutures. The sutures are cut as they are tied. A flap of pericardial fat or omentum is used to wrap the anastomosis and separate it from the adjacent pulmonary artery. An intercostal or other muscle flap may also be used. Bronchoscopy is performed to suction secretions and assure a proper anastomosis was performed. Ideally, postoperative ventilation will be avoided. Routine postoperative bronchoscopy on postoperative day 7 is done to confirm normal healing.

Although any lobe may be resected by bronchoplasty, the most common "sleeve" resections are the right upper lobe followed by left upper lobe sleeve resections. The bronchoplasty may also require tangential or sleeve resections of the pulmonary artery, if the tumor cannot be dissected away or invades it. The reader is referred to texts and publications that review the specific bronchoplasties and adjunctive techniques that have been developed [23].

There are several large series of bronchoplastic resections from a variety of centers. Recently, MGH published a retrospective review of 196 bronchoplastic resections performed between 1980 and 2007 [24]. In this series, the mean age of the patients was 54 years, with the range being 13–87 years. The overall mortality in this series was 2%, while the morbidity rate was 37%. Five-year survival for non-small-cell lung cancer patients undergoing bronchoplasty was 44%. The local recurrence rate was 17%. A multivariate analysis was performed looking for risk factors for all complications and anastomotic complications specifically. In this analysis, age greater than 70 years was an independent risk factor for complications, although not for anastomotic complications. Anastomotic complications were more likely in patients receiving neoadjuvant therapy, although this contradicts several other studies that found no such association. At MGH, we do not believe neoadjuvant therapy should be considered a contraindication. Rather, we believe that meticulous technique and flap coverage of the anastomosis are even more important in these cases. Other studies have also found that while overall morbidity, including complications such as pneumonia and need for bronchoscopy, may be higher in the elderly, anastomotic complications themselves are not more likely in the elderly.

Conclusion

Airway surgery requires mature surgical judgment and excellent technique in order to be performed safely and to ensure good outcomes. There are a number of principles applicable to surgery on any segment of the airway. The elderly offer no specific challenges that cannot be surmounted by attention to detail in patient evaluation, operating, and postoperative care.

References

1. Grillo H. Surgery of the trachea and bronchi. Hamilton: BC Decker; 2004.

2. Grillo HC, Dignan EF, Miura T. Extensive resection and reconstruction of mediastinal trachea without prosthesis or graft: an anatomical study in man. J Thorac Cardiovasc Surg. 1964;48:741–9.

3. Salassa JR, Pearson BW, Payne WS. Gross and microscopical blood supply of the trachea. Ann Thorac Surg. 1977;24(2):100–7.

4. Grillo HC, Mathisen DJ. Primary tracheal tumors – treatment and results. Ann Thorac Surg. 1990;49(1):69–77.

5. Gaissert HA, Grillo HC, Shadmehr B, et al. Long-term survival after resection of primary adenoid cystic and squamous cell carcinoma of the trachea and carina. Ann Thorac Surg. 2004;78(6):1889–96.

6. Heitmiller RF, Mathisen DJ, Ferry JA, Mark EJ, Grillo HC. Mucoepidermoid lung-tumors. Ann Thorac Surg. 1989;47(3):394–9.

7. Kim AW, Maxhimer JB, Quiros RM, Weber K, Prinz RA. Surgical management of well-differentiated thyroid cancer locally invasive to the respiratory tract. J Am Coll Surg. 2005;201(4):619–27.

8. Gaissert HA, Honings J, Grillo HC, et al. Segmental laryngotracheal and tracheal resection for invasive thyroid carcinoma. Ann Thorac Surg. 2007;83(6):1952–9.

9. Shin DH, Mark EJ, Suen HC, Grillo HC. Pathological staging of papillary carcinoma of the thyroid with airway invasion based on the anatomic manner of extension to the trachea – a clinicopathological study based on 22 patients who underwent thyroidectomy and airway resection. Hum Pathol. 1993;24(8):866–70.

10. Mitchell JD, Mathisen DJ, Wright CD, et al. Resection for bronchogenic carcinoma involving the carina: long-term results and effect of nodal status on outcome. J Thorac Cardiovasc Surg. 2001;121(3):465–71.

11. Grillo HC, Donahue DM, Mathisen DJ, Wain JC, Wright CD. Postintubation tracheal stenosis – treatment and results. J Thorac Cardiovasc Surg. 1995;109(3):486–93.

12. Macchiarini P, Verhoye JP, Chapelier A, Fadel E, Dartevelle P. Evaluation and outcome of different surgical techniques for postintubation tracheoesophageal fistulas. J Thorac Cardiovasc Surg. 2000;119(2):268–74.

13. Mathisen DJ, Grillo HC, Wain JC, Hilgenberg AD. Management of acquired nonmalignant tracheoesophageal fistula. Ann Thorac Surg. 1991;52(4):759–65.

14. Wright CD, Grillo HC, Hammoud ZT, et al. Tracheoplasty for expiratory collapse of central airways. Ann Thorac Surg. 2005;80(1):259–67.

15. Greene R, Lechner G. "Saber-sheath" trachea: a clinical and functional study of marked coronal narrowing of the intrathoracic trachea. Radiology. 1975;115(2):265–8.

16. Katlic MR, Grillo HC, Wang CA. Substernal goiter – analysis of 80 patients from Massachusetts General Hospital. Am J Surg. 1985;149(2):283–7.

17. Baskin JZ, Panagopoulos G, Parks C, Rothstein S, Komisar A. Clinical outcomes for the elderly patient receiving a tracheotomy. Head Neck. 2004;26(1):71–5.

18. Gaissert H, Grillo H, Mathisen D, Wain J. Temporary and permanent restoration of airway continuity with the tracheal T-tube. J Thorac Cardiovasc Surg. 1994;107(2):600–6.

19. Wright CD, Grillo HC, Wain JC, et al. Anastomotic complications after tracheal resection: prognostic factors and management. J Thorac Cardiovasc Surg. 2004;128(5):731–9.

20. Grillo H. Primary reconstruction of airway after resection of subglottic laryngeal and upper tracheal stenosis. Ann Thorac Surg. 1982;33(1):3–18.

21. Mangi AA, Giassert HA, Wright CD, et al. Benign broncho-esophageal fistula in the adult. Ann Thorac Surg. 2002;73(3):911–5.

22. Mitchell JD, Mathisen DJ, Wright CD, et al. Clinical experience with carinal resection. J Thorac Cardiovasc Surg. 1999;117(1):39–52.

23. Rendina EA, Venuta F, de Giacomo T, Rossi M, Coloni GF. Parenchymal sparing operations for bronchogenic carcinoma. Surg Clin North Am. 2002;82(3):589–609.

24. Merritt RE, Mathisen DJ, Wain JC, et al. Long-term results of sleeve lobectomy in the management of non-small cell lung carcinoma and low-grade neoplasms. Ann Thorac Surg. 2009;88(5):1574–82.

Activities of Daily Living (ADL)

Katz index of independence in activities of daily living

Activities Points (1 or 0)	Independence (1 point) NO supervision, direction or personal assistance	Dependence (0 points) WITH supervision, direction, personal assistance or total care
BATHING Points: _____	(1 POINT) Bathes self completely or needs help in bathing only a single part of the body such as the back, genital area or disabled extremity.	(0 POINTS) Need help with bathing more than one part of the body, getting in or out of the tub or shower. Requires total bathing.
DRESSING Points:_____	(1 POINT) Gets clothes from closets and drawers and puts on clothes and outer garments complete with fasteners. May have help tying shoes.	(0 POINTS) Needs help with dressing self of needs to be completely dressed.
TOILETING Points: _____	(1 POINT) Goes to toilet, gets on and off, arranges clothes, cleans genital area without help.	(0 POINTS) Needs help transferring to the toilet, cleaning self or uses bedpan or commode.
TRANSFERRING Points: _____	(1 POINT) Moves in and out of bed or chair unassisted. Mechanical transfer aids are acceptable.	(0 POINTS) Needs help moving from bed to chair or requires complete transfer.
CONTINENCE Points: _____	(1 POINT) Exercises complete self control over urination and defecation.	(0 POINTS) Is partially or totally incontinent of bowel or bladder.
FEEDING Points: _____	(1 POINT) Gets food from plate into mouth without help. Preparation of food may be done by another person.	(0 POINTS) Needs partial or total help with feeding or required parenteral feeding.

Total points: _____

Score of 6 = High, patient is independent

Score of 0 = Low, patient is very dependent

Source: Adapted from Katz S, Down TD, Cash HR, et al. Progress in the development of index of ADL. **Gerontologist**. 1970;10:20–30. Copyright © The Gerontological Society of America. Used by permission of Oxford University Press

Instrumental Activities of Daily Living (IADL)

INSTRUMENTAL SCTIVITEIES OF DAILY LIVING SCALE (IADL)
M.P. Lawton and E.M. Brody

A. Ability to use telephone
1. Operates telephone on own initiative; looks up and dials numbers, etc.   1
2. Dials a few well-known numbers.   1
3. Answers telephone but does not dial.   1
4. Does not use telephone at all.   0

B. Shopping
1. Takes care of all shopping needs independently.   1
2. Shops independently for small purchases.   0
3. Needs to be accompanied on any shopping trip.   0
4. Completely unable to shop.   0

C. Food preparation
1. Plans, prepares, and serves adequate meals independently.   1
2. Prepares adequate meals if supplied with ingredients.   0
3. Heats serves and prepares meals or prepares meals but does not maintain adequate diet.   0
4. Needs to have meals prepared and served.   0

D. Housekeeping
1. Maintains house alone or with occasional assistance (e.g., "heavy work domestic help").   1
2. Performs light daily tasks such as dish washing, bed making.   1
3. Performs light daily tasks but cannot maintain acceptable level of cleanliness.   1
4. Needs help with all home maintenance tasks.   1
5. Does not participate in any housekeeping tasks.   0

E. Laundry
1. Does personal laundry completely.   1
2. Launders small items; rinses stockings, etc.   1
3. All laundry must be done by others.   0

F. Mode of transportation
1. Travels independently on public transportation or drives own car.   1
2. Arranges own travel via taxi, but does not otherwise use public transportation   1
3. Travels in public transportation when accompanied by another.   1
4. Travel limited to taxi or automobile with assistance of another.   0
5. Does not travel at all.   0

G. Responsibility for own medications
1. Is responsible for taking medication in correct dosages at correct time.   1
2. Takes responsibility if medication is prepared in advance in separate dosage.   0
3. Is not capable of dispensing own medication.   0

H. Ability to handle finances
1. Manages financial matters independently (budgets, writes checks, pays rent, bills, goes to bank), collects and keeps track of income.   1
2. Manages day-to-day purchases, but needs help with banking, major purchases, etc.   1
3. Incapable of handling money.   0

Source: Lawton MP, Brody EM. Assessment of older people; self-maintaining and instrumental activities of daily living. **Gerontologist**. 1969;9:179–86. Copyright © The Gerontological Society of America. Used by permission of Oxford University Press

Karnofsky Score

- 100% – normal, no complaints, no sign of disease.
- 90% – capable of normal activity, few symptoms or signs of disease.
- 80% – normal activity with some difficulty, some symptoms or signs.
- 70% – caring for self, not capable of normal activity or work.
- 60% – requiring some help, can take care of most personal requirements.
- 50% – requires help often, requires frequent medical care.
- 40% – disabled, requires special care and help.
- 30% – severely disabled, hospital admission indicated but no risk of death.
- 20% – very ill, urgently requiring admission, requires supportive measures or treatment.
- 10% moribund, rapidly progressive fatal disease processes.
- 0% – death.

Source: From Karnofsky DA, Burchenal JH. The clinical evaluation of chemotherapeutic agents in cancer. In: MacLeod CM, editor. **Evaluation of chemotherapeutic agents**. Columbia: Columbia University Press; 1949. p. 196. Copyright © 1949 Columbia University Press. Reprinted with permission of the publisher.

Eastern Cooperative Oncology Group (ECOG)/Zubrod Score

- 0 – Asymptomatic (fully active, able to carry on all pre-disease activities without restriction).
- 1 – Symptomatic but completely ambulatory (restricted in physical strenuous activity but ambulatory and able to care out work of a light or sedentary nature (for example, light housework, office work)).
- 2 – Symptomatic, <50% in bed during the day (ambulatory and capable of all self-care but unable to carry out any work activities. Up and about more than 50% of waking hours).
- – Symptomatic, >50% in bed, but not bedbound (capable of only limited self-care, confined to bed or chair 50% or more of waking hours).
- – Bedbound (completely disabled; cannot carry on any self-care; totally confined to bed or chair).
- – Death.

Source: Oken MM, Creech RH, Tormey DC, et al. Toxicity and response criteria of the Eastern Cooperative Oncology Group. **Am J Clin Oncol**. 1982;5(6):649–66.

Appendix C: Physiologic

Six-Minute Walk Test

Standardization of the six-minute walk test (6MWT) is very important.

At the commencement of pulmonary rehabilitation, the 6MWT must be performed on *two occasions* to account for a learning effect. Please note that:

- The best distance walked in meters is recorded.
- If the two tests are performed on the same day, at least 30 min rest should be allowed between tests. Debilitated individuals may require tests to be performed on separate days, preferably less than one week apart.

  - The walking track should be the same layout for all tests for a patient:
  - The track may be a continuous track (oval or rectangular) or a point-to-point (stop, turn around, go) track.
  - The minimum recommended length for a center-based walking track is 25 m and could be marked in meter increments.

Note: If you do not have access to a 25 m track, make sure you use the same track for all tests and be aware that the distance walked may be less due to the patient having to slow down and turn more often in six minutes.

- A comfortable ambient temperature and humidity should be maintained for all tests.
- The information from the 6MWT can be used to prescribe the intensity of walking exercise.

6MWT Equipment

The equipment needed to conduct the 6MWT is described in the below checklist.

What do I need for the six-minute walk test?	Yes	No
Do I have access to a health professional trained in CPR and with the expertise to run the test?		
Do I have access to a flat continuous (oval or rectangular) or point-to-point (stop, turn around, go) walking track at least 25 m in length?		

(continued)

Is the walking track clear of hospital traffic and obstacles, with minimal blind turns?
Can the walking test be conducted in a comfortable ambient temperature and humidity?
Do I have a stethoscope?
Do I have a sphygmomanometer?
Do I have a pulse oximeter?
Do I have a stopwatch?
Do I have a portable oxygen delivery system?
Do I have chairs positioned to allow for patient rest?
Do I have a dyspnea scale?
Do I have measuring tape or can the walking track be marked in 1 m ingrements?

Before the 6MWT

- Ensure that you have already obtained a medical history of the patient and have taken into account any precautions or contraindications to exercise testing.
- Instruct the patient to dress comfortably, wear appropriate footwear and to avoid eating for at least two hours before the test (where possible or appropriate).
- Any prescribed inhaled bronchodilator medication should be taken within one hour of testing or when the patient arrives for testing.
- The patient should rest for at least 15 min before beginning the 6MWT.
- Record:

  - Blood pressure
  - Heart rate
  - Oxygen Saturation
  - Dyspnea score.*

Note: Show the patient the dyspnea scale (i.e., Borg scale) and give standardized instructions on how to obtain a score.

Instructions for the 6MWT

Instructions and encouragement must be standardized.

Tip: Put the instructions on a laminated card and read them out to each patient

Before the Test

Describe the walking track to the patient and then give the patient the following instructions:

> "You are now going to do a six-minute walk test. The object of the test is to walk as quickly as you can for 6 min (around the track; up and down the corridor, etc. depending on your track set up) so that you cover as much ground as possible."
>
> You may slow down if necessary. If you stop, I want you to continue to walk again as soon as possible. You will be regularly informed of the time and you will be encouraged to do your best. Your goal is to walk as far as possible in 6 min.
>
> Please do not talk during the test unless you have a problem or I ask you a question. You must let me know if you have any chest pain or dizziness.
>
> When the 6 min is up, "I will ask you to stop wherever you are. Do you have any questions?"
>
> Begin the test by instructing the patient to:
>
> "Start walking now."

During the Test

Monitor the patient for untoward signs and symptoms.
Use the following standard encouragements during the test:

- At minute one: "Five minutes remaining (*patient name*). Do your best!"
- At minute two: "Four minutes remaining (*patient name*). You're doing well, keep it up!"
- At minute three: "Half way – 3 min remaining (*patient name*). Do your best!"
- At minute four: "Two minutes remaining (*patient name*). You're doing well – keep it up!"
- At minute five: "One minute remaining (*patient name*). Do your best!"

At the End of the 6MWT

- Put a marker on the distance walked.
- Seat the patient or, if the patient prefers, allow the patient to stand.

Note: The measurements taken before and after the test should be taken with the patient in the same position.

- Immediately record oxygen saturation (SpO_2%, heart rate, and dyspnea rating on the *6MWT recording sheet*.
- Measure the excess distance with a tape measure and tally up the total distance.

The patient should remain in a clinical area for at least 15 min following an uncomplicated test.

Clinical Notes

Normally, the clinician does not walk with the patient during the test to avoid the problem of setting the walking pace. The pulse oximeter should be applied immediately if the patient chooses to rest, and at the completion of the 6-min walking period. Any delay may result in readings being recorded that are not representative of maximum exercise response.

In some instances, the clinician may choose to walk with the patient for the entire test (e.g., if continuous oximetry is desired). If this is the case, the clinician should try to walk slightly behind the patient to avoid setting the walking pace. Alternatively, if the oximeter is small and lightweight, it may be attached to the patient and checked throughout the test without interfering with walking pace.

If the Patient Stops During the Six Minutes

- Allow the patient to sit in a chair if they wish.
- Measure the SpO_2% and heart rate.
- Ask patient why they stopped.
- Record the time the patient stopped (but keep the watch running).
- Give the following encouragement (repeat this encouragement every 15 s if necessary):
- "Begin walking as soon as you feel able."
- Monitor the patient for untoward signs and symptoms.

Stop the Test in the Event of Any of the Following

- Chest pain suspicious for angina.
- Evolving mental confusion or lack of coordination.
- Evolving light-headedness.
- Intolerable dyspnea.
- Leg cramps or extreme leg muscle fatigue.
- Persistent $SpO_2 < 85\%$.
- Any other clinically warranted reason.

Predicted Normal Values for the 6MWT

The following predictive equations use the reference values determined from a study that performed two 6MWTs according to the above protocol (for further details see Jenkins S, Cecins N, Camarri B, Williams C, Thompson P, Eastwood P. Regression equations to predict 6 min walk distance in middle-aged and elderly adults. Physiother Theory Pract. 2009;25(7):1–7).

- Predictive equation for males: $6MWD(m) = 867 - (5.71\ age,\ yrs) + (1.03\ height,\ cm)$
- Predictive equation for females: $6MWD(m) = 525 - (2.86\ age,\ yrs) + (2.71\ height,\ cm)$

Source: American Thoracic Society Board of Directors. ATS statement: guidelines for the six-minute walk test. Am J Respir Crit Care Med. 2002;166:111–7. Reprinted with permission of the American Thoracic Society. Copyright © American Thoracic Society.

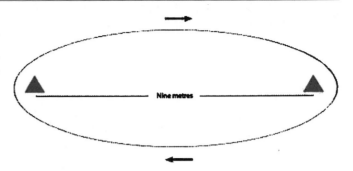

Shuttle Walk Test

Incremental Shuttle Walking Test

The incremental shuttle walking test (ISWT) was developed to simulate a cardiopulmonary exercise test using a field walking test.

Note: The ISWT is available from Dr Sally Singh, Department of Respiratory Medicine, Glenfield Hospital NHS Trust, Groby Road, Leicester LE3 9QP, UK or email: leslie.shortt@uhl-tr.nhs.uk.

- The patient is required to walk between two cones in time to a set of auditory beeps played on a CD.
- Initially, the walking speed is very slow, but each minute the required walking speed progressively increases.
- The patient walks for as long as they can until they are either too breathless or can no longer keep up with the beeps at which time, the test ends.
- The number of shuttles (laps between the cones) is recorded. Each shuttle represents a distance of 10 m.
- The results of the ISWT can be used to prescribe the intensity of walking exercise.

Standardization

Standardization of the ISWT is very important for obtaining meaningful outcomes.

The ISWT must be measured on *two occasions* to account for a learning effect. Please note that:

- The best result is recorded.
- If the repeat test is performed on the same day, 30 min rest should be allowed between tests.
- Debilitated individuals may require tests to be performed on separate days, but aim for tests to be less than 1 week apart.
- Only standardized instructions from the CD should be used. In contrast to the six-minute walking test, no encouragement should be given throughout the ISWT.
- A comfortable ambient temperature and humidity should be maintained for all tests.
- The walking track must be the same for all tests for a patient:

  o Cones are placed 9 m apart.
  o The distance walked around the cones is 10 m.

ISWT Equipment

The equipment needed to conduct the ISWT is identified in the below checklist.

What do I need for the incremental shuttle walking test?	Yes	No
Do I have access to a health professional trained in CPR and with the expertise to run the test?		
Do I have access to a flat, straight walking track at least 10 m in length?		
Is the walking track clear of hospital traffic and obstacles?		
Can the walking test be conducted in a comfortable ambient temperature and humidity?		
Do I have a stethoscope?		
Do I have a sphygmomanometer?		
Do I have a pulse oximeter?		
Do I have two cones?		
Do I have a cassette tape or CD of the test?		
Do I have a cassette or DC player?		
Do I have access to a main power source?		
Do I have a stopwatch?		
Do I have access to a portable oxygen delivery system?		
Do I have a dyspnea scale?		
Do I have chairs positioned to allow for patient rest at the end of the test?		

Before the ISWT

- Ensure that you have obtained a medical history of the patient and have taken into account any precautions or contraindications to exercise testing.
- Instruct the patient to dress comfortably and to wear appropriate footwear.
- Any prescribed inhaled bronchodilator medication should be taken within 1 h of testing or when the patient arrives for testing.
- The patient should rest for at least 15 min before beginning the ISWT.
- Record:

  o Blood pressure.
  o Heart rate.
  o Oxygen saturation.
  o Dyspnea score.*

Note: Show the patient the dyspnea scale (e.g., Borg scale) and give standardized instructions on how to obtain a score.

During the ISWT

Follow the instructions on the CD, and use the following standard prompts:

- Each time the beep sounds:
- "Increase your speed now."
- Use the following prompt if the patient is less than 0.5 m away from the cone when the beep sounds.
- "You're not going fast enough; try to make up the speed this time."
- Record each shuttle that is completed on the ISWT recording sheet.
- Monitor the patient for untoward signs and symptoms.

Ending the ISWT

The ISWT ends if any one of the following occurs:

- The patient is *more than* 0.5 m away from the cone when the beep sounds (allow one lap to catch up).
- The patient reports that they are too breathless to continue.
- The patient reaches 85% of predicted maximum heart rate (maximum heart rate $= 210 - 0.65 \times$ age)
- The patient exhibits any of the following signs and symptoms:

  - Chest pain that is suspicious of angina.
  - Evolving mental confusion or lack of coordination.
  - Evolving light-headedness.
  - Intolerable dyspnea.
  - Leg cramps or extreme leg muscle fatigue.
  - Persistent $SpO_2 \leq 85\%$.
  - Any other clinically warranted reason.

At the End of the ISWT

- Seat the patient or, if the patient prefers, allow to the patient to stand.
  Note: The measurements taken before and after the test should be taken with the patient in the same position.

- Immediately record oxygen saturation (SpO_2)%, heart rate, and dyspnea rating.
- Two minutes later, record SpO_2% and heart rate to assess the recovery rate.
- Record the total number of shuttles.
- Record the reason for terminating the test. The patient can be asked:

"What do you think stopped you from keeping up with the beeps?"

The patient should remain in a clinical area for at least 15 min following an uncomplicated test.

Source: From Singh SJ, Morgan MDL, Scott S, Walter D, et al. The development of the shuttle walking test of disability in patients with chronic airway obstruction. Thorax. 1992;47:1019–24. © 1992 with permission from BJM Publishing Group, Ltd.

Metabolic Equivalent (MET)

Physical Activity	MET
Light intensity activities	**<3**
Sleeping	0.9
Watching television	1.0
Writing, desk work, typing	1.8
Walking, less than 2.0 mph (3.2 km/h), level ground, strolling, very slow	2.0
Moderate intensity activities	**3–6**
Bicycling, stationary, 50 W, very light effort	3.0
Calisthenics, home exercise, light or moderate effort, general	3.5
Bicycling, <10 mph (16 km/h), leisure, to work or for pleasure	4.0
Bicycling, stationary, 100 W, light effort	5.5
Vigorous intensity activities	**>6**
Jogging, general	7.0
Calisthenics (e.g., pushups, situps, pullups, jumping jacks), heavy, vigorous effort	8.0
Running jogging, in place	8.0
Rope jumping	10.0

Source: Ainsworth BE, et al. Compendium of physical activities: an update of activity codes and MET intensities. **Med Sci Sports Exerc**. 2000;32(9 Suppl):S498–504

Appendix D: References

Books

Rosenthal RA, Zenilman M, Katlic MR, editors. Principles and practice of geriatric surgery. 2nd ed. New York: Springer; 2010.

LoCicero J, Rosenthal RA, Katlic MR, editors. New frontiers in geriatrics research: an agenda for surgical and related medical specialties. 2nd ed. New York: American Geriatrics Society; 2007.

Silverstein JH, Rooke GA, Reeves JG, McLesky CH, editors. Geriatric anesthesiology. 2nd ed. New York: Springer; 2008.

Sieber F. Geriatric anesthesiology. New York: McGraw-Hill; 2007.

Reuben DB, Herr KA, Pacala JT, et al. Geriatrics at your fingertips. 11th ed. New York: American Geriatrics Society; 2009.

Durso S, Bowker L, Price J, Smith S. Oxford American handbook of geriatric medicine. Oxford: Oxford University Press; 2010.

Fillit HM, Rockwood K, Woodhouse K. Brocklehurst's textbook of geriatric medicine and gerontology. New York: Saunders; 2010.

Gershman K. Little black book of geriatrics. 4th ed. Sudbury: Jones & Bartlett Publishers; 2009.

Sinclair AJ. Principles and practice of geriatric medicine. New York: Wiley; 2006.

Cassel CK, Leipzig RM, Cohen HJ, et al., editors. Geriatric medicine. 4th ed. New York: Springer; 2003.

Kane R. Essentials of clinical geriatrics. 5th ed. New York: McGraw-Hill; 2004.

Hazzard WR, Blass JP, Ouslander JG, et al., editors. Principles of geriatric medicine & gerontology. 5th ed. New York: McGraw-Hill; 2003.

Landefeld CS. Current geriatric diagnosis and treatment. New York: McGraw-Hill; 2004.

Historical

Katlic MR, editor. Geriatric surgery; Comprehensive care of the elderly patient. Baltimore: Williams & Wilkins; 1990.

Websites

Administration on Aging	http://www.aoa.gov
Alzheimer's Association	http://www.alz.org
American Association for Thoracic Surgery	http://www.aats.org
American Association of Retired Persons	http://www.aarp.org
American Board of Surgery	http://www.absurgery.org
American Board of Thoracic Surgery	http://www.abts.org
American College of Cardiology	http://www.acc.org
American College of Chest Physicians	http://www.chestnet.org
American College of Surgeons	http://www.facs.org
American Geriatric Society	http://www.americangeriatrics.org
American Heart Association	http://www.americanheart.org
American Hospital Association	http://www.aha.org
American Medical Directors Association	http://www.amda.com
American Society of Anesthesiologists	http://www.asahq.org
American Society on Aging	http://www.asaging.org
American Surgical Association	http://www.americansurgical.info
Association of Program Directors in Surgery	http://www.apds.org
Cardiothoracic Surgery Network	http://www.ctsnet.org
Centers for Medicare and Medicaid Services	http://www.cms.hhs.gov
Donald W. Reynolds Foundation	http://www.dwreynolds.org
Geriatrics for Specialists Initiative	http://www.americangeriatrics.org/specialists
Gerontological Society of America	http://www.geron.org
International Association of Gerontology and Geriatrics	http://www.iagg.org
John A. Hartford Foundation	http://www.jhartford.org
Medscape Geriatric Resource	http://www.medscape.com/resource/geriatric
National Association of Area Agencies on Aging	http://www.n4a.org
National Council on Aging	http://www.ncoa.org
National Institute on Aging	http://www.nia.nih.gov
Nurses Improving Care for Healthsystem Elders	http://www.nicheprogram.org
Society of Thoracic Surgeons	http://www.sts.org
Surgical Council on Resident Education	http://www.surgicalcore.org
Thoracic Surgery Directors Association	http://www.tsda.org

Index